Krieglstein · Klumpp

Pharmacology of Cerebral Ischemia

Pharmacology of Cerebral Ischemia 2000

Edited by Josef Krieglstein and Susanne Klumpp

Institut für Pharmakologie und Toxikologie und Abt. Biochemie
im Fachbereich Pharmazie der Philipps-Universität, Marburg

With 165 figures and 23 tables

medpharm Scientific Publishers Stuttgart 2000

Prof. Dr. Dr. Josef Krieglstein
Institut für Pharmakologie und Toxikologie
Ketzerbach 63
D-35032 Marburg (FRG)

Prof. Dr. Susanne Klumpp
Abt. Biochemie des Fachbereiches Pharmazie
Marbacher Weg 6
D-35032 Marburg (FRG)

Die Deutsche Bibliothek – CIP-Einheitsaufnahme

Pharmacology of cerebral ischemia ...
Stuttgart : Medpharm Scientific Publ.
1992 –; 1994 – (Verlagswechsel
ISBN 3–88763–087–4

Printed in F. R. Germany
Typesetting: DTP + TEXT Eva Burri, Stuttgart
Printing and binding: Hofmann, Schorndorf
Cover design: Atelier Schäfer, Esslingen

Preface

"Books must follow sciences, and not sciences books." (Francis Bacon)

The proceedings of our symposia series fulfill this demand. Since 1986 eight volumes have been published and they describe impressively the development in the field of cerebral ischemia, neurodegeneration and -protection.

At the first meeting in 1986 there was little pharmacology to discuss but at that time the field was hastily starting to develop. At the next symposium in 1988 calcium and NMDA antagonists played a great role, in 1990 studies on oxygen free radicals, platelet activating factor, adenosine and monoamine transmitters were added. In 1992 successful attempts to protect neurons by pharmacologically modifying the NO system were presented and nerve growth factors were described as neuroprotectants. In 1994, molecular biology techniques were starting to influence the field. Gene expression was a relevant topic and the question arised whether cell death after ischemia could be of apoptotic type. Two years later, gene expression, transgenic animals, gene therapy, apoptosis, growth factors, cytokines, inflammatory mechanisms and the mitochondrial function in neurodegeneration after cerebral ischemia moved more and more into the centre of the field. At the 8th International Symposium on the Pharmacology of Cerebral Ischemia in July 2000 these topics were still highly actual. Stem cell therapy and neurogenesis were additionally stressed. Since many drugs were experimentally shown to protect neurons and brain tissue against damage, but on the other hand the breakthrough in clinical therapy still was not achieved, the question was discussed whether the animal models used could predict clinical efficacy of drugs.

The publication of this volume enabled us again to describe the state of the art. We are very grateful to all authors who promptly delivered their manuscripts, being the prerequisite for this fast publication. Most important for the scientific standard of the meeting were the valuable suggestions of the members of the advisory board. We are deeply grateful for their support and cooperation. We would like to thank the official sponsors of the symposium, as well as the pharmaceutical companies listed in this book for their financial support. Many thanks also to the publishing house who guaranteed the speedy publication of the proceedings. And last, but not least, we are indebted to our co-workers without their help and cooperation a smooth running of the meeting would not have been possible.

The editors

Invited speakers

Koji Abe, Okayama (Japan)
Stuart M. Allan, Manchester (UK)
R. David Andrew, Kingston (Canada)
Paolo Bernardi, Padova (Italy)
Alastair M. Buchan, Calgary (Canada)
Pak H. Chan, Palo Alto (USA)
Jun Chen, Pittsburgh (USA)
Michael Chopp, Detroit (USA)
Valina L. Dawson, Baltimore (USA)
Gregory J. del Zoppo, La Jolla (USA)
Ulrich Dirnagl, Berlin (Germany)
Ella W. Englander, Galveston (USA)
Seth P. Finklestein, Boston (USA)
Gary Fiskum, Baltimore (USA)
James L. Franklin, Madison (USA)
David D. Gilboe, Madison (USA)
Myron D. Ginsberg, Miami (USA)
James Grotta, Houston (USA)
W.-D. Heiss, Köln (Germany)
K.-A. Hossmann, Köln (Germany)
Constantin Iadecola, Minneapolis (USA)
Umeo Ito, Tokyo (Japan)
Christian Kaltschmidt, Witten (Germany)
Susanne Klumpp, Marburg (Germany)
Jari Koistinaho, Kuopio (Finland)
Kerstin Krieglstein, Homburg (Germany)
Hans Lehrach, Berlin (Germany)
Baowan Lin, Miami (USA)
Sarah A. Loddick, Manchester (UK)
John P. MacManus, Ottawa (Canada)
Michael A. Moskowitz, Boston (USA)
Pierluigi Nicotera, Konstanz (Germany)
Tiho P. Obrenovitch, Bradford (UK)
David S. Park, Ottawa (Canada)
Wulf Paschen, Köln (Germany)
Miguel A. Pérez-Pinzón, Miami (USA)
Elizabeth Pinard, Paris (France)
Jochen H. M. Prehn, Münster (Germany)
Gennadij Raivich, Martinsried (Germany)
Nancy J. Rothwell, Manchester (UK)
Timothy Schallert, Austin (USA)
Markus Schwaninger, Heidelberg (Germany)
Frank R. Sharp, Cincinnati (USA)
Bo K. Siesjö, Honululu (USA)
Roger P. Simon, Portland (USA)
Evan Snyder, Boston (USA)
Gary K. Steinberg, Stanford (USA)
Clive N. Svendsen, Cambridge (UK)
Denis Vivien, Caen Cedex (France)
Eberhard Weihe, Marburg (Germany)
John H. Zhang, Jackson (USA)
Yuan Zhu, Marburg (Germany)

Sponsors of the symposium

Official sponsors

Deutsche Forschungsgemeinschaft
International Society for Cerebral Blood Flow and Metabolism
International Society for Neurochemistry
Philipps-Universität Marburg

Financial support was provided by the following companies:

Arzneimittelwerk Dresden GmbH, Radebeul
Aventis Behring GmbH, Marburg
Bayer AG, Wuppertal
Boehringer Ingelheim GmbH, Biberach an der Riss
Chiron-Behring GmbH & Co., Marburg
Eppendorf-Netheler-Hinz GmbH, Hamburg
Forschungsinstitut Angewandte Neurowissenschaften, Magdeburg
Janssen-Cilag, Neuss
Lichtwer Pharma AG, Berlin
E. Merck, Darmstadt
PHOENIX Pharmahandel AG & Co., Hanau
Pfizer GmbH, Karlsruhe
Schering AG, Berlin
Dr. Willmar Schwabe GmbH & Co., Karlsruhe
SmithKline Beecham Pharma GmbH, München
Carl Zeiss Jena, Jena

Contents

Apoptosis and necrosis after ischemia

Receptors and intracellular signaling

Role of mitochondria in neuronal cell death

Inflammation and neuronal cell death

Circulation

Repair, recovery and neuroprotection

Growth factors and cytokines

Genes and gene therapy

Stem cell therapy and neurogenesis

Predictiveness of animal models for clinical trials

Apoptosis and necrosis after ischemia

Apoptosis and neurodegeneration: the role of caspases

P. Nicotera

Summary

The execution of the apoptotic programme involves a relatively limited number of pathways that converge on the activation of the caspase family of proteases (Villa et al. 1997). However, there is increasing evidence that apoptotic-like features can be found also when cells are treated with inhibitors of caspases such as the cell permeable tripeptide, Z-Val-Ala-Asp-fluoromethyl-ketone (Z-VAD-fmk), or similar compounds. This has posed the question as to whether death with apoptotic features can still occur in a caspase independent way, and whether caspase inhibitors may then be used to treat diseases characterised by excessive apoptosis. In several neurodegenerative diseases metabolic defects are often linked to the loss of neuronal connectivity and cell loss. The resulting ATP depletion can preclude caspase activation, and consequently switch execution of cell death towards necrosis. A block or partial inhibition of the typical apoptotic demise may have profound implications *in vivo*, as persistence within the nervous system of damaged, but "undead" cells, followed by delayed lysis may favour neuroinflammatory reactions. Furthermore, caspases may be involved in loss of neurons, but not in the loss of connectivity that seems to initiate degenerative processes in the nervous system. Some recent findings, which suggest that degenerating neurons may use multiple execution pathways will be discussed.

Introduction

During development, genetically encoded programmes decide the fate of individual cells or organs. The term "programmed cell death" has therefore been used primarily to describe the co-ordinated series of events leading to controlled cell demise in developing organisms (Schwartz and Osborne 1993). Because of this definition, the term "physiological cell death" has been associated to that of "programmed cell death." Cells, however, execute a biochemical programme (i.e., a controlled sequence of biochemical events) of cell death also in pathological conditions. The consequence for the individual cell may be practically indistinguishable from those observed during developmental demise. In many cases, developmental cell death as well as pathological cell death have the classical morphological characteristics described by Kerr, Wyllie and Currie and termed apoptosis (Kerr et al. 1972). The morphological appearance, however, is also not necessarily

Keywords: apoptosis/caspases/neurodegeneration/ATP

Faculty of Biology, University of Konstanz, Box X911, D-78457 Konstanz, Germany.
e-mail: Pierluigi.Nicotera@uni-konstanz.de

associated to the execution of a death programme. For example, in non-vertebrate systems, programmed cell death does not always display an apoptotic-like morphology (Yuan and Horvitz 1990; Schwartz et al. 1993). The discovery that both developmental and non-developmental death can share similar execution systems and controlling proteins has then finally blurred the boundary between developmental cell death and cell demise in adult tissues. In particular the characterisation of the main executioners of apoptosis, the caspases, has linked the physiological type of death encountered in development with that observed in pathological situations through the whole life span.

Caspases and cell death

One class of death-related genes, those expressing caspases (cysteine aspartases) (Yuan et al. 1993), can mediate cell death in genetically distant organisms. Most of the typical features of apoptosis (i.e., cleavage of nuclear substrates, DNA fragmentation) are the consequence of caspase activation. Consequently, there is a tendency to conceptually identify apoptosis with its main execution system (Samali et al. 1999). Caspases are constitutively expressed in mammals, similar to *ced-3* in *C. elegans* (Weil et al. 1996; Shaham and Horvitz 1996). To date 14 mammalian caspases have been identified. They are expressed as inactive pro-enzymes and proteolytically activated to form active tetramers. A recent classification divides them in three different groups based on the tetrapeptide recognition sequence (DExDases, WEHDases, (IVL)ExDases). Caspases participate in the signalling and execution of apoptosis (Nicholson and Thornberry 1997) with the exception of WEHDases, which are implicated in inflammatory processes. Substrates include cytoskeletal proteins, nuclear structural proteins and enzymes, and some controllers of caspase activation (i.e., Bcl-2) (Nicholson and Thornberry 1997). Caspase multiplicity likely reflects their diverse roles in pathophysiological conditions. For example, caspases degrade amyloid precursor protein (APP), presenilins (PS1, PS2), tau, huntingtin, atrophin-1, ataxin-3, and the androgen receptor (Weidemann et al. 1999; Ellerby et al. 1999; Kobayashi et al. 1998; Wellington et al. 1998; Gervais et al. 1999). On the other hand, cleavage of relevant substrates does not necessarily imply that caspase activation has the predominant pathogenetic role in neurodegeneration (van den Craen et al. 1999), and it does not prove that neuronal apoptosis is the basis for neurodegeneration.

It is indeed unlikely that a single execution system, even as diversified as the one involving caspases, is the sole responsible for the loss of neuronal connectivity and death execution. Should this be the case, viruses and transformed cells could have easily escaped or shut-down a programme converging on a single execution pathway. Also, it is difficult to conceive how the plethora of signals causing mammalian cell death would converge on a single linear pathway. Thus, in higher organisms, additional interrelated or independent pathways may have developed to regulate death.

These considerations may help to understand why different sets of caspases are recruited in different paradigms of mammalian cell death, and also why deletion of single caspases has only localised and partial effects on cell death (Kuida et al. 1995, 1996). Moreover, several forms of demise seem to be caspase-independent (Hirsch et al. 1997; Sarin et al. 1997; Xiang et al. 1997) or even be accelerated by caspase inhibitors (Vercammen et al. 1998). Indeed, other protease families have been implicated in apoptosis (Adjei et al. 1996; Grimm et al. 1996), while caspases can be activated without causing cell death (Jaattela et al. 1998). In some cases, caspase inhibition does not alter the extent of death, but rather the shape of demise (Leist et al. 1997; Hirsch et al. 1997).

The major evidence for a central role of caspases in apoptosis has come from experiments in which caspase inhibitors, including small peptide inhibitors such as Z-VAD-fmk block apoptosis. However, using the same caspase inhibitors, other studies have suggested that apoptosis can occur in a caspase-independent manner (for review see Borner and Monney

1999). Part of the problem may be due to the fact that caspase inhibitors can prevent the appearance of certain, but not all features of apoptosis in certain model systems (McCarthy et al. 1997). In this context, caution should be exerted, because of possible non-specific effects of caspase inhibitors. Although generally considered specific for the caspase family, these inhibitory peptides may in fact block only some, but not all caspases. It is also clear that caspase inhibitors can also inhibit unrelated proteases, whose activity may be necessary for survival.

While the existence of alternative pathways may be conceivable, to date, the evidence for effective alternative execution systems is limited. One candidate protein is the apoptosis-inducing factor (AIF) (Susin et al. 1997). This 57 kDa protein can directly cause some of the apoptotic features. Apoptosis may also involve activation of other protease families including serine proteases, cathepsin and calpains. This raises the question as to whether every protease (i.e., even proteinase K) may indeed trigger apoptotic-like changes. This was the conclusion of an early study (Williams and Henkart 1994, 1996). Dysregulation of proteolysis may indeed be a general mechanism to dispose of aging cells, where intracellular deposition of misfolded proteins is a powerful stimulus for protease activation (Johnston et al. 1998). Interestingly, the concept that oxidatively-modified proteins can be degraded more effectively has been around for quite a while (Levine et al. 1981), along with the notion that oxidative stress may eliminate cells by activating proteases (Nicotera et al. 1986).

Energy requirement for the shape of cell death

While the occurrence of caspase-independent apoptosis is strongly debated, it is instead widely accepted that, in some cases, caspase inhibition can only delay cell demise. Cells eventually die with morphologically different features (Hirsch et al. 1997; Leist et al. 1997). Evidence that cells triggered to undergo apoptosis are instead forced to die by necrosis when intracellular ATP is depleted has been recently provided (Leist et al. 1997).

In vivo, under pathological conditions, apoptosis and necrosis may often coexist (Leist et al. 1995) and it is apparent that when intracellular energy levels are compromised early in dying neurons, death progresses in a caspase-3 independent way (Volbracht et al. 1999). This, in neuronal cultures, takes the appearance of necrosis (Ankarcrona et al. 1995), or of a death with mixed features of apoptosis and necrosis.

Energy-requiring steps for the execution of the apoptotic programme are at the level of the formation of the protein complex between Apaf-1, cyt-c and procaspases (Liu et al. 1996), and possibly at other steps upstream to the event leading to cyt-c release by mitochondria. Lack of ATP at this step would prevent the resulting downstream degradative processes including caspase-3 activation, poly-(ADP-ribose)-polymerase cleavage and lamin cleavage, and exposure of phosphatidylserine (PS) on the outer membrane.

Energy deprivation and caspase inhibition in neuronal cell death

The implications of energy deprivation for the final outcome, apoptosis or necrosis, may be particularly relevant in the nervous system. An increased rate of apoptosis has been suggested to be a feature of several neurodegenerative diseases, although its role in the manifestation and progression of disease is still unclear. Apoptotic features are elicited in cultured neurons by β-amyloid and prion proteins, or by expressing a mutated Huntingtin protein (Forloni et al. 1993, 1996; Saudou et al. 1998; Kim et al. 1999). Nevertheless, it is unclear whether the onset of the pathological manifestations *in vivo* it is due to neuronal loss by apoptosis, or to functional neuronal damage. A common feature of neurodegenerative disorders is the accumulation of intracellular inclusions mostly formed by protein aggregates that are usually difficult to unfold or degrade (Johnston et al. 1998). The potentially pathogenic consequences of accumulation of misfolded proteins include alterations of axonal transport, cytoskeletal damage, and finally loss of connectivity with target cells. Thus, it appears reasonable that apoptosis would be triggered to dispose of these dysfunctional neurons. However, if apoptosis is blocked, for example by a concomitant defect in energy metabolism, injured cells may persist and later lyse. A defect in energy metabolism may derive either from mitochondrial genetic alterations, as suggested for some neuropathological syndromes (Shoubridge 1998), or from generation of mediators in injured areas.

To address the role of ATP in neuronal apoptosis, and the possible role of signalling molecules such as nitric oxide (NO) in modulating apoptosis, cerebellar granule neurons (CGC) were exposed to apoptosis inducing conditions under normal or depressed energy levels. Neurons were treated with the microtubule-disassembling agent, colchicine to model the cytoskeletal damage and axonal loss seen in neurodegenerative conditions (Volbracht et al. 1999). This treatment induced activation of caspases and classical apoptosis. However, if ATP was depleted by mitochondrial poisons, the execution of apoptosis was blocked. Lowering of neuronal ATP could also be elicited by NO, suggesting that local production of NO can interfere with the execution of apoptosis by impairing energy metabolism. ATP depletion prevented both the activation of caspases and the exposure of phagocytosis-recognition molecules. However, caspase inhibition did not prevent the initial cytoskeletal damage and neurite loss, whereas recognition molecules for phagocytosis, such as PSs were not displayed on the neuronal surface. Notably, when caspase inhibitors such as Z-VAD-fmk where used to block apoptosis, neurons with a damaged cytoskeleton went on to die, with slowed-down kinetics, but still exhibiting some morphological apoptotic features, including chromatin condensation and fragmentation of DNA in high molecular weight fragments.

Consequently, we may speculate that *in vivo*, a partial execution of apoptosis, lacking phagocyte recognition molecules may result in the persistence of damaged cells within the tissue.

Therapeutic implications of a branched death program

The observation that caspase inhibition hindered PS exposure, but did not prevent late lysis in colchicine-treated neurons raises the question as to whether inhibition of caspases is always desirable. Caspase inhibitors have been shown to be effective in acute liver injury (Künstle et al. 1997) and in models of stroke (Fink et al. 1998; Schulz et al. 1999). The efficacy of caspase inhibitors to treat slow-progressing neurodegenerative diseases may be more problematic. The pathogenesis of Alzheimer's, Huntington's and Parkinson's disease may be independent from neuronal loss at least in early stages. For example, motor alterations are observed in transgenic mice overexpressing the mutated Huntingtin protein, prior to any major pathological evidence of death (Carter et al. 1999). Similarly, deficits in synaptic activity are accompanied by minimal loss of presynaptic or postsynaptic elements or cell death in mice overexpressing the amyloid precursor protein (Chapman et al. 1999). Notably, mice expressing exon 1 of the human huntingtin gene with an expanded CAG/polyglutamine repeat exhibit a significant decrease in striatal volume without any detectable neuronal loss or the appearance of any disease sign (Hansson et al. 1999). This suggests that loss of connectivity or changes in extracellular matrix occur before cell death.

Nevertheless, during disease progression, apoptosis would be activated in affected neurons (i.e., in neurons expressing long-polyglutamine stretches for Huntington's disease) as shown in several model systems (Kim et al. 1999; Sanchez et al. 1999; Miyashita et al. 1999). Then, while pharmacological inhibition of caspases would prolong neuronal survival (Sanchez et al. 1999), it may also allow the persistence of functionally damaged neurons. Unless strategies to promote regeneration and re-establishment of connectivity are implemented concomitantly, caspase-inhibited neurons or neurons unable of completing the apoptotic execution would eventually lyse and, paradoxically, promote the onset of inflammatory responses, with further progression of disease. This potential vicious loop may be interrupted more efficiently by interfering with activation of the pro-inflammatory caspases, rather than inhibiting those involved in the execution of apoptosis. This may account, at least in part, for the protective effect of dominant-negative caspase-1 mutants in mice expressing exon 1 of the human huntingtin gene with an expanded CAG/polyglutamine repeat (Ona et al. 1999).

Clearly, caspase-based therapeutic strategies alone or in combination with other agents may be useful in stroke. Observations in stroke models suggest that apoptosis occurs mainly in the border regions (penumbra), while necrosis dominates in the more severely stressed areas of the ischemic core (Charriaut-Marlangue et al. 1996). Apoptosis of penumbral neurons may be due both to a mild direct excitotoxic-ischemic insult, but also to secondary mediators such as oxygen radicals, cytokines and lipid peroxidation products from the necrotic core (Mattson 1998; Lipton and Rosenberg 1994). Intervention, a few hours after the ischemic insults, is normally aimed to reduce spreading of the lesion and to inhibit delayed cell death in the border areas. If the level of injury decides the activation of different pathways for the execution of cell death, it is apparent that caspase inhibitors may be most effective in areas where the intensity of the excitotoxic insult is low, and positive feedback loops between different execution subroutines are not fully established. In the regions where the stress is more intense, inhibition of caspases alone may not prevent cell death (Green and Kroemer 1998). Thus, strategies that combine agents to reduce the overall intensity of the insult and the overall lesion size (i.e., N-methyl-D-aspartate (NMDA)-antagonists and other ion channel blockers or selective bNOS inhibitors), with agents that block execution of apoptosis (caspase inhibitors) has proven more successful than individual treatments (Schulz et al. 1999). Finally, caspase inhibition has been recently proven to be effective in improving survival of nigral transplants in hemiparkinsonian rats and thereby improving functional recovery (Schierle et al. 1999).

Conclusions

It is not surprising that initially simple death programs, developed early during phylogeny, undergo complex modifications in mammalian cells. Large gene families have evolved to provide a more intricate control of cell death in higher organisms, in part perhaps to accommodate the need of individual organ differentiation. Some characteristics of the original cell death machinery that would affect predominantly the shape of death may have become more significant or predominant in some subsets of mammalian cells. A further consequence of the increased complexity may be that an increasing number of feed-back loops gives rise to multiple possibilities of initiation, control and execution .

In our view, stimulation of self-feeding loops, which maintain both the activation of executioners and the neutralisation of anti-apoptotic defence systems, is necessary for the completion of most death programs. The main implication of this standpoint is the exclusion of a single, predominant and molecularly-defined commitment step. It seems likely that accumulation of damage incompatible with cell survival would require disruption of several vital functions. Once such a threshold is trespassed, multiple positive feed-back loops would ensure the progression of the death programme to the end, and the safe disposal of the injured cell. This also implies that the morphological appearance of cell death (apoptosis or necrosis) is not linked to a single commitment point, but rather is the result of a more or less complete execution of subroutines deciding on the shape of dying cells.

Acknowledgements

This work has been supported by grants from Deutsche Forschungsgemeinshaft (DFG), the European Community and the POP European Fund for Regional Development 94–99.

References

1. Adjei PN, Kaufmann SH, Leung W-Y, Mao F, Gores GJ (1996) Selective induction of apoptosis in Hep 3B cells by toposiomerase I inhibitors: evidence for a protease-dependent pathway that does not activate cysteine protease P32. J Clin Invest 98:2,588–2,596
2. Ankarcrona M, Dypbukt JM, Bonfoco E, Zhivotovsky B, Orrenius S, Lipton SA, Nicotera P (1995) Glutamate-induced neuronal death: a succession of necrosis or apoptosis depending on mitochondrial function. Neuron 15:961–973
3. Borner C, Monney L (1999) Apoptosis without caspases: an inefficient molecular guillotine? Cell Death & Differ 6:497–507
4. Carter RJ, Lione LA, Humby T, Mangiarini L, Mahal A, Bates GP, Dunnett SB, Morton AJ (1999) Characterization of progressive motor deficits in mice transgenic for the human Huntington's disease mutation. J Neurosci 19:3,248–3,257
5. Chapman PF, White GL, Jones MW, Cooper-Blacketer D, Marshall VJ, Irizarry M, Younkin L, Good MA, Bliss TV, Hyman BT, Younkin SG, Hsiao KK (1999) Impaired synaptic plasticity and learning in aged amyloid precursor protein transgenic mice. Nat Neurosci 2:271–276
6. Charriaut-Marlangue C, Aggoun-Zouaoui D, Represa A, Ben-Ari Y (1996) Apoptotic features of selective neuronal death in ischemia, epilepsy and gp120 toxicity. Trends Neurosci 19:109–114
7. Ellerby LM, Andrusiak RL, Wellington CL, Hackam AS, Propp SS, Wood JD, Sharp AH, Margolis RL, Ross CA, Salvesen GS, Hayden MR, Bredesen DE (1999) Cleavage of atrophin-1 at caspase site aspartic acid 109 modulates cytotoxicity J Biol Chem 274:8,730–8,736
8. Fink K, Zhu J, Namura S, Shimizu-Sasamata M, Endres M, Ma J, Dalkara T, Yuan J, Moskowitz MA (1998) Prolonged therapeutic window for ischemic brain damage caused by delayed caspase activation. J Cereb Blood Flow Metab 18:1,071–1,076
9. Forloni G, Angeretti N, Chiesa R, Monzani E, Salmona M, Bugiani O, Tagliavini F (1993) Neurotoxicity of a prion protein fragment. Nature 362:543–546
10. Forloni G, Bugiani O, Tagliavini F, Salmona M (1996) Apoptosis-mediated neurotoxicity induced by beta-amyloid and PrP fragments. Mol Chem Neuropathol 28:163–171
11. Gervais FG, Xu D, Robertson GS, Vaillancourt JP, Zhu Y, Huang J, LeBlanc A, Smith D, Rigby M, Shearman MS, Clarke EE, Zheng H, Van Der Ploeg LH, Ruffolo SC, Thornberry NA, Xanthoudakis S, Zamboni RJ, Roy S, Nicholson DW (1999) Involvement of caspases in proteolytic cleavage of Alzheimer's amyloid-beta precursor protein and amyloidogenic A beta peptide formation. Cell 97:395–406
12. Green D, Kroemer G (1998) The central executioners of apoptosis: caspases or mitochondria? Trends Cell Biol 8:267–271
13. Grimm LM, Goldberg AL, Poirier GG, Schwartz LM, Osborne BA (1996) Proteasomes play an essential role in thymocyte apoptosis. EMBO J 15:3,835–3,844
14. Hansson O, Petersen A, Leist M, Nicotera P, Castilho RF, Brundin P (1999) Transgenic mice expressing a Huntington's disease mutation are resistant to quinolinic acid-induced striatal excitotoxicity. Proc Natl Acad Sci USA 96:8,727–8,732
15. Hirsch T, Marchetti P, Susin SA, Dallaporta B, Zamzami N, Marzo I, Geuskens M, Kroemer G (1997) The apoptosis-necrosis paradox. Apoptogenic proteases activated after mitochondrial permeability transition determine the mode of cell death. Oncogene 15:1,573–1,581
16. Jaattela M, Wissing D, Kokholm K, Kallunki T, Egeblad M (1998) Hsp70 exerts its anti-apoptotic function downstream of caspase-3-like proteases. EMBO J 17:6,124–6,134
17. Johnston JA, Ward CL, Kopito RR (1998) Aggresomes: a cellular response to misfolded proteins. J Cell Biol 143:1,883–1,898
18. Kerr JF, Wyllie AH, Currie AR (1972) Apoptosis: A basic biological phenomenon with wide ranging implications in tissue kinetics. Br J Cancer 26:239–247
19. Kim M, Lee HS, LaForet G, McIntyre C, Martin EJ, Chang P, Kim TW, Williams M, Reddy PH, Tagle D, Boyce FM, Won L, Heller A, Aronin N, DiFiglia M (1999) Mutant huntingtin expression in clonal striatal cells: dissociation of inclusion formation and neuronal survival by caspase inhibition. J Neurosci 19:964–973
20. Kobayashi Y, Miwa S, Merry DE, Kume A, Mei L, Doyu M, Sobue G (1998) Caspase-3 cleaves the expanded androgen receptor protein of spinal and bulbar muscular atrophy in a polyglutamine repeat length-dependent manner. Biochem Biophys Res Commun 252:145–150
21. Künstle G, Leist M, Uhlig S, Revesz L, Feifel R, MacKenzie A, Wendel A (1997) ICE-protease inhibitors block murine liver injury and apoptosis caused by CD95 or by TNF-α. Immunol Lett 55:5–10
22. Kuida K, Lippke JA, Ku G, Harding MW, Livingston DJ, Su MS, Flavell RA (1995) Altered cytokine export and apoptosis in mice deficient in interleukin-1beta converting enzyme. Science 267:2,000–2,003
23. Kuida K, Zheng TS, Na S, Kuan C-y, Yang D, Karasuyama H, Rakic P, Flavell RA (1996) Decreased apoptosis in the brain and premature lethality in CPP32-deficient mice. Nature 384:368–372
24. Leist M, Gantner F, Bohlinger I, Tiegs G, Germann PG, Wendel A (1995) Tumor necrosis factor-induced hepatocyte apoptosis precedes liver failure in experimental murine shock models. Am J Pathol. 146:1,220–1,234
25. Leist M, Single B, Castoldi AF, Kühnle S, Nicotera P (1997) Intracellular ATP concentration: a switch deciding between apoptosis and necrosis. J Exp Med 185:1,481–1,486
26. Levine RL, Oliver CN, Fulks RM, Stadtman ER (1981) Turnover of bacterial gluatmine synthase: oxidative inactivation precedes proteolysis. Proc Natl Acad Sci USA 78:2,120–2,125
27. Lipton SA, Rosenberg PA (1994) Excitatory amino acids as a final common pathway for neurologic disorders. New Engl J Med 330:613–622
28. Liu X, Kim CN, Yang J, Jemmerson R, Wang X (1996) Induction of apoptotic program in cell-free extracts: requirement for dATP and cytochrome c. Cell 86:147–157
29. Mattson MP (1998) Modification of ion homeostasis by lipid peroxidation: roles in neuronal degerneation and adaptive plasticity. TINS 21:53–57
30. McCarthy NJ, Whyte MKB, Gilbert CS, Evan GI (1997) Inhibition of Ced-3/ICE-related proteases does not prevent cell death induced by oncogenes, DNA damage, or the bcl-2 homologue bak. J Cell Biol 136:215–227
31. Miyashita T, Matsui J, Ohtsuka Y, Mami U, Fujishima S, Okamura-Oho Y, Inoue T, Yamada M (1999) Expression of extended polyglutamine sequentially activates initiator and effector caspases. Biochem Biophys Res Commun 257:724–730
32. Nicholson D, Thornberry NA (1997) Caspases: killer proteases. Trends Biochem 22:299–306
33. Nicotera P, Hartzell P, Baldi C, Svensson S-A, Bellomo G, Orrenius S (1986) Cystamine induces toxicity in hepatocytes through the elevation of cytosolic Ca^{2+} and the stimulation of a nonlysosomal proteolytic system. J Biol Chem 261:14,628–14,635
34. Ona VO, Li M, Vonsattel JP, Andrews LJ, Khan SQ, Chung WM, Frey AS, Menon AS, Li XJ, Stieg PE, Yuan J, Penney JB, Young AB, Cha JH, Friedlander RM (1999) Inhibition of

caspase-1 slows disease progression in a mouse model of Huntington's disease. Nature 399:263–267

35. Samali A, Zhivotovsky B, Jones D, Nagata S, Orrenius S (1999) Apoptosis: Cell death defined by caspase activation. Cell Death & Differ 6:495–496
36. Sanchez I, Xu CJ, Juo P, Kakizaka A, Blenis J, Yuan J (1999) Caspase-8 is required for cell death induced by expanded polyglutamine repeats. Neuron 22:623–633
37. Sarin A, Williams MS, Alexander-Miller MA, Berzofsky JA, Zacharchuk CM, Henkart PA (1997) Target cell lysis by CTL granule exocytosis is independent of ICE/Ced-3 family proteases. Immunity 6:209–215
38. Saudou F, Finkbeiner S, Devys D, Greenberg ME (1998) Huntingtin acts in the nucleus to induce apoptosis but death does not correlate with the formation of intranuclear inclusions. Cell 95:55–66
39. Schierle GS, Hansson O, Leist M, Nicotera P, Widner H, Brundin P (1999) Caspase inhibition reduces apoptosis and increases survival of nigral transplants. Nat Med 5:97–100
40. Schulz JB, Weller M, Moskowitz MA (1999) Caspases as treatment targets in stroke and neurodegenerative diseases. Ann Neurol 45:421–429
41. Schwartz LM, Osborne BA (1993) Programmed cell death, apoptosis and killer genes. Immunol Today 14:582–590
42. Schwartz LM, Smith SW, Jones MEE, Osborne BA (1993) Do all programmed cell deaths occur via apoptosi? Proc Natl Acad Sci USA 90:980–984
43. Shaham S, Horvitz HR (1996) Developing caenorhabditis elegans neurons may contain both cell-death protective and killer activities. Genes & Develop 10:578–591
44. Shoubridge EA (1998) Mitochondrial encephalomyopathies. Curr Opin Neurol 11:491–496
45. Susin SA, Zamzami N, Castedo M, Daugas E, Wang H-G, Geley S, Fassy F, Reed JC, Kroemer G (1997) The central executioner of apoptosis: multiple connections between protease activation and mitochondria in Fas/APO-1/CD95- and ceramide-induced apoptosis. J Exp Med 186:25–37
46. Van de Craen M, de Jonghe C, van den Brande I, Declercq W, van Gassen G, van Criekinge W, Vanderhoeven I, Fiers W, van Broeckhoven C, Hendriks L, Vandenabeele P (1999) Identification of caspases that cleave presenilin-1 and presenilin-2. Five presenilin-1 (PS1) mutations do not alter the sensitivity of PS1 to caspases. FEBS Lett 445:149–154
47. Vercammen D, Beyaert R, Denecker G, Goossens V, Van Loo G, Declercq W, Grooten J, Fiers W, Vandenabeele P (1998) Inhibition of caspases increases the sensitivity of L929 cells to necrosis mediated by tumor necrosis factor. J Exp Med 187:1,477–1,485
48. Villa P, Kauffmann SH, Earnshaw WC (1997) Caspases and caspase inhibitors. Trends Biochem Sci 22:388–393
49. Volbracht C, Leist M, Nicotera P (1999) ATP controls neuronal apoptosis triggered by microtubule breakdown or potassium depravation. Mol Med 5:477–489
50. Weidemann A, Paliga K, D rrwang U, Reinhard FB, Schuckert O, Evin G, Masters CL (1999) Proteolytic processing of the Alzheimer's disease amyloid precursor protein within its cytoplasmic domain by caspase-like proteases. J Biol Chem 274:5,823–5,829
51. Weil M, Jacobson MD, Coles HSR, Davies TJ, Gardner RL, Raff KD, Raff MC (1996) Constitutive expression of the machinery for programmed cell death. J Cell Biol 133:1,053–1,059
52. Wellington CL, Ellerby LM, Hackam AS, Margolis RL, Trifiro MA, Singaraja R, McCutcheon K, Salvesen GS, Propp SS, Bromm M, Rowland KJ, Zhang T, Rasper D, Roy S, Thornberry N, Pinsky L, Kakizuka A, Ross CA, Nicholson DW, Bredesen DE, Hayden MR (1998) Caspase cleavage of gene products associated with triplet expansion disorders generates truncated fragments containing the polyglutamine tract. J Biol Chem 273:9,158–9,167
53. Williams MS, Henkart PA (1994) Apoptotic cell death induced by intracellular proteolysis. J Immunol 153:4,247–4,255
54. Williams MS, Henkart PA (1996) Role of reactive oxygen intermediates in TCR-induced death of T cell blasts and hybridomas. J Immunol 157:2,395–2,402
55. Xiang J, Chao DT, Korsmeyer SJ (1997) BAX-induced cell death may not require interleukin 1 beta-converting enzyme-like proteases. Proc Natl Acad Sci USA 93:14,559–14,563
56. Yuan J, Horvitz HR (1990) The caenorhabditis elegans genes ced-3 and ced-4 act cell autonomously to cause programmed cell death. Develop Biol 138:33–41
57. Yuan J, Shaham S, Ledoux S, Ellis HM, Horvitz HR (1993) The C. elegans cell death gene ced-3 encodes a protein similar to mammalian interleukin-1beta-converting enzyme. Cell 75:641–652

Apurinic/apyrimidinic endonuclease expression and oxidative stress in apoptosis after transient focal cerebral ischemia

M. Fujimura, Y. Morita-Fujimura, M. Kawase, Y.-Y. Chang, P. H. Chan

Abstract

We examined the protein expression of apurinic/apyrimidinic endonuclease (APE/Ref-1), a multifunctional protein in the DNA base excision repair pathway, in mice after transient focal cerebral ischemia. Immunohistochemistry showed nuclear expression of this enzyme in the entire region of the control brains. Immunoreactivity and Western analysis showed an early and rapid decrease in APE/Ref-1 in the entire middle cerebral artery. A similar level was detected in the control brains of both transgenic mice that overexpress human CuZn-superoxide dismutase (SOD1) and wild-type littermates. While APE/Ref-1 was significantly reduced 1 hour after transient focal cerebral ischemia in both groups, the SOD1 transgenic mice has less reduction than the wild-type mice. The delayed occurrence of DNA laddering was also significantly reduced in the transgenic mice. Double staining with APE/Ref-1 and TUNEL showed that neurons that lost APE/Ref-1 immunoreactivity became TUNEL-positive. Finally, treatment with the antioxidant 21-aminosteroid also prevented the early decrease of APE/Ref-1 expression after photothrombotic cortical cerebral ischemia in mice. These results suggest that reactive oxygen species contribute to the early decrease of APE/Ref-1 and thereby exacerbate DNA fragmentation after transient focal cerebral ischemia in mice.

The DNA repair enzyme apurinic/apyrimidinic endonuclease (APE/Ref-1) is a multifunctional protein in the DNA base excision repair pathway, which is responsible for repairing apurinic/apyrimidinic sites in DNA (Bennett et al. 1997). DNA base excision repair is known to require two types of enzymes, such as DNA glycosylases and APEs (Sancar and Sancar 1988; Doetsch and Cunningham 1990; Lindahl 1990; Demple and Harrison 1994). DNA glycosylases remove a damaged base, which could be caused by various kinds of insults, such as oxidative stress in particular, creating an apurinic/apyrimidinic site in the DNA that is then acted on by an APE (Doetsch and Cunningham 1990; Demple and Harrison 1994). The DNA repair is completed by abasic residue followed by synthesis of a new base by DNA polymerase and ligation. Incomplete repair of apurinic/apyrimidinic sites is reported to cause mutagenesis and genetic instability (Loeb and Preston 1986). DNA damage and repair is drawing more attention in the field of central nervous system injuries, including cerebral ischemia and brain trauma (Chopp et al.

Keywords: APE/Ref-1; DNA repair enzymes; CuZn; Apptosis; Oxidative stress; Transgenic mice

Neurosurgical Laboratories, Stanford University, MSLS #P304, 1201 Welch Rd., Stanford, CA 94305–5487, USA

J. Krieglstein, S. Klumpp (Eds.) Pharmacology of Cerebral Ischemia 2000

1996). Liu and colleagues (1996) have suggested that free radicals could attack the nuclear genes and cause genetic instability after mouse forebrain ischemia. As for the relationship of the DNA base excision repair pathway to necrosis and/or apoptosis, recent evidence suggests that down-regulation of APE expression is associated with apoptosis in cells of the myeloid lineage (Robertson et al. 1997). We have shown that the loss of APE/Ref-1 is closely associated with the occurrence of DNA fragmentation in hippocampal CA_1 neurons after transient global ischemia (Kawase et al. 1999). However, the mechanism by which these early modifications of APE/Ref-1 expression after focal cerebral ischemia/reperfusion injury is regulated *in vivo* is unknown.

Antioxidant enzymes and DNA repair proteins are thought to be two major mechanisms by which cells counteract the deleterious effects of reactive oxygen species (ROS), however, little is known about the interaction between them. Moreover, there is no report that indicates the direct correlation between ROS and the expression of DNA repair enzymes including APE/Ref-1, *in vivo*. To address this critical issue *in vivo*, we examined APE/Ref-1 expression after transient focal cerebral ischemia (FCI) in both wild-type mice and transgenic (Tg) mice that overexpress human CuZn-superoxide dismutase (SOD1), and with the treatment of a known antioxidant, 21-aminosteroid, in mice after photothrombotic cerebral ischemia.

Physiological data and cerebral infarction in mice after transient FCI

Physiological parameters showed no significant differences in mean arterial blood pressure and arterial blood gas analysis between each group. The pre-ischemic physiological values are as follows (wild-type/SOD1 Tg): mean arterial blood pressure, 71.5 ± 3.4/72.5 ± 6.6 mm Hg; PaO2, 157.2 ± 20.1/169.5 ± 7.0 mm Hg; PaCO2, 33.0 ± 4.6/31.5 ± 3.5 mm Hg; pH, 7.33 ± 0.06/7.36 ± 0.02 (values are mean ± SD, n = 4). There was no deviation from these values over the period of assessment. An ischemic lesion of the core of the caudate putamen was visible as a pale, slightly stained area in the ischemic hemisphere as early as 1 hour after reperfusion, and extended to the entire middle cerebral artery (MCA) territory at 4 hours by cresyl violet staining (data not shown). The time-dependent increase of infarction in mouse brain using the intraluminal suture blockade is consistent with previous reports that used the same focal stroke model in mice (Yang et al. 1994; Kondo et al. 1997).

APE/Ref-1 Immunohistochemistry of wild-type and SOD1 Tg mice before and after transient FCI

The APE/Ref-1 protein was constitutively expressed in the entire region of the normal mouse brain in both wild-type and SOD1 Tg mice. It was mainly expressed in the nucleus, which is consistent with previous reports (Ono et al. 1995; Wilson et al. 1996). We observed regional predominance in the hippocampus compared with the cortex and the caudate putamen from wild-type animals as well as from SOD1 Tg mice. This regional predominance was confirmed by Western blot analysis. After 1 hour of reperfusion, following 60 minutes of ischemia, a significant reduction of APE/Ref-1 immunoreactive cells was observed in the caudate putamen from both groups. Four hours after ischemia, the number of APE/Ref-1-positive cells was significantly decreased in the entire MCA territory including the caudate putamen and cortex, and was sustained 24 hours after ischemia. As shown in Figure 1, the percentage of APE/Ref-1-positive cells was not significantly different in the non-ischemic brain between the wild-type and SOD1 Tg mice, however, the percentage of APE/Ref-1-positive cells was significantly lower in the wild-type animals in the lateral caudate putamen 1 and 4 hours after ischemia, and in the MCA territory cortex 4 hours after ischemia (Fujimura et al. 1999a). Most, if not all of the APE/Ref-1-positive cells were stained with NeuN, a neuronal marker (Fujimura et al. 1999b).

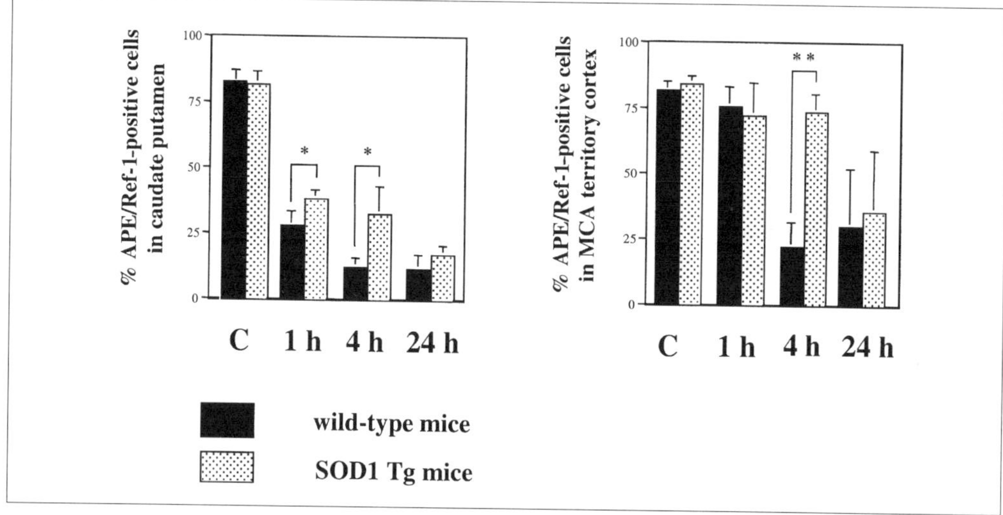

Fig. 1. Results of immunohistochemical analysis. There was no significant difference in the percentage of APE/Ref-1-positive cells between wild-type and SOD1 Tg mice before ischemia. In the wild-type mice, the percentage of APE/Ref-1-positive cells significantly decreased as early as 1 hour after ischemia in the lateral caudate putamen, while it began decreasing 4 hours after ischemia in the MCA territory cortex. The percentage of APE/Ref-1-positive cells was significantly lower in the wild-type mice after 1 and 4 hours in the lateral caudate putamen and after 4 hours in the MCA territory cortex compared with the SOD1 Tg mice. All values shown are mean ± SD (n = 5 to 6). C, non-ischemic control. * $P = 0.01$; ** $P = 0.001$. Results are from Fujimura et al. (1999b).

Western blot analysis

As shown in Figure 2, APE/Ref-1 immunoreactivity was evident as a single band of molecular mass 37 kDa of a whole cell fraction from the non-ischemic striatum in both wild-type mice (lane 1, upper panel) and SOD1 Tg mice (lane 2, upper panel), and was reduced 4 hours after ischemia in both groups (lanes 3–6, upper lane panel). SOD1 Tg mice showed much less reduction in APE/Ref-1 protein levels (lanes 5 and 6, upper panel; mean optical density = 0.191) than wild-type littermates (lanes 3 and 4, upper panel; mean optical density = 0.098). On the other hand, a consistent amount of β-actin immunoreactivity between each lane is seen in the lower panel, suggesting that the amount of the loaded protein was consistent. These data not only confirm the specificity of the antibody for APE/Ref-1 used in this study, but also suggest that there was more reduction of APE/Ref-1 after transient focal ischemia in wild-type animals than in SOD1 Tg mice.

Double labeling with APE/Ref-1 expression and TUNEL staining

Constitutive expression of APE/Ref-1 was detected in the non-ischemic caudate putamen, in which there were no TUNEL-positive cells. TUNEL-positive cells were barely recognized 4 hours after FCI, while a marked reduction of APE/Ref-1-positive cells was seen at this time point. Twenty-four hours after FCI, a significant amount of TUNEL-positive cells with the characteristic features of apoptosis (densely labeled in their nuclei, accompanied by apoptotic bodies) were seen. None of these cells showed APE/Ref-1 immunoreactivity. On the other hand, none of the cells with APE/Ref-1 immunoreactivity were TUNEL-positive 24 hours after FCI. To quantify the temporal profile of DNA fragmentation after FCI, the number of TUNEL-positive cells in the caudate putamen was counted 4 and 24 hours after FCI as well as in the control specimens, as previously described (Fujimura et al. 1998). Only a small

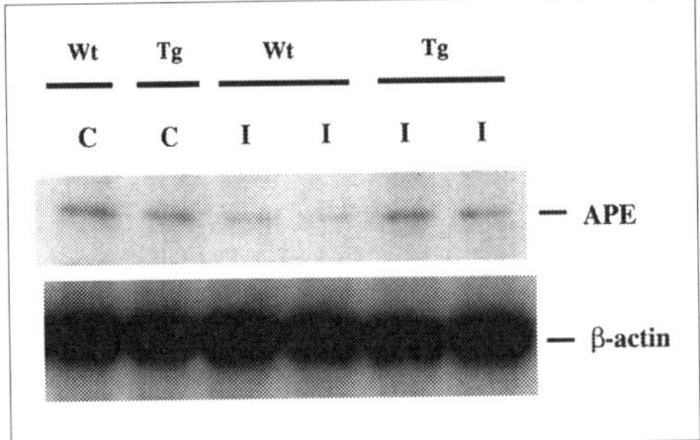

Fig. 2. Western blot analysis of the APE/Ref-1 protein and β-actin protein as an internal control. APE/Ref-1 immunoreactivity is evident as a single band of molecular mass 37 kDa of the whole cell fraction from the non-ischemic brain (lanes 1 and 2, top panel) and was significantly decreased 4 hours after 60 minutes of MCA occlusion (lanes 3 to 6). More reduction was seen in the wild-type animals (lanes 5 and 6, top panel) than in the SOD1 Tg mice (lanes 3 and 4, top panel). On the other hand, a consistent amount of β-actin immunoreactivity is shown in the lower panel. Wt, wild-type; C, non-ischemic control; I, ischemic brain. Results are from Fujimura et al. (1999b).

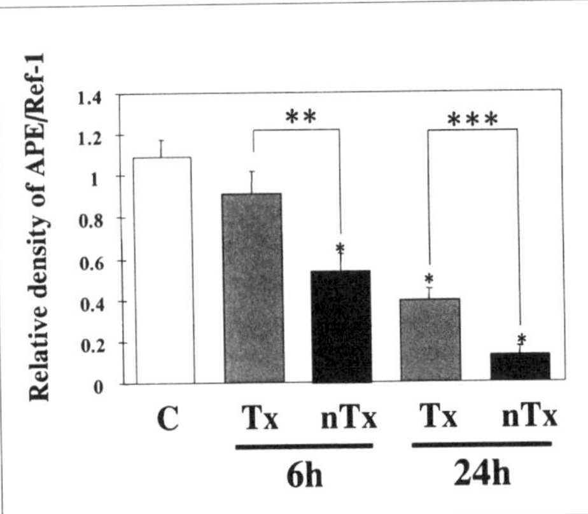

Fig. 3. APE/Ref-1 expression in mice after photothrombotic cortical cerebral ischemia, the result of the densitometric analysis. Apart from the group treated 6 hours after ischemia, the difference between the sham and other ischemic groups is significant (*$P < 0.001$, $n = 4$). When analyzing the differences between the treated and vehicle control groups, the levels of APE/Ref-1 protein were significantly preserved in the treated group 6 hours (**$P < 0.005$) and 1 day (*** $P < 0.001$) after ischemia. C, sham-operated control; Tx, treated with 21-aminosteroid; nTx, vehicle-treated group. Results are from Chang et al. (1999).

number of TUNEL-positive cells was detected in the control specimens and in the brain 4 hours after FCI, while they significantly increased 24 hours after FCI.

DNA laddering was detected by genomic DNA gel electrophoresis

To detect the occurrence of apoptosis as characterized by intranucleosomal DNA fragmentation, we analyzed DNA from both the ischemic brain and the homologous sample on the contralateral side. DNA laddering was absent in the control tissue from both wild-type and SOD1 Tg mice. No DNA laddering was detected in either the SOD1 Tg mice or the wild-type mice 4 hours after FCI. However, a significant amount of DNA laddering was detected 24 hours after ischemia. The level of DNA laddering (Fujimura et al. 1999b) was significantly decreased in the SOD1 Tg mice.

Ischemia-induced reduction in APE/Ref-1 expression is prevented in antioxidant-treated mice

We further examined the effects of the free radical scavenger, 21-aminosteroid, on APE/Ref-1 protein expression and subsequent infarction volume after photothrombotic cortical cerebral ischemia in mice. Immunohistochemistry and Western blot analysis showed a significant reduction in APE/Ref-1 expression 6 and 24 hours after ischemia in untreated animals, whereas in drug-treated animals the reduction was much less at the same time points (Fig. 3). The administration of 21-aminosteroid significantly decreased subsequent infarction volume 3 days after ischemia (Chang et al. 1999). These data suggest that 21-aminosteroid prevents the early decrease in APE/Ref-1 expression, thereby reducing cortical infarction after photothrombotic cerebral ischemia.

Discussion

The present study provides the first evidence that ROS contribute to the early decrease of the DNA repair enzyme APE/Ref-1 and subsequent DNA fragmentation after focal ischemia/reperfusion injury. Our observations were that the early decrease of APE/Ref-1 has a role in the apoptotic cell death pathway in transient FCI, and that this reduction in Tg mice is prevented in part by the overexpression of the antioxidant enzyme SOD-1. These observations derive from the following findings. First, a marked reduction of APE/Ref-1 was seen in the entire ischemic area in wild-type mice as early as 1 hour after ischemia, and preceded the occurrence of DNA fragmentation. Second, double staining with APE/Ref-1 and TUNEL clearly showed that the neurons that lost APE/Ref-1 immunoreactivity became TUNEL-positive, indicating the spatial relationship between APE/Ref-1 expression and DNA damage after transient FCI. Third, despite the decrease in APE/Ref-1 expression following transient FCI in SOD1 Tg mice, its reduction was significantly less than that in wild-type mice as shown by both immunohistochemistry and Western blot analysis. Finally, nucleosomal DNA fragmentation was seen 24 hours after transient FCI and was reduced in SOD1 Tg mice, suggesting the possibility that a lesser reduction of APE/Ref-1 in Tg mice may contribute to the smaller amount of nucleosomal DNA fragmentation compared to that of the wild-type mice. Taken together, this suggests that overexpression of SOD1 in Tg mice may prevent the early decrease of APE/Ref-1 after transient FCI, and could thereby contribute to reducing the amount of DNA fragmentation.

Antioxidant enzymes and DNA repair proteins are thought to be two major mechanisms by which cells counteract the deleterious effects of ROS, and we have shown evidence that antioxidant enzymes such as SOD play a protective role in ischemia/reperfusion injury in the mouse brain (Kinouchi et al. 1991; Chan et al. 1995, 1998; Chan 1996; Kondo et al. 1997). SOD1 Tg mice had a significant reduction in infarct volume after transient FCI (Kinouchi et al. 1991), whereas infarction was increased in SOD1 knockouts after transient ischemia (Kondo et al. 1997). Furthermore, a marked increase in DNA damage was seen in SOD1 knockout mice after transient FCI compared with the wild-type mice (Kondo et al. 1997). In the present study, nucleosomal DNA fragmentation was detected 24 hours after transient FCI and was decreased in Tg mice that overexpress SOD1, again suggesting that SOD1 has a protective role against DNA-damaged cell death after transient FCI. We do not completely rule out the possibility that SOD1 delayed but did not prevent the decrease of APE/Ref-1 expression at later time points since there was a *in vitro* report showing that the injection or transfection of SOD1 into cultured sympathetic neurons delayed apoptosis induced by nerve growth factor deprivation (Greenlund et al. 1995). Nevertheless, we do believe that ROS play a major role in the rapid reduction of APE/Ref-1 in the ischemic brain. This additional and unequivocal proof was obtained from the 21-aminosteroid treatment study showing that the antioxidant prevented the early decrease of APE/Ref-1 expression, thereby reducing cortical infarction in mice after photothrombotic cerebral ischemia. We propose that the level of APE/Ref-1 expression may serve as an early molecular marker for oxidative DNA damage in transient FCI.

Acknowledgments

This study was supported by National Institutes of Health grants NS14543, NS25372, NS36147, NS38653 and NO1 NS82386. We thank Cheryl Christensen for editorial assistance.

References

1. Bennett RAO, Wilson DM III, Wong D, Demple B (1997) Interaction of human apurinic endonuclease and DNA polymerase beta in the base excision repair pathway. Proc Natl Acad Sci USA 94:7166–7169
2. Chan PH (1996) Role of oxidants in ischemic brain damage. Stroke 27:1124–1129
3. Chan PH, Epstein CJ, Li Y, Huang T-T, Carlson E, Kinouchi H, Yang G, Kamii H, Mikawa S, Kondo T, Copin J-C, Chen SF, Chan T, Gafni J, Gobbel G, Reola L (1995) Transgenic mice and knockout mutants in the study of oxidative stress in brain injury. J Neurotrauma 12:815–824

4. Chan PH, Kawase M, Murakami K, Chen SF, Li Y, Calagui B, Reola L, Carlson E, Epstein CJ (1998) Overexpression of SOD1 in transgenic mice protects vulnerable neurons against ischemic damage after global cerebral ischemia and reperfusion. J Neurosci 18:8292–8299
5. Chang Y-Y, Fujimura M, Morita-Fujimura Y, Kim GW, Huang C-Y, Wu H-S, Kawase M, Copin J-C, Chan PH (1999) Neuroprotective effects of an antioxidant in cortical cerebral ischemia: Prevention of early reduction of the apurinic/apyrimidinic endonuclease DNA repair enzyme. Neurosci Lett 277:61–64
6. Chopp M, Chan PH, Hsu CY, Cheung ME, Jacobs TP (1996) DNA damage and repair in central nervous system injury: National Institute of Neurological Disorders and Stroke workshop summary. Stroke 27:363–369
7. Demple B, Harrison L (1994) Repair of oxidative damage to DNA: enzymology and biology. Annu Rev Biochem 63:915–948
8. Doetsch PW, Cunningham RP (1990) The enzymology of apurinic/apyrimidinic endonucleases. Mutat Res 236:173–201
9. Fujimura M, Morita-Fujimura Y, Murakami K, Kawase M, Chan PH (1998) Cytosolic redistribution of cytochrome c following transient focal cerebral ischemia in rats. J Cereb Blood Flow Metab 18:1239–1247
10. Fujimura M, Morita-Fujimura Y, Kawase M, Chan, PH (1999a) Early decrease of apurinic/apyrimidinic endonuclease expression after transient focal cerebral ischemia in mice. J Cereb Blood Flow Metab 19:495–501
11. Fujimura M, Morita-Fujimura Y, Narasimhan P, Copin J-C, Kawase M, Chan PH (1999b) Copper-zinc superoxide dismutase prevents the early decrease of apurinic/apyrimidinic endonuclease and subsequent DNA fragmentation after transient focal cerebral ischemia in mice. Stroke 30:2408–2415
12. Greenlund LJS, Deckwerth TL, Johnson EM Jr (1995) Superoxide dismutase delays neuronal apoptosis: a role for reactive oxygen species in programmed neuronal death. Neuron 14:303–315
13. Kawase M, Fujimura M, Morita-Fujimura Y, Chan PH (1999) Reduction of apurinic/apyrimidinic endonuclease expression after transient global cerebral ischemia in rats. Implication of the failure of DNA repair in neuronal apoptosis. Stroke 30:441–449
14. Kinouchi H, Epstein CJ, Mizui T, Carlson EJ, Chen SF, Chan PH (1991) Attenuation of focal cerebral ischemic injury in transgenic mice overexpressing CuZn superoxide dismutase. Proc Natl Acad Sci USA 88:11158–11162
15. Kondo T, Reaume AG, Huang T-T, Carlson E, Murakami K, Chen SF, Hoffman EK, Scott RW, Epstein CJ, Chan PH (1997) Reduction of CuZn-superoxide dismutase activity exacerbates neuronal cell injury and edema formation after transient focal cerebral ischemia. J Neurosci 17:4180–4189
16. Lindahl T (1990) Repair of intrinsic DNA lesions. Mutat Res 238:305–311
17. Liu PK, Hsu CY, Dizdaroglu M, Floyd RA, Kow YW, Karakaya A, Rabow LE, Cui J-K (1996) Damage, repair, and mutagenesis in nuclear genes after mouse forebrain ischemia-reperfusion. J Neurosci 16:6795–6806
18. Loeb LA, Preston BD (1986) Mutagenesis by apurinic/apyrimidinic sites. Annu Rev Genet 20:201–230
19. Ono Y, Watanabe M, Inoue Y, Ohmoto T, Akiyama K, Tsutsui K, Seki S (1995) Developmental expression of APEX nuclease, a multifunctional DNA repair enzyme, in mouse brains. Brain Res Dev Brain Res 86:1–6
20. Robertson KA, Hill DP, Xu Y, Liu L, Van Epps S, Hockenbery DM, Park JR, Wilson TM, Kelley MR (1997) Down-regulation of apurinic/apyrimidinic endonuclease expression is associated with the induction of apoptosis in differentiating myeloid leukemia cells. Cell Growth Differ 8:443–449
21. Sancar A, Sancar GB (1988) DNA repair enzymes. Annu Rev Biochem 57:29–67
22. Wilson TM, Rivkees SA, Deutsch WA, Kelley MR (1996) Differential expression of the apurinic/apyrimidinic endonuclease (APE/ref-1) multifunctional DNA base excision repair gene during fetal development and in adult rat brain and testis. Mutat Res 362:237–248
23. Yang G, Chan PH, Chen J, Carlson E, Chen SF, Weinstein P, Epstein CJ, Kamii H (1994) Human copper-zinc superoxide dismutase transgenic mice are highly resistant to reperfusion injury after focal cerebral ischemia. Stroke 25:165–170

A role for the transcription factor E2F1 in experimental stroke damage

J. P. MacManus, S. T. Hou, M. Jian, E. Preston, J. Webster, B. Zurakowski

Summary

E2F1 +/+ and –/– mice had similar brain areas supplied by the middle cerebral artery (MCA), similar intra- and post-ischemic reductions in cerebral blood flow after occlusion of the MCA, and similar areas of hypoxic brain tissue. However the E2F1 –/– mice had less infarcted brain, especially in littermates at 7 d of reperfusion after 20 min of MCA occlusion where the infarct volume was 6.5 ± 4.9 mm^3 ($\pm$ SD, n = 9) compared to 27.6 ± 5.4 mm^3 ($\pm$ SD, n = 8) in wild-type mice. Cultured cortical neurons from E2F1 –/– mice had an increased resistance to induction of apoptosis. On the other hand, overexpression of E2F1 by means of adenoviral vectors in cultured cortical neurons led to the appearance of many hallmarks of apoptosis. It is concluded that the transcription factor E2F1 has a role in neuronal death following ischemia and other insults.

Introduction

The delayed neuronal cell death occurring in experimental stroke models is regarded as gene directed (Lipton 1999; MacManus and Linnik 1997; MacManus and Buchan 2000). Such an active mechanism of cell death may also underlie neurodegeneration in chronic disease states (Michel et al. 1999; Tatton 1999). Some of these activated genes are associated with apoptosis such as Bax, Bcl2 or members of the caspase family of protease particularly caspase-3. Others are transcription factors such as p53 or Myc. Another transcription factor implicated in apoptosis is E2F1, but which like a number of molecules involved in cell death also functions in control of cell cycle progression (Dyson 1998; Nevins 1998).

Evidence for a role for E2F1 in apoptosis has been mounting. For example, overexpression of E2F1 in quiescent cells by viral recombinants (Kowalik et al. 1995; DeGregori et al. 1997) or in transgenic mice (Holmberg et al. 1998; Pierce et al. 1998) can trigger apoptosis. Further evidence of E2F1's role in induction of apoptosis came from E2F1-deficient mice where decreased cell death in thymocytes was observed (Field et al. 1996; Yamasaki et al. 1996). However, these mutant mice develop and reproduce normally for up to six months with no apparent morphological effects in many organs including brain presumably because of the ability of other E2F family members to compensate for the absence of E2F1.

Keywords: stroke, apoptosis, ischemia, E2F1, transcription factor

Apoptosis Research Group, Institute for Biological Sciences M54, National Research Council Canada, Ottawa, ON, K1A 0R6.
e-mail: John.MacManus@NRC.CA

The mechanism of induction of cell death by E2F1 in non-neuronal cells may involve p53 (Nevins 1998; Kowalik et al. 1998). Increased p53 has been described in neuronal death following focal ischemia and also following kainic acid treatment (Li et al. 1994; Sakhi et al. 1994). In other studies, gene knock-out of p53 decreased ischemic brain damage or cerebellar granule cell loss due to γ-radiation (Crumrine et al. 1994; Wood and Youle 1995). An alternate, p53-independent, view of the proapoptotic action of E2F1 involves the blockage of antiapoptotic signal pathways leading to NFkB (Phillips et al. 1999). E2F1 is expressed during neurogenesis as might be expected (Dagnino et al. 1997) but can still be detected in adult mouse brain (Helin et al. 1992; Dupont et al. 1998). Because of the presence of E2F1 in neurons and involvement in cell death, and the fact that E2F1-null cells may be viewed as being deficient in p53 function, we surmised that E2F1-deficient mice would have attenuated brain damage following an ischemic insult.

Materials and methods

All procedures using animals were approved by a local committee for the Canadian Council on Animal Care. Our first series of experiments used mice obtained from Jackson Laboratories (Bar Harbor, MA, USA) bred locally. The E2F1–/– (Stock 2785) (Field et al. 1996) and the E2F1+/+ mice (Stock 101045) are a cross between C57B/6 and SV129 strains. In our second series of experiments we used F2 generation littermates produced from interbreeding the F1 generation of E2F1 –/– stock crossed with purebred C57B/6 mice. F2 generation animals were genotyped by PCR as described (Field et al. 1996). The mice (20–23 g) were subjected to occlusion of the middle cerebral artery (MCAO) under isoflurane anaesthesia by an intraluminal filament (Hara et al. 1996) for either 20 min or 2 h of ischemia, the animals briefly reanaesthetized with isoflurane and the filament withdrawn. Regional cerebral blood flow, blood pressure and blood gases were measured as previously described (MacManus et al. 1999). To measure ischemic damage 24 h or 7 d post MCAO, the brains were removed from euthanized animals, and the forebrain cut into five 2 mm thick coronal slices which were stained with 2% 2,3,5-triphenyltetrazolium chloride (TTC), photographed with a mm-scale and the images were digitized. Infarct areas were obtained by digital planimetry of the slices using ImagePro software (Media Cybernetics, Silver Spring MD) and normalized for edema as described (MacManus et al. 1999). In other experiments, the bioreductive pentaflouro-2-nitroimidazole, EF5, was used to directly delineate hypoxic territory by immunohistochemistry using ELK3.51 Cy3-conjugated monoclonal antibody (Evans et al. 1997; MacManus et al. 1999).

Primary fetal cortical mouse neuronal cells deficient in E2F1 (Jackson Laboratories and bred locally) were cultured from E18 brain tissue (Hou et al. 2000). Primary cortical neuronal cells were cultured from E18 Sprague-Dawley rats as previously described (MacManus et al. 1997), and overexpression of E2F1 was achieved by using adenoviral vectors. Replication defective wild-type free adenovirus containing either cDNA coding for E2F1 under the CMV promoter/enhancer (AdCMV-E2F1), β-galactosidase (AdCMV-LacZ), or green fluorescent protein (AdCMV5-GFP_Q) were constructed and propagated in E1-complementing 293 cells (Kowalik et al. 1995; Massie et al. 1998) and used as described previously (Hou et al. 2000).

Results and discussion

Decreased ischemic damage in E2F1-null mice

When E2F1+/+ mice were subjected to 2 h of MCAO an infarct was produced in the ischemic hemisphere at 24 h of reperfusion of 77.0 ± 12.3 mm^3 (± SD, n = 15) whereas a significantly smaller infarct volume of 58.8 ± 18.5 mm^3 (± SD, n = 15) ($p < 0.01$) was found in the E2F1–/– animals (Fig. 1A). This reduction in infarct volume was most apparent in the anterior brain

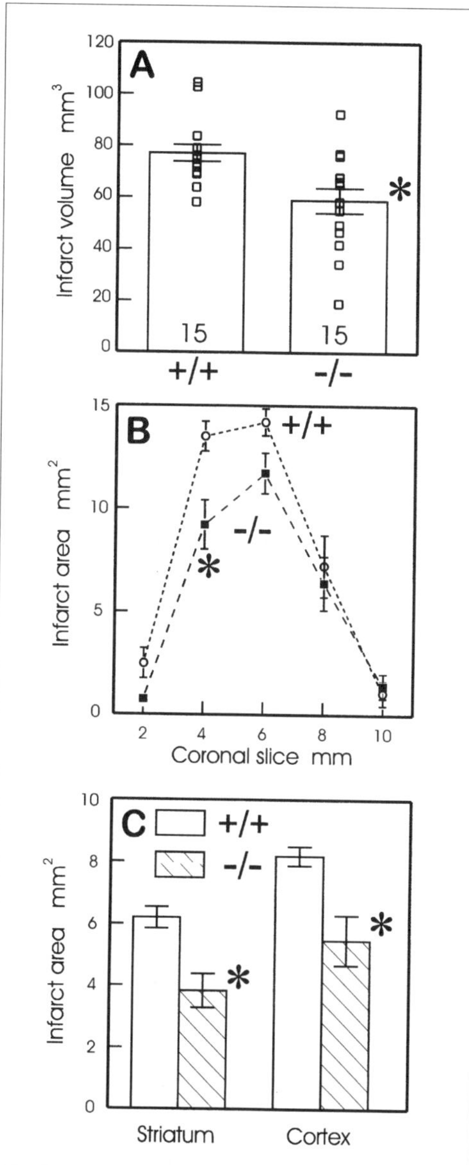

Fig. 1. Decreased ischemic brain damage at 24 h of reperfusion in E2F1-deficient mice following 2 h MCAO based on TTC staining (mean ± SEM). **A:** Decreased infarct volume in E2F1–/– mice. $^*p < 0.01$ on non-paired t test ($n = 15$). **B**: Decreased infarct areas in coronal slices of E2F1–/– mice. $^*p < 0.002$ on non-paired t test ($n = 15$) in second coronal slice. **C**: Decreased infarct areas in striatum and cortex in second coronal slice in B. $^*p < 0.001$ on ANOVA ($n = 15$). *Reproduced with permission of the publisher from MacManus et al. 1999.*

slices particularly in the second slice from the frontal pole (Fig. 1B). The reduction of damage in this slice was seen in both cortex and striatum (Fig. 1C). No differences were found in mean arterial blood pressure, or in arterial pO_2, pCO_2 or pH between E2F1+/+ and –/– mice during ischemia or reperfusion (data not shown).

There is current awareness that differences in infarct volume in mutant mice could be wrongly attributed to specific genes when in fact anatomical or physiological differences due to the genetic background of normal and knockout animals are at play as seen in neurotrauma models (Steward et al. 1999). Clear evidence of angioarchitectural differences between the strains C57B/6 and SV129 has been reported (Maeda et al. 1998), in line with reported variable sensitivities of mouse strains to ischemia (Barone et al. 1993; Connolly et al. 1996; Fujii et al. 1997; Yang et al. 1997). However, in our case no obvious difference was seen in the extent of the supplying territory of the MCA between the E2F1+/+ and–/– mice after visualization of the cerebrovasculature with india ink. An analysis similar to that of Maeda and colleagues (1998) was made of the distance from the midline to the line of anastomoses between the MCA and the ACA, and no significant difference was found between the two groups of mice (MacManus et al. 1999).

In addition to this visualization of the angioarchitecture of mouse brain, we also visualized the hypoxic territory using immunohistochemical localization of the bioreductive compound EF5 (Evans et al. 1997). EF5 is a pentafluorinated derivative of 2-nitroimidazole which is reduced by hypoxia leading to the formation of covalent macromolecular adducts detectable with a specific antibody, and which has been used to localize hypoxic brain tissue in a neonatal model of ischemia (Evans et al. 1997). In mice subjected to 2 h of MCAO and 15 min of reperfusion, EF5 immunolocalisation clearly distinguished hypoxic tissue of the ischemic hemisphere of normal and mutant mice in contrast to the very faint adjacent background staining similar to that seen in the contralateral hemisphere (Fig. 2A, B). A measurement of the EF5 stained area in brain sections at the level of greatest protection in the

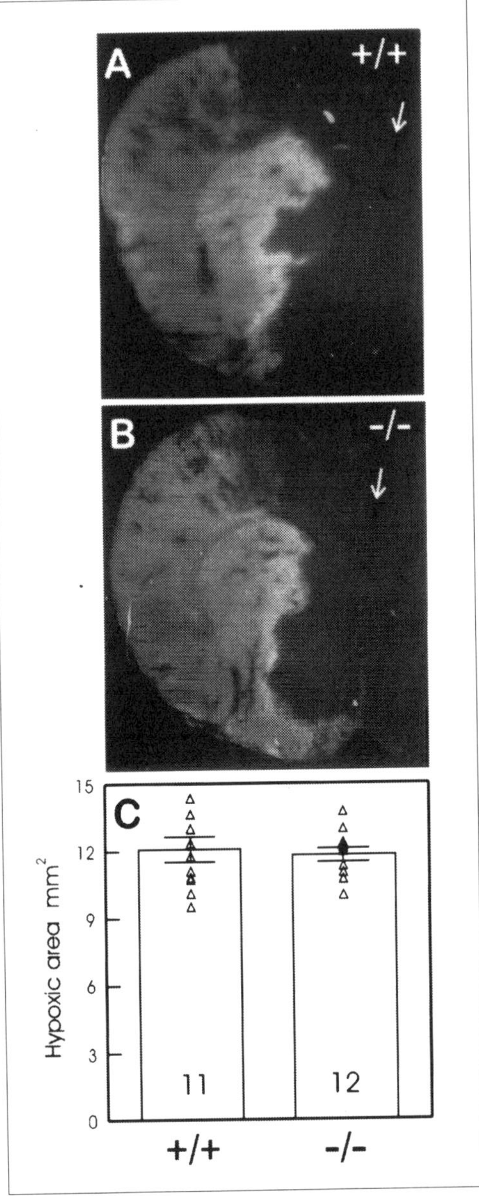

Fig. 2. Similar areas of hypoxia in ischemic E2F1+/+ and –/– mice at 15 min of reperfusion following 2 h of MCAO. **A** & **B**: Hypoxic territory was stained for EF5 in brain sections approximating the second coronal slice in Fig. 1B (approximately +1.0 mm from bregma). The arrow indicates the midline. **C**: No significant difference in hypoxic areas of E2F1+/+ (n = 11) or E2F1–/– (mean ± SEM, n = 12) mice: p > 0.05 on paired t test. *Reproduced with permission of the publisher from MacManus et al. 1999.*

E2F1–/– mice (eg about 4 mm from frontal pole in Fig. 1B) showed that the hypoxic territory was equivalent to that in E2F1 +/+ animals (Fig. 2C). It was therefore concluded that both mutant and wildtype animals became equally hypoxic in response to the ischemic insult.

Although we interpreted these results to indicate that the E2F1 gene was modulating ischemic damage, we remained concerned that the decrease in infarct in the E2F1-null animals was only 25%. We considered it possible that a subtle metabolic effect of genetic background, which was not evident as a difference in cerebrovasculature or hypoxia, was the underlying cause of the smaller infarct in the E2F1-null mice and not the absence of the E2F1 gene itself. We therefore undertook to repeat the experiment in interbred littermates. After 24 h of reperfusion following 2 h of MCAO, no difference in infarct size was observed in E2F1 +/+ compared to E2F1 +/– littermate animals. However, again in the E2F1 –/– mice a decrease infarct of 25% was observed (data not shown). This result suggested that genetic background could be eliminated as the cause of the smaller infarct size in E2F1-null mice. Because the 2 h MCAO essentially destroys 30% of the ischemic hemisphere after 24 h, we proceeded to ask whether this prolonged occlusion was too severe an insult to permit more robust resistance in the mutant animals. We undertook to examine the infarct volume in littermates at 7 d of reperfusion after only 20 min of MCAO which typically results in about 10–15% infarction of the ischemic hemisphere. Again no significant difference in the volume of injured brain was observed in E2F1 +/+ mice [27.6 ± 5.4 mm^3 (± SD, n = 8)] compared with the heterozygous animals [28.6 ± 5.5 mm^3 (± SD, n = 11)] (Fig. 3). However, a striking decrease in infarct volume of 77% [6.5 ± 4.9 mm^3 (± SD, n = 9; p < 0.001)] was observed in the E2F1-null animals after this milder ischemic injury (Fig. 3). This suggests that if the injury is not too severe, the resistance due to the absence of the E2F1 gene is quite striking.

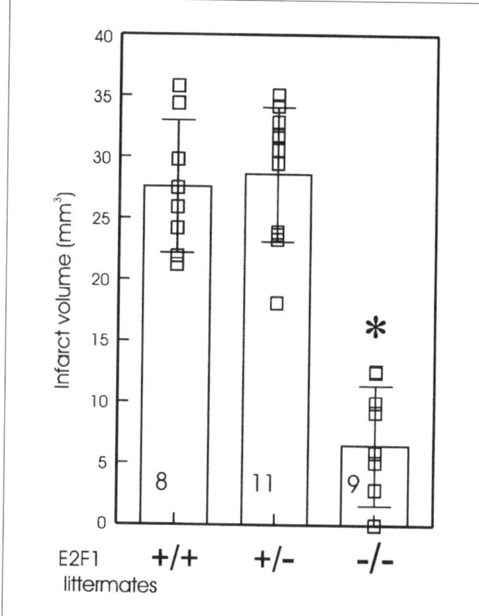

Fig. 3. Decrease of 77% in infarct volume at 7 d of reperfusion following 20 min of MCAO in E2F1-deficient mice compared to wild-type and heterozygous littermates (mean ± SD) *$p < 0.001$ on ANOVA ($n = 8–11$). Measurements of infarct volume in individual animals based on TTC staining are shown.

Decreased apoptosis in E2F1-null cultured neurons

Experimental stroke studies in mutant animals are fraught with both technical and interpretative difficulties, and we therefore also performed parallel studies using cultured neurons. Cortical neuronal cultures derived from E2F1 +/+ and E2F1 –/– mice were identical in their morphology, expression of NMDA receptors, and proportion of cells staining for the neuronal markers NeuN & Hu (Hou et al. 2000). When treated with 1 μM staurosporine the E2F1 +/+ mouse neurons died by apoptosis with significantly increased caspase 3-like activity and punctate nuclear chromatin (Fig. 4B). By comparison, E2F1 –/– neuronal cells had five-fold lower caspase 3-like proteolytic activity (Fig. 4A), and three-fold less cells with apoptotic morphology (Fig. 4C) in comparison with E2F1 +/+ cells after staurosporine treatment. While caspase 3-like activity from E2F1 +/+ cortical cultures continued to increase at 12 h, both caspase 3-like activity and the number of apoptotic cells reached a plateau in E2F1 –/– cultures after 12 h staurosporine treatment (Fig. 4C).

Increased apoptosis in cultured neurons overexpressing E2F1

Rat cortical neurons infected with 400 MOI AdCMV-E2F1 exhibited signs of cell death after 72 h post-infection, whereas neurons infected with control recombinant adenoviral vectors such as AdCMV-GFP remained viable (Hou et al. 2000). Several hallmarks of apoptosis such as increased caspase 3-like proteolytic activity, TUNEL staining, and DNA fragmentation were examined after AdCMV-E2F1 infection (Fig. 5). In conjunction with marked reduction in cellular viability, a 3 to 5-fold increase in caspase 3-like activity was measured 72 h to 96 h after AdCMV-E2F1 infection in comparison with mock-infected cells or cells infected with AdCMV5-GFP_Q (Hou et al. 2000). TUNEL positive cells increased after 72 h post-infection with AdCMV-E2F1 in comparison with controls (Fig. 5B, D, F) and such TUNEL positive cells also had typical punctate nuclei upon staining with Hoechst 33258 (Fig. 5A, C, E), indicative of apoptosis. Cells with both TUNEL positive staining and with punctate nuclear morphology increased by 2.5-fold and 6 fold in comparison with controls (i.e. uninfected or AdCMV5-GFP_Q infected cells) after 72 h or 96 h infection respectively (Fig. 5G). Increased DNA fragmentation in the form of oligonucleosomal DNA ladders was detected in the 72 and 96 h AdCMV-E2F1 infected cortical cells (Fig. 5H).

Conclusions

E2F1 is present during mouse neurogenesis (Dagnino et al. 1997), decreases in P19 embry-

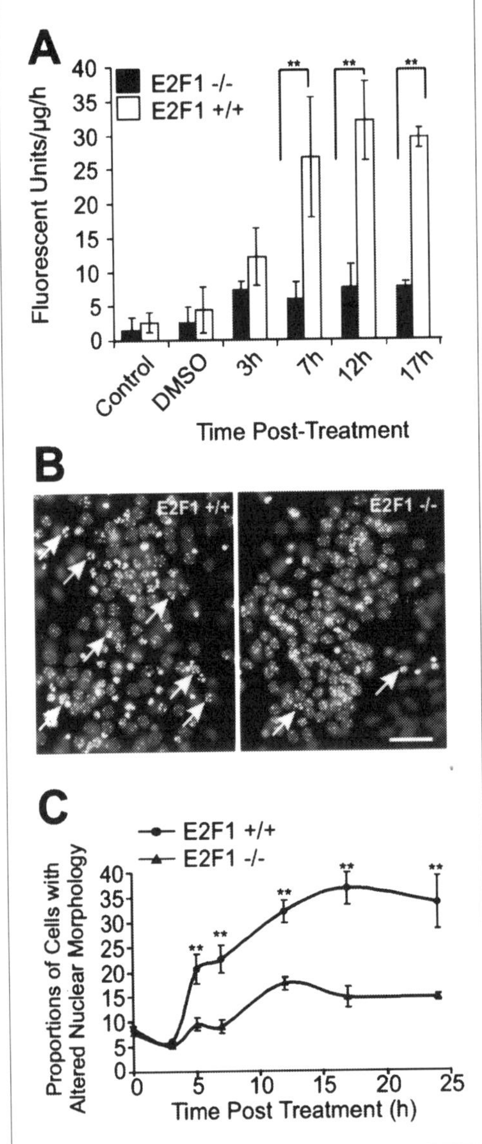

Fig. 4. E2F1 –/– cortical cultures were protected from staurosporine-induced apoptosis. Cortical cultures 14 DIV were treated with 1 µM staurosporine for 3, 7, 12, or 17 h, and cytosolic extracts were prepared and evaluated for Ac-DEVD-AFC cleavage activity (**A**). Caspase 3-like activity in E2F1 +/+ cortical cultures increased more than 5-fold after 3 h treatment with 1 µM staurosporine and continued to increase to more that 10-fold after 12 h in comparison with untreated or DMSO-treated controls. In contrast, caspase-3-like activity in E2F1 –/– cortical cultures increased only about 2-fold after 3 h treatment in comparison with the untreated or DMSO-treated E2F1 –/– cortical cultures. Furthermore, caspase 3-like activity level had no further significant increase after 3 h treatment with staurosporine in E2F1 –/– cultures. At 7, 12, and 17 h points, caspase 3-like activity of E2F1 +/+ cortical cultures were significantly higher than that from the E2F1 –/– cultures (** $p < 0.001$, ANOVA). E2F1 +/+ and –/– cortical cultures treated with 1 µM staurosporine for 3, 7, 12, 17, or 24 h were also fixed with 2% paraformaldehyde, stained with Hoechst 33258 and photographed. Examples of the microphotographs are shown in **B**. Note there were markedly more cells with punctate nuclei (arrows) in E2F1 +/+ than E2F1 –/– cortical cultures. More than 1000 cells were counted and the proportions of apoptotic cells plotted as shown in **C**. A significant increase of apoptotic cells in E2F1 +/+ cortical cultures in comparison with E2F1 –/– cultures was evident after 5 h treatment (** $p < 0.001$, Student's t-test). While the number of apoptotic cells continued to increase even after 12 h in E2F1 +/+ cells, the number reached a plateau in E2F1 –/– cortical cultures (**C**). All data are the mean ± SEM of at least five separate experiments. Scale bar = 50 µM. *Reproduced with permission of the publisher from Hou et al. 2000.*

onal carcinoma cells differentiated into a neuronal lineage (Azuma-Hara et al. 1999), but remains postmitotically detectable in adult mouse brain (Helin et al. 1992; Dupont et al. 1998). E2F1 mRNA and protein increases in dying neurons (Giovanni et al. 2000; Hou et al. 2000; O'Hare et al. 2000) and ischemic brain (Hou et al. unpublished observations). Our finding that cortical neurons devoid of the transcription factor E2F1 are resistant to induction of cell death *in vitro* (Hou et al. 2000) is in accord with our studies on experimental stroke in the E2F1-deficient mice (MacManus et al. 1999). Our finding that cortical neurons enriched with E2F1 succumb to cell death supports a role for this transcription factor in modulating cellular decisions in response to injury. There are now several other studies with similar conclusions which utilize cultured neurons induced to die in various ways, ie differentiated neurons obtained from embryonal carcinoma P19 (Azuma-Hara et al. 1999), cerebellar granule neurons treated with β-amyloid (Giovanni et al. 2000) or low potassium (O'Hare et al. 2000). All of these neuronal studies arrive at similar conclusions to the studies which used either proliferating or quiescent cells (Kowalik et al. 1995; Dyson 1998; Nevins 1998).

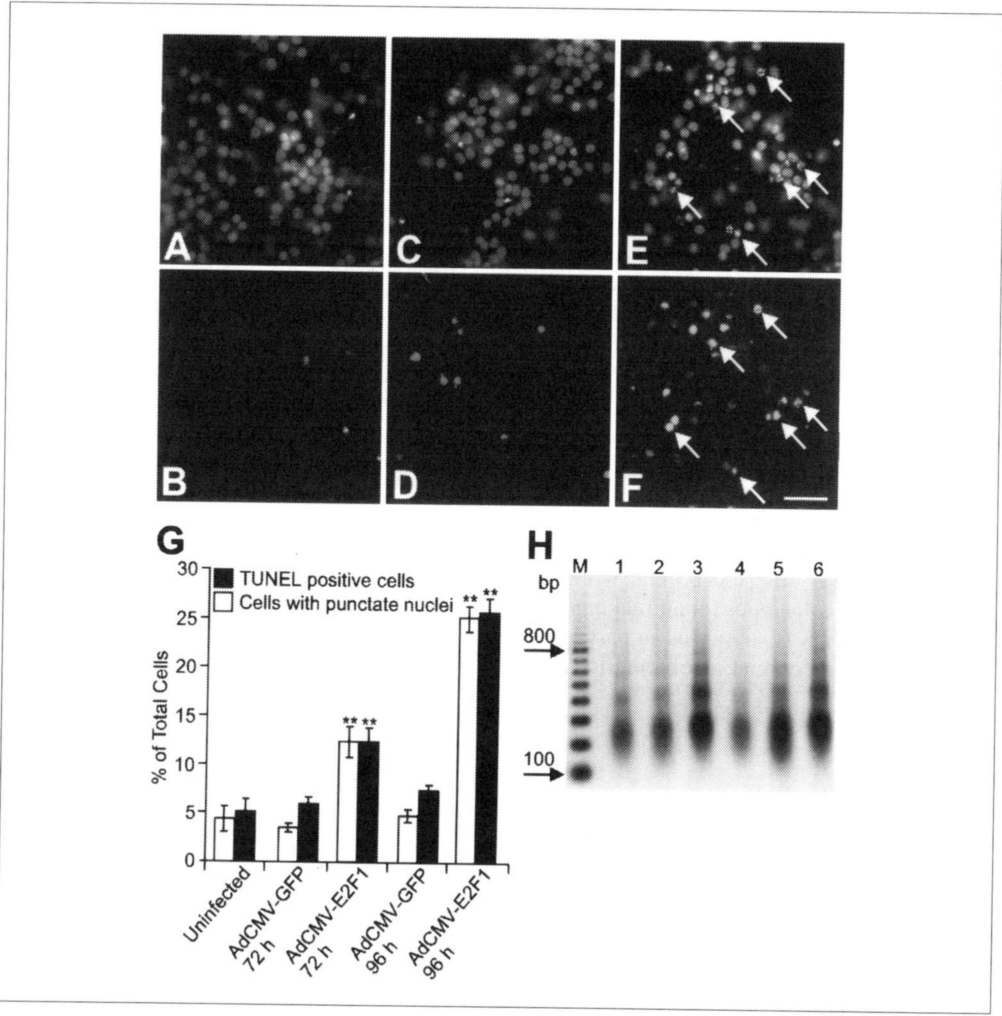

Fig. 5. Significant increase in apoptosis and DNA fragmentation in cultures overexpressing E2F1. After 72 h infection with AdCMV-E2F1, cells both TUNEL positive and with punctate nuclei significantly increased in comparison with cells infected with AdCMV5-GFP_Q (**A-F**), indicating increased apoptosis (**$p < 0.001$, ANOVA). More than a 6-fold increase in the number of cells both TUNEL positive and with punctate nuclei appeared after 96 h infection with AdCMV-E2F1 in comparison with cells uninfected or AdCMV5-GFP_Q infected (**G**). Increased DNA fragmentation in the form of oligonucleosomal DNA ladders occurred after 72 h or 96 h infection with AdCMV-E2F1 (lane 3 and 6, respectively) as detected by gel electrophoresis (**H**). Much lower level of background DNA fragmentation was also detectable in untreated cells (Lane 1, 4) or AdCMV5-GFP_Q infected cells for 72 h or 96 h (lane 2 and 5, respectively), due to natural occurrence of cell death in cultured cells. Data are presented as mean ± SEM. *Reproduced with permission of the publisher from Hou et al. 2000.*

The mechanism whereby the transcription factor E2F1 modulates cellular decisions to die are unknown. There is evidence that another transcription factor p53 may be involved (Nevins 1998; Kowalik et al. 1998), and thus p53 downstream target genes such as the proapoptotic Bax gene may be the instigator of entry into the cell death pathway (MacManus and

Buchan 2000). However, not all E2F1 induced cell death, including that of neurons is p53 dependent (Phillips et al. 1997; Giovanni et al. 2000) and other mechanisms of cellular destruction must be involved. Mutants of E2F1 which are missing the transactivation domain can still induce cell death (Phillips et al. 1997), and may do so by blocking anti-apoptotic signaling pathways (Phillips et al. 1999). Clearly while these p53 dependent and independent mechanisms may play a role in ischemic cell death in the brain, much work will be needed to investigate the possibilities.

Acknowledgements

Our thanks are due D Callaghan, J Daoust, MC Fournier, I Rasquinha, T Walker for technical assistance with various aspects of the work, and to J Daoust and colleagues for animal management. This study was supported in part by the Heart and Stroke Foundation of Ontario (grant A3457 to JPM).

References

1. Azuma-Hara M, Taniura H, Uetsuki T, Niinobe M, Yoshikawa K (1999) Regulation and deregulation of E2F1 in postmitotic neurons differentiated from embryonal carcinoma P19 cells. Exper Cell Res 251:442–451
2. Barone FC, Knudsen DJ, Nelson AH, Feuerstein GZ, Willette RN (1993) Mouse strain differences in susceptibility to cerebral ischemia are related to cerebral vascular anatomy. J Cerebral Blood Flow Metab 13:683–692
3. Connolly ES, Winfree CJ, Stern DM, Solomon RA, Pinsky DJ (1996) Procedural and strain-related variables significantly affect outcome in a murine model of focal cerebral ischemia. Neurosurgery 38:523–532
4. Crumrine RC, Thomas AL, Morgan PF (1994) Attenuation of p53 expression protects against focal ischemic damage in transgenic mice. J Cerebral Blood Flow Metab 14:887–891
5. DeGregori J, Leone G, Miron A, Jakoi L, Nevins JR (1997) Distinct roles for E2F proteins in cell growth control and apoptosis. Proc Natl Acad Sci USA 94:7245–7250
6. Dagnino L, Fry CJ, Bartley SM, Farnham P, Gallie BL, Phillips RA (1997) Expression patterns of the E2F family of transcription factors during mouse nervous system development. Mech Dev 66:13–25
7. Dupont E, Sansal I, Evrard C, Rouget P (1998) Developmental pattern of expression of NPDC-1 and its interaction with E2F1 suggest a role in the control of proliferation and differentiation of neural cells. J Neurosci Res 51:257–267
8. Dyson N (1998) The regulation of E2F by pRB-family proteins. Genes & Dev 12:2245–2262
9. Evans SM, Bergeron M, Ferriero DM, Sharp FR, Hermeking H, Kitsis RN, Geenen DL, Bialik S, Lord EM, Koch CJ (1997) Imaging hypoxia in diseased tissue. Adv Exp Med 428:595–603
10. Field SJ, Tsai FY, Kuo F, Zubiaga AM, Kaelin WG, Livingston DM, Orkin SH, Greenberg ME (1996) E2F1 functions in mice to promote apoptosis and suppress proliferation. Cell 85:549–561
11. Fujii M, Hara H, Meng W, Vonsattel JP, Huang Z, Moskowitz MA (1997) Strain-related differences in susceptability to transient forebrain ischemia in SV-129 and C57Black/6 mice. Stroke 28:1805–1811
12. Giovanni A, Keramaris E, Morris EJ, Hou ST, O'Hare M, Dyson N, Robertson GS, Slack RS, Park DS (2000) E2F1 mediates death of β-amyloid-treated cortical neurons in a manner independent of p53 and dependent on bax and caspase-3. J Biol Chem 275:11553–11560
13. Hara H, Huang P, Panahian N, Fishman MC, Moskowitz MA (1996) Reduced brain edema and infarction volume in mice lacking the neuronal isoform of nitric oxide synthase after transient MCA occlusion. J Cereb Blood Flow Metab 16:605–611
14. Helin K, Lees JA, Vidal M, Dyson N, Harlow E, Fattaey A (1992) A cDNA encoding a pRb-binding protein with properties of the transcription factor E2F. Cell 70:337–350
15. Holmberg C, Helin K, Sehested M, Karlstrom O (1998) E2F-1-induced p53-independent apoptosis in transgenic mice. Oncogene 17:143–155
16. Hou ST, Callaghan D, Fournier MC, Hill I, Kang L, Massie B, Morley P, Murray C, Rasquinha I, Slack R, MacManus JP (2000) The transcription factor E2F1 modulates apoptosis of neurons. J Neurochem 75:91–100
17. Kowalik TF, DeGregori J, Schwarz JK, Nevins JR (1995) E2F1 overexpression in quiescent fibroblasts leads to induction of cellular DNA synthesis and apoptosis. J Virol 69:2491–2500
18. Kowalik TF, DeGregori J, Leono G, Jakoi L, Nevins JR (1998) E2F1-specific induction of apoptosis and p53 accumulation, which is blocked by Mdm2. Cell Growth & Diff 9:113–118
19. Li Y, Chopp M, Zhang ZG, Zaloga C, Niewenhuis L, Gautam S (1994) p53 immunoreactive protein and p53 mRNA expression after transient middle cerebral artery occlusion in rats. Stroke 25:849–856
20. Lipton P (1999) Ischemic cell death in brain neurons. Physiol Rev 79:1431–1568
21. MacManus JP, Buchan AM (2000) Apoptosis following experimental stroke: fact or fashion? J NeuroTrauma 17:899–914
22. MacManus JP, Koch CJ, Jian M, Walker T, Zurakowski B (1999) Decreased brain infarct following focal ischemia in mice lacking the transcription factor E2F1. NeuroReport 10:2711–2714
23. MacManus JP Linnik MD (1997) Gene expression induced by cerebral ischemia: an apoptotic perspective. J Cereb Blood Flow Metab 17:815–832
24. MacManus JP, Rasquinha I, Black MA, Laferriere NB, Monette R, Walker T, Morley P (1997) Glutamate-treated rat cortical neuronal cultures die in a way different from the classical apoptosis induced by staurosporine. Exp Cell Res 233:310–320
25. Maeda K, Hata R, Hossmann KA (1998) Differences in the cerebrovascular anatomy of C57Black/6 and SV129 mice. NeuroReport 9:1317–1319
26. Massie B, Mosser DD, Koutroumanis M, Vitte-Mony I, Lamoureux L, Couture F, Paquet L, Guilbault C, Dionne J, Chahla D, Jolicoeur P, Langelier Y (1998) New adenovirus vectors for protein production and gene transfer. Cytotech 28:53–64
27. Michel PP, Lambeng N, Ruberg M. (1999) Neuropharmacological aspects of apoptosis: significance for neurodegenerative diseases. Clin Neuropharmacol 22:137–150
28. Nevins JR (1998) Towards an understanding of the functional complexity of the E2F and retinoblastoma families. Cell Growth & Diff 9:585–593

29. O'Hare MJ, Hou ST, Morris EJ, Cregan SP, Xu Q, Slack RS, Park DS (2000) Induction and modulation of cerebellar granule neuron death by E2F1. J Biol Chem 275:25358–25364
30. Phillips AC, Bates S, Ryan KM, Helin K, Vousden KH (1997) Induction of DNA synthesis and apoptosis are separable functions of E2F1. Genes Dev 11:1853–1863
31. Phillips AC, Ernst MK, Bates S, Rice NR, Vousden KH (1999) E2F1 potentiates cell death by blocking antiapoptotic signaling pathways. Mol Cell 4:771–781
32. Pierce AM, Gimenez-Conti IB, Schineider-Broussard R, Martinez LA, Conti CJ, Johnson DG (1998) Increased E2F1 activity induces skin tumors in mice heterozygous and nullizygous for p53. Proc Natl Acad Sci USA 95:8858–8863
33. Sakhi S, Bruce A, Sun N, Tocco G, Baudry M, Schreiber SS (1994) p53 induction is associated with neuronal damage in the central nervous system. Proc Natl Acad Sci USA 91:7525–7529
34. Steward O, Schauwecker PE, Guth L, Zhang Z, Fujiki M, Inman D, Wrathall J, Kempermann G, Gage FH, Saatman KE, Raghupathi R, McIntosh T. (1999) Genetic approaches to neurotrauma research: opportunities and potential pitfalls of murine models. Exper Neurol 157:19–42
35. Tatton WG (1999) Apoptotic mechanisms in neurodegeneration: possible relevance to glaucoma. Eur J Opthalmol 9:Suppl 1, S22–S29
36. Wood KA, Youle RJ (1995) The role of free radicals and p53 in neuron apoptosis in vivo. J Neurosci 15:5851–5857
37. Yamasaki L, Jacks T, Bronson R, Goillot E, Harlow E, Dyson NJ (1996) Tumor induction and tissue atrophy in mice lacking E2F1. Cell 85:537–548
38. Yang G, Kitagawa K, Matsushita K, Mabuchi T, Yagita Y, Yanagihara T, Matsumoto M (1997) C57BL/6 strain is most susceptible to cerebral ischemia following bilateral common carotid occlusion among seven mouse strains: selective neuronal death in the murine transient forebrain ischemia. Brain Res 752:209–218

Reactive oxygen and cytochrome c release in neuronal apoptosis

R. A. Kirkland, J. L. Franklin

Abstract

Release of cytochrome c from the mitochondrial intermembrane space into the cytoplasm is central to the apoptotic death of many types of cells including neurons. Once in the cytoplasm, cytochrome c activates caspase proteases, the executioners of the apoptotic process. We investigated mechanisms of cytochrome c release during the apoptotic death of nerve growth factor-deprived sympathetic neurons in cell culture. A large burst in production of reactive oxygen species occurred at about the same time as redistribution of cytochrome c from the mitochondria into the cytoplasm of these cells. Increasing cellular glutathione concentration by any of several means blocked this reactive oxygen burst, potently inhibited cytochrome c release, and blocked apoptosis. Treatment of cells with hydrogen peroxide caused rapid and complete release of cytochrome c into the cytoplasm without disrupting mitochondrial membrane potential. These findings suggest that cytochrome c redistribution during the apoptotic death of neurotrophin-deprived sympathetic neurons is regulated by cellular redox state. We suggest that a similar effect may contribute to cytochrome c release and induction of apoptosis in pathological states, such as ischemia, where increased production of reactive oxygen is known to occur.

Introduction

All cells are subject to oxidative damage. However, neurons, particularly those in the brain, are especially sensitive to such damage. This, likely, results from the very high O_2 consumption of neural tissue, and the subsequent excessive production of O_2-derived reactive oxygen species (ROS; Halliwell and Gutteridge 1999). ROS, which include superoxide (O_2^-), singlet oxygen, and hydroxyl radicals ($OH^•$), along with related species (e.g., oxides of nitrogen), are the principal biological free radicals. The primary source of ROS is the mitochondrial electron transport chain where approximately 1–6% of O_2 consumed is reduced to O_2^- by electrons leaked from the respiratory complexes (Turrens 1997; Halliwell and Gutteridge 1999). The O_2^- produced is rapidly converted to hydrogen peroxide (H_2O_2) by the dismutation reaction which is catalyzed by superoxide dismutase: $O_2^- + O_2^- + 2H^+ \rightarrow H_2O_2 + O_2$. The H_2O_2

Keywords: cytochrome c, reactive oxygen species (ROS), mitochondria, nerve growth factor, apoptosis, programmed cell death

Department of Neurological Surgery, University of Wisconsin Medical School, 4640 MSC, 1300 University Avenue, Madison, WI 53706. e-mail: jlfrankl@facstaff.wisc.edu

J. Krieglstein, S. Klumpp (Eds.) Pharmacology of Cerebral Ischemia 2000

can subsequently be converted to H_2O by oxidation of the small tripeptide glutathione (GSH) via a reaction catalyzed by the enzyme glutathione peroxidase: $H_2O_2 + 2GSH \rightarrow GSSG + 2H_2O$. Reduction of the oxidized glutathione (GSSG) in a reaction catalyzed by glutathione reductase creates more GSH that then converts more H_2O_2 to H_2O. In this way, GSH neutralizes the potentially damaging effects of these ROS. In the presence of iron H_2O_2, can also undergo Fenton chemistry to produce hydroxyl ($OH^{\bullet}$) radicals: $Fe^{2+} + H_2O_2 \rightarrow Fe^{3+} + OH^{\bullet} + OH^-$. The $OH^{\bullet}$ radicals produced are among the most reactive chemical species known, reacting at a high rate constant with almost every type of molecule in a cell. Indeed, the $OH^{\bullet}$ radical is so reactive that, upon formation, it almost immediately attacks nearby molecules and, thus, cannot diffuse far from its point of origin.

Increased ROS production has been observed in many disparate pathological conditions, including ischemia. Much evidence suggests that the elevated ROS have important roles in the etiology of these pathological states (Beal et al. 1997; Reynolds and Hastings 1995; Halliwell and Gutteridge 1999). Most past work devoted to understanding how ROS cause cellular injury has focused on direct free-radical damage to cellular constituents (membranes, proteins, etc.). While such injury is likely to be part of the story, recent evidence suggests more subtle and, perhaps, more important ways in which ROS contribute to pathological states (Fujimura et al. 1999). There is strong evidence that elevation of ROS levels during the apoptotic death of many types of cells contributes to the apoptotic process (Hockenbery et al. 1993; Kane et al. 1993; Ratan et al. 1994; Ferrari et al. 1995; Greenlund et al. 1995; Dugan et al. 1997; Murphy and Bredesen 1997; Polyak et al. 1997; Troy et al. 1997; Tan et al. 1998). How these ROS affect apoptosis is unknown. Here we describe some of our recent findings that suggest mitochondrial-produced ROS influence the apoptotic death of neurons, at least in part, by regulating release of cytochrome c from the mitochondria into the cytoplasm where it then activates caspase proteases (Kirkland and Franklin, submitted; Alnemri et al. 1996).

ROS in programmed neuronal death

During metazoan development and tissue turnover in mature multicellular organisms, a great many cells die via programmed cell death PCD; Kerr et al. 1972), a process first described well over a hundred years ago (Clarke and Clarke 1996). This death is physiologically appropriate, serving distinct functions in different tissues. PCD is particularly prominent in the developing nervous system (Oppenheim 1991; Pettman and Henderson 1998). About half of all neurons produced during neurogenesis die during a period of development corresponding approximately to the time at which synaptic contact with target tissue is established. Evidence suggests that the result of this death is appropriate matching of innervation density with target size. The primary determinant of which neurons survive developmental apoptosis is attainment of a sufficient quantity of neurotrophic substance from their target or other tissues (Purves and Lichtman 1985). Only neurons obtaining adequate amounts of neurotrophic factor survive the period of PCD.

The best-characterized model of neuronal PCD is that of immature sympathetic neurons deprived of nerve growth factor (NGF). When this trophic factor is removed from these cells, either *in vitro* or *in vivo*, they die with many of the morphological, genetic, and biochemical features common to many other types of cells undergoing apoptotic death. Among these features are atrophy, sustained induction of several "immediate early genes", condensation of nuclear chromatin, degradation of DNA into oligonucleosomal-sized fragments, (multiples of about 200 bp), fragmentation of the nucleus, and activation of caspase family proteases (Deckwerth and Johnson 1993; Edwards and Tolkovsky 1994; Deshmukh et al. 1996; Troy et al. 1997; Franklin and Johnson 1998). Increasing evidence demonstrates a central role for mitochondria in the apoptotic death of many types of cells, including NGF-deprived sympathetic neurons and other types of neurons (Deckwerth et al. 1993; Greenlund et al. 1995; Dugan et al. 1997; Neame et al. 1998; Deshmukh and

Johnson 1998; Pettman and Henderson 1998; Martinou et al. 1999). A principal means by which mitochondria influence apoptosis is by release of pro-apoptotic agents from the mitochondrial intermembrane space into the cytoplasm (Yang et al. 1997; Reed 1997). Prominent among these agents is cytochrome c. This protein is encoded as apocytochrome c by a nuclear gene. After translation by cytosolic ribosomes, apocytochrome c translocates into the mitochondrial intermembrane space where the enzyme heme lyase covalently attaches a heme group onto it. The resultant protein folds to form the mature protein, holocytochrome c (van Loon and Schatz 1987; Mayer et al. 1995; Komiya and Mihara 1996; Reed 1997). All holocytochrome c is normally found between the inner and outer mitochondrial membranes where it functions in the electron transport chain to carry electrons from respiratory complex III to respiratory complex IV (Radi et al. 1997). Holocytochrome c induces apoptotic death when released from the mitochondria into the cytoplasmic compartment of many cell types (Krippner et al. 1996; Liu et al. 1996; Kluck et al. 1997; Reed 1997; Deshmukh and Johnson 1998; Neame et al. 1998). The pro-apoptotic activity of cytochrome c requires that it bind onto the protein, apoptosis protease activating factor 1 (Apaf-1). A number of molecules of Apaf-1, holocytochrome c, and caspase 9 then form a large oligomeric complex known as an apoptosome. In the presence of dATP, the caspase 9 in the complex is activated (Zou et al. 1997; Li et al. 1997; Zou et al. 1999). The activated caspase 9 then cleaves and activates other downstream caspases that kill cells by destroying (or activating) many important cellular protein substrates.

Greenlund et al. (1995) and Dugan et al. (1997) found that removal of NGF from sympathetic neurons in culture causes a transient increase of ROS production in these cells. This ROS burst reaches a peak within a few hours after deprivation and by 8 hours after withdrawal returns to control levels. Several antioxidant compounds have also been demonstrated to have a potent anti-apoptotic effect on these cells, suggesting a central role for ROS production in the death process (Ferrari et al. 1995). Because no sympathetic neurons die until about 18 hours after NGF withdrawal (Deckwerth and Johnson 1993; Franklin et al. 1995), these data suggest that the ROS burst is an early and important part of the apoptotic cascade. Indeed, increased ROS production is the earliest cellular change detected to date after inactivation of the NGF tyrosine kinase receptor, TrkA, by NGF removal (Franklin et al. 1995; Greenlund et al. 1995). This early increase in ROS production after NGF deprivation has been suggested to cause induction of stress-activated genes such as the transcription factor, *c-jun*. Subsequent to this induction, it was postulated that other, downstream, "killer" genes are induced. The protein products of these genes then cause cell death. Consistent with this hypothesis, sustained induction of *c-jun* occurs early after depriving sympathetic neurons of NGF (Estus et al. 1994). The induction appears to be important for apoptotic death because direct injection of antibodies that block the transcriptional activity of *c-jun* slows apoptosis in these cells. Figure 1 illustrates a temporal sequence of some events that are either known, or are hypothesized, to be mechanistically important components of the apoptotic process in NGF-deprived sympathetic neurons. Many other cellular events are also known to occur after NGF deprivation. For example, greatly decreased glucose uptake and reduced protein and RNA synthesis occur within a few hours of NGF withdrawal (Deckwerth and Johnson 1993; Franklin and Johnson 1998). However, the relevance of these events to the apoptotic process is unknown.

A more direct role for ROS in PCD: Redox regulation of cytochrome c release

We have recently discovered evidence that the model of the mechanisms underlying apoptotic death in NGF-deprived sympathetic neurons presented in Figure 1 is in need of revision. Previous work concerned with ROS levels and the role of ROS in the apoptotic death of these

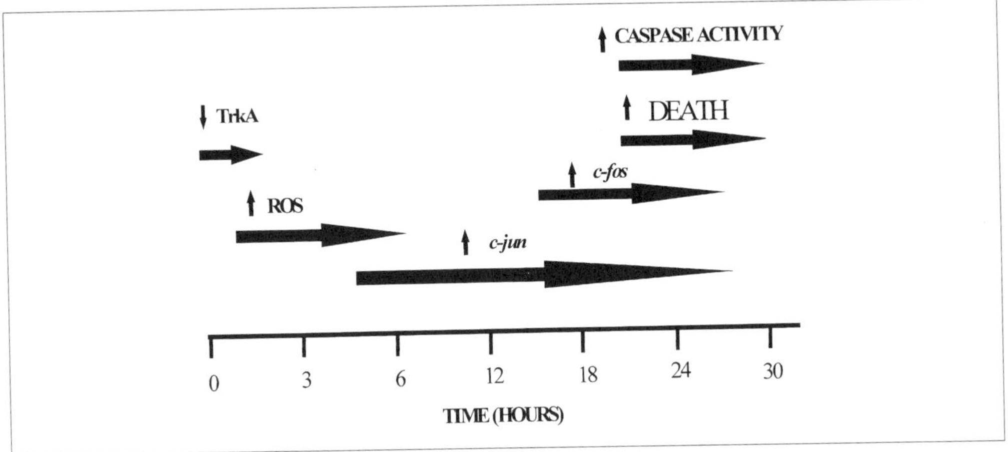

Fig. 1. Summary of events occurring after NGF withdrawal from sympathetic neurons that have been proposed to be a part of the apoptotic cascade in these cells. Forward-pointing arrows indicate times at which the event occurs after deprivation. Arrows pointing up or down indicate increase or decrease. Time is in hours after NGF withdrawal at t_0. Time-courses of the individual events are taken from Franklin et al. (1995), Greenlund et al. (1995), Estus et al. (1994), and Deshmukh et al. (1996).

cells after NGF deprivation did not take into account ROS production later that about 8 hours after NGF withdrawal. None of these cells are committed to apoptotic death until about 18 hours after NGF removal (Deckwerth and Johnson 1993). Therefore, ROS production during the intervening 10 hours, as well as during the 6–12 hours it takes for most of the cells to die, has not been explored. Presumably, the truncated time-courses reported for ROS production after NGF withdrawal were due to the lack of availability of adequate ROS-sensitive dyes for a more complete temporal analysis. For example, Dugan et al. (1997) used the dye, dihydrorhodamine, whose fluorescence depends not only on oxidation but also on a stable mitochondrial membrane potential. Because mitochondrial membrane potential depolarizes during the apoptotic process of these cells (Neame et al. 1998), the dye cannot be used at later time-points. Other available redox-sensitive dyes have similar short comings.

We have found that the new fluorescence-based, redox-sensitive dye, 5-(and-6)-chloromethyl-2', 7'-dichlorodihydrofluoresceindiacetate (CM-H_2 DCFDA), is vastly superior to the earlier redox-sensitive dyes used to study ROS in sympathetic neurons and other cell types (Nedergaard et al. 1990; Greenlund et al. 1995; Dugan et al. 1997). This dye is non-fluorescent in reduced form and is readily membrane-permeant. Once in a cell, esterases cleave its acetate groups. The thiol-reactive chloromethyl group then binds to cellular thiols trapping the dye inside the cell where oxidation converts it to the fluorescent form. CM-H_2 DCFDA is oxidized by cellular hydrogen peroxide, hydroxyl radicals, and various free radical products lying downstream from H_2O_2. It is relatively insensitive to oxidation by superoxide (Royall and Ischiropoulos 1993). We found that this dye was well retained by cells and was resistant to photo-oxidation. Earlier versions of the same dye, such as one used by Greenlund et al. (1995), rapidly leaked out of cells and were extremely sensitive to photo-oxidation. Using CM-H_2DCFDA, we generated a complete time-course (0–30 hours) of ROS production in sympathetic neurons after NGF deprivation. This was accomplished with semi-quantitative laser scanning confocal microscopy of NGF-deprived rat sympathetic neurons loaded with CM-H_2 DCFDA (Kirkland and Franklin, submitted). We found that, in addition to the early ROS burst, there was also a later ROS burst that occurred at about the same time as redistribution of cytochrome c from the mitochondria into the cytoplasm and of commitment of the cells to apoptotic death (Fig. 2). We also found that the apparent transience of the early increase of ROS production after NGF deprivation is illusory. Beginning about 3 hours after NGF withdrawal, GSH concentration increased. This, effectively, neutralized elevated H_2O_2 levels but did not decrease upstream O_2^- production. Buthionine sulfoximine, an inhibitor of GSH production, prevented the transience of the early ROS burst indicating that it was the increased GSH concentration rather than alteration in O_2^- production that caused the transience. Thus, the early increase of ROS after NGF deprivation appeared to stimulate the cells to mount an antioxidant defense. Experiments with selective inhibitors of electron flow through mitochondrial respiratory complexes suggested that the source of all increased ROS after NGF deprivation was mitochondrial respiratory complex 2 (coenzyme-Q-cytochrome c reductase). Therefore, ROS production increased long before any cytochrome c was released and continued throughout the time-course of the apoptotic process.

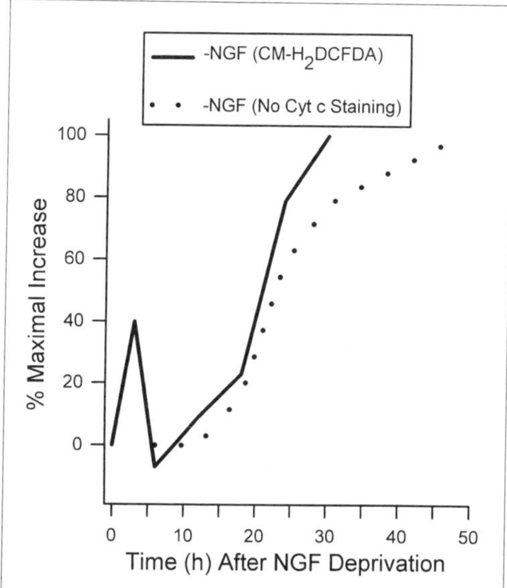

Fig. 2. Comparison of the time-course of cellular redox changes with the time-course of cytochrome c release and death after NGF deprivation. ROS were determined by confocal microscopic imaging of CM-H_2DCFDA-stained cells. Increased ROS are indicated by increased CM-H_2DCFDA intensity. Relative intensities were normalized to those measured in NGF-replete cells. Cellular cytochrome c status (mitochondrial or cytoplasmic) was determined by confocal microscopic imaging of immuno-stained cells. Illustration of time-courses is adapted from Kirkland and Franklin (submitted).

Cai and Jones (1998) reported that increased O_2^- production during the apoptotic death of HL60 cells is caused by a shift from 4-electron reduction of O_2 to 1-electron reduction subsequent to cytochrome c release. This shift causes increased leakage of electrons to O_2 to form O_2^-. The early component of the ROS burst in NGF-deprived sympathetic neurons could not be explained by such a shift because it occurred hours before any cytochrome c redistribution. However, the time-course of the late burst was closely associated with the time-course of cytochrome c release. Thus, it was possible that loss of cytochrome c after NGF deprivation was responsible for the late burst. Arguing against this possibility, the peak of the late burst coincided with the appearance of cytochrome c in the cytoplasm but preceded total depletion of cytochrome c from mitochondria.

We found that several antioxidants promoted survival when added to NGF-deprived cells well after the end of the early ROS burst, implying that the late, but not the early, burst was important for death. These data suggested that, regardless of the source of the late burst, it was an integral part of the apoptotic process. The close association of the late ROS burst with cytochrome c redistribution suggested that the survival-promoting effects of antioxidants might be mediated by suppression of an oxidation-sensitive step in cytochrome c release. The membrane permeant analog of cysteine, N-acetyl-L cysteine (L-NAC), a potent antioxidant, exerts a strong survival-promoting effect on NGF-deprived sympathetic neurons (Ferrari et al. 1995). We found that this compound caused a dose-dependent suppression of the late ROS burst and that this suppression was mediated by an increase of GSH concentration. L-NAC also blocked cytochrome c release (Fig. 3).

A membrane-permeant analog of GSH, GSH ethyl ester, had a similar survival-promoting effect and also potently inhibited cytochrome c release (Fig. 3). Surprisingly, the protein synthesis inhibitor cycloheximide (CHX), a potent anti-apoptotic agent for these cells (Martin et al. 1988), also elevated GSH levels. Blocking this elevation with BSO blocked the ability of CHX to prevent apoptosis (not shown). This finding is consistent with that of Ratan et al. (1994) who reported that CHX prevents oxidative stress-induced apoptosis of cortical neurons by increasing GSH levels. The elevated GSH concentration in cells in which protein synthesis is suppressed, apparently, derives from a shunting of cysteine from protein production into GSH synthesis. Therefore, the well-known anti-apoptotic effects of protein synthesis inhibitors on these cells appears to be, at least partially, mediated via antioxidant effects rather than by suppression of production of pro-apoptotic proteins as is often assumed.

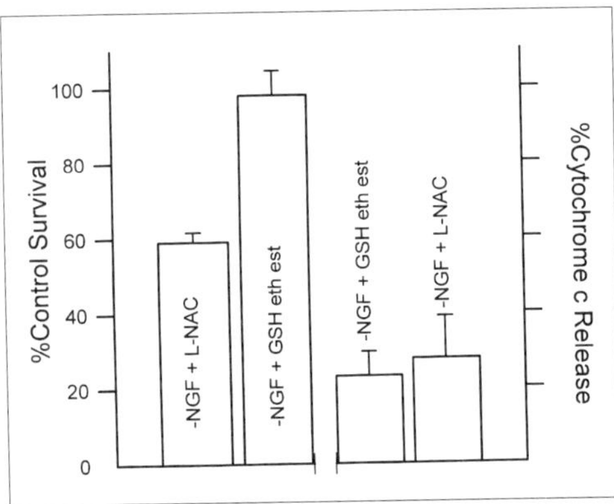

Fig. 3. Effects of the antioxidants, L-NAC (30 mM), and GSH ethyl ester (10 mM) on cytochrome c release and survival of NGF-deprived neurons. Survival was determined 2–3 days after NGF-deprived cells were treated with the compounds (see Franklin et al. 1995 for survival assay). Survival is normalized to that of cells maintained for the same period in NGF-containing medium. Cytochrome c status was determined 48 hours after NGF deprivation in cells that had been saved from apoptotic death by including a pan-caspase inhibitor (boc-aspartyl (Ome)-fluoromethylketone, 30 µM) in the culture medium. Inhibition of caspases had no effect on rate of cytochrome c redistribution. As with figure 2, illustration is derived from data presented in Kirkland and Franklin (submitted).

These data suggest a role for cellular redox state, as determined by mitochondrial ROS production and cellular GSH concentration, in release of cytochrome c during the PCD of NGF-deprived sympathetic neurons. More direct proof that redox state can regulate cytochrome c release in these cells is shown in Figure 4. Direct application of H_2O_2 to cultures of sympathetic neurons maintained either in the presence of NGF or deprived of NGF for 24 h and kept alive with CHX, L-NAC, or GSH ethyl ester caused almost complete loss of cytochrome c from mitochondria within an hour of treatment. This release occurred with no change in mitochondrial membrane potential, indicating that the H_2O_2 did not cause non-specific disruption of mitochondria. In cells maintained alive by CHX, L-NAC, or GSH ethyl ester, H_2O_2 treatment also caused rapid fragmentation of nuclei characteristic of apoptotic death. In NGF-maintained cells, on the other hand, such treatment did not induce apoptotic nuclei even though it caused complete redistribution of cytochrome c from the mitochondria into the cytoplasm. This finding is consistent with the report of Deshmukh and Johnson (1998) that sympathet-

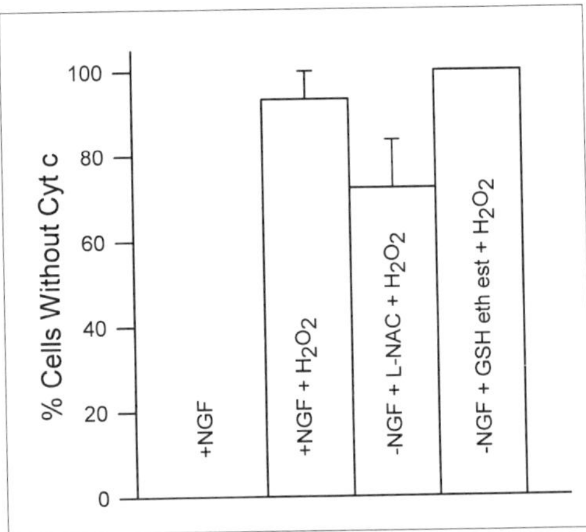

Fig. 4. Complete release of cytochrome c in sympathetic neurons exposed for 1 hour to 10 mM H_2O_2. The L-NAC (30 mM)- and GSH ethyl ester (10 mM)-treated cells, were exposed for 24 hours to medium containing the compounds and lacking NGF before treatment with H_2O_2. Again, illustration is adapted from data presented in Kirkland and Franklin (submitted).

ic neurons exposed to NGF are not competent to die when microinjected with cytochrome c. Rather, several hours of NGF deprivation are required before cytoplasmic cytochrome c could induce death. The mechanism underlying development of "competence to die" is unknown. These findings show that a pro-oxidant state can directly cause cytochrome c redistribution and apoptosis in cells that have developed competence to die after NGF deprivation. They also strongly suggest that the late ROS burst in NGF-deprived cells regulates cytochrome c release in naturally occurring PCD.

Discussion

We have provided evidence that cellular redox state, as determined primarily by mitochondrial ROS production and cellular GSH concentration, regulates cytochrome c redistribution during the apoptotic death of NGF-deprived sympathetic neurons. Growing evidence suggests that apoptosis is the means by which cells die in certain diseases (Gougeon and Montagnier 1993; Mountz et al. 1994) including some neurodegenerative diseases such as Alzheimer's disease and Amyotrophic Lateral Sclerosis (Altman 1992; Su et al. 1994; Yoshiyama et al. 1994; LaFerla et al. 1995; Murphy and Bredesen 1997). It is also apparent that at least some of the molecular machinery of apoptosis is activated in neurons following ischemia (Lipton 1999). For example Fujimura et al. (1999) recently demonstrated that cytochrome c is released following permanent focal ischemia in mice. This redistribution appears to be regulated, at least in part, by cellular redox state. Therefore, understanding mechanisms of redox-regulated cytochrome c release in NGF-deprived sympathetic neurons may be relevant not only to elucidating the basic biology of developmental death but may also aid in understanding pathological states.

How alterations of cellular redox state could control cytochrome c release is unknown. Members of the Bcl-2 family of proteins are central regulators of cytochrome c redistribution. However, despite a great deal of work, the mechanism of action of these proteins and the means by which they regulate cytochrome c release during apoptosis remains something of a mystery. Some Bcl-2 family members have pro-apoptotic effects (e.g., Bax, Bad, Bak, Bcl-x_s, Bik) while others have anti-apoptotic activity (e.g., Bcl-2, Bcl-x_L; Deckwerth et al. 1996; Kroemer 1997). A major clue as to their possible mode of action is that Bcl-2 family members are found, primarily, in mitochondrial membranes (OM; Hockenbery et al. 1993; Monaghan et al. 1992; Nakai et al. 1993). This localization suggests a role for these proteins in control of mitochondrial function. Anti-apoptotic Bcl-2 family proteins maintain mitochondrial integrity and retain cytochrome c within the intermembrane space (Kharbanda et al. 1997; Yang et al. 1997). The exact means by which this takes place remains undetermined. In the case of NGF-deprived sympathetic neurons, it is clear that the pro-apopotic member of the Bcl-2 family, Bax, is central to death. Sympathetic neurons from Bax-knockout (KO) mice do not die in culture when deprived of NGF. This protection against apoptosis derives solely from retention of cytochrome c in the mitochondrial intermembrane space of the Bax-KO cells (Deshmukh and Johnson 1998). When cytochrome c is microinjected into NGF-deprived sympathetic neurons from Bax-KO mice, the cells undergo rapid apoptotic death. During the time-course of death in neurons from wild-type animals, Bax translocates from a, primarily, cytoplasmic location to the mitochondria. This translocation occurs concurrently with commitment to death, suggesting that it is the primary determining factor for when the cells die (Putcha et al. 1999). One conceivable mechanism by which an antioxidant state blocks cytochrome c release in these cells is by inhibition of this translocation. In this scenario, the Bax translocation lies downstream from increased mitochondrial ROS production after NGF deprivation. However, our preliminary findings concerning ROS production in Bax-KO mice are inconsistent with this hypothesis. We have discovered that, while NGF-deprived sympathetic neurons from wild type mice have increased ROS levels similar to what we found in NGF-deprived sympathetic neurons from rats, that sympathetic neurons from Bax-KO animals exhibit no increase in ROS production at all (not shown). This finding implies that the increased ROS after NGF deprivation lies downstream from Bax. Should this be true, Bax may, at least in part, regulate cytochrome c release by controlling cellular redox state. Only further work can resolve this issue.

Several reports suggest that regulation of ROS production, or its effects on cells, may be a mechanism by which Bcl-2 family members influence cellular survival. Both Hockenbery et al. (1993) and Kane et al. (1993) found that Bcl-2 could block lipid peroxidation in several types of cells undergoing apoptosis, suggesting that it functions upstream of free radical-mediated events. However, Jacobson and Raff (1995) found that some cell types die by apoptosis under hypoxic conditions that should have lowered the amount of ROS produced in cells. Bcl-2 blocked this death. These seemingly contradictory findings have not yet been resolved. However, it is clear that increased ROS production is an important part of the apoptotic cascade in sympathetic neurons (Greenlund et al. 1995) and other cell types as well (Polyak et al. 1997). Likely explanations for this apparent discrepancy is that ROS are important in the apoptotic death of some cell types but not others, and/or that there are multiple apoptotic pathways, some involving ROS and others that are ROS-independent (Park et al. 1998). Bcl-2 family members interact with a number of proteins (Wang et al. 1996) and, thus, may effect apoptosis via several mechanisms in addition to regulation of redistribution of cytochrome c (Chinnaiyan et al. 1997; Xue and Horvitz 1997; Clem et al. 1998; Rossé et al. 1998).

Acknowledgments

This work was supported by a grant to the University of Wisconsin Medical School under the Howard Hughes Medical Institute Research Resources Program for Medical Schools and by National Institutes of Health grant NS37110.

References

1. Alnemri ES, Livingston DJ, Nicholson DW, Salvesen G, Thornberry NA, Wong WW, Yuan J (1996) Human ICE/CED-3 protease nomenclature. Cell 87:171
2. Altman J (1992) Programmed cell death: the paths to suicide. Trends Neurosci 15:278–280
3. Beal MF, Howell N, Bodis-Wollner I (1997) Mitochondria and Free Radicals in Neurodegenerative Diseases. New York, NY: Wiley-Liss
4. Cai J, Jones DP (1998) Superoxide in apoptosis: mitochondrial generation triggered by cytochrome c loss. J Biol Chem 273:11401–11404
5. Chinnaiyan AM, O'Rourke K, Lane BR, Dixit VM (1997) Interaction of CED-4 with CED-3 and CED-9: a molecular framework for cell death. Science 275:1122–1126
6. Clarke PGH, Clarke S (1996) Nineteenth century research on naturally occurring cell death and related phenomena. Anat Embryol 193:81–99
7. Clem RJ, Cheng EHY, Karp CL, Kirsch DG, Ueno K, Takahashi A, Kastan MB, Griffin DE, Earnshaw WC, Veliuona MA, Hardwick JM (1998) Modulation of cell death by Bcl-x_L through caspase interaction. Proc Natl Acad Sci 95:554–559
8. Deckwerth TL, Johnson EM Jr (1993) Temporal analysis of events associated with programmed cell death (apoptosis) of sympathetic neurons deprived of nerve growth factor. J Cell Biol 123:1207–1222
9. Deckwerth TL, Elliot JL, Knudson CM, Johnson EM Jr, Snider WD, Korsmeyer SJ (1996) BAX is required for neuronal death after trophic factor deprivation and during (1997) development. Neuron 17:401–411
10. Deshmukh M, Johnson EM Jr (1998) Evidence of a novel event during neuronal death: development of competence-to-die in response to cytoplasmic cytochrome c. Neuron 21:695–705
11. Deshmukh M, Vasilakos J, Deckwerth TL, Lampe PA, Shivers BD, Johnson EM Jr (1996) Genetic and metabolic status of NGF-deprived sympathetic neurons saved by an inhibitor of ICE-family proteases. J Cell Biol 135:1341–1354
12. Dugan LL, Creedon DJ, Johnson EM Jr, Holtzman DM (1997) Rapid suppression of free radical formation by nerve growth factor involves the mitogen-activated protein kinase pathway. Proc Natl Acad Sci USA 94:4086–4091
13. Edwards SN, Tolkovsky AM (1994) Characterization of apoptosis in cultured rat sympathetic neurons after nerve growth factor withdrawal. J Cell Biol 124:537–546
14. Estus S, Zaks WJ, Freeman RS, Gruda M, Bravo R, Johnson EM Jr (1994) Altered gene expression in neurons during programmed cell death: Identification of *c-jun* as necessary for neuronal apoptosis. J Cell Biol 127:1717–1727
15. Ferrari G, Yan CYI, Greene LA (1995) N-acetylcysteine (D- and L-stereoisomers) prevents apoptotic death of neuronal cells. J Neurosci 15:2857–2866
16. Franklin JL, Johnson EM Jr (1998) Control of neuronal size homeostasis by trophic factor-mediated coupling of protein degradation to protein synthesis. J Cell Biol 142:1313–1324
17. Franklin JL, Sanz-Rodriguez C, Juhasz A, Deckwerth TL, Johnson EM Jr (1995) Chronic depolarization prevents programmed death of sympathetic neurons *in vitro* but does not support growth: Requirement for Ca^{2+} influx but not Trk activation. J Neurosci 15:643–664
18. Fujimura M, Morita-Fujimura Y, Kawase M, Copin JC, Calagui B, Epstein CJ, Chan PH (1999) Manganese superoxide dismutase mediates the early release of mitochondrial cytochrome c and subsequent DNA fragmentation after permanent focal cerebral ischemia in mice. J Neurosci 19:3414–3422
19. Gougeon ML, Montagnier L (1993) Apoptosis in aids. Science 260:1269–1270

20. Greenlund LJS, Deckwerth TL, Johnson EM Jr (1995) Superoxide dismutase delays neuronal apoptosis: a role for reactive oxygen species in programmed neuronal death. Neuron 14:303–315
21. Halliwell B, Gutteridge JMC (1999) Free radicals in biology and medicine third edition. Oxford, UK: Oxford University Press
22. Hockenbery DM, Oltvai ZN, Yin X -M, Milliman CL, Korsmeyer SJ (1993) Bcl-2 functions in an antioxidant pathway to prevent apoptosis. Cell 75:241–251
23. Jacobson MD, Raff MC (1995) Programmed cell death and Bcl-2 protection in very low oxygen. Nature 374:814–816
24. Kane DJ, Sarafian TA, Anton R, Hahn H, Gralla EB, Valentine JS, Örd T, Bredesen DE (1993) Bcl-2 inhibition of neural death: decreased generation of reactive oxygen species. Science 262:1274–1277
25. Kerr JFR, Wyllie AH, Currie AR (1972) Apoptosis: a basic biological phenomenon with wide-ranging implications in tissue kinetics. Br J Cancer 26:239–257
26. Kharbanda S, Pandey P, Schofield L, Israels S, Roncinske R, Yoshida K, Bharti A, Yuan Z, Saxena S, Weichselbaum R, Nalin C, Kufe D (1997) Role for Bcl-x_L as an inhibitor of cytosolic cytochrome c accumulation in DNA damage-induced apoptosis. Proc Natl Acad Sci USA 94:6939–6942
27. Kluck RM, Bossy-Wetzel E, Green DR, Newmeyer DD (1997) The release of cytochrome c from mitochondria: a primary site for Bcl-2 regulation of apoptosis. Science 275:1132–1136
28. Komiya T, Mihara K (1996) Protein import into mammalian mitochondria. J Biol Chem 271:22105–22110
29. Krippner A, Matsuno-Yagi A, Gottlieb RA, Babior BM (1996) Loss of function of cytochrome c in jurkat cells undergoing fas-mediated apoptosis. J Biol Chem 271:21629–21636
30. Kroemer G (1997) The proto-oncogene Bcl-2 and its role in regulating apoptosis. Nature Med 3:614–620
31. LaFerla FM, Tinkle BT, Bieberich CJ, Haudenschild CC, Jay G (1995) The Alzheimer's a-β peptide induces neurodegeneration and apoptotic cell death in transgenic mice. Nature Gen 9:21–30
32. Li P, Nijhawan D, Budihardjo I, Srinivasula SM, Ahmad M, Alnemri ES, Wang X (1997) Cytochrome c and dATP-dependent formation of Apaf-1/caspase-9 complex initiates an apoptotic protease cascade. Cell 91:479–489
33. Lipton P (1999) Ischemic cell death in brain neurons. Physiol Rev 79:1431–568
34. Liu X, Kim CN, Yang J, Jemmerson R, Wang X (1996) Induction of apoptotic program in cell-free extracts: requirement for dATP and cytochrome c. Cell 86:147–157
35. Martin DP, Schmidt RE, DiStefano PS, Lowry OH, Carter JG, Johnson EM Jr (1988) Inhibitors of protein synthesis and RNA synthesis prevent neuronal death caused by nerve growth factor deprivation. J Cell Biol 106:829–844
36. Martinou I, Desagher S, Eskes R, Antonsson B, André E, Fakan S, Martinou JC (1999) The release of cytochrome c from mitochondria during apoptosis of NGF-deprived sympathetic neurons is a reversible event. J Cell Biol 144:883–889
37. Mayer A, Neupert W, Lill R (1995) Translocation of apocytochrome c across the outer membrane of mitochondria. J Biol Chem 270:12390–12397
38. Monaghan P, Robertson D, Amos TAS, Dyer MJS, Mason DY, Greaves MF (1992) Ultrastructural localization of Bcl-2 protein. J Histochem and Cytochem 40:1819–1825
39. Mountz JD, Wu J, Cheng J, Zhou T (1994) Autoimmune disease. A problem of defective apoptosis. Arth and Rheum 37:1415–1420
40. Murphy AN, Bredesen DE (1997) Mitochondria, reactive oxygen species, and apoptosis. In Mitochondria and Free Radicals in Neurodegenerative Diseases. Beal MF, Howell N, and Bodis-Wollner I, eds. Wiley-Liss. NY
41. Nakai M, Takeda A, Cleary ML, Endo T (1993) The Bcl-2 protein is inserted into the outer membrane but not into the inner membrane of rat liver mitochondria *in vitro*. Biochem Biophys Res Comm 196:233–239
42. Neame SJ, Rubin LL, Philpott KL (1998) Blocking cytochrome c activity within intact neurons inhibits apoptosis. J Cell Biol 142:1583–1593
43. Nedergaard M, Desai S, Pulsinelli W (1990) Dicarboxy-dichlorofluorescein: a new fluorescent probe for measuring acidic intracellular pH. Anal Biochem 187:109–114
44. Oppenheim RW (1991) Cell death during development of the nervous system. Ann Rev Neurosci 14:453–501
45. Pettman B, Henderson CE (1998) Neuronal cell death. Neuron 20:633–647
46. Park DS, Morris EJ, Stefanis L, Troy CM, Shelanski ML, Geller HM, Greene LA (1998) Multiple pathways of neuronal death induced by DNA-damaging agents, NGF-deprivation, and oxidative stress. J Neurosci 18:830–840
47. Polyak K, Xia Y, Zweier JL, Kinzler KW, Vogelstein B (1997) A model for p53-induced apoptosis. Nature 389:300–305
48. Purves D, Lichtman JW (1985) Principles of Neural Development. Sinauer. Sunderland, MA
49. Putcha GV, Deshmukh M, Johnson EM Jr (1999) BAX translocation is a critical event in neuronal apoptosis: regulation by neuroprotectants, BCL-2, and caspases. J Neurosci 19:7476–7485
50. Radi R, Castro L, Rodríguez M, Cassina A, Thomson L (1997) Free radical damage to mitochondria. In Mitochondria and Free Radicals in Neurodegenerative Diseases. Beal MF, Howell N, and Bodis-Wollner I, eds. Wiley-Liss. NY
51. Ratan RR, Murphy TH, Baraban JM (1994) Macromolecular synthesis inhibitors prevent oxidative stress-induced apoptosis in embryonic cortical neurons by shunting cysteine from protein synthesis to glutathione. J Neurosci 14:4385–4392
52. Reed JC (1997) Cytochrome c: can't live with it-can't live without it. Cell 91:559–562
53. Reynolds IJ, Hastings TG (1995) Glutamate induces the production of reactive oxygen species in cultured forebrain neurons following NMDA receptor activation. J Neurosci 15:3318–3327
54. Rossé T, Olivier R, Monney L, Rager M, Conus S, Fellay I, Jansen B, Borner C (1998) Bcl-2 prolongs cell survival after Bax-induced release of cytochrome c. Nature 391:496–499
55. Royall JA, Ischiropoulis H (1993) Evaluation of 2', 7'-dichlorofluorescin and dihydrorhodamine123 as fluorescent probes for intracellular H_2O_2 in cultured endothelial cells. Arch Biochem Biophys 302:348–355
56. Su JH, Anderson AJ, Cummings BJ, Cotman C (1994) Immunohistochemical evidence for apoptosis in Alzheimer's disease. Neuroreport 5:2529–2533
57. Tan S, Sagara Y, Liu Y, Maher P, Schubert D (1998) The regulation of reactive oxygen species production during programmed cell death. J Cell Biol 141:1423–1432
58. Troy CM, Stefanis L, Greene LA, Shelanski ML (1997) Nedd2 is required for apoptosis after trophic factor withdrawal but not superoxide dismutase (SOD1) downregulation, in sympathetic neurons and PC12 cells. J Neurosci 17:1911–1918
59. Turrens JF (1997) Superoxide production by the mitochondrial respiratory chain. Bioscience Rep 17:3–8
60. van Loon APGM, Schatz G (1987) Transport of proteins to the mitochondrial intermembrane space: the "sorting domain" of the cytochrome c_1 presequence is a stop-transfer sequence specific for the mitochondrial inner membrane. EMBO 6:2441–2448
61. Wang H, Rapp UR, Reed JC (1996) Bcl-2 targets the protein kinase Raf-1 to mitochondria. Cell 87:629–638
62. Xue D, Horvitz HR (1997) Caenorhabditis elegans Ced-9 protein is a bifunctional cell-death inhibitor. Nature 390:305–308

63. Yang J, Liu X, Bhalla K, Kim CN, Ibrado AM, Cai J, Peng T, Jones DP, Wang X (1997) Prevention of apoptosis by Bcl-2: release of cytochrome c from mitochondrial blocked. Science 275:1129–1132
64. Yoshiyama Y, Yamada T, Asanuma K, Asahi T (1994) Apoptosis-related antigen Le^{e} and nick-end labeling are positive in spinal motor neurons in amyotrophic lateral sclerosis. Acta Neuropathol 88:207–211
65. Zou H, Henzel WJ, Liu X, Lutschg A, Wang X (1997) Apaf-1, a human protein homologous to C. elegans CED-4, participates in cytochrome c-dependent activation of caspase-3. Cell 90:405–413
66. Zou H, Li Y, Liu X, Wang X (1999) An APAF-1 cytochrome c multimeric complex is a functional apoptosome that activates procaspase-9. J Biol Chem 274:11549–11556

The roles of beta-amyloid precursor protein and amyloid beta peptide in ischemic brain injury

B. Lin, M. D. Ginsberg

Introduction

β-amyloid precursor protein (βAPP) is a transmembrane protein. Amyloid beta peptide (Aβ), a fragment derived from βAPP, plays a crucial role in the pathogenesis of Alzheimer's disease (AD). Recently, both the overexpression of βAPP and the deposition of Aβ have been described in cortical and subcortical areas and in the hippocampal CA1 sector of human brains of non-demented patients affected by ischemia (Wisniewski and Maslinska 1996; Jendroska et al. 1995; Sparks 1996). In experimental studies, both global and focal ischemic insults induce βAPP upregulation in brain. βAPP expression is particularly strong in areas showing pathological evidence of injury after ischemia (Baiden-Amissah et al. 1998). Aβ deposits are also found in the rat brain after ischemia (Pluta 1997; Popa-Wagner et al. 1998). These observations have given rise to the speculation that ischemia may contribute to pathogenesis of AD.

βAPP, a 110- to 135-kDa glycoprotein, is normally present in neuronal and non-neuronal tissues at low levels (Selkoe et al. 1988; Nishimoto 1998). Similar-sized proteins occur in rat, cow and monkey (Selkoe et al. 1988; Mori et al. 1992). βAPP accumulation is highest in the cytoplasm of neuronal cell bodies and their processes (Coria et al. 1992; Palacios et al. 1992; Martin et. al. 1994), as well as in non-neural tissues as a normal protein synthesized by chromosome 21 (Kang et al. 1987; Selkoe 1999; Mazur-Kolecka et al. 1997). This protein has a large extracellular N-terminus and a short cytoplasmic C-terminus, and resembles a cell-surface glycosylated membrane receptor (Kang et al. 1987). βAPP has four isoforms: APP_{770} and APP_{751}, which contain the Kunitz protease inhibitor (KPI) (whose function is unknown); and APP_{695} and APP_{714}, which lack KPI (Mattson et al. 1993a; Selkoe 1999). Neurons express exclusively APP_{695}, while glial cells mainly express APP_{770} and APP_{751}. APP_{695} is expressed almost entirely in brain and is more abundant than APP_{770} and APP_{751} (Selkoe et al. 1988; Beeson et al. 1994; Checler 1995; Kim et al. 1998).

Previous studies employing labeling of the N-terminal portion of βAPP_{695} have found that forebrain ischemia induces its accumulation and upregulation in pyramidal *neurons* in layers III, IV, V of cortex and in hippocampal CA3 (Wakita et al. 1992; Stephenson et al. 1992; Tomimoto et al. 1994 1995; Pluta et al. 1994; Yokota et al. 1996; Hall et al. 1995; Horsburgh and Nicoll 1996); and their *axons* (Stephenson et al. 1992); and in *white matter* (Dietrich et al. 1998). Ischemia also leads to expression of the *C-terminus* in neurons (Yokota et al. 1996) and macrophages (Popa-Wagner et al. 1998) in the

Cerebral Vascular Disease Research Center, University of Miami School of Medicine, Miami, PO Box 016960, Miami, Florida, USA 33101.
e-mail: lin@stroke.med.miami.edu

J. Krieglstein, S. Klumpp (Eds.) Pharmacology of Cerebral Ischemia 2000

acute stage. Increases in the C-terminus in CA1 pyramidal neurons occur very early, prior to morphological evidence of neuronal death at 3 days (Saido et al. 1994; Yokota et al. 1996). The C-terminus of APP, as visualized by immunostaining, is evident in the perikarya of degenerating CA1 neuronal soma and processes, whereas the N-terminal portion of APP is not (Palacios et al. 1995; Horsburgh and Nicoll 1996). Global ischemia also leads to increases in the C-terminus in hyperplastic astrocytes at 7–28 days but not at earlier stages (Palacios et al. 1995; Yokota et al. 1996).

βAPP is degraded by the endosomal/lysosomal system (Munger et al. 1995; Koo et al. 1996; Yamazaki et al. 1996), as well as by the secretory pathway in the Golgi complex, at the cell surface (Busciglio et al 1993). The release of non-amyloidogenic peptide results from proteolytic cleavage of βAPP within Aβ region. α-secretase cleaves βAPP between amino acids 612–613 (based on the APP_{695} sequence), corresponding to amino acids 16 and 17 of Aβ, to release one of secreted forms (sAPP) of APP, sAPPα, from the cell. β-secretase cleaves βAPP at the N-terminus of Aβ and releases a C-terminally truncated form of sAPP (sAPPβ), and Aβ (Furukawa et al. 1996). The activity of sAPPα is localized to amino acids 591–612 at its C-terminus. The secreted form, sAPP, plays excitoprotective and neuromodulatory roles (Mattson et al. 1993b). While sAPPβ is weakly neuroprotective, sAPPα exhibits 100-fold more potent neuroprotectant properties than sAPPβ (Furukawa et al. 1996). By contrast, Aβ is neurotoxic.

Processing of βAPP can be influenced by environmental signals, including ischemia (Wakita et al. 1992; Mattson et al. 1993b; Baiden-Amissah 1998; Dietrich et al. 1998), hypoxia (Ghribi 1999), chronic hypoperfusion (Kalaria et al. 1993), subarachnoid hemorrhage (Ryba et al. 1999), and brain trauma (Smith et al. 1999). Aberrant or altered βAPP processing results in neurodegeneration by impeding the neuroprotective action of sAPP and by inducing Aβ accumulation, which destabilizes calcium homeostasis (Mattson et al. 1993c; Mattson 1994; Furukawa et al. 1996).

β-amyloid peptide (Aβ) refers to 40–42 amino acid peptide fragments of βAPP termed Aβ(1–40) or Aβ(1–42) (Beeson et al. 1994). Aβ is a normal secretory product of cells that express APP. Aβ is normally and continuously secreted at low levels and is released from healthy neural and non-neural cells in vivo and in vitro; it accumulates in the plasma membrane (Haass et al. 1992; Seubert et al. 1992; Busciglio et al. 1993; Mattson et al. 1993a). Aβ is derived from APP by proteolytic truncation (Koo et al. 1996; Citron et al. 1996; Yamazaki et al. 1996), and is degraded by a metalloprotease secreted by microglia and other neural and non-neural cells (Qiu et al. 1997). Neurons play a central role in the processing of Aβ (Wertkin et al. 1993; Simons et al. 1996). Glial cells also produce Aβ. In the rat, neurons secrete higher levels of Aβ than astrocytes, while human astrocytes generate higher levels of Aβ than other cells (Busciglio et al. 1993). Macrophages phagocytose Aβ (Akiyama et al. 1996). The N-terminus of Aβ is neurotoxic and is critical for the cellular binding, as well as activation of macrophages (Freek et al. 1999). Aggregated Aβ is neurotoxic by a mechanism related to *peptide fibril formation, generation of free radicals, impairment of membrane transport system, and disruption of ion homeostasis* (Mattson et al. 1993a, Mattson 1997; Behl et al. 1994; Goodman and Mattson 1994; Yankner 1996). Aβ is capable of interaction with extracellular matrix components such as laminin or fibronectin to promote neurite outgrowth and to exert either trophic or toxic effects (Selkoe 1993). Its neurotoxicity is via the activation of Ca^{2+} channels linked to excitatory amino acid receptors (Selkoe 1993). Aggregated Aβ may also damage the membrane transport systems, mitochondrial enzymes and increase the generation of free radicals (Iversen et al. 1995; Yankner 1996, Mattson 1997). This leads to endothelial necrosis in vitro (Sutton et al. 1997), and neurodegeneration in vivo (Migul-Hidalgo and Cacabelos 1998). In addition, Aβ(1–42) can pass through the BBB and enter into rat brain parenchyma from the circulation as early as 15 min after cardiac arrest (Pluta et al. 1996, 1997).

Aβ release from βAPP is susceptible to environmental stressors (Querfurth et al. 1997;

Sparks 1996). Ischemia and cerebral hypoperfusion lead directly to amyloid formation (Meier-Ruge and Bertoni-Freddari 1997; de la Torre 1999). In vitro hypoxia induces the progressive over-accumulation of the N-terminal portion of Aβ (Taylor et al. 1999). Severe head injury induces Aβ deposition in the brain (Graham et al. 1995; Smith et al. 1999). Brain injury and inflammation induce the activation and release of IL-1 and -6, which encourage βAPP and Aβ increases in the brain (Araujo and Cotman 1992; Vasilakos et al. 1994; Griffin et al. 1994, 1998; Sheng et al. 1996). Inflammation stimulates 1000-fold increases in serum amyloid-associated protein within 24 hours (Kumar et al. 1997).

Despite these investigations, our understanding of the adaptive and/or destructive sequelae of APP upregulation, and the mechanisms of Aβ production and plaque formation after cerebral ischemia, remains incomplete. Recent studies conducted in our laboratory have provided new evidence of delayed, secondary injury emerging in the chronic stage after brief global ischemia (Lin et al. 1998b); and of an influence of pre-ischemic hyperglycemia in enhancing and accelerating this secondary injury (Lin et al 1998a). Since APP_{695} plays an important role in neuronal metabolism, and since all isoforms of APP have the same C-terminus, we conducted immunohistochemical studies using an antibody to the *N-terminus* of APP_{695} [Anti-Alzheimer Precursor Protein A4 (clone 22C11)] to investigate the postischemic behavior of APP_{695}. In addition, to explore the role of Aβ in ischemic brains, we employed the antibody NCL-B-Amyloid (clone 6F/3D) to detect residues 8–17 of Aβ. This antibody stains human senile plaque cores, plaque periphery, and diffuse plaques, and is very useful in the diagnosis of human Alzheimer's disease (AD) (Ikeda et al. 1989; Allsop et al. 1986; Thal et al. 1997). Anti-$A\beta_{8-17}$ (6F/3D) also has high-affinity binding sites in rat brain (Allsop et al. 1991).

Immunohistochemical studies of βAPP and Aβ in forebrain ischemia

Materials and Methods

Animal preparation:

Male Wistar rats weighing 265–370 g were studied following an overnight fast. Anesthesia was induced with 3% halothane and 70% nitrous oxide. Rats were intubated endotracheally and ventilated mechanically on mixtures of 0.5% halothane, 70% nitrous oxide and a balance of oxygen. The femoral arteries were catheterized to permit blood pressure monitoring and arterial sampling for blood-gas and glucose measurement. Arterial PCO_2 and PO_2 were maintained in the normal ranges by ventilatory adjustments. Animals were immobilized by pancuronium bromide, 0.75 mg/kg i.v. Rectal temperature was measured continually and maintained at 37.0–37.5 °C by a warming lamp above the rat's body. Cranial temperature was separately monitored by a 29-gauge thermocouple implanted into the left temporalis muscle and was maintained at 36.0–36.5 °C throughout the experiment by a small warming lamp above the rat's head. In the hyperglycemia group, rats receive 25% dextrose, 2.5 ml i.p., 30 min prior to ischemia. Preischemic serum glucose was 340 ± 66 mg/dl in hyperglycemia group, and 133 ± 21 mg/dl in normoglycemic group.

Production of forebrain ischemia:

Transient forebrain ischemia was produced by the method of bilateral carotid artery occlusions plus systemic hypotension. Blood was withdrawn gradually into a heparinized syringe to reduce systemic blood pressure to 50 mmHg. The carotid ligatures were then tightened bilaterally for 7-, or 10-, or 12.5-min depending upon the specific protocol, and mean blood pressure (MAP) was held at 40–50 mmHg by controlled arterial exsanguination. The ischemic insult was terminated by removing the ligatures and reinfusing the shed blood to restore MAP to 100–120 mmHg. After catheters were removed and incisions closed, rats were returned to their cages and were allowed free access to food and water.

Histological studies:

In our chronic protocols to study βAPP, rats exposed to 10-min ischemia were killed at the end of 1, 2, 4, 6, 8, and 10 weeks (n = 5,4,4,5,5,6, respectively). In the hyperglycemia protocol, rats subjected to a 12.5-min ischemic insult were sacrificed at 24 h (hyperglycemic group, n = 6; normoglycemic group, n = 6) or 3 days (n = 5 in each group). In the Aβ study, rats with 7- and 12.5-min ischemia were killed on the 3rd day (12.5-min ischemia, n = 5) or at the end of 2 months (n = 5 in each group). Rats were reanesthetized with halothane and perfused via the ascending aorta with FAM (a mixture of 40% formaldehyde, glacial acetic acid and methanol, 1:1:8 by volume) for 19 min at a pressure of 100–120 mmHg following a 1-min perfusion with physiological saline. The heads were immersed in FAM at 4 °C for 1 day. The brains then were removed and placed in FAM for an additional day. Coronal brain blocks were embedded in paraffin for tissue sectioning. Ten-μm-thick brain sections were prepared at 250-μm intervals. Sections were stained with hematoxylin and eosin (H&E); selected sections were also stained with *Cresyl echt Violett*. Adjacent sections were reacted with a monoclonal antibody to the N-terminal portion of βAPP_{695} (clone 22C11, 0.1 μg/ml, Boehringer Mannheim, dilution 1:500); or with the monoclonal antibody, NCL-B-Amyloid (clone 6F/3D), 1:50, to the N-terminus of Aβ (Vector Lab). Human brains, formalin-fixed and paraffin embedded, from AD and stroke patients (n = 3 in each group, offered by Dr. Deborah Mash, Director of the Brain Bank, University of Miami) were also examined with these 2 antibodies. To enhance immunoreactivity, sections were heated with a microwave oven in 0.01 M citrate buffer pH 6.0 (Egensperger et al. 1999; Lin et al. 1999). To test for non-specific staining, negative controls were conducted in which the primary antibodies were omitted and, instead, mouse IgG (1:500 for βAPP, 1:50 for Aβ) was used during tissue processing.

Results

βAPP in the early and chronic stages after forebrain ischemia:

1. βAPP reactivity in the early stage after ischemia: intraneuronal deposition

In 3 sham brains studied at 3 days, scattered faintly stained extracellular foci of βAPP immunoreactivity were observed on non-counterstained sections, randomly distributed within the middle layers of neocortex. These foci, however, lacked both a dark-brown appearance and a punctate or granular texture in hemotoxylin-counterstained sections and were only rarely intraneuronal.

In all 6 rats studied at 24 h after 12.5 min forebrain ischemia, βAPP immunoreactivity was noted in large pyramidal neurons, within the dorsolateral and lateral regions of frontoparietal neocortex (Fig. 1). This immunopositivity involved the cytoplasm but not the nuclear region and was punctate or granular in texture. βAPP-positive neurons appeared morphologically normal, with intact nuclear morphology, a visible nucleolus, and no cellular shrinkage. The CA1 sector of hippocampus showed faint βAPP reactivity within normal-appearing neurons in 2 of 6 brains. The cingulate gyrus and thalamus contained no βAPP reaction. βAPP reactivity became weaker at 3 days after ischemia and was observed only in occasional neurons of parietal neocortex in 4 of 5 brains, with normal morphology by H&E stain. Very mild βAPP immunoreaction was present in corpus callosum at 3 days. No reactivity was present in thalamus, striatum, or hippocampus. No extracellular βAPP immunoreactivity was observed.

2. βAPP reactivity in subacute and chronic stages – extra- and intra-neuronal deposition

In sham brains studied at 1 and 10 weeks, neurons were not immunostained. Only 1 brain in each group showed infrequent small, low-density spots of cortical βAPP immunopositiv-

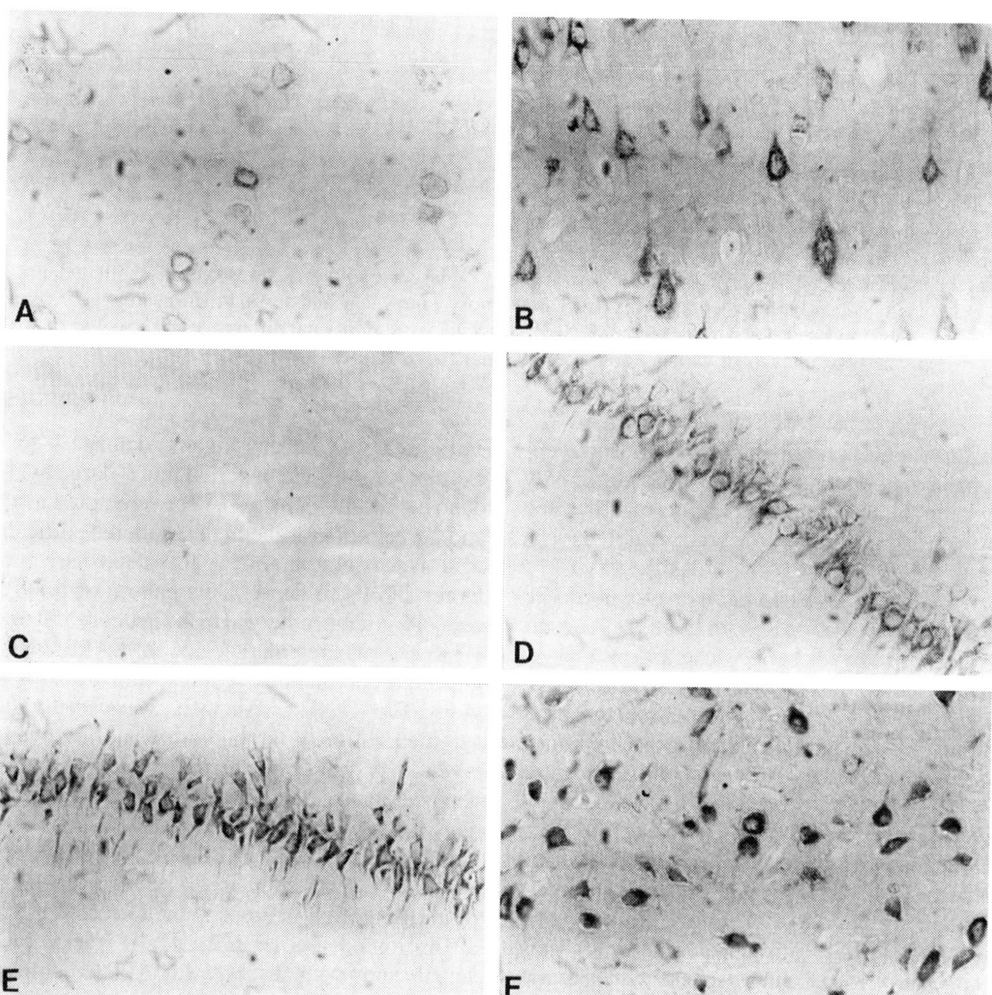

Fig. 1 A–F. βAPP immunohistochemistry of necortex (A, B), hippocampal CA1 (C–E) and ventrolateral thalamus (F) at 24 hours after 12.5-min global ischemia, without hematoxylin counterstain (A–F). Panels A and C, preischemic normoglycemia. Panels B and D–F, preischemic hypergycemia. A: Low-intensity, intraneuronal cytoplasmic βAPP immunoreactivity is present in a few cortical neurons, which appear morphologically intact. B: Strong βAPP immunostaining is evident in morphologically relatively normal-appearing neurons of cortical layers 3–5. C: βAPP immunostaining is very weak after normoglycemic ischemia. D, E: By contrast, striking βAPP immunoreactivity is induced by hyperglycemic ischemia. (D and E are from the same rat, in which necrosis is present in one hippocampal CA1 sector (E) but not in the other hippocampus (D) by H&E stain [not shown].) F: Robust βAPP immunoreactivity of large numbers of neurons having normal morphology. A, B, D–F, x1000; C, x500.

ity. In marked contrast to the findings in sham-operated rats, striking βAPP_{695} immunoreactivity was observed in rats recovering from ischemia (Table 1). Two distinct patterns of βAPP immunoreactivity were noted: (1) a diffuse punctate pattern of tiny round βAPP-labeled granules distributed in cells of those areas of the hippocampal CA1 sector, stiatum, and thalamus identified in our previous study as ischemically lesioned; and (2) a pattern of non-

Table 1. Extraneuronal APP_{695} deposits in cortex at 1–10 weeks after 10-min global ischemia

	Shams 1 week $n = 4$	*Shams* 10 weeks $n = 4$	*Ischemia* 1 week $n = 5$	2 weeks $n = 4$	4 weeks $n = 4$	6 weeks $n = 5$	8 weeks $n = 5$	10 weeks $n = 6$
Small deposits	7 ± 7	1.25 ± 1.25	22 ± 15	60 ± 10*	10 ± 10	37 ± 17	50 ± 17*	34 ± 15
Large ovoid deposits	0	0	2 ± 1	3 ± 1	0.5 ± 0.5	4 ± 3	14 ± 5*	5 ± 3

Numbers of small (< 15 um) beta-APP deposits and of larger ovoid structures were quantitated in a standardized region of inferomedial cortex (inferior auditory, entorhinal, and dorsal piriform areas at bregma level –3.6 mm) and are shown as means ± S.E.M. Asterisks denote significant difference from pooled shams ($p < 0.05$, one-way analysis of variance followed by Dunnett's test).

diffuse, large, non-punctate extra- and intraneuronal foci of βAPP deposition, most commonly in ventral cortical regions – zones not affected by necrosis in our previous study (Table 1) (Lin et al. 1999).

In the areas of ischemic damage, no βAPP accumulation was present in brains of rats surviving 1 or 2 weeks after ischemia. With 4- to 10-week survival, however, numerous tiny granular deposits were observed within those regions of striatum and thalamus that exhibited well-demarcated foci of necrosis when stained by H&E or by GFAP or isolectin immunochemistry (Lin et al. 1998b). At 8 weeks, dense intracellular βAPP accumulated at the borders of large striatal lesions, while the lesion centers contained no immunolabeling. In hippocampal sector CA1, βAPP immunostaining was absent at the end of 1 week but was present in all brains by 2 weeks. Numerous tiny granular deposits were present throughout the strata radiatum and oriens but not in the pyramidal cell layer. By 4 weeks, in three of four rats, these granules enlarged, became rounded, and occupied the pyramidal cell layer. At 6 weeks, the punctate immunostaining became more intense but was confined only to cells of the pyramidal layer. At 8 and 10 weeks, injured neurons were densely immunostained (Fig. 2). This staining only affected the subgroup of rats that exhibited a more severe pattern of ischemic injury by H&E (Lin et al. 1998b). In some brains, neurons in hippocampal CA3 showed very mild βAPP immunostaining at 1 week.

In areas devoid of ischemic damage – for example, cortex and hypothalamus – large oval deposits of low-density βAPP were noted at 1 and 2 weeks after ischemia in scattered cortical neurons of some brains. A few deposits were larger and more dense. This pattern of βAPP deposition again emerged in the neocortex at 6–10 weeks, where enlarged foci of βAPP were located predominantly in the basal cortical regions (Fig. 2). These deposits were scattered symmetrically within the cortex and involved layers II–VI. By 8 weeks, the number of these deposits had increased, their immunostaining density was more pronounced, and the deposits were associated with neuronal enlargement or karyolysis. Extracellular βAPP deposits appeared to entrap neurons so as to form large, diffuse ovoid foci (Fig. 2). At 10 weeks, the density and size of these ovoid βAPP structures increased, and in many instances their cores disappeared. The size of these structures in cortical layers II–V was larger than that in layer VI; however, these foci were more numerous in the deeper cortical layers. By 8 weeks, these structures were present in dendritic areas of hippocampus in most rats. Temporally, there were two peaks of βAPP ovoid structures: the first at 2 weeks, the second at 6–10 weeks. Ovoid structures were observed in hypothalamus, but not in striatum or thalamus. Occasional small intraneuronal βAPP deposits were noted in thalamus, which peaked at 2 weeks after ischemia. A few small oval immunoreactive profiles were present in the corpus callosum

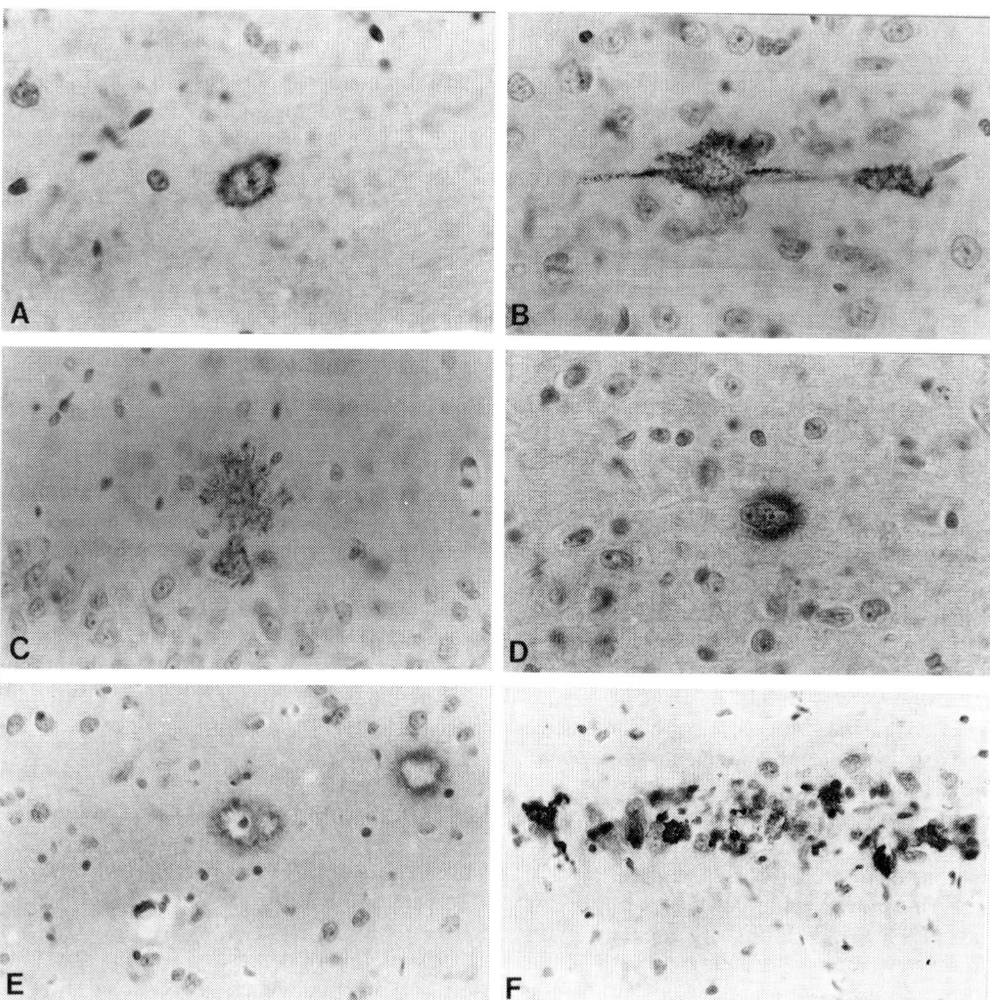

Fig. 2 A–F. βAPP immunoreactivity in cortex (A–E) and hippocampal CA1 (F) after 10-min global ischemia. A–D, 8-week survival; E, F, 10-week survival; with hematoxylin counterstain (A–F). A: Neuronal perikarya is immunolabeled for βAPP. Note enlarged neuron and nucleus as well abnormal immunopositive nucleolus. B: βAPP is contained within dendrites and axon as well in the cytoplasm of a cell, which has a neuronal shape but is enlarged. C: Diffuse extraneuronal βAPP deposit. D: Cortical pyramidal neuron partially surrounded by extracellular βAPP deposit. Karyorrhexis is evident. E: Large, dense ovoid structures resembling the plaques of Alzheimer's disease. F: βAPP immunoreactivity within cells of CA1 pyramidal layer. A, B, D x1500, C, E, F x1000.

and external capsule at 1 week in a few cases, but these changes disappeared by 2 weeks. Glia and endothelium showed no βAPP immunostaining. No relationship between blood vessels and sites of ovoid βAPP deposits was noted.

3. *Pre-ischemic hyperglycemia enhances βAPP immunoreactivity in the absence of Aβ*

Pre-ischemic hyperglycemia dramatically and robustly enhanced N-terminal βAPP immunoreactivity (Fig. 1, Table 2). The striking finding was the presence of prominent high-density intraneuronal βAPP immunoreactivity involving neurons throughout the neocortex, hipocampus, and dorsal and ventrolateral thalamus at 24 h in all 6 rats. In neocortex, robust intraneuronal βAPP immunostaining consistently involved neurons of the cingulate gyrus and all layers of dorsolateral and lateral neocortex. Large pyramidal neurons were the most consistently affected. In hippocampus, all 6 brains revealed prominent βAPP immunoreactivity involving all sectors and extending into the dentate hilus (Fig. 1). On H&E and *Cresyl echt Violett* sections, the hippocampal CA1 sector of these brains contained extensive bilateral ischemic necrosis of pyramidal neurons in 2 of 6 brains; predominantly unilateral alterations in 2 brains; and an absence of ischemic neuronal changes in the remaining 2 rats. In all brains, the dorsal and ventrolateral regions of thalamus also contained extensive zones of markedly βAPP-positive neurons (Fig. 2). H&E and *Cresyl echt Violett* staining of adjacent sections revealed that the strong βAPP immunoreactivity existed in both necrotic and *normal-appearing* neurons.

At 3 days, 4 of 5 brains contained intraneuronal βAPP immunoreactivity within necrotic neurons of frontoparietal neocortical layer V. Fewer neurons were affected than on the first day (Table 2). Neurons of cingulate gyrus, however, were typically uninvolved. All 4 brains with cortical βAPP immunoreactivity also contained prominent βAPP reactivity throughout the entire pyramidal layer of the hippocampal CA1 sector and subiculum; βAPP immunopositive neurons appeared necrotic. By contrast, neurons of the CA3 sector were immunonegative. One brain displayed CA1 necrosis and βAPP immunopositivity on one side, but normal CA1 morphology and βAPP immunoreactivity on the other. The thalamus contained βAPP-positive neurons in only 2 cases. Quantitative analysis of βAPP-positive neurons in parietal neocortex part 2 of hyperglycemic-ischemic rats revealed 5.9-fold mean elevations at 24 h, and 10.6-fold elevations at 3 days, compared to counts in animals with normoglycemic ischemia. These differences were highly significant. Infarcted areas showed no βAPP immunoreactivity on either the 1st or 3rd day after ischemia. Since infarcts failed to show positive immunostaining, and morphologically normal neurons in the CA1 sector were strongly immunostained in hyperglycemic rats, we conclude that the strongly positive immunostaining in hyperglycemic rats is *not* a false-positive result of absorption of the antibody by necrotic tissue. Aβ immunoreactivity was absent in necrotic regions of cortex, CA1, and thalamus despite the persistence of robust βAPP immunoreactivity.

4. *Aβ immunoreactivity after ischemia*

A. *Extracellular deposition in the early stages and in the chronic stage*

Extracellular Aβ deposition was the only pattern of Aβ immunoreactivity observed (Fig. 3). Small numbers of cortical extracellular Aβ deposits were present in sham rats (n = 8). Aβ deposits were also noted in rats with 3-day survival after 12.5-min ischemia (n = 5); the

Table 2. APP_{695}-positive neurons.

	Shams (*n* = 6)	Normoglycemic ischemia 24 h (*n* = 6)	Hyperglycemic ischemia 24 h (*n* = 6)	Normoglycemic ischemia 3 days (*n* = 5)	Hyperglycemic ischemia 3 days (*n* = 5)
Cortex	0	76 ± 19	445 ± 70*	15 ± 5	157 ± 53*

APP-positive cell counts, area Par2 of parietal cortex (bilateral pooled values) (mean ± S.E.M).
*, different from corresponding normoglycemic-ischemic value, Mann-Whitney rank sum test, p < 0.01.

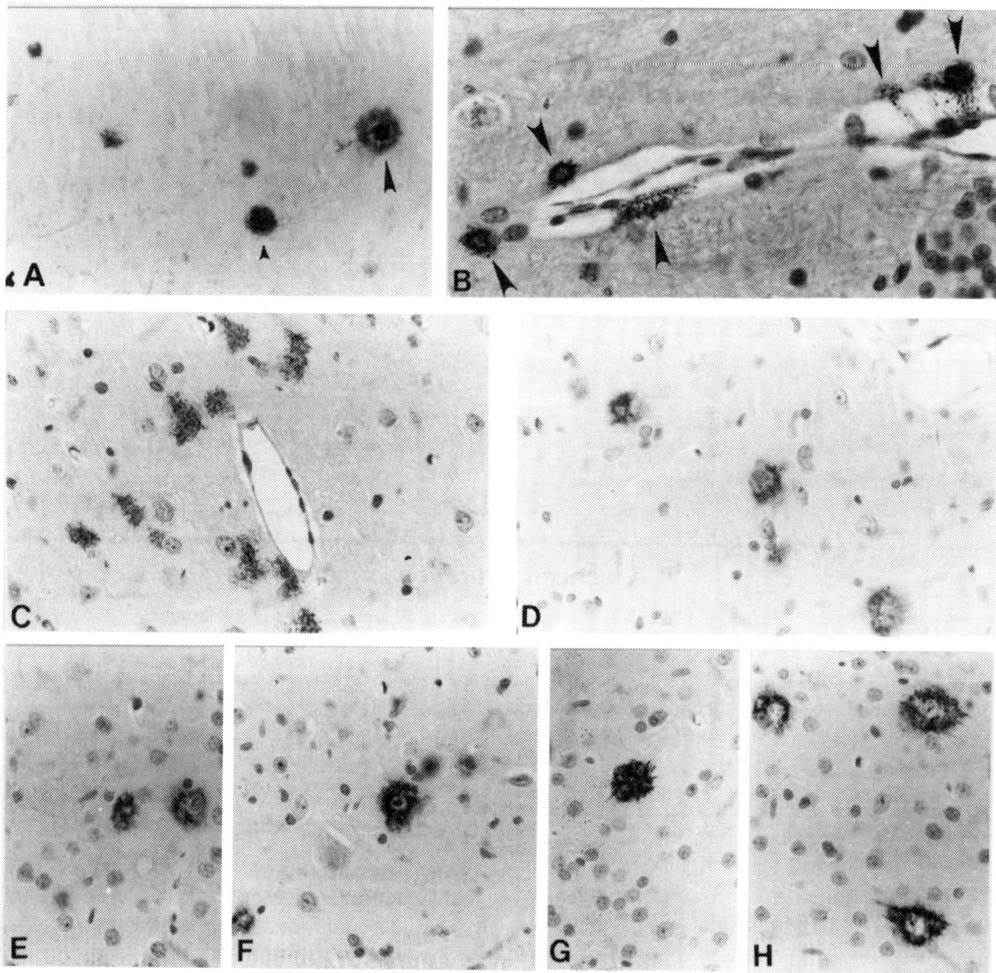

Fig. 3 A–H. Aβ immunostaining in cortex of a stroke patient (A) and in neocortex of rats after 12.5-min global ischemia (B–H), without (A) and with (B–H) hematoxylin counterstain. Panel B: Third day after ischemia. Panels C–H: 2 months' survival. A: Intense Aβ(8–17) immunoreactivity in human brain in a mature plaque (large arrowhead) and immature plaque (small arrowhead) as well as diffuse plaques. B: Numerous round and granular Aβ deposits in close relationship to a blood vessel, thus suggesting a vascular origin. C–H: Extraneuronal Aβ deposition showing three plaque-patterns which resemble human plaques (cf. A). Note that some neurons are partially or totally surrounded by diffuse plaques (C–E). Neurons surrounded by Aβ deposits appear shrunken (D, E). Panel F shows a mature plaque. In panel H, neurons in the plaque-center have disappeared (H). A, x250; B, x2000; C–H, x1000.

numbers of cortical Aβ deposits at this time point were close to sham levels. However, the numbers of deposits increased at 2 months after the ischemic insult (Figs. 3, 4). Increasing duration of ischemia, and in particular the 12.5-min insult, led to large numbers of Aβ deposits at the end of 2 months, while the 7-min ischemic insult failed to induce Aβ, and a 10-min insult induced fewer deposits ($p = 0.0007$) (Fig. 4). Aβ immunoreactivity was present in both gray matter and white matter. The Aβ deposits resembled all three types of human Aβ plaques –

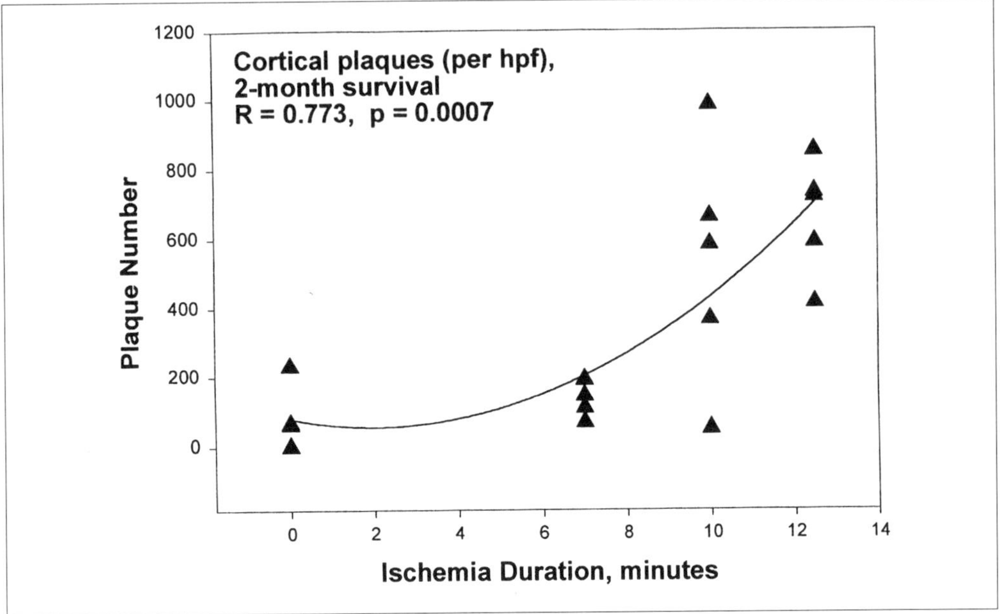

Fig. 4. Numbers of Aβ plaques per standard high-power microscopic regions of neocortex in sham rats (= 0 min) and in rats with 7, 10, and 12.5 minutes of global forebrain ischemia. The curve is a second-order least-squares fit to the data. Numbers of Aβ plaques increase significantly with increasing duration of ischemia.

diffuse, immature, and mature – that are observed in the brains of stroke and AD patients (Fig. 3) (Masliah et al. 1990; Iwatsubo et al. 1994). The Aβ deposits were morphologically similar to the extraneuronal βAPP deposits described above. The initial deposits of amyloid appeared around cell bodies and processes of neurons (Dickson 1997). It appeared that some neurons became gradually surrounded by Aβ deposits and eventually disappeared. In addition, some Aβ deposits exhibited a close relationship to blood vessels, suggestive of a vascular origin. However, no Aβ (6F/3D) immunoreactivity was observed in the regions of the cell layer of CA1 that exhibited intracellular βAPP deposits. Abundant Aβ deposits were noted in white matter, including corpus callosum and internal and external capsule at 2 months, while βAPP immunostaining was absent in these areas.

Discussion

In the present studies, we have demonstrated that ischemia induces intra- and extra-neuronal βAPP accumulation, as well as Aβ expression, in the rat brain in both the acute and chronic stages. The extracellular deposits of βAPP and Aβ in the chronic stage after experimental forebrain ischemia resemble the plaques seen in human AD. Hyperglycemia strikingly enhances the acute upregulation of intraneuronal βAPP (in the absence of Aβ) prior to or coincident with morphological evidence of neuronal death. As the length of the ischemic insult is increased, more Aβ is deposited in the brain at 2 months after the insult.

1. βAPP after ischemia

Our data confirm postischemic βAPP upregulation in the acute stage. The increased immunoreactivity of N-terminal portion of βAPP_{695}

in pyramidal neurons of the cortex and hippocampal CA3 sector and in white matter, but not in the hippocampal CA1 sector, at 1–3 days after forebrain ischemia is similar to the findings of other investigators (Wakita et al. 1992; Pluta et al. 1994; Tomimoto et al. 1995; Horsburgh and Nicoll 1996; Dietrich et al. 1998). Upregulation of βAPP in these regions is common. Hypoxia (Ghribi 1999), chronic hypoperfusion (Kalaria et al. 1993), and subarachnoid hemorrhage (Ryba et al. 1999) all lead to upregulation of βAPP in the same regions. The function of βAPP in these settings, however, is not clear. As the majority of neurons intensely immunoreactive to βAPP survive after ischemia (Tomimoto et al. 1994), it is possible that its normal accumulation in the acute stage after ischemia is beneficial. sAPP, the N-terminus of βAPP, protects neurons against ischemic insults by stabilizing intracellular Ca^{2+} concentration in vivo and vitro (Selkoe et al. 1988; Mattson et al. 1993b; Robison et al. 1993; Smith-Swintosky et al. 1994).

2. *Influence of hyperglycemia on βAPP expression after brief ischemia*

For the first time, we have reported that brief global ischemia under hyperglycemic conditions induces the robust overexpression of βAPP, prior to or coincident with morphological signs of neuronal necrosis. This implies that the overexpression of βAPP in this context may contribute to the hyperglycemic accentuation on ischemic brain injury. βAPP expression is particularly strong in the areas showing histological evidence of injury but is also seen in apparently undamaged areas (Baiden-Amissah et al. 1998). Thus, βAPP upregulation may be both positively adaptive or destructive, depending upon its quantity.

3. *βAPP in the chronic stage after global ischemia*

This is the first description of βAPP immunoreactivity between 7 days and 10 weeks after global ischemia. In other studies, the total amount of βAPP mRNA in brain did not change over a 21-day period after global ischemia (Abe et al. 1991b), suggesting that neuronal βAPP synthesis did not increase during this period. As βAPP is present in plasma, it is possible that it may have entered the brain via a leaky BBB (Martins et al. 1993), aided by cerebrovascular endothelial injury, which exists at this time (Lin et al. 1998b). On the other hand, the increased βAPP accumulation may reflect altered protein metabolism or decreased removal of βAPP. It is possible that ischemia, even if insufficient to induce neuronal necrosis, might impair the lysosomal system and Golgi apparatus, slowing the neuronal degradation of βAPP and promoting its accumulation.

Since almost all βAPP deposits in the present study were plaque-like, it is appropriate to question whether chronic neuronal degeneration after brief global ischemia might be triggered by adjacent βAPP accumulation. Not only did we find βAPP deposits adjacent to and entrapping neurons, but we also noted that the neurons in contact with βAPP deposits exhibited cellular injury in the form of karyorrhexis and/or cellular enlargement.

The mechanism of destruction induced by βAPP may involve apoptosis. In recent studies, APP was found to be an intrinsic activator of caspase-3-mediated death machinery in neurons (Barnes et al. 1998; Uetsuki et al. 1999). Intracellular accumulation of APP_{695} causes a specific "shrinkage-type" of neuronal degeneration in vivo in the absence of extracellular Aβ deposition (Nishimura et al. 1998). Other workers have suggested that intense βAPP immunoreactivity connotes neuronal injury (Tomimoto et al. 1995), and/or delayed degeneration (Saido et al. 1994; Pluta et al. 1994; Pluta 1997; Hall et al. 1995). Recent studies have noted that high βAPP expression coincides with cNOS after cortical injury in the rat (Luth and Arendt 1997), and that the overexpression of $βAPP_{695}$ results in *more severe ischemic neuronal injury* (Zhang et al. 1997; Kim et al. 1998) and *apoptosis in neurons* (Barnes et al. 1998). Most importantly, βAPP regulates intracellular signals and behaves as a signaling receptor (Nishimoto 1998).

The punctate βAPP deposits accumulating in the border zone of a chronic infarct in the present study resembled those observed in acute focal ischemia (Stephenson et al. 1992; Popa-Wagner et al. 1998). The exact mechanism of upregulation of βAPP is unknown because the expression of βAPP mRNAs did not emerge at an early stage after ischemia (Abe et al.1991a). Some studies have shown that IL-1 and -6 released by glia stimulate βAPP synthesis in neurons (Donnelly et al. 1990; Gray and Patel 1993). This cannot explain the overexpression of $βAPP_{695}$ in hyperglycemic ischemia, however, because a glial reaction was just beginning at 24 h. In the chronic stage after normoglycemic ischemia, the $βAPP_{695}$ increases may be due to glial proliferation, however.

In conclusion, the present studies provide evidence that βAPP is a protein involved in ischemic damage and repair. In the acute stage, lesser degrees of βAPP upregulation may be neuroprotective while frank overexpression of APP may be destructive. In the chronic stage after ischemia, βAPP deposition may contribute to a gradual process of neuronal degeneration – i.e., to slowly evolving neuronal death. Thus, βAPP deposition may convert an acute-phase injury response into chronic injury.

4. *Aβ after ischemia*

Our study is the first to report increasing Aβ deposition in the ischemic brain at 2 months. Longer periods of ischemia induced more extensive Aβ deposits. These Aβ deposits gradually surrounded neurons to form plaques before these cells disappeared. Some Aβ appeared to enter the parenchyma from blood vessels. In the white matter, numbers of Aβ deposits increased distinctly at chronic time-points while βAPP deposits were absent.

It has been reported that Aβ deposits are derived from βAPP, then condense to form primitive plaques and, later, mature plaques (Cotman et al. 1996). Usually, punctuate Aβ deposits coexist with plaques and diffuse infiltrates (Wisniewski et al. 1989). In the Alzheimer's brain, some apparently normal neurons are entrapped by amyloid protein deposits (Wisniewski et al. 1989). Unfortunately, the mechanistic links interrelating Aβ, plaque formation, neuronal degeneration and cell death are still incomplete (Burns 1997).

Our study suggests that some Aβ accumulating after cerebral ischemia may arise from the blood. Previous studies have found that soluble Aβ is present in the blood of healthy humans and animals. The level of Aβ in blood is higher than that in the nervous system (Seubert et al. 1992; Selkoe 1993). Serum Aβ levels are elevated in patients suspected to have early-onset AD (Reagan Research Institute 1998). Human Aβ(1–42) is also deposited in organs beyond the brain in transgenic mice (Kawarabayashi et al. 1996). This implies that some cerebral Aβ probably arises from outside the brain, e.g., vascular source or from hepatic synthesis (Selkoe 1989). As early as 15 min after ischemia in the rat, human Aβ injected prior to ischemia is able to cross the BBB and enter the brain parenchyma (Pluta et al. 1996, 1997). However, prior to our study, direct evidence of a vascular origin of Aβ in plaques was lacking.

Endothelial damage persists for long periods after ischema (Lin et al. 1998b; Lin and Ginsberg, 2000); BBB dysfunction allows plasma proteins to escape into the brain parenchyma. Our results show that some of this Aβ partially surrounds neurons or totally entraps them to form plaques, and some of the neurons so entrapped by Aβ eventually disappear. Caspases may be involved in this process (LeBlanc et al. 1999).

Glial reactions might contribute to cerebral Aβ deposition. Glia produce APP after global ischemia (Siman et al. 1989; Kalaria et al. 1993; Palacios et al. 1995; Banati et al. 1995). IL-1 and -6 released by glia stimulate βAPP synthesis in neurons (Donnelly et al. 1990; Gray and Patel 1993). Glial proliferation was observed at 10 weeks after global ischemia (Lin et al. 1998b). Thus, increased cerebral Aβ deposition may result in part from upregulation of βAPP by glia.

Inflammatory processes in the brain have also been thought to contribute to AD in recent years (Eckert et al. 1997; Eikelenboon et al. 1998; Hauss-Wegrzyniak et al. 1998). In our previous study (Lin et al. 1998b), we noted postischemic inflammation persisting over a long time period in the brain. Inflammation stimulates Aβ production in brain via cytokine mechanisms (Araujo and Cotman 1992; Griffin et al. 1994, 1998; Sheng et al. 1996, 1999). Interleukin-1 (IL-1), -6, -10 are released in response to ischemia and enter the circulation (Seekamp et al. 1998). This might possibly encourage Aβ formation by other organs. AD is the most common cause of dementia in the elderly, with cerebrovascular dementia accounting for most of the remaining cases (Burns 1997). Our study has shown that Aβ, which dominates the pathological picture of AD, is also involved in the pathology of cerebral ischemia.

Conclusion

In summary, the information presented above strongly suggests that amyloid peptide and its precursor protein are involved both acutely and chronically in ischemic brain injury. The plaque-like deposits resemble the plaques of human AD. It is possible that not only Aβ, but also βAPP overexpression and chronic βAPP deposition, may be harmful to neuronal cells. Their abnormal metabolism after ischemia may contribute to chronic pathological changes. Questions raised by our studies include the following: 1) Do Aβ and βAPP initiate neuronal degeneration after brain ischemia? 2) Does abnormal βAPP expression exacerbate secondary injury?

Acknowledgment

These studies were supported by NIH Grant NS 05820. The contributions of Raul Busto, Isabel Saul, Guillermo Rodriquez, and Lin Li are gratefully acknowledged.

References

1. Abe K, Tanzi RE, Kogure K (1991a) Selective induction of Kunitz-type protease inhibitor domain-containing amyloid precursor protein mRNA after persistent focal ischemia in rat cerebral cortex. Neurosci Lett 125:172–174
2. Abe K, Tanzi RE, Kogure K (1991b) Induction of HSP70 mRNA after transient ischemia in gerbil brain. Neurosci Lett 125:166–168
3. Akiyama H, Kondo H, Mori H, Kametani F, Nishimura T, Ikeda K, Kato M, MeGeer PL (1996) The amino-terminally truncated forms of amyloid beta-protein in brain macrophages in the ischemic lesions of Alzheimer's disease patients. Neurosci Lett 219:115–118
4. Allsop D, Landon M, Kidd M, Lowe JS, Reynolds GP, Gardner A (1986) Monoclonal antibodies raised against a subsequence of senile plaque core protein react with plaque cores, plaque periphery and cerebrovascular amyloid in Alzheimer's disease. Neurosci Lett 68:252–256
5. Allsop D, Yamamoto T, Kametani F, Miyazaki N, Ishii T (1991) Alzheimer amyloid beta/A4 peptide binding sites and a possible 'APP-secretase' activity associated with rat brain cortical membranes. Brain Res 551:1–9
6. Araujo DM, Cotman CW (1992) β-amyloid stimulates glial cells in vitro to produce growth factors that accumulate in senile plaques in Alzheimer's disease. Brain Res 569:141–145
7. Baiden-Amissah K, Joashi U, Blumberg R, Mehmet H, Edwards AD, Cox PM (1998) Expression of amyloid precursor protein (beta-APP) in the neonatal brain following hypoxic ischemic injury. Neuropathol Appl Neurobiol 24:346–352
8. Banati RB, Gehrmann J, Wiessner C, Hossmann KA, Kreutzberg GW (1995) Glial expression of the beta-amyloid precursor protein (βAPP) in global ischemia. J Cereb Blood Flow Metab 15:647–654
9. Barnes NY, Li L, Yoshikawa K, Schwartz ML, Oppenheim RW, Milligan CE (1998) Increased production of amyloid precursor protein provides a substrate for caspase-3 in dying motoneurons. J Neurosci 18:5,869–5,880
10. Beeson JG, Shelton ER, Chan HW, Gage FH (1994) Differential distribution of amyloid protein precursor immunoreactivity in the rat brain studied by using five different antibodies. J Comp Neurol 342:78–96
11. Behl C, Davis JB, Lesley R, Schubert D (1994) Hydrogen peroxide mediates amyloid beta protein toxicity. Cell 77:817–827
12. Burns DK (1997). The nervous system. In: Basic Pathology, 6th edn (Kumar V, Cotran RS, Robbins SL, eds). Philadelphia, Saunders, pp 739–740
13. Busciglio J, Gabuzda DH, Matsudaira P, Yankner BA (1993) Generation of β-amyloid in the secretory pathway in neuronal and nonneuronal cells. Proc Natl Acad Sci USA 90:2092–2096
14. Checler F (1995) Processing of the β-amyloid precursor protein and its regulation in Alzheimer's disease. J Neurochem 65:1431–1444
15. Citron M, Diehl TS, Gordon G, Biere AL, Seubert P, Selkoe DJ (1996) Evidence that the 42- and 40-amino acid forms of amyloid beta protein are generated from the beta-amyloid precursor protein by different protease activities. Proc Natl Acad Sci USA 93:13170–13175
16. Coria F, Moreno A, Torres A, Ahmad I, Ghiso J (1992) Distribution of Alzheimer's disease amyloid protein precursor in normal human and rat nervous system. Neuropathol Appl Neurobiol 18:27–35
17. Cotman CW, Tenner AJ, Cummings BJ. (1996) β-amyloid converts an acute phase injury response to chronic injury responses. Neurobiol Aging 17:723–731
18. de la Torre JC (1999) Review: Critical threshold cerebral hypoperfusion causes Alzheimer's disease? Acta Neuropathol 98:1–8
19. Dickson DW (1997) The pathogenesis of senile plaques. J Neuropathol Exp Neurol 56:321–339
20. Dietrich WD, Kraydieh S, Prado R, Stagliano NE (1998) White matter alterations following thromboembolic stroke: a β-amy-

loid protein precursor immunocytochemical study in rats. Acta Neuropathol 95:524–531

21. Donnelly RJ, Friedhoff AJ, Beer B, Blume AJ, Vitek MP (1990) Interleukin-1 stimulates the beta-amyloid precursor protein promoter. Cell Mol Neurobiol 10:485–495
22. Eckert A, Oster M, Forstl H, Hennerici M, Muller WE (1997) Impaired calcium regulation in subcortical vascular encephalopathy. Stroke 28:1351–1356
23. Egensperger R, Weggen S, Ida N, Multhaup G, Schnabel R, Beyreuther K, Bayer TA (1999) Reverse relationship between β-amyloid precursor protein and β-amyloid peptide plaques in Down's syndrome versus sporadic/familial Alzheimer's disease. Acta Neuropathol 97:113–118
24. Eikelenboom P, Rozemuller JM, van Muiswinkel FL (1998) Inflammation and Alzheimer's disease: relationships between pathogenic mechanisms and clinical expression. Exp Neurol 154:89–98
25. Freek L, Van Muiswinkel FL, Raupp SF, de Vos NM, Smits HA, Verhoef J, Eikelenboom P, Nottet HS (1999) The amino-terminus of the amyloid-β protein is critical for the cellular binding and consequent activation of the respiratory burst of human macrophages. J Neuroimmunol 96:121–130
26. Furukawa K, Sopher BL, Rydel RE, Begley JG, Pham DG, Martin GM, Fox M, Mattson MP (1996) Increase activity-regulating and neuroprotective efficacy of α-secretase-derived secreted amyloid precursor protein conferred by a C-terminal heparin-binding domain. J Neurochem 67: 1882–1896
27. Ghribi O, Lapierre L, Girard M, Ohayon M, Nalbantoglu J, Massicotte G (1999) Hypoxia-induced loss of synaptic transmission is exacerbated in hippocampal slices of transgenic mice expressing C-terminal fragments of Alzheimer amyloid precursor protein. Hippocampus 9:201–205
28. Goodman Y, Mattson MP (1994) Secreted forms of beta-amyloid precursor protein protect hippocampal neurons against amyloid beta-peptide-induced oxidative injury. Exp Neurol 128:1–12
29. Graham DI, Gentleman SM, Lynch A, Roberts GW (1995) Distribution of β-amyloid protein in the brain following severe head injury. Neuropathol Appl Neurobiol 21:27–34
30. Gray CW, Patel AJ (1993) Regulation of beta-amyloid precursor protein isoform mRNAs by transforming growth factor-beta 1 and interleukin-1 beta in astrocytes. Mol Brain Res 19:251–256
31. Griffin WS, Sheng JG, Gentleman SM, Graham DI, Mrak RE, Roberts GW (1994) Microglial interleukin-1 alpha expression in the human head injury: correlations with neuronal and neuritic beta-amyloid precursor protein expression. Neurosci Lett 176:133–136
32. Griffin WS, Sheng JG, Royston MC, Gentleman SM, McKenzie JE, Graham DI, Roberts GW, Mrak RE (1998) Glial-neuronal interactions in Alzheimer's disease: the potential role of a "cytokine cycle" in disease progression. Brain Pathol 8:65–72
33. Haass C, Schlossmacher MG, Hung AY, Vigo-Pelfrey C, Mellon A, Ostaszewski BL, Lieberburg I, Koo EH, Schenk D, Teplow DB, Selkoe DJ (1992) Amyloid β-peptide is produced by cultured cells during normal metabolism. Nature 359:322–325
34. Hall ED, Oostveen JA, Dunn E, Carter DB (1995) Increased amyloid protein precursor and apolipoprotein E immunoreactivity in the selectively vulnerable hippocampus following transient forebrain ischemia in gerbils. Exp Neurol 135:17–27
35. Hauss-Wegrzyniak B, Dobrzanski P, Stoehr JD, Wenk GL (1998) Chronic neuroinflammation in rats reproduces components of the neurobiology of Alzheimer's disease. Brain Res 780:294–303
36. Horsburgh K, Nicoll JAR (1996) Selective cellular alterations in amyloid precursor protein and apolipoprotein E following transient cerebral ischemia in the rat. Alzheimer's Res 2:37–42
37. Ikeda S, Allsop D, Glenner GG (1989) Morphology and distribution of plaque and related deposits in the brains of Alzhemer's disease and control cases. An immunohistochemical study using amyloid beta-protein antibody. Lab Invest 60:113–122
38. Iversen LL, Mortishire-Smith RJ, Pollack SJ, Shearman MS (1995) The toxicity in vitro of β-amyloid protein. Biochem J 311:1–16
39. Iwatsubo T, Odaka A, Suzuki N, Mizusawa H, Nukina N, Ihara Y (1994) Visualization of Aβ42(43) and Aβ40 in senile plaques with end-specific Aβ monoclonals: Evidence that an initially deposited species is Aβ 42(43). Neuron 13:45–53
40. Jendroska K, Poewe W, Daniel SE, Pluess J, Iwerssen-Schmidt H, Paulsen J, Barthel S, Schelosky L, Cervos-Navarro J, DeArmond SJ (1995) Ischemic stress induces deposition of amyloid β immunoreactivity in human brain. Acta Neuropathol 90:461–466
41. Kalaria RN, Bhatti SU, Palatinsky EA, Pennington DH, Shelton ER, Chan HW, Perry G, Lust WD (1993) Accumulation of the beta amyloid precursor protein at sites of ischemic injury in rat brain. Neuroreport 4:211–214
42. Kang J, Lemaire HG, Unterbeck A, Salbaum JM, Masters CL, Grzeschik KH, Multhaup G, Beyreuther K, Muller-Hill B (1987) The precursor of Alzheimer's disease amyloid A4 protein resembles a cell-surface receptor. Nature 325:733–736
43. Kawarabayashi T, Shoji M, Sato M, Sasaki A, Ho L, Eckman CB, Prada C-M, Younkin SG, Kobayashi T, Tada N, Matsubara E, Iizuka T, Harigaya Y, Kasai K, Hirai S (1996) Accumulation of β-amyloid fibrils in pancreas of transgenic mice. Neurobiol Aging 17:215–222
44. Kim HS, Lee SH, Kim SS, Kim YK, Jeong SJ, Ma J, Han DH, Cho BK, Suh YH (1998) Post-ischemic changes in the expression of Alzheimer's APP isoforms in rat cerebral cortex. Neuroreport 9:533–537
45. Koo EH, Squazzo SL, Selkoe DJ, Koo CH (1996) Trafficking of cell-surface amyloid β-protein precursor. I. Secretion, endocytosis and recycling as detected by labeled monoclonal antibody. J Cell Sci 109:991–998
46. Kumar V, Cotran RS, Robbins SL (1997) Disorders of the immune system. In Basic Pathology, 6th edition. (Kumar V, Cotran RS, Robbins SL, eds), Philadelphia, W.B. Saunders Co., pp 126–131
47. LeBlanc A, Liu H, Goodyer C, Bergeron C, Hammond J (1999) Caspase-6 role in apoptosis of human neurons, amyloidogenesis, and Alzheimer's disease. J Biol Chem 274:23,426–23,436
48. Lin B, Ginsberg MD (2000) Quantitative assessment of normal microvascular morphology by endothelial barrier antigen (EBA) immunohistochemistry: application to cerebral ischemia. Brain Res 865:237–244
49. Lin B, Schmidt-Kastner R, Busto R, Ginsberg MD (1999) Progressive parenchymal deposition of beta-amyloid precursor protein in rat brain following global cerebral ischemia. Acta Neuropathol 97:359–368
50. Lin B, Ginsberg MD, Busto R (1998a) Hyperglycemic exacerbation of neuronal damage following forebrain ischemia: microglial, astrocytic and endothelial alterations. Acta Neuropathol 96:610–620
51. Lin B, Ginsberg MD, Busto R, Dietrich WD (1998b) Sequential analysis of subacute and chronic neuronal, astrocytic and microglial alterations after transient global ischemia in rats. Acta Neuropathol 95:511–523
52. Luth HJ, Arendt T (1997) Co-expression of APP with cNOS but not iNOS after cortical injury in rat. Neuroreport 8:2321–2324
53. Martins RN, Muir J, Brooks WS, Creasey H, Montgomery P, Sellers P, Broe GA (1993) Plasma amyloid precursor protein is decreased in Alzheimer's disease. Neuroreport 4:757–759
54. Martin LJ, Pardo CA, Cork LC, Price DL (1994) Synaptic pathology and glial responses to neuronal injury precede the

formation of senile plaques and amyloid deposits in the aging cerebral cortex. Am J Pathol 145:1358–1381
55. Masliah E, Terry RD, Mallory M, Alford M, Hansen LA (1990) Diffuse plaques do not accentuate synapse loss in Alzheimer's disease. Am J Pathol 137:1293–1297
56. Mattson MP, Barger SW, Cheng B, Lieberburg I, Smith-Swintosky VL, Rydel RE (1993a) β-Amyloid precursor protein metabolites and loss of neuronal Ca^{2+} homeostasis in Alzheimer's disease. TINS 16:409–414
57. Mattson MP, Cheng B, Culwell AR, Esch F, Lieberburg I, Rydel RE, (1993b) Evidence for excitoprotective and intraneuronal calcium-regulation roles for secreted forms of the β-amyloid precursor protein. Neuron 10:243–254
58. Mattson MP, Rydel RE, Lieberburg I, Smith-Swintosky VL (1993c) Altered calcium signaling and neuronal injury: stroke and Alzheimer's disease as examples. Ann NY Acad Sci 679:1–21
59. Mattson MP (1994) Calcium and neuronal injury in Alzheimer's disease. Contributions of beta-amyloid precursor protein mismetabolism, free redicals, and metabolic compromise. Ann NY Acad Sci 747:50–76
60. Mattson MP (1997) Cellular actions of beta-amyloid precursor protein and its soluble and fibrillogenic derivatives. Physiol Rev 77:1081–1132
61. Mazur-Kolecka B, Frackowiak J, Carroll RT, Wisniewski HM (1997) Accumulation of Alzheimer amyloid-β peptide in cultured myocytes is enhanced by serum and reduced by cerebrospinal fluid. J Neuropathol Exp Neurol 56: 263–272
62. Meier-Ruge WA, Bertoni-Freddari C (1997) Pathogenesis of decreased glucose turnover and oxidative phosphorylation in ischemic and trauma-induced dementia of the Alzheimer type. Ann NY Acad Sci 826:229–241
63. Miguel-Hidalgo JJ, Cacabelos R (1998) β-Amyloid(1–40)-induced neurodegeneration in the rat hippocampal neurons of the CA1 subfifeld. Acta Neuropathol 95:455–465
64. Mori RD, Martins RN, Bush AI, Small DH, Milward EA, Rumble BA, Multhaup G, Beyreuther K, Masters CL (1992) Human brain beta A4 amyloid protein precursor of Alzheimer's disease: purification and partial characterization. J Neurochem 59:1,490–1,498
65. Munger JS, Hass C, Lemere CA, Shi GP, Wong WS, Teoplow DB, Selkoe DJ (1995) Lysosomal processing of amyloid precursor protein to a beta peptides: a distinct role for cathepsin S. Biochem J 311(Pt 1):299–305
66. Nishimoto I (1998) A new paradigm for neurotoxicity by FAD mutants of βAPP: a signaling abnormality. Neurobiol Aging 19:S33–S38
67. Nishimura I, Uetsuki T, Dani SU, Ohsawa Y, Saito I, Okamura H, Uchiyama Y, Yoshikawa K (1998) Degeneration in vivo of rat hippocampal neurons by wild-type Alzheimer amyloid precursor protein overexpressed by adenovirus-mediated gene transfer. J Neurosci 18:2387–2398
68. Palacios G, Mengod G, Tortosa A, Ferrer I, Palacios JM (1995) Increased β-Amyloid precursor protein expression in astrocytes in the gerbil hippocampus following ischemia: association with proliferation of astrocytes. Eur J Neurosci 7:501–510
69. Palacios G, Palacios JM, Mengod G, Frey P (1992) Beta-amyloid precursor protein localization in the Golgi apparatus in neurons and oligodendrocytes. An immunocytochemical structural and ultrastructural study in normal and axotomized neurons. Brain Res Mol Brain Res 15:195–206
70. Pluta R (1997) Experimental model of neuropathological changes characteristic for Alzheimer's disease. Folia Neuropathol 35:94–98
71. Pluta R, Misicka A, Januszewski S, Barcilowska M, Lipkowski AW (1997) Transport of human beta-amyloid peptide through the rat blood-brain barrier after global cerebral ischemia. Acta Neurochir Suppl (Wien) 70: 247–249
72. Pluta R, Barcikowska M, Januszewski S, Misicka A, Lipkowski AW (1996) Evidence of blood-brain barrier permeability/leakage for circulating human Alzheimer's β-amyloid-(1–42)-peptide. Neuroreport 7:1261–1265
73. Pluta R, Kida E, Lossinski AS, Golabek AA, Mossakowski MJ, Wisniewski HM (1994) Complete cerebral ischemia with short-term survival in rats induced by cardiac arrest. I. Extracellular accumulation of Alzheimer's beta-amyloid protein precursor in the brain. Brain Res 649:323–328
74. Popa-Wagner A, Schroder E, Walker LC, Kessler C (1998) β-Amyloid precursor protein and ss-amyloid peptide immunoreactivity in the rat brain after middle cerebral artery occlusion: effect of age. Stroke 29:2196–2202
75. Querfurth HW, Jiang J, Geiger JD, Selkoe DJ (1997) Caffeine stimulates amyloid beta-peptide release from beta-amyloid precursor protein-transfected HEK 293 cells. J Neurochem 69:1580–1591
76. Qiu WQ, Ye Z, Kholodenko D, Seubert P, Selkoe DJ (1997) Degradation of amyloid beta-protein by a metalloprotease secreted by microglia and other neural and non-neural cells. J Biol Chem 272:6641–6646
77. RE and N Reagan Research Institute of the Alzheimer's Association and the National Institute on Aging Working Group (1998) Consensus report of the working group on: "Molecular and biochemical markers of Alzheimer's disease". Neurobiol Aging 19:109–116
78. Robison PM, Clemens JA, Smalstig EB, Stephenson D, May PC (1993) Decrease in amyloid precursor protein precedes hippocampal degeneration in rat brain following transient global ischemia. Brain Res 608:334–337
79. Ryba MS, Gordon-Krajcer W, Walski M, Chalimoniuk M, Chrapusta SJ (1999) Hydroxylamine attenuates the effects of simulated subarachnoid hemorrhage in the rat brain and improves neurological outcome. Brain Res 850:225–233
80. Saido TC, Yokota M, Maruyama K, Yamao-Harigaya W, Tani E, Ihara Y, Kawashima S (1994) Spatial resolution of the primary β-amyloidogenic process induced in postischemic hippocampus. J Biol Chem 269:15,253–15,257
81. Seekamp A, Jochum M, Ziegler M, van Griensven M, Martin M, Regel G (1998) Cytokines and adhesion molecules in elective and accidental trauma-related ischemia/reperfusion. J Trauma: Injury, Infection Critical Care 44:874–882
82. Selkoe DJ (1999) Translating cell biology into therapeutic advances in Alzheimer's disease Nature 399 (Supp):A23–31
83. Selkoe DJ (1993) Physiological production of the β-amyloid protein and the mechanism of Alzheimer's disease. TINS 16:403–409
84. Selkoe DJ (1989) Amyloid β protein precursor and the pathogenesis of Alzheimer's disease. Cell 58:611–612
85. Selkoe DJ, Podlinsny MD, Joachim CL, Vickers EA, Lee G, Fritz LC, Oltersdorf T (1988) Beta-amyloid precursor protein of Alzheimer's disease occurs as 110- to 135-kilodalton membrane-associated proteins in neural and nonneunal tissues. Proc Natl Acad Sci USA 85:7341–7345
86. Seubert P, Vigo-Pelfrey C, Esch F, Lee M, Dovey H, Davis D, Sinha S, Schlossmacher M, Whaley J, Swindlehurst C, McCormack R, Wolfert R, Selkoe D, Lieberburg I, Schenk D (1992) Isolation and quantification of soluble Alzheimer's β-peptide from biological fluids. Nature 359:325–327
87. Sheng JG, Griffin WS, Royston M, Mrak RE (1998) Distribution of interleukin-1-immunoreactive microglia in cerebral cortical layers: implications for neuritic plaque formation in Alzheimer's disease. Neuropathol Appl Neurobiol 24:278–283
88. Sheng JG, Ito K, Skinner RD, Mrak RE, Rovnaghi CR, Van Eldik LJ, Griffin WS (1996) In vivo and in vitro evidence supporting a role for the inflammatory cytokine interleukin-1 as a driving force in Alzheimer's pathogenesis. Neurobiol Aging 17:761–766

89. Siman R, Card JP, Nelson RB, Davis LG (1989) Expression of beta-amyloid precursor protein in reactive astrocytes following neuronal damage. Neuron 3:275–285
90. Simons M, Strooper BD, Multhaup G, Tienari P, Dotti CG (1996) Amyloidogenic processing of the human amyloid precursor protein in primary cultures of rat hippocampal neurons. J Neurosci 16:899–906
91. Smith DH, Chen XH, Nonaka M, Trojanowski JQ, Lee VM, Saatman KE, Leoni MJ, Xu BN, Wolf JA, Meaney DF (1999) Accumulation of amyloid β and tau and the formation of neural filament inclusions following diffuse brain injury in pig. J Neuropathol Exp Neurol 58:982–992
92. Smith-Swintosky VL, Pettigrew LC, Craddock SD, Culwell AR, Ryded RE, Mattson MP (1994) Secreted forms of β-amyloid precursor protein protect against ischemic brain injury. J Neurochem 63:781–784
93. Sparks DL (1996) Intraneuronal β-amyloid immunoreactivity in the CNS. Neurobiol Aging 17:291–299
94. Stephenson DT, Rash K, Clemens JA (1992) Amyloid precursor protein accumulates in regions of neurodegeneration following focal cerebral ischemia in the rat. Brain Res 593:128–135
95. Sutton ET, Hellermann GR, Thomas T (1997) β-amyloid-induced endothelial necrosis and inhibition of nitric oxide production. Exp Cell Res 230:368–376
96. Taylor SC, Batten TFC, Peers C (1999) Hypoxic enhancement of quantal catecholamine secretion: evidence for the involvement of amyloid β-peptides. J Biol Chem 274:31,217–31,222
97. Thal DR, Glas A, Schneider W, Schober R (1997) Differential pattern of β-amyloid, amyloid precursor protein and apolipoprotein E expression in cortical senile plaques. Acta Neuropathol 94:255–265
98. Tomimoto H, Akiguchi I, Wakita H, Nakamura S, Kimura J (1995) Ultrastructural localization of amyloid protein percursor in the normal and postischemic gerbil brain. Brain Res 672:187–195
99. Tomimoto H, Wakita H, Akiguchi I, Nakamura S, Kimura J (1994) Temporal profiles of accumulation of amyloid β/A4 protein precursor in the gerbil after graded ischemic stress. J Cereb Blood Flow Metab 14:565–573
100. Uetsuki T, Takemoto K, Nishimura I, Okamoto M, Niinobe M, Momoi T, Miura M, Yoshikawa K (1999) Activation of neuronal caspase-3 by intracellular accumulation of wild-type Alzheimer amyloid precursor protein. J Neurosci 19:6955–6964
101. Vasilakos JP, Carroll RT, Emmerling MR, Doyle PD, Davis RE, Kim KS, Shivers BD (1994) Interleukin-1 beta dissociates beta-amyloid precursor protein and beta-amyloid peptide secretion. FEBS Lett 354:2889–2892
102. Wakita H, Tomimoto H, Akiguchi I, Ohnishi K, Nakamura S, Kimura J (1992) Regional accumulation of amyloid β/A4 protein precursor in the gerbil brain following transient cerebral ischemia. Neurosci Lett 146:135–138
103. Wertkin AM, Turner RS, Pleasure SJ, Golde TE, Younkin SG, Trojanowski JQ, Lee VM (1993) Human neurons derived from a teratocarcinoma cell line express solely the 695-amino acid amyloid precursor protein and produce intracellular beta-amyloid or A4 peptides. Porc Natl Acad Sci USA 90:9513–9517
104. Wisniewski HM, Bancher C, Barcikowska M, Wen GY, Currie J (1989) Spectrum of morphological appearance of amyloid deposits in Alzheimer's disease. Acta Neuropathol 78:337–347
105. Wisniewski HM, Maslinska D (1996) Beta-protein immunoreactivity in the human brain after cardiac arrest. Folia Neuropathol 34:65–71
106. Yamazaki T, Koo EH, Selkoe DJ (1996) Trafficking of cell-surface amyloid β-protein precursor. II. Endocytosis, recycling, and lysosomal targeting detected by immunolocalization. J Cell Sci 109:999–1008
107. Yankner BA (1996) Mechanisms of neuronal degeneration in Alzheimer's disease. Neuron 16:921–932
108. Yokota M, Saido TC, Tani E, Yamaura I, Minami N (1996) Cytotoxic fragment of amyloid precursor protein accumulates in hippocampus after global forebrain ischemia. J Cereb Blood Flow Metab 16:1219–1223
109. Zhang F, Eckman C, Younkin S, Hsiao KK, Iadecola C (1997) Increased susceptibility to ischemic brain damage in transgenic mice overexpressing the amyloid precursor protein. J Neurosci 17:7655–7661

Receptors and intracellular signaling

A possible role for tachykinins in stroke

R. K. Stumm[1], C. Culmsee[2], C. Schaper[2], M. K.-H. Schäfer[1], J. Krieglstein[2], E. Weihe[1]

Abstract

Evidence is emerging that tachykinins participate in excitotoxic and inflammatory processes in the central nervous system. To test the hypothesis whether tachykinins may play a role in stroke, we analyzed at the mRNA and protein level cell-type specific expressional changes of the tachykinin neuropeptides substance P (SP) and neurokinin B (NKB) and of the respective receptors NK1 and NK3 at different stages after middle cerebral artery occlusion (MCAO) in the rat. The changes after MCAO revealed by quantitative in situ hybridization, double in situ hybridization, immunohistochemistry and double fluorescence confocal microscopy were compared to changes after transient forebrain ischemia in the rat. After MCAO, NK1 was transiently de novo expressed in the endothelium of blood vessels running in the meninges covering the infarct, within the infarct, and especially in the periinfarct border region. Here, NK1 expression was induced in the endothelium of activated venules. In contrast, there was no evidence for ischemia-induced induction of NK1 in reactive microglia or astrocytes. After transient forebrain ischemia, induction of NK1 in cerebrovascular endothelium did not occur. After MCAO, neuronal gene expression in the infarct was lost due to early neuronal death. In the cerebrocortical periinfarct area SP and NK1 expression was enhanced in GABAergic neurons and ectopically induced in glutamatergic pyramidal cells. After transient forebrain ischemia, the mRNA encoding SP was ectopically expressed in the CA1 pyramidal cell layer. After MCAO, the expression of NKB in the periinfarct cortex was increased in GABAergic neurons while NK3 receptor expression was decreased in pyramidal cells. Transient forebrain ischemia caused major downregulation of NK3 in pyramidal cells of the cerebral cortex with no obvious change in NKB expression.

Our results indicate that NK1 receptor induction in the endothelium may contribute to the impairment of the blood brain barrier after focal cerebral ischemia resulting in edema formation and leukocyte infiltration. The ischemia-induced changes in neuronal tachykinin and NK receptor expression after focal and transient forebrain ischemia may cause imbalance between GABAergic and glutamatergic neurotransmission in the post-ischemic cerebral cortex or CA1 regions resulting in stage-and region-specific excitotoxicity. We postulate that NK1 and NK3 receptors are novel targets for pharmacological intervention in stroke.

[1]Dept. of Molecular Neuroscience, Institute of Anatomy and Cell Biology, Philipps University Marburg, Robert-Koch-Straße 6, D-35033 Marburg, Germany
[2]Institute of Pharmacology and Toxicology, Philipps University Marburg, Ketzerbach 63, D-35032 Marburg, Germany

J. Krieglstein, S. Klumpp (Eds.) Pharmacology of Cerebral Ischemia 2000

Introduction

The pathophysiology of stroke is characterized by complex neuroglial reactions in the brain (Dirnagl et al. 1999). Primary and secondary neuronal cell death is accompanied by neuroinflammatory reactions such as astrogliosis, microgliosis, impairment of the blood brain barrier, and leukocyte invasion. Tachykinin neuropeptides and tachykinin receptors (NK receptors) are widely distributed in the central and peripheral nervous systems where they serve a variety of functions (Warden and Young 1988; Nakaya et al. 1994; Ding et al. 1996), including modulation of GABAergic and glutamatergic neurotransmission, pain signalling, neurogenic inflammation and neuroimmune interaction (Weihe et al. 1991; Weihe et al. 1994; Maubach et al. 1998; Quartara and Maggi 1998). The mammalian tachykinins (see Fig. 1) are encoded by preprotachykinin A (PPT-A) and preprotachykinin B (PPT-B). The alternatively spliced PPT-A mRNAs encode for substance P (SP) and neurokinin A (NKA), which have the high affinites for the NK1 and NK2 receptors, respectively (Carter and Krause 1990; Hershey et al. 1991; Sasai and Nakanishi 1991). Neurokinin B (NKB) is derived from the PPT-B gene and binds with high affinity to the NK3 receptor (Bonner et al. 1987; Shigemoto et al. 1990).

Recent evidence suggests a major role for tachykinins in excitotoxic neurological disorders and neuroinflammatory brain injury. The NK1 antagonist CP-122,721-1 reduces excitotoxin-induced seizures (Zachrisson et al. 1998) and PPT-A-deficient mice are resistant to kainate-induced seizures and apoptotic neuronal death (Liu et al. 1999). Application of NKB increases frequency and duration of epileptiform discharges (Maubach et al. 1998). Astrocyte activation and brain inflammation during trypanosoma-induced meningoencephalitis are reduced by the NK1 receptor antagonist RP-67,580 (Kennedy et al. 1997) suggesting the possibility of a role of tachykinins in CNS inflammation and glial function. In addition, neuronal injury induces binding sites for SP in reactive astrocytes as shown in a model of optic nerve lesion (Mantyh et al. 1989). Moreover, SP enhances the secretion of the pro-inflammatory cytokine TNF-alpha from astrocytes and microglial cells (Luber-Narod et al. 1994), hence is likely to stimulate inflammatory responses.

These data in the literature lead to the hy-

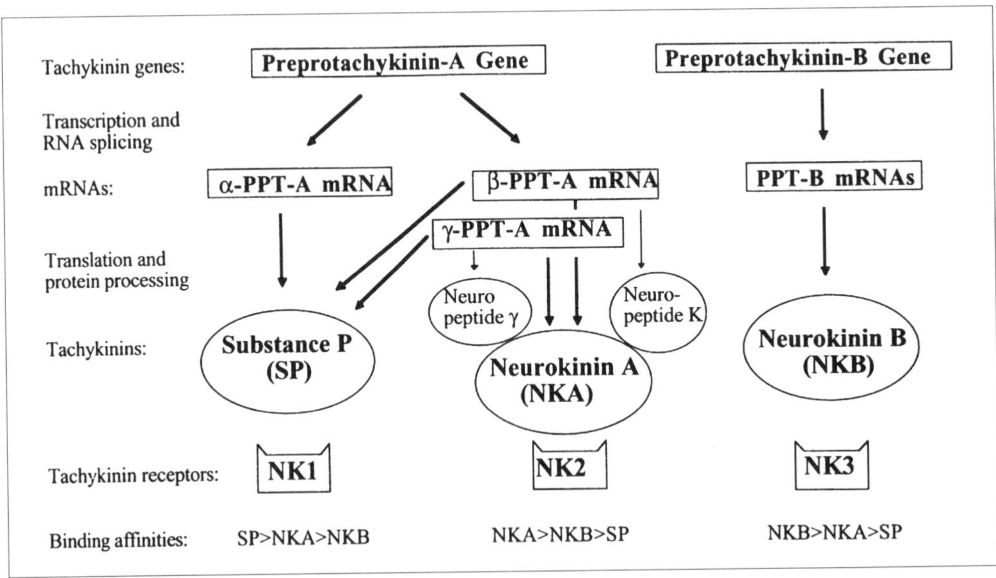

Fig. 1. Schematic diagram of the tachykinin system.

pothesis that tachykinins may play a dual role in the pathophysiology of stroke, i.e., regulation of ischemia-induced neuronal hyperexcitability and modulation of neuro-inflammatory events in the brain. To test this hypothesis, we investigated the spatio-temporal and specific neuronal and non-neuronal cellular expression patterns of tachykinin and tachykinin receptor genes in an established animal model of stroke, the permanent middle cerebral artery occlusion (MCAO) in the rat , and compared it to changes after transient forebrain ischemia.

Materials and methods

Experimental groups and tissue preparation. Middle cerebral artery occlusion (MCAO) was performed in the rat as introduced by Tamura et al. (1981) and modified by Culmsee et al. 1999. Transient forebrain ischemia was employed by clamping both common carotid arteries and reducing the blood pressure (Zhu et al. 1998). For qualitative and quantitative radioactive *in situ* hybridization (ISH), brains (n = 6 per group) were collected and frozen at 6 h, 2 d and 7 d after sham operation and MCAO, respectively. For qualitative ISH and subjective rating of hybridization signals, brains (n = 2–3) were collected and frozen at 6 h, 1 d, 2 d, 4 d and 7 d after transient forebrain ischemia and sham operation. For immunohistochemistry, 2 animals per group were perfused transcardially with 10 mM PBS containing 20 units/ml heparin followed by Bouin Hollande fixative. The postfixed brains were washed in 70% 2-propanol prior to routine paraffin embedding.

Immunohistochemistry. Single enzyme and fluorescence immunohistochemistry was performed on deparaffinized sections according to a standard protocol including antigen retrieval as described (Röhrenbeck et al. 1999; Schäfer et al. 2000). The following polyclonal rabbit antibodies were used. An antiserum against the rat NK1 was generously provided by R. Shigemoto (Shigemoto et al. 1993). The antiserum against SP was a gift of R.L. Eskay, (NIDA, Bethesda) and that against a 30-residue fragment of the protein precursor to NKB was provided by J.E. Krause (Lucas et al. 1992). An antibody against CD62P (P-selectin), a marker of activated venular endothelium after MCAO (Suzuki et al. 1998), was purchased from Pharmingen (San Diego, USA). Sections were incubated with primary antibodies overnight. Species-specific biotinylated secondary antibodies (Dianova, Hamburg, Germany) were applied and detected with the ABC reagents (Vectastain ABC-Kit, Vector Laboratories, Burlingame USA) followed by a nickel-enhanced diaminobenzidine reaction. *Double-immunofluorescence and confocal laser scanning microscopy.* Using the Olympus Fluoview confocal laser scanning microscope (Olympus Optical Co., Hamburg, Germany), the coexpression of NK1 and glial fibrillary acidic protein (GFAP, a marker for astrocytes) as well as of NK1 and C1q (a marker for microglia) was performed as described (Dietzschold et al. 1995; Schäfer et al. 2000).

Single and double in situ hybridization histochemistry. Plasmids containing cDNAs of the rat PPT-A gene (Carter and Krause 1990) and of the three tachykinin receptors NK1 (Hershey et al. 1991), NK2 (Sasai et al. 1989) and NK3 (Shigemoto et al. 1990), were provided by J.E. Krause. The PPT-A specific cDNA was homologous to the α-, β- and γ-PPT-A mRNAs (Carter and Krause 1990). Specific cDNAs of rat PPT-B (Bonner et al. 1987), rat glutamic acid decarboxylase $M_{(r)}$ 67,000 (GAD, EC 4.1.1.15, Wyborski et al. 1990) and rat phosphate activated glutaminase (PAG, EC 3.5.1.2, Shapiro et al. 1991) were generated by RT-PCR cloning. GAD was used as a marker for GABAergic neurons and PAG as a marker for glutamatergic cerebrocortical neurons (Kaneko et al. 1994; Najlerahim et al. 1990). In vitro transcription (Melton et al. 1984) was employed to generate ^{35}S-labelled or digoxigenin-labelled probes. Radioactive and double labelling ISH was performed as described previously (Schäfer et al. 1993; Schäfer and Day 1995; Schäfer et al. 2000). After hybridization, slides were exposed to X-ray films. Emulsion coating was used to detect the cellular localization of hybridization signals.

Semiquantitative image analysis of changes in PPT-A, PPT-B, NK1 and NK3 mRNA expres-

sion after MCAO. Densitometry for semiquantitative analysis of ISH autoradiograms was conducted as described (Schäfer et al. 1993; Schäfer et al. 2000). The ipsilateral and contralateral cingulate/frontal cortex were measured. Mean values of the hybridization signals were determined for each brain-region from three sections per animal. The mRNA levels were compared between animals after MCAO (n = 6) and the stage-matched sham-operated animals (n = 6) using a non-paired two-way Student's t-test (P-values < 0.05 were labelled by *, p-values < 0.01 were labelled by **).

Subjective rating of changes in PPT-A, PPT-B, NK1 and NK3 mRNA expression after transient forebrain ischemia and comparison to MCAO. Comparative subjective rating of the intensity of hybridization signals was performed at peak stages of expressional changes after MCAO (day 2) and global cerebral ischemia (day 1). We compared tachykinin and tachykinin receptor expression in GABAergic and glutamatergic neurons in the frontocingulate cortex and hippocampal CA1 region of animals subjected to MCAO, transient forebrain ischemia and respective sham treatment. After MCAO and sham operation to MCAO, only the ipsilateral regions were rated.

Results

Transient induction of NK1 at the blood brain barrier endothelium but absence of NK1 expression in reactive microgliosis and astrogliosis after MCAO

To test whether PPT or NK receptor genes were regulated on mRNA and protein levels in the endothelium at the blood brain barrier and in activated microglial or astroglial cells, we analyzed their expression in the infarct and periinfarct areas exhibiting blood brain barrier impairment, microgliosis and astrogliosis. NK1 mRNA and protein was transiently de novo expressed in the endothelium of blood vessels running in the meninges covering the infarct, within the infarct, and especially in the periinfarct border region (Fig. 2). Here, NK1 expression was induced in the endothelium of activated venules. However, no induction of NK1 in cerebrovascular endothelium was seen after transient forebrain ischemia. The selectivity of *de novo* expression of NK1 in the endothelium after MCAO was confirmed by co-staining of endothelial cells for the endothelial activation marker P-selectin. Double immunofluorescence confocal microscopy demonstrated absence of NK1 from GFAP-positive astrocytes or C1q-positive microglial cells and revealed that in both models of cerebral ischemia areas of microgliosis and astrogliosis exhibited no induction of NK1.

Specific changes of PPT and NK receptor expression in glutamatergic and GABAergic cerebrocortical neurons after MCAO

Constitutive pattern. In sham operated animals, PPT-A, PPT-B and NK1 expression was restricted to subpopulations of GABAergic neurons. PPT-A and PPT-B expression was strictly segregated in two different subpopulations of GABAergic neurons. PPT-A and NK1 were

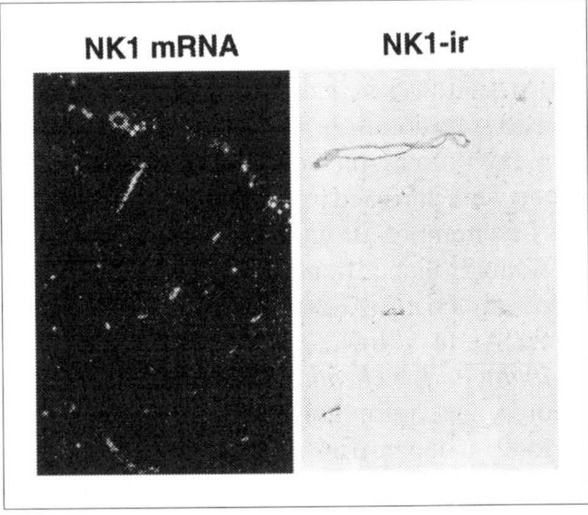

Fig. 2. Induction of NK1 expression in endothelial cells at 2 d post MCAO. Dark field micrograph of the infarct/periinfarct border and leptomeninx covering the infarct (left panel) demonstrating strong signals for NK1 mRNA in blood vessel endothelium and some pravacular cells. Bright field micrograph of the periinfarct cerebral cortex (right panel) demonstrating NK1 immunoreactivity (NK1-ir) in endothelial cells of venules.

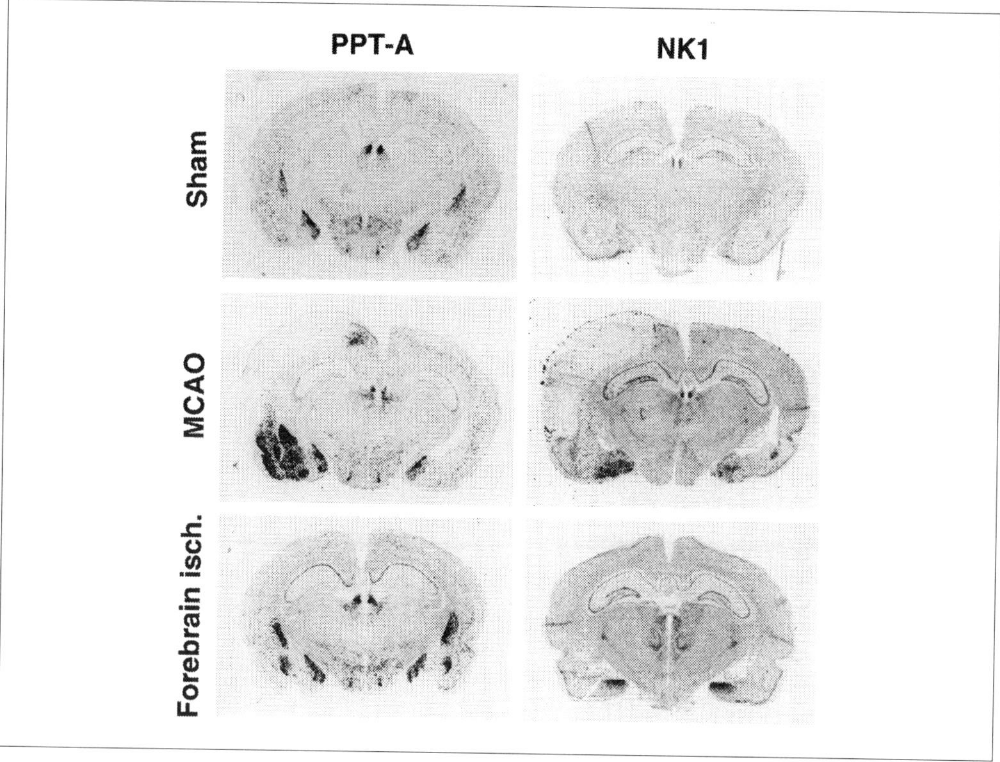

Fig. 3. Differential changes in PPT-A and NK1 mRNA expression after MCAO and transient forebrain ischemia as compared to sham treatment. *Sham:* Low PPT-A and NK1 mRNA levels in single scattered cells in the cerebral cortex and hippocampus (CA1 region). *MCAO:* Marked increase in PPT-A and NK1 mRNA levels in the periinfarct cortex at 2 d post injury but no obvious change in CA1. Note also a dramatic increase of PPT-A and NK1 in ipsilateral amygdaloid nuclei. *Transient forebrain ischemia:* Induction of PPT-A mRNA in the pyramidal cell layer of CA1 but no obvious change in hippocampal NK1 mRNA levels. No change in PPT-A and NK1 mRNA levels in the cerebral cortex and amygdaloid nuclei.

mostly segregated with only very occasional co-expression. NK3 expression was restricted to pyramidal cells, presumably glutamatergic neurons and not found in GABAergic neurons. Cerebral NK2 expression was neither detectable in sham operated rats nor after MCAO.

Postischemic pattern in the periinfarct area. In the infarct core, neuronal gene expression of tachykinins and NK receptors was abolished from 6 h up to 7 d. In the periinfarct area, MCAO caused dramatic changes in PPT-A/PPT-B and NK1/NK3 receptor expression levels (Fig. 3, 4, 5) which were most pronounced at 2 d post MCAO. At this stage, the expression of PPT-A, PPT-B and NK1 in GABAergic neurons was markedly increased as shown by quantitative ISH and immunohistochemical estimation of protein levels. In addition, PPT-A and NK1 expression was induced in non-GABAergic neurons which were identified as glutamatergic pyramidal cells (Fig. 6, 7). A high proportion of NK1 receptor expressing neurons exhibited receptor internalization indicating enhanced tachykininergic neurotransmission. Increased PPT-B expression remained confined to GABAergic neurons. NK3 expression in glutamatergic pyramidal cells was dramatically down-regulated. Changes in PPT-A/PPT-B and NK1/NK3 expression started to be detectable at 1 d post MCAO but were absent at 6 h post MCAO.

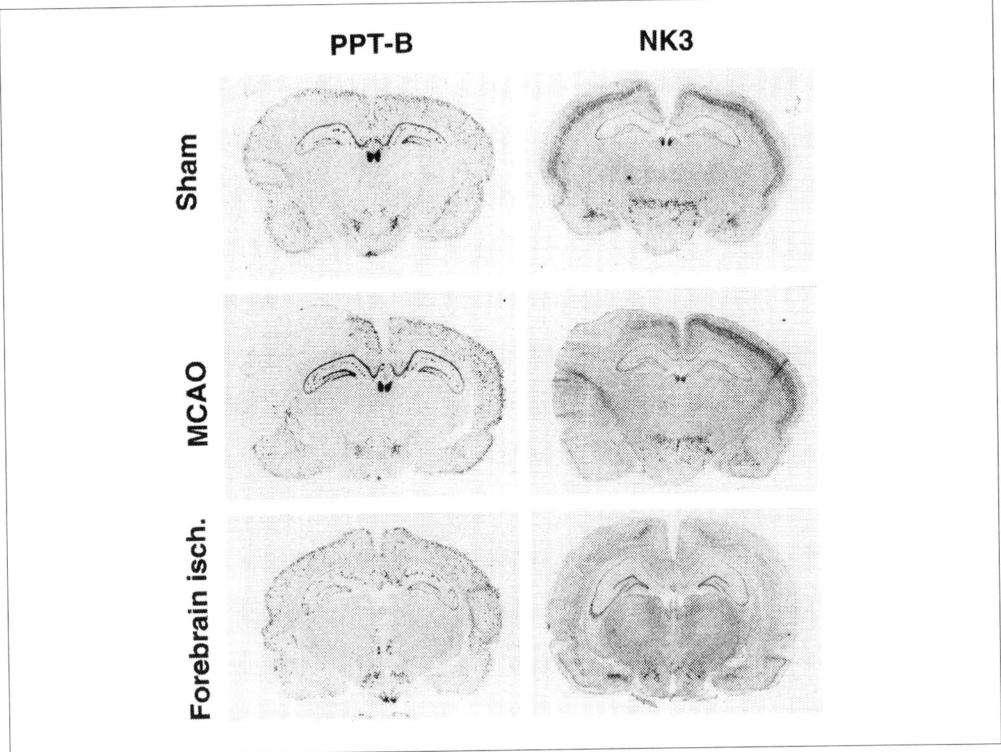

Fig. 4. Differential changes in PPT-B and NK3 mRNA expression after MCAO and transient forebrain ischemia as compared to sham treatment. *Sham:* Moderate levels of PPT-B mRNA in scattered neurons of the cerebral cortex and hippocamus; high levels of NK3 mRNA in the pyramidal cells of cortical layer V and low levels of NK3 mRNA in the pyramidal layer of CA1. *MCAO:* Marked increase in PPT-B mRNA levels in the periinfarct cortex and in the ipsilateral pyramidal cell layer of CA1 and dramatic decrease in NK3 mRNA levels in the periinfarct cortex. *Transient forebrain ischemia:* Dramatic decrease in NK3 mRNA levels in the cerebral cortex. No obvious change in PPT-B mRNA levels in the cortex and in NK3 mRNA levels in the hippocampus.

Table 1. Comparison of changes in tachykinin and NK receptor mRNA expression after MCAO and transient forebrain ischemia

	cerebral cortex						hippocampus (CA1)					
	GABAergic			glutamatergic			GABAergic			glutamatergic		
	sham	MCAO	TFI	sham	MCAO	TFI	sham	MCAO	TFI	sham	MCAO	TFI
PPT-A	++	+++	+/++	–	+++	–	+	+/++	+/++	–	–	++
NK1	++	+++	+/++	–	+	–	+	+	+	–	–	–
PPT-B	++	+++	++	–	–	–	++	++	++	++	+++	–
NK3	–	–	–	+++	+	+	+	+	+	+	+	+

Subjective rating of the relative intensity of in situ hybridization signals at 2 days post MCAO and 1 day (PPT-A, NK1) or 2 days (PPT-B, NK3) post transient forebrain ischemia (TFI). GABAergic and glutamatergic neurons were identified by neuronal cell size and shape (pyramidal vs. non-pyramidal) and co-hybridization for the GABAergic marker GAD or the glutamatergic marker PAG. (–) no signal; (+) low, (++) moderate, (+++) high signal intensities.

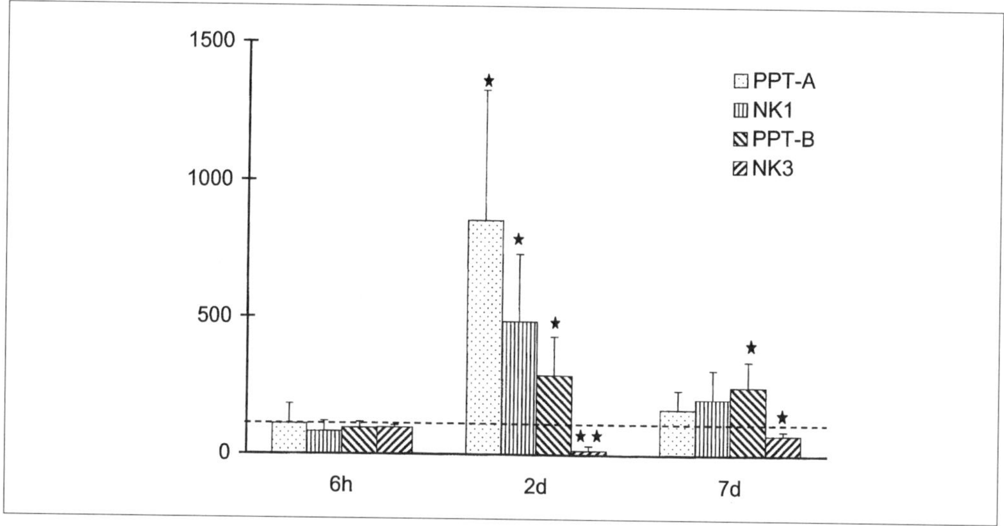

Fig. 5. Changes in tachykinin and NK receptor mRNA levels in the periinfarct cingulate and frontal cortex at different stages after MCAO as measured by quantitative radioactive in situ hybridization. Mean values and standard deviation (n = 6) after MCAO are expressed as percent of mean values (n = 6) after sham operation of the respective time points. The dotted line indicates 100% values of sham operated animals for orientation.

While changes in PPT-A and NK1 were no longer evident at 7 d post MCAO, the increase in PPT-B and, to a lesser extent, the decrease in NK3 expression levels were sustained up to 7 d post MCAO.

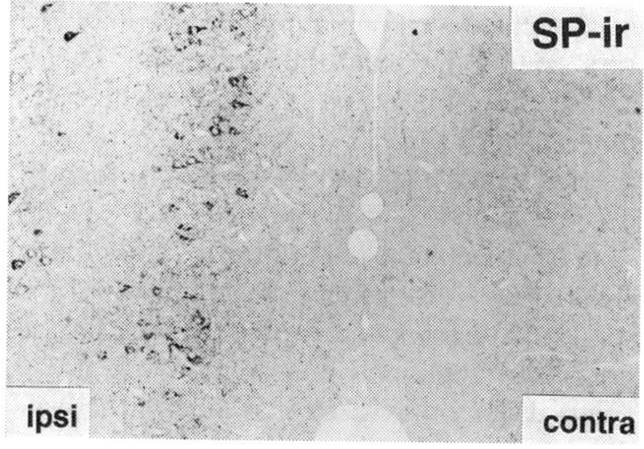

Fig. 6. Upregulation of SP immunoreactivity (ir) in interneurons and induction of SP in pyramidal neurons of the periinfarct cingulate cortex 2 d after MCAO. Note induction of SP-ir in many small interneurons and larger pyramidal neurons ipsilateral to the infarct as compared to contralateral side (corresponding to sham treatment).

Comparison of neuronal changes after transient forebrain ischemia and MCAO

Changes in PPT and NK expression after MCAO and transient forebrain ischemia were compared 1 d and 2 d after the respective insults. At this time point virtually all neurons in the primary infarct region of the cortex after MCAO are dead while after transient forebrain ischemia, neuronal damage (apoptosis) in the most vulnerable CA1 region of the hippocampus is in its early stages with still many viable neurons present in CA1.

MCAO and transient forebrain ischemia exhibited some similarities but also profound differences in their adaptive plasticity patterns of PPT and NK receptor expression (Fig. 3 and 4; Table 1). In contrast to MCAO, the expression of PPT-A, PPT-B and NK1 mRNAs in GABAergic neurons was not altered after transient forebrain ischemia. NK3 mRNA expression in cerebrocortical glutamatergic neurons was transiently downregulated, both after MCAO and transient forebrain ischemia. In both models, GABAergic hippocampal neurons showed a slight in-

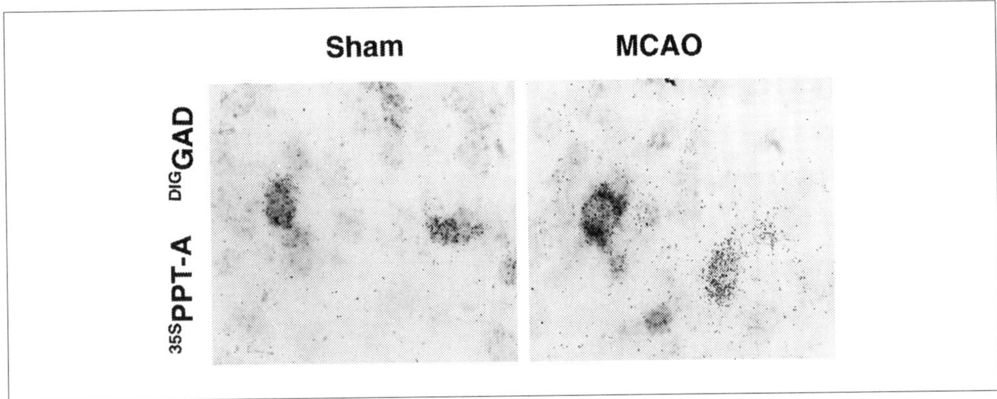

Fig. 7. Induction of PPT-A mRNA expression in non-GABAergic neurons of the periinfarct cortex 2d after MCAO. Colocalization of PPT-A mRNA (silver grains) in GABAergic neurons (gray/dark reaction products of DIG-labeled glutamic acid decarboxylase, GAD) after sham treatment (left panel). After MCAO (right panel), note *de novo* expression of PPT-A mRNA (silver grains) in non GABAergic neurons in addition to colocalization in a subpopulation of GABAergic neurons.

crease in PPT-A expression but, as a rule, no prominent other changes. The hippocampal increase in NK1 mRNA expression seen at 2 d post MCAO was variable. In hippocampal glutamatergic neurons, PPT-A mRNA was induced after transient forebrain ischemia but not after MCAO. In contrast, PPT-B mRNA expression in glutamatergic hippocampal neurons was increased after MCAO but markedly decreased – to virtually undetectable levels – in transient forebrain ischemia. In both forms of ischemia, hippocampal NK3 mRNA expression was essentially unaffected.

Discussion

In confirmation and extension of our rcecent study (Stumm et al. 2000), the present investigation reveals marked and differential changes in PPT-A, PPT-B, NK1 and NK3 gene expression in GABAergic and/or glutamatergic neurons of the viable cerebral cortex and/or hippocampus after focal and transient forebrain ischemia. NK1 was induced in endothelium of the blood brain barrier after MCAO but not after transient forebrain ischemia. The upregulation of NK1 in the endothelium after MCAO suggests that NK1 may specifically contribute to blood brain barrier dysfunction in the course of focal ischemic damage (see also schematic diagram, Fig. 8). NK1 is likely to interact with cell adhesion molecules, cytokines and prostaglandins to facilitate transendothelial migration of leukocytes and local plasma extravasation (Weihe et al. 1991; Shepheard et al. 1993; Bowden et al. 1994; Nakagawa et al. 1995; Maggi 1997; Saban et al. 1997; Quinlan et al. 1999a, 1999b). This may be an important mechanism in the development of ischemia-induced brain edema and neuroinflammation. Therefore, the recently reported effect of the NK1 antagonist SR140333 to reduce ischemia-induced damage in a model of transient focal cerebral ischemia in the rat (Yu et al. 1997) could be attributable to inhibiton of endothelial NK1 receptors resulting in stabilization of the blood brain barrier and reduction of leukocyte egress from the blood stream into the brain.

The absence of NK1 expression from activated microglia or astroglia precludes a direct role of NK1 in ischemia-induced microgliosis and astrogliosis. This is in contrast to other conditions of neurodegeneration and neuroinflammation where NK1 and SP have been suggested to be directly involved in gliosis (Kennedy et al. 1997).

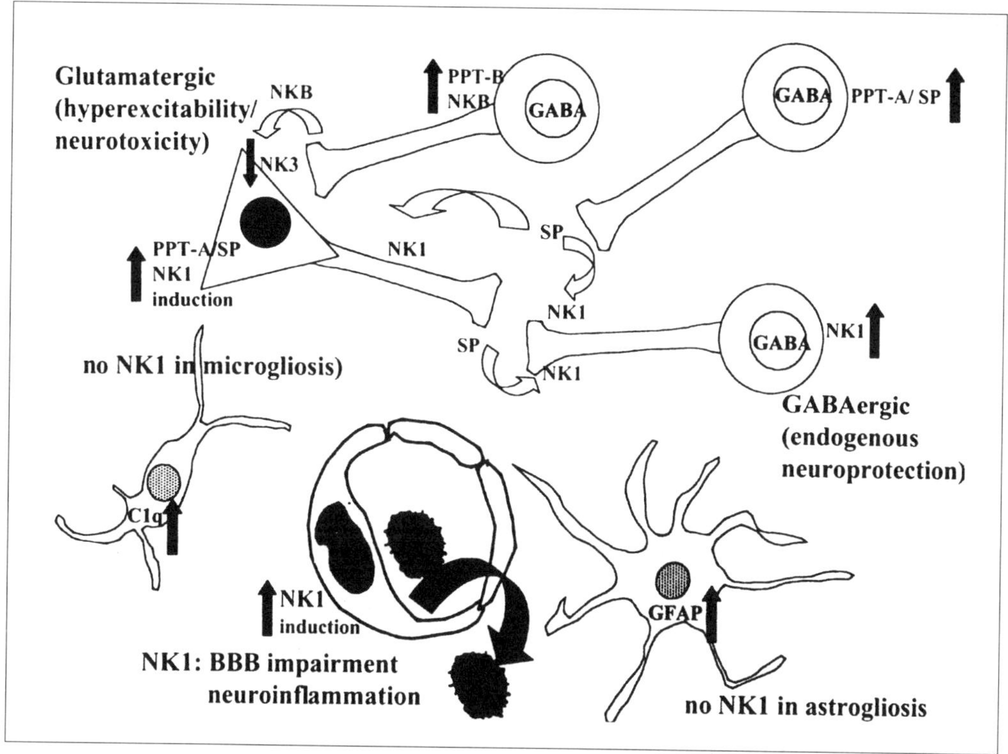

Fig. 8. Schematic diagram summarizing the possible scenario of tachykinin and NK receptor involvement in focal cerebral ischemia (MCAO). *Non-neuronal functions:* At the blood brain barrier (BBB), the transient induction of NK1 in endothelial cells is postulated to transiently (1 to 2 d post MCAO) contribute to protein extravasation and brain edema and leukocyte invasion into the lesioned brain. Absence of NK1 from activated microglial cells (C1q complement positive) and astrocytes (GFAP positive) indicates that NK1 has no direct role in microgliosis or astrogliosis. *Neuronal functions:* The increase of PPT-A/SP and NK1 expression in separate GABAergic neurons and the induction or co-induction of PPT-A/SP and NK1 in glutamatergic pyramidal cells (with signs of NK1 receptor internalization) is postulated to have the following consequences. The physiological function of SP to enhance GABAergic neurotransmission via NK1 is likely to be enhanced after MCAO. This may represent a defense reaction of the brain to reduce glutamate-mediated excitotoxicity. In contrast, the ectopic induction of NK1 in glutamatergic pyramidal neurons would drive glutamate release and excitotoxicity. Increased PPT-B/NKB expression in GABAergic neurons and a presumed increase of NKB release is likely to transiently excite pyramidal cells via NK3 and to enhance excitotoxicity. Excitoxicity may depend on the balance between tachykinin and NK 1 or NK3 receptor-mediated GABAergic inhibition (neuroprotection) and glutamatergic excitation (neurotoxicity).

The neuronal changes indicate a profound role of specific tachykinin and NK receptor genes in the balance of excitatory and inhibitory cortical and hippocampal neurotransmission under conditions of cerebral ischemia as schematically summarized in Fig. 8. We suggest that the MCAO-induced increase of NK1 in GABAergic neurons in conjunction with increased availability of SP may amplify inhibitory circuits which could result in endogenous neuroprotection by reducing hyperexcitability. On the other hand, increased cerebrocortical SP expression in GABAergic and glutamatergic neurons and the parallel induction of NK1 in glutamatergic cerebrocortical pyramidal cells after MCAO recruits novel circuits allowing direct activation of glutamatergic pyramidal neurons via NK1. Given the role of NK1 and SP to wind up NMDA receptor mediated excitability (Lieberman and Mody 1998), this is likely to further enhance hyperexcitability and excitotoxicity in the course of ischemia. Thus, inhibition of NK1-mediated hyperexcitability is a likely mechanism of action by which the synthetic NK1 antagonist SR140333 reduces ischemia-induced damage (Yu et al. 1997). The induction of PPT-A expression in CA1 pyramidal cells after transient forebrain ischemia may lead to increased release of SP resulting in hippocampal excitotoxicity and delayed pyramidal cell death. In this process, NK-1 mediated imbalance between inhibitory and disinhibitory GABAergic circuits in the hippocampus may occur. In the cerebral cortex, the ischemia-induced sustained increase in PPT-B/NKB expression in GABAergic neurons is accompanied by a downregulation of NK3 expression in glutamatergic pyramidal neurons. We postulate that the increase in PPT-B expression causes increased synthesis and release of NKB which would stimulate glutamatergic neurotransmission and, consequently, postischemic glutamate-mediated hyperexcitability and excitotoxicity. The downregulation of NK3 may reflect receptor downregulation/desensitization upon activation of NK3 by NKB to limit glutamate excitability. In any case, the reciproke regulation of NKB and NK3 expression are signs of postischemic functional plasticity of NKB/NK3-mediated neuromodulation.

We conclude that NK1 and NK3 receptors are promising novel targets for the pharmacotherapy of stroke and other cerebrovascular disorders.

References

1. Bonner TI, Affolter HU, Young AC, Young WD (1987) A cDNA encoding the precursor of the rat neuropeptide, neurokinin B. Brain Res 388:243–249
2. Bowden JJ, Garland AM, Baluk P, Lefevre P, Grady EF, Vigna SR, Bunnett NW, McDonald DM (1994) Direct observation of substance P-induced internalization of neurokinin 1 (NK1) receptors at sites of inflammation. Proc Natl Acad Sci USA 91:8964–8968
3. Carter MS, Krause JE (1990) Structure, expression, and some regulatory mechanisms of the rat preprotachykinin gene encoding substance P, neurokinin A, neuropeptide K, and neuropeptide gamma. J Neurosci 10:2203–2214
4. Culmsee C, Stumm RK, Schäfer MK, Weihe E, Krieglstein J (1999) Clenbuterol induces growth factor mRNA, activates astrocytes, and protects rat brain tissue against ischemic damage. Eur J Pharmacol 379:33–45
5. Dietzschold B, Schwaeble W, Schafer MK, Hooper DC, Zehng YM, Petry F, Sheng H, Fink T, Loos M, Koprowski H, et al. (1995) Expression of C1q, a subcomponent of the rat complement system, is dramatically enhanced in brains of rats with either Borna disease or experimental allergic encephalomyelitis. J Neurol Sci 130:11–16
6. Ding YQ, Shigemoto R, Takada M, Ohishi H, Nakanishi S, Mizuno N (1996) Localization of the neuromedin K receptor (NK3) in the central nervous system of the rat. J Comp Neurol 364:290–310
7. Dirnagl U, Iadecola C, Moskowitz MA (1999) Pathobiology of ischaemic stroke: an integrated view. Trends Neurosci 22:391–397
8. Hershey AD, Dykema PE, Krause JE (1991) Organization, structure, and expression of the gene encoding the rat substance P receptor. J Biol Chem 266:4366–4374
9. Kaneko T, Mizuno N (1994) Glutamate-synthesizing enzymes in GABAergic neurons of the neocortex: a double immunofluorescence study in the rat. Neuroscience 61:839–849
10. Kennedy PG, Rodgers J, Jennings FW, Murray M, Leeman SE, Burke JM (1997) A substance P antagonist, RP-67,580, ameliorates a mouse meningoencephalitic response to Trypanosoma brucei brucei. Proc Natl Acad Sci USA 94:4167–4170
11. Lieberman DN, Mody I (1998) Substance P enhances NMDA channel function in hippocampal dentate gyrus granule cells. J Neurophysiol 80:113–119
12. Liu H, Cao Y, Basbaum AI, Mazarati AM, Sankar R, Wasterlain CG (1999) Resistance to excitotoxin-induced seizures and neuronal death in mice lacking the preprotachykinin A gene. Proc Natl Acad Sci USA 96:12096–12101
13. Luber-Narod J, Kage R, Leeman SE (1994) Substance P enhances the secretion of tumor necrosis factor-alpha from neuroglial cells stimulated with lipopolysaccharide. J Immunol 152:819–824
14. Lucas LR, Hurley DL, Krause JE, Harlan RE (1992) Localization of the tachykinin neurokinin B precursor peptide in rat brain by immunocytochemistry and in situ hybridization. Neuroscience 51:317–345
15. Maggi CA (1997) The effects of tachykinins on inflammatory and immune cells. Regul Pept 70:75–90
16. Mantyh PW, Johnson DJ, Boehmer CG, Catton MD, Vinters HV, Maggio JE, Too HP, Vigna SR (1989) Substance P receptor binding sites are expressed by glia in vivo after neuronal injury. Proc Natl Acad Sci USA 86:5193–5197
17. Maubach KA, Cody C, Jones RS (1998) Tachykinins may modify spontaneous epileptiform activity in the rat entorhinal cortex in vitro by activating GABAergic inhibition. Neuroscience 83:1047–1062
18. Melton DA, Krieg PA, Rebagliati MR, Maniatis T, Zinn K, Green MR (1984) Efficient in vitro synthesis of biologically active RNA and RNA hybridization probes from plasmids containing a bacteriophage SP6 promoter. Nucleic Acids Res 12:7035–7056
19. Najlerahim A, Harrison PJ, Barton AJ, Heffernan J, Pearson RC (1990) Distribution of messenger RNAs encoding the enzymes glutaminase, aspartate aminotransferase and glutamic acid decarboxylase in rat brain. Brain Res Mol Brain Res 7:317–333
20. Nakagawa N, Sano H, Iwamoto I (1995) Substance P induces the expression of intercellular adhesion molecule-1 on vascular endothelial cells and enhances neutrophil transendothelial migration. Peptides 16:721–725
21. Nakaya Y, Kaneko T, Shigemoto R, Nakanishi S, Mizuno N (1994) Immunohistochemical localization of substance P receptor in the central nervous system of the adult rat. J Comp Neurol 347:249–274
22. Quartara L, Maggi CA (1998) The tachykinin NK1 receptor. Part II: Distribution and pathophysiological roles. Neuropeptides 32:1–49

23. Quinlan KL, Song IS, Naik SM, Letran EL, Olerud JE, Bunnett NW, Armstrong CA, Caughman SW, Ansel JC (1999a) VCAM-1 expression on human dermal microvascular endothelial cells is directly and specifically up-regulated by substance P. J Immunol 162:1656–1661
24. Quinlan KL, Naik SM, Cannon G, Armstrong CA, Bunnett NW, Ansel JC, Caughman SW (1999b) Substance P activates coincident NF-AT- and NF-kappa B-dependent adhesion molecule gene expression in microvascular endothelial cells through intracellular calcium mobilization. J Immunol 163:5656–5665
25. Röhrenbeck AM, Bette M, Hooper DC, Nyberg F, Eiden LE, Dietzschold B, Weihe E (1999) Upregulation of COX-2 and CGRP expression in resident cells of the Borna disease virus-infected brain is dependent upon inflammation. Neurobiol Dis 6:15–34
26. Saban MR, Saban R, Bjorling D, Haak FM (1997) Involvement of leukotrienes, TNF-alpha, and the LFA-1/ICAM-1 interaction in substance P-induced granulocyte infiltration. J Leukoc Biol 61:445–451
27. Sasai Y, Nakanishi S (1989) Molecular characterization of rat substance K receptor and its mRNAs. Biochem Biophys Res Commun 165:695–702
28. Schäfer MK, Nohr D, Krause JE, Weihe E (1993) Inflammation-induced upregulation of NK1 receptor mRNA in dorsal horn neurones. Neuroreport 4:1007–1010
29. Schäfer MK, Day R (1995) In situ hybridization techniques to map processing enzymes. In: AI Smith (ed.) Methods in Neurosciences 23: Peptidases and Neuropeptide processing, Academic Press, San Diego, pp. 16–44
30. Schäfer MK, Schwaeble WJ, Post C, Salvati P, Calabresi M, Sim RB, Petry F, Loos M, Weihe E (2000) Complement C1q is dramatically upregulated in brain microglia in response to transient global cerebral ischemia. J Immunol 164:5446–5452
31. Shapiro RA, Farrell L, Srinivasan M, Curthoys NP (1991) Isolation, characterization, and in vitro expression of a cDNA that encodes the kidney isoenzyme of the mitochondrial glutaminase. J Biol Chem 266:18792–18796
32. Shepheard SL, Williamson DJ, Hill RG, Hargreaves RJ (1993) The non-peptide neurokinin1 receptor antagonist, RP 67580, blocks neurogenic plasma extravasation in the dura mater of rats. Br J Pharmacol 108:11–12
33. Shigemoto R, Yokota Y, Tsuchida K, Nakanishi S (1990) Cloning and expression of a rat neuromedin K receptor cDNA. J Biol Chem 265:623–628
34. Shigemoto R, Nakaya Y, Nomura S, Ogawa MR, Ohishi H, Kaneko T, Nakanishi S, Mizuno N (1993) Immunocytochemical localization of rat substance P receptor in the striatum. Neurosci Lett 153:157–160
35. Stumm RK, Culmsee C, Schäfer MK-H, Krieglstein J, Weihe E (2000) Adaptive plasticity in tachykinin and tachykinin receptor expression after focal cerebral ischemia is differentially linked to GABAergic and glutamatergic cerebrocortical circuits and cerebrovenular endothelium. J Neurosci (in press)
36. Suzuki H, Abe K, Tojo S, Kimura K, Mizugaki M, Itoyama Y (1998) A change of P-selectin immunoreactivity in rat brain after transient and permanent middle cerebral artery occlusion. Neurol Res 20:463–469
37. Tamura A, Graham DI, McCulloch J, Teasdale GM (1981) Focal cerebral ischaemia in the rat: 1. Description of technique and early neuropathological consequences following middle cerebral artery occlusion. J Cereb Blood Flow Metab 1:53–60
38. Warden MK, Young WD (1988) Distribution of cells containing mRNAs encoding substance P and neurokinin B in the rat central nervous system. J Comp Neurol 272:90–113
39. Weihe E, Nohr D, Muller S, Buchler M, Friess H, Zentel HJ (1991) The tachykinin neuroimmune connection in inflammatory pain. Ann NY Acad Sci 632:283–295
40. Weihe E, Schäfer MK-H, Nohr D, Persson S (1994) Expression of neuropeptides, neuropeptide receptors and neuropeptide processing enzymes in spinal neurons and peripheral nonneuronal cells and plasticity in models of inflammatory pain. In: Neuropeptides, Nociception and Pain (Hökfelt T, Schmidt RF, Schaible HG, ed.), pp. 43–69. Weinheim: Chapman & Hall
41. Wyborski RJ, Bond RW, Gottlieb DI (1990) Characterization of a cDNA coding for rat glutamic acid decarboxylase. Brain Res Mol Brain Res 8:193–198
42. Yu Z, Cheng G, Huang X, Li K, Cao X (1997) Neurokinin-1 receptor antagonist SR140333: a novel type of drug to treat cerebral ischemia. Neuroreport 8:2117–2119
43. Zachrisson O, Lindefors N, Brene S (1998) A tachykinin NK1 receptor antagonist, CP-122,721-1, attenuates kainic acid-induced seizure activity. Brain Res Mol Brain Res 60:291–295
44. Zhu Y, Culmsee C, Semkova I, Krieglstein J (1998) Stimulation of beta2-adrenoceptors inhibits apoptosis in rat brain after transient forebrain ischemia. J Cereb Blood Flow Metab 18:1032–1039

New insights into the role of NMDA-receptors and nitric oxide formation in the genesis of spreading depression

T. P. Obrenovitch

Abstract

Recurrent spreading depression (SD, i.e. transient, propagating disruption of local brain ionic homeostasis) may contribute to lesion progression in focal brain ischaemia. The purpose of this chapter is to provide new insights into the contribution of *N*-methyl-D-aspartate (NMDA)-receptor activation, and that of nitric oxide (NO) formation, to SD genesis. Application of NMDA to the cerebral cortex of anaesthetised rats, at concentrations selected to effectively activate NMDA-receptors but below the threshold for NMDA-induction of SD, concentration-dependently inhibited K^+-induced SD elicitation. From this finding and previous data, we propose that functional NMDA-receptor-ionophores are required for SD initiation, but that widespread, increased NMDA-receptor activation is not the cause for the elicitation of SD by elevated extracellular K^+. With regard to NO, local inhibition of NO synthesis did not alter the elicitation of SD by high extracellular K^+, but markedly delayed the initiation phase of repolarisation, i.e. the recovery from SD. This new finding indicates that NO formation during SD contributes to the inactivation of ion channels and/or gap junctions that contribute to the normalisation of ion homeostasis after each SD wave.

Spreading depression (SD) is a transient suppression of neuronal activity, resulting from a temporary disruption of local brain ionic homeostasis that propagates slowly across the cerebral cortex and other regions of grey matter (Bures et al. 1974; Martins-Ferreira et al. 2000). Spreading depression is attracting renewed attention because it has become clear that this phenomenon contributes to the pathophysiology of experimental cerebral ischaemia. In particular, recurrent SD in regions surrounding the ischaemic core promote lesion progression and worsen the outcome in models of stroke (Mies et al. 1993; Chen et al. 1993; Back et al. 1996; Bush et al. 1996). Despite over 50 years of research since the discovery of SD by Leão (1944), the cascade of events leading to SD initiation and/or its propagation remains unclear (Martins-Ferreira et al. 2000). The primary purpose of this chapter is to bring new insights into the suspected contribution of two important biological processes to SD genesis; i.e. *N*-methyl-D-aspartate (NMDA)-receptor activation, and nitric oxide (NO) formation.

Key words: Spreading depression – glutamate – high extracellular potassium – nitric oxide – *N*-methyl-D-aspartate

School of Pharmacy, Pharmacology, University of Bradford, Bradford, BD7 1DP, England.
e-mail: t.obrenovitch@bradford.ac.uk

J. Krieglstein, S. Klumpp (Eds.) Pharmacology of Cerebral Ischemia 2000

NMDA-receptor activation and spreading depression

Three complementary lines of evidence may be used to support the hypothesis that *abnormally high* NMDA-receptor activation is a key contributor to SD initiation, but the validity of each corresponding argument can be questioned through a reassessment of the initial data and/or more recent experimental data.

1. SD could be triggered by application of excitatory amino acids to some preparations (Curtis and Watkins 1961; Lauritzen et al. 1988). However, the threshold concentration for glutamate-induced SD elicitation appears far above the extracellular concentrations that may occur in the living brain, even if one accounts for the efficacy of glutamate uptake. For example, at least 10 mM of L-glutamic acid had to be applied to the exposed cortex of pentobarbital-anaesthetised cats to elicit SD within 2 min (Curtis and Watkins 1961). In rats anaesthetised with halothane (1.5% in N_2O:O_2, 2:1), SD could be consistently elicited by perfusion of 400 μM NMDA for 2 min through a microdialysis probe inserted in the frontoparietal cortex, but perfusion of up to 500 mM glutamate failed to elicit any propagating SD despite the production of a much larger negative shift of the extracellular direct current (DC) potential at the site of glutamate application (Fig. 1).
2. A marked efflux of glutamate in the extracellular space is associated with SD (Van Harreveld and Fifková 1970; Obrenovitch and Zilkha 1995a). However, this change is not specific to glutamate (Moghaddam et al. 1987; Fabricius et al. 1993), and we have demonstrated that high extracellular glutamate contributes neither to K^+-induced SD elicitation nor to SD propagation (Obrenovitch and Zilkha 1995b; Obrenovitch et al. 1996). With regard to our data on high extracellular glutamate and SD, it is important to stress that they do not rule out the possibility of increased glutamate exocytosis contributing to SD genesis, because the monitoring of extracellular glutamate does not provide reliable information on the presynaptic vesicular release of glutamate (Obrenovitch 1999).
3. Both elicitation and propagation of SD are inhibited by NMDA-receptor antagonists (Hernandez-Caceres et al. 1987; Obrenovitch and Zilkha 1996; Tatlisumak et al. 1998; Menniti et al. 2000). This demonstrates that functional NMDA-receptor ionophore complexes are required for SD genesis, but does not necessarily imply that *excessive* stimulation of NMDA-receptors is the cause of, or a critical contributor to, SD initiation.

In order to clarify whether or not abnormally high activation of NMDA-receptors promotes SD elicitation, we have examined how increasing NMDA concentrations, added to the high-K^+ medium used to elicit repetitive SD, alters their latency, frequency and magnitude. Repetitive SD, high extracellular K^+, and increased NMDA-receptor activation, are abnormalities that are all relevant to focal brain ischaemia, especially at the interface between irreversibly damaged tissue and surrounding viable regions.

Two microdialysis electrodes (Obrenovitch et al. 1993) were implanted symmetrically into the frontoparietal cortex of halothane-anaesthetised rats and used for (i) elicitation of repetitive SD by perfusion of 130 mM K^+ through the probe for 20 min, (ii) recording of SD as a negative shift of the extracellular DC potential, and (iii) co-perfusion of NMDA with high K^+ medium on one side. All experiments were performed at least 2 h after electrode implantation. Each K^+ stimulus was followed by 40 min of recovery, i.e. perfusion of the microdialysis probe/electrode with normal artificial CSF. Preliminary experiments allowed us to determine the suitable range of NMDA concentrations for this study, i.e. perfusion of NMDA through a cortical microdialysis electrode which, by itself, induces neither SD nor excessive negative shifts of the local DC potential (see: Fig. 1, and Obrenovitch et al. 1994). Five separate episodes of repetitive SD were produced by perfusion of 130 mM K^+ alone on the control side. Contralaterally, the K^+ medium was supplemented with 25, 50 and 75 μM NMDA for the 2nd, 3rd and 4th SD episodes (Fig. 2). No NMDA was applied during the 1st SD episode because

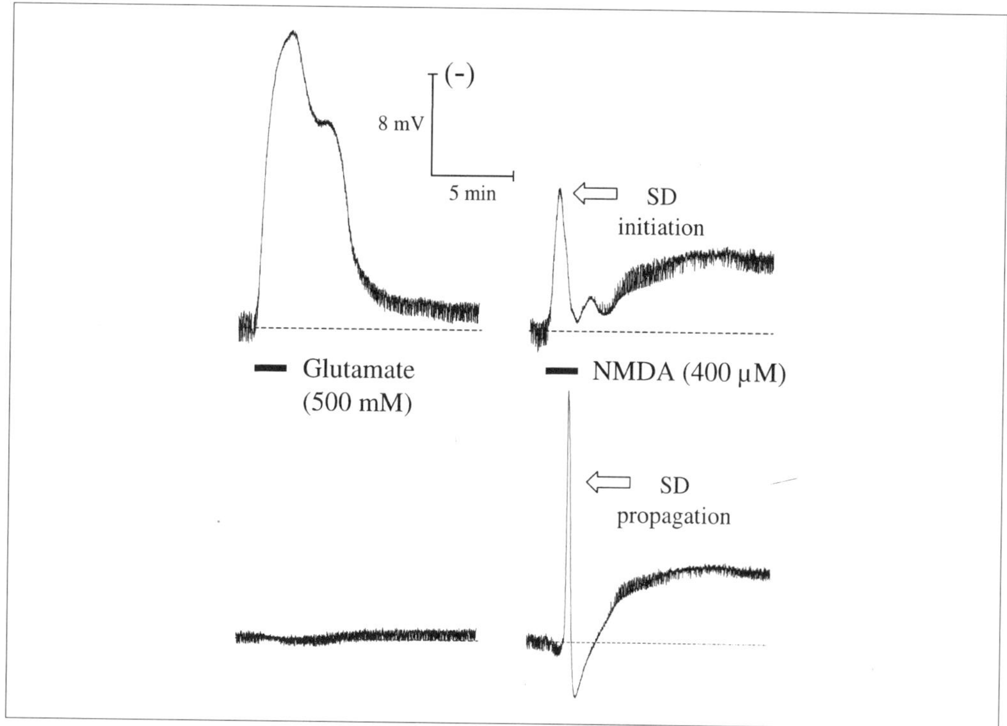

Fig. 1. Negative shifts of the extracellular DC potential recorded from the cerebral cortex of anaesthetised rats (halothane 1.5% in N_2O:O_2 2:1), at the site of application of glutamate or NMDA (top traces) and 2 mm posterior from this site (bottom traces). Note the characteristic pattern of the DC-potential negative shift produced by 400 µM NMDA at the site of application (upper trace), i.e. negative shift with repolarisation as NMDA was still applied, followed by secondary, sustained negative shift; and the subsequent, remote transient depolarisation (bottom trace). These features, which demonstrate effective SD elicitation, were not observed with glutamate, tested up to 500 mM in 4 separate experiments. Elicitation and propagation of SD was recorded with a microdialysis electrode and a glass capillary electrode, respectively, inserted 2 mm apart in the frontoparietal cortex (Obrenovitch and Zilkha 1996). In agreement with previous reports, the polarity of the DC potential was reversed so that negative shifts of the DC potential (i.e. depolarisation) produce an upward deflection. Filled horizontal bars indicate 2-min perfusion of glutamate or NMDA through the microdialysis probe.

the magnitude of the resulting SD is consistently much larger than the subsequent ones. The 5th SD episode was used to assess the reversibility of the NMDA effects. From the *in vitro* microdialysis recovery/delivery for NMDA (~23% at 1 µl/min, i.e. the perfusion rate used in this study), the calculated extracellular concentrations of NMDA tested were 5.7, 11.4 and 17.0 µM.

Application of 130 mM K^+ for 20 min through the cortical microdialysis electrode consistently produced a sustained negative shift of the DC potential, onto which were superimposed between 4 to 6 peaks of further depolarisation (Fig. 2, left trace). Each of these peaks indicated the elicitation of a SD wave (Obrenovitch et al. 1993). The latency for elicitation of the first SD was 1.7 ± 0.3 min (mean ± standard deviation; n = 12).

Application of NMDA, at concentrations that effectively activate NMDA-receptors but below the threshold for NMDA-induction of SD, concentration-dependently inhibited K^+-induced SD elicitation (Figs. 2, 3). The latency for the occurrence of 1st SD was markedly prolonged, whereas the number of SD during the 20-min perfusion of K^+-medium was reduced. Perfusion of 75 µM NMDA through the

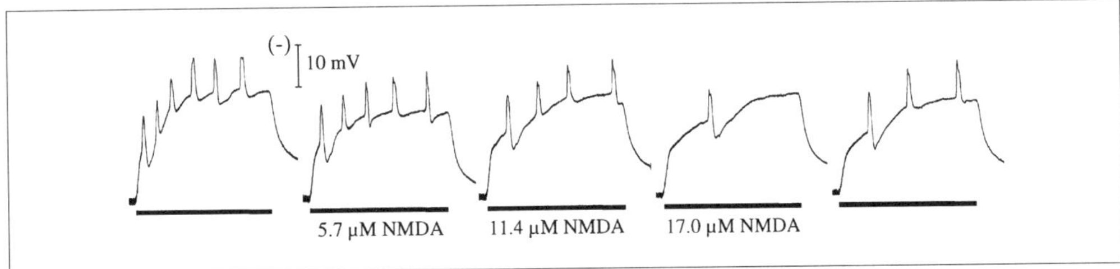

Fig. 2. Representative effects of NMDA on K⁺-induced SD recorded at the elicitation site. Five separate episodes of repetitive SD were produced by perfusion of 130 mM K⁺ for 20 min through a cortical microdialysis probe, with each SD episode followed by 40 min of recovery. During the 2nd, 3rd and 4th SD elicitation periods, 25, 50 and 75 μM of NMDA was co-perfused with K⁺, in respective order. The 'true' extracellular NMDA concentrations that are given under the traces were calculated from the dialysate concentrations and the *in vitro* microdialysis recovery/delivery for NMDA. Filled horizontal bars indicate perfusion of high K⁺ for 20 min.

probe abolished K⁺-induced SD in 2 of the 6 experiments. The parallel reduction in the overall SD peak area (i.e. magnitude of SD, Fig. 3) suggested that NMDA inhibited SD without any marked change in their pattern. However, the rate of maximal recovery from individual SD showed a tendency to be reduced in the presence of NMDA. All these effects of NMDA

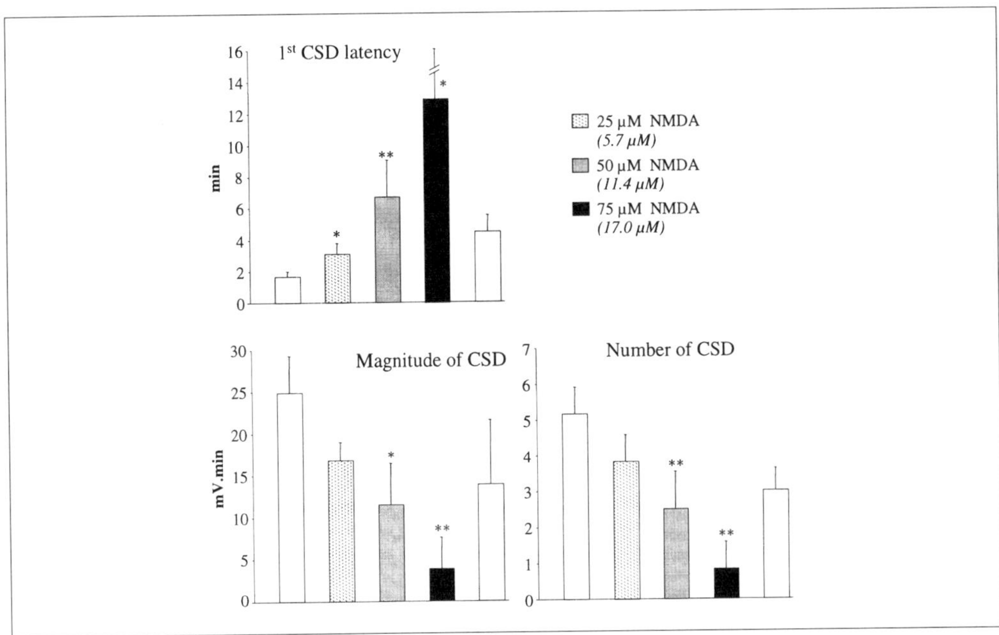

Fig. 3. Effects of co-application of NMDA on K⁺-induced SD; i.e. latency for 1st SD (min), magnitude of SD (mV.min), and number of SD. Increasing concentrations of NMDA (25, 50 and 75 μM) were co-perfused with 130 mM K⁺-medium during the 2nd, 3rd and 4th SD elicitation periods; calculated, *'true' extracellular NMDA concentrations* were 5.7, 11.4, and 17.0 μM. Note the concentration-dependent suppression of SD by NMDA, and the reversibility of this effect. Values are means ± standard deviation; $^{*}p<0.05$ and $^{**}p<0.01$, comparison to corresponding control data (i.e. obtained contralaterally with 5 repeated applications of K⁺-medium alone; data not shown) by Mann-Whitney test (n = 6).

were fully reversible (Figs. 2, 3; comparison to control side, data not shown).

This inhibition of K^+-induced SD by NMDA may be a direct consequence of the sustained presence of NMDA-receptor-ionophore agonist, through the following cascade of events: Ca^{2+}-influx through these cation channels ⇒ intracellular Ca^{2+}-loading and/or altered Ca^{2+}-buffering ⇒ alteration in the pattern of intra- and intercellular Ca^{2+} waves involved in SD initiation. Several lines of evidence suggest strongly that Ca^{2+} waves play a pivotal role in the initiation of SD (Wang et al. 1997): (i) the presence of extracellular Ca^{2+} is prerequisite for SD elicitation (Bures et al. 1974); (ii) Ca^{2+} waves preceded the electrophysiological changes associated with SD in hippocampal organ cultures (Kunkler and Kraig 1998); (iii) intercellular Ca^{2+} waves may be generated primarily by the propagation of depolarisation through gap junctions (Charles et al. 1996); and (iv) both Ca^{2+} waves and SD are blocked by pharmacological uncoupling of gap junctions (Nedergaard et al. 1995; Kunkler and Kraig 1998). Increased intracellular Ca^{2+} associated with the sustained presence of agonist (i.e. NMDA) may also lead, paradoxically, to glycine-insensitive desensitisation of NMDA-receptors (Tong and Jahr 1994).

Another, more indirect contributing mechanism for the observed inhibition of SD may be a reduction in the capacity of the cortex to cope with SD when NMDA-receptor activation was superimposed on high K^+ (Riepe et al. 1995). This potential mechanism for SD inhibition is especially relevant to repetitive SD, because each individual SD is followed by a refractory period that may be prolonged by alterations in the brain tissue condition (Brand et al. 1998). Indeed, both the amplitude and duration of elicited SD depend on the efficiency of the brain tissue homeostatic mechanisms (Koroleva and Bures 1980, 1996), and separate experiments confirmed that perfusion of 25–75 μM of NMDA through the implanted microdialysis probe led to cation flux across the cellular membrane with associated increased energy demand, detected as small negative shifts of the DC potential and increased extracellular lactate, respectively.

Conclusion

This study demonstrates that sustained, moderate NMDA-receptor activation inhibits K^+-SD. It confirms and extends our previous demonstration that high extracellular glutamate does not promote the initiation of SD by high extracellular K^+, nor its propagation (Obrenovitch and Zilkha 1995b; Obrenovitch et al. 1996). Together with the well established notion that both SD elicitation and propagation are very sensitive to NMDA-receptor block, these data indicate that functional NMDA-receptor-ionophores are required for SD initiation, but that widespread, increased NMDA-receptor activation is not the cause for the elicitation of SD by elevated extracellular K^+.

Inhibition of NO synthesis and spreading depression

Several lines of evidence have suggested a possible relationship between NO synthesis and SD: (i) Both SD initiation and propagation require functional NMDA-receptor-ionophore complexes (see previous section), and Ca^{2+}-influx through these ion channels stimulates NO synthesis (Garthwaite and Boulton 1995); (ii) direct amperometric measurements of NO showed a multiphasic release of NO associated with SD elicitation in the cerebral cortex of cats (Read et al. 1997); and (iii) NO decreased concentration-dependently the velocity of retinal SD waves, an effect that could be mimicked partially by membrane-permeable cGMP derivatives (Ulmer et al. 1995). However, whether endogenous NO formation associated with SD contributes to the genesis of SD or its modulation remains unclear. This issue was addressed by investigating the effects of pharmacological inhibition of NO synthesis on K^+-induced SD.

As it is described in the previous section, recurrent SD were elicited by perfusion of high-K^+ medium through a microdialysis probe implanted in the cerebral cortex of anaesthetised rats, and recorded at the site of elicitation with a microelectrode placed within the probe. The NO synthase (NOS) inhibitor (Nω-nitro-L-arginine methyl ester, L-NAME) was administered through the microdialysis probe to rule out any possible interference of peripheral NOS inhibition. In this study, a single microdialysis electrode was implanted in each animal and used for the following procedures: (i) elicitation of 5 episodes of repetitive SD by perfusion of 160 mM K^+ through the probe for 20 min, with 40 min of recovery after each SD episode; and (ii) perfusion of 0.3, 1 and 3 mM L- or D-NAME (inactive isomer of NAME) for the 2nd, 3rd and 4th SD episode (in respective order) for 60 min, starting 20-min before the K^+-application.

Inhibition of NOS with L-NAME had no effect on the 1st SD latency. The number of SD elicited during each K^+ stimulus was dose-dependently reduced (e.g. 3.1 ± 0.6 under 1 mM L-NAME versus 5.0 ± 0.9 in controls; mean ± standard deviation; $n = 6$–8, $p < 0.01$, Student's *t*-test), but this change was associated with a marked increase in the cumulative SD peak area (e.g. 23.5 ± 4.5 mV.min under 1 mM L-NAME versus 16.7 ± 4.2 in controls, $p < 0.05$), suggesting that under NOS inhibition SD waves are fewer but larger. Indeed, L-NAME markedly, and concentration-dependengly broadened the SD peaks (53.2 ± 7.0 s under 1 mM L-NAME versus 25.0 ± 6.2 in controls; $p < 0.001$) (Fig. 4), primarily by delaying the repolarisation phase (Fig. 4, right upper trace). In comparison to L-NAME, D-NAME only slightly reduced both the number and magnitude of SD at the highest dose tested (3mM).

This study demonstrates that NOS inhibition does not alter the initiation of SD by high extracellular K^+ (latency for 1st SD was unchanged), but markedly alters its pattern by delaying the initiation of repolarisation. The reduction in the frequency of SD observed with L-NAME (i.e. fewer peaks during the corresponding K^+-stimuli) was likely a consequence of the delayed repolarisation increasing the duration of the refractory period after each individual SD.

A deficient coupling of local blood flow to energy demand under NOS inhibition is unlikely to be a major contributor to the delayed initiation of repolarisation such as that showed in Fig. 4 (upper traces). Firstly, because energy demand appears to be maximum during repolarisation (Taylor et al. 1994), and the rate of repolarisation was only slightly reduced under L-NAME (data not shown). Secondly, because the increase in local cerebral blood flow that is closely associated with SD does not appear to be NO-mediated in rats (Zhang et al. 1994; Fabricius et al. 1995; Wolf et al. 1996; Read and Parsons 1998). Therefore, the delayed repolarisation-phase of SD under NOS inhibition is probably linked to the suppression of a direct action of NO on brain cells. One such action may be the inhibitory effects of NO on NMDA-receptor function that was demonstrated in rat cortical neurones in vitro (Hoyt et al. 1992). These effects of NO are not mediated by neuronal cGMP production (Hoyt et al. 1992), but through direct S-nitrosylation of free sulfhydryl groups on the NMDA-receptor-ionophore complex by NO (Aizenman and Potthoff 1999; Choi et al. 2000). Another possibility may be the down-modulation of gap junctions. Indeed, NO was found to modulate gap junction conductance in both turtle retina and rat neocortex via stimulation of the cGMP pathway (Miyachi et al. 1990; Rorig and Sutor 1996), and gap junctions are necessary for the propagation of SD (Martins-Ferreira et al. 1995; Nedergaard et al. 1995).

Conclusion

Whatever the mechanism(s) underlying this delayed initiation of repolarisation under NOS inhibition, our data imply that NO formation during SD contributes to the inactivation of ion channels and/or gap junctions that initiates the recovery from SD, i.e. normalisation of ion homeostasis. Selective pharmacological and genetic manipulations have showed that the pathogenesis of neuronal ischaemic injury can be altered by NO, either positively or negatively, depending on the stage of evolution of ischaemic injury and on the cellular source of NO (Iadecola 1997). The current consensus is that NO produced by endothelial NOS (eNOS) is beneficial by favouring blood supply to vulnerable regions (e.g. the penumbra), whereas post-

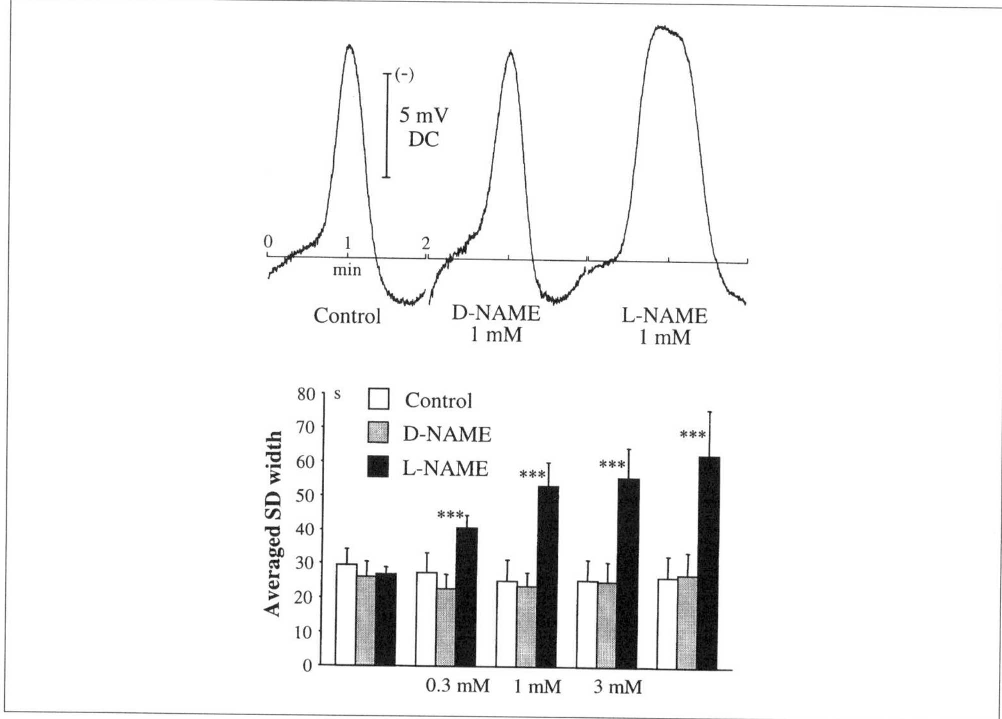

Fig. 4. Effects of local NOS inhibition with L-NAME on the pattern of the 1st individual SD (upper traces), and comparison with the inactive stereoisomer D-NAME. The upper traces are representative recording of the 1st SD elicited in control, and under 1 mM D- or L-NAME. In the bar chart below, values are means ± standard deviation of the width at mid-height of the 1st SD wave occurring with each of the K^+ applications. In the control group, 5 separate episodes of repeated SD were produced by perfusion of 160 mM K^+ for 20-min; In the D- and L-NAME group, 0.3, 1.0 and 3.0 mM of the drug were co-perfused with high K^+ during the 2nd, 3rd, and 4th challenge, in respective order. Note the marked increase in the width of individual SD under NOS inhibition (L-NAME), primarily due to delayed repolarisation. Note also that this effect persisted when L-NAME was omitted from the last K^+-stimulus. $^{***}p < 0.001$, comparison of the L-NAME group to the D-NAME group; Student's *t*-test (n = 6 to 8).

ischaemic production of NO by neuronal NOS (nNOS) may be neurotoxic. The finding that NO production may be part of a feedback control mechanism that promotes the recovery phase of SD adds a new degree of complexity to this already complicated picture.

References

1. Aizenman E, Potthoff WK (1999) Lack of interaction between nitric oxide and the redox modulatory site of the NMDA receptor. Br J Pharmacol 126:296–300
2. Back T, Ginsberg MD, Dietrich WD, Watson BD (1996) Induction of spreading depression in the ischemic hemisphere following experimental middle cerebral artery occlusion: effect on infarct morphology. J Cereb Blood Flow Metab 16:202–213
3. Brand S, Fernandes de Lima VM, Hanke W (1998) Pharmacological modulation of the refractory period of retinal spreading depression. Naunyn-Schmiedeberg's Arch Pharmacol 357:419–425
4. Bures J, Buresová O, Krivánek J (1974) The mechanisms and applications of Leao's spreading depression of electroencephalographic activity. New York: Academic Press
5. Busch E, Gyngel ML, Eis M, Hoehn-Berlage M, Hossmann KA (1996) Potassium-induced cortical spreading depressions during focal cerebral ischemia in rats: contribution to lesion growth assessed by diffusion-weighted NMR and biochemical imaging. J Cereb Blood Flow Metab 16:1,090–1,099
6. Charles AC, Kodali SK, Tyndale RF (1996) Intercellular calcium waves in neurons. Mol Cell Neurosci 7:337–353
7. Chen Q, Chopp M, Bodzin G, Chen H (1993) Temperature modulation of cerebral depolarization during focal cerebral ischemia in rats: correlation with ischemic injury. J Cereb Blood Flow Metab 13:389–394

8. Choi YB, Tenneti L, Le DA, Ortiz J, Bai G, Chen HS, Lipton SA (2000) Molecular basis of NMDA receptor-coupled ion channel modulation by S-nitrosylation. Nat Neurosci 3:15–21
9. Curtis DR, Watkins JC (1961) Analogues of glutamic and γ-amino-*n*-butyric acids having potent actions on mammalian neurones. Nature 191:1,010–1,011
10. Fabricius M, Akgoren N, Lauritzen M (1995) Arginine-nitric oxide pathway and cerebrovascular regulation in cortical spreading depression. Am J Physiol 269:H23–H29
11. Fabricius M, Jensen LH, Lauritzen M (1993) Microdialysis of interstitial amino acids during spreading depression and anoxic depolarization in rat neocortex. Brain Res 612:61–69
12. Garthwaite J, Boulton CL (1995) Nitric oxide signalling in the central nervous system. Ann Rev Neurosci 57:683–706
13. Hernandez-Caceres J, Macias-Gonzalez R, Brozek G, Bures J (1987) Systemic ketamine blocks cortical spreading depression but does not delay the onset of terminal anoxic depolarization in rats. Brain Res 437:360–364
14. Hoyt KR, Tang LH, Aizenmann E, Reynolds IJ (1992) Nitric oxide modulates NMDA-induced increases in intracellular Ca^{2+} in cultured rat forebrain neurons. Brain Res 592:310–316
15. Iadecola C (1997) Bright and dark sides of nitric oxide in ischemic brain injury. Trends Neurosci 20:132–139
16. Koroleva VI, BuresJ (1980) Blockade of cortical spreading depression in electrically and chemically stimulated areas of cerebral cortex in rats. Electroencephalogr Clin Neurophysiol 48:1–15
17. Koroleva VI, Bures J (1996) The use of spreading depression waves for acute and long-term monitoring of the penumbra zone of focal ischemic damage in rats. Proc Natl Acad Sci USA 93:3,710–3,714
18. Kunkler PE, Kraig RP (1998) Calcium waves precede electrophysiological changes of spreading depression in hippocampal organ cultures. J Neurosci 18:3,416–3,425
19. Lauritzen M, Rice ME, OkadaY, Nicholson C (1988) Quisqualate, kainate and NMDA can initiate spreading depression in the turtle cerebellum. Brain Res 475:317–327
20. Leão APP (1944) Further observations on spreading depression of activity in the cerebral cortex. J Neurophysiol 7:359–390
21. Martins-Ferreira H, Nedergaard M, Nicholson C (2000) Perspectives on spreading depression. Brain Res Brain Res Rev 32:215–234
22. Martins-Ferreira H, Ribeiro LJ (1995) Biphasic effects of gap junctional uncoupling agents on the propagation of retinal spreading depression. Braz J Med Biol Res 28:991–994
23. Menniti FS, Pagnozzi MJ, Butler P, Chenard BL, Jaw-Tsai SS, Frost White W (2000) CP-101,606, and NR2B subunit selective NMDA receptor antagonist, inhibits NMDA and injury induced c-fos expression and cortical spreading depression in rodents. Neuropharmacology 39:1,147–1,155
24. Mies G, Iijima T, Hossmann K-A (1993) Correlation between peri-infarct DC shifts and ischemic neuronal damage in rat. Neuroreport 4:709–711
25. Miyachi E, Murakami M, Nakaki T (1990) Arginine blocks gap junctions between retinal horizontal cells. Neuroreport 1:107–110
26. Moghaddam B, Schenk JO, Stewart WB, Hansen AJ (1987) Temporal relationship between neurotransmitter release and ion flux during spreading depression and anoxia. Can J Physiol Pharmacol 65:1,105–1,110
27. Nedergaard M, Cooper AJ, Goldman SA (1995) Gap junctions are required for the propagation of spreading depression. J Neurobiol 28:433–444
28. Obrenovitch TP (1999) High extracellular glutamate and neuronal death in neurological disorders: Cause, contribution, or consequence. Ann NY Acad Sci 890:273–286
29. Obrenovitch TP, Zilkha E (1995a) Changes in extracellular glutamate concentration associated with propagating cortical spreading depression. In: Olesen J, Moskowitz MA Eds. Experimental headache models. New York: Raven Press. pp 113–117
30. Obrenovitch TP, Zilkha E (1995b) High extracellular potassium, and not extracellular glutamate, is required for the propagation of spreading depression. J Neurophysiol 73:2,107–2,114
31. Obrenovitch TP, Zilkha E (1996) Inhibition of cortical spreading depression by L-701,324, a novel antagonist at the glycine site of the N-methyl-D-aspartate receptor complex. Br J Pharmacol 117:931–937
32. Obrenovitch TP, Richards DA, Sarna GS, Symon L (1993) Combined intracerebral microdialysis and electrophysiological recording: Methodology and applications. J Neurosci Meth 47:139–145
33. Obrenovitch TP, Urenjak J, Zilkha E (1994) Intracerebral microdialysis combined with recording of extracellular field potential: A novel method for investigation of depolarizing drugs in vivo. Br J Pharmacol 113:1,295–1,302
34. Obrenovitch TP, Zilkha E, Urenjak J (1996) Evidence against high extracellular glutamate promoting the elicitation of spreading depression. J Cereb Blood Flow Metab 16:923–931
35. Read SJ, Parsons AA (1998) Nitric oxide does not mediate cerebral blood flow changes during cortical spreading depression in the anaesthetised rat. Neurosci Lett 250:115–118
36. Read SJ, Smith MI, Hunter AJ, Parsons AA (1997) The dynamics of nitric oxide release measured directly and in real time following repeated waves of cortical spreading depression in the anaesthetised cat. Neurosci Lett 232:127–130
37. Riepe MW, Hori N, Ludolph AC, Carpenter DO (1995) Failure of neuronal ion exchange, not potentiated excitation, causes excitotoxicity after inhibition of oxidative phosphorylation. Neuroscience 64:91–97
38. Rorig B, Sutor B (1996) Nitric oxide-stimulated increase in intracellular cGMP modulates gap junction coupling in rat neocortex. Neuroreport 31:569–572
39. Tatlisumak T, Takano K, Meiler MR, Fisher M (1998) A glycine site antagonist, ZD9379, reduces number of spreading depressions and infarct size in rats with permanent middle cerebral artery occlusion. Stroke 29:190–195
40. Taylor DL, Richards DA, Obrenovitch TP, Symon L (1994) Time course of changes in extracellular lactate evoked by transient K^+-induced depolarisation in the rat striatum. J Neurochem 62:2,368–2,374
41. Tong G, Jahr CE (1994) Regulation of glycine-insensitive desensitization of the NMDA receptor in outside-out patches. J Neurophysiol 72:754–761
42. Ulmer HJ, de Lima VM, Hanke W (1995) Effects of nitric oxide on the retinal spreading depression. Brain Res 691:239–242
43. Van Harreveld A, Fifková E (1970) Glutamate release from the retina during spreading depression. J Neurobiol 2:13–29
44. Wang Z, Tymianski M, Jones OT, Nedergaard M (1997) Impact of cytoplasmic calcium buffering on the spatial and temporal characteristics of intercellular calcium signals in astrocytes. J Neurosci 17:7,359–7,371
45. Wolf T, Lindauer U, Obrig H, Dreier J, Back T, Villringer A, Dirnagl U (1996) Systemic nitric oxide synthase inhibition does not affect brain oxygenation during cortical spreading depression in rats: a noninvasive near-infrared spectroscopy and laser-Doppler flowmetry study. J Cereb Blood Flow Metab 16:1,100–1,107
46. Zhang ZG, Chopp M, Maynard KI, Moskowitz MA. (1994) Cerebral blood flow changes during cortical spreading depression are not altered by inhibition of nitric oxide synthesis. J Cereb Blood Flow Metab 14:939–943

Imaging the anoxic depolarization, a multifocal and propagating event

R. D. Andrew, T.R. Anderson, A.J. Biedermann, I. Joshi, C.R. Jarvis

Abstract

For more than 15 years extracellular glutamate accumulation has been suspected as the initiator of immediate and delayed neuronal death following stroke. However all induced responses leading to damage are downstream from an initial mass depolarization of neurons and glia which is termed the anoxic depolarization (AD). During focal or global ischemia, the AD is sustained in cerebral regions where blood flow is severely restricted. However AD generation neither requires glutamate nor elicits a maintained level of extracellular glutamate. The AD and the acute neuronal damage that follows it are notoriously difficult to prevent, resisting channel blockade and glutamate receptor antagonists. In the ischemic core adjacent to regions of intermediate blood flow (the penumbra) the maintained depolarization can repeatedly initiate peri-infarct depolarization (PID). Unlike AD, a PID repolarizes but then recurs, increasing the metabolic load and promoting damage over the first 3–4 h following stroke onset. PIDs are thought to propagate into regions of normal blood flow as classic spreading depression (SD) where repolarization is rapid compared to the PID. By imaging intrinsic optical signals (IOSs) and recording extracellularly from neocortical brain slices, we show that the AD induced by O_2/glucose deprivation or ouabain exposure is a propagating event that initiates multi-focally and is not blocked by glutamate receptor (GluR) antagonists. Neither do GluR antagonists slow AD propagation or reduce acute neuronal damage that follows in the wake of the AD. In contrast, certain sigma receptor ligands at micromolar concentrations (with or without NMDA receptor affinity) block AD initiation, thereby preventing acute neuronal damage. Surprisingly then, sigma receptors ligands can uncouple the AD from O_2/glucose deprivation thereby lowering metabolic demand.

The multi-focal and propagating nature of the anoxic depolarization is similar to spreading depression as imaged in normoxic neocortical slices. In vivo, the PID represents an event intermediary along a continuum between AD and SD. Unlike SD, PID repolarization is delayed by lowered energy reserves and serves to further reduce these stores, promoting neuronal damage. We propose that in vivo, $sigma_1$ receptor ligands may block AD and PID initiation and so reduce acute and delayed stroke damage.

Keywords: spreading depression, excitotoxicity, anoxic depolarization, stroke, intrinsic optical signals, sigma receptors

Department of Anatomy & Cell Biology, Queen's University, Kingston, Ontario, Canada, K7L 3N6.
e-mail: andrewd@post.queensu.ca

Introduction

The concept of excitotoxicity

'Excitotoxicity' refers to nerve cell depolarization and the resultant death arising from excess release and accumulation of the excitatory amino acid neurotransmitter L-glutamate (Choi 1991; 1994; Haddad and Jiang 1992; Limbrick et al. 1995). The concept arose from the finding that large amounts of injected glutamate (or its receptor agonists) killed nerve cells, a process subsequently observed in cultured neurons. The damage could be blocked by glutamate receptor (GluR) antagonists, later proposed as protective in animal models of stroke. Thus the 'textbook' description of excitotoxicity is as follows. During metabolic compromise (brain trauma, ischemia, carbon monoxide poisoning) ATP resources decline. With failure of the Na^+/K^+ pump, neurons depolarize and release glutamate. Reuptake mechanisms also fail and accumulating glutamate binds to its receptors, inducing further depolarization and more release. An influx of Na^+ and Cl^- is osmotically followed by water, causing neurons to swell and die (termed *acute* or *early* excitotoxic cell death). Elevated levels of extracellular glutamate is considered the trigger of acute ischemic injury.

Surviving neurons may continue to die over many hours or days because increased intracellular $[Ca^{2+}]$ or other second messenger systems initiate cascades that activate various proteases, lipases and nucleases. Together with free radical formation, these enzymes cause *delayed* (or *late*) neuronal death, a consequence nevertheless of the initial ischemic insult. In the hippocampal CA1 region, mild ischemia activates programmed neuronal death (apoptosis) whereas severe ischemia leads to necrosis (Dragunow et al. 1994; Schreiber and Baudry 1995). Both processes contribute to stroke damage (Lee et al. 1999).

Despite almost universal acceptance of this scenario, no effective stroke therapy has emerged based on GluR blockade using established receptor antagonists or through enhancement of glutamate reuptake (Goldberg 2000). Direct observation of the earliest events of excitotoxicity (neuronal swelling and elevated Ca^{2+}) has been limited to cultured or acutely dissociated neuronal cell bodies. However, there are also concomitant volume increases and 'beading' by the dendritic tree as observed in metabolically stressed neurons in culture (Park et al. 1996; Faddis et al. 1997), in situ (Hori and Carpenter 1994) and in live brain slices (Obeidat et al. 2000). Dendritic beading, which can occur within minutes, is the basis for our imaging of acute neuronal damage as described later.

Excitotoxicity: Some serious problems

As noted by Obrenovitch and Urenjak (1997a), three influential discoveries in 1984 encouraged the idea that excess glutamate release resulting from stroke could kill neurons in ischemia: 1) extracellular glutamate levels increased during ischemia; 2) blockade of glutamate receptors protected cultured neurons from glutamate toxicity; 3) antagonists of NMDA receptors reduced ischemia-induced neuronal damage in vivo. However, these three findings are open to re-interpretation.

First, increased extracellular glutamate levels as measured in experimental models of neurological disorders (ischemia, trauma, epilepsy) do not necessarily produce neuronal dysfunction and death in vivo. This issue is reviewed elsewhere (Obrenovitch et al. 1996; Obrenovitch 1999) and will not be detailed here except to note the important observation by several groups that a progressive increase in dialysate glutamate does not occur until *after* the onset of the anoxic depolarization (e.g. Zilkha et al. 1995). Cho et al. (1992) showed no correlation between glutamate levels during and shortly after ischemia and CA1 cell injury. Benveniste et al. (1984) showed that 10 min of global ischemia elevated $[\text{glutamate}]_o$ from 2 to 16 μM, returning to near baseline 15 min later. It is arguable that such a small increase alone can account for the ensuing damage. Even 30 min of focal ischemia results in only minor efflux of neuroactive neurotransmitters in the penumbra (Obrenovitch et al. 1993) and with 2 hours of focal ischemia, penumbral levels of glutamate return to baseline in the first hour (Takagi et al. 1993). The global brain depolarization that follows cardiac arrest must be sustained in order to evoke glutamate release in large amounts.

Second, it has been argued that cultured brain cells do not provide reliable models of neurological disorders. One important reason is the reduction of the astrocyte population which normally removes extracellular glutamate, and so attenuates excitotoxic death of nerve cells (Rosenberg and Aizenman 1989; Dugan et al. 1995). Other problems include altered intrinsic, receptor and synaptic properties of neurons in prolonged culture, the loss of the finite and tortuous extracellular space, and glutamate contamination of the culture media (Ye and Sontheimer 1998). The lack of damage in brain slices exposed to levels of glutamate that kill cultured neurons is attributable to the intact neuron-glia relationship maintained in slices (Obeidat and Andrew 1998).

A third problem is that the sensitivity of an event (e.g., ischemia, trauma) to glutamate receptor antagonists does not necessarily indicate high extracellular glutamate levels as the generator of the event. There is no question that glutamate antagonists are protective in animal models of focal ischemia (McCulloch et al. 1993). However, Obrenovitch and Urenjak (1997a, 1997b) have argued that glutamate antagonists work because they *preserve energy* which is the bottom line determining neuronal protection. Brain energy demand increases dramatically with sustained depolarization, a result of the opening of voltage-sensitive Na^+ channels and to a lesser extent GluR mediation (Taylor and Narasimhan 1997). But GluR antagonists, glutamate release inhibitors or glutamate uptake inhibitors will be of little help if the energy pool is insufficient to re-establish the resting membrane potential of severely depolarized neurons (Obrenovitch et al. 1993). We suggest in this article that in regions sufficiently removed from the ischemic core where ATP levels are only moderately reduced, GluR antagonists can be partly protective.

Some experts in the field have abandoned the original excitotoxic basis of ischemic damage, but the central role of NMDA receptors and glutamate continues. Thus more recent studies have focused on AMPA receptors or Zn^{2+} or pH as activators of NMDARs (Lee et al. 1999) and on failure of glutamate re-uptake mechanisms (Rossi et al. 1999). The argument has been made that the minimal therapeutic benefits of GluR antagonists in human studies are "too little, too late" and therefore cannot replicate animal models where some ischemic protection has been shown. The possibility that glutamate is simply not the key to unlocking the enigma of acute stroke damage is rarely discussed.

Three alternative mechanisms depend on maintained depolarization

There is no doubt that excessive opening of GluRs contributes to ischemic brain damage, but that simple accumulation of glutamate in the extracellular space is probably not the initiator as argued by Obrenovitch and Urenjak (1997a). Excessive depolarization during ischemia will release the Mg^{2+} block of NMDA activated channels, causing further depolarization and Ca^{2+} influx (Turski and Turski 1993). It follows that potential modulation of NMDA receptor function by glycine, polyamides, redox changes or phosphorylation is important in ischemia, as are endogenous excitotoxins such as quinolinic acid. But the key excitoxic factor is relief of the Mg^{2+} block by *sustained depolarization*.

In cultured neurons, omitting oxygen/glucose or adding metabolic inhibitors to block ATP as an energy source means that the membrane potential cannot be maintained and sustained depolarization ensues (Beal et al. 1993). It is the K^+gradient across cellular membrane that primarily determines the membrane potential and any treatment reducing sustained depolarization (including GluR antagonists) can be protective to some extent. In contrast to cultured neurons, Riepe et al. (1995) found that GluR-mediated electrophysiological responses were *not* enhanced in CA1 neurons or glia during metabolic inhibition of brain slices. They proposed that failure of Na^+ extrusion and declining ionic concentration gradients were the excitotoxic culprits rather than glutamate accumulation.

A third proposed excitotoxic mechanism that is probably important in delayed neuronal death is a persistent and widespread synaptic enhancement. This is essentially an ischemia-induced long term potentiation (LTP) which requires NMDA receptors and involves second messenger pathways (Hammond et al. 1994). It is thought that peri-infarct depolarization (which are essentially repeated periods of spreading depression in ischemic tissue) leads to a widespread and generalized LTP that can be hazardous to neurons possessing GluRs (Edwards 1995).

Note that for all three potentially destructive mechanisms noted above (i.e. loss of Mg^{2+} block, Na^+ influx, ischemic LTP), a strong and maintained membrane depolarization is prerequisite. In fact all three are direct consequences of what we propose is the initial and fundamental mechanism leading to stroke damage: prolonged depolarization. In the penumbra, the mass depolarization can recover and recur. The recurrent event has been called transient anoxic depolarization, peri-infarct spreading depression, transient ischemic depolarization, or peri-infarct depolarization (PID), or ischemic spreading depression (Fig. 1).

The penumbra and recurring depolarization

Where blood flow is most reduced there is a single anoxic depolarization (AD), which is recorded extracellularly as a negative voltage

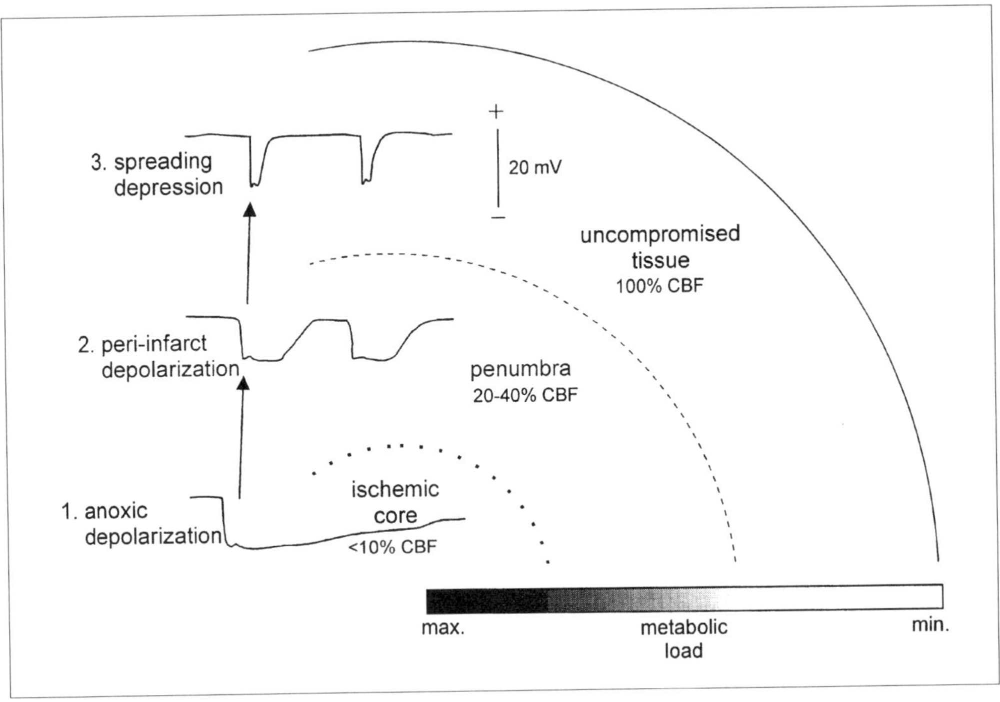

Fig. 1. In the ischemic core, depolarization measured as a negative shift in extracellular voltage is maintained because loss of energy resources prevents repolarization. Elevated $[K^+]_0$ at the edge of the core may promote PID initiation in the penumbra where improved blood flow provides energy for the tissue to repolarize. Depolarization can then recur. Each PID, we propose, propagates into more peripheral regions where repolarization is quickly established by adequate energy reserves. Here, the metabolic demand created by what is essentially classic spreading depression does not cause neuronal damage. In well vascularized regions directly adjacent to the ischemic core, SD may also arise but again is not damaging (not shown).

shift of 10–30 mV. Leao (1947) first recorded this "anemic" depolarization as a propagating signal. The maintained depolarization and near absence of both O_2 and glucose quickly damages neurons, forming the ischemic core. The penumbra, a rim of gray matter that surrounds the ischemic core, is viable but suffers reduced blood flow, so the neurons can eventually undergo infarct *or* recovery. This uncertainty arises partly from the variable number and duration of peri-infarct depolarizations (PIDs) which initiate at the edge of the ischemic core and propagate through the penumbra (Fig. 1). *These ischemic spreading depression events are themselves metabolically compromising due to the mismatch of energy supply with the demands of repolarization.* Each PID is probably initiated by elevated $[K^+]_o$, a product of terminal depolarization and necrosis within the core (Nedergaard 1996). It propagates away from the core along a decreasing gradient of metabolic stress and into healthy tissue where it does no harm because energy resources are not compromised. Here, it is essentially classic spreading depression (SD). During the first 3 to 4 h following stroke, recurring PIDs expand the core into the penumbra (Back et al. 1996) where SD duration can be up to five times longer than in normal tissue (Nedergaard 1996). There is a linear relationship between the number of PIDs and infarct volume (Mies et al. 1994; Otsuka et al. 2000), although PID duration rather than frequency is reported as a critical factor in early damage (Dijkhuisen et al. 1999). Note that more compromised tissue will lack the metabolic reserves to repolarize quickly so PID duration and tissue damage are not simply 'cause and effect'. Rather one promotes the other.

More recent studies using DWI or MRI (Busch et al. 1996; Takano et al.1996; Dijkhuisen et al. 1999) indicate that PIDs indeed expand the focal lesion. A transient ADC (apparent diffusion coefficient) signal represents SD or PID (as correlated with the negative voltage shift), whereas a prolonged ADC reduction measures cellular swelling. Recurrent PIDs are observed during the first 3 hours post-MCA occlusion, the time when lesion expansion is most rapid (see Dijkhuisen et al. 1999).

It is noteworthy that human neocortical slices support repeated SD events following a brief period of mild hypoxia at 33 °C (Kohling et al. 1996). There is little doubt that SD in humans underlies the aura of migraine headache (Welsh 1997). In this case SD is not damaging because the tissue is not stressed by both SD *and* reduced energy stores.

Prolonged depolarization and glutamate antagonists

In regions of metabolic compromise the AD and PIDs are remarkably difficult to block. Several intact animal studies show that AD is different from normoxic SD induced by focal K^+ application or by mechanical or tetanic stimulation in at least one important property (Hernandez-Caceres et al. 1987; Marranes et al. 1988; Lauritzen and Hansen 1992; Nellgard and Wieloch 1992; Koroleva et al. 1998). Each group has consistently observed that the AD arising from *ischemia* is *not* blocked by NMDA receptor (or non-NMDAR) antagonists. These same studies show that SD in *normoxic* tissue *is* blocked by NMDAR antagonists, but not non-NMDAR antagonists. The PIDs are more problematic. A high dose of the NMDAR antagonist MK-801 has been reported to reduce cortical SD events (Iijima et al 1992; Gill et al 1992; Koroleva et al. 1998) possibly because the drug is more effective in regions of less severe ischemia (Yao et al. 1994) which are distant from the ischemic core. MK-801 may also reduce cortical SDs by improving blood flow (Buchan et al. 1992).

Recent brain slice studies support these in vivo findings but terminology is confusing. Brain slice studies suggest AD is actually a spreading signal, termed an 'anoxic', 'hypoxic' or 'ischemic' spreading depression which returns to near baseline even as metabolic stress continues. We previously referred to the AD imaged in the hippocampal slice as an 'ischemic' SD (Obeidat and Andrew 1998). GluR antagonists do *not* block OGD – or ouabain – induced AD (ischemic SD) in the rat hippocampal slice (Balestrino 1995; Obeidat et al. 2000), in the rat neocortical slice (Footit and Newberry 1998; Jarvis et al.1999; Anderson et al. 1999) or in the mouse neocortical slice (Joshi and Andrew, in press). Ischemic SD induced by ouabain is not blocked by known GluR antagonists (Balestrino et al. 1999; Jarvis et al. in press; Joshi and Andrew, in press). In contrast, NMDAR antagonists are effective in blocking *normoxic* SD as tested in the rat neocortical slice (Anderson et al. 1999). Apparently glutamate receptors drive a larger proportion of the underlying depolarization in normoxic situations.

Drugs reducing Na^+ influx delay the anoxic depolarization both in vivo (Xie et al. 1995) and in brain slices (Aitken et al. 1991; Taylor et al. 1999). The latter study also showed that in half the slices there was no effect. A Na^+ channel antagonist fosphenytoin had no therapeutic efficacy in clinical trials (Lee et al. 1999). With K^+ channel blockers, there are potential cardiac and brain penetration problems and the standard Na^+ channel blockers can also have cardiac effects. Voltage-gated Ca^{2+} channel blockers or low Ca^{2+} aCSF do not block the AD in brain slices (Jing et al. 1993; Basarsky et al. 1998). No neurotransmitter receptor antagonists block ischemic SD in brain slices or have yet proved effective against stroke in humans (Lee et al. 1999; Goldberg 2000). *We propose that acute stroke damage is difficult to prevent (other than by restoring blood supply) because AD in the ischemic coare and recurrent PIDs near the core resist pharmacological blockade.* As such there can be no relief from these events during the first 3–4 hours following stroke. Therefore, we found it significant that 10–100 μM dextromethorphan (DM) blocked ischemic *or* normoxic SD while maintaining brain slice function (Anderson et al. in press). DM has been used a non-prescription cough suppressant for over 20 years, acting centrally by inhibiting the expiratory motor drive (Bolser et al. 1999).

Sigma receptor ligands and ischemia

Several studies using intact animals have shown neuroprotection by DM, usually attributed to NMDAR inhibition (Wong et al. 1988; Church et al. 1991). DM pretreatment reduced damage caused by arterial occlusion in rabbit (George et al. 1988; Steinberg et al.1988a) or in young rats with MCA occlusion (Prince and Feeser 1988). Similar results were found in rat following MCA occlusion with DM treatment delayed by 10 min (Steinberg et al. 1991) or by one h post-ischemia (Steinberg et al. 1988b), well within the 3 h period of recurring PIDs. A period of 12–48 h prior to DM treatment was not protective in a human study (Albers et al. 1995), but this was well after recurrent PID would subside.

Because DM blocked the AD whereas NMDAR antagonists did not, we suspected a mechanism independent of NMDARs. DM is also a sigma receptor ligand. *"The mysteries of sigma receptors"* is an apt title of a recent review (Moebius et al. 1997), given how little is known about the biological role of these receptors, with the exception of their influence on NMDARs. Sigma receptors differ from phencyclidine (PCP) binding sites, NMDA receptors and opioid receptors (Quirion et al. 1992; Ferris et al. 1991; Chou et al. 1999). Two subtypes of the receptor exist (Quirion et al. 1992). The σ_1R sub-type binds (+)-pentazocine, (+) NANM, carbetapentane and dextromethorphan with high affinity whereas the σ_2R subtype shows very low affinity. Most high affinity ligands specific to σ_2R also bind σ_1R in a like fashion but recently a specific σ_2R antagonist has been reported (Vilner et al. 1999). Sigma receptors have a regional distribution with the highest concentration in hindbrain and intermediate densities in neocortex and hippocampus (Tortella et al. 1989; Leitner et al. 1994). Sigma$_1$ receptors are found almost exclusively in neurons. Pyramidal cells, the cortical output neurons, possess significant σ_1R numbers (Gundlach et al. 1986; Phan et al. 1999). Bouchard and Quirion (1996) have autoradiographically mapped σ_1 and σ_2 receptor sites, the former high in dentate gyrus and the latter high in motor cortex and other motor-related areas. The amino acid sequence of σ_1R shows no homology to known mammalian proteins (Hanner et al. 1996), displaying one transmembrane domain (Seth et al. 1998). There is no evidence as yet that the monomer can oligimerize into a functional receptor. Despite cDNA cloning of σ_1R (Hanner et al. 1996), the second messenger pathways are unclear, although σ_1R (but not σ_2) binding is sensitive to GTP and its analogues (see Ferris et al. 1991). There appears to be no direct coupling between σ_1R and G proteins (Hong and Werling 1999). Rather, intracellular signalling components (as yet undescribed) mediate GTP$_\gamma$S binding to G proteins (Joseph and Bowen 1998).

Recently neuroprotection by other sigma receptor ligands in addition to DM has been investigated. Senda et al. (1998) showed that two σ receptor ligands protected against glutamate toxicity in cultured retinal neurons and that NE-100, a σ receptor antagonist, eliminated protection. Whittemore et al. (1997) showed that seventeen σ R ligands bound NMDAR subunits, but that there was no correlation between σ site affinity and potency of NMDAR antagonism measured by inhibition of NMDA-activated currents. Klette et al. (1997) showed protection by σR ligands including DM in primary cultured neurons. However (+)-3-PPP, a σ_1R antagonist, was ineffective even though it displays NMDAR antagonism (Whittemore et al. 1997). Lockhart et al. (1995) showed σR ligand protection from hypoxia or NMDA toxicity in neuronal cultures by σ ligands with σ/PCP receptor affinity but not by σ ligands without such affinity (e.g. DTG or 3-PPP). Most importantly following 2 h of focal ischemia, (+)-pentazocine (a specific σ_1R ligand) but not (–)-pentazocine (a non-specific opioid R ligand) greatly reduced infarct size (Takahashi et al. 1997). Note that both isomers antagonize NMDARs (Whittemore et al. 1997) so the protection does not appear to be NMDAR-mediated. Takahashi et al. (1996, 1997) have shown that the σR ligand PPBP reduces infarct volume, not simply the rate of injury development. Moreover protecton was not through changes in blood flow. PPBP acts through σ_2R, has no cross-reactivity with NMDARs and has minimal side effects (Takahashi 1996).

Hypothesis

Excess glutamate release and accumulation is not the primary cause of acute neuronal death in focal ischemia. Instead we hypothesize that prolonged depolarization in the form of AD and PIDs in metabolically compromised gray matter is a major determinant of neuronal damage. Optically mapping prolonged depolarization reveals its genesis, propagation and destructive consequences in brain slice preparations. Studying pharmacological strategies to block or inhibit sustained depolarization should help prevent or lessen its considerable impact in stroke. This is because all acute *and* delayed neuronal death is essentially downstream from the initial AD and the subsequent PIDs that expand the ischemic core.

Objective

Assessing acute neuronal damage requires an experimental approach to simulated stroke that is both accessible and manipulable. Cell cultures do not replicate the complexity of the brain nor do they generate SD. We have established a brain slice paradigm suitable both for imaging the optical wave front and for recording the negative field shift during simulated stroke. Both techniques display the distinct signatures of AD or SD which can be recorded across a an entire live cerebral brain slice. Potentially useful therapeutics can be assessed in terms of whether they block the AD, slow its propagation or reduce post-AD damage.

Methods

Developing an 'Ischemic' Brain Slice Model for Imaging and Electrophysiology

Stroke-related studies utilizing brain slices have been on-going for 30 years but experimental paradigms have varied considerably in the following aspects:

1) Hypoxia vs. O_2/glucose deprivation (OGD).

A brain slice does not recover very well

when deprived of both O_2 *and* glucose because once AD occurs, the neurons are too stressed by the combination of slicing, the AD and energy deprivation at 35–37 °C to expect a return to the health of pre-OGD conditions. Therefore many electrophysiological studies have used very brief exposure to OGD to avoid AD generation; alternately they simply lower O_2 (but not glucose) to promote recovery from 'hypoxic' SD. However hypoxia, while useful for studying the effects of pulmonary edema, asphyxiation or altitude sickness, inadequately simulates stroke where both O_2 *and* glucose levels drop precipitously.

2) *Submersion vs. interface.* Slices submerged in flowing aCSF do not support SD as readily as 'interface' slices where the top surface is exposed to a O_2/CO_2 atmosphere and aCSF flows beneath. We discovered that a fast superfusion rate of 3–4 ml/min helps overcome this discrepancy. Brief exposure to aCSF containing 26 mM KCl initiates SD onset and the slices recover from repeated bouts of SD without damage, as detailed in Results.
3) *Simplifying the light path for intrinsic optical signal (IOS) imaging.* The most straightforward configuration for IOS imaging involves collecting light that is transmitted, rather than reflected, by a tissue slice. Moreover scattering at the air/slice interface further complicates the light path. We have reviewed the basic biophysics involved and the benefits of utilizing submerged slices in this regard (Jarvis et al. 1999).

Experimental Rationale

The brain slice preparation avoids several experimental difficulties associated with the intact animal. In the past, acute stroke damage has been assessed based on histopathological evidence many hours post-insult. Cortical SD is usually extracellularly recorded from only 1 or 2 sites, although more recent studies have used several electrodes to demonstrate propagation (Nallet et al. 1999; Dijkhuisen et al. 1999). The penumbra is a narrow and unstable rim whose location cannot be accurately predicted in individual experiments in situ (Obrenovitch and Urenjak 1997a). Local changes in blood flow may affect neuronal discharge. The inability to induce SD 'on command' in patients limits the testing of potential therapeutic agents to block SD during migraine aura or stroke.

Unlike neuronal cultures or dissociated neurons, the brain slice preparation offers several experimental advantages:

- it supports the anoxic depolarization or repeatedly evoked spreading depression
- it avoids long-term changes to neurons that occur under cultured conditions
- the neuron/glia relationship remains reasonably intact
- functional synapses are retained with their endogenous transmitters, receptors and 2nd messengers
- electrical synapses (gap junctions) are maintained
- stimulating electrodes can be visually placed into intact local synaptic pathways
- up to 10 mm^2 of cortical tissue can be imaged to reveal population-wide events
- distinct brain regions or neuronal populations can be imaged and assessed side-by-side.

Tissue Preparation

Live coronal brain slices are prepared from 3–4 week old male Sprague-Dawley rats or C57 black/6 mice. Slices are cut at 400 μm in artificial CSF (aCSF) and gassed with 95% O_2, 5% CO_2. For O_2/glucose deprivation (OGD), N_2 replaces O_2 and [glucose] is lowered from 11 to1 mM. The aCSF contains (in mM): NaC1 126, KC1 3.3, $NaHCO_3$ 26, $MgC1_2$ 1.3, D-glucose 11 and $CaC1_2$ 1.8. A slice is submerged at 35–37 °C in flowing aCSF and viewed through an Zeiss inverted Axiovert microscope with only a coverslip between the slice and the objective.

Electrophysiology

The electrophysiological hallmark of the AD or SD is the 'negative shift', a voltage deflection of 5–30 mV recorded extracellularly that reflects local neuronal and glial depolarization to near zero mV. Neurons depolarize with more variability and longer duration than glia (Higashida et al. 1974; Sugaya et al. 1975). For extracellular recordings, a 5–15 MΩ micropipette filled with 2 M NaCl is placed in layers II–III of neocortex. The viability of the slice is monitored by recording the field potential evoked by stimulation to layer VI immediately beneath the recording site in II/III.

Imaging Intrinsic Optical Signals (IOSs)

IOSs represent alterations in the way biological tissue scatters or absorbs light (Sick and LaManna 1995; Andrew et al. 1999). Change in the amount of light reflected from the brain surface or transmitted through the brain slice is detected with a charge coupled device (CCD camera). Swollen cells scatter less light, resulting in greater light transmittance. IOS imaging permits the monitoring of second-by-second volume changes in 10 mm^2 of cortical tissue over periods of up to two hours with spatial resolution limited only by the objective lens. We have shown (Basarsky et al. 1998; Obeidat and Andrew 1998) that *cell swelling* generated in real time can be imaged during AD (ischemic SD) initiation and propagation in the cortical brain slice. IOS imaging also reveals *dendritic damage* in the form of a reduction in LT which overrides the LT increase caused by cell swelling. LT is reduced by the formation of dendritic beads (Polischuk et al. 1998; Jarvis et al. 1999; Obeidat et al. 2000) which are highly efficient in scattering light. We have recently described in detail several biophysical principles underlying IOS generation (Jarvis et al. 1999). Frames are acquired at 30 Hz, digitized and averaged using a frame grabber in a Pentium computer controlled by Axon Imaging Workbench software. Essentially, evolving changes in gray level of the subtracted images represent regional change in slice transparency.

Results

SD Induced by Oxygen/Glucose Deprivation (OGD) or Ouabain Exposure

In hemi-brain slices from rat or mouse at 35–37 °C, a signal is initiated within 5 min of OGD onset (Fig. 2A). Faster superfusion of aCSF delayed the signal onset (Fig. 4C). There was a dramatic focal increase in LT in layers II/III of the mouse neocortex (n = 18) which expanded concentrically. The LT peak (Fig. 2B) was followed by a marked *decrease* in LT, resulting in a wave-like front propagating across the brain slice. The route of signal propagation was usually inferiorly through the neocortex and inferiorly through the striatum towards the anterior commissure, averaging 1.8 mm/min. The signal first ignited in the neocortex, followed 2 to 3 min later by independent initiation in the striatum. There was some variation. In 6 of 18 slices, a single focus spread in opposite directions along the neocortex. In 3 slices, the signal arose near the anterior commissure and propagated laterally in neocortex. In 2 slices it initiated in the striatum *before* initiation in the neocortex. In all areas where it had just passed, the LT front returned to baseline within 5 minutes followed by a progressive decrease in LT.

The LT decrease developed exclusively in regions that supported the LT front. To confirm that the front represented a mass cellular depolarization, the negative shift was recorded. First, the evoked extracellular field potential was recorded in layers II/III of the neocortex (n = 7). Stimulation evoked a mixed antidromic/orthodromic response, confirming that the electrode was in a viable region (top trace, Fig. 2C). Occasionally one recording electrode was placed in layers II/III of the neocortex and another in the striatum. A negative shift of 10 mV recorded in the neocortex was followed by a negative shift of 15 mV in the striatum 1.5 minutes later (Fig. 2D). Similarly, Figure 2E shows initiation, propagation, and negative transmittance change first in neocortex and then in striatum. At 20 minutes and thereafter no evoked response could be recorded in layers II/III, indicating that the tissue was functionally compromised (bottom trace, Fig. 2C).

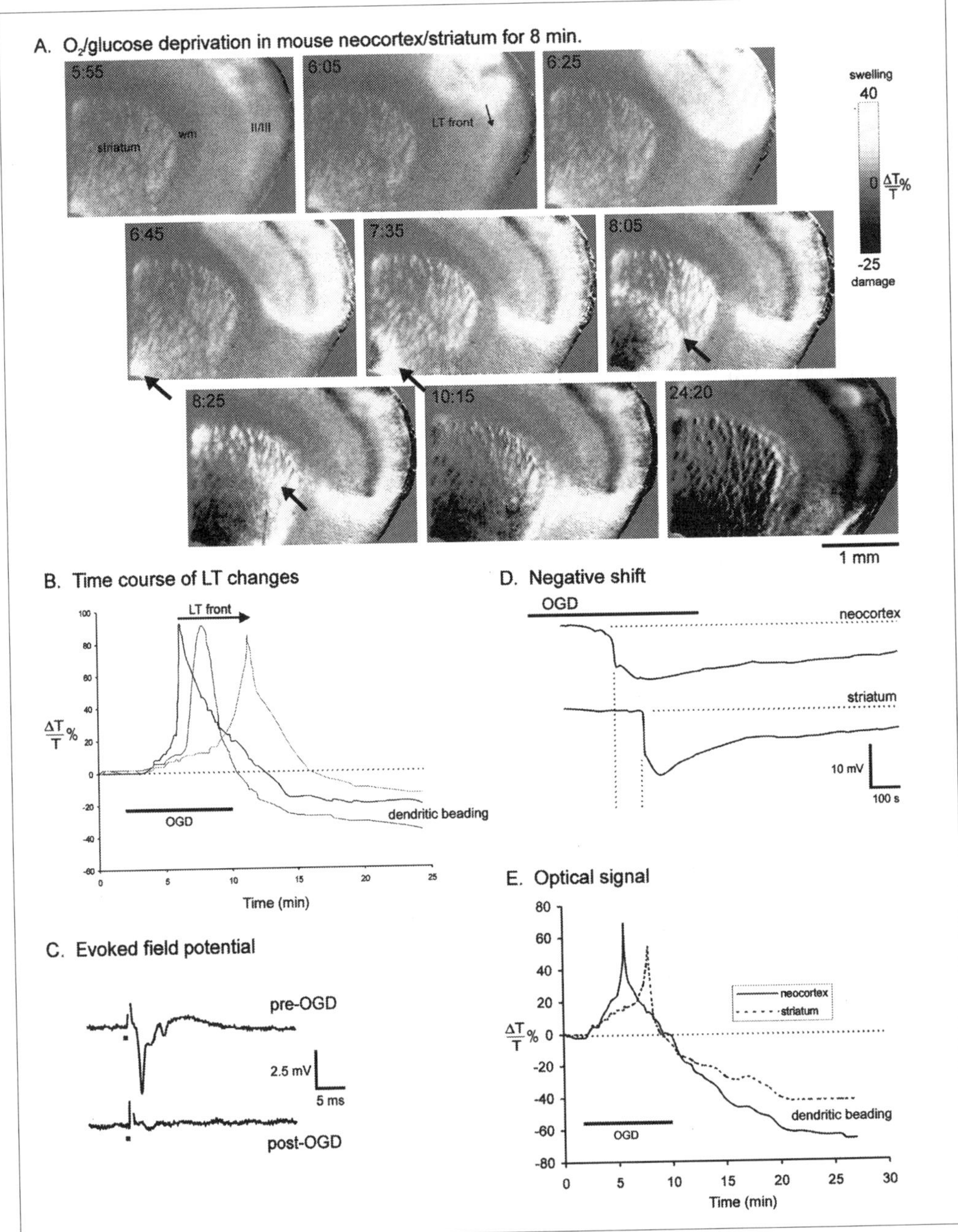

Fig. 2. Spreading signal induced by O_2/glucose deprivation (OGD) for 8 minutes at 35 °C in the mouse neocortex/striatum. *A*. The focal white signal increase represents AD onset, first in layers II/III in the neocortex (5:55, upper right) and then in the striatum near anterior commissure (6:45, lower right). A wave of elevated LT propagates through the neocortex (5:55 to 6:45) and later through the striatum (arrow, 6:45 to 8:25). Where the white signal has passed, there is a delayed and irreversible decrease (black signal) representing dendritic damage. *B*. Time course of signal change in three zones of interest

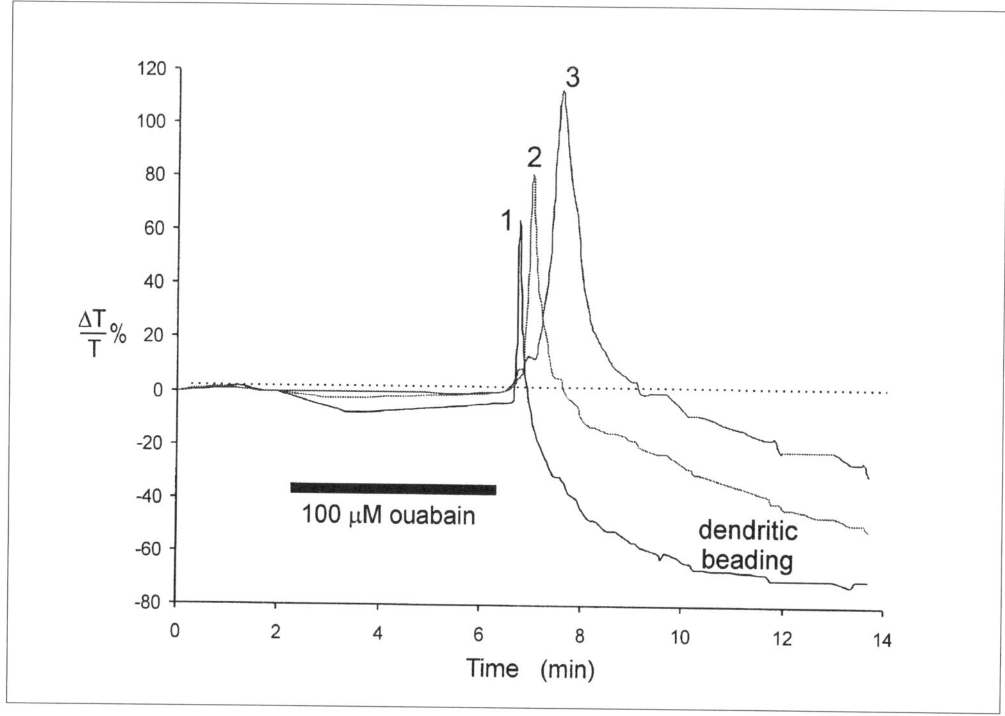

Fig. 3. Spreading AD induced in mouse neocortex by bath application of ouabain at 35 °C. *A*. Time course of light transmittance changes in three zones of interest in layers II/III. The peak transmittance values in each zone represents propagation of the AD front along the neocortex. The graph also shows a quick return to baseline which then evolves into an irreversible transmittance decrease, denoting damage.

Brief bath application of 100 μM ouabain, a Na^+/K^+ ATPase inhibitor, elicited a spreading signal that was remarkably similar to that induced by OGD. In all 14 mouse slices tested at 35 °C, it ignited in layers II/III of the neocortex after approximately 4 min of ouabain exposure. Again, a focal LT increase expanded and migrated as a front across the neocortex (and later in the striatum) at about 2.5 mm/min (Fig. 3). In some cases, there were two sites of ignition in the neocortex that propagated and collided (not shown). As with OGD, propagation was immediately followed by an irreversible decrease in LT only in regions where the signal front had passed.

It could be argued that the slicing procedure stresses the tissue to the point that the metabolic demands of the spreading signal provides a 'death blow'. However our slices support *repeated* spreading depression induced by briefly elevated K^+ under a normal metabolic regime (Fig. 4A). Note that while a secondary swelling followed each episode, there was no ensuing damage (i.e. no negative LT values). Thus the SD event itself is not damaging. However when

along the neocortex. By 17 minutes, all zones display an irreversible decrease in LT, representing neuronal damage. *C*. The evoked field potential, recorded prior to AD, is permanently lost following AD. *D*. Extracellular field recordings in response to OGD. A negative shift recorded in the neocortex is followed by a second negative shift in the striatum 1.5 minutes later. *E*. In another slice, the front in neocortex propagates ~3 min earlier than in striatum. In both regions, the propagating signal leads to irreversible decreases in light transmittance.

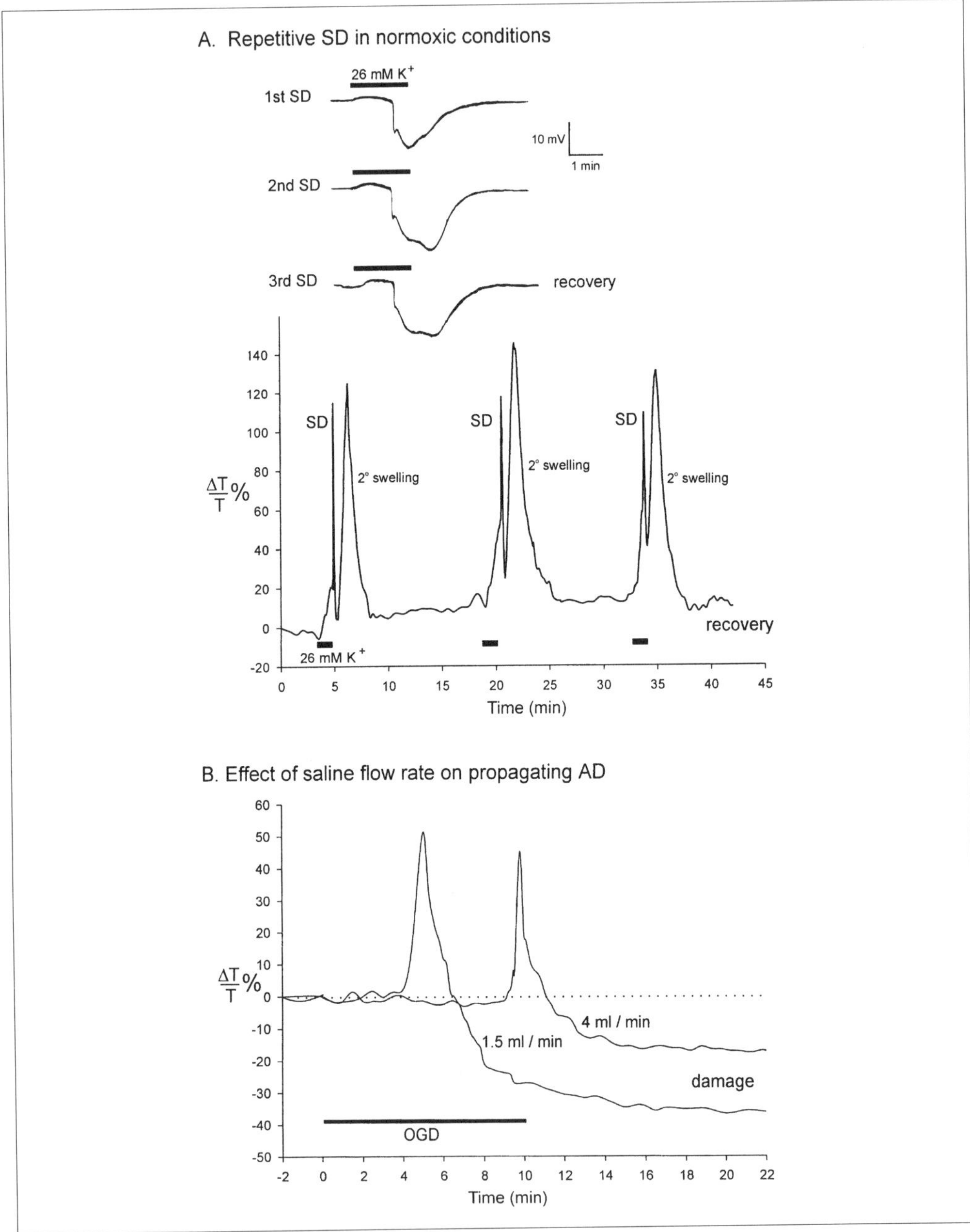

Fig. 4A. Classic spreading depression (SD) can be repeatedly induced in the rat neocortical slice by briefly elevating extracellular [K^+] in the superfusate. Secondary swelling follows each SD event but may be an effect from elevated K^+ rather than from the SD itself. No tissue damage follows SD as shown by a lack of negative light transmittance developing post-SD. Also, SD can be repeatedly evoked unlike the AD. B. AD onset is delayed and post-AD damage can be reduced by increasing the superfusion rate of the aCSF. Both observations imply that the slice is initially healthier at the fast rate and that post-SD damage can be modulated by the less stressful conditions of a 'fast flow' regime.

combined with a metabolic deficit, the slice becomes more compromised. When the flow rate of the aCSF over the slice is slowed (Fig. 4B), the signal initiates sooner and results in more damage. This is denoted by the greater negative optical value, implicating that more dendritic beading develops under the slower superfusion regime.

Anoxic Depolarization or Spreading Depression?

In normal metabolic conditions there is no doubt that the response in Figure 4A is classic spreading depression (SD) because the signal is propagating, repeatable and does not cause tissue damage. Moreover the negative shift is brief (~90s) and returns to baseline. This 'normoxic' SD contrasts with the negative shift during OGD (or ouabain exposure) which is more prolonged and often does not return to baseline (Fig. 1D). On this basis we propose that the AD in vivo is a focally initiating and propagating signal, not unlike classic SD. We have previously termed it 'ischemic-SD' in our hippocampal studies (Obeidat and Andrew 1998; Obeidat et al. 2000). We envision AD as being the 'ischemic' extreme of normal SD where post-signal damage increases with regional metabolic demand (Fig. 1).

Glutamate Receptors and Anoxic Depolarization

To test the potential role of glutamate receptors in the SD-like response to OGD, the non-specific glutamate antagonist kynurenate (2 mM) was applied 15–40 min before, during and after OGD at 37.5 °C. Treatment with kynurenate did not prevent the initiation and propagation of AD induced by 10 min of OGD in 9 of 9 rat neocortical slices tested (not shown). Moreover, kynurenate did not significantly alter the AD onset time nor the propagation rate (Jarvis et al. in press). The negative shift recorded extracellularly in layers II/III was similar in waveform to slices without kynurenate (n = 6, not shown). In support of these findings, treatment of slices with a combination of an NMDA and a non-NMDA receptor antagonist, AP-5 (D-isomer, 25 μM) and CNQX (10 μM) respectively, did not prevent OGD-induced SD in 5 of 5 slices tested (Fig. 5). Neither the time to onset nor the propagation rate were altered by AP-5/CNQX treatment (Jarvis et al. in press). Likewise treatment with 50 μM of the D-isomer of AP-5 alone was ineffective in 5 of 5 slices tested (not shown).

Ischemic SD could also be generated by OGD in the underlying hippocampus (Fig. 5 arrow). The signal usually spread from CA1 to dentate gyrus, but never into CA3. As such the CA3 region was always spared from post signal damage (Obeidat and Andrew 1998). The latency to signal onset in the CA1 region was 7:45 ± 1:27 (n = 7), an average of 3 min after SD onset in neocortex. The onset time was in keeping with that reported in isolated hippocampal slices (Obeidat and Andrew 1998) and so was independent of the signal in the overlying neocortex. The propagation rate in the hippocampus ranged between 0.6 and 2 mm/min. In the hippocampus (n = 6), the AD was delayed in the presence of kynurenate, in agreement with previous observations (Obeidat et al. 2000) and persisted in the presence of AP-5/CNQX (n = 3). Most importantly in both neocortex and hippocampus, treatment with glutamate receptor antagonists did not affect the subsequent reduction in LT which represents neuronal damage (Fig. 5).

If extracellular glutamate accumulation has a role in OGD-induced AD, then glutamate receptor agonists should elicit a propagating signal in a pattern similar to OGD. However, the application of 100 μM NMDA at 37.5 °C (n = 8, not shown) first produced a generalized, not focal, elevation in LT which developed more slowly and did not propagate (Jarvis et al. in press).

Sigma Receptor (σR) Ligands and Ischemic SD

We have carried out a preliminary study of the effects of σ_1R ligands (10–100 uM) upon the AD induced by OGD or ouabain treatment as summarized in the following table:

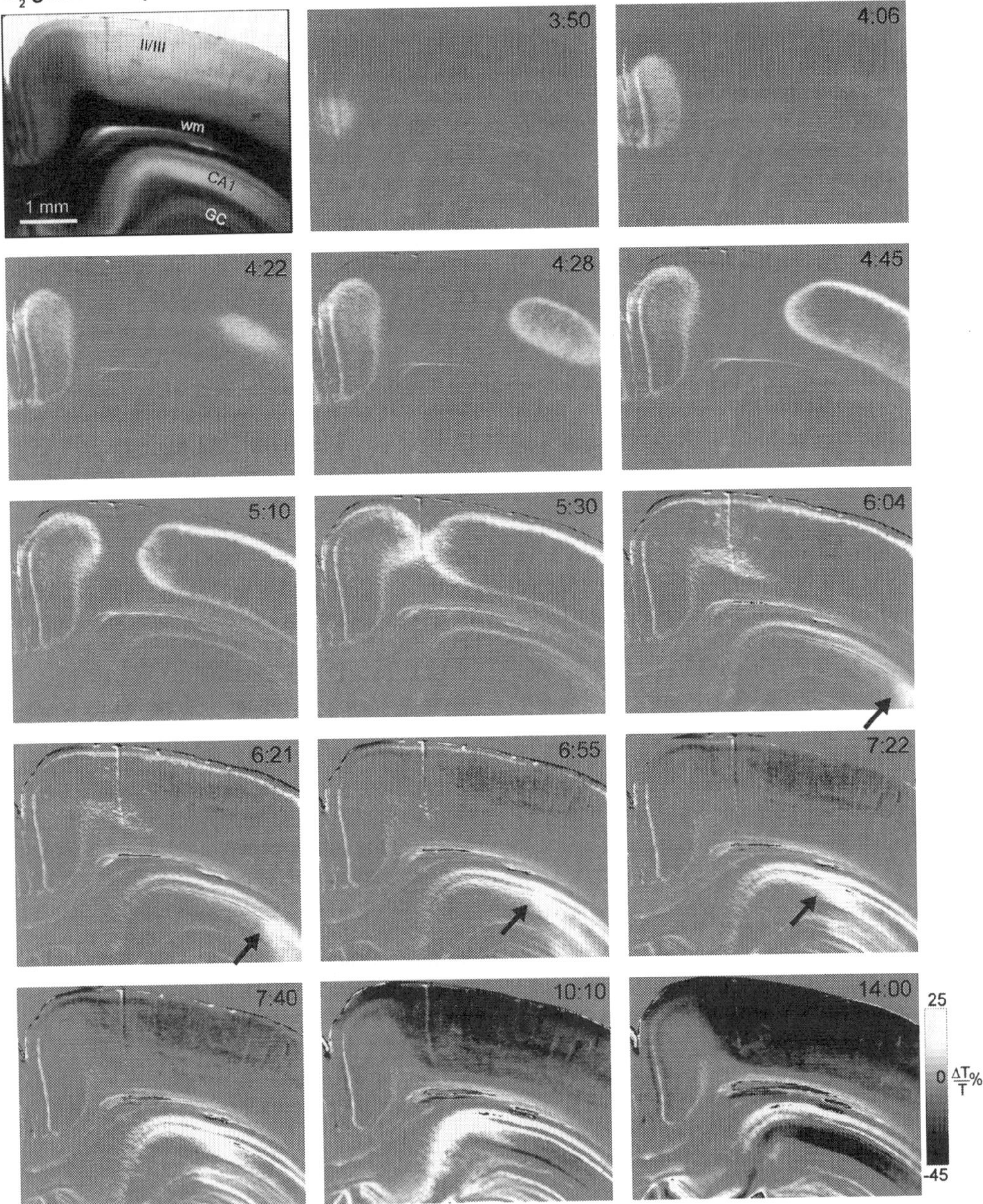

Fig. 5. OGD-induced spreading depression in neocortical gray is not altered by glutamate receptor antagonists. Bath application of AP-5 (25 µM) and CNQX (10 µM) applied 15 min before, during and after OGD does not block the spreading AD front (white signal) or slow migration of the AD front across neocortical grey and the hippocampus. AD initiates later in the CA1 region (arrow, 6:04), and in underlying granule cells (GC) but not in the CA3 region (not shown). Neuronal damage slowly arises in the wake of AD (black signal).

R ligand	binds	agonist/antag	binding to NMDAR	reference	action upon AD*
DM	σ_1R	agonist	+++	Quirion et al. 1992	blocks
CP	σ_1R	agonist	+	Quirion et al. 1992	blocks
DTG	σ_1R,σ_2R	agonist	+	Kobayashhi et al. 1997	blocks
4-IBP	σ_1R?	agonist	–	Whittemore et al. 1997	blocks
(+)-3PPP	σ_1R	antagonist	+	Watling 1998	opposes block

* unpublished data; 10–20 min OGD at 35 °C

In striking contrast to GluR antagonists, σR ligands such as dextromethorphan (DM) and carbetapentane (CP) inhibit ischemic AD initiation, thereby protecting the slice from post-AD damage. The exception is (+)-3PPP which does not inhibit AD. However in slices pretreated with (+)-3PPP, DM inhibition of the AD is lost, presumably because (+)-3PPP occupies, but does not activate, the σ_1 receptor. Since only DM has a high affinity for NMDA receptors, these effects appear to be acting through the σ_1 receptor. We have also found that DM and CP block classic SD in normoxic neocortical slices (Anderson et al. 2000).

Discussion

Measuring intrinsic optical signals (IOSs) provides a means of monitoring cell swelling and the ensuing acute neuronal damage induced by stroke-like conditions (Obeidat and Andrew 1998; Obeidat et al. 2000). Light transmittance increases across submerged brain slices when cells swell (reviewed by Jarvis et al. 1999; Andrew et al. 1999; Aitken et al. 1999). Hippocampal slices acutely damaged by excitotoxic stress (Polischuk et al. 1998; Jarvis et al. 1999) or by OGD (Obeidat et al. 2000) develop a *reduced* light transmittance (LT) in dendritic regions, the result of dendritic "beading". Varicosities form along dendrites in response to brief but acute metabolic stress. The beading of hundreds of dendrites across the thickness of the slice is of an ideal configuration to scatter light, reducing LT even as the tissue continues to swell (Jarvis et al. 1999). In hippocampal slices, an acutely damaged cell body layer displays permanently *increased* LT because dendrites are sparce. In neocortex, dendrites are distributed across all layers so early neuronal cell body and glial swelling (which increases LT) is eventually overwhelmed by beading (which decreases LT). As observed in vivo (Nedergaard and Hansen 1998) and in neocortical slices (Footit and Newberry 1998), repeated SD under *normoxic* conditions causes no damage to rat neocortical slices in the form of reduced LT or loss of the evoked field potential (Anderson et al. 1999). The current study of the spreading signal evoked by ischemia-like conditions in the brain slice demonstrates that acute neuronal damage in neocortex and striatum is caused by the high metabolic demand created by both the spreading signal *and* O_2/glucose deprivation. This signal apparently represents the anoxic depolarization (AD) because it arises concurrently with the negative voltage shift and is followed by acute neuronal damage. Our experiments show that the AD is 'SD-like' in that it arises suddenly, is multifocal and propagates.

We found that depriving the rat or mouse neocortical brain slice of oxygen/glucose, or inhibiting Na^+/K^+ ATPase with ouabain induces the spreading signal in neocortex and independently in striatum or hippocampus. A single extracellular electrode records the AD, but misses the spreading nature of the signal. The negative shift and the LT front are correlated in time and space. Only in areas where AD passed did an irreversible decrease in LT develop within 10 minutes of the insult. Several lines of evidence indicate that this represents neuronal damage. Obeidat et al. (2000) showed that a similar LT reduction was associated with damage to CA1 dendrites in the wake of AD. Filling single CA1 neurons with the fluorescent dye lucifer yellow post-AD revealed extensive dendritic beading not observed in control tissue. Likewise in the present study, irreversible decreases in LT occurred only where AD propagated; the evoked field potential was lost in these areas. Our results indicate that irreversible neuronal damage is not due to metabolic compromise of OGD alone, but is contingent upon AD occurring concurrently which increases energy demand (Obrenovitch and Urenjak 1997a).

Blocking the Anoxic Depolarization

We found no significant difference in the peak LT values (i.e. cell swelling) at the AD front between control slices and those pretreated with glutamate antagonists such as 2 mM kynurenate. In addition, there was no significant difference in the time of AD onset, propagation rate or the extent of LT reversal in hippocampus (Obeidat et al. 2000) or in neocortex (Joshi and Andrew in press; Jarvis et al. in press). Kynurenate (2 mM) abolished the evoked field potential when bath applied to the hippocampal slice, indicating that this dose effectively antagonized NMDA receptors.

These results are consistent with several electrophysiological studies of intact animals. Competitive and non-competitive NMDA antagonists (but not non-NMDA receptor antagonists) block normoxic SD but are ineffective against the AD (see Introduction). MK-801 reduces the number of SD events and infarct size possibly by inhibiting SD onset in tissue away from the core where conditions are less ischemic (Fig. 6). The implication is that accumulating extracellular glutamate is only one of the several factors that contribute to AD and PID genesis and to the ischemic damage (Obrenovitch and Urenjak 1997). Our slice studies suggest that during global ischemia in vivo, AD initiates at multiple sites and propagates out-

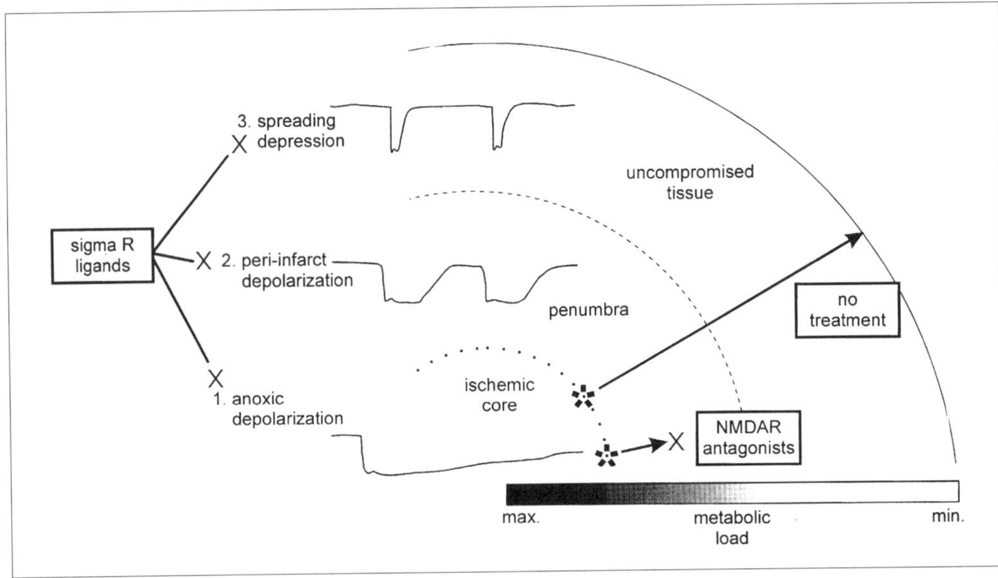

Fig. 6. NMDA antagonists, which block SD in normoxic regions may partly protect from acute stroke damage by blocking PIDs (and resultant damage) in the penumbra regions well removed from the core. In contrast, we hypothesize that certain sigma receptor (σR) ligands may be protective even in regions of high metabolic stress (i.e. the ischemic core and inner penumbra) by blocking AD onset and/or recurring PIDs. We propose that the AD, PID and SD represent a response continuum whereby the ability to quickly repolarize (and so lower metabolic demand) is determined by the available energy stores.

wards from each focus, like the ripples from several stones thrown in a pond. In their wake the ripples leave further energetically compromised gray matter.

An important reason why acute stroke damage is difficult to prevent (other than by restoring blood supply or lowering temperature) is because the AD and PIDs are so resistant to pharmacological blockade. However $sigma_1$ receptor ligands such as dextromethorphan or carbetapentane block ischemic and normoxic SD in neocortical slice preparations (Anderson et al. 2000). Our findings presented here suggest that an ideal stroke treatment would uncouple AD and PIDs from ischemia yet be clinically tolerable. Sigma receptor ligands may prove useful in this regard. A recent study by During et al. (2000) has demonstrated the possibility of inducing NMDAR autoantibody production by an oral adeno-associated virus vaccine. Antibodies penetrate into the brain only in the ischemic region where the blood-brain barrier breaks down. A similar approach to the sigma1 receptor might prove protective during stroke.

To conclude, the anoxic depolarization and peri-infarct depolarization within brain regions of severely reduced blood flow promote neuronal damage at the onset of ischemia. Glutamate receptor antagonists have no effect on this process, indicating that glutamate neither triggers nor significantly drives the depolarization. In contrast, the inhibition of recurrent PIDs by $sigma_1R$ ligands might reduce stroke damage if they prove clinically tolerable and if administered during the 3 hour period following stroke when PID recurs. These drugs might also be effective in blocking the AD if taken prophylactically.

Acknowledgements

This work was supported by the Heart and Stroke Foundation of Ontario (Grant B-4003) and the Canadian Institutes for Health Research.

References

1. Aitken PG, Fayuk D, Somjen GG, Turner DA (1999) Use of intrinsic optical signals to monitor physiological changes in brain tissue slices. Methods: A Companion to Methods in Enzymology 18:91–103
2. Aitken PG, Jing J, Young J, Somjen GG (1991) Ion channel involvement in hypoxia-induced spreading depression in hippocampal slices. Brain Res 541:7–11
3. Albers GW, Atkinson RP, Kelley RE, Rosenbaum DM (1995) Safety, tolerability, and pharmacokinetics of the N-methyl-D-aspartate antagonist dextrorphan in patients with acute stroke. Stroke 26:254–258
4. Anderson TA, Biedermann AJ, Andrew RD (2000) Sigma receptor ligands block spreading depression in rat neocortical slices. Soc. Neurosci. Abstr. 26, in press
5. Anderson, TA, Jarvis CR, Andrew RD (1999) Imaging repetitive spreading depression in submerged neocortical slices. Soc. Neurosci. Abstr. 25:740
6. Andrew RD, Jarvis CR, Obeidat AS (1999) Potential sources of intrinsic optical signals imaged in live brain slices. Methods: A Companion to Methods in Enzymology 18:185–196
7. Back T, Ginsberg MD, Dietrich WD, Watson BD (1996) Induction of spreading depression in the ischemic hemisphere following experimental middle cerebral artery occlusion: Effect on infarct morphology. J Cereb Blood Flow Metab 16:202–213
8. Balestrino M (1995) Studies on anoxic depolarization. In: Brain Slices in Basic and Clinical Research. Eds: (Shurr A, Rigor BM, eds), CRC Press, London pp 273–293
9. Balestrino M, Young J, Aitken P (1999) Block of (Na^+, K^+) ATPase with ouabain induces spreading depression-like depolarization in hippocampal slices. Brain Res. 838:37–44
10. Basarsky TA, Duffy SN, Andrew RD, MacVicar BA (1998) Imaging spreading depression and associated intracellular calcium waves in brain slices. J Neurosci 18:7189–7199
11. Beal MF, Hyman BT, Koroshetz W (1993) Do defeats in mitochondrial energy metabolism underlie the pathology of neurodegenerative diseases? Trends Neurosci 16:125–131
12. Benveniste H, Drejer J, Schousboe A, Diemer NH (1984) Elevation of the extracellular concentrations of glutamate and aspartate in the rat hippocampus during transient focal ischemia monitored by intracerebral microdialysis. J Neurochem 43:1369–1374
13. Bolser CD, Hey JA, Chapman RW (1999) Influence of central antitussive drugs on the cough motor pattern. J Appl Physiol 86:1017–1024
14. Bouchard P, Quirion R (1996) [^{3}H]1,2-Di(2-tolyl)guanidine and [^{3}H](+)Pentazocine binding sites in the rat brain: autoradiographic visualization of the putative $sigma_1$ and $sigma_2$ receptor subtypes. Neuroscience 76:467–477
15. Buchan AM, Slivka A, Xue D (1992) The effect of the NMDA receptor antagonist MK-801 on cerebral blood flow and infarct volume in experimental focal stroke. Brain Res 574:171–177
16. Busch E, Gyngell ML, Eis M, Hoehn BM, Hossman KA (1996) Potassium-induced cortical spreading depressions during focal cerebral ischemia in rats: Contributioni to lesion growth assessed by diffusion-weighted NMR and biochemical imaging. J Cerb Blood Flow Metab 16:1090–1099
17. Cho S, Takeda Y, Pulsinelli W (1992) Ischemic damage to CA1 hippocampus correlates poorly with glutamate release during ischemia. Soc Neurosci Abstr 18:570
18. Choi DE (1991) Excitotoxicity. In: Excitatory amino acid antagonists (Meldum BS, ed), Oxford, Blackwell Scientific Publications, pp 216–236
19. Choi DW (1994) Glutamate receptors and the induction of excitotoxic neuronal death. Prog Brain Res 100:47–51

20. Chou YC, Liao JF, Chang WY, Lin MF, Chen CF (1999) Binding of dimemorfan to sigma-a receptor and its anticonvulsant and locomotor effects in mice, compared with dextromethorphan and dextrorphan. Brain Res 821:516–519
21. Church J, Shacklock JA, Baimbridge KG (1991) Dextromethorphan and phencyclidine receptor ligands: Differential effects on K^+- and NMDA-evoked increases in cytosolic free Ca^{2+} concentration. Neurosci Lett 124:232–234
22. Dijkhuizen RM, Beekwilder JP, van der Worp HB, van der Sprenkel JWB, Tulleken KAF, Nicolay K (1999) Correlation between tissue depolarizations and damage in focal ischemic rat brain. Brain Res 840:194–205
23. During MJ, Symes CW, Lawlor PA (2000) An oral vaccine against NMDAR1 with efficacy in experimental stroke and epilepsy. Science 287:1453–1460
24. Dragunow M, Beilharz E, Sirimanne E, Lawlor P, Williams C, Bravo R, Gluckman P (1994) Immediate-early gene protein expression in neurons undergoing delayed death, but not necrosis, following hypoxic-ischaemic injury to the young rat brain. Mol Brain Res 25:19–33
25. Dugan LL, Bruno VMG, Amagasu SM, Gifford RG (1995) Glia modulate the response of murine cortical neurons to excitotoxicity: glia exacerbate AMPA neurotoxicity. J Neurosci 15:4545–4555
26. Edwards FA (1995) Anatomy and electrophysiology of fast central synapses lead to a structural model for long-term potentiation. Physiol Rev 75:59–787
27. Faddis BT, Hasbani MJ, Goldberg MP (1997) Calpain activation contributes to dendritic remodeling after brief excitotoxic injury in vitro. J Neurosci 17:951–959
28. Ferris CD, Hirsch DJ, Brooks BP, Snyder SH (1991) $\sigma\sigma$ Receptors: From Molecule to Man. J Neurochem 57:729–737
29. Footit DR, Newberry NR (1998) Cortical spreading depression induces an LTP-like effect in rat neocortex in vivo. Brain Res 781:339–34
30. George CP, Goldberg MP, Choi DW, Steinberg GK (1988) Dextromethorphan reduces neocortical ischemic neuronal damage in vivo. Brain Res 440:375–379
31. Gill R, Andiné P, Hillered L, Persson L, Hagberg H. (1992) The effect of MK-801 on cortical spreading depression in the penumbral zone following focal ischaemia in the rat. J Cereb Blood Flow and Metab 12:371–379
32. Goldberg MP (2000) Stroke Trials Database, Internet Stroke Center, Wash U (*http://www.neuro.wustl.edu/stroke*)
33. Gundlach AL, Largent BL, Snyder SH (1986) Autoradiographic localization of sigma receptor binding sites in guinea pig and rat central nervous system with (+)^{3}H-3-(3-hydroxyphenyl)-N-(1-propyl)piperdine. J Neurosci 6:1757–1779
34. Haddad GG, Jiang C (1992) O_2 deprivation in the central nervous system: on mechanisms of neuronal response, differential sensitivity, and injury. Prog Neurobiol 40:277–318
35. Hammond C, Crepel V, Gozlan H, Ben AY (1994) Anoxic LTP sheds light on the multiple facets of NMDA receptors. Trends Neurosci 17:497–503
36. Hanner M, Moebius FF, Flannorfer A, Knaus HG, Striessnig J, Kempner E, Glossman H (1996) Purification, molecular cloning, and expression of the mammalian sigma$_1$-binding site. Proc Natl Acad Sci 93:8072–8077
37. Hernandez-Caceres J, Maclas-Gonzales K, Brozek G, Bures J (1987) Systemic ketamine blocks cortical spreading depression but does not delay the onset of terminal anoxic depression. Brain Res 437:360–364
38. Higashida H, Mitarai G, Watanabe S (1974) A comparative study of membrane potential changes in neurons and neuroglial cells during spreading depression in the rabbit. Brain Res 65:411–425
39. Hong W, Werling LL (1998) Investigation of the involvement of heterotrimeric guanine nucleotide regulatory proteins in sigma$_1$ receptor signaling in rodent brain. Soc Neurosci Abstr 24, 1593
40. Hori N, Carpenter DO (1994) Functional and morphological changes induced by transient in vivo ischemia. Exptl Neurol 129:279–289
41. Iijima T, Mies G, Hossman KA (1992) Repeated negative DC deflections in rat cortex following middle cerebral artery occlusion are abolished by MK-801: effect on volume of ischemic injury. J Cereb Blood Flow Metab 12:727–733
42. Jarvis CR, Lilge L, Vipond GJ, Andrew RD (1999) Interpretation of intrinsic optical signals and calcein fluorescence during acute excitotoxic insult in the hippocampal slice. NeuroImage 10:357–372
43. Jarvis CR, Anderson TR, Andrew RD (2000) The anoxic depolarization mediates acute damage independent of glutamate in neocortical brain slices. Cerebral Cortex (in press)
44. Jing J, Aitken PG, Somjen GG (1993) Role of calcium channels in spreading depression in rat hippocampal slices. Brain Res 604:251–259
45. Joseph DB, Bowen WE (1998) Sigma receptor ligands robustly stimulate [^{35}S]GTP$\gamma\gamma$S binding to intact sk-n-sh neuroblastoma cells but not to sk-n-sh cell membrane preparations. Soc Neurosci Abstr 24:1594
46. Joshi I, Andrew RD (2000) Imaging anoxic depolarization during ischemia-like conditions in the mouse hemi-brain slice. J Neurophysiol (in press)
47. Klette KL, DeCoster MA, Moreton JE, Tortella FC (1995) Role of calcium in sigma-mediated neuroprotection in rat primary cortical neurons. Brain Res 704:31–41
48. Klette KL, Lin Y, Clapp LE, DeCoster MA, Moreton JE, Tortella FC (1997) Neuroprotective sigma ligands attenuate NMDA and trans-ACPD-induced calcium signalling in rat primary neurons. Brain Res 756:231–240
49. Kohling R, Schmidinger A, Hulsmann S, Vanhatalo S, Luke A, Straub H, Speckman E-J, Tuxhorn I, Wolf P, Lahl R, Pannek H, Oppel F, Griener C, Moskopp D, Wassmann H (1996) Anoxic terminal negative DC-shift in human neocoritcal slices in vitro. Brain Res 741:174–179
50. Koroleva VI, Korolev OS, Loseva E, Bures J. (1998) The effect of MK-801 and of brain-derived polypeptides on the development of ischemic lesion induced by photothrombotic occlusion of the distal middle cerebral artery in rats. Brain Res 786:104–114
51. Lauritzen M, Hansen AJ (1992) The effect of glutamate receptor blockade on anoxic depolarization and cortical spreading depression. J Cereb Blood Flow Metab 12:223–229
52. Leao AAP (1947) Further observations on the spreading depression of activity in the cerebral cortex. J Neurophysiol 10:409–414
53. Lee JM, Zipfel GJ, Choi DW (1999) The changing landscape of ischaemic brain injury mechanisms. Nature 399:A7–A14
54. Leitner Ml, Hohmann AG, Patrick SL, Walker JM (1994) Regional variation in the ratio σ_1 to σ_2 binding in rat brain. Euro J Pharmacol 259:65–69
55. Limbrick DD, Churn SB, Sombati S, Delorenzo RJ (1995) Inability to restore resting intracellular calcium levels as an early indicator of delayed neuronal cell death. Brain Res 690:145–156
56. Lockhart BP, Soulard P, Benicourt C, Privat A, Junien J-L (1995) Distinct neuroprotective profiles for $\sigma\sigma$ ligands against N-methyl-D-aspartate (NMDA), and hypoxia-mediated neurotoxicity in neuronal culture toxicity studies. Brain Res 675:110–120
57. Marrannes R, Willems R, DePrins E (1988) Evidence for a role of the NMDA receptor in cortical spreading depression in the rat. Brain Res 457:226–240
58. McCulloch J, Ozyurt E, Park CK, Nehls DG, Teasdale GM, Graham DI (1993) Glutamate receptor antagonists in experi-

mental focal cerebral ischaemia. Acta Neurochir Suppl 57:73–79
59. Mies G, Kohno K, Hossmann KA (1994) Prevention of periinfarct direct current shifts with glutamate antagonist NBQX following occlusion of the middle cerebral artery in the rat. J Cereb Blood Flow Metab 14:802–807
60. Moebius FF, Streissnig J, Glossmann H (1997) The mysteries of sigma receptors: new family members reveal a role in cholesterol synthesis. Trends Pharmacol Sci 18:67–70
61. Nallet H, MacKenzie ET, Roussel S (1999) The nature of penumbral depolarizations following focal cerebral ischemia in the rat. Brain Res 842:148–158
62. Nedergaard M, Hansen AJ (1988) Spreading depression is not associated with neuronal injury in the normal brain. Brain Res 449:395–398
63. Nedergaard M. (1996) Spreading depression as a contributor to ischemic brain damage. Advan Neurobiol 71:75–84
64. Nellgard B, Wieloch T (1992) NMDA-receptor blockers but not NBQX, an AMPA-receptor antagonist, inhibit spreading depression in the rat brain. Acta Physiol Scand 146:497–503
65. Obeidat A, Jarvis CR, Andrew RD (2000) Glutamate does not mediate acute neuronal damage following spreading depression induced by O_2/glucose deprivation in the hippocampal slice. J Cereb Blood Flow Metab 20:412–422
66. Obeidat A, Andrew RD (1998). Spreading depression determines acute cellular damage in the hippocampal slice during oxygen/glucose deprivation. Euro J Neurosci 10:3451–3461
67. Obrenovitch TP (1999) High extracellular glutamate and neuronal death in neurological disorders: Cause, contribution, or consequence. Ann NY Acad Sci 890:273–286
68. Obrenovich TP, Urenjak J, Richards DA, Euda Y, Curzon G, Symon L (1993) Extracellular neuroactive amino acids in the rat stratum during ischemia: Comparison between penumbral conditions and ischemia with sustained anoxic depolarization. J Neurochem 61:178–186
69. Obrenovitch TP, Urenjak J (1997a) Altered glutamatergic transmission in neurological disorders: from high extracellular glutamate to excessive synaptic efficacy. Progr Neurobiol 51:37–87
70. Obrenovitch TP, Urenjak J (1997b) Is high extracellular glutamate the key to excitotoxicity in traumatic brain injury? J Neurotrauma 14:677–697
71. Obrenovitch TP, Zilkha E, Urenjak J (1996) Evidence against high extracellular glutamate promoting the elicitation of spreading depression by potassium. J Cereb. Blood Flow Metab 16:923–931
72. Otsuka H, Ueda K, Heimann A, Kempski O (2000) Effects of cortical spreading depression on cortical blood flow, impedance, DC potential and infarct size in a rat venous infarct model. Exptl Neurol 162:201–214
73. Park JS, Bateman MC, Goldberg MP (1996) Rapid alterations in dendrite morphology during sublethal hypoxia or glutamate receptor activation. Neurobiol Disease 3:215–227
74. Phan VL, Alonso G, Legrand A, Anoal M, Urani A, Maurice T (1999) Immunocytochemical localization of the $sigma_1$ receptor in the central nervous system of the adult rat and mouse. Soc Neurosci Abstr 25, 1473
75. Polischuk TM, Jarvis CR, Andrew RD (1998) Intrinsic optical signaling denoting neuronal damage in response to acute excitotoxic insult in the hippocampal slice. Neurobiol Disease 4:423–437
76. Prince DA, Feeser HR (1988) Dextromethorphan protects against cerebral infarction in a rat model of hypoxia-ischemia. Neurosci Lett 85:291–296
77. Quirion R, Bowen WD, Itzhak Y, Junien JL, Musacchio JM, Rothman RB, Tam SW, Taylor DP (1992) A proposal for the classification of sigma binding sites. Trends Pharmacol Sci 13:85–86
78. Riepe MW, Hori N, Ludolph AC, Carpenter DO (1995) Failure of neuronal ion exchange, not potential excitation, causes excitotoxicity after inhibition of oxidative phosphorylation. Neuroscience 64:91–97
79. Rosenberg PA, Aizenman E. (1989) Hundred-fold increase in neuronal vulnerability to glutamate toxicity in astrocyte-poor cultures of rat cerebral cortex. Neurosci Lett 103:162–168
80. Rossi DJ, Oshima T, Attwell D (1999) Glutamate release in severe brain ischemia is mainly by reversed uptake. Nature 403:316–321
81. Schreiber SS, Baudry M (1995) Selective neuronal vulnerability in the hippocampus – a role for gene expression? Trends Neurosci 18:446–451
82. Senda T, Mita S, Kaneda K, Kikuchi M, Akaike A (1998) Effect of SA4503, a novel σσ, receptor agonist, against glutamate neurotoxicity in cultured rat retinal neurons. Euro J Pharmacol 342:105–111
83. Seth P, Fei YJ, Li HW, Huang W, Leibach FH, Ganapathy V (1998) Cloning and Functional Characterization of a σ Receptor from Rat Brain. J Neurochem 70:922–931
84. Sick TJ, LaManna LC (1995) Intrinsic optical properties of brain slices: useful indices of electrophysiology and metabolism. In: Brain Slices in Basic and Clinical Research. (Schurr A, Rigor BM, eds), CRC Press Inc, London, pp 47–63
85. Steinberg GK, George CP, DeLaPaz R, Shibata DK, Gross T (1988a) Dextromethorphan Protects Against Cerebral Injury Following Transient Focal Ischemia in Rabbits. Stroke 29:1112–1118
86. Steinberg GK, Lo EH, Kunis DM, Grant GA, Poljak A, DeLaPaz R (1991) Dextromethorphan alters cerebral blood flow and protects against cerebral injury following focal ischemia. Neurosci Lett 133:225–228
87. Steinberg GK, Saleh J, Kunis D (1988b) Delayed treatment with dextromethorphan and dextrorphan reduces cerebral damage after transient focal ischemia. Neurosci Lett 89:193–197
88. Sugaya E, Takato M, Noda Y (1975) Neuronal and Glial Activity During Spreading Depression in Cerebral Cortex of Cat. J Neurophysiol 38:822–841
89. Takagi K, Ginsberg MD, Globus MY-T, Dietrich WD, Martinez E, Kraydieh S, Busto R (1993) Changes in amino acid neurotransmitters and cerebral blood flow in the ischemic penumbral region following middle cerebral artery occlusion in the rat: correlation with histopathology. J Cereb Blood Flow Metab 13:575–585
90. Takano K, Latour LL, Formato JE, Carano RA , Helmer KG, Hasegawa Y, Sotak CH, Fisher M (1996) The role of spreading depression in focal ischemia evaluated by diffusion mapping. Annals Neurol 39:308–318
91. Takahashi H, Traystman RJ, Hashimoto K, London ED, Kirsch JR (1997) Postischemic Brain Injury Is Affected Stereospecifically by Pentazocine in Rats. Anesth Analg 85:353–357
92. Takahashi H, Kirsch JR, Hashimoto K, London ED, Koehler RC, Traystman RJ (1996) PPBP[4-Phenyl-1-(4-Decreases Brain Injury After Transient Focal Ischemia in Rats. Stroke 27:2120–2123
93. Taylor CP, Narasimhan LS (1997) Sodium channels and therapy of central nervous system diseases. Advan Pharmacol 39:47–98
94. Taylor CP, Weber ML, Gaughan CL, Lehning EJ, LoPachin RM (1999) Oxygen/glucose deprivation in hippocampal slices: altered intraneuronal elemental composition predicts structural and functional damage. J Neurosci 19:619–629
95. Tortella FC, Pellicano M, Bowery NG (1989) Dextromethorphan and neuromodulation: old drug coughs up new activities. Trends Pharmacol Sci 10:501–507
96. Turski L, Turski WA (1993) Towards an understanding of the role of glutamate in neurodegenerative disorders: energy metabolism and neuropathology. Experientia 49:1064–1072

97. Vilner BJ, Coop A, Williams S, Bowen WD (1999) Sigma-2 receptor antagonists: Inhibition of agonist-induced calcium release and cytotoxicity in sk-n-sk neuroblastoma. Soc Neurosci Abstr 25:1475
98. Watling KJ (1998) The RBI Handbook, 3rd ed., RBI, Natick, MA.
99. Welsh KMA (1997) Pathogenesis of migraine. Seminars Neurol 17:335–341
100. Whittemore ER, Ilyin VI, Woodward RM (1997) Antagonism of N-methul-D-aspartate receptors by sigma site ligands: Potency, subtype – selectivity and mechanisms of inhibition. J Pharmacol Exptl Therapeut 282:326–338
101. Wong BY, Coulter DA, Choi DW, Prince DA (1988) Dextrorphan and dextromethorphan, common antitussives, are antiepileptic and antagonize N-methyl-D-aspartate in brain slices. Neurosci Lett 85:261–266
102. Xie Y, Zacharias E, Hoff P, Tegtmeier F (1995) Ion channel involvement in anoxic depolarization induced by cardiac arrest in rat brain. J Cereb Blood Flow Metab 15:587–594
103. Ye Z-C, Sontheimer H (1998) Astrocytes protect neurons from neurotoxic injury by serum glutamate. Glia 22:237–248
104. Yao H, Markgraf CG, Fietrich WD, Prado R, Watson BD, Ginsberg MD (1994) Glutamate antagonist MK-801 attenuates incomplete but not complete infarction in thrombotic distal middle cerebral artery occlusion in Wistar rats. Brain Res 642:117–122
105. Zilka E, Obrenovich TP, Koshy A, Kusakabe H, Bennetto HP (1995) Extracellular glutamate: On-line monitoring using microdialysis coupled to enzyme-amperometric analysis. J Neurosci Meth 60:1–9

Protein phosphatases and neuronal apoptosis

S. Klumpp[1*], D. Selke[1], J. Krieglstein[2]

Abstract

Phosphorylation and dephosphorylation touch on most aspects of cell physiology. It is the function of the vertebrate central nervous system where studies of reversible phosphorylation seem likely to have great impact in the near future. The majority of kinases and phosphatases are expressed in the brain, and many of the novel vertebrate kinases and phosphatases revealed by genomic sequencing will probably function in specific neurons. Transcriptional control and apoptosis are emergent areas. One can foresee that the accumulating knowledge about signaling networks and the proteins involved will permit development of potent and specific pharmacological modulators that can be used therapeutically.

Phosphorylation and dephosphorylation of proteins

Reversible phosphorylation represents the most common post-translational modification of proteins. As much as 30–40% of eukaryotic proteins are subject to reversible, often multiple and interdependent phosphorylation at serine, threonine and tyrosine residues. It is long known that classical metabolic functions and signal transduction pathways involving second messengers like Ca^{2+} and cyclic nucleotides are regulated by reversible phosphorylation. The last decade revealed that, in addition, kinases and phosphatases also integrate and regulate signaling cascades at the level of growth factors and receptors, transcription factors and gene expression.

The dynamic nature of protein phosphorylation implies that phosphorylation levels can be modulated by changes in the activities of protein kinases and/or protein phosphatases. Sequencing of *Saccharomyces cerevisiae* and *Caenorhabditis elegans* genomes revealed that genes encoding protein kinases are abundant and outnumbered only by genes encoding G-protein coupled receptors. For a mammalian genome of 50,000 genes, one can extrapolate and estimate that it contains ~1200 protein kinases and 300–400 protein phosphatases. Since a single protein phosphatase catalytic subunit often associates with several different regulatory subunits, the number of functional phosphatase holoenzymes finally is expected to end up relatively equal to the number of func-

Keywords: Cell death, dephosphorylation, fatty acids, ginkgolic acid, oleic acid, PP2C

[1]Abt. Biochemie, Institut für Pharmazeutische Chemie, Philipps-Universität, Marbacher Weg 6, D-35032 Marburg, Germany, [2]Institut für Pharmakologie und Toxikologie, Philipps-Universität, Ketzerbach 63, D-35037 Marburg, Germany
e-mail: Klumpp@mailer.uni-marburg.de

tional protein kinases. Traditionally much attention has been focused on the role of protein kinases. This is also true for the field of neurochemistry, as exemplified in the chapters of this volume: Cyclin dependent kinases are involved in death signaling (D. S. Park), phosphorylations in the Raf/Mek signaling cascade are important in the mechanisms leading to ischemic tolerance (Dawson and Dawson), activation of NF-κB is induced by phosphorylation (Schneider et al.), and many more contributions. Knowledge about the phosphatases involved is fairly limited. But one can anticipate the dephosphorylating enzymes being as important and representing novel targets.

Protein phosphatases (PP)

The field of protein phosphatases is exciting and moves rapidly. Much ground has been covered since the first identification, isolation and classification of serine/threonine protein phosphatases (Ingebritsen and Cohen 1983) and tyrosine phosphatases (Tonks et al. 1988a, 1988b). In the meantime, the crystal structures of at least 20 phosphatases have been determined yielding important insights into mechanisms of substrate recognition and catalysis.

Serine/threonine protein phosphatases were initially divided according to biochemical parameters into two classes: Type-1 protein phosphatases are inhibited by heat-stable inhibitor-proteins and preferentially dephosphorylate the β-subunit of phosphorylase kinase; whereas type-2 phosphatases are insensitive to these inhibitors and preferentially dephosphorylate the α-subunit of phosphorylase kinase. Type-2 protein phosphatases can be further subdivided into spontaneously active PP2A, Ca^{2+}-dependent PP2B (calcineurin) and Mg^{2+}-dependent PP2C (for review see Wera and Hemmings 1995). Later on, primary structure information of the catalytic subunits, deduced from cDNA cloning, has revealed that PP1, 2A and 2B belong to the same gene family PPP (Barton et al. 1994). Currently, four PP1, two PP2A, three PP2B and five PP2C catalytic subunit isoforms have been identified. Molecular biology has revealed several additional enzymes in the PPP family: PP4, PP5, PP6 and PP7 (Cohen 1997). The latest entry – August 2000 – in the database is PP12 for mammals, and PP16 in *arabidopsis thaliana*. PP2C is structurally different. Five PP2C isoforms together with the pyruvate dehydrogenase phosphatase constitute a distinct gene family, PPM.

Non-catalytic targeting subunits of ser/thr protein phosphatases identified for PP1, 2A and 2B serve to mediate substrate specificity and to regulate the activity of the catalytic moiety. Such adaptor proteins also allow localization to distinct intracellular sites and in some cases even co-localization of kinases and phosphatases on the same protein but at different docking sites (Klauck et al. 1996; Pawson and Scott 1997; for review see Sim and Scott 1999). For instance, Yatiao, an NMDA receptor associated protein, is a scaffold protein that physically attaches protein phosphatase type-1 and cAMP-dependent protein kinase to NMDA receptors to regulate channel activity (Westphal et al. 1999).

Protein *tyrosine* phosphatases (PTP) are another expanding field. They can be divided into three groups: Receptor-like, non-transmembrane cytoplasmic and dual-specificity (acting on P-ser/thr *and* P-tyr) phosphatases. Interest was pushed by the discovery that CD45, a prototype for the family of receptor-linked PTPs plays a direct role in modulating cellular signaling responses through ligand-regulated *dephosphorylation* of tyrosyl residues on proteins (Tonks et al. 1988c). Intriguingly, further studies of CD45 have shown that the same tyrosine phosphatase can have different effects on cell signaling, depending on the cellular context and the particular pathway under investigation: CD45 is a positive regulator of Src family protein tyrosine kinase activity in thymocytes, whereas CD45 negatively regulates macrophage Src family protein tyrosine kinases (Roach et al. 1997). One of the most spectacular recent discoveries within the dual-specificity (ser/thr *and* tyr) tyrosine phosphatases was that PTEN has protein phosphatase as well as lipid phosphatase activitiy (Maehama and Dixon 1998). It has been shown to dephosphorylate phosphoinositides; to act on 3´phospholipids which are generated in response to the PI-3 kinase. It now seems clear that it is the lipid phosphatase activity of the PTEN gene product which is relevant to its tumor suppressor function.

Protein phosphatase type-2C (PP2C)

PP2C was originally identified as a Mg^{2+}-dependent protein phosphatase. Dephosphorylation of [^{32}P]casein in the presence of 20 mM Mg^{2+} is considered the standard technique to determine PP2C activity in vitro (McGowan and Cohen 1988). It is probably the least well characterized member of the ser/thr protein phosphatases. Unlike PP1, 2A and 2B, targeting subunits of PP2C have not been identified. Studying the function of PP2C is further hampered by the fact that no inhibitor is available. Okadaic acid, known to inhibit PP1, 2A and 2B, does not affect the activity of PP2C. The enzyme has a marked preference for phosphothreonyl- over phosphoseryl residues (Pinna and Donella-Deana 1994).

Mammalian PP2C is representative of a large and varied family of protein phosphatases. The two isoforms α and β are most prominent, mainly cytosolic and ubiquitously expressed. They share 75% sequence identity and are enzymatically indistinguishable. They are monomers with an apparent molecular mass of 43–48 kDa. The crystal structure of human PP2Cα revealed a protein fold with a catalytic domain composed of a central β-sandwich that binds two manganese ions, which is surrounded by α-helices (Das et al. 1996). In eukaryotes, PP2Cα and 2Cβ have been implicated in a number of cellular processes including reversal of protein kinase cascades that become activated as a result of stress. PP2C inhibited activation of the p38 and JNK cascades by dephosphorylation and inactivation of MAPKKs and MAPK p38 (Takekawa et al. 1998). PP2C could dephosphorylate Ca^{2+}/calmodulin-dependent protein kinase (CaM kinase II), leading to the generation of Ca^{2+}-independent activity and inhibition of the total activity (Fukunaga et al. 1993). In mammalian hepatocytes, inhibition of cholesterol and fatty acid biosynthesis mediated by activation of the AMP-stimulated protein kinase (AMPK) is reversed by PP2C-catalyzed dephosphorylation of AMPK (Moore et al. 1991). PP2Cα was furthermore found to dephosphorylate and to inactivate cystic fibrosis transmembrane conductance regulator (CFTR) Cl^--channels in epithelia (Travis et al. 1997).

The occurrence of sequences related to PP2C within proteins of diverse functions and origins suggests that the PP2C protein emerged early in evolution. In addition to the α- and β-isoforms described above, sequence related to their catalytic moiety of ~300 amino acids is found in PP2Cγ(FIN13), PP2Cδ and Wip1. These members of the PP2C-family also display Mg^{2+}-dependent, okadaic acid insensitive dephosphorylation. PP2Cγ(FIN13) is localized in nuclei. It is a growth factor-inducible phosphatase of 75 kDa which can inhibit cell cycle progression (Guthridge et al. 1997). The protein is 35% identical to PP2Cα and 2Cβ. It contains an additional highly acidic domain. PP2Cγ (FIN 13) recently had been reported to act as pre-mRNA splicing factor essential for the formation of the spliceosome (Murray et al. 1999). Wip1 is another member of the PP2C family localized in the nucleus. Expression of the 60 kDa Wip1 protein is induced in response to ionising radiation in a p53-dependent manner (Fiscella et al. 1997). PP2Cδ has 30% sequence identity in its catalytic domain with PP2Cα and 2Cβ, lacking a 90-residue carboxy-terminal sequence conserved in the classical PP2C isozymes. It has been suggested that PP2Cδ plays a role in regulation of cell cycle progression (Tong et al. 1998). These examples described PP2C as part of proteins displaying phosphatase activity. In addition, however, amino acid sequence of PP2C is also observed as building block in proteins that lack the capacity of dephosphorylation, e.g. fungal adenylyl cyclase (Bork et al. 1996).

Apoptosis in context with ser/thr protein phosphatases

To investigate how pertubation of phosphorylation and dephosphorylation processes might affect neuronal behavior and survival, it is popular to search for effects of okadaic acid, microcystin, tautomycin or calyculin and conclude about a possible involvement of ser/thr protein phosphatases 1 and 2A. Indeed, nanomolar concentrations of these compounds are inhibitory for PP1 and PP2A. The sensitivity of the enzymes differs by a factor of 10. Literature on that topic will not be discussed herein. One has to be aware, however, that at least PP4 and PP5 are also inhibited by those compounds – in exactly the same concentration range as described for PP1 and 2A. Calcineurin (PP2B) is much less sensitive to inhibition by okadaic acid. Instead, PP2B is inhibited by cyclosporin and FK506. PP2C is insensitive to any of these inhibitors (for review of phosphatase inhibitors see Sheppeck et al. 1997). Four examples will follow presenting more and direct convincing evidence that phosphatases play an important role in apoptotic pathways and interact with different players on distinct levels.

(I) Phosphatases are crucial for the function of the proto-oncogene Bcl-2 to suppress apoptosis (Deng et al. 1998). Bcl-2 is post-translationally modified by phosphorylation via protein kinase C alpha on an evolutionary conserved serine site (ser-70). Phosphorylation of Bcl-2 is required for maximal and potent suppression of apoptosis. Interleukin-3 induces and increases phosphorylation at serine 70. Dephosphorylation is carried by PP2A. In addition, the death action of ceramide has been shown to involve and activate mitochondrial PP2A (Ruvolo et al. 1999) causing more dephosphorylation thus inactivation of Bcl-2 and finally cell death.

(II) There is also evidence for a link to proteases. PP2A was found to be a substrate for caspase-3 (Santoro et al. 1998). Apoptosis involves caspase-3 activation. This enzyme then cleaves the regulatory subunit A_{α} of PP2A thereby increasing the activity of the catalytic moiety of PP2A and finally leading to a decrease in the amount of phosphorylated forms of MAP-kinase.

(III) A phosphatase cascade sequentially involving PP2C, PP2B and PP1 has been reported (Desdouits et al. 1998). The dopamine- and cAMP-regulated phosphoprotein of 32 kDa (DARP-32) is highly expressed in striatonigral neurons. Physiological targets for regulation via DARP-32/PP1 include Ca^{2+}-channels, Na^{+}-channels and Na^{+}, K^{+}-ATPase. DARP-32 becomes a potent inhibitor of PP1 when it is phosphorylated on thr-34 by cAMP- and cGMP-dependent kinases. DARP-32 is also phosphorylated on ser-137 by casein kinase-1. The latter phosphorylation has an important regulatory role since it inhibits dephosphorylation of thr-34 by PP2B. Furthermore, dephosphorylation of ser-137 by PP2C facilitates dephosphorylation of thr-34 thereby removing the cyclic nucleotide induced inhibition of PP1.

(IV) The Ca^{2+}/calmodulin-dependent protein phosphatase calcineurin (PP2B) had been purified for the first time from brain (Klee et al. 1988; for review see Guerini 1997). Afterwards it was shown that it is expressed in a wide range of tissues. PP2B has a relatively narrow substrate specificity, including Ca^{2+}-channels, NMDA- and IP_3-receptors. Immunosuppressants like cyclosporine A and FK506 inhibit PP2B-activity. PP2B triggers dephosphorylation and translocation of the cytosolic subunit of the transcription factor NF-AT into the nucleus, where it induces expression of the interleukin-2 gene, one of the early genes in the T-cell-activation pathway (Luo et al. 1996).

Calcineurin also is a major player in neurochemical processes. PP2B is involved in the regulation of long-term depression (Mulkey et al. 1994). Superoxide dismutase has been shown to prevent inactivation of PP2B – damage to its Fe-Zn active center – by oxidizing agents (Wang et al. 1996). PP2B facilitates or even induces apoptosis in neuronal cells; inhibitors of PP2B-activity are protective. PP2B activity was reported to decrease to about 50% of control in rat hippocampus immediately after 20 min transient forebrain ischemia (Morioka et al. 1999). Activity of PP2B recovered within 12 hours; the amount of PP2B protein remained constant.

So far, two proteins of the complex apoptotic signal transduction have been shown to directly interact with calcineurin: (i) Caspase-3 removes the C-terminal calmodulin-binding and autoinhibitory regions from the catalytic domain of PP2B (Mukerjee et al. 2000). This results in loss of the Ca^{2+}- and calmodulin-dependency and increases phosphatase activity. (ii) PP2B dephosphorylates Bad, a pro-apoptotic member of the Bcl-2 family (Wang et al. 1999). The resulting reduced phosphorylation level of Bad causes its dissociation from 14-3-3 in the cytosol and translocation of Bad to mitochondria where Bcl-xl resides. Subsequent heterodimerization of Bad with Bcl-xl promotes apoptosis.

Activation of PP2C and induction of apoptosis

The cellular lipid composition and free fatty acid levels affect cell proliferation and survival. Literature of the influence of fatty acids added to neuronal cells is contradictory; it varies from protection to degeneration. The outcome depends on the assay system, cell type, chemical nature and concentration of the fatty acid used: Linolenic acid has been reported to prevent neuronal cell death (Lauritzen et al. 2000), whereas apoptosis could be induced by an increase in the concentration of palmitic acid (Shimabukuro et al. 1988) or arachidonic acid (Surette et al. 1999).

Among a number of other essential functions for life, phospholipids and fatty acids are also known to act as second messengers. Precursors and metabolites of arachidonic acid (20:4) are embedded in Ca^{2+}- and G-protein coupled pathways. Ion channels and enzymes are affected. Regulation via cellular lipids extends to the field of phosphorylation and dephosphorylation. Activation of protein kinase C by diacylglycerol is the most famous example on the kinase site. Several protein phosphatases are affected by fatty acids: Arachidonic acid has been reported to activate PP5 (Chen and Cohen 1997) and to inhibit myosin light chain phosphatase activity (Gailly et al. 1996). Phospholipids stimulate PP2B activity upon interaction with its Ca^{2+}-binding subunit (Politino and King 1990). Short and long chain natural ceramides increase the activities of PP1 and PP2A (Chalfant et al. 1999). Unsaturated fatty acids stimulate PP2C activity (Klumpp et al. 1998a). Those studies have been continued and part of it is presented here.

Activity of PP2C increases at a physiological concentration of 0.5–1.5 mM free Mg^{2+} by the addition of unsaturated fatty acids 10–15 fold (Klumpp et al. 1998a). Stimulation was found to depend on the chain length of the fatty acid. A minimum backbone of 15 C-atoms is required (Table 1). The number of double-bonds, in contrast, is not decisive. Single unsaturated fatty acids are as potent as multiple unsaturated ones (Klumpp et al. 1998a). Non-lipophilic antioxidants such as ascorbic acid had no effect on PP2C activity, suggesting that radical scavenging most likely is not involved (Table 1). Surprisingly, testing the adduct of ascorbic acid with palmitic acid (16:0) – both by itself not affecting PP2C activity – revealed that palmitoyl-ascorbic acid increased PP2C activity (Table 1). We therefore conclude that in addition to a certain degree of lipophilicity an oxidizable component is essential as well. It is the combination of both that is necessary for stimulation of PP2C. A third requirement for the activation of PP2C is that the fatty acid carries a free, negatively charged carboxy-group. Lipophilic compounds of sufficient chain length that can be oxidized but lack – COOH or where it had been modified (e.g. methyl ester derivative) failed to stimulate PP2C activity.

Table 1. Schematic representation of the correlation of activation of PP2C with induction of apoptosis. Activity of PP2C was determined in vitro using casein as a substrate. Induction of apoptosis was evaluated in primary cultures of neurons obtained from chick embryo telencephalons by nuclei staining with Hoechst 33258.

Compound		Activation of PP2C	Induction of apoptosis
Saturated fatty acid		no	no
Unsaturated fatty acid	< C-15	no	no
	> C-15	YES	YES
Ascorbic acid		no	no
Palmitic acid (16:0)		no	no
Palmitoyl-ascorbic acid		YES	YES

Figure 1 shows the effect of the physiological fatty acid oleic acid (18:1 cis-9) on PP2C activity. Maximal stimulation (14-fold) was observed at 500 μM. Activation could be shifted to lower concentrations of the fatty acid when bovine serum albumin – necessary as carrier for the TCA precipitation step – was added after the assay. Leaving out serum albumin shifted the dose-response curve by 200 μM to the left (data not shown). Knowing that the substrate casein also chelates free fatty acids, the concentration required for stimulation of PP2C under physiological conditions will be even less.

The extract of the leaves from *Ginkgo biloba* (EGb 761) is used worldwide for treatment of dementia (Le Bars et al. 1997; Ahlemeyer and Krieglstein 1998). Ginkgolic acids are excluded from Egb 761 because they might cause allergy and toxic side effects. They fulfill the chemical requirements to theoretically increase the activity of PP2C. The mixture of ginkgolic acids used in this study consisted of three 6-alkyl (n-tridecyl-, n-pentadecyl- and n-pentadecenyl-) salicylates. Salicylic acid and the ginkgolic fatty acid side chains 13:0 and 15:0 each by itself did not stimulate PP2C activity. The third fatty acid side chain 15:1 had a slightly stimulating effect. In contrast, ginkgolic acid potently increased the activity of PP2Cα (Fig. 1) and PP2Cβ (data not shown). Stimulation was found to be specific for PP2C (Fig. 2): Alkaline phosphatase was not affected; the activity of acid phosphatase strongly decreased; PP2A activity was reduced by 50%; PP1 and PP2B were potently inhibited; and tyrosine phosphatase was most sensitive and completely blocked. In summary, having tested representatives from various categories of phosphatases (ser/thr, tyr, universal) we discovered a striking specificity. Activity of PP2C increased by ginkgolic acid severalfold, whereas the activity of six other phosphatases was either not affected or inhibited.

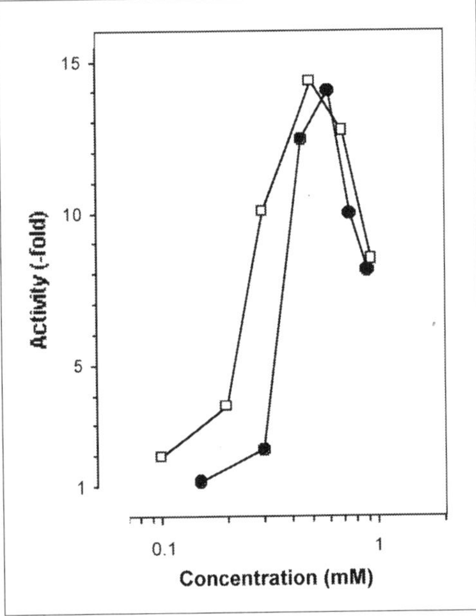

Fig. 1. Effect of oleic acid and ginkgolic acid on PP2C activity. PP2Cα was assayed as described in detail (Klumpp et al. 1998b) at 30 °C for 10 min in 30 μl containing 20 mM Tris/HCl pH 7.5, 0.1% 2-mercaptoethanol, 1.3 mg/ml BSA, 0.7 mM magnesium-acetate, lipid as indicated (in 10% DMSO) and 1 μM [^{32}P]casein (5 x 10^4 cpm). Reactions were terminated by the addition of 200 μl 20% trichloroacetic acid. After centrifugation at 10,000 *g* (5 min), 200 μl of the supernatant was analysed for [^{32}P]phosphate content. Oleic acid (□), ginkgolic acid (●).

Very little is known about PP2C in brain and neuronal tissues. DARP-32 has been suggested as a substrate for PP2C (see above), and mRNA for PP2C was observed in various brain regions (Abe et al. 1992). In the meantime, we were able to measure PP2C activity (in vitro assays) and to detect PP2C protein (western blotting) in rat brain and in neuronal cells. The next logical consequence, therefore, was to see whether the fatty acids specifically stimulating PP2C do have an effect on cultured neurons. For that purpose, 5-day old chick embryonic neuronal cultures were seeded in serum free medium for 24 hours prior to treatment with ginkgolic acid or other compounds for another 24 hours. These conditions yielded 15–20% apoptotic neurons for control. Addition of ginkgolic acid had great impact on cell viability. Reduction of the nucleus size and chromatin condensation (Fig. 3) as well as TUNEL-labelling (data not shown) were strong indicators for apoptosis. This process was dose-dependent. Incubation with 100 μM (250 μM) ginkgolic acid caused apoptosis of

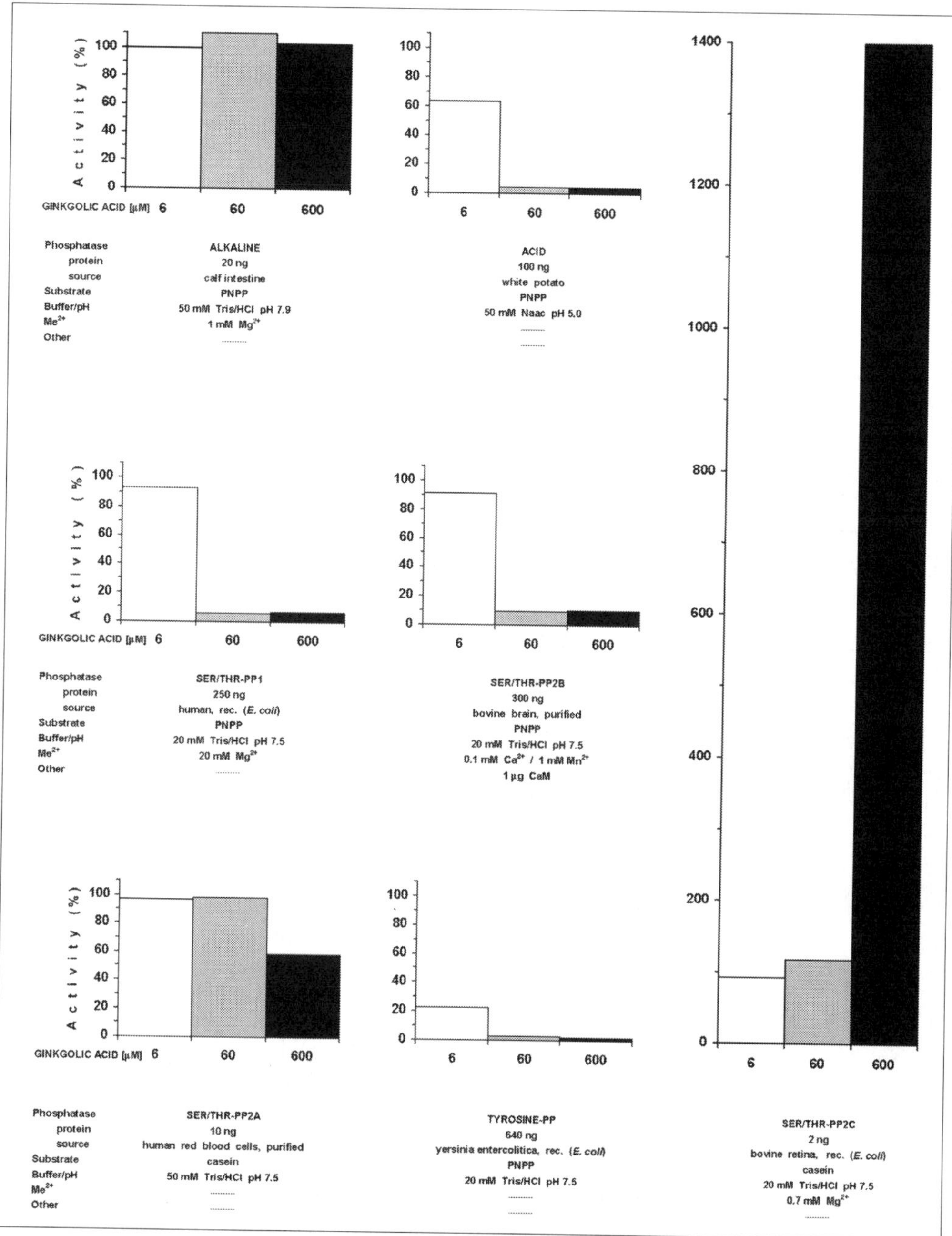

Fig. 2. Effect of ginkgolic acid on phosphatase activities. Assay conditions and information on enzyme sources are summarized below the bar graphs, respectively. Incubation time was chosen so that phosphate release was kept within the linear range. 100% = specific activitiy in the absence of ginkgolic acid, respectively. The final concentration of DMSO used as solvent was maximally 10%. Abbreviations: PNPP, *p*-nitrophenyl phosphate; rec., recombinant.

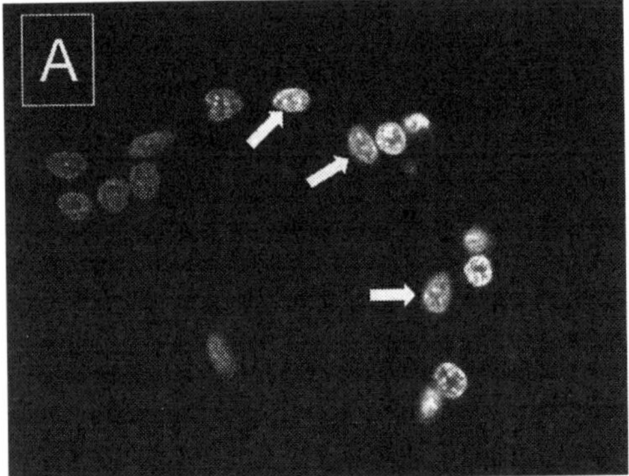

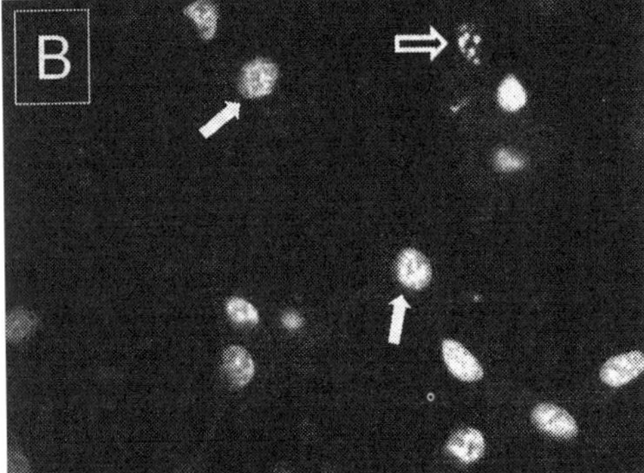

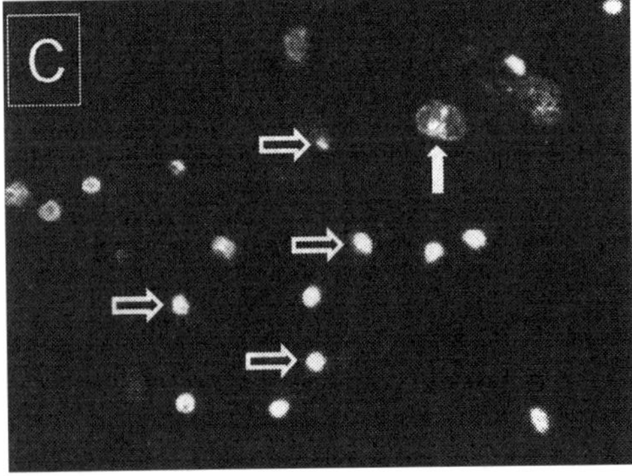

Fig. 3. Nuclear staining with Hoechst 33258. Chick embryonic neurons were treated for 24 hours with vehicle (A), 1 μM ginkgolic acid (B), and 250 μM ginkgolic acid (C). Subsequent incubation with the DNA fluorochrome (10 μg/ml) at 37 °C for 15 min was followed by two washing steps (methanol and phosphate-buffered saline). Cells were examined under a fluorescence microscope. Filled arrows indicate intact nuclei; empty arrows point to the fluorescence typical for apoptotic nuclei with condensed chromatin.

80% (95%) of the cultured neurons. Cycloheximide abolished the apoptotic effect of ginkgolic acid (data not shown).

These studies have been extended. Fatty acids that had been tested for an effect on PP2C activity systematically were analysed in the neuronal cell culture assay. The results were quite striking (Table 1). Compounds of sufficient lipophilicity carrying at least one function for oxidation and equipped with a free carboxygroup not only stimulated PP2C activity but were also found to induce apoptosis (Table 1). This correlation still holds on going deeper into chemistry – location of the double-bond and cis/trans configuration (submitted).

Conclusions

PP2C is as abundant and has the same specific activity as other protein phosphatases, yet, much less is known about its function. The discovery that compounds stimulating PP2C activity in vitro are causing induction of apoptosis in neuronal cells suggests PP2C as novel player in apoptotic signaling. We were able to detect specificity on two levels: (i) chemistry of the compounds activating PP2C, and (ii) type of phosphatase, the effector enzyme. Searching for the neuronal substrate of PP2C is warranted. It might be rewarding.

Acknowledgment

We thank Schwabe GmbH&Co, Karlsruhe, for ginkgolic acid, and K. Eger, Leipzig, for palmitoyl-ascorbic acid. This work was supported by grants from the Deutsche Forschungsgemeinschaft to J.K. and to S.K. (KR 354/16-4).

References

1. Abe H, Tamura S, Kondo H (1992) Localization of mRNA for protein phosphatase 2C in the brain of adult rats. Mol Brain Res 13:283–288
2. Ahlemeyer B, Krieglstein J (1998) Neuroprotective effects of ginkgo biloba extract. In: Phytomedicines of Europe (Lawson LD, Bauer R, eds) ACS Symposium Series 691:210–220

3. Barton GJ, Cohen PT, Barford D (1994) Conservation analysis and structure prediction of the protein serine/threonine phosphatases. Sequence similarity with diadenosine tetraphosphatase from Escherichia coli suggests homology to the protein phosphatases. Eur J Biochem 220:225–237
4. Bork P, Brown NP, Hegyi H, Schultz J (1996) The protein phosphatase 2C superfamily: Detection of bacterial homologues. Protein Sci 5:1,421–1,425
5. Chalfant CE, Kishikawa K, Mumby MC, Kamibayashi C, Bielawska A, Hannun YA (1999) Long chain ceramides activate protein phosphatase-1 and protein phosphatase-2A. J Biol Chem 274:20,313–20,317
6. Chen MX, Cohen PTW (1997) Activation of protein phosphatase 5 by limited proteolysis or the binding of polyunsaturated fatty acids to the TPR domain. FEBS Lett 400:136–140
7. Cohen PTW (1997) Novel protein serine/threonine phosphatases: variety is the spice of life. Trends in Biochem Sci 22:245–251
8. Das AK, Helps NR, Cohen PTW, Barford D (1996) Crystal structure of the protein serine/threonine phosphatase 2C at 2.0 Å resolution. EMBO J 15:6,798–6,809
9. Deng X, Ito T, Carr B, Mumby M, May WS (1998) Reversible phosphorylation of Bcl-2 following interleukin 3 or bryostatin 1 is mediated by direct interaction with protein phosphatase 2A. J Biol Chem 273:34,157–34,163
10. Desdouits F, Siciliano JC, Nairn AC, Greengard P, Girault J-A (1998) Dephosphorylation of Ser-137 in DARPP-32 by protein phosphatases 2A and 2C: different roles *in vitro* and in striatonigral neurons. Biochem J 330:211–216
11. Fiscella M, Zhang HL, Fan S, Sakaguchi K, Shen S, Mercer WE, vande Woude GF, O'Connor PM, Appella E (1997) Wip1, a novel human protein phosphatase that is induced in response to ionizing radiation in a p53-dependent manner. Proc Natl Acad Sci USA 94:6,048–6,053
12. Fukunaga K, Kobayashi T, Tamura S, Miyamoto E (1993) Dephosphorylation of autophosphorylated Ca^{2+}/Calmodulin-dependent protein kinase II by protein phosphatase 2C. J Biol Chem 268:133–137
13. Gailly P, Wu X, Haystead T, Somlyo AP, Cohen PTW, Cohen P, Somlyo AV (1996) Regions of the 110-kDa regulatory subunit M110 required for regulation of myosin-light-chain-phosphatase activity in smooth muscle. Eur J Biochem 239:326–332
14. Guerini D (1997) Calcineurin: Not just a simple protein phosphatase. Biochem Biophys Res Commun 235:271–275
15. Guthridge MA, Bellosta P, Tavoloni N, Basilico C (1997) FIN13, a novel growth factor-inducible serine-threonine phosphatase which can inhibit cell cycle progression. Mol Cell Biol 17:5,485–5,498
16. Ingebritsen TS, Cohen P (1983) Protein phosphatases: Properties and role in cellular regulation. Science 221:331–338
17. Klauck TM, Faux MC, Labudda K, Langeberg LK, Jaken S, Scott JD (1996) Coordination of three signaling enzymes by AKAP79, a mammalian scaffold protein. Science 271:1,589–1,592
18. Klee CB, Draetta GF, Hubbard MJ (1988) Calcineurin. Adv Enzymol Relat Areas Mol Biol 61:149–200
19. Klumpp S, Selke D, Hermesmeier J (1998a) Protein phosphatase type 2C active at physiological Mg^{2+}: Stimulation by unsaturated fatty acids. FEBS Lett 437:229–232
20. Klumpp S, Selke D, Fischer D, Baumann A, Müller F, Thanos S (1998b) Protein phosphatase type 2C isozymes present in vertebrate retinae: Purification, characterization and localization in photoreceptors. J Neurosci Res 51:328–338
21. Lauritzen I, Blondeau N, Heurteaux C, Widmann C, Romey G, Lazdunski M (2000) Polyunsaturated fatty acids are potent neuroprotectors. EMBO J 19:1,784–1,793
22. Le Bars PL, Katz MM, Berman N, Itil TM, Freedman AM, Schatzberg AF (1997) A placebo-controlled, double-blind, randomized trial of an extract of ginkgo biloba for dementia. JAMA 278:1,327–1,332
23. Luo C, Shaw KT, Raghavan A, Aramburu J, Cozar G, Perrino BA, Hogan PG, Rao A (1996) Interaction of calcineurin with a domain of the transcription factor NFAT1 that controls nuclear import. Proc Natl Acad Sci USA 93:8,907–8,912
24. Maehama T, Dixon JE (1998) The tumor suppressor PTEN/MMAC1 dephosphorylates the lipid second messenger, phosphatidylinositol 3,4,5-trisphosphate. J Biol Chem 273:13,375–13,378
25. McGowan CH, Cohen P (1988) Protein phosphatase 2C from rabbit skeletal muscle and liver: A Mg^{2+}-dependent enzyme. Meth Enzymol 159:416–426
26. Moore F, Weekes J, Hardie DG (1991) Evidence that AMP triggers phosphorylation as well as direct allosteric activation of rat liver AMP-activated protein kinase. Eur J Biochem 199:691–697
27. Morioka M, Fukunaga K, Hasegawa S, Okamura A, Korematsu K, Kai Y, Hamada J, Nagahiro S, Miyamoto E, Ushio Y (1999) Activities of calcineurin and phosphatase 2A in the hippocampus after transient forebrain ischemia. Brain Res 828:135–144
28. Mukerjee N, McGinnis KM, Park YH, Gnegy ME, Wang KK (2000) Caspase-mediated proteolytic activation of calcineurin in thapsigargin-mediated apoptosis in SH-SY5Y neuroblastoma cells. Arch Biochem Biophys 379:337–343
29. Mulkey RM, Endo S, Shenolikar S, Malenka RC (1994) Involvement of a calcineurin/inhibitor-1 phosphatase cascade in hippocampal long-term depression. Nature 369:485–488
30. Murray MV, Kobayashi R, Krainer AR (1999) The type 2C Ser/Thr phosphatase PP2Cγ is a pre-mRNA splicing factor. Genes Dev 13:87–97
31. Pawson T, Scott JD (1997) Signaling through scaffold, anchoring, and adaptor proteins. Science 278:2,075–2,080
32. Pinna LA, Donella-Deana A (1994) Phosphorylated synthetic peptides as tools for studying protein phosphatases. Biochim Biophys Acta 1222:415–431
33. Politino M, King MM (1990) Calcineurin-phospholipid interactions. Identification of the phospholipid-binding subunit and analyses of a two-stage binding process. J Biol Chem 265:7,619–7,622
34. Roach T, Slater S, Koval M, White L, McFarland EC, Okumura M, Thomas M, Brown E (1997) CD45 regulates Src family member kinase activity associated with macrophage integrin-mediated adhesion. Curr Biol 7:408–417
35. Ruvolo PP, Deng X, Ito T, Carr BK, May WS (1999) Ceramide induces Bcl-2 dephosphorylation via a mechanism involving mitochondrial PP2A. J Biol Chem 274:20,296–20,300
36. Santoro MF, Annand RR, Robertson MM, Peng Y-W, Brady MJ, Mankovich JA, Hackett MC, Ghayur T, Walter G, Wong WW, Giegel DA (1998) Regulation of protein phosphatase 2A activity by caspase-3 during apoptosis. J Biol Chem 273:13,119–13,128
37. Sheppeck JE, Gauss C-M, Chamberlin AR (1997) Inhibition of the Ser-Thr phosphatases PP1 and PP2A by naturally occurring toxins. Bioorg Med Chem 5:1,739–1,750
38. Shimabukuro M, Zhou Y-T, Levi M, Unger RH (1998) Fatty acid-induced β cell apoptosis: A link between obesity and diabetes. Proc Natl Acad Sci USA 95:2,498–2,502
39. Sim ATR, Scott, JD (1999) Targeting of PKA, PKC and protein phosphatases to cellular microdomains. Cell Calcium 26:209–217
40. Surette ME, Fonteh AN, Bernatchez C, Chilton FH (1999) Pertubations in the control of cellular arachidonic acid levels block cell growth and induce apoptosis in HL-60 cells. Carcinogenesis 20:757–763

41. Takekawa M, Maeda T, Saito H (1998) Protein phosphatase 2Cα inhibits the human stress-responsive p38 and JNK MAPK pathways. EMBO J 17:4,744–4,752
42. Tong Y, Quirion R, Shen S-H (1998) Cloning and characterization of a novel mammalian PP2C isozyme. J Biol Chem 273:35,282–35,290
43. Tonks NK, Diltz CD, Fischer EH (1988a) Characterization of the major protein tyrosine phosphatases of human placenta. J Biol Chem 263:6,731–6,737
44. Tonks NK, Diltz CD, Fischer EH (1988b) Purification of the major protein-tyrosine phosphatases of human placenta. J Biol Chem 263:6,722–6,730
45. Tonks NK, Charbonneau H, Diltz CD, Fischer EH, Walsh KA (1988c) Demonstration that the leukocyte common antigen CD45 is a protein tyrosine phosphatase. Biochemistry 27:8,695–8,701
46. Travis SM, Berger HA, Welsh MJ (1997) Protein phosphatase 2C dephosphorylates and inactivates cystic fibrosis transmembrane conductance regulator. Proc Natl Acad Sci USA 94:11,055–11,060
47. Wang HG, Pathan N, Ethell IM, Krajewski S, Yamaguchi Y, Shibasaki F, McKeon F, Bobo T, Franke TF, Reed JC (1999) Ca^{2+}-induced apoptosis through calcineurin dephosphorylation of BAD. Science 284:339–343
48. Wang XT, Culotta VC, Klee CB (1996) Superoxide dismutase protects calcineurin from inactivation. Nature 383:434–437
49. Wera S, Hemmings BA (1995) Serine/threonine protein phosphatases. Biochem J 311:17–29
50. Westphal RS, Tavalin SJ, Lin JW, Alto NM, Fraser IDC, Langeberg LK, Sheng M, Scott JD (1999) Regulation of NMDA receptors by an associated phosphatase-kinase signaling complex. Science 285:93–96

Role of cyclin dependent kinases in neuronal death

D. S. Park

Regulation of neuronal death is complex and likely dependent upon multiple signalling components. Growing evidence suggests that one such death signal involves the activation of cyclin dependent kinases. In this review, the potential importance of cyclin dependent kinases and its relationship to other death components will be discussed in the context of neuronal death evoked by DNA damage in vitro and during stroke induced injury *in vivo*.

It is now clear that neuronal death is regulated by multiple death signals which depend upon cell type and stress/death stimuli. In the classic model of death, numerous upstream regulatory signals (both pro and anti apoptotic) are modulated upon a death stimuli. These signals are integrated to control the commitment of death. Growing evidence suggests that one upstream signal which contributes to the death signal in some paradigms of neuronal death is the activation of cyclin dependent kinases (CDKs). The evidence for the involvement of CDKs and the mechanisms by which events downstream of CDK activation may regulate neuronal death will be reviewed. In addition, the potential relevance of CDK activation in animal models of stroke will be discussed in the following sections.

CDK

CDKs are a group of related kinases which have homologies to its prototypic member, cdc2 (Cdk1). They share common motifs consisting of PSTAIRE theme or related derivatives thereof (Pines 1993a, 1993b). In general, the best recognized role of the CDKs is in cell cycle control. In this regard, the regulation of CDKs is complex. As the name implies, activity of CDKs are dependent upon bindings to its appropriate cyclin partner (Pines 1993a, 1993b). CDKs are also regulated through both activating and inhibitory phosphorylations and endogenous inhibitors of CDK activity such as those of the INK and KIP/Waf family (Morgan 1995). Different members of the CDK family regulate cell cycle progression. In general, it is thought that cyclin D1/cdk4/6, Cdk3, and cyclinE/cdk2 complexes regulate G1, while Cdk2/cyclinA regulate S phase progression. CyclinB/cdc2 complexes mediate M phase progression (Pines 1993a, 1993b).

While the role of CDK activity in cell cycle regulation is best characterized, it must be noted that not all members of the CDK family are involved in cell cycle control. One clear example of this is Cdk5 which utilizes p35 as its activating partner. Cdk5 is reported to be required for neuronal development and process outgrowth (Nikolic et al. 1996; Patrick et al. 1999). Other members of the family include

Neuroscience Research Institute, University of Ottawa, 451 Smyth Rd., Ottawa, ON, K1H 8M5, Canada.
e-Mail: dpark@uottawa.ca

J. Krieglstein, S. Klumpp (Eds.) Pharmacology of Cerebral Ischemia 2000

PIFTAIRE (Lazzaro et al. 1997), which is located primarily in the brain, and PISTLRE. Some isoforms of PISTLRE have been associated with apoptosis (Beyaert et al. 1997; Lahti et al. 1995a, 1995b; Tang et al. 1998).

CDKs and neuronal death

The involvement of cell cycle related CDKs in neuronal death is supported by 1) reports from several groups indicating the association of increased CDK and cyclin levels/activity with neuronal death; and 2) that inhibition of this activity by both pharmacological and molecular means inhibits neuronal death under certain conditions. For example, cyclin D1 transcripts and Cdk4/Cdc2 protein levels are upregulated during death of sympathetic neurons and neuronal PC12 cells deprived of NGF (Freeman et al. 1994; Gao and Zelenka 1995). In addition, increase in cyclin D1, cyclin B, and Cdk4 levels are upregulated in brains of AD patients and during stroke (Busser et al. 1998; Li et al. 1997; McShea et al. 1997; Nagy et al. 1997; Timsit et al. 1999; Vincent et al. 1997). In certain cases of neuronal death, increased CDK activity has been reported. For example, pRb, a critical target of Cdk 2 and 4, is phosphorylated on a CDK consensus site during neuronal injury evoked by stroke (Osuga et al. 2000), DNA damage (Park et al. 2000), B-amyloid (Copani et al. 1999; Giovanni et al. 1999), cisplatinum toxicity (Gill and Windebank 1998) and K^+ deprivation (Padmanabhan et al. 1999). Cyclin D1 associated kinase activity is also observed during death of cortical neurons evoked by DNA damage (Park et al. 1998a).

The requirement/importance of cell cycle related CDKs in death is supported by neuroprotection studies. For example, expression of DN Cdk4 have been shown to be neuroprotective against B-amyloid evoked toxicity (Copani et al. 1999; Giovanni et al. 1999) and DNA damage (Park et al. 1998a). In addition, pharmacological inhibitors of CDKs are protective in models of low K+ (Padmanabhan et al. 1999), B-amyloid (Giovanni et al. 1999), DNA damage, and trophic factor deprivation (Park et al. 1996).

Cell cycle related CDKs may not be the only CDKs important for regulation of neuronal death. In this regard, p35, the required activator of Cdk5, has been shown to be cleaved and activated during neuronal death (Patrick et al. 1999). While the target of Cdk5 activity mediating neuronal death is unclear, Cdk5 is known to phosphorylate Tau, an event which has been implicated in the neurodegeneration of Alzheimer's disease (Patrick et al. 1999).

The above evidence, while intriguing, raises important questions. How does CDK activation mediate neuronal death and what are its downstream targets? How does the presumed activation of CDKs regulate the more conserved death pathways involving proteins like Bax and caspases? Finally, are CDKs relevant to neuronal injury or neurodegeneration of mature adult neurons *in vivo*? We have addressed some of these questions in an *in vitro* model of neuronal death evoked by DNA damage and in *in vivo* stroke models of neuronal injury.

CDKs, DNA damage and neuronal death

Previous work by ourselves and others demonstrate that DNA damage activates the apoptotic process in neurons. For example, irradiation (Enokido et al. 1996), the chemotherapeutic agents, cytosine arabinoside (AraC) (Martin et al. 1990; Park et al. 1998b; Tomkins et al. 1994; Wallace and Johnson 1989; Winkelman and Hines 1983), and cisplatin (Gill and Windebank 1998), the DNA topoisomerase-II inhibitors etoposide, teniposide, and mitoxanthrone (Nakajima et al. 1994; Tomkins et al. 1994), all induce apoptotic neuronal cell death. Interestingly, a number of these agents cause peripheral neuropathies and neurodegeneration (for example Winkelman and Hines 1983). DNA damage may also participate in initiating cell death in neuropathological conditions. For example, early formation of DNA strand breaks have been reported in ischemia well before the occurrence of DNA fragmentation resulting from apoptosis (Chen et al. 1997). Given these observations, it has become increasingly important to understand the downstream signalling events which control DNA damage-evoked neuronal cell death.

Embryonic cultured cortical neurons undergo apoptosis when exposed to the topoisomerase I inhibitor, camptothecin (Morris and Geller 1996). DNA strand breaks are detected within 10 minutes of exposure (as detected by the comet assay). Morphological characteristics of death appear 8–10 hrs after 10 μM camptothecin treatment. What are the signals that mediate this apoptotic death? Interestingly, cyclin D1 associated kinase activity increases within 1 h after initiation of camptothecin treatment (Park et al. 1998a). The notion that this signal may be required for death derives from two lines of evidence. First, pharmacological CDK inhibitors, flavopiridol and olomoucine, block neuronal death evoked by DNA damage (Park et al. 1997; Park et al. 1998b). Importantly, the concentrations required for protection correlate well with the ability of the CDK inhibitors to inhibit DNA synthesis in proliferating PC12 cells (Park et al. 1996; Park et al. 1997). In addition, the CDK inhibitor flavopiridol is effective only if added within 1–2 hrs after camptothecin treatment (D.S. Park, unpublished data). This correlates well with the early rise in cyclin D1 associated kinase activity (Park et al. 1998a). Second, expression of kinase dead dominant negative (DN) forms of Cdk4/and 6 are efficient at protecting neurons from DNA damage evoked death (Park et al. 1998a). Expression of DN cdk2 and 3 were less effective (Park et al. 1998a). Taken together, these results suggest the activation and requirement of CDKs, particularly CDK4/6, in neuronal death evoked by DNA damage.

CDK activity and Bax mediated caspase activation

As with other models of apoptotic death, Bax is translocated to the mitochondria (D.S. Park, unpublished data) and cytochrome C is released from the mitochondria upon camptothecin treatment (Keramaris et al. 2000; Stefanis et al. 1999). In addition, caspase 3-like activity begins to increase 4 hrs after camptothecin treatment (Stefanis et al. 1999). We and others have shown that Bax is absolutely required for cytochrome C release (Keramaris et al. 2000), caspase activation (Park et al. unpublished data), and apoptotic death (Park et al. unpublished data; Xiang et al. 1998) in this death paradigm. In addition, inhibition of caspases, either by general caspase inhibitors (Stefanis et al. 1999) or by caspase 3 deficiency (Keramaris et al. 2000), protects neurons from apoptotic death. However, this protection is only transient (12 hrs vs the sustained 2–3 day protection one observes with Bax deficiency). Cytochrome C release is not inhibited in neurons protected by caspase inhibition (Keramaris et al. 2000; Stefanis et al. 1999). Accordingly, we have hypothesized that the transient protection afforded by caspase inhibition may be the result of mitochondrial defects.

Where does the involvement of CDKs relate biochemically to this mitochondrially-related pathway of death? Inhibition of CDK by flavopiridol blocks Bax translocation, and cytochrome C release and caspase activity (D.S. Park unpublished data; Stefanis et al. 1999). As with Bax deficiency, sustained protection is observed. Taken together, along with the early rise in cyclin D1 associated kinase activity, we propose that CDKs are upstream death mediators that act to regulate the mitochondrial-related pathway of death.

CDKs and p53

The tumor suppressor p53 is also required for death evoked by camptothecin (Giovanni et al. 2000; Johnson et al. 1999). An increase in p53 protein levels as well as DNA binding is detectable approximately two hours after addition of camptothecin (D.S. Park; unpublished results). In addition, p53 deficient neurons are resistant to DNA damage (Giovanni et al. 2000; Johnson et al. 1999). The observation that p53 deficient neurons treated with camptothecin do not show Bax translocation, cytochrome C release and caspase activity (D.S. Park unpublished results) indicate that like CDKs, p53 is an upstream regulator of death.

What is the relationship between p53 and CDKs? Inhibition of CDKs by flavopiridol has no effect on the increase in p53 levels, DNA binding or p53 translocation to the nucleus (D.S. Park unpublished results). Conversely, Rb was still phosphorylated in p53 deficient neurons treated with camptothecin. These results suggest that p53 and CDK act on separate parallel pathways to mediate death. However, inhibition of either pathway alone inhibits Bax mediated cytochrome C release and caspase activity (Stefanis et al. 1999) (D.S. Park unpublished results). Accordingly, we hypothesize that the downstream effectors of p53 and CDK must cooperate to mediate Bax activity.

Substrates of CDK which may mediate death

The immediate downstream effectors of the CDKs are not clear. As of yet, the only well characterized target of Cdk4 is the tumor suppressor Rb (Chellappan et al. 1991; Weinberg 1995). In a hypophosphorylated state, Rb members are known to interact with members of the E2F transcription factor family (Chellappan et al. 1991; Suzuki-Takahashi et al. 1995; Weinberg 1995). Once phosphorylated by CDKs, Rb is release from E2F which can then mediate transcription. In regards to cell cycle control, E2F members are thought to activate genes required for S phase progression. The role of Rb is complex and is known to interact with numerous proteins other than the E2F members.

Interestingly, both Rb and E2F members seem to regulate cell death as well as cell cycle control. Numerous reports in proliferating systems has suggested that expression of Rb is protective while expression of E2F members, in particular, E2F1, induces death (Hiebert et al. 1995; Qin et al. 1994). In neurons, it is particularly relevant that Rb deficient neurons show inappropriate neuronal death which is dependent upon E2F1 in the CNS (Jacks et al. 1992; Lee et al. 1992; Tsai et al. 1998). In addition, inactivation of Rb by large T antigen expression causes death of purkinje neurons (Feddersen et al. 1997).

In cortical neurons treated with DNA damage, Rb is phosphorylated on a CDK phosphorylation consensus site (Park et al. 2000). This phosphorylation is inhibited by flavopiridol treatment and occurs at approximately the same time as cyclin D1 associated kinase activity (Park et al. 2000). Expression of a mutant of Rb which lacks this phosphorylation site partially protects neurons from death (Park et al. 2000). This suggests that Cdk4 may transduce its signal, in part, through Rb phosphorylation.

A logical hypthesis is that phosphorylation and inactivation of Rb may lead to increase in activity of E2F members. In support of this, expression of a DN form of DP1, an obligate binding partner to the E2F members, partially inhibits death evoked by DNA damage (Park et al. 2000). Which E2F member(s) play an important role in this neuronal death? E2F1 has been most associated with death and expression of E2F1 in cortical and cerebellar granule neurons induces apoptosis (O'Hare et al. 2000). In addition, recent reports from our group and others suggest that E2F1 deficiency is partially neuroprotective from insults such as B-amyloid toxicity (Giovanni et al. 2000), K+ deprivation (O'Hare et al. 2000), staurosporine (Hou et al. 2000), and ischemic damage (MacManus et al. 1999). However, in the paradigm of DNA damage, E2F1 deficient neurons are not resistant to death (D.S. Park, unpublished data). Accordingly, we predict that multiple Rb interacting factors, including several E2F members, may mediate the CDK associated death signal. In support of this, E2F2 and 3 has been also shown to evoke death when overexpressed (Dirks et al. 1998; Vigo et al. 1999).

In summary, we believe that at least two pathways are activated upon DNA damage in neurons. CDKs and p53 are activated in parallel to mediate Bax mediated translocation, cytochrome C release, and caspase activation (see Fig. 1 for summary). We are currently examining the involvement of other potential death effectors such as calpains and the JNK pathway.

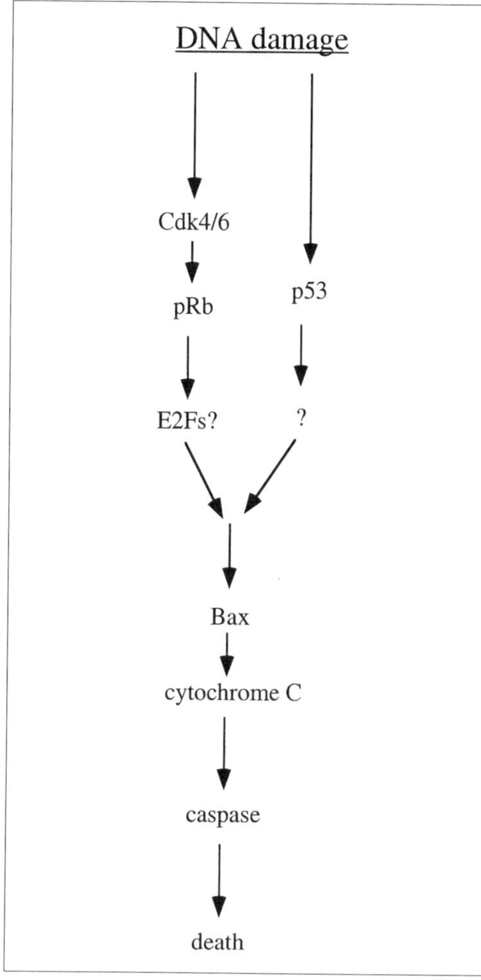

Fig. 1. Schematic model of neuronal death evoked by DNA damage.

CDKs and ischemic damage

While the above death pathways involving CDKs in *in vitro* models of death are intriguing, the relevance to neuropathological conditions in adult neurons *in vivo* is unclear. Several reports have suggested increases in activity and levels of CDKs and cyclins in brains from AD patients and in *in vivo* models of excitotoxic death (Busser et al. 1998; Li et al. 1997; McShea et al. 1997; Nagy et al. 1997; Timsit et al. 1999; Vincent et al. 1997). However, the requirement of these death signals is unknown.

To address these questions, we examined whether CDKs were activated in animal models of stroke and whether this signal might be required for neuronal death. Upon short term focal occlusion in the rat, we have observed increases in cyclin D1 and Cdk4 protein levels in neurons of the ischemic regions of the cortex by immunohistochemical analyses (Osuga et al. 2000). We believe that the CDK complexes are active since we observed phosphoRb positive neurons in the same region utilizing an antibody specific for CDK phosphorylated Rb. In addition, increased E2F1 levels, an expected consequence of deregulated Rb, is also observed in the ischemic core region. Finally, cell cycle related activity increases in neurons which are TUNEL positive (Osuga et al. 2000). Accordingly, we hypothesized that the cell cycle pathway is a pro-death signal in neurons following stroke. To test this, we examined whether the CDK inhibitor, flavopiridol would be protective from ischemic damage. Flavopiridol was administered ICV 24 hrs prior to focal insult and continuously afterwards via Alza pump. Flavopiridol treatment reduced infarct volume by approximately 70% 6 days post reperfusion (Osuga et al. 2000). These results are intriguing in light of published findings which suggest that E2F1 deficient mice also have reduced infarct volume after focal stroke (MacManus et al. 1999). These observations suggest that signals mediated through CDK activation, Rb phosphorylation, and increased E2F1 levels may regulate neuronal death after ischemic insult.

Conclusion

Data from *in vitro* and *in vivo* models of death suggest that CDK activity is an important regulator of neuronal death. However, it would be simplistic to think that CDK or any other single signal is the primary event which regulates death. We require a comprehensive picture of how multiple signals interact and integrate to control the ultimate death phenotype. In this way, perhaps, a more realistic approach to therapeutic intervention for a variety of neuropathologies including stroke may be developed.

Acknowledgements

This work was supported by grants from the Medical Research Council of Canada and the Heart Stroke Foundation of Canada.

References

1. Beyaert R, Kidd VJ, Cornelis S, Van de Craen M, Denecker G, Lahti JM, Gururajan R, Vandenabeele P, Fiers W (1997) Cleavage of PITSLRE kinases by ICE/CASP-1 and CPP32/CASP-3 during apoptosis induced by tumor necrosis factor. J Biol Chem 272:11694–11697
2. Busser J, Geldmacher DS, Herrup K (1998) Ectopic cell cycle proteins predict the sites of neuronal cell death in Alzheimer's disease brain. J Neurosci 18:2801–2807
3. Chellappan SP, Hiebert S, Mudryj M, Horowitz JM, Nevins JR (1991) The E2F transcription factor is a cellular target for the RB protein. Cell 65:1053–1061
4. Chen J, Jin K, Chen M, Pei W, Kawaguchi K, Greenberg DA, Simon RP (1997) Early detection of DNA strand breaks in the brain after transient focal ischemia: implications for the role of DNA damage in apoptosis and neuronal cell death. J Neurochem 69:232–245
5. Copani A, Condorelli F, Caruso A, Vancheri C, Sala A, Giuffrida Stella AM, Canonico PL, Nicoletti F, Sortino MA (1999) Mitotic signaling by beta-amyloid causes neuronal death [published erratum appears in FASEB J 2000 Jan;14(1):220]. Faseb J 13:2225–2234
6. Dirks PB, Rutka JT, Hubbard SL, Mondal S, Hamel PA (1998) The E2F-family proteins induce distinct cell cycle regulatory factors in p16-arrested, U343 astrocytoma cells. Oncogene 17:867–876
7. Enokido Y, Araki T, Tanaka K, Aizawa S, Hatanaka H (1996) Involvement of p53 in DNA strand break-induced apoptosis in postmitotic CNS neurons. Eur J Neurosci 8:1812–1821
8. Feddersen RM, Yunis WS, O'Donnell MA, Ebner TJ, Shen L, Iadecola C, Orr HT, Clark HB (1997) Susceptibility to cell death induced by mutant SV40 T-antigen correlates with Purkinje neuron functional development. Mol Cell Neurosci 9:42–62
9. Freeman RS, Estus S, Johnson EM, Jr (1994) Analysis of cell cycle-related gene expression in postmitotic neurons: selective induction of Cyclin D1 during programmed cell death. Neuron 12:343–355
10. Gao CY, Zelenka PS (1995) Induction of cyclin B and H1 kinase activity in apoptotic PC12 cells. Exp Cell Res 219:612–618
11. Gill JS, Windebank AJ (1998) Cisplatin-induced apoptosis in rat dorsal root ganglion neurons is associated with attempted entry into the cell cycle. J Clin Invest 101:2842–2850
12. Giovanni A, Keramaris E, Morris EJ, Hou ST, O'Hare M, Dyson N, RG S, Slack R, Park DS (2000) E2F1 mediates death of B-amyloid treated cortical neurons in a manner independent of p53 and depended on Bax and caspase 3. J Biol Chem. in press
13. Giovanni A, Wirtz-Brugger F, Keramaris E, Slack R, Park DS (1999) Involvement of cell cycle elements, cyclin-dependent kinases, pRb, and E2F x DP, in B-amyloid-induced neuronal death. J Biol Chem 274:19011–19016
14. Hiebert SW, Packham G, Strom DK, Haffner R, Oren M, Zambetti G, Cleveland JL (1995) E2F-1:DP-1 induces p53 and overrides survival factors to trigger apoptosis. Mol Cell Biol 15:6864–6874
15. Hou ST, Callaghan D, Fournier MC, Hill I, Kang L, Massie B, Morley P, Murray C, Rasquinha I, Slack R, MacManus JP (2000) The transcription factor E2F1 modulates apoptosis of neurons. J Neurochem 75:91–100
16. Jacks T, Fazeli A, Schmitt EM, Bronson RT, Goodell MA, Weinberg RA (1992) Effects of an Rb mutation in the mouse. Nature 359:295–300
17. Johnson MD, Kinoshita Y, Xiang H, Ghatan S, Morrison RS (1999) Contribution of p53-dependent caspase activation to neuronal cell death declines with neuronal maturation. J Neurosci 19:2996–3006
18. Keramaris E, Stefanis L, Maclaurin J, Harada N, Takaku K, Ishikawa T, Taketo MM, Robertson GS, Nicholson DW, Slack RS, Park DS (2000) Involvement of caspase 3 in apoptotic death of cortical neurons evoked by DNA damage. Mol Cell Neurosci 15:368–379
19. Lahti JM, Xiang J, Heath LS, Campana D, Kidd VJ (1995a) PITSLRE protein kinase activity is associated with apoptosis. Mol Cell Biol 15:1–11
20. Lahti JM, Xiang J, Kidd VJ (1995b) The PITSLRE protein kinase family. Prog Cell Cycle Res 1:329–338
21. Lazzaro MA, Albert PR, Julien JP (1997) A novel cdc2-related protein kinase expressed in the nervous system. J Neurochem 69:348–364
22. Lee EY, Chang CY, Hu N, Wang YC, Lai CC, Herrup K, Lee WH, Bradley A (1992) Mice deficient for Rb are nonviable and show defects in neurogenesis and haematopoiesis [see comments]. Nature 359:288–294
23. Li Y, Chopp M, Powers C, Jiang N (1997) Immunoreactivity of cyclin D1/cdk4 in neurons and oligodendrocytes after focal cerebral ischemia in rat. J Cereb Blood Flow Metab 17:846–856
24. MacManus JP, Koch CJ, Jian M, Walker T, Zurakowski B (1999) Decreased brain infarct following focal ischemia in mice lacking the transcription factor E2F1. Neuroreport 10:2711–2714
25. Martin DP, Wallace TL, Johnson EM, Jr (1990) Cytosine arabinoside kills postmitotic neurons in a fashion resembling trophic factor deprivation: evidence that a deoxycytidine-dependent process may be required for nerve growth factor signal transduction. J Neurosci 10:184–193
26. McShea A, Harris PL, Webster KR, Wahl AF, Smith MA (1997) Abnormal expression of the cell cycle regulators P16 and CDK4 in Alzheimer's disease. Am J Pathol 150:1933–1939
27. Morgan DO (1995) Principles of CDK regulation. Nature 374:131–134
28. Morris EJ, Geller HM (1996) Induction of neuronal apoptosis by camptothecin, an inhibitor of DNA topoisomerase-I: evidence for cell cycle-independent toxicity. J Cell Biol 134:757–770
29. Nagy Z, Esiri MM, Cato AM, Smith AD (1997) Cell cycle markers in the hippocampus in Alzheimer's disease. Acta Neuropathol (Berl) 94:6–15
30. Nakajima M, Kashiwagi K, Ohta J, Furukawa S, Hayashi K, Kawashima T, Hayashi Y (1994) Etoposide induces programmed death in neurons cultured from the fetal rat central nervous system. Brain Res 641:350–352
31. Nikolic M, Dudek H, Kwon YT, Ramos YF, Tsai LH (1996) The cdk5/p35 kinase is essential for neurite outgrowth during neuronal differentiation. Genes Dev 10:816–825
32. O'Hare MJ, Hou ST, Morris EJ, Cregan SP, Xu Q, Slack RS, Park DS (2000) Induction and modulation of cerebellar granule neuron death by E2F1. J Biol Chem. in press

33. Osuga H, Osuga S, Wang F, Fetni R, Hogan MJ, Slack RS, Hakim AM, Ikeda J, Park DS (2000) Cyclin dependent kinases as a therapeutic target for stroke. Proc Natl Acad Sci 97:10254–10259
34. Padmanabhan J, Park DS, Greene LA, Shelanski ML (1999) Role of cell cycle regulatory proteins in cerebellar granule neuron apoptosis. J Neurosci 19:8747–8756
35. Park DS, Farinelli SE, Greene LA (1996) Inhibitors of cyclin-dependent kinases promote survival of post-mitotic neuronally differentiated PC12 cells and sympathetic neurons. J Biol Chem 271:8161–8169
36. Park DS, Morris EJ, Bremner R, Keramaris E, Padmanabhan J, Rosenbaum M, Shelanski ML, Geller HM, Greene LA (2000) Involvement of Retinoblastoma Family Members and E2F/DP Complexes in the Death of Neurons Evoked by DNA Damage. J Neurosci 20:3104–3114
37. Park DS, Morris EJ, Greene LA, Geller HM (1997) G1/S cell cycle blockers and inhibitors of cyclin-dependent kinases suppress camptothecin-induced neuronal apoptosis. J Neurosci 17:1256–1270
38. Park DS, Morris EJ, Padmanabhan J, Shelanski ML, Geller HM, Greene LA (1998a) Cyclin-dependent kinases participate in death of neurons evoked by DNA-damaging agents. J Cell Biol 143:457–467
39. Park DS, Morris EJ, Stefanis L, Troy CM, Shelanski ML, Geller HM, Greene LA (1998b) Multiple pathways of neuronal death induced by DNA-damaging agents, NGF deprivation, and oxidative stress. J Neurosci 18:830–840
40. Patrick GN, Zukerberg L, Nikolic M, de la Monte S, Dikkes P, Tsai LH (1999) Conversion of p35 to p25 deregulates Cdk5 activity and promotes neurodegeneration [see comments]. Nature 402:615–622
41. Pines J (1993a) Cyclins and cyclin-dependent kinases: take your partners. Trends Biochem Sci 18:195–197
42. Pines J (1993b) Cyclins and their associated cyclin-dependent kinases in the human cell cycle. Biochem Soc Trans 21:921–925
43. Qin XQ, Livingston DM, Kaelin WG, Jr, Adams PD (1994) Deregulated transcription factor E2F-1 expression leads to S-phase entry and p53-mediated apoptosis. Proc Natl Acad Sci USA 91:10918–10922
44. Stefanis L, Park DS, Friedman WJ, Greene LA (1999) Caspase-dependent and -independent death of camptothecin-treated embryonic cortical neurons. J Neurosci 19:6235–6247
45. Suzuki-Takahashi I, Kitagawa M, Saijo M, Higashi H, Ogino H, Matsumoto H, Taya Y, Nishimura S, Okuyama A (1995) The interactions of E2F with pRB and with p107 are regulated via the phosphorylation of pRB and p107 by a cyclin-dependent kinase. Oncogene 10:1691–1698
46. Tang D, Gururajan R, Kidd VJ (1998) Phosphorylation of PITSLRE p110 isoforms accompanies their processing by caspases during Fas-mediated cell death. J Biol Chem 273:16601–16607
47. Timsit S, Rivera S, Ouaghi P, Guischard F, Tremblay E, Ben-Ari Y, Khrestchatisky M (1999) Increased cyclin D1 in vulnerable neurons in the hippocampus after ischaemia and epilepsy: a modulator of in vivo programmed cell death? Eur J Neurosci 11:263–278
48. Tomkins CE, Edwards SN, Tolkovsky AM (1994) Apoptosis is induced in post-mitotic rat sympathetic neurons by arabinosides and topoisomerase II inhibitors in the presence of NGF. J Cell Sci 107:1499–1507
49. Tsai KY, Hu Y, Macleod KF, Crowley D, Yamasaki L, Jacks T (1998) Mutation of E2f-1 suppresses apoptosis and inappropriate S phase entry and extends survival of Rb-deficient mouse embryos. Mol Cell 2:293–304
50. Vigo E, Muller H, Prosperini E, Hateboer G, Cartwright P, Moroni MC, Helin K (1999) CDC25A phosphatase is a target of E2F and is required for efficient E2F-induced S phase. Mol Cell Biol 19:6379–6395
51. Vincent I, Jicha G, Rosado M, Dickson DW (1997) Aberrant expression of mitotic cdc2/cyclin B1 kinase in degenerating neurons of Alzheimer's disease brain. J Neurosci 17:3588–3598
52. Wallace TL, Johnson EM, Jr (1989) Cytosine arabinoside kills postmitotic neurons: evidence that deoxycytidine may have a role in neuronal survival that is independent of DNA synthesis. J Neurosci 9:115–124
53. Weinberg RA (1995) The retinoblastoma protein and cell cycle control. Cell 81:323–330
54. Winkelman MD, Hines JD (1983) Cerebellar degeneration caused by high-dose cytosine arabinoside: a clinicopathological study. Ann Neurol 14:520–527
55. Xiang H, Kinoshita Y, Knudson CM, Korsmeyer SJ, Schwartzkroin PA, Morrison RS (1998) Bax involvement in p53-mediated neuronal cell death. J Neurosci 18:1363–1373

p21^{ras}/Erk-dependent signaling activates ischemic tolerance

V. L. Dawson[1–3], T. M. Dawson[1,2]

1. Abstract

The mechanisms underlying neuronal ischemic preconditioning, a phenomenon in which brief episodes of ischemia protect against the lethal effects of subsequent periods of prolonged ischemia, are poorly understood. We report that preconditioning induces p21^{ras} (Ras) activation in a NMDA receptor- and NO-dependent, but cGMP-independent manner. Ras activity is both necessary and sufficient for ischemic tolerance in neurons. Genetic and chemical inhibition of Ras blocks ischemic preconditioning, whereas a constitutively active form of Ras promotes neuroprotection against lethal ischemic insults. In contrast, the activity of phosphatidyl inositol 3-kinase (PI3K), essential for survival of various cell lines and cultured primary neurons, is not required for ischemic preconditioning as pharmacological and genetic inhibition of PI3K does not have any effect on the development of ischemic tolerance. Furthermore, using recombinant adenoviruses and pharmacological inhibitors, we show that downstream of Ras the extracellular regulated kinase (Erk) cascade is required for ischemic preconditioning. Our observations implicate activation of the Ras/Erk cascade by NO as a crucial mechanism in the development of ischemic tolerance in cortical neurons.

2. Introduction

Preconditioning to ischemic tolerance is a phenomenon in which brief episodes of a subtoxic insult induce a robust protection against the deleterious effects of subsequent, prolonged, lethal ischemia. The subtoxic stimuli which constitutes the preconditioning event are quite diverse ranging from brief ischemic episodes, spreading depression or potassium depolarization, chemical inhibition of oxidative phosphorylation (Riepe et al. 1997), exposure to excitotoxins and cytokines. The beneficial effects of preconditioning were first demonstrated in the heart; it is now clear that preconditioning can induce ischemic tolerance in a variety of organ systems including brain, heart, liver, small intestine, skeletal muscle, kidney and lung (Ishida et al. 1997).

2.1 Neuronal ischemic tolerance

In the brain, ischemic preconditioning is mediated largely by the activation of the N-methyl-D-aspartate (NMDA) glutamate receptors

Departments of Neurology[1], Neuroscience[2] and Physiology[3], Johns Hopkins University School of Medicine, 600 N. Wolfe St., Carnegie 2–214, Baltimore, MD 21287, USA.
e-mail: vdawson@jhmi.edu

J. Krieglstein, S. Klumpp (Eds.) Pharmacology of Cerebral Ischemia 2000

through increases in intracellular calcium and requires new protein synthesis (Gonzalez-Zulueta et al. 2000; Grabb and Choi 1999; Kasischke et al. 1996; Kato et al. 1992; Roth et al. 1998). While the importance of ischemic preconditioning in providing profound protection against ischemic injury has been established (Ferrari et al. 1999; Ishida et al. 1997; Murry et al. 1986; Tomai et al. 1999), the intracellular signaling mechanisms accounting for this phenomenon are still very poorly understood. In part, the requirements for the induction of tolerance depend on the experimental model, whether it is global or focal ischemia. While there are a number of descriptive papers detailing changes in protein modifications, protein expression or gene transcription, there are few functional studies that address whether any of these changes mediate the development of tolerance.

2.2 Global ischemia preconditioning

In the two-vessel occlusion model of global ischemia in the rat, PKCγ is translocated to cell membranes during ischemic preconditioning and is rapidly removed or degraded during the second otherwise lethal ischemic insult (Shamloo and Wieloch 1999b). Preconditioning selectively induces a decrease in the levels of the NMDA receptor NR2A and NR2B subunits and a modest decrease in the levels of NR1 subunit proteins in the synaptosomal fraction of the neocortex, but not in the hippocampus (Shamloo and Wieloch 1999a). There is increased phosphorylation of the extracellular signal-regulated protein kinase kinase and extracellular signal-regulated protein kinase (Shamloo et al. 1999). Additionally preconditioning markedly reduces the activation of p53 and its response genes p21(WAF1/Cip1) and PAG608/Wig-1 (Tomasevic et al. 1999). Following transient global ischemia in rats and gerbils the stress proteins hsp 27 (Kato et al. 1994) and hsp70 are induced in hippocampus, neocortex and thalamic nuclei (Aoki et al. 1993; Liu et al. 1993). Expression of the neuroprotective protein bcl-2 is increased in the CA1 area of the hippocampus (Shimazaki et al. 1994). Since ischemic tolerance is calcium dependent it is possible that some of the protective effect may be due to restricted Ca^{2+} influx through Ca^{2+} channels. RNA editing of the GluR2 subunit of alpha-amino-3-hydroxy-5-methyl-4-isoxazole propionic acid (AMPA) receptor, determines receptor desensitization and Ca^{2+} permeability. Following ischemic tolerance RNA editing of Q/R of GluR2 subunit in hippocampus is not altered but the R/G editing is reduced approximately 20% (Yamaguchi et al. 1999). The effect of this editing on the induction and maintenance of tolerance is not known. The expression profile of the fos, jun and Krox immediate early gene transcription factor families have also been examined. Only c-jun expression is induced following the ischemic preconditioning stimulus (Sommer et al. 1995). All these data suggest dynamic and possibly extensive alterations in cell signaling, but the data is descriptive and the role of these changes in the development of tolerance is still conjecture.

2.3 Focal ischemia preconditioning

In the focal ischemia model in the adult rat, tolerance can be induced in cortex (Barone et al. 1998; Chen et al. 1996) using the middle cerebral artery (MCA) suture method. This preconditioning ischemia substantially reduces the volume of infarction 72 h after subsequent 100-min MCA occlusion. This approach does not induce significant changes in regional cerebral blood flow in the tolerant regions. In this model, hsp70 protein is expressed in neurons in the tolerant regions. Other stress proteins, grp75 and grp78, were not altered significantly (Chen et al. 1996). Induction of hsp72 is also observed in hippocampal slices exposed to a preconditioning stimulus (Pringle et al. 1999).

3. Functional analysis of OGD (ischemic) tolerance in cortical cultures

Ischemia can be mimicked *in vitro* by combined oxygen and glucose deprivation (OGD) of primary neuronal cultures (Monyer et al. 1992). Tolerance can be induced *in vitro* by brief OGD followed 24 h later by a lethal insult (Gonzalez-Zulueta et al. 2000; Grabb and Choi 1999). In this culture model system the key features of ischemic tolerance observed *in vivo* can be replicated. Tolerance is dependent on NMDA receptor activation, but not AMPA or kainate receptor activation. Tolerance is dependent on calcium influx (Gonzalez-Zulueta et al. 2000; Grabb and Choi 1999) and new protein synthesis (Gonzalez-Zulueta et al. 2000).

There is a developing literature in the cardiac field for a requirement for NO in the development of tolerance. There are also several provocative functional experiments in the postnatal hypoxia model (Gidday et al. 1999) and hippocampal slice model (Centeno et al. 1999) demonstrating a functional dependence on NO for the development of tolerance. Since nNOS is activated during OGD, we wondered whether NO may be mediating tolerance in the OGD model and if so, how?

3.1 Nitric oxide

We investigated the signaling pathways that are stimulated during the 5 min preconditioning exposure to OGD and determined the functional significance of these signaling events (Fig. 1) (Gonzalez-Zulueta et al. 2000). To evaluate the role of NO we examined the effect of inhibition of nNOS during the preconditioning episode on ischemic tolerance. Nitro-L-arginine (100 μM) blocks the protective actions of preconditioning by approximately 70%, and coadministration of an excess of the NOS substrate, L-arginine (1 mM) restores protection. If OGD preconditioning induces tolerance via NO, then application of NO donors should also induce tolerance against lethal OGD applied 24 h later. Three different NO donors (sodium nitroprusside, DETA/NO and NOR-3) induced tolerance in primary cortical cultures in a dose-dependent manner. These data functionally implicate NO as a key mediator in processes leading to tolerance against lethal ischemia. OGD and NO are not inducing neuroprotection by altering calcium entry into cells (Gonzalez-Zulueta et al. 2000). Since a well-known target of NO signaling is activation of guanylyl cyclase we investigated the actions of guanylyl cyclase on tolerance. The potent and selective inhibitor of guanylyl cyclase, 1H-[1,2,4] oxidiazolo [4,3-alpha] quinoxalin-1-one (ODQ) had no effect on ischemic preconditioning, nor did the cell permeable cGMP analog, 8Br-cGMP elicit tolerance. These data rule out a role for guanylyl cyclase in the signaling pathways induced by OGD preconditioning (Gonzalez-Zulueta et al. 2000).

3.2 p21ras (Ras) Activation induces tolerance

Ras was identified through its ability to transform cells and it has been extensively studied as a mediator of oncogenesis. Ras has been shown to regulate cell growth, differentiation and ap-

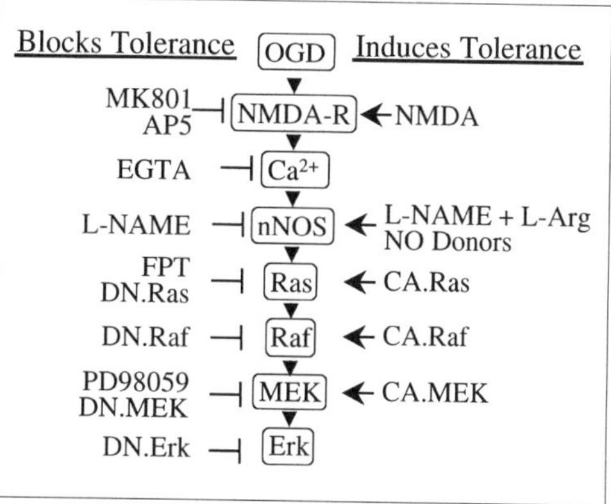

Fig. 1. Ischemia can be mimicked *in vitro* by combined oxygen and glucose deprivation (OGD). Tolerance can be induced *in vitro* by brief OGD followed 24 h later by a lethal insult. In this culture model system the key features of ischemic tolerance observed *in vivo* can be replicated. Tolerance is dependent on NMDA receptor activation and new protein synthesis. Our studies identified NMDA receptor/NO activation of the Ras/Erk signaling cascade as an essential early intracellular mediator of ischemic preconditioning in cortical neurons. By using activators and inhibitors of each step in this signaling pathway, we were able to systematically dissect the role of each intermediate of the NMDA receptor/NO to Ras/Erk cascade in neuronal ischemic tolerance. Our results indicate that all of these signaling mediators, Ras, Raf, Mek and Erk, are required for the development of tolerance to ischemia.

optosis, as well as influencing processes such as cell migration and neuronal activity. Most importantly there is emerging evidence for a key role for Ras activation in the development of neuronal plasticity. Since ischemic preconditioning is a form of neuronal plasticity that results in long-term cellular changes, activation of Ras is an intriguing cellular target. Ras acts as a branch point in signal transduction orchestrating the activity of multiple signaling pathways to regulate diverse cellular activities (Fig. 2). The various activators of Ras are still under investigation as are the mechanisms that control the selectivity of Ras activation of select signaling pathways.

NO activates $p21^{ras}$ (Ras) following NMDA receptor activation in primary neuronal cultures (Yun et al. 1998). Lander and colleagues have also observed NO activation of Ras in cell lines (Lander et al. 1995). How NO activates Ras is not known. It is possible that NO nitrosylates a critical cysteine and directly activates Ras (Lander et al. 1995) or NO nitrosylation of Ras could promote an interaction with a critical GEF that leads to Ras activation. Ras is rapidly activated during the 5 min preconditioning exposure to OGD in a NMDA receptor- and NO-dependent, but cGMP-independent manner. Inhibition of Ras during the preconditioning event both pharmacologically or with dominant negative mutants to Ras completely abolishes the development of tolerance. Expression of a constitutively active form of Ras is sufficient to induce protection against lethal OGD. These data provide functional evidence for activation of Ras in the development of tolerance (Gonzalez-Zulueta et al. 2000).

Ras acts on multiple signaling pathways to regulate diverse cellular activities. Ras signaling mediates cell survival of cerebellar granule cell neurons or peripheral neurons through activation of the PI3K/Akt or Raf/Erk effector cascades (Bading and Greenberg 1991; Downward 1998; Rosen et al. 1994). The PI3K/Akt

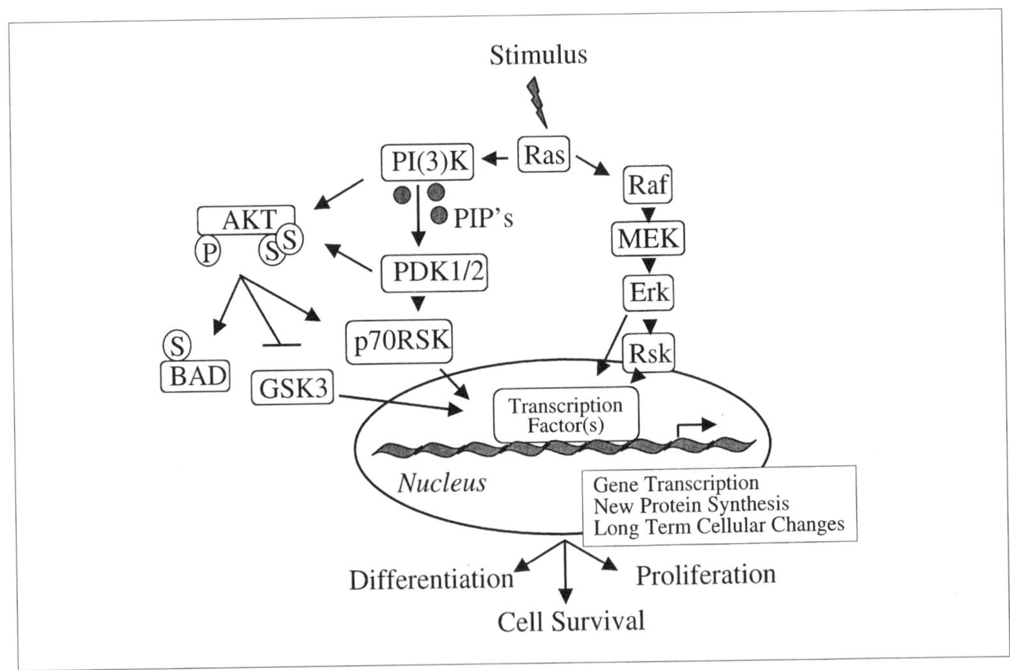

Fig. 2. Ras activation can result in gene transcription, new protein synthesis and cell survival through several different pathways. In OGD induced preconditioning and tolerance the Ras/Erk signaling pathway is predominant over the PI3K pathway as inhibitors of PI3K have no effect on reversing preconditioning.

pathway has been implicated in anti-apoptotic signaling in neurons (Dudek et al. 1997). However, neither pharmacologic inhibition nor dominant negative mutants to PI3K had any effect on the development of tolerance to OGD in primary cortical neurons, indicating that PI3K activity is not required for ischemic preconditioning in these cells (Gonzalez-Zulueta et al. 2000). Thus, we turned our attention to the Ras/Raf/Mek/Erk signaling cascade.

3.3 Raf/Mek Signaling induces tolerance

The Ras/Erk pathway is a hierarchical cascade. Ras activates Raf, a serine threonine kinase, which activates MEK (MAPK/ERK kinase). MEK, in turn, phosphorylates and activates Erk1 and Erk2 (Tibbles and Woodgett 1999). To evaluate a functional role for the Ras/Raf/Mek signaling cascade we tested dominant negative mutants to Raf and Mek. All dominant negative mutants were able to block the development of tolerance to OGD and these dominant negative mutants to Raf and Mek blocked OGD activation of Erk. Conversely, constitutively active (CA) Raf and Mek induced neuroprotection against 60 min of OGD. The CA mutants were capable of activating similar levels of Erk phosphorylation. These results strongly suggest that the Ras effector Raf and Mek are important in the mechanisms leading to ischemic tolerance.

3.4 Erk (Extracellular signal-Regulated Kinase) Signaling

Erk's are members of the mitogen-activated protein kinases (MAPK), a family of serine-threonine protein kinases that phosphorylate many cytoplasmic and nuclear target proteins. The MAPK/Erk signaling cascades are crucial regulators and mediators responsible for transducing extracellular stimuli. In addition to acting as cytoplasmic relay molecules by regulating downstream signaling proteins, the Erk's can directly phosphorylate and activate a number of transcription factors. The MAPK/Erk signaling cascades have been linked to diverse neuronal processes including long-term potentiation, consolidation of memory, development and cell survival and cell death (Impey et al. 1999). The sequential nature of the Erk signaling allows for regulation, integration and amplification of the original signals. The first suggestion that ERK cascade could participate in neuronal plasticity came from long-term facilitation studies in the invertebrate *Aplysia* (Bailey et al. 1997; Martin et al. 1997). Supporting evidence was subsequently gathered in *Drosophila* and in rodent models (Brambilla et al. 1997; Broadie et al. 1997; Li et al. 1997; Orban et al. 1999; Skoulakis and Davis 1996). Additionally, *in vitro* studies of long-term potentiation (LTP) and long-term depression (LTD), which are thought to be cellular models of learning and memory, also indicate a role for Erk in the formation of LTP (Winder et al. 1999) and LTD (Norman et al. 2000). Interestingly, Erk can mediate LTP through post-translational modification of proteins and at the transcriptional level (Winder et al. 1999).

Preconditioning is another form of neuronal plasticity and Erk may play an important role. Hypoxia stimulates Erk phosphorylation within minutes in the cortex of rats in a NMDA receptor mediated manner (Gozal et al. 1999). In primary cortical neurons both isoforms of Erk (42- and 44-kDa) are phosphorylated within 10 minutes of a 5 min OGD preconditioning stimulus (Gonzalez-Zulueta et al. 2000). Activation of Erk was NMDA receptor, NO, Ras and Mek dependent. Dominant negative mutants to Erk2 block the development of tolerance to OGD and activation of Erk, implicating a role for Erk in the mechanisms leading to ischemic tolerance.

How activation of the Ras/Erk pathway results in preconditioning and leads to resistance against neuronal ischemic damage is not yet known. Recently, stimulation of Erk signaling has been associated with different models of neuronal survival. BDNF protects cortical neurons against camptothecin or serum deprivation induced apoptosis and activates Erk and the phosphatidylinositol 3-kinase (PI3K) pathways (Hetman et al. 1999). However, in primary cortical neurons exposed to OGD, BDNF and PI3K do not mediate OGD tolerance (Gonzalez-Zulueta et al. 2000). Nerve growth factor (NGF) induced survival of sympathetic neurons involves Erk activation and Rsk stimulation leading to bcl-2 expression (Riccio et al. 1999). However, cycloheximide induces bcl-2 (Furukawa et al. 1997), but blocks tolerance in primary cortical neurons suggesting bcl-2 does not play a necessary role in OGD tolerance in these cells (Gonzalez-Zulueta et al. 2000). In cerebellar granule neurons treated with neurotrophins, Erk is activated leading to survival by both post-translational modification of BAD and transcriptional activation of CREB (Bonni et al. 1999). In ischemic tolerance it is unlikely that phosphorylation of BAD plays a role in the long-term neuroprotection, but it might play a role in acute protection. Since ischemic tolerance is dependent on new protein synthesis, activation of transcriptional elements is a strong possibility. Erk itself can activate gene transcription. Activation of the Ras/Erk can lead to the phosphorylation and activation of transcription factors in the nucleus such as the cyclic AMP response element binding protein (CREB), and Elk-1, which are attractive candidates. Identification of which transcriptional elements are activated will allow for a more directed search for the proteins responsible for the profound neuroprotection observed following ischemic or OGD preconditioning.

4. Summary

Preconditioning sets in motion a series of signaling cascades that ultimately result in profound neuroprotection due to expression of newly synthesized proteins. Preconditioning leading to tolerance is a novel form of neuronal plasticity that may share common signaling pathways. We have identified one signal cascade that is critical to the development of tolerance following OGD preconditioning. OGD stimulates the NMDA receptor allowing the influx of calcium to the cell. The NMDA receptor is tethered to nNOS via PSD95. Thus, a major calcium activated response to OGD and NMDA receptor activation is production of NO. Since OGD induced Ras activation is dependent on the activity of nNOS we conclude that NO production stimulates Ras activation. However, the exact mechanism by which NO activates Ras is not clear. Additionally, it is possible and likely that Ras is activated by other calcium dependent mechanisms. nNOS positive neurons comprise only 1–2% of the adult neuronal population. Although they project diffusely, the majority of neurons with NMDA receptors do not express nNOS. While activation of nNOS mediates a large component of tolerance, inhibitors and dominant negative mutants of the Ras/Erk signaling cascade are more potent in reversing preconditioning and tolerance then NOS inhibition, suggesting that additional calcium mediated pathways of activation of Ras/Erk signaling may occur (Curtis and Finkbeiner 1999). These other calcium dependent mechanisms may be more important in K^+-depolarization induced preconditioning, a model of cortical spreading depression. And it is possible that other calcium dependent pathways may play a key role *in vivo* in the development of tolerance. We also need to understand the transcriptional elements responsible for preconditioning and tolerance. This will point the direction towards the proteins and cellular changes which mediate tolerance. Until these pathways are identified and understood we will not be able to fully understand the phenomena of tolerance or harness its powerful neuroprotective strategies.

Acknowledgments

This work was supported by the following: V.L.D. by USPHS NS39148, AHA, MDA, and ALSA and T.M.D. by the AHA and USPHS NS37090.

5. References

1. Aoki M, Abe K, Kawagoe J, Sato S, Nakamura S, Kogure K (1993) Temporal profile of the induction of heat shock protein 70 and heat shock cognate protein 70 mRNAs after transient ischemia in gerbil brain. Brain Res 601:185–192

2. Bading H, Greenberg ME (1991) Stimulation of protein tyrosine phosphorylation by NMDA receptor activation. Science 253:912–914
3. Bailey CH, Kaang BK, Chen M, Martin KC, Lim CS, Casadio A, Kandel ER (1997) Mutation in the phosphorylation sites of MAP kinase blocks learning-related internalization of apCAM in Aplysia sensory neurons. Neuron 18:913–924
4. Barone FC, White RF, Spera PA, Ellison J, Currie RW, Wang X, Feuerstein GZ (1998) Ischemic preconditioning and brain tolerance: temporal histological and functional outcomes, protein synthesis requirement, and interleukin-1 receptor antagonist and early gene expression. Stroke 29:1937–50; discussion 1950–1951
5. Bonni A, Brunet A, West AE, Datta SR, Takasu MA, Greenberg ME (1999) Cell survival promoted by the Ras-MAPK signaling pathway by transcription-dependent and -independent mechanisms. Science 286:1358–1362
6. Brambilla R, Gnesutta N, Minichiello L, White G, Roylance AJ, Herron CE, Ramsey M, Wolfer DP, Cestari V, Rossi-Arnaud C et al. (1997) A role for the Ras signalling pathway in synaptic transmission and long-term memory. Nature 390:281–286
7. Broadie K, Rushton E, Skoulakis EM, Davis RL (1997) Leonardo, a Drosophila 14-3-3 protein involved in learning, regulates presynaptic function. Neuron 19:391–402
8. Centeno JM, Orti M, Salom JB, Sick TJ, Perez-Pinzen MA (1999) Nitric oxide is involved in anoxic preconditioning neuroprotection in rat hippocampal slices. Brain Res 836:62–69
9. Chen J, Graham SH, Zhu RL, Simon RP (1996) Stress proteins and tolerance to focal cerebral ischemia. J Cereb Blood Flow Metab 16:566–577
10. Curtis J, Finkbeiner S (1999) Sending signals from the synapse to the nucleus: possible roles for CaMK, Ras/ERK, and SAPK pathways in the regulation of synaptic plasticity and neuronal growth. J Neurosci Res 58:88–95
11. Downward J (1998) Mechanisms and consequences of activation of protein kinase B/Akt. Curr Opin Cell Biol 10:262–267
12. Dudek H, Datta SR, Franke TF, Birnbaum MJ, Yao R, Cooper GM, Segal RA, Kaplan DR, Greenberg ME (1997) Regulation of neuronal survival by the serine-threonine protein kinase Akt. Science 275:661–665
13. Ferrari R, Ceconi C, Curello S, Percoco G, Toselli T, Antonioli G (1999) Ischemic preconditioning, myocardial stunning, and hibernation: basic aspects. Am Heart J 138:61–68
14. Furukawa K, Estus S, Fu W, Mark RJ, Mattson MP (1997) Neuroprotective action of cycloheximide involves induction of bcl-2 and antioxidant pathways. J Cell Biol 136:1137–1149
15. Gidday JM, Shah AR, Maceren RG, Wang Q, Pelligrino DA, Holtzman DM, Park TS (1999) Nitric oxide mediates cerebral ischemic tolerance in a neonatal rat model of hypoxic preconditioning. J Cereb Blood Flow Metab 19:331–340
16. Gonzalez-Zulueta M, Feldman AB, Klesse LJ, Kalb RG, Dillman JF, Parada LF, Dawson TM, Dawson VL (2000) Requirement for nitric oxide activation of p21(ras)/extracellular regulated kinase in neuronal ischemic preconditioning. Proc Natl Acad Sci USA 97:436–441
17. Gozal E, Simakajornboon N, Dausman JD, Xue YD, Corti M, El-Dahr SS, Gozal D (1999) Hypoxia induces selective SAPK/JNK-2-AP-1 pathway activation in the nucleus tractus solitarii of the conscious rat. J Neurochem 73:665–674
18. Grabb MC, Choi DW (1999) Ischemic tolerance in murine cortical cell culture: critical role for NMDA receptors. J Neurosci 19:1657–1662
19. Hetman M, Kanning K, Cavanaugh JE, Xia Z (1999) Neuroprotection by brain-derived neurotrophic factor is mediated by extracellular signal-regulated kinase and phosphatidylinositol 3-kinase. J Biol Chem 274:22569–22580
20. Impey S, Obrietan K, Storm DR (1999) Making new connections: role of ERK/MAP kinase signaling in neuronal plasticity. Neuron 23:11–14
21. Ishida T, Yarimizu K, Gute DC, Korthuis RJ (1997) Mechanisms of ischemic preconditioning. Shock 8:86–94
22. Kasischke K, Ludolph AC, Riepe MW (1996) NMDA-antagonists reverse increased hypoxic tolerance by preceding chemical hypoxia. Neurosci Lett 214:175–178
23. Kato H, Liu Y, Araki T, Kogure K (1992) MK-801, but not anisomycin, inhibits the induction of tolerance to ischemia in the gerbil hippocampus. Neurosci Lett 139:118–121
24. Kato H, Liu Y, Kogure K, Kato K (1994) Induction of 27-kDa heat shock protein following cerebral ischemia in a rat model of ischemic tolerance. Brain Res 634:235–244
25. Lander HM, Ogiste JS, Pearce SF, Levi R, Novogrodsky A (1995) Nitric oxide-stimulated guanine nucleotide exchange on p21ras. J Biol Chem 270:7017–7020
26. Li W, Skoulakis EM, Davis RL, Perrimon N (1997) The Drosophila 14-3-3 protein Leonardo enhances Torso signaling through D-Raf in a Ras 1-dependent manner. Development 124:4163–4171
27. Liu Y, Kato H, Nakata N, Kogure K (1993) Temporal profile of heat shock protein 70 synthesis in ischemic tolerance induced by preconditioning ischemia in rat hippocampus. Neuroscience 56:921–927
28. Martin KC, Michael D, Rose JC, Barad M, Casadio A, Zhu H, Kandel ER (1997) MAP kinase translocates into the nucleus of the presynaptic cell and is required for long-term facilitation in Aplysia. Neuron 18:899–912
29. Monyer H, Giffard RG, Hartley DM, Dugan LL, Goldberg MP, Choi DW (1992) Oxygen or glucose deprivation-induced neuronal injury in cortical cell cultures is reduced by tetanus toxin. Neuron 8:967–973
30. Murry CE, Jennings RB, Reimer KA (1986) Preconditioning with ischemia: a delay of lethal cell injury in ischemic myocardium. Circulation 74:1124–1136
31. Norman ED, Thiels E, Barrionuevo G, Klann E (2000) Long-term depression in the hippocampus in vivo is associated with protein phosphatase-dependent alterations in extracellular signal-regulated kinase. J Neurochem 74:192–198
32. Orban PC, Chapman PF, Brambilla R (1999) Is the Ras-MAPK signalling pathway necessary for long-term memory formation? Trends Neurosci 22:38–44
33. Pringle AK, Thomas SJ, Signorelli F, Iannotti F (1999) Ischaemic pre-conditioning in organotypic hippocampal slice cultures is inversely correlated to the induction of the 72 kDa heat shock protein (HSP72). Brain Res 845:152–164
34. Riccio A, Ahn S, Davenport CM, Blendy JA, Ginty DD (1999) Mediation by a CREB family transcription factor of NGF-dependent survival of sympathetic neurons. Science 286:2358–2361
35. Riepe MW, Esclaire F, Kasischke K, Schreiber S, Nakase H, Kempski O, Ludolph AC, Dirnagl U, Hugon J (1997) Increased hypoxic tolerance by chemical inhibition of oxidative phosphorylation: "chemical preconditioning". J Cereb Blood Flow Metab 17:257–264
36. Rosen LB, Ginty DD, Weber MJ, Greenberg ME (1994) Membrane depolarization and calcium influx stimulate MEK and MAP kinase via activation of Ras. Neuron 12:1207–1221
37. Roth S, Li B, Rosenbaum PS, Gupta H, Goldstein IM, Maxwell KM, Gidday JM (1998) Preconditioning provides complete protection against retinal ischemic injury in rats. Invest Ophthalmol Vis Sci 39:777–785
38. Shamloo M, Rytter A, Wieloch T (1999) Activation of the extracellular signal-regulated protein kinase cascade in the hippocampal CA1 region in a rat model of global cerebral ischemic preconditioning. Neuroscience 93:81–88
39. Shamloo M, Wieloch T (1999a) Changes in protein tyrosine

phosphorylation in the rat brain after cerebral ischemia in a model of ischemic tolerance. J Cereb Blood Flow Metab 19:173–183
40. Shamloo M, Wieloch T (1999b) Rapid decline in protein kinase Cgamma levels in the synaptosomal fraction of rat hippocampus after ischemic preconditioning. Neuroreport 10:931–935
41. Shimazaki K, Ishida A, Kawai N (1994) Increase in bcl-2 oncoprotein and the tolerance to ischemia-induced neuronal death in the gerbil hippocampus. Neurosci Res 20:95–99
42. Skoulakis EM, Davis RL (1996) Olfactory learning deficits in mutants for leonardo, a Drosophila gene encoding a 14-3-3 protein. Neuron 17:931–944
43. Sommer C, Gass P, Kiessling M (1995) Selective c-JUN expression in CA1 neurons of the gerbil hippocampus during and after acquisition of an ischemia-tolerant state. Brain Pathol 5:135–144
44. Tibbles LA, Woodgett JR (1999) The stress-activated protein kinase pathways. Cell Mol Life Sci 55:1230–1254
45. Tomai F, Crea F, Chiariello L, Gioffre PA (1999) Ischemic preconditioning in humans: models, mediators, and clinical relevance. Circulation 100:559–563
46. Tomasevic G, Shamloo M, Israeli D, Wieloch T (1999) Activation of p53 and its target genes p21(WAF1/Cip1) and PAG608/Wig-1 in ischemic preconditioning. Brain Res Mol Brain Res 70:304–313
47. Winder DG, Martin KC, Muzzio IA, Rohrer D, Chruscinski A, Kobilka B, Kandel ER (1999) ERK plays a regulatory role in induction of LTP by theta frequency stimulation and its modulation by beta-adrenergic receptors. Neuron 24:715–726
48. Yamaguchi K, Yamaguchi F, Miyamoto O, Hatase O, Tokuda M (1999) The reversible change of GluR2 RNA editing in gerbil hippocampus in course of ischemic tolerance. J Cereb Blood Flow Metab 19:370–375
49. Yun HY, Gonzalez-Zulueta M, Dawson VL, Dawson TM (1998) Nitric oxide mediates N-methyl-D-aspartate receptor-induced activation of $p21^{ras}$. Proc Natl Acad Sci USA 95:5773–5778

Neuroprotective potency of activated NF-κB

C. Kaltschmidt, B. Kaltschmidt

Abstract

Nuclear factor kappa B (NF-κB) is a transcription factor crucially involved in glial and neuronal function. Within the nervous system NF-κB is ubiquitously distributed and inducible activity can be discerned from constitutive activity. Prototypic inducible NF-κB in the nervous system is composed of the DNA-binding subunits p50 and p65 complexed with an inhibitory IκB-α molecule. A number of signals from the cell surface can lead to rapid activation of NF-κB. Thus releasing the inhibition by IκB. Several pathways such as cytokine- and neurotophin-mediated activation, glutamatergic signal transduction and various diseases with crucial ROI involvement (e.g. Alzheimer disease, Parkinson, experimental autoimmune encephalomyelitis, multiple sclerosis, ALS and injury) activate NF-κB in neurons. Here some of our findings on the role of NF-κB mediated neuroprotection in Alzheimer disease and the modulatory role of glia on neuronal NF-κB activation are discussed.

Introduction

The NF-κB system and the nervous system

NF-κB is an inducible transcription factor, which is present in many neuronal cell types (for review see O'Neill and Kaltschmidt 1997, 1999a). Five mammalian NF-κB DNA-binding subunits where investigated in some depth: p50, p52, p65 (RelA), c-Rel and RelB. The p65 subunit is somewhat unique in that it contains some extremely strong transactivation domains (Schmitz and Baeuerle 1991). Consequently knock out of p65 results in embryonic lethality, a phenotype, that is not associated with knockouts of the other DNA-binding or inhibiting NF-κB subunits. This finding might underscore the immanent role of the transactivating p65 subunit. Well characterized inhibitory proteins are known as IκB-α, IκB-β, IκB-γ(p105), IκB-δ (p100), and IκB-ε. (Whiteside and Israel 1997). Within the nervous system heteromeric NF-κB is most frequently composed of two DNA-binding subunits (e.g. p50 or p65/RelA), which are either constitutively active or are complexed with the inhibitory subunit IκB-α (Kaltschmidt et al. 1993b; Rattner et al. 1993; Kaltschmidt et al. 1994b, 1995a, 1995b; Guerrini et al. 1995; Kaltschmidt et al. 1997). Interaction of ankyrin repeats are covering the nuclear localization signal of p65 and p50 (Malek et al. 1998; Jacobs and Harrison 1998), thus keeping the complex in the cytoplasm. Activation of NF-κB results in the degradation of IκB, which in turn exposes the nuclear localization signals, resulting in a nuclear import of NF-κB.

Institut für Neurobiochemie, Universität Witten/Herdecke, Sockumer Str. 10, D-58448 Witten, Germany.
e-mail: c.kaltschmidt@uni-wh.de

J. Krieglstein, S. Klumpp (Eds.) Pharmacology of Cerebral Ischemia 2000

In neurons NF-κB can be either activated by stimuli such as glutamate (Kaltschmidt et al. 1995a; Guerrini et al. 1995) or NGF (Wood 1995), which can involve activation of p75NTR (Carter et al. 1996). In some subtypes of neurons NF-κB is constitutively activated (Rattner et al. 1993; Kaltschmidt et al. 1994b; Schmidt-Ullrich et al. 1996). The specific post-translational regulation qualifies NF-κB as immediate signal transducer for transmitting short-term external signals to the nucleus. Thus NF-κB is a transcription factor, which was found in synaptic compartments (Kaltschmidt et al. 1993b; Guerrini et al. 1995; Meberg et al. 1996; Suzuki et al. 1997) and in Aplysia axoplasm (Povelones et al. 1997). Localization and signals which activate NF-κB qualify this factor as ideal candidate to transport information from synapse to nucleus. We have suggested that NF-κB functions as retrograde signal transducer which unifies both signal perception at distant sites (dendrites, axons, synapses) together with an effector function as a molecular switch for turning on gene expression (Kaltschmidt et al. 1993a; O'Neill and Kaltschmidt 1997; Kaltschmidt and Kaltschmidt 1998; Kaltschmidt et al. 2000a).

Signal transduction via tumor necrosis factor activates NF-κB

In terms of understanding NF-κB relevant signal transduction pathways, most progress was achieved with tumor necrosis factor (TNF). Therefore we will try to briefly summarize current knowledge. TNF receptors (p55 and p75) are expressed in the nervous system both in neurons and glia. Recent findings suggest a role for TNF in the nervous system on modulating neuronal responses to excitotoxic and hypoxic insults (see O'Neill and Kaltschmidt 1997 for review). In contrast to the protective effects of TNF there are also reports that identify TNF-α as potent mediator of microgliosis, astrogliosis and cell death (Feuerstein et al. 1997). Neuronal cell death and breakdown of blood brain barrier and demyelination was described in a transgenic model expressing TNF in astrocytes (Probert et al. 1997). Hence TNF might play an important role in the nervous system, most signal transduction pathways were characterized in the immune system (for review see Ashkenazi and Dixit 1998). Binding of soluble TNF to the trimeric TNF-receptor triggers the recruitment of various adapter molecules. For clarity the TNF-dependent caspase pathway will not be discussed in this context. NF-κB activation could be mediated via the interaction of the adapter TRAF-2 with the kinase RIP. This in turn activates the kinase NIK that is part of a high molecular weight complex. Homo- or heterodimeric complexes of Ikkα or Ikkβ are activated via the action of NIK. The Ikk complex can phosphorylate IκB bound by NF-κB more efficiently than free IκB. Thus this preference for bound IκB provides a mechanism to turn off activated NF-κB via the accumulation of unphosphorylated free IκB. Recently a modifier protein (NEMO/IKKγ, Yamaoka et al. 1998) was discovered, which must be expressed to transduce NF-κB activation by TNF, and Interleukin-1. Therefore NEMO/IKKγ might function as to physically link the IκB kinases to upstream activators. Several inhibitors of TNF-mediated signaling were recently identified such as the zinc finger protein A20 (Song et al. 1996), TRIP (TRAF-interacting protein) which contains a RING finger motif and FIP-3 containing a zinc finger and multiple leucin zippers. In contrast to the other inhibitors FIP-3 expression induces apoptosis on its own in HEK 293 cells presumably due to inhibition of NF-κB. In contrast the proteins cIAP and TRAF were recently identified as NF-κB target genes mediating the anti-apoptotic action of activated NF-κB (Wang et al. 1998).

Recent Results:

Role of NF-κB in Alzheimer Disease

Primary cerebellar granule cell cultures were used as a convenient well established culture system with a high content (> 95%) of neurons. Using this culture paradigm we have previously shown, that 0.1 μM Aβ (1–40) activates NF-κB, whereas the neurotoxic dose of 10 μM Aβ (1–40) does not (Kaltschmidt et al. 1997). We have tested the physiological significance of this observation using cerebellar granule cells pre-treated with 0.1 μM Aβ (1–40) for 24 h or left untreated (Kaltschmidt et al. 1999a). Cultures without pretreatment (0.1 μM Aβ (1–40)) did not survive an insult with 10 μM Aβ (1–40) for 24 h (Kaltschmidt et al. 1999b), as apparent from the large number of pyknotic nuclei. In contrast, cultures pretreated with 0.1 μM Aβ (1–40) did survive very well after treatment. This survival effect correlates with a long lasting activation of NF-κB p65. Quantitative analysis showed a significant protection of neurons with activated NF-κB (92% alive) in comparison to neurons without pretreatment (38% alive), whereas a concentration of 0.1 μM Aβ is not neurotoxic (92% alive; see Kaltschmidt et al.

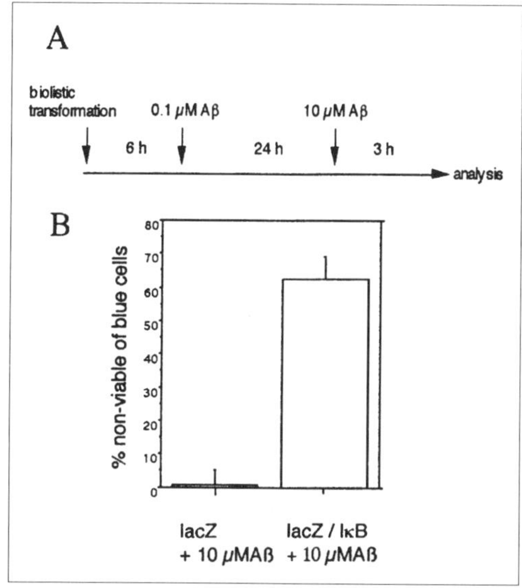

Fig. 1. Overexpression of IκB reverses the neuroprotective effect of pre-treatment with a low dose of Aβ peptide. **A,** Experimental setup for the treatment and biolistic transfection of primary cerebellar granule cells. Primary granule cells were transfected with the expression vectors by the gene gun, after 6 hours the cells were pre-treated with 0.1 μM Aβ (1–40) for 24 h to activate NF-κB and after 3 h the survivors were counted. **B,** Quantification of cell death in LacZ positive cells. Means (7 independent determinations) of dying cells were depicted (± SEM, $p < 0.001$) Modified from Kaltschmidt et al. 1999b.

1999b). To further corroborate the pharmacological data we specifically inhibited NF-κB, using overexpression of a transdominant negative super-repressor mutant of IκB in cerebellar granule cells. This mutant misses phosphorylation sites for IκB-kinases, which transforms this molecule in a constitutive repressor. We used biolistic transfection to express either E. coli beta-galactosidase (LacZ) or LacZ together with super-repressor IκB in cerebellar granule cells. These cells were as shown in Figure 1A (see Kaltschmidt et al. 1999b). LacZ expressing cells depicted a viable nuclear morphology, in contrast transfection of neurons with the IκB expression vector resulted in a high amount of cell death after the addition of 10 μM Aβ as apparent by the large amount of pyknotic cell nuclei (Fig. 1B). These data point to a critical role of NF-κB in activating a gene-expression program with neuroprotective function.

We have noted earlier that NF-κB is activated in neurons around early plaque stages (Kaltschmidt et al. 1997) presumably activating a neuroprotective gene-expression program as well. Based on our in vitro data discussed above we quantified the NF-κB activation in cells around different plaque types of Alzheimer's disease patients and healthy controls (Fig. 2). We found (Kaltschmidt et al. 1999b), that the earliest plaque stage, the diffuse plaque was most abundant (80%) in healthy controls (Fig. 2), whereas mature plaque types such as primitive, classical and compact plaques were typical for Alzheimer's disease patients (Fig. 2). Thus primitive, classical and compact types are accounting for up to 70% of all plaques in disease patients. Taken together a quantitative analysis of plaque types could distinguish between healthy (predominantly diffuse plaques) and Alzheimer's disease patients (predominantly primitive and classical plaques). We found a high amount of nuclear immunoreactivity in cells surrounding diffuse, primitive and classical plaques of healthy controls (Fig. 3, see Kaltschmidt et al. 1999b). In contrast to healthy controls many of the cells surrounding plaques of AD-patients show a vastly reduced NF-κB activity (Fig. 3, see Kaltschmidt et al. 1999b). Taken together data from 11 AD cases point to gradual loss of

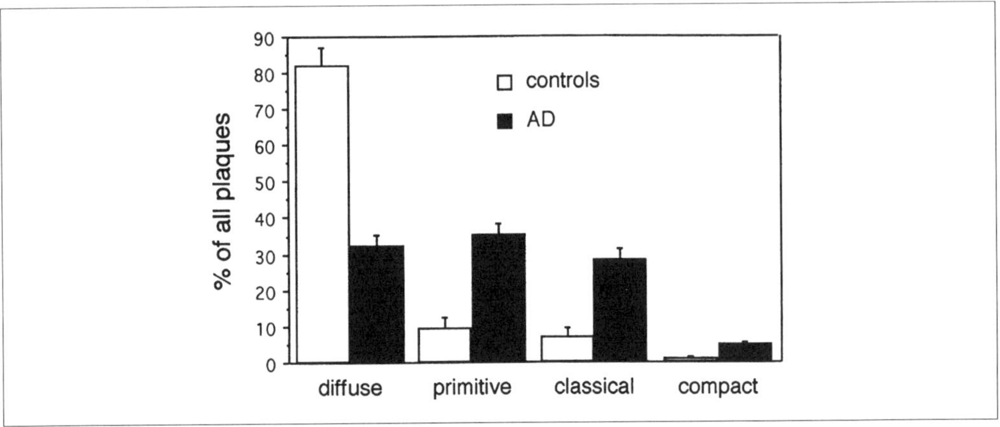

Fig. 2. Quantification of plaque types in AD-patients and controls. Means (n = 15 for AD; n = 15 for controls) expressing a percentage of the total plaque numbers in 98,175 mm[2] (5 randomly selected microscopic views) were depicted (Kaltschmidt et al. 1999b).

nuclear NF-κB immunoreactivity during plaque maturation. In comparison to controls the NF-κB activity in cells around all plaque types is reduced at least for 50% in AD patients (Fig. 3).

Our observations lend crescence to the idea that NF-κB activation is part of an important counteracting stress-response of neurons. Taken together this study shows that preactivation by low amounts of Aβ and TNF protects neurons through the activation of a NF-κB dependent gene-expression program. This effect can be blocked by overexpression of the specific NF-κB inhibitor IκB. Data from pathological and control material suggest that a protective effect is also operative in cells around plaques of healthy controls. As shown in vitro in cerebellar granule cells NF-κB can be activated by low amounts of Aβ and this activation leads to a neuroprotective gene-expression program. This might be due to an increased production of ROIs e.g. H_2O_2, since the antioxidant PDTC can inhibit the Aβ induced NF-κB activation.

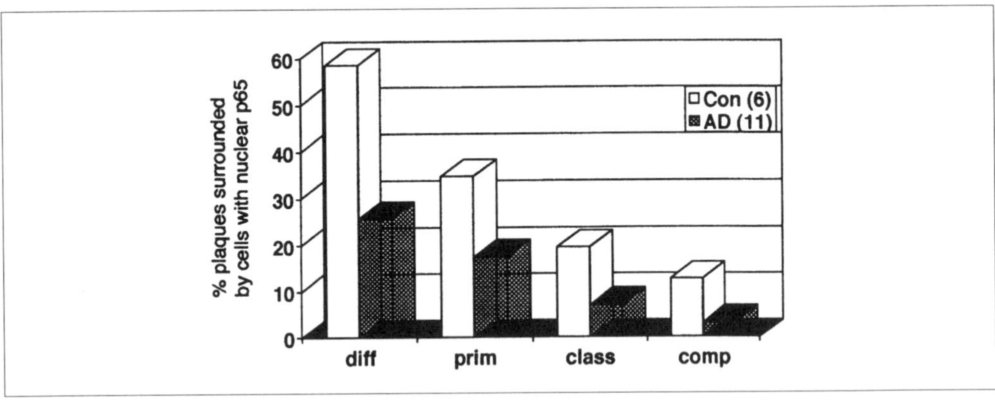

Fig. 3. Immunohistochemical analysis of nuclear NF-κB in cells around plaques. Note the reduced nuclear NF-κB immunoreactivity around plaques of AD patients in comparison to healthy controls (data from Kaltschmidt et al. 1999b).

Since astrocytes are absent in some plaques they seem not directly involved in plaque formation, but the loss of their neuromodulatory influence might be relevant for AD. Therefore we have analyzed the role of neuron glia interaction on NF-κB activation in an *in vitro* paradigm developed by Banker and colleagues. In this paradigm neurons cultivated on coverslips can be removed from the co-cultured astrocytes on the buttom of the petri dish. This allowed us, to compare cultures at various times post disassembly with control cultures of the same age and preparation, which were not disassembled. Figure 4 shows a time course of NF-κB activation after astroglia removal. The neurons adhering to a glass coverslip were fixed at various time points (0 h, 1 h and 6 h) after removal of astroglia. Intracellular labeling for NF-κB was performed with a monoclonal antibody recognizing exclusively the activated form of NF-κB. This form of analysis faithfully correlates with data obtained with other assays e.g. gelshift experiments (Kaltschmidt et al. 1995b) or reporter gene assays (Kaltschmidt et al. 1994b), but provides the advantages of single cell analysis. Under control conditions, that is with cocultured astrocytes in the assembled coculture (see Fig. 4), barely any NF-κB immunoreactivity was detectable. In contrast NF-κB activation was strongly enhanced after 6 h post astrocyte removal (Fig. 4). This increase was significantly different ($p < 0.001$) to the numbers of nuclear immunoreactive cells obtained after 0 h and 1 h post astrocyte removal. In order to define a potential signal transduction pathway for this activation, we were interested to determine if NF-κB could be activated in this coculture paradigm by glutamate or agonists. Since we have found in the previous experiments, that after 1 h of disassembly the separately cultured neurons do not show any NF-κB activation, we used this time frame of 1 h for further investigations. Cultures of hippocampal neurons were separated from the cocultured astrocytes and treated with kainate. After the 5 min. pulse with kainate cultures were either reassembled with astroglia or left disassembled for 1 h. Interestingly a 5 min. kainate treatment triggered a strong increase in NF-κB activation, in cultures without the astrocyte feeder layer. The same result was achieved when the cultures were treated with glutamate (data not shown). Surprisingly the coculture with astrocytes strongly suppressed the activation of NF-κB. Kainate could activate NF-κB in up to 90% of all pyramidal neurons of separated cultures, whereas reassembling of the neuron-astrocyte coculture resulted in a highly significant repression of NF-κB activation (Kaltschmidt and Kaltschmidt 2000). It was surprising that the repressing action of astrocytes is able to inhibit the kainate-mediated NF-κB activation down to basal levels (Kaltschmidt and Kaltschmidt 2000). Therefore, we conclude that astrocytes might provide means to inhibit an already triggered signal cascade in neurons, when added after the stimulation. In a broader sense one reason for the activation of NF-κB in neurons araound early plaque stages might be the failure of neuromodulatory glia.

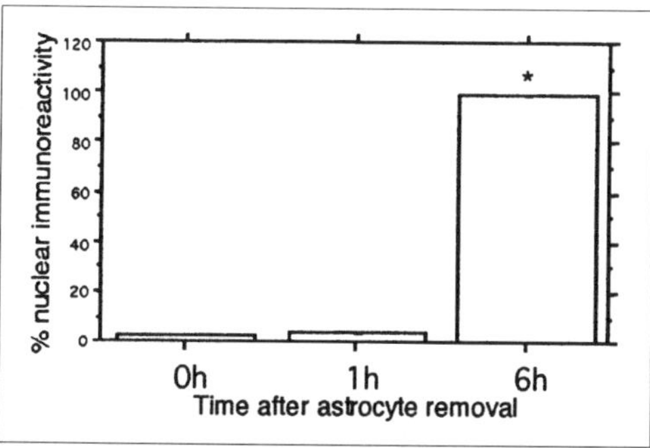

Fig. 4. Kinetic of NF-κB activation after separation from astroglia. Cocultures were separated and neurons were fixed and stained with an antibody specific for activated NF-κB. Pyramidal neurons were scored using a 40 x objective as nuclear positive or cytoplasmic positive by comparison with DAPI images. Counting was done in five fixed fields/chamber of up to 5 separate cultures. Values present the means ± SEM. * $p < 0.001$ compared with each of the other values; ANOVA with Scheffé post hoc test. Modified from Kaltschmidt and Kaltschmidt 2000.

Discussion

What could connect several signal transduction pathways?

Molecular evidence for redox-sensitive NF-κB activation?

Redox regulation of DNA-protein interaction could play an important role in controlling the actions of many mammalian transcription factors and thus providing means to control gene expression. Two eminent transcription factors regulated by redox-changes were described: AP-1 (Abate et al. 1990) and NF-κB (Staal et al. 1990; Schreck et al. 1991). The DNA-binding activity of AP-1 (e.g. Fos-Jun heterodimers) is also regulated by a redox mechanism. NF-κB is an example of a transcription factor activated by reactive oxygen intermediates (ROIs) (Schreck et al. 1991)), whereas AP-1 DNA-binding and AP-1 dependent transcription could be activated by antioxidants e.g. PDTC (Meyer et al. 1993). NF-κB binding activity is stimulated by reducing agents (Zabel et al. 1991; Schenk et al. 1994; Mihm et al. 1995) (e.g. dithiothreitol, 2-mercaptoethanol, thioredoxin). DNA-binding is abolished by sulfhydryl-modifying agents e.g. diamide, N-ethylmaleimide) (Toledano and Leonard 1991). In contrast, to the activation process the requirements for DNA-binding are demanding a reducing environment. Similarly later it was shown that the inhibition of DNA-binding by increased amounts of oxidants could be rescued via reduction with β-mercaptoethanol in extracts derived from intact cells (Brennan and O'Neill 1996; Toledano and Leonard 1991). Thus pointing to a role of reactive cysteins in DNA-binding. Using recombinant p50 R. Hay and coworkers have shown a crucial role for Cys 62 as a redox-sensitive site. Mutation of this aminoacid rendered the protein insensitive to the inactivating action of thiol-group modifiers. Similarly thioredoxin was able to stimulate DNA-binding of wt p50 in vitro and enhance HIV-LTR driven reporter gene expression in vivo (Matthews et al. 1992). In this line it was shown that cys 59 of (mouse sequence) p50 and cysteine 38 of p65 subunit (mouse sequence) are probably the two most critical for redox controlled cysteine residues involved in DNA-binding (Toledano et al. 1993). Acetylation of cys59 inhibits DNA-binding of p50 but not its mutation to serine. All redox-sensitive cysteins are found in conserved sequence motif present in all Rel-proteins (Toledano et al. 1993). Interestingly p50 from man and mouse contain the same critical sequence motif as p65 from man and mouse (see Kaltschmidt et al. 1999b). Recent progress in solving the molecular structures of p50 and p65 bound to DNA (Chen et al. 1998) explains the data obtained from mutational analysis where two redox sensitive cysteins are making key backbone contacts to DNA. Identical contacts in the homodimer structures (p50/DNA and p65/DNA complexes, (Ghosh et al. 1995; Chen et al. 1998)) were also observed (G. Ghosh, personal communication). Within the nervous system a considerable amount of knowledge was gathered about ROI-dependent pathways leading to NF-κB activation (see O'Neill and Kaltschmidt 1997). When starting our analysis of the NF-κB system in the nervous system, we made some predictions about a potential involvement of NF-κB in several ROI-dependent neurological diseases such as Alzheimer disease, Parkinson, multiple sclerosis and amyotropic lateral sclerosis (Kaltschmidt et al. 1993a). Due to work of many colleagues these predictions were now proven in great detail (see below). Recent data about the nuclear import as second redox-checkpoint were gathered using an activity specific monoclonal antibody. This antibody recognizes the activated form of NF-κB due to interaction with its nuclear localization signal (see Kaltschmidt et al. 1999b for detailed discussion). Using the neurotoxic amyloid beta peptide (Aβ) an inverted U-shaped dose dependence of NF-κB activation could be shown (Kaltschmidt et al. 1997), using this antibody. Interestingly high amounts of Aβ still activated the degradation of IκB and thus allowed the antibody to bind, but all p65 immunoreactivity was now concentrated in perinuclear aggregates (Kaltschmidt et al. 1997). This finding suggests that massive overoxidation interferes with nuclear import. It was reported that both activation and nuclear import are inhibited in T47D cells overexpressing glutathione peroxidase (Kretz-Remy et al. 1996). The oxidative ROIs could be either applied extracellularly as H_2O_2, or the ROI production could be induced via Aβ. This translated to a dose-dependent activation of NF-κB, were increasing amounts inhibited nuclear import and/or activation of NF-κB. For primary cerebellar granule cells a concentration of 10 μM H_2O_2 or 0.1 μM Aβ resulted in an optimal activation of NF-κB which was abolished with higher concentrations (Kaltschmidt et al. 1997). In this line it was previously reported that cholinergic stimulation could activate NF-κB, and that this activation could be blocked by H_2O_2 (Li et al. 1996). Cholinergic system deficits are reported in Alzheimer disease and are also detected during normal aging. In this line the constitutively activated form of NF-κB was analysed during aging in rat hippocampus and basal forebrain. Surprisingly an increase of NF-κB specific binding activity was detected (Toliver-Kinsky et al. 1997), perhaps suggesting an increase of NF-κB-activating ROI during aging. Similarly a ROI production by TNF could be abolished by PDTC pre-treatment in primary cerebellar granule cells and TNF showed a similar dose-dependence (Kaltschmidt et al. 1999b). Interestingly these dose-dependent effects translate in physiological relevant responses (see Fig. 5): Pre-activation of NF-κB with

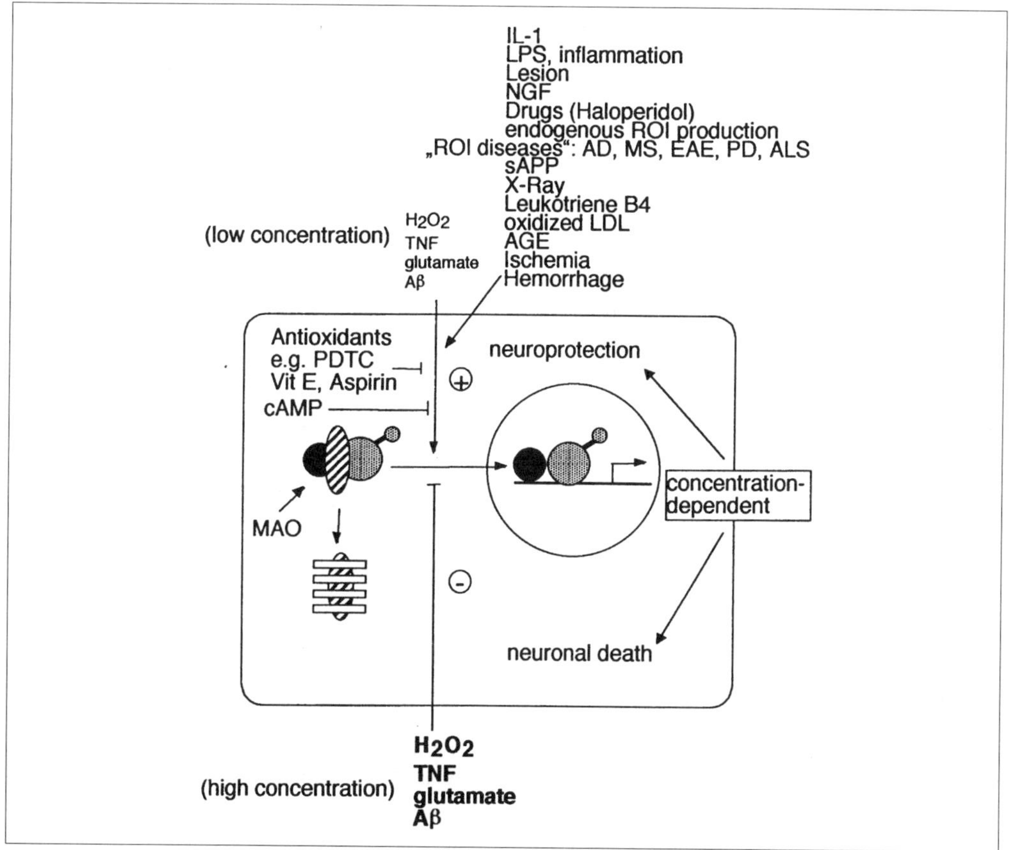

Fig. 5. Concentration dependent NF-κB activation via ROI-dependent pathways. Note that the same stimulus can either activate or inhibit NF-κB, depending on the concentration. In addition NF-κB activation can lead to stimulus dependent neuronal death or neuronal survival, which might also depend on the cell type with activated NF-κB.

low doses Aβ or TNF translated in a neuroprotection against high amounts of Aβ whereas pre-activation with a non-NF-κB-activating dose did not induce neuroprotection (Kaltschmidt et al. 1999b). Similarly it was found that NF-κB could be very efficiently activated with nano-molar doses of glutamate in cerebellar granule cells via the NMDA-receptor (Guerrini et al. 1995); but higher amounts (500 μM) resulted in only a weak NF-κB activation in the same culture paradigm (Kaltschmidt et al. 1995a). In contrast the glutamate agonist kainate, specific for non-NMDA receptors resulted in a concentration of 100 μM in a very efficient activation of NF-κB (Kaltschmidt et al. 1995a). NF-κB activation induced by ceramide was protective against glutamate mediated excitotoxicity (Goodman and Mattson 1996). In contrast in a quinolinic acid induced model of striatal excitotoxicity inhibition of NF-κB via striatal administration of an NLS peptide decoy reduced apoptotic cell death (Qin et al. 1998). In this respect a recent study showed NF-κB activation via kainate in the hippocampal fields CA1/CA3 and in the pyriform/entorhinal cortex sensitive to neurotoxicity (Perez et al. 1996), albeit in astrocytes. Behl and coworkers have shown that several antioxidants including α-tocopherol (vitamine E) act as neuroprotective agents (Behl et al. 1992). Similarly the anti-inflammatory agent aspirin, which can either act as an antioxidant or as a specific inhibitor of IKKβ (Yin et al. 1998) was shown to be neuroprotective in an excitotoxicity paradigm presumably due to inhibition of NF-κB (Grilli et al. 1996). It could be shown that Aβ toxicity is mediated by the production of H_2O_2, which could activate NF-κB (Behl et al. 1994). This H_2O_2 neurotoxic action of Aβ could be inhibited by antioxidants. PC-12 cell clones resistant to Aβ could be isolated (Behl et al. 1994). These PC-12 cell clones were shown (Mazziotti and Perlmutter 1998) to withstand the apoptotic effects of ROI-generation (hydroxyl radical or H_2O_2) via Aβ, amylin, 6-hydroxydopamine and H_2O_2, but show no resistance to other forms of apoptotic cell death or to necrotic cell death. Interestingly the molecular mechanisms of Aβ resistance relies on the constitutive activation of NF-κB (Lezoualc'h et al. 1998). Resistance to H_2O_2 was abolished via overexpression of a transdominant negative IκB or by the synthetic glucocorticoid dexamethasone, leading to increased expression of endogenous IκB. These data point to a crucial role of NF-κB in protecting neurons from the neurotoxic action of Aβ. In this line analysis of Alzheimer patients brains have shown that neurons located in concentric rings around early plaque stages contain constitutively activated NF-κB, in contrast to neurons in plaque-free regions (Kaltschmidt et al. 1997). Constitutively activated NF-κB was also shown to mediate neuronal survival of cortical cultures when challenged with Aβ (Bales et al. 1998). Oxidative stress induced by overexpression of the mutated presenillin-1 could be counteracted by treatment with the soluble form of APP. This counteraction could be blocked in PC-12 cells with decoy oligonucleotides comprising κB motifs (Guo et al. 1998). Similarly it was shown that TNF-mediated neuroprotection involves a NF-κB dependent increase in Ca^{2+} buffering (Barger et al. 1995). Reduction of protein nitration was correlated with a NF-κB-dependent increase in MnSOD expression (Mattson et al. 1997). Despite of the large amount of evidence for a role of NF-κB in neuroprotection there is also the notion that NF-κB activation is linked to neurodegeneration. In astrocytes NF-κB can be also activated by Aβ, which in turn activates the expression of iNOS. The iNOS induced NO production might contribute to the oxidative stress known to play a crucial role in Alzheimer's disease. On the other hand the autoregulatory loop present in astrocytic iNOS expression might also switch off increased iNOS production. Similarly LPS and cytokine-mediated NF-κB-dependent iNOS regulation in astrocytes is blocked by cAMP in contrast to macrophages were NF-κB can be activated by cAMP (Pahan et al. 1997). It was shown that Haloperidol, a dopamine receptor antagonist, is cytotoxic to mouse clonal hippocampal HT22 cells and causes cell death by oxidative stress (Post et al. 1998). Consequently NF-κB was activated by haloperidol and blocking of NF-κB was partially cytoprotective. Furtheron it was shown that dopaminergic cell death was ROI dependent apoptosis (Hunot et al. 1997). NF-κB was found to be constitutively activated in dopaminergic neurons of Parkinson patients. In primary cultures ROI dependent apoptosis induced via C2-ceramide correlated with NF-κB activation. On the other hand ceramide induced NF-κB activation was protective in hippocampal neurons – against excitotoxic and oxidative insults (Goodman and Mattson 1996). Other diseases with increased ROI amounts include experimental autoimmune encephalomyelitis (EAE) which is an animal model of multiple sclerosis. Increased ROIs are also found in multiple sclerosis (MS) itself. In these diseases with mainly inflammatory character microglia and macrophages might be crucially important for the increased ROI production and cytotoxicity (for review see Banati et al. 1993). In this line constitutively activated NF-κB could be detected in EAE, which correlated with the height of disease (Kaltschmidt et al. 1994a). Similarly activated NF-κB was found in macrophages present in actively demyelinating plaques of MS patients brains (Gveric et al. 1998). Interestingly NF-κB is activated in astrocytes and not in motor neurons in amyotropic lateral sclerosis (Migheli et al. 1997), suggesting that ROI dependent cell death of motor neurons is the consequence of missing NF-κB directed neuroprotection. Ionising radiation also increases ROI production and leads to NF-κB activation in PC12 cells, which in turn might activate IL-6 production (Abeyama et al. 1995). Interestingly this radiation induced IL-6 can act as differentiating agent. Previously we have shown that nerve growth factor (NGF) activates NF-κB via the $p75^{NTR}$ (Carter et al. 1996). NGF has multiple functions e.g. it can act to induce the differentiation of the pheochromocytoma cell line PC12 or induce cell death. Deprivation of NGF results in increased ROI production. Interestingly inhibition of NF-κB in PC12 cells induces apoptosis which was resistant to NFG (Taglialatela et al. 1997). Similarly inhibition of NF-κB in the central nervous system via proteasome inhibitors results in increased apoptosis (Taglialatela et al. 1998), speaking for an essential role of constitutively activated NF-κB (Kaltschmidt et al. 1994b) for neuronal survival in vivo. Inflammatory responses are a major component of secondary injury and ROI-mediated NF-κB activation might be crucially involved. In this line, using the activity-dependent monoclonal antibody specific for p65, it was found that activated NF-κB is present within the nuclei of macrophages/microglia, endothelial cells and neurons of traumatic spinal cord injury (Bethea et al. 1998). In addition upregulation of the NF-κB target gene iNOS was detected in this model of traumatic injury. Similarly increased NF-κB binding activity was detected in a cortical trauma paradigm (Yang et al. 1995). Surprisingly another report presents data on a downregulation of p65 immunoreactivity after crush-lesion of the rat sciatic nerve (Doyle and Hunt 1997). Similarly crush lesion of Aplysia pedal neurons results in a downregulation of axoplasmic NF-κB binding activity (Povelones et al. 1997). We have suggested that this might be a consequence of ROI-mediated NF-κB activation (Kaltschmidt and Kaltschmidt 1998), but so far there is no direct experimental proof. In the aspect of relevant target gene expression recently a NF-κB dependent enhancer was identified on an intronic enhancer regulating the TNF- and IL-1 induced expression of MnSOD (Jones et al. 1997). Moreover recently it was shown that MnSOD overexpression in liver resulted in a repression of NF-κB binding-activity (Zwacka et al. 1998) suggesting an autoregulatory loop. Other NF-κB target genes which itself contribute to ROI production include the NO-producing enzyme iNOS, Cyclooxygenase 2, 12-Lipooxygenase, Phospholipase A_2, the iron-binding protein Ferritin H-chain and NAD(P)H: quinone oxidoreductase. An important NF-κB target gene with direct link to apoptosis is CD95L (Fas Ligand), which can be induced via ROI-dependent NF-κB activation (H_2O_2 or hypoxia/reoxygenation) in microglial cells (Vogt et al. 1998). An important in vivo model for hypoxia is forebrain ischemia, using this model ROI dependent NF-κB activation could be detected (Salminen et al. 1995; Clemens et al. 1997). This ROI induced NF-κB activity could be repressed by the disease ameliorating antioxidants LY231617 (Clemens et al. 1998) and N-acetylcysteine (NAC)

(Carroll et al. 1998) or α-Lipoic acid (Packer 1998). Thus a large body of evidence accumulated on a crucial role of ROI mediated activation of NF-κB in the nervous system. While data are available for disease models such as Alzheimer disease, Parkinson, EAE, MS and inflammation, in vitro studies have shown a wealth of specific activators known to rely on oxidative stress both for neurons and glia. Conflicting results about the role of NF-κB in neuroprotection or neurodegeneration (Fig. 5) might either reflect a stimulus specific complexity or could be due to different experimental paradigms. Moreover recent interest has been focused on the length of the NF-κB activation (short term protective versus long-term destructive and on the cell type (protective in neurons versus degenerative in glia). In this respect recent data point to the importance of the stimulus, determining the contribution of NF-κB in both pro- or anti-apoptotic action (Kaltschmidt et al. 2000b). An easy explanation for this paradox janus-faced action of NF-κB might be the module character of regulatory cis-elements, were NF-κB acts in concert with other transcription factors. Taken together the exquisite sensitivity of NF-κB to various stimuli during ischemia qualifies this factor as a key regulator mediating either normal physiological signals or triggering a pathological gene expression program. Future studies will concentrate on the gene expression program defining neuroprotection versus neurodegeneration.

Acknowledgement

We are grateful to M. Frotscher for continuous support and to the Deutsche Forschungsgemeinschaft, Volkswagen Stiftung and European Community for generous funding.

References

1. Abeyama K, Kawano K, Nakajima T, Takasaki I, Kitajima I, Maruyama I (1995) Interleukin 6 mediated differentiation and rescue of cell redox in PC12 cells exposed to ionizing radiation. FEBS Lett 364:298–300
2. Ashkenazi A, Dixit VM (1998) Death receptors: signaling and modulation. Science 281:1305–1308
3. Bales KR, Du Y, Dodel RC, Yan GM, Hamilton-Byrd E, Paul SM (1998) The NF-kappaB/Rel family of proteins mediates Abeta-induced neurotoxicity and glial activation. Brain Res Mol Brain Res 57:63–72
4. Banati RB, Gehrmann J, Schubert P, Kreutzberg GW (1993) Cytotoxicity of microglia. Glia 7:111–118
5. Barger SW, Horster D, Furukawa K, Goodman Y, Krieglstein J, Mattson MP (1995) Tumor necrosis factors alpha and beta protect neurons against amyloid beta-peptide toxicity: evidence for involvement of a kappa B-binding factor and attenuation of peroxide and Ca2+ accumulation. Proc Natl Acad Sci USA 92:9328–9332
6. Behl C, Davis J, Cole GM, Schubert D (1992) Vitamin E protects nerve cells from amyloid beta protein toxicity. Biochem Biophys Res Commun 186:944–950
7. Behl C, Davis JB, Lesley R, Schubert, D (1994) Hydrogen peroxide mediates amyloid beta protein toxicity. Cell 77:817–827
8. Bethea JR, Castro M, Keane RW, Lee TT, Dietrich WD, Yezierski RP (1998) Traumatic spinal cord injury induces nuclear factor-kappaB activation. J Neurosci 18:3251–3260.
9. Brennan P, O'Neill LA (1996) 2-mercaptoethanol restores the ability of nuclear factor kappa B (NF kappa B) to bind DNA in nuclear extracts from interleukin 1-treated cells incubated with pyrollidine dithiocarbamate (PDTC). Evidence for oxidation of glutathione in the mechanism of inhibition of NF kappa B by PDTC. Biochem J 320:975–981
10. Carroll JE, Howard EF, Hess DC, Wakade CG, Chen Q, Cheng C (1998) Nuclear factor-kappa B activation during cerebral reperfusion: effect of attenuation with N-acetylcysteine treatment. Brain Res Mol Brain Res 56:186–191
11. Carter BD, Kaltschmidt C, Kaltschmidt B, Offenhauser N, Bohm-Matthaei R, Baeuerle PA, Barde YA (1996) Selective activation of NF-κB by nerve growth factor through the neurotrophin receptor p75. Science 272:542–545
12. Chen FE, Huang DB, Chen YQ, Ghosh G (1998) Crystal structure of p50/p65 heterodimer of transcription factor NF-kappaB bound to DNA. Nature 391:410–413
13. Chen YQ, Ghosh S, Ghosh G (1998) A novel DNA recognition mode by the NF-kappa B p65 homodimer. Nat Struct Biol 5:67–73
14. Clemens JA, Stephenson DT, Smalstig EB, Dixon EP, Little SP (1997) Global ischemia activates nuclear factor-kappa B in forebrain neurons of rats. Stroke 28:1073–1080
15. Clemens JA, Stephenson DT, Yin T, Smalstig EB, Panetta JA, Little SP (1998) Drug-induced neuroprotection from global ischemia is associated with prevention of persistent but not transient activation of nuclear factor-kappaB in rats. Stroke 29:677–682
16. Doyle CA, Hunt SP (1997) Reduced nuclear factor kappaB (p65) expression in rat primary sensory neurons after peripheral nerve injury. Neuroreport 8:2937–2942
17. Feuerstein GZ, Wang X, Barone FC (1997) Inflammatory gene expression in cerebral ischemia and trauma. Potential new therapeutic targets. Ann NY Acad Sci 825:179–193
18. Ghosh G, van Duyne G, Ghosh S, Sigler PB (1995) Structure of NF-kappa B p50 homodimer bound to a kappa B site. Nature 373:303–310
19. Goodman Y, Mattson MP (1996) Ceramide protects hippocampal neurons against excitotoxic and oxidative insults, and amyloid beta-peptide toxicity. J Neurochem 66:869–872
20. Grilli M, Pizzi M, Memo M, Spano P (1996) Neuroprotection by aspirin and sodium salicylate through blockade of NF-kappaB activation. Science 274:1383–1385
21. Guerrini L, Blasi F, Denis DS (1995) Synaptic activation of NF-κB by glutamate in cerebellar granule neurons in vitro. Proc Natl Acad Sci USA 92:9077–9081

22. Guo Q, Robinson N, Mattson MP (1998) Secreted beta-amyloid precursor protein counteracts the proapoptotic action of mutant presenilin-1 by activation of NF-kappaB and stabilization of calcium homeostasis. J Biol Chem 273:12341–12351
23. Gveric D, Kaltschmidt C, Cuzner ML, Newcombe J (1998). Transcription factor NF-kappaB and inhibitor I kappaBalpha are localized in macrophages in active multiple sclerosis lesions. J Neuropathol Exp Neurol 57:168–178
24. Hunot S, Brugg B, Ricard D, Michel PP, Muriel MP, Ruberg M, Faucheux BA, Agid Y, Hirsch EC (1997) Nuclear translocation of NF-kappaB is increased in dopaminergic neurons of patients with Parkinson disease. Proc Natl Acad Sci USA 94:7531–7536
25. Jacobs MD, Harrison SC (1998) Structure of an IkappaBalpha/NF-kappaB complex. Cell 95:749–758
26. Jones PL, Ping D, Boss JM (1997) Tumor necrosis factor alpha and interleukin-1beta regulate the murine manganese superoxide dismutase gene through a complex intronic enhancer involving C/EBP-beta and NF-kappaB. Mol Cell Biol 17:6970–6981
27. Kaltschmidt B, Baeuerle PA, Kaltschmidt C (1993a) Potential involvement of the transcription factor NF-kappa B in neurological disorders. Mol Aspects Med 14:171–190
28. Kaltschmidt C, Kaltschmidt B, Baeuerle PA (1993b) Brain synapses contain inducible forms of the transcription factor NF-κB. Mech Dev 43:135–147
29. Kaltschmidt C, Kaltschmidt B, Lannes-Vieira J, Kreutzberg GW, Wekerle H, Baeuerle PA, Gehrmann J (1994a) Transcription factor NF-kappa B is activated in microglia during experimental autoimmune encephalomyelitis. J Neuroimmunol 55:99–106
30. Kaltschmidt C, Kaltschmidt B, Neumann H, Wekerle H, Baeuerle PA (1994b) Constitutive NF-κB activity in neurons. Mol Cell Biol 14:3981–3992
31. Kaltschmidt C, Kaltschmidt B, Baeuerle PA (1995a) Stimulation of ionotropic glutamate receptors activates transcription factor NF-κB in primary neurons. Proc Natl Acad Sci USA 92:9618–9622
32. Kaltschmidt C, Kaltschmidt B, Henkel T, Stockinger H, Baeuerle PA (1995b) Selective recognition of the activated form of transcription factor NF-kappa B by a monoclonal antibody. Biol Chem Hoppe Seyler 376:9–16
33. Kaltschmidt B, Uherek M, Volk B, Baeuerle PA, Kaltschmidt C (1997) Transcription factor NF-κB is activated in primary neurons by amyloid β peptides and in neurons surrounding early plaques from patients with Alzheimer disease. Proc Natl Acad Sci USA 94:2642–2647
34. Kaltschmidt C, Kaltschmidt B (1998) A novel signaling system from the synapse to the nucleus. Trends Neurosci 21:106
35. Kaltschmidt B, Sparna T, Kaltschmidt C (1999a) Activazion of NF-κB via reactive oxygen intermediates in the nervous system. Antioxidants & Redox Signaling 1:129–144
36. Kaltschmidt B, Uherek H, Wellmann B, Volk B, Kaltschmidt C (1999b) Inhibition of NF-κB potentiates amyloid-β-mediated neuronal apoptosis. Proc Natl Acad Sci USA 96:9409–9414
37. Kaltschmidt B, Kaltschmidt C (2000) Constitutive NF-κB activity is modulated via neuron-astroglia interaction. Exp Brain Res 130:100–104
38. Kaltschmidt B, Deller T, Frotscher M, Kaltschmidt C (2000a) Ultrastructural localization of activated NF-κB in granule cells of the fascia dentata. Neuroreport 11:839–844
39. Kaltschmidt B, Kaltschmidt C, Hofmann TG, Hehner SP, Dröge W, Schmitz ML (2000b) The pro- or anti-apoptotic function of NF-κB is determined by the nature of the apoptotic stimulus. Eur J Biochem 267:3828–3835
40. Kretz-Remy C, Mehlen P, Mirault ME, Arrigo AP (1996) Inhibition of I kappa B-alpha phosphorylation and degradation and subsequent NF-kappa B activation by glutathione peroxidase overexpression. J Cell Biol 133:1083–1093
41. Lezoualc'h F, Sagara Y, Holsboer F, Behl C (1998) High constitutive NF-kappaB activity mediates resistance to oxidative stress in neuronal cells. J Neurosci 18:3224–3232
42. Li X, Song L, Jope RS (1996) Cholinergic stimulation of AP-1 and NF kappa B transcription factors is differentially sensitive to oxidative stress in SH-SY5Y neuroblastoma: relationship to phosphoinositide hydrolysis. J Neurosci 16:5914–5922
43. Malek S, Huxford T, Ghosh G (1998) Ikappa Balpha functions through direct contacts with the nuclear localization signals and the DNA binding sequences of NF-kappaB. J Biol Chem 273:25427–25435
44. Matthews JR, Botting CH, Panico M, Morris HR, Hay RT (1996) Inhibition of NF-kappaB DNA binding by nitric oxide. Nucleic Acids Res 24:2236–2242
45. Matthews JR, Wakasugi N, Virelizier JL, Yodoi J, Hay RT (1992) Thioredoxin regulates the DNA binding activity of NF-kappa B by reduction of a disulphide bond involving cysteine 62. Nucleic Acids Res 20:3821–3830
46. Mattson MP, Goodman Y, Luo H, Fu W, Furukawa K (1997) Activation of NF-kappaB protects hippocampal neurons against oxidative stress-induced apoptosis: evidence for induction of manganese superoxide dismutase and suppression of peroxynitrite production and protein tyrosine nitration. J. Neurosci. Res. 49:681–697
47. Mazziotti M, Perlmutter DH (1998) Resistance to the apoptotic effect of aggregated amyloid-beta peptide in several different cell types including neuronal- and hepatoma-derived cell lines. Biochem J 332:517–524
48. Meberg PJ, Kinney WR, Valcourt EG, Routtenberg A (1996). Gene expression of the transcription factor NF-κB in hippocampus: regulation by synaptic activity. Mol Brain Res 38:179–190
49. Meyer M, Schreck R, Baeuerle PA (1993) H_2O_2 and antioxidants have opposite effects on activation of NF-kappa B and AP-1 in intact cells: AP-1 as secondary antioxidant-responsive factor. Embo J 12:2005–2015
50. Migheli A, Piva R, Atzori C, Troost D, Schiffer D (1997) c-Jun, JNK/SAPK kinases and transcription factor NF-kappa B are selectively activated in astrocytes, but not motor neurons, in amyotrophic lateral sclerosis. J Neuropathol Exp Neurol 56:1314–1322
51. Mihm S, Galter D, Droge W (1995) Modulation of transcription factor NF kappa B activity by intracellular glutathione levels and by variations of the extracellular cysteine supply. Faseb J 9:246–252
52. O'Neill LAJ, Kaltschmidt C (1997) NF-κB: a crucial transcription factor for glial and neuronal cell function. Trends Neurosci. 20:252–258
53. Packer L (1998) alpha-Lipoic acid: a metabolic antioxidant which regulates NF-kappa B signal transduction and protects against oxidative injury. Drug Metab Rev 30:245–275
54. Pahan K, Namboodiri AM, Sheikh FG, Smith BT, Singh I (1997) Increasing cAMP attenuates induction of inducible nitric-oxide synthase in rat primary astrocytes. J Biol Chem 272:7786–7791
55. Perez OI, McMillian MK, Chen J, Bing G, Hong JS, Pennypacker KR (1996) Induction of NF-kB-like transcription factors in brain areas susceptible to kainate toxicity. Glia 16:306–315
56. Post A, Holsboer F, Behl C (1998) Induction of NF-kappaB activity during haloperidol-induced oxidative toxicity in clonal hippocampal cells: suppression of NF-kappaB and neuroprotection by antioxidants. J Neurosci 18:8236–8246
57. Povelones M, Tran K, Thanos D, Ambron RT (1997) An NF-kappaB-like transcription factor in axoplasm is rapidly inactivated after nerve injury in Aplysia. J Neurosci 17:4915–4920
58. Probert L, Akassoglou K, Kassiotis G, Pasparakis M, Alexopoulou L, Kollias G (1997) TNF-alpha transgenic and knock-

out models of CNS inflammation and degeneration. J Neuroimmunol 72:137–141

59. Qin ZH, Wang Y, Nakai M, Chase TN (1998) Nuclear factor-kappa B contributes to excitotoxin-induced apoptosis in rat striatum. Mol Pharmacol 53:33–42
60. Rattner A, Korner M, Walker MD, Citri Y (1993) NF-kappa B activates the HIV promoter in neurons. EMBO J 12:4261–4267
61. Salminen A, Liu PK, Hsu CY (1995) Alteration of transcription factor binding activities in the ischemic rat brain. Biochem Biophys Res Commun 212:939–944
62. Schenk H, Klein M, Erdbrugger W, Droge W, Schulze-Osthoff K (1994) Distinct effects of thioredoxin and antioxidants on the activation of transcription factors NF-kappa B and AP-1. Proc Natl Acad Sci USA 91:1672–1676
63. Schmidt-Ullrich R, Memet S, Lilienbaum A, Feuillard J, Raphael M, Israel A (1996) NF-κB activity in transgenic mice: developmental regulation and tissue specificity. Development 122:2117–2128
64. Schmitz ML, Baeuerle PA (1991) The p65 subunit is responsible for the strong transcription activating potential of NF-kappa B. Embo J 10:3805–3817
65. Schreck R, Baeuerle PA (1991) A role for oxygen radicals as second messengers. Trends Cell Biol 1:39–42
66. Schreck R, Meier B, Mannel DN, Droge W, Baeuerle PA (1992) Dithiocarbamates as potent inhibitors of nuclear factor kappa B activation in intact cells. J Exp Med 175:1181–1194
67. Schreck R, Rieber P, Baeuerle PA (1991) Reactive oxygen intermediates as apparently widely used messengers in the activation of the NF-kappa B transcription factor and HIV-1. Embo J 10:2247–2258
68. Song HY, Rothe M, Goeddel DV (1996) The tumor necrosis factor-inducible zinc finger protein A20 interacts with TRAF1/TRAF2 and inhibits NF-kappaB activation. Proc Natl Acad Sci USA 93:6721–6725
69. Staal FJ, Roederer M, Herzenberg LA (1990) Intracellular thiols regulate activation of nuclear factor kappa B and transcription of human immunodeficiency virus. Proc Natl Acad Sci USA 87:9943–9947
70. Suzuki T, Mitake S, Okumura-Noji K, Yang JP, Fujii T, Okamoto T (1997) Presence of NF-κB-like and IκB-like immunoreactivities in postsynaptic densities. Neuroreport 8:2931–2935
71. Taglialatela G, Kaufmann JA, Trevino A, Perez-Polo JR (1998) Central nervous system DNA fragmentation induced by the inhibition of nuclear factor kappa B. Neuroreport 9:489–493
72. Taglialatela G, Robinson R, Perez PJ (1997) Inhibition of nuclear factor kappa B (NFkappaB) activity induces nerve growth factor-resistant apoptosis in PC12 cells. J Neurosci Res 47:155–162
73. Toledano MB, Ghosh D, Trinh F, Leonard WJ (1993) N-terminal DNA-binding domains contribute to differential DNA-binding specificities of NF-kappa B p50 and p65. Mol Cell Biol 13:852–860
74. Toledano MB, Leonard WJ (1991) Modulation of transcription factor NF-kappa B binding activity by oxidation-reduction in vitro. Proc Natl Acad Sci USA 88:4328–4332
75. Toliver-Kinsky T, Papaconstantinou J, Perez-Polo JR (1997) Age-associated alterations in hippocampal and basal forebrain nuclear factor kappa B activity. J Neurosci Res 48:580–587.
76. Vogt M, Bauer MK, Ferrari D, Schulze-Osthoff K (1998) Oxidative stress and hypoxia/reoxygenation trigger CD95 (APO-1/Fas) ligand expression in microglial cells. FEBS Lett 429:67–72
77. Wang CY, Mayo MW, Korneluk RG, Goeddel DV, Baldwin AS, Jr (1998) NF-kappaB antiapoptosis: induction of TRAF1 and TRAF2 and c-IAP1 and c-IAP2 to suppress caspase-8 activation. Science 281:1680–1683
78. Whiteside ST, Israel A (1997) I kappa B proteins: structure, function and regulation. Semin Cancer Biol 8:75–82
79. Wood JN (1995) Regulation of NF-kappa B activity in rat dorsal root ganglia and PC12 cells by tumour necrosis factor and nerve growth factor. Neurosci Lett 192:41–44
80. Yamaoka S, Courtois G, Bessia C, Whiteside ST, Weil R, Agou F, Kirk HE, Kay RJ, Israel A (1998) Complementation cloning of NEMO, a component of the IkappaB kinase complex essential for NF-κB activation. Cell 93:1231–1240
81. Yang K, Mu XS, Hayes RL (1995) Increased cortical nuclear factor-kappa B (NF-kappa B) DNA binding activity after traumatic brain injury in rats. Neurosci Lett 197:101–104
82. Yin MJ, Yamamoto Y, Gaynor RB (1998) The anti-inflammatory agents aspirin and salicylate inhibit the activity of I(kappa)B kinase-beta. Nature 396:77–80
83. Zabel U, Schreck R, Baeuerle PA (1991) DNA binding of purified transcription factor NF-kappa B. Affinity, specificity, Zn2+ dependence, and differential half-site recognition. J Biol Chem 266:252–260
84. Zwacka RM, Zhou W, Zhang Y, Darby CJ, Dudus L, Halldorson J, Oberley L, Engelhardt JF (1998) Redox gene therapy for ischemia/reperfusion injury of the liver reduces AP1 and NF-kappaB activation. Nat Med 4:698–704

NF-κB is activated and promotes cell death in focal cerebral ischemia

A. Schneider*, A. Martin-Villalba, F. Weih, J. Vogel, T. Wirth, M. Schwaninger

In cerebral ischemia numerous genes are expressed that modulate inflammation, apoptosis, and neural plasticity. A better knowledge of the molecular mechanisms of transcription in cerebral ischemia may allow us to interfere with gene expression at a higher level of regulation and to influence several pathogenic pathways at a time. Therefore, many investigators of cerebral ischemia have focussed on the role of transcription factors including CREB (Hata et al. 1998), AP1 (Kiessling and Gass 1994), or NF-κB. NF-κB is known as a key regulator of genes that are activated in inflammation and apoptosis. Many genes that are induced in cerebral ischemia have been shown to be regulated in vitro by NF-κB. Examples include TNFα, IL-1β, IL-6, Fas-L, iNOS, COX-2, ICAM-1, MMP-9, p53, bcl-2, and bcl-x (Baeuerle and Henkel 1994). This has suggested that NF-κB may be activated in cerebral ischemia.

However, naturally occuring promoters always bind several transcription factor and their induction cannot conclusively show the activity of an individual factor. To avoid this problem we have used transgenic mice that contain a transgene that is under exclusive transcriptional control of NF-κB (Lernbecher et al. 1993). A transient cerebral ischemia in these animals was induced with the filament model. 20 h after a MCAO for 2 h the expression of the transgene was induced 3-fold on the ischemic side (Schneider et al. 1999). This demonstrates that NF-κB activates transcription after cerebral ischemia. NF-κB is a preformed transcription factor that resides in the cytosol in its inactive state. It is a dimer that is complexed to its inhibitor IκB (Fig. 1). IκBα covers the nuclear translocation domain of NF-κB. Activation is due to degradation of the inhibitor IκB. Thereby, the nuclear translocation domain is uncovered and NF-κB is translocated to the nucleus where it binds to the promoter of multiple genes and activates their transcription (Baeuerle and Henkel 1994). Activation of NF-κB can be localized in situ with an antibody that detects the nuclear translocation domain of the subunit RelA (Kaltschmidt et al. 1995). With this antibody we obtained evidence that NF-κB is translocated to the cell nucleus in the striatum, the thalamus, the hippocampus, and the cerebral cortex in the ischemic cortex (Schneider et al. 1999). Double-staining with the neuronal marker neurofilament-200 kD demonstrated that NF-κB is activated in neurons. We could not detect activation of NF-κB in astrocytes. A neuronal localization has also been described by Clemens and colleagues (Clemens et al. 1997; Stephenson et al. 2000) while others could detect NF-κB in astrocytes after focal cerebral ischemia (Gabriel et al. 1999).

Department of Neurology, University of Heidelberg, Im Neuenheimer Feld 400, D-69120 Heidelberg; *BASF-LYNX Bioscience AG, Im Neuenheimer Feld 515, D-69120 Heidelberg.
e-mail: markus.schwaninger@med.uni-heidelberg.de

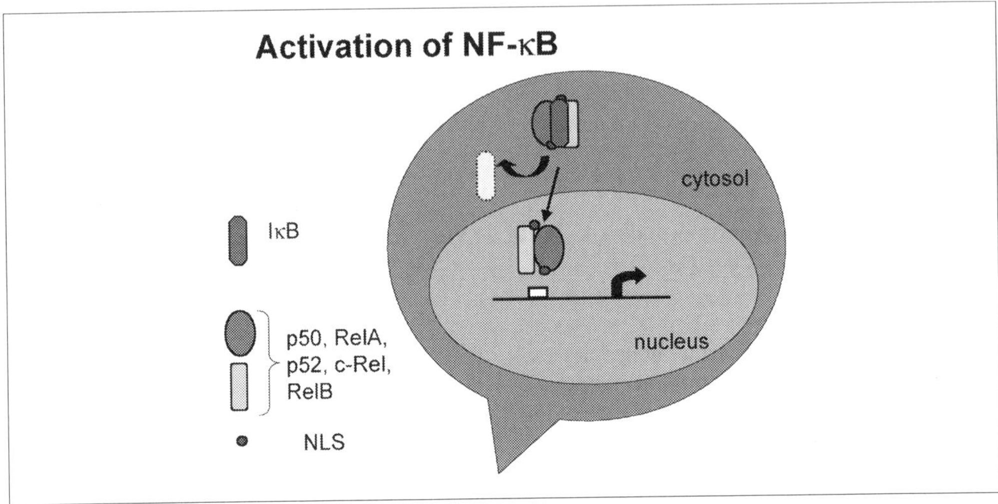

Fig. 1. The preformed transcription factor NF-κB is a dimer. There are five subunits (p50, RelA, p52, c-Rel, RelB) that can dimerize in various combinations. In its inactivated state the dimer is complexed with the inhibitor IκB in the cytosol. IκB covers the nuclear localization sequence (NLS). Activation of NF-κB is induced by phosphorylation and subsequent degradation of IκB. The NLS is uncovered and NF-κB translocates to the nucleus where it binds to the promoter of various genes involved in inflammation and apoptosis.

To analyze which subunits of NF-κB other than RelA are translocated to the nucleus we performed electrophoretic mobility shift assays of tissue extracts from the ischemic and non-ischemic hemisphere after 2 h MCAO and 30 min of reperfusion. Two bands bound in sequence specific manner to a typical NF-κB binding site. Both bands were increased in the ischemic compared with the non-ischemic hemisphere (Schneider et al. 1999). With antibodies against four subunits of NF-κB we found that one band consists of the p50 homodimer and the other of the p50/RelA heterodimer. An increase in the DNA binding activity of NF-κB after cerebral ischemia has been supported by others (Salminen et al. 1995; Clemens et al. 1997; Carroll et al. 1998).

As both NF-κB complexes contain the subunit p50 we used p50 deficient mice to approach the functional significance of NF-κB activation. p50 deficient mice had smaller infarcts than control animals (Schneider et al. 1999). The infarct spared the upper thalamus and the hippocampus where we found evidence for the activation of NF-κB by immunohistochemistry. From these data we concluded that NF-κB is activated in cerebral ischemia by translocation of p50 homodimers and p50/RelA heterodimers and that the activation of NF-κB contributes to the ischemic damage. As NF-κB is activated in neurons and neurons die by apoptosis after cerebral ischemia, an implicit conclusion from these data would be that NF-κB contributes to apoptosis in cerebral ischemia. Indeed, glutamate-induced apoptosis of the neuron-like hNT cells could be reduced by an NF-κB decoy oligo nucleotide that competes with natural promoters for DNA binding of NF-κB (Fig. 2). However, this view is controversial as will be outlined by Christian Kaltschmidt in this symposium. He and other investigators have obtained evidence that NF-κB may have a protective role in neurons that were treated with TNFα or amyloid β-peptide (Kaltschmidt et al. 1999; Mattson et al: 2000).

This apparent discrepancy could have several causes. A very interesting explanation comes from a recent paper by Ryan and colleagues (Ryan et al. 2000). These authors showed very convincingly that activation of NF-κB has op-

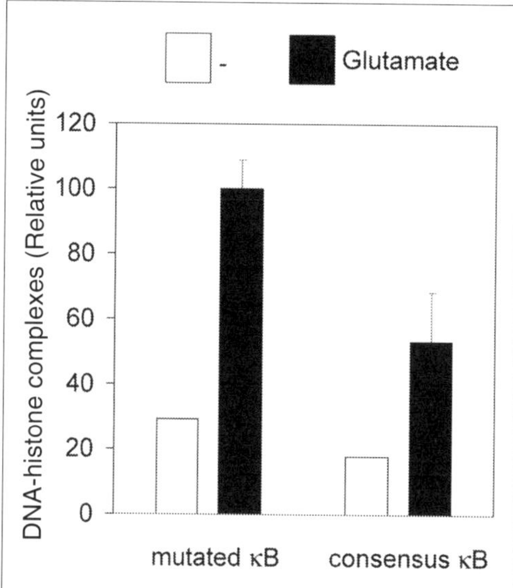

Fig. 2. An NF-κB decoy oligonucleotide inhibits glutamate-induced apoptosis in the neuron-like cell line hNT. Apoptosis was measured by an ELISA for DNA-histone complexes (Roche Diagnostics). Glutamate, 1 mM. Double-stranded phosphothioate oligonucleotides, 12.5 μM.

posite effects on apoptosis triggered either by p53 or by TNFα. If the effect of NF-κB on apoptosis depends on the stimulus, it will be a challenge for the future to define the mechanism of NF-κB activation that is relevant for cerebral ischemia.

Acknowledgment

We thank P. Chan for help with establishing the filament model in mice; and S. Prinz, N. Attigah, Y. Xu for their help at various stages of the project. This work was supported by a grant of the DFG to M. S.

References

1. Baeuerle P, Henkel T (1994) Function and activation of NF-κB in the immune system. Annu Rev Immunol 12:141–179
2. Carroll JE, Howard EF, Hess DC, Wakade CG, Chen Q, Cheng C (1998) Nuclear factor-kappa B activation during cerebral reperfusion: effect of inhibiton with N-acetylcystein treatment. Mol Brain Res 56:186–191
3. Clemens JA, Stephenson DT, Smalstig EB, Dixon EP, Little SP (1997) Global ischemia activates nuclear Factor-κB in forebrain neurons of rats. Stroke 28:1073–1081
4. Gabriel C, Justicia C, Camins A, Planas AM (1999) Activation of nuclear factor-kB in the rat brain after transient focal ischemia. Mol Brain Res 65:61–69
5. Hata R, Gass P, Mies G, Wiessner C, Hossmann K-A (1998) Attenuated c-fos mRNA induction after middle cerebral artery occlusion in CREB knockout mice does not modulate focal ischemic injury. J Cereb Blood Flow Metab 18:1325–1335
6. Kaltschmidt B, Uherek M, Wellmann H, Volk B, Kaltschmidt C (1999) Inhibition of NF-κB potentiates amyloid β-mediated neuronal apoptosis. Proc Natl Acad Sci USA 96:9409–9414
7. Kaltschmidt C, Kaltschmidt B, Henkel T, Stockinger H, Baeuerle PA (1995) Selective recognition of the activated form of transcription factor NF-kappa B by a monoclonal antibody. Biol Chem Hoppe Seyler 376:9–16
8. Kiessling M, Gass P (1994) Stimulus-transcription coupling in focal cerebral ischemia. Brain Pathol 4:77–83
9. Lernbecher T, Müller U, Wirth T (1993) Distinct NF-κB/Rel transcription factors are responsible for tissue-specific and inducible gene activation. Nature 365:767–770
10. Mattson MP, Culmsee C, Yu ZF, Camandola S (2000) Roles of nuclear factor κB in neuronal survival and plasticity. J Neurochem 74:443–456
11. Ryan KM, Ernst MK, Rice NR, Vousden KH (2000) Role of NF-κB in p53-mediated programmed cell death. Nature 404:892–897
12. Salminen A, Liu PK, Hsu CY (1995) Alteration of transcription factor binding activities in the ischemic rat brain. Biochem Biophys Res Comm 212:939–944
13. Schneider A, Martin-Villalba A, Weih F, Wirth T, Schwaninger M (1999) NF-κB is activated and promotes cell death in focal cerebral ischemia. Nat Med 5:554–559
14. Stephenson D, Yin T, Smalstig EB, Hsu MA, Panetta J, Little S, Clemens J (2000) Transcription factor nuclear factor-kappa B is activated in neurons after cerebral ischemia. J Cereb Blood Flow Metab 20:592–603

Caspases in cerebral ischemia

N. Plesnila, M. A. Moskowitz

Introduction

Ischemic neurons die acutely by a process called necrosis. However, many groups have now shown that cell death also occurs in a delayed manner during ischemia, dependent upon the synthesis and/or activation of proteins. One family of proteins, cysteine proteases named caspases, is of particular interest, because family members mediate programmed cell death and apoptosis in multiple organs and cell types.

At least 14 caspases have been identified to date, designated caspase-1 to 14 according to their date of discovery. Although most caspases are constitutively expressed in humans, two caspases, 11 and 12 are found only in mice. Caspases 1,2,3,7,8, and 9 are constitutively expressed in brain. Caspases 1,4 and 5 (caspase 1 family members) lead to cytokine maturation and mediate inflammation while caspases 2,3,6,7,8, and 9 (caspase 3 family members) promote apoptotic cell death. Upon activation, murine caspase 11 promotes both cytokine maturation and apoptosis.

The highly regulated and cascade-like cleavage of caspases resembles the complement or the coagulation system. Caspases are synthesized as inactive proenzymes and contain three subunits, an N-terminal prodomain, a large (~20 kD) and a small subunit (~10 kD). Upon cleavage they form heterotetramers and are thus activated. Family members show a near absolute specificity for cleavage at the N-terminal of aspartic acid residues; its catalytic site contains a highly conserved sequence (QACXG). Caspases are functionally divided into two groups, caspases regulating and cleaving other caspases (1–5 and 8–10) and caspases cleaving non-caspase substrates (3, 6, 7, 14), depending upon their substrate specificities.

In this review, we will briefly summarize the evidence implicating caspases in global and focal brain ischemia. Caspase involvement in ischemic cell death may have important therapeutic implications as well as for other acute and chronic CNS conditions in which cell death is prominent.

Global ischemia

Early evidence suggesting the involvement of caspases in global ischemia came from two simultaneously published studies showing upregulation of caspase-1 mRNA by RT-PCR (Bhat et al. 1996) and in situ hybridization (Honkaniemi et al. 1996) beginning 24 h after forebrain ischemia in the gerbil (see also Table 1). The

Stroke and Neurovascular Regulation Laboratory, Massachusetts General Hospital, Harvard Medical School, 149 13th Street, Room 6403, Charlestown, MA 02129 USA.
e-mail: Moskowitz@helix.mgh.harvard.edu

J. Krieglstein, S. Klumpp (Eds.) Pharmacology of Cerebral Ischemia 2000

Table 1. Caspases in ischemic brain injury

Global ischemia						
Author	**Caspase**	**Species**	**Strain**	**Ischemia**	**Model**	**Finding**
Bhat et al.	Caspase-1	Gerbil	Mong	7'	BCAO	+
Honkaniemi et al.	Caspase-1	Gerbil	Mong	5 or 10'	BCAO	+
Nakatsuka et al.	Caspase-3	Gerbil	Mong	5'	BCAO	–
Gillardon et al.	Caspase-3	Rat	SD	10'	Cardiac arrest	+
Chen et al.	Caspase-3	Rat	SD	15'	4 VO	+
Xu et al.	Caspase-3	Rat	Wistar	12'	4 VO	+
Ni et al.	Caspase-3	Rat	Wistar	30'	4VO	+
Gillardon et al.	Caspase-3	Rat	Wistar	15'	4VO	+
Ouyang et al.	Caspase-3	Rat	Wistar	15'	BCAO/Hypot	+
Krajevski et al	Caspase-9	Dog	Beagle	10'	Cardiac arrest	+
Focal ischemia						
Author	**Caspase**	**Species**	**Strain**	**Ischemia**	**Model**	**Finding**
Hara et al.	Caspase-1	Mouse	Transg	3 h MCAO	Filament	+
Schielke et al.	Caspase-1	Mouse	KO	Perm MCAO	Filament	+
Asahi et al.	Caspase-3	Rat	SD	Perm MCAO	Filament	+
Namura et al.	Caspase-3	Mouse	SV129	2 h MCAO	Filament	+
Ḟink et al.	Caspase-3	Mouse	SV129	30' MCAO	Filament	+
Guegan et al.	Caspase-3	Mouse	C57bl	Perm MCAO	Distal	+
Velier et al.	Caspase-3 and 8	Rat	SH	Perm MCAO	Distal	+
Kang et al.	Caspase-11	Mouse	KO	Perm MCAO	Filament	+

SD = Sprague Dawley; BCAO = Bilateral carotic artery occlusion; Hypot = Hypotension; Transg = Transgenic; KO = Knock out; SH = Spontaneously hypertensive; MCAO = Middle cerebral artery occlusion; Perm = permanent.

protein was found at 48 h (Bhat et al. 1996). Upregulation of caspase-3 mRNA (in situ hybridization) plus a 2-fold increase in DEVD cleaving activity was identified at 24 h in rat CA1 hippocampal neurons after 10 min of cardiac arrest (Gillardon et al. 1997). These findings were later confirmed (Chen et al. 1998; Ni et al. 1998; Gillardon et al. 1999; Ouyang et al. 1999), along with additional evidence for increased caspase-3 protein and enzyme activity within hippocampus after global ischemia. One report, however, failed to show active caspase-3 after global ischemia in the gerbil by immunohistochemistry, although the constitutive proform was widely expressed in CA1 hippocampus (Nakatsuka et al. 2000). More recently, caspase 9 release from mitochondria was documented after canine cardiac arrest (Krajewski et al. 1999). Under basal conditions, caspase-9 was localized within mitochondria by electron microscopy and fluorescence microscopy. In cultured cells, caspase-9 forms a complex with APAF-1 (apoptosis activating factor-1) plus cytochrome c and deoxy-ATP within the cytosol, and thereby promotes downstream caspase cleavage and activation. Cytochrome c release was detected in hippocampal neurons up to 2 h after a global ischemic insult (Nakatsuka et al. 1999) and thereafter (Antonawich 1999; Sugawara et al. 1999). Hence, this pathway may possibly be involved in caspase-9 activation by formation of a mitochondrial death complex (apoptosome) (Perez-Pinzon et al. 1999).

Table 2. Caspase inhibitors in cerebral ischemia

Global ischemia						
Author	**Species**	**Strain**	**Ischemia**	**Model**	**Inhibitor and dosasge**	**Protection**
Hirni et al.	Gerbil	Mong	5'	BCAO	zD (1 μmol) intrahippocampally (CA1); 0', 12 h, 24 h	+
Chen et al.	Rat	SD	15'	4 VO	zDEVD (1.5 μg) icv; –30, 2, 24 h	+
Gillardon et al.	Rat	Wistar	15'	4VO	zDEVD icv; cont 0' to 24 h (50 pmol/h)	+
Rami et al.	Rat	Wistar	10'	BCAO/Hypo	zVAD (200 μg) icv; 60'	+
Li et al.	Rat	Wistar	10'	4 VO	zVAD (200ng)/DEVD (200ng) icv; –15', 10'	–
Focal ischemia						
Author	**Species**	**Strain**	**Ischemia**	**Model**	**Inhibitor and dosage**	**Protection**
Loddick et al.	Rat	SD	Per MCAO	Distal	zVAD (1 pmol) icv; –30', 15', 2,4,6,8 h	+
Wiessner et al.	Rat	Fisher	Per MCAO	Distal	zVAD icv; –30' (120 ng), cont for 24 h (40 ng/h)	+
Li et al.	Rat	SH	90' MCAO	Distal	zVAD (200 ng)/DEVD (200 ng) icv; –30, 30', 60', 2 h	+
Hara et al.	Rat	SD	2 h MCAO	Filament	zVAD (160 ng) icv; –15', 2 h 10'	+
Hara et al.	Mouse	SV129	2 h MCAO	Filament	zVAD (80 ng)/DEVD (240 ng)/YVAD (400ng) icv; –15', 2 h	+
Endres et al.	Mouse	SV129	30' MCAO	Filament	zVAD (120 ng)/DEVD (480 ng) icv; –10', or 3 or 6 h	+
Fink et al.	Mouse	SV129	30' MCAO	Filament	zDEVD (480 ng) icv; –10', or 6 or 9 h	+

SD = Sprague Dawley; BCAO = Bilateral carotic artery occlusion; Hypot = Hypotension; SH = Spontaneously hypertensive; MCAO = Middle cerebral artery occlusion; Per = permanent.

The importance of caspases after global ischemia was further established by pharmacological evidence showing enhanced resistance to ischemic injury following caspase inhibition (Table 2). Himi et al. (1998) injected in the gerbil hippocampus an irreversible pancaspase inhibitor, benzyloxycarbonyl-Asp-CH2-dichlorobenzene (zD), and showed nearly complete rescue of CA1 neurons after 8 days. Performance on memory tests was better and cleavage of a caspase 3 substrate, PARP was inhibited. Several other groups confirmed that rat hippocampal neurons were resistant after similar treatment protocols using different global ischemia models (Chen et al. 1998; Gillardon et al. 1999; Rami et al. 2000). For example, Chen et al. and Gillardon et al. showed that cell death was decreased by 30–85% in the CA1 region after inhibition of caspase-3. However, not all studies agree. Li and colleagues injected zVAD.FMK or zDEVD.FMK both as a pre- and postreatment but did not find protection (Li et al. 2000), possibly because a 10-fold lower dose (2 x 200 ng vs. 3 x 1.5 µg) was used in their global ischemia model.

Focal ischemia

The evidence establishing the significance of caspases is strong not only in global but also in focal ischemia. This is based on pharmacological and biochemical data plus findings from experiments in transgenic and knockout mice. Early evidence came from a preliminary study using repeated administration of a pancaspase inhibitor, z-VAD before and after permanent focal ischemia in the rat. 24 h later, a 50% reduction of total infarct volume was observed (Loddick et al. 1996) (Table 2). Hara et al. (1997) confirmed these findings in models of transient focal ischemia (2 h) in mice and rats and showed 25% protection at 24 hours after zDEVD.FMK, a more selective caspase inhibitor without inhibition of IL-1beta formation. Another study by the same group demonstrated the importance of caspase-1 by showing neuroprotection (45% decrease of infarct volume) using transgenic mice expressing a dominant negative inhibitor of caspase-1 (Hara et al. 1997). A similar infarct reduction (–50%) was also found in caspase-1 deficient animals (Schielke et al. 1998). However, as shown recently, caspase-1 deficient mice do not express caspase-11 (Kang et al. 2000), which is also cleaved and activated during cerebral ischemia (see below). Therefore it is not entirely clear if the neuroprotection seen in these animals is only due to lack of caspase 1.

Caspase 3 has been particularly implicated in focal ischemic brain damage. Asashi et al. (1997) demonstrated upregulation of rat caspase-3 mRNA already 1 h after the induction of permanent ischemia. Namura et al. detected constitutive expression of caspase 3 within neurons. Upregulation of murine caspase-3 protein plus increased enzyme activity was shown by Namura et al. (1998) and Fink et al. (1998), respectively after severe and mild focal ischemia. After severe ischemia (2 h), caspase-3 was maximally active shortly after reperfusion, whereas after mild ischemia (30 min) the enzyme was maximally active after 12 h. Consistent with these results, infarct volume decreased by 60% at 3 days when zDEVD was given up to 9 h after mild ischemia (30 min), consistent with previous findings (Endres et al. 1998).

Severe injury (> 2 h) is less responsive to delayed application of caspase inhibitors (Hara et al. 1997; Li et al. 2000; Wiessner et al. 2000), in contrast to models using mild cerebral ischemia (30 min) (Fink et al. 1998; Endres et al. 1998). For example, Li et al. (2000) found that pre- and post treatment together afforded neuroprotection but not when given only during (30 and 60 min) and after (120 min) 90 min ischemia. Similarly, when given as a bolus 30 min before ischemia and as a continuous icv infusion over 24 h thereafter, brain damage was reduced by 30% (Wiessner et al. 2000), albeit less than the 55–70% in models using mild ischemic injury (Fink et al. 1998; Endres et al. 1998).

In addition to caspase-1 and 3, caspases 7, 8, 11 and cytochrome c, a coactivator of caspase-9, have been implicated in ischemic brain injury (Fujimura et al. 1998; Velier et al. 1999; Kang et al. 2000). Caspase 11 for example was upregulated and cleaved 12 h after permanent ischemia. Caspase-11 knock out mice exhibit a 75% reduction in TUNEL positive cells and had reduced caspase-3 cleavage within the ischemic cortex (Kang et al. 2000), although the relative importance of caspase 11 or caspase 1 remains to be determined (see above). Caspase 8 was cleaved in ischemic cortex beginning 6 h after permanent MCA occlusion (Velier et al. 1999). Because caspase 8 processing is coupled to activation of TNF-like receptors, cell surface receptors (e.g. Fas, TNF-R1) may promote ischemic neuronal cell death (Matsuyama et al. 1994, 1995; Martin-Villalba et al. 1999; Harrison et al. 2000; Felderhoff-Mueser et al. 2000). Recently we showed constitutive caspase 7 mRNA and caspase 7 protein expression in mouse brain. After 2 h distal MCAO and 24 h reperfusion, caspase 7 mRNA is upregulated and the proform decreased, suggesting increased caspase 7 turnover (Y. Wu, personal communication).

There are also reports about caspases which are not involved in ischemic brain injury. For example, caspase 2 protein levels are unchanged after cerebral ischemia in the mouse and mice deficient in caspase 2 are not protected from ischemic brain damage, at least 24 h after 2 h MCAO model (Bergeron et al. 1998).

Neonatal hypoxic-ischemic brain injury

In rodent models, neuronal cell death develops after a delay of 6 to 12 h and is paralleled by activation of downstream caspases, as shown by DEVD cleavage activity (Cheng et al. 1998), the appearance of active caspase 3 (Hee et al. 2000), and cleavage of actin, a caspase substrate (Pulera et al. 1998). Caspase 1 deficient neonatal mice are more resistant to 70 min but not 120 min ischemia/hypoxia (Liu et al. 1999), again indicating a role for caspases in milder forms of cerebral ischemia. Finally, pancaspase inhibitors (BAF) reduced injured brain tissue by > 50% even when given systemically 3 h after the insult (Cheng et al. 1998).

Spinal cord ischemia

Motorneurons die selectively and in a delayed manner after spinal cord ischemia (Hayashi et al. 1998). During this time window caspases 1, 3 and 8 are activated and the FAS death receptor is detected by immunohistochemistry and Western Blot analysis (Hayashi et al. 1998; Matsushita et al. 2000). Processed caspase 8 precedes the activation of caspase 3 and colocalizes with FAS on motorneurons possibly by formation of a death inducing signaling complex (DISC) (Matsushita et al. 2000).

Conclusion

There is already sufficient evidence to implicate caspases in ischemic pathophysiology and to suggest their targeting for treatment of acute CNS injury. Together, the data suggest that caspases are constitutively expressed in adult nervous system and become activated after brain and spinal cord injury. The onset and extent of cleavage depends to some degree, upon the magnitude and duration of insult with evidence favoring a greater role for caspase-mediated cell death under briefer and milder-moderate ischemic injury. The mechanisms appear distinct from necrotic cell death mediated by excitotoxicity, and there is in vivo and in vitro evidence to suggest synergistic effects which may have important implications for combination therapy (Schulz et al. 1998; Ma et al. 1998). The two mechanisms of cell death are not mutually exclusive however. The use of caspase inhibitors for human stroke will depend upon the successful development of drugs which cross the blood brain barrier and penetrate CNS cells at sufficient levels to achieve enzyme inhibition. The expression and activation of other caspases (e.g., caspase 8 and caspase 7) suggest advantages of developing pancaspase inhibitors.

Acknowledgements

The current work was supported by the NIH (NS10828 and NS374141-02 to MAM) and the Deutsche Forschungsgemeinschaft (Pl 249/5-1 to NP).

References

1. Antonawich FJ (1999) Translocation of cytochrome c following transient global ischemia in the gerbil. Neurosci Lett 274: 123–126
2. Asahi M, Hoshimaru M, Uemura Y, Tokime T, Kojima M, Ohtsuka T, Matsuura N, Aoki T, Shibahara K, Kikuchi H (1997) Expression of interleukin-1 beta converting enzyme gene family and bcl-2 gene family in the rat brain following permanent occlusion of the middle cerebral artery. J Cereb Blood Flow Metab 17:11–18
3. Bergeron L, Perez GI, MacDonald G, Shi L, Sun Y, Jurisicova A, Varmuza S, Latham KE, Flaws JA, Salter JC, Hara H, Moskowitz MA, Li E, Greenberg A, Tilly JL, Yuan J (1998) Defects in regulation of apoptosis in caspase-2-deficient mice. Genes Dev 12:1304–1314
4. Bhat RV, DiRocco R, Marcy VR, Flood DG, Zhu Y, Dobrzanski P, Siman R, Scott R, Contreras PC, Miller M (1996) Increased expression of IL-1beta converting enzyme in hippocampus after ischemia: selective localization in microglia. J Neurosci 16:4146–4154
5. Chen J, Nagayama T, Jin K, Stetler RA, Zhu RL, Graham SH, Simon RP (1998) Induction of caspase-3-like protease may mediate delayed neuronal death in the hippocampus after transient cerebral ischemia. J Neurosci 18:4914–4928
6. Cheng Y, Deshmukh M, D'Costa A, Demaro JA, Gidday JM, Shah A, Sun Y, Jacquin MF, Johnson EM, Holtzman DM (1998) Caspase inhibitor affords neuroprotection with delayed administration in a rat model of neonatal hypoxic-ischemic brain injury. J Clin Invest 101:1992–1999
7. Endres M, Namura S, Shimizu-Sasamata M, Waeber C, Zhang L, Gomez-Isla T, Hyman BT, Moskowitz MA (1998) Attenuation of delayed neuronal death after mild focal ischemia in mice by inhibition of the caspase family. J Cereb Blood Flow Metab 18:238–247
8. Felderhoff-Mueser U, Taylor DL, Greenwood K, Kozma M, Stibenz D, Joashi UC, Edwards AD, Mehmet H (2000) Fas/CD95/APO-1 can function as a death receptor for neuronal cells in vitro and in vivo and is upregulated following cerebral hypoxic-ischemic injury to the developing rat brain. Brain Pathol 10:17–29
9. Fink K, Zhu J, Namura S, Shimizu-Sasamata M, Endres M, Ma J, Dalkara T, Yuan J, Moskowitz MA (1998) Prolonged therapeutic window for ischemic brain damage caused by delayed caspase activation. J Cereb Blood Flow Metab 18:1071–1076
10. Fujimura M, Morita-Fujimura Y, Murakami K, Kawase M, Chan PH (1998) Cytosolic redistribution of cytochrome c after transient focal cerebral ischemia in rats. J Cereb Blood Flow Metab 18:1239–1247
11. Gillardon F, Bottiger B, Schmitz B, Zimmermann M, Hossmann KA (1997) Activation of CPP-32 protease in hippocampal neurons following ischemia and epilepsy. Brain Res Mol Brain Res 50:16–22
12. Gillardon F, Kiprianova I, Sandkuhler J, Hossmann KA, Spranger M (1999) Inhibition of caspases prevents cell death of hippocampal CA1 neurons, but not impairment of hippocampal long-term potentiation following global ischemia. Neuroscience 93:1219–1222
13. Hara H, Fink K, Endres M, Friedlander RM, Gagliardini V, Yuan J, Moskowitz MA (1997) Attenuation of transient focal cerebral ischemic injury in transgenic mice expressing a mutant ICE inhibitory protein. J Cereb Blood Flow Metab 17:370–375
14. Harrison DC, Roberts J, Campbell CA, Crook B, Davis R, Deen K, Meakin J, Michalovich D, Price J, Stammers M, Maycox PR (2000) TR3 death receptor expression in the normal and ischaemic brain. Neuroscience 96:147–160
15. Hayashi T, Sakurai M, Abe K, Sadahiro M, Tabayashi K, Itoyama Y (1998) Apoptosis of motor neurons with induction of caspases in the spinal cord after ischemia. Stroke 29:1007–1012
16. Hee HB, D'Costa A, Back SA, Parsadanian M, Patel S, Shah AR, Gidday JM, Srinivasan A, Deshmukh M, Holtzman, DM (2000) BDNF blocks caspase-3 activation in neonatal hypoxia-ischemia. Neurobiol Dis 7:38–53
17. Himi T, Ishizaki Y, Murota S (1998) A caspase inhibitor blocks ischaemia-induced delayed neuronal death in the gerbil. Eur J Neurosci 10:777–781
18. Honkaniemi J, Massa SM, Breckinridge M, Sharp FR (1996) Global ischemia induces apoptosis-associated genes in hippocampus. Brain Res Mol Brain Res 42:79–88
19. Kang SJ, Wang S, Hara H, Peterson EP, Namura S, Amin-Hanjani S, Huang Z, Srinivasan A, Tomaselli KJ, Thornberry NA, Moskowitz MA, Yuan J (2000) Dual role of caspase-11 in mediating activation of caspase-1 and caspase-3 under pathological conditions. J Cell Biol 149:613–622
20. Krajewski S, Krajewska M, Ellerby LM, Welsh K, Xie Z, Deveraux QL, Salvesen GS, Bredesen DE, Rosenthal RE, Fiskum G, Reed JC (1999) Release of caspase-9 from mitochondria during neuronal apoptosis and cerebral ischemia. Proc Natl Acad Sci USA 96:5752–5757
21. Li H, Colbourne F, Sun P, Zhao Z, Buchan AM, Iadecola C (2000) Caspase inhibitors reduce neuronal injury after focal but not global cerebral ischemia in rats. Stroke 31:176–182
22. Liu XH, Kwon D, Schielke GP, Yang GY, Silverstein FS, Barks JD (1999) Mice deficient in interleukin-1 converting enzyme are resistant to neonatal hypoxic-ischemic brain damage. J Cereb Blood Flow Metab 19:1099–1108
23. Loddick SA, MacKenzie A, Rothwell NJ (1996) An ICE inhibitor, z-VAD-DCB attenuates ischaemic brain damage in the rat. Neuroreport 7:1465–1468
24. Ma J, Endres M, Moskowitz MA (1998) Synergistic effects of caspase inhibitors and MK-801 in brain injury after transient focal cerebral ischaemia in mice. Br J Pharmacol 124:756–762
25. Martin-Villalba A, Herr I, Jeremias I, Hahne M, Brandt R, Vogel J, Schenkel J, Herdegen T, Debatin KM (1999) CD95 ligand (Fas-L/APO-1L) and tumor necrosis factor-related apoptosis-inducing ligand mediate ischemia-induced apoptosis in neurons. J Neurosci 19:3809–3817
26. Matsushita K, Wu Y, Qui J, Lang-Landunski L, Hirt L, Waeber C, Hyman BT, Yuan J, Moskowitz MA (2000) Fas receptor and neuronal cell death after spinal cord ischemia. J Neurosci 20:6879–6887
27. Matsuyama T, Hata R, Tagaya M, Yamamoto Y, Nakajima T, Furuyama J, Wanaka A, Sugita M (1994) Fas antigen mRNA induction in postischemic murine brain. Brain Res 657:342–346
28. Matsuyama T, Hata R, Yamamoto Y, Tagaya M, Akita H, Uno H, Wanaka A, Furuyama J, Sugita M (1995) Localization of Fas antigen mRNA induced in postischemic murine forebrain by in situ hybridization. Brain Res Mol Brain Res 34:166–172
29. Nakatsuka H, Ohta S, Tanaka J, Toku K, Kumon Y, Maeda N, Sakanaka M, Sakaki S (1999) Release of cytochrome c from mitochondria to cytosol in gerbil hippocampal CA1 neurons after transient forebrain ischemia. Brain Res 849:216–219
30. Nakatsuka H, Ohta S, Tanaka J, Toku K, Kumon Y, Maeda N, Sakanaka M, Sakaki S (2000) Histochemical cytochrome c

oxidase activity and caspase-3 in gerbil hippocampal CA1 neurons after transient forebrain ischemia. Neurosci Lett 285:127–130

31. Namura S, Zhu J, Fink K, Endres M, Srinivasan A, Tomaselli KJ, Yuan J, Moskowitz MA (1998) Activation and cleavage of caspase-3 in apoptosis induced by experimental cerebral ischemia. J Neurosci 18:3659–3668
32. Ni B, Wu X, Su Y, Stephenson D, Smalstig EB, Clemens J, Paul SM (1998) Transient global forebrain ischemia induces a prolonged expression of the caspase-3 mRNA in rat hippocampal CA1 pyramidal neurons. J Cereb Blood Flow Metab 18:248–256
33. Ouyang YB, Tan Y, Comb M, Liu CL, Martone ME, Siesjo BK, Hu BR (1999) Survival- and death-promoting events after transient cerebral ischemia: phosphorylation of Akt, release of cytochrome C and Activation of caspase-like proteases. J Cereb Blood Flow Metab 19:1126–1135
34. Perez-Pinzon MA, Xu GP, Born J, Lorenzo J, Busto R, Rosenthal M, Sick TJ (1999) Cytochrome C is released from mitochondria into the cytosol after cerebral anoxia or ischemia. J Cereb Blood Flow Metab 19:39–43
35. Pulera MR, Adams LM, Liu H, Santos DG, Nishimura RN, Yang F, Cole GM, Wasterlain CG (1998) Apoptosis in a neonatal rat model of cerebral hypoxia-ischemia. Stroke 29:2622–2630
36. Rami A, Agarwal R, Botez G, Winckler J (2000) mu-Calpain activation, DNA fragmentation, and synergistic effects of caspase and calpain inhibitors in protecting hippocampal neurons from ischemic damage. Brain Res 866:299–312
37. Schielke GP, Yang GY, Shivers BD, Betz AL (1998) Reduced ischemic brain injury in interleukin-1 beta converting enzyme-deficient mice. J Cereb Blood Flow Metab 18:180–185
38. Schulz JB, Weller M, Matthews RT, Heneka MT, Groscurth P, Martinou JC, Lommatzsch J, von CR, Wullner U, Loschmann PA, Beal MF, Dichgans J, Klockgether T (1998) Extended therapeutic window for caspase inhibition and synergy with MK-801 in the treatment of cerebral histotoxic hypoxia. Cell Death Differ 5:847–857
39. Sugawara T, Fujimura M, Morita-Fujimura Y, Kawase M, Chan PH (1999) The mitochondrial release of cytochrome c corresponds to the selective vulnerability of hippocampal CA1 neurons in rats after transient global cerebral ischemia. J Neurosci (Online) 19:RC39
40. Velier JJ, Ellison JA, Kikly KK, Spera PA, Barone FC, Feuerstein GZ (1999) Caspase-8 and caspase-3 are expressed by different populations of cortical neurons undergoing delayed cell death after focal stroke in the rat. J Neurosci 19:5932–5941
41. Wiessner C, Sauer D, Alaimo D, Allegrini PR (2000) Protective effect of a caspase inhibitor in models for cerebral ischemia in vitro and in vivo. Cell Mol Biol 46:53–62

Intrinsic and extrinsic pathways of caspase activation in cerebral ischemia

K. Jin[1], J. Chen[2], R. P. Simon[3]

It is now clear that ischemic injury to the brain activates the gene based substrate of program cell death and that this process, of apoptosis, constitutes a major mechanism of brain injury in the setting of ischemia. Thus the prospect of therapeutic intervention in regard to modulating the phenomenon of apoptosis is a new potential direction for therapy. Mechanisms of apoptotic cell death are, to a substantial degree, known in other biological systems including those of primitive organisms as well as higher animals, particularly in the area of developmental neurobiology (Green 1998). This basic neurobiology is then available to be used as a template for the phenomenon of apoptosis in brain ischemia. From this work two pathways of apoptotic initiation have evolved: the intrinsic and the extrinsic.

The *intrinsic pathway* of initiation of apoptosis begins with the mitochondria. The integrity of the mitochondrial membrane is altered with release of intramitochondrial contents, particularly cytochrome c, into the cytosol where activation of the caspase cascade is initiated. Among the factors which may be responsible for the loss of mitochondrial membrane integrity include the insertion of pore forming proteins in the outer membrane, particularly those proteins of the Bcl-2 family. The mitochondria based pathophysiologic phenomenon particularly referable to ischemia, which produces loss of mitochondrial membrane integrity and cytochrome c release, is intramitochondrial calcium loading, which is a prominent event early after ischemia (Simon et al. 1984). For these reasons the intrinsic pathway of induction of apoptosis and the caspase cascade has received early attention in the study of ischemic injury and was the topic of a number of presentations at the previous Marburg symposia. Cytochrome c release in the presence of apoptosis activating factor-1 (Apaf-1) then binds to and initiates the cleavage of caspase-9 to its active component. Activated caspase-9 initiates the cleavage of caspase-3 and apoptosis commences.

The *extrinsic* system in apoptosis initiation has no clear links to the glutamate-calcium-excitotoxicity story which forms the central core of the modern understanding of the cellular mechanism of ischemic cell death. This system revolves around the transmembrane death receptor protein (Fas) which, in the presence of a ligand, traditionally tumor necrosis factor (TNF) or Fas ligand (FasL) also initiates the apoptotic cascade of caspase activation. In this setting, ligand binding to the Fas death receptor initiates the binding of an adaptor protein to the intracytoplasmic portion of the death receptor. The adaptor protein, FADD (Fas activating death domain), then binds procaspase-8 which is cleaved to its active form which initiates cas-

[1]Buck Center for Aging, Novato, California; [2]Department of Neurology, University of Pittsburgh, Pittsburgh, Pennsylvania; [3]R.S. Dow Laboratories for Neurobiology, Portland, Oregon

J. Krieglstein, S. Klumpp (Eds.) Pharmacology of Cerebral Ischemia 2000

pase-3 cleavage and takes apoptosis to completion.

We recently studied both the intrinsic and extrinsic systems in cerebral ischemia and defined their respective roles.

The intrinsic pathway

The intrinsic pathway is initiated by pro-apoptotic Bcl-2 family genes acting at the mitochondrial membrane and/or by calcium. Intracellular calcium loading is a early and prominent event in the cellular mechanism of ischemia being driven by increased concentrations of extracellular glutamate. As calcium moves down its 1,000:1 gradient through mainly NMDA gated channels, it must be sequestered inside the cell. While to some extent this is accomplished in the golgi apparatus, the majority of the calcium sequestration occurs as mitochondrial calcium loading (Simon et al. 1984). Such mitochondria swell and have structural deformities. The release of cytochrome c in this setting has been recently demonstrated (Fujimura et al. 2000).

We have modeled this phenomenon using recombinant proteins in vitro. As apoptosis inducers we used recombinant Bax protein or calcium; as apoptosis suppressor we used the Bcl-2 family gene Bcl-w. We then purified mitochondria from normal nonischemic rat brain by the method of Berman and Hastings (1999). The mitochondria were then incubated either in recombinant Bax or calcium in the presence or absence of recombinant Bcl-w. Mitochondria were then pelleted by centrifugation and subjected to immunoblotting with antibodies to Bax or Bcl-w. The resulting supernatants were analyzed by immunoblotting with a monoclonal antibody against cytochrome c. Both recombinant rat Bcl-2 protein and truncated Bax protein were expressed in E-coli DL21 cells. The incubation of mitochondria without the addition of Bax resulted in no release of cytochrome c into the supernatant (defined as the α tubulin positive compartment). Incubation with the addition of Bax or calcium resulted in a redistribution of cytochrome c from the mitochondrial compartment into the supernatant. In the presence of Bcl-w protein, however, the release of cytochrome c induced by either Bax (in a dose-dependent manner) or calcium was inhibited (Fig. 1a). Western blot analysis detect an increased amount of Bcl-w protein in the mitochondrial pellet from ischemic whole brain homogenates, which suggests that this protein was incorporated into the mitochondrial membrane in the setting of cytochrome c release (Fig. 1b).

We next looked for evidence in in vivo ischemia of involvement of the intrinsic system. Immunocytochemistry demonstrated Bcl-w expression in ischemic cortex and in the caudate putamen. The pattern of the immunoreactivity was that of a punctate appearance in the cytoplasm of ischemic neurons. Double labeling with TUNEL and Bcl-w showed that the Bcl-w expression was not seen in cells with

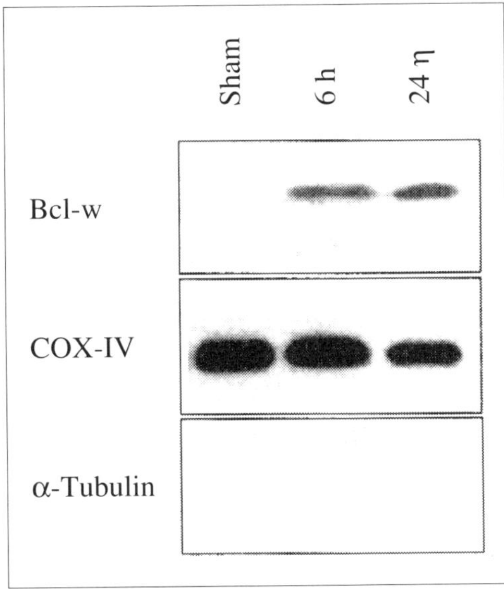

Fig. 1a. Representative western blots show increases of Bcl-w immunoreactivity in the mitochondrial fraction after ischemia. Mitochondrial protein was purified from the cortex at 6 or 24 hours after ischemia or 24 hours after sham operation and subjected to western blot analysis. Control western blots show that the purified protein fraction is enriched in the mitochondrial membrane-bound protein cytochrome c oxidase IV (COX-IV) but does not contain the cytosolic protein α-tubulin.

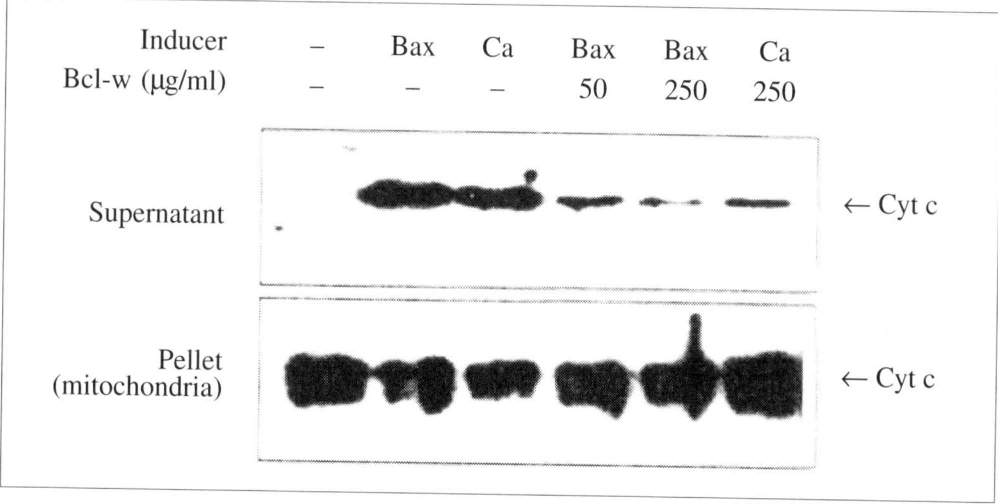

Fig. 1b. Effects of Bcl-w on cytochrome c release from isolated brain mitochondria induced by Bax or calcium (Ca). Mitochondria were incubated with the recombinant Bax protein (50 μg/mL) or calcium (100 μmol/L) for 1 hour in the presence or absence of Bcl-w at the indicated concentrations and then centrifuged. The supernatant and pellet were subjected to western blot analysis for cytochrome c. Note that Bcl-w inhibits Bax- or calcium-induced cytochrome c release. Results are representative of two independent experiments.
Data for Figure 1a and 1b from: Yan C., Chen J., Chen, D. et al. Overexpression of the cell death suppressor Bcl-w in ischemic brain: Implications for a neuroprotective role via the mitochondrial pathway. J Cereb Blood Flow and Metab 20:620, 2000.

DNA damage recognized by TUNEL labeling. Immunoreactivity in the caudate putamen also demonstrated Bcl-w expression but here it was localized to endothelial cells. In the transition zone between the infracted core and the cortex the Bcl-2 immunoreactivity was mainly seen in astrocytes. In cortical neurons (and to a lesser degree in astrocytes) the punctate expression of Bcl-w in the cytoplasm was very clear. This suggested that the protein was membrane-bound in the cytoplasm of these ischemic cells. Such a localization would be in keeping with the hydrophobic C-terminal domain of Bcl-w. Accordingly, double labeling for Bcl-w and the mitochondrial membrane bound protein COX-IV was performed. The double label showed that most areas of Bcl-w immunoreactivity co-localized with COX-IV.

The extrinsic pathway

The extrinsic pathway (Fig. 2) has no clear link to the glutamate excitotoxicity cascade, except that through TNFα and the inflammatory pathways. Thus its role in acute ischemia, if present, is less obvious than that of the mitochondrial pathway. We chose to investigate the possibility of involvement of the extrinsic system in a model of global ischemia with reperfusion. We used a model of transient global ischemia (15 minutes duration) with a four-vessel occlusion technique.

At 4, 8, 24, and 72 hours of reperfusion, brains were removed and analyzed by Northern blot hybridization using a ^{32}P-labeled Fas oligonucleotide probe. A single band of the predicted size for Fas was detected in each of the ischemic samples but not in the controls. The experiment was repeated using a ^{32}P-labeled oligonucleotide probe for the Fas ligand (Fas-L). Again, a single hybridizing transcript of the

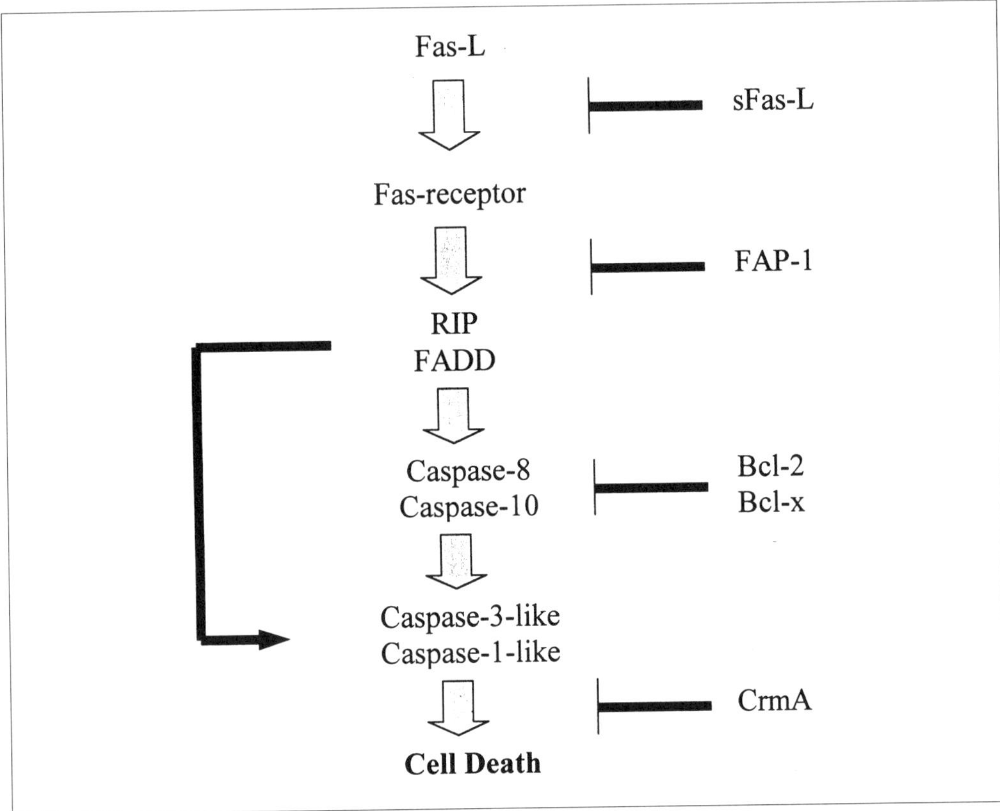

Fig. 2. The extrinsic pathway:
- Bcl (B cell lymphoma oncogenic protein)
- CrmA (cytokine response modifier A)
- Caspase (aspartate-specific cysteinyl proteases)
- Fas (CD95/APO-1)
- Fas-L (Fas ligand)
- sFas (soluble Fas)
- FADD (Fas-associated death domain)
- FAP-1 (Fas-associated phosphatase-1)
- RIP (receptor-interacting protein)

predicted size for Fas-L was detected at 4, 8, 24, and 72 hours, but not detected in the control material. The distribution of Fas and Fas-L mRNA expression was then studied by in situ hybridization analysis. Fas and Fas-L mRNA were barely detectable in sham operated hippocampus, but were significantly induced in the CA-1 sector at 72 hours after ischemia.

At the protein level, the expression and distribution of Fas in the hippocampus was studied using Western blotting. Protein was extracted from control hippocampus or hippocampi removed 8 hours, 24 hours, or 72 hours after 15 minutes of transient focal ischemia. There was slight constitutive expression of the protein which was substantially upregulated at 8 hours and was maximal at 24 hours and 72 hours of reperfusion. Immunocytochemical staining showed an absence of immunoreactivity in the control material, but positive staining in the

CA-1 pyramidal cells at both 24 and 72 hours of reperfusion. Repeating the experiment to look at Fas-L protein in hippocampus produced similar results to those of Fas in regard to immunoreactivity but at Western blotting there was a bold band in the control samples and no change at 8, 24, and 72 hours of reperfusion. The Western data may be contaminated by cellular elements in these brains.

If the Fas ligand binds to the Fas receptor in ischemic brain then there should be binding, intracellularly, to the Fas activated death domain (FADD). Western blotting for FADD was therefore performed. A band of the predicted molecular weight was seen faintly in control material at 4 hours of reperfusion but was boldly demonstrated at 8, 24, and 72 hours of reperfusion. Immunoprecipitation with FADD and blotting with Fas showed that FADD co-immunoprecipitated with Fas, suggesting that the FADD protein, in ischemic brain, does indeed interact with the Fas receptor. Double label fluorescent microscopy in the CA-1 sector showed co-localization of Fas with FADD in the same CA-1 sector neurons.

With activation of the extrinsic pathway and activation of the death domain, caspase-3 activation is accomplished via the activation of caspase-8. Accordingly, Western blots for caspase-8 were done at 0, 4, 8, 24, and 72 hours following reperfusion. Bold bands were seen at each time point without the change in ischemic samples. We then performed immunoprecipitation of FADD and blotting with caspase-8. A faint band was seen in the control material, which was less apparent in the ischemic material. We then measured the activity of caspase-8 with the colorimetric substrate IETD-pNA. There was very modest and insignificant increase in immunoreactivity in the ischemic samples versus the sham. We then used the specific peptide inhibitor for caspase-8 (Z-IETD-MFK) injected into the left lateral ventricle of the rat brain beginning 30 minutes before the induction of ischemia. Morphologic assessment was performed at 72 hours. There was no inhibition of neuronal cell death in CA-1 neurons in animals treated with the caspase-8 inhibitor. We have previously shown (Chen et al. 1998) that the caspase-3 inhibitor (Z-YVAD-MFK) substantially reduces cell death in the CA-1 sector following global ischemia. Presuming that the extrinsic system is involved in such caspase-3 activity, caspase-8 activation might not be necessary for Fas mediated cell death signaling.

An additional link between FADD and caspase-3 activation is the activation of caspase-10. Caspase-10 is a close structural homologue of caspase-8 which also encodes two functional death effector domains. One of these domains binds to the corresponding domain in the adaptor molecule FADD, and in turn activates the Fas mediated death cascade in a manner similar to that of caspase-8 (Boldin et al. 1996). We therefore performed Western blotting for caspase-10 in brain following global ischemia. Using an affinity-purified polyclonal antibody, a 58kDa band of the predicted molecular weight for the parent protein was seen at 0, 4, 8, 24, and 72 hours of ischemia/reperfusion without change. However, at 4, 8, 24, and especially 72 hours, the cleaved P-20 fragment was seen. In addition, immunoprecipitation with FADD and blotting with caspase-10 showed co-immunoprecipitation of caspase-10 and FADD which increased with increasing durations of reperfusion. Further, double labeling of CA-1 neurons with caspase-10 and FADD antibodies showed co-localization in these cells following ischemic injury.

Thus, both the intrinsic and extrinsic systems of apoptosis initiation via caspase-3 are induced in ischemic brain. Caspase-3 then cleaves caspase activated DNAase (CAD) from its inhibitory protein (ICAD) to execute nuclear fragmentation. The relative importance of the extrinsic versus intrinsic pathway is an important new area to be pursued in the quest for novel mechanisms of protection for ischemic brain.

References

1. Green DR (1998) Apoptotic pathways: the roads to ruin. Cell 94(6):695
2. Simon RP, Griffiths T, Evans MC, Swan JH, Meldrum BS (1984) Calcium overload in selectively vulnerable neurons of the hippocampus during and after ischemia: an electron microscopy study in the rat. J Cereb Blood Flow Metab 4(3):350

3. Fujimura M, Morita-Fujimura Y, Noshita N, Yoshimoto T, Chan PH (2000) The cytosolic antioxidant copper/zinc-superoxide dismutase prevents the early release of mitochondrial cytochrome c in ischemic brain after transient focal cerebral ischemia in mice. J Neurosci 20(8):2817
4. Berman SB, Hastings TG (1999) Dopamine oxidation alters mitochondrial respiration and induces permeability transition in brain mitochondria: implications for Parkinson's disease. J Neurochem 73(3):1127
5. Chen J, Nagayama T, Jin K, Statler RA, Zhu RL, Graham SH, Simon RP (1998) Induction of caspase-3-like protease may mediate delayed neuronal death in the hippocampus after transient cerebral ischemia. J Neurosci 18(13):4914
6. Boldin MP, Goncharov TM, Goltsev YV, Wallach D (1996) Involvement of MACH, a novel MORT1/FADD-interacting protease, in Fas/APO-1- and TNF receptor-induced cell death. Cell 85(6):803

Mechanisms of neuronal cell injury: does endoplasmic reticulum dysfunction play a special role?

W. Paschen

Introduction

Disturbance of calcium homeostasis has been considered a central mechanism underlying neuronal cell injury in various pathological states of the brain. Three different subcellular compartments are thought to be involved in calcium-related neuronal cell injury, the cytoplasm (Siesjö 1981), mitochondria (Kristian and Siesjö 1998) and the endoplasmic reticulum (ER) (Paschen 1996; Paschen and Doutheil 1999). The traditional calcium hypothesis holds that the pathological process culminating in ischemic cell death is triggered by high cytoplasmic calcium activity during ischemia (Siesjö 1981). In the physiological state, calcium ions are highly compartimentalized, calcium activity being in the mM range in the extracellular space and in the ER, and about 100 nM in the cytoplasm. This calcium gradient is maintained by pumping calcium ions from the cytoplasm into the ER and to the extracellular space in an energy-requiring reaction. During ischemia, cells are depleted of high energy phosphates which leads to a suppression of calcium pump activity. In addition, calcium influx is induced by activation of agonist-dependent and voltage-gated calcium channels. High cytoplasmic calcium activity during ischemia is thought to trigger cell injury by activating various calcium-dependent enzymes, including proteases, lipases and nitric oxide synthase.

The traditional calcium hypothesis has been modified, taking into account that cell death induced by transient cerebral ischemia is a reperfusion injury, since pathological disturbances occurring during ischemia are potentially reversible. It has been suggested that mitochondria are targets of calcium-related processes leading to neuronal cell injury (Kristian and Siesjö 1998). Mitochondria take up calcium ions during reperfusion, and evidence suggests that an excessive uptake of calcium ions into mitochondria could play a key role in ischemic cell death by activating the production of oxygen free radicals and blocking the synthesis of high energy phosphates. Disturbance of mitochondrial function is thought to cause opening of the mitochondrial transition pore, release of cytochrome-c and cytochrome-c-induced activation of caspase 3. Cell injury induced by transient ischemia or hypoglycemia can indeed be suppressed by cyclosporine A (Uchino et al. 1995; Friberg et al. 1998; Uchino et al. 1998; Yoshimoto and Siesjö 1999), which blocks the opening of the mitochondrial transition pore (Duchen et al. 1993).

Recently, it has been proposed that disturbances of ER calcium homeostasis contributes to the pathological process leading to ischemic cell injury (Paschen and Doutheil 1999). The

Department of Experimental Neurology, Max-Planck-Institute for Neurological Research, Gleuelerstr. 50, D-50931 Köln, Germany.
E-mail: Paschen@mpin-koeln.mpg.de

J. Krieglstein, S. Klumpp (Eds.) Pharmacology of Cerebral Ischemia 2000

basis for this hypothesis is that the response of cells to transient ischemia is in many respects identical to the response of neurons to an isolated disturbance of ER calcium homeostasis, implying common underlying mechanisms. In contrast to the situation in cytoplasm and mitochondria, it is a decrease and not an increase in ER calcium activity which is thought to trigger cell death.

Control of ER calcium homeostasis

The ER plays a central role in cellular calcium signaling and calcium storage (Garaschuk et al. 1997; Berridge 1998). ER calcium levels are high, being in the high micromolar or even millimolar range (Hofer and Machen 1993; Chen et al. 1996; Pozzomiller et al. 1997). ER calcium homeostasis is controlled by the ryanodine receptor (RyaR) and the IP_3 receptor (IP_3R) which upon activation induce release of calcium ions, and by a calcium pump (*s*arcoplasmic/*e*ndoplasmic *r*eticulum Ca^{2+}-ATPase; SERCA) which pumps back calcium ions against a concentration gradient of several orders of magnitude. In the physiological state, the extent of IP_3-induced ER calcium release varies with cytoplasmic calcium activity, leading to a bell-shaped cytoplasmic calcium activity-calcium release curve (Bezprozvanny et al. 1991), and inducing increased IP_3-induced calcium release when neurons are in their active state. With respect to calcium, the ER is divided into subcompartments which have been identified by using compounds known to influence ER calcium homeostasis (Gosh et al. 1989; Verma et al. 1990; Bian et al. 1991; Fasolato et al. 1991; Tanaka and Tashjian 1993; Pizzo et al. 1997). About 80% of ER calcium is released when the uptake is blocked by thapsigargin (Tg, a specific, irreversible inhibitor of ER Ca^{2+}-ATPase; (Inesi and Sagara 1994)). A subset of the Tg-sensitive calcium store responds to IP_3. Another subset of the Tg-sensitive store, which does not respond to IP_3, can be transformed into a IP_3-sensitive pool in the presence of GTP. ER calcium stores are completely depleted by calcium ionophores. The observation that Tg exposure does not induce a total depletion of ER calcium stores points to the existence of a subset of the calcium pool which is filled by a calcium pump other than the Tg-sensitive SERCA.

In addition to receptors which upon activation induce release of calcium from the ER lumen, and calcium pumps which pump back calcium ions, two ER-resident proteins seem to play an important role in the control of ER calcium homeostasis, the glucose-regulated protein 78 (GRP78) and the protooncogene Bcl-2. The ER calcium homeostasis stabilizing effect of GRP78 is indicated by the observation that in cells with down-regulated GRP78 levels ER calcium release, induced by glutamate exposure, is markedly increased (Yu et al. 1999) while it is reduced in cells where GRP78 synthesis was activated (Lee et al. 1999). Overexpression of Bcl-2, on the other hand, inhibits ER calcium pool depletion in a variety of pathological conditions, including exposure to glucocorticoids, growth factor withdrawal, and peroxidative damage (Baffy et al. 1993; Lam et al. 1994; Distelhorst et al. 1996; He et al. 1997). Bcl-2 has indeed been found in the ER membrane (Reed et al. 1996). The observation that Bcl-2 and related proteins form ion channels in synthetic lipid membranes (Minn et al. 1997; Schendel et al. 1997) implies that this protein may facilitate calcium fluxes between different ER subcompartments. Furthermore, Bcl-2 overexpression up-regulates expression and levels of ER calcium pump protein and increases ER calcium uptake (Kuo et al. 1998). A calcium homeostasis stabilizing effect of Bcl-2 has also been found in mitochondria: Bcl-2 over-expression induces an increase in mitochondrial calcium load (Zhu et al. 1999) and an inhibition of calcium efflux (Chakraborti et al. 1999). Recently, it has been shown that over-expression of Bcl-2 induces a decrease in total ER calcium levels and an increase in calcium leak currents across the ER membrane (Foyouzi-Youssefi et al. 2000; Pinton et al. 2000), an observation divergent to those cited above. Thus, the exact role of Bcl-2 in ER calcium homeostasis still remains to be established.

ER stress response – unfolded protein response

Beside its function in cellular calcium signaling and calcium storage, the ER plays a fundamental role in protein folding and processing. In this subcellular compartment newly synthesized membrane and secretory proteins are folded and processed, reactions which are strictly calcium dependent (Lodish and Kong 1990; Gosh et al. 1991; Kutznetsov et al. 1992; Lodish et al. 1992). Conditions associated with disturbance of ER calcium homeostasis, or a direct blocking of the protein folding and processing reactions, induce the activation of two different, highly conserved stress responses, the ER overload response (EOR; for review see: Pahl and Baeuerle 1997) and the unfolded protein response (UPR; for recent reviews see: Gething 1999; Kaufman 1999; Pahl 1999). Induction of EOR results in activation of the transcription factor NFkB, and a corresponding rise in mRNA levels of NFkB-dependent target genes, such as interferone and cytokines. Induction of UPR, on the other hand, results in the induction of various kinases: Ire1p, which upon activation induces the expression of genes coding for ER-resident stress proteins (such as: erp72, grp78, grp94) and the transcription factor gadd153 (Shamu and Walter 1996), and the kinases PERK and PKR, which upon activation induce the phosphorylation of the eukaryotic translation initiation factor 2α (eIF-2α) (Prostko et al. 1995; Srivastava et al. 1995; Harding et al. 1999), resulting in a disaggregation of polyribosomes (Wong et al. 1993; Doutheil et al. 1999) and a suppression of protein synthesis (Brostrom and Brostrom 1990; Wong et al. 1993; Paschen et al. 1996).

Activation of UPR is an indication that ER function is disturbed under the experimental conditions under investigation, because this response is specifically induced under pathological conditions associated with an accumulation of unfolded proteins in the ER lumen (for review see: Kaufman 1999). As will be discussed below, severe disturbance of ER function is sufficient to induce a pathological process culminating in cell death. The molecular mechanisms underlying ER dysfunction-induced cell injury have still to be established and it has yet not been elucidated whether activation of UPR contributes to this process. In experimental conditions associated with programed cell death, suppression of protein synthesis is thought to protect cells from injury by blocking the formation of "killer" proteins. This view is supported by the observation that PERK over-expressing cells are more vulnerable to conditions associated with ER dysfunction (Harding et al. 2000). On the other hand, suppression of protein synthesis is always closely related to the extent of neuronal cell injury in models of transient ischemia (Bodsch et al. 1985; Thilmann et al. 1986; Hata et al. 2000), and therapeutic interventions which suppress the development of ischemic cell death also activate the recovery of protein synthesis (Xie et al. 1989; Bonnekoh et al. 1992; Widmann et al. 1991, 1993). Furthermore, activation of PKR induces cell injury and this process is blocked by over-expression of an PKR inhibitor (Srivastava et al. 1998; Tang et al. 1999). Apoptosis can also be induced by expressing a mutant eIF-2α (S51D) that mimics phosphorylated eIF2α (Srivastava et al. 1998). All these observations point to an involvement of protein synthesis suppression in the pathological process leading to neuronal cell injury.

Expression of genes (e.g. erp72, grp78, grp94) coding for ER-resident stress proteins or the transcription factor gadd153 may have divergent effects on cells in which UPR is activated. Over-expression of GADD153 activates programed cell death (Friedman 1996), suggesting that activated UPR-induced gadd153 expression may contribute to the pathological process leading to cell injury, providing that activation of transcription is followed by translation. Activation of grp78 expression, in contrast, is thought to be a protective response, as indicated by the observation that cell injury is enhanced after down-regulation of grp78 expression (Lee et al. 1999) and cells are less vulnerable to various pathological conditions after up-regulation of grp78 expression (Liu et al. 1998; Bush et al. 1999; Lee et al. 1999; Yu et al. 1999). Furthermore, induction of grp78 expression by a non-lethal form of ER stress renders cells tolerant to an otherwise lethal form of ER stress (Brostrom et al. 1990), and transfection of cells with grp78 antisense vector eliminates resistance to lethal stress (Li and Lee 1999), indicating that GRP78 protein plays a central role in the accommodation of cells to a severe form of stress.

Indications that ER function is disturbed in pathological states of the brain

An up-regulation of the unfolded protein response (UPR) can be used as evidence that ER function is disturbed in the pathological process under investigation, as discussed above. The suppression of the initiation process of protein synthesis after transient cerebral ischemia resembles that observed after an isolated depletion of ER calcium stores, implying common underlying mechanisms. Under both conditions protein synthesis is suppressed by increased phosphorylation of eIF-2α, leading to a disaggregation of polyribosomes (Cooper et al. 1977; Prostko et al. 1995; Srivastava et al. 1995; DeGracia et al. 1996; Doutheil et al. 1999). This pattern of protein synthesis inhibition is different to that induced by an increase in cytoplasmic calcium activity, where it is the elongation step that is blocked, leading to a maximal aggregation of polyribosomes (Wong et al. 1991). The initiation process of protein synthesis is controlled by calcium levels of the ER subcompartment sensitive to an activation of the ryanodine receptor, but not by calcium levels of the subset of ER stores depleted by an activation of the IP_3 receptor (Preston and Berlin 1992; Alcázar et al. 1997). This observation is of particular interest, because blocking the ryanodine receptor has proven to be neuroprotective in various pathological states including ischemia (Frandsen and Schousboe 1992; Wei and Perry 1996; Zhang et al. 1993; Berg et al. 1995; Mody and McDonald 1995).

Up-regulation of UPR is also indicated by a rise in mRNA levels of genes coding for ER-resident stress proteins and the transcription factor gadd153. Results from various experimental studies do indeed indicate that transient cerebral ischemia induces a rise in mRNA levels of grp78, gadd153, erp72, and heme oxygenase 1 (Wang et al. 1993; Lowenstein et al. 1994; Paschen et al. 1994; Wiessner et al. 1994; Paschen et al. 1998a, 1998b). Expression of these genes is activated under conditions associated with depletion of ER calcium stores, even when the ER-calcium store depletion-induced rise in cytoplasmic calcium activity is prevented by pre-loading cells with the calcium chelator BAPTA, indicating that it is a decrease in ER calcium levels and not a corresponding increase in cytoplasmic calcium activity which triggers the genomic response (Linden et al. 1998; Paschen et al. 1998b).

ER calcium pools are depleted in cultured neurons after oxygen/glucose deprivation and this process is blocked by the ryanodine receptor antagonist dantrolene, an observation emphasizing the role of the RyaR-activation-sensitive subset of ER calcium pools in the pathological process leading to neuronal cell injury (Pisani et al. 2000). Depletion of ER calcium stores has also been observed after transient forebrain ischemia in-vivo in vulnerable neurons of the hippocampal CA1 subfield (Kohno et al. 1997). Restoration of ER calcium stores of CA1 subfield neurons was observed only in animals pretreated with a neuroprotective dose of an nitric oxide synthase (NOS) inhibitor, implying a role of ischemia-induced NOS activation in this pathological process. NO exposure of cells has indeed been shown to suppress ER Ca^{2+}-ATPase activity, to deplete ER calcium stores and to inhibit the initiation process of protein synthesis (Willmott et al. 1995; Pernolett et al. 1996; Kim et al. 1998; Doutheil et al. 2000), suggesting that ischemia-induced activation of nitric oxide formation may contribute to the development of ER dysfunction.

A new type of ER dysfunction, a down-regulation of UPR, has been identified recently in cells over-expressing mutant presenilin-1 (Katayama et al. 1999). In cultures over-expressing mutant presenilin-1, an experimental model of familial Altheimer's disease, cells did not respond to ER dysfunction with an upregulation of grp78 expression, and these cells also had a reduced resistance to conditions inducing ER stress (Katayama et al. 1999). The reduced tolerance to conditions associated with impaired ER functions was almost completely restored by grp78 over-expression, pointing to a central role of GRP78 protein in inducing cellular resistance to a severe form of stress. The observation that GRP78 protein levels are reduced in Alzheimer's disease patients suggests that ER dysfunction may play a central role in the pathological process underlying this disease.

Presenilins are ER membrane proteins (Kovacs et al. 1996) and are thought to be involved in the processing of amyloid precursor protein (Weidemann et al. 1997; Refolo et al. 1999). Depending on the cleavage site, two different amyloid β-peptides are produced, Aβ(1–40) and the highly neurotoxic Aβ(1–42) (Younkin 1995; Hardy 1997). Presenilin mutations associated with familial Alzheimer's disease disturbe cellular calcium homeostasis (enhanced calcium release from IP_3- and ryanodine-sensitive stores) and sensitize cells to the toxic effects of amyloid β-peptide (Guo et al. 1996, 1999a, 1999b).

ER dysfunction and cell injury

Depending on the extent and severity of the insult, cell injury is induced under conditions associated with disturbance of ER function. The pathological process is activated by agents blocking ER-resident processes (Goss et al. 1995; Chang and Korolev 1996; Gow et al. 1998; Lin et al. 1999; Häcki et al. 2000), or by depleting ER calcium stores through inhibition of the ER calcium pump with thapsigargin (Tsukamoto and Kaneko 1993; Furuya et al. 1994; Kaneko and Tsukamoto 1994; Lam et al. 1994; Takei and Endo 1994; Waring and Beaver 1996; Bian et al. 1997; He et al. 1997; McCormick et al. 1997; Nath et al. 1997; Preston et al. 1997; Qi et al. 1997; Takadera and Ohyashiki 1998; Wei et al. 1998; Zhou et al. 1998). Under these experimental conditions, cell injury is induced by a decrease of ER calcium levels and not by a corresponding increase in cytoplasmic calcium activity: removal of extracellular calcium augments the pathological process and cell death is blocked by raising ER calcium levels (Bian et al. 1997; He et al. 1997; Preston et al. 1997). Thus, impairment of ER function is sufficient to activate a pathological process culminating in cell death.

Summary and conclusions

Disturbances of calcium homeostasis are thought to be the trigger of neuronal cell injury in various pathological states of the brain. Three different subcellular compartments have been considered as contributors to this pathological process, the cytoplasm, mitochondria and the endoplasmic reticulum (ER). As discussed above, depletion of ER calcium stores even in the absence of changes in cytoplasmic calcium activity is sufficient to induce cell injury. A high ER calcium activity is needed for the ER to fulfill important cellular functions, the folding and processing of newly synthesized membrane and secretory proteins. Any experimental conditions leading to severe impairment of ER function (disturbance of calcium homeostasis or blocking the folding or glycolyzation reactions) can cause cell injury. Severe disturbance of ER function may also cause secondary mitochondrial failure. Brefeldin A or tunicamycin, agents known to interfere with ER functions by blocking the secretion or glycolyzation of proteins, induce a release of cytochrom-c from mitochondria and a cytochrom-c-induced activation of caspase 3 (Häcki et al. 2000), and both these changes are heavily implicated in neuronal cell injury in various pathological states of the brain. The observation that ER dysfunction-induced cytochrom-c release and caspase 3 activation can be blocked by Bcl-2 targeted on the ER points to a causal relationship between impairment of ER function and the release of apoptotic signals from mitochondria (Häcki et al. 2000). Thus, a large body of evidence is accumulating pointing to a central role of ER dysfunction in the induction of neuronal cell injury in various pathological states of the brain.

Acknowledgement

This work was supported by the Deutsche Forschungsgemeinschaft, Grant Pa 266/13-1.

References

1. Alcázar A, de la Vega CM, Bazán E, Fando JL, Salinas M (1997) Calcium mobilization by ryanodine promotes the phosphorylation of initiation factor 2α subunit and inhibits protein synthesis in cultured neurons. J Neurochem 69:1703–1708
2. Baffy G, Miyashita T, Williamson JR, Reed JC (1993) Apoptosis induced by withdrawal of interleukin-3 (IL-3) from an IL-3-dependent hematopoietic cell line is associated with repartitioning of intracellular calcium and is blocked by enforced BCl-2 oncoprotein production. J Biol Chem 268:6511–6519
3. Berg M, Bruhn T, Frandsen A, Schousboe A, Diemer NH (1995) Kainic acid-induced seizures and brain damage in the rat – role of calcium homeostasis. J Neurosci Res 40:641–646
4. Berridge MJ (1998) Neuronal Calcium signaling. Neuron 21:13–26
5. Bezprozvanny I, Watras J, Ehrlich BE (1991) Bell-shaped calcium release-response curves of Ins(1,4,5)P_3- and calcium-gated channels from endoplasmic reticulum of cerebellum. Nature 351:751–754
6. Bian JH, Ghosh TK, Wang JC, Gill DL (1991) Identification of intracellular calcium pools. Selective modification by thapsigargin. J Biol Chem 266:8801–8806
7. Bian X, Hughes FM, Huang Y, Sidlowski JA, Putney JW (1997) Roles of cytoplasmic Ca^{2+} and intracellular Ca^{2+} stores in induction and suppression of apoptosis in S49 cells. Am J Physiol Cell Physiol Cell Physiol 41:C1241–C1249
8. Bodsch W, Takahashi K, Barbier A, Grosse Ophoff B, Hossmann K-A (1985) Cerebral protein synthesis and ischemia. Progr Brain Res 63:197–210
9. Bonnekoh P, Kuroiwa T, Oschlies U, Hossmann K-A (1992) Barbiturate promotes post-ischemic reaggregation of polyribosomes in gerbil hippocampus. Neurosci Lett 146:75–78
10. Brostrom MA, Brostrom CO (1990) Calcium dependent regulation of protein synthesis in intact mammalian cells. Ann Rev Physiol 52:557–590
11. Brostrom MA, Cade C, Prostko CR, Gmitter-Yellen D, Brostrom CO (1990) Accomodation of protein synthesis to chronic deprivation of intracellular sequestered calcium. J Biol Chem 265:20539–20546
12. Bush KT, George SK, Zhang PL, Nigam SK (1999) Pretreatment with inducers of ER molecular chaperones protects epithelial cells subjected to ATP depletion. Am J Physiol 277:F211–F218
13. Chakraborti T, Das S, Mondal M, Roychoudhury S, Chakraborti S (1999) Oxidant, mitochondria and calcium: an overview. Cell Signalling 11:77–85
14. Chang JY, Korolev VV (1996) Specific toxicity of tunicamycin in induction of programmed cell death of sympathetic neurons. Exp Neurol 137:201–211
15. Chen W, Steenbergen C, Levy LA, Vance J, London RE, Murphy E (1996) Measurement of free Ca^{2+} in sarcoplasmic reticulum in perfused rabbit heart loaded with 1,2-Bis(2-amino-5,6-difluorophenoxy)ethane-N,N,N',N'-tetraacetic acid by ^{19}F NMR. J Biol Chem 271:7398–7403
16. Cooper HK, Zalewska T, Kawakami S, Hossmann K-A (1997) The effect of ischemia and recirculation on protein synthesis in the brain. J Neurochem 28:929–934
17. DeGracia DJ, Neumar RW, White BC, Krause GS (1996) Global brain ischemia and reperfusion: modifications in eukaryotic initiation factors associated with inhibition of translational initiation. J Neurochem 67:2005–2012
18. Distelhorst CW, Lam M, McCormick TS (1996) Bcl-2 inhibits hydrogen peroxide-induced ER Ca^{2+} pool depletion. Oncogene 10:2051–2055
19. Doutheil J, Althausen S, Treiman M, Paschen W (1999) Effect of nitric oxide on endoplasmic reticulum calcium homeostasis, protein synthesis and energy metabolism. Cell Calcium 27:107–115.
20. Doutheil J, Althausen S, Treiman M, Paschen W (2000) Effect of nitric oxide on endoplasmic reticulum calcium homeostasis, protein synthesis and energy metabolism. Cell Calcium 27:107–115
21. Duchen M, McGuinness O, Brown L, Crompton M (1993) On the involvement of a cyclosporin A sensitive mitochondrial pore in myocardial reperfusion injury. Cardiovasc Res 27: 1790–1794
22. Fasolato C, Zottini M, Clementi E, Zacchetti D, Meldolesi J, Possan TI (1991) Intracellular Ca^{2+} pools in PC12 cells. Three intracellular pools are distinguished by their turnover and mechanisms of Ca^{2+} accumulation, storage and release. J Biol Chem 266: 20159–20167
23. Foyouzi-Youssefi R, Arnaudeau S, Borner C, Kelley WL, Tschopp J, Lew DP, Demaurex N, Krause K-H (2000) Bcl-2 decreases the free Ca^{2+} concentration within the endoplasmic reticulum. Proc Natl Acad Sci USA 97:5723–5728
24. Frandsen A, Schousboe A (1992) Mobilization of dantrolene-sensitive intracellular calcium pools is involved in the cytotoxicity induced by quisqualate and N-methyl-D-aspartate but not by 2-amino-3-(3-hydroxy-5-methylisoxaxol-4-yl)propionate and kainate in cultured cerebral cortical neurons. Proc Natl Acad Sci USA 89:2590–2594
25. Friberg H, Ferrand-Drake M, Bengtsson F, Halestrap AP, Wieloch T (1998) Cyclosporin A, but not FK506, protects mitochondria and neurons against hypoglycemic damage and implicates the mitochondrial permeability transition in cell death. J Neurosci 18:5151–5159
26. Friedman AD (1996) GADD153/CHOP, a DNA damage-inducible protein, reduced CAAT/enhancer binding protein activities and increased apoptosis in 32D c13 myeloid cells. Cancer Res 56:3250–3256
27. Furuya Y, Lundmo P, Short AD, Gill DL, Isaacs JT (1994) The role of calcium, pH, and cell proliferation in the programmed (apoptotic) death of androgen-independent prostatic cancer cells induced by thapsigargin. Cancer Res 54: 6167–6175
28. Garaschuk O, Yaari Y, Konnerth A (1997) Release and sequestration of calcium by ryanodine-sensitive stores in hippocampal neurons. J Physiol 502:13–20
29. Gething MJ (1999) Role and regulation of the ER chaperone BiP. Sem Cell Dev Biol 10:465–472
30. Gosh TK, Mullaney JM, Tarazi FI, Gill DL (1989) GTP-activated communication between distinct inositol 1,4,5-triphosphate-sensitive and -insensitiv calcium pools. Nature 340:236–239
31. Gosh TK, Bian J, Short AD, Rybak SL, Gill DL (1991) Persistent intracellular calcium pool depletion by thapsigargin and its influence on cell growth. J Biol Chem 266:24690–24697
32. Goss PE, Baker MA, Carver JP, Dennis JW (1995) Inhibitors of carbohydrate processing – a new class of anticancer agents. Clin Cancer Res 1:935–944
33. Gow A, Southwood CM, Lazzarini RA (1998) Disrupted proteolipid protein trafficking results in oligodendrocyte apoptosis in an animal model of Pelizaeus-Merzbacher-Disease. J Cell Biol 140:925–934
34. Guo Q, Furukawa K, Sopher BL, Pham DG, Xie J, Robinson N, Martin GM, Mattson MP (1996) Alheimers PS-1 mutations

perturbs calcium homeostasis and sensitizes PC12 cells to death induced by amyloid beta-peptide. NeuroReport 8:379–383
35. Guo Q, Fu WM, Sopher BL, Miller MW, Ware CB, Martin GM, Mattson MP (1999a) Increased vulnerability of neurons to excitotoxic necrosis in presenilin-1 mutant knock-in mice. Nature Med 5:101–106
36. Guo Q, Sebastian L, Sopher BL, Miller MW, Ware CB, Martin GM, Mattson MP (1999b) Increased vulnerability of hippocampal neurons from presenilin-1 mutant knock-in mice to amyloid beta-peptide toxicity: central roles of superoxide production and caspase activation. J Neurochem 72:1019–1029
37. Häcki J, Egger L, Monney L, Conus S, Rosse T, Fellay I, Borner C (2000) Apoptotic crosstalk between the endoplasmic reticulum and mitochondria controlled by Bcl-2. Oncogene 19:2286–2295
38. Harding HP, Zhang Y, Ron D (1999) Protein translation and folding are coupled by an endoplasmic-reticulum-resident kinase. Nature 397:271–274
39. Harding HP, Zhang YH, Bertolotti A, Zeng HQ, Ron D (2000) Perk is essential for translational regulation and cell survival during the unfolded protein response. Mol Cell 5:897–904
40. Hardy J (1997) Amyloid, the presenilins and Alzheimer's Disease. Trends Neurosci 20:154–159
41. Hata R, Maeda K, Hermann D, Mies G, Hossmann K-A (2000) Dynamics of regional brain metabolism and gene expression after middle cerebral artery occlusion in mice. J Cereb Blood Flow Metabol 20:306–315
42. He H, Lam M, McCormick TS, Diestelhorst CW (1997) Maintenance of calcium homeostasis in the endoplasmic reticulum by Bcl-2. J Cell Biol 138: 1219–1228
43. Hofer AM, Machen TE (1996) Technique for in situ measurement of calcium in in-tracellular inositol 1,4,5,-trisphosphate-sensitive stores using the fluorescent indicator mag-fura-2. Proc Natl Acad Sci 90:2598–2602
44. Inesi G, Sagara Y (1994) Specific inhibitors of intracellular Ca^{2+} ATPases. J Membr Biol 141:1–6
45. Kaneko Y, Tsukamoto A (1994) Thapsigargin-induced persistent intracellular calcium pool depletion and apoptosis in human hepatoma cells. Cancer Lett 97:147–155
46. Katayama T, Imaizumi K, Sato N, Miyoshi K, Kudo T, Hitomi J, Morihara T, Yoneda T, Gomi F, Mori Y, Nakano J, Takeda J, Tsuda T, Itoyama Y, Murayama O, Takashima A, St George-Hyslop P, Takeda M, Tohyama M (1999) Presenilin-1 mutations downregulate the signalling pathway of the unfolded protein response. Nature Cell Biol. 1:479–485
47. Kaufman RJ (1999) Stress signaling from the lumen of the endoplasmic reticulum: coordination of gene transcriptional and translational controls. Genes Dev 13:1211–1233
48. Kim Y-M, Son K, Hong S-J, Green A, Chen J-J, Tzeng E, Hierholzer C, Billiar TR (1998) Inhibition of protein synthesis by nitric oxide correlates with cytostatic activity: nitric oxide induces phosphorylation of initiation factor eIF-2α. Mol Med 4:179–190
49. Kohno K, Higuchi T, Ohta S, Kohno K, Kumon Y, Sakaki S (1997) Neuroprotective nitric oxide synthase inhibitor reduces intracellular calcium accumulation following transient global ischemia in the gerbil. Neurosci Lett 224:17–20
50. Kovacs DM, Fausett HJ, Page KJ, Kim TW, Moir RD, Merriam DE, Hollister RD, Hallmark OG, Mancini R, Felsenstein KM, Hyman BT, Tanzi RE, Wasco W (1996) Alzheimer-associated presenilins 1 and 2: neuronal expression in brain and localization to intracellular membranes in mammalian cells. Nature Med 2:224–229
51. Kristian T, Siesjö BK (1998) Calcium in ischemic cell death. Stroke 29: 705–718
52. Kuo TH, Kim HRC, Zhu LP, Yu YJ, Lin HM, Tsang W (1998) Modulation of endoplasmic reticulum calcium pump by Bcl-2. Oncogene 17:1903–1910
53. Kuznetsov G, Brostrom MA, Brostrom CO (1992) Demonstration of a calcium requirement for secretory protein processing and export. Differential effects of calcium and dithiothreitol. J Biol Chem 265:3932–3939
54. Lam M, Dubyak G, Chen L, Nunez G, Miesfeld RL, Distelhorst CW (1994) Evidence that Bcl-2 represses apoptosis by regulating endoplasmic reticulum-associated Ca^{2+} fluxes. Proc Natl Acad Sci USA 91:6569–6573
55. Lee J, Bruce-Keller AJ, Kruman Y, Chan SL, Mattson MP (1999) 2-deoxy-D-glucose protects hippocampal neurons against excitotoxic and oxidative injury: Evidence for the involvement of stress proteins. J Neurosci Res 57:48–61
56. Li X, Lee AS (1991) Competitive inhibition of a set of endoplasmic reticulum proteins (grp78, grp94 and erp72) retards cell growth arrest and lowers viability after ionophore treatment. Mol Cell Biol 11:3446–3453
57. Lin TY, Wang SM, Fu WM, Chen YH, Yin HS (1999) Toxicity of tunicamycin to cultured brain neurons: ultrastructure of the degenerating neurons. J Cell Biochem 74:638–647
58. Linden T, Doutheil J, Paschen W (1998) Role of calcium in the activation of erp72 and heme oxygenase-1 expression on depletion of endoplasmic reticulum calcium stores in rat neuronal cell culture. Neurosci Lett 247:1–4
59. Liu H, Miller E, Vandewater B, Stevens JL (1998) Endoplasmic reticulum stress proteins block oxidant-induced Ca^{2+} increases and cell death. J Biol Chem 273:12858–12862
60. Lodish HF, Kong N (1990) Perturbation of cellular calcium blocks exit of secretory proteins from rough endoplasmic reticulum. J Biol Chem 265:10893–10899
61. Lodish HF, Kong N, Wikström L (1992) Calcium is required for folding of newly made subunits of the asialoglycoprotein receptor within the endoplasmic reticulum. J Biol Chem 267:12753–12760
62. Lowenstein DH, Gwinn RP, Seren MS, Simon RP, McIntosh TK (1994) Increased expression of mRNA encoding calbindin-D28K, the glucose regulated proteins, or the 72 kDa heat-shock protein in three models of acute CNS injury. Brain Res Mol Brain Res 22:299–308
63. McCormick TS, McColl KS, Distelhorst CW (1997) Mouse lymphoma cells destined to undergo apoptosis in response to thapsigargin treatment fail to generate a calcium-mediated grp78/grp94 stress response. J Biol Chem 272:6087–6092
64. Minn AJ, Velez P, Schendel SL, Liang H, Muchmore SW, Fesik SW, Fill M, Thompson CB (1997) Bcl-X(L) forms an ion channel in synthetic lipid membranes. Nature 385:353–357
65. Mody I, Macdonald JF (1995) NMDA receptor-dependent excitotoxicity – the role of intracellular Ca^{2+} release. Trends Pharmacol Sci 16:356–359
66. Nath R, Raser KJ, Hajimohammadreza I, Wang KK (1997) Thapsigargin induces apoptosis in SH-SY5Y neuroblastoma cells and cerebrocortical cultures. Biochem Mol Biol Int 43:197–205
67. Pahl HL (1999) Signal transduction from the endoplasmic reticulum to the cell nucleus. Physiol Rev 79:683–701
68. Pahl HL, Baeuerle PA (1997) The ER-overload response: activation of NF-κB. Trends Biochem Sci 1997; 22:63–67
69. Paschen W (1996) Disturbances in calcium homeostasis within the endoplasmic reticulum may contribute to the development of ischemic cell damage. Med Hypoth 47:283–288
70. Paschen W, Uto A, Djuricic B, Schmitt J (1994) Hemeoxygenase expression after reversible ischemia of rat brain. Neurosci Lett 180:5–8
71. Paschen W, Doutheil J, Gissel C, Treiman M (1996) Depletion of neuronal endoplasmic reticulum calcium stores by thapsigargin: effect on protein synthesis. J Neurochem 67:1735–1743
72. Paschen W, Gissel C, Linden T, Doutheil J (1998a) Erp72 expression activated by transient cerebral ischemia or distur-

bances of neuronal endoplasmic reticulum calcium stores. Metabol Brain Dis 13:55–68
73. Paschen W, Gissel C, Linden T, Althausen S, Doutheil J (1998b) Activation of gadd153 expression through transient cerebral ischemia: evidence that ischemia causes endoplasmic reticulum dysfunction. Mol Brain Res 60:115–122
74. Paschen W, Doutheil J (1999) Disturbances of the functioning of endoplasmic reticulum: a key mechanism underlying neuronal cell injury? J Cereb Blood Flow Metabol 19:1–18
75. Pernollet M-G, Lantoine F, Devynck M-A (1996) Nitric oxide inhibits ATP-dependent Ca^{2+} uptake into platelet membrane vesicles. Biochem Biophys Res Comm 222:780–785
76. Pinton P, Ferrari D, Magashaes P, Schulze-Osthoff K, Di Virgilio F, Pozzan T, Rizzuto R (2000) Reduced loading of intracellular Ca^{2+} stores and downregulation of capacitative Ca^{2+} influx in Bcl-2-overexpressing cells. J Cell Biol 148:857–862
77. Pisani A, Bonsi P, Centonze D, Giacomini P, Calabresi P (2000) Involvement of intracellular calcium stores during oxygen/glucose deprivation in striatal large aspiny interneurons. J Cereb Blood Flow Metabol 20:839–846
78. Pizzo P, Fasolato C, Pozzan T (1997) Dynamic properties of an inositol 1,4,5-triphosphate- and thapsigargin-insensitive calcium pool in mammalian cell lines. J Cell Biol 136:355–366
79. Pozzomiller LD, Pivovarova NB, Leapman RD, Buchanan RA, Reese TS, Andrews SB (1997) Activity-dependent calcium sequestration in dendrites of hippocampal neurons in brain slices. J Neurosci 17:8729–8738
80. Preston SF, Berlin RD (1992) An intracellular calcium store regulates protein synthesis in HeLa cells, but it is not the hormone-sensitive store. Cell Calcium 13:303–312
81. Preston GA, Barrett JC, Biermann JA, Murphy E (1997) Effects of alterations in calcium homeostasis on apoptosis during neoplastic progression. Cancer Res 57:537–542
82. Prostko CR, Dholakia JN, Brostrom MA, Brostrom CO (1995) Activation of the double-stranded RNA-regulated protein kinase by depletion of endoplasmic reticulum calium stores. J Biol Chem 270:6211–6215
83. Qi X-M, He H, Zhong H, Distelhorst CW (1997) Baculovirus p35 and Z-VAD-fmk inhibit thapsigargin-induced apoptosis of breast cancer cells. Oncogene 15:1207–1212
84. Reed JC, Miyashita T, Takayama S, Wang HJ, Sato T, Krajewski S, Aime-Sempe C, Bodrug S, Kitada S, Hanada M (1996) BCL-2 family proteins: regulators of cell death involved in the pathogenesis of cancer and resistance to therapy. J Cell Biochem 60:23–32
85. Refolo LM, Eckman C, Prada C-M, Yager D, Sambamurti K, Mehta N, Hardy J, Younkin SG (1999) Antisense-induced reduction of presenilin 1 expression selectively increases the production of amyloid β42 in transfected cells. J Neurochem 73:2382–2388
86. Schendel SL, Xie Z, Montal MO, Matsuyama S, Montal M, Reed JC (1997) Channel formation by antiapoptotic protein Bcl-2. Proc Natl Acad Sci USA 94:5113–5118
87. Shamu CE, Walter P (1996) Oligomerization and phosphorylation of the Ire1p kinase during intracellular signaling from the endoplasmic reticulum to the nucleus. EMBO J 15:3028–3039
88. Siesjö BK (1981) Cell damage in the brain: a speculative synthesis. J Cereb Blood Flow Metabol 1:155–185
89. Srivastava SP, Davies MV, Kaufman RJ (1995) Calcium depletion from the endoplasmic reticulum activates the double-stranded RNA-dependent protein kinase (PKR) to inhibit protein synthesis. J Biol Chem 270:16619–16624
90. Srivastava SP, Kumar KU, Kaufman RJ (1998) Phosphorylation of eukaryotic translation initiation factor 2 mediates apoptosis in response to activation of the double-stranded RNA-dependent protein kinase. J Biol Chem 273:2416–2423
91. Takadera T, Ohyashiki T (1998) Apoptotic cell death and CPP32-like activation induced by thapsigargin and their prevention by nerv growth factor in PC12 cells. Biochim Biophys Acta – Mol Cell Res 1401:63–71
92. Takei N, Endo Y (1994) Ca^{2+}-induced apoptosis on cultured embryonic rat cortical neurons. Brain Res 652:65–70
93. Tanaka Y, Tashjian Jr AH (1993) Functional identification and quantification of three intracellular calcium pools in GH_4C_1 cells – evidence that the caffeine-responsive pool is coupled to a thapsigargin-resistant, ATP-dependent process. Biochemistry USA 32:12062–12073
94. Tang NM, Korth MJ, Gale MJr, Wambach M, Der SD, Bandyopadhyay SK, Williams BR, Katze MG (1999) Inhibition of double-stranded RNA- and tumor necrosis factor alpha-mediated apoptosis by tetratricopeptide repeat protein and cochaperone P58 (IPK). Mol Cell Biol 19:4757–4765
95. Thilmann R, Xie Y, Kleihues P, Kiessling M (1986) Persistent inhibition of protein synthesis precedes delayed neuronal death in postischemic gerbil hippocampus. Acta Neuropathol (Berl.) 71:88–93
96. Tsukamoto A, Kaneko Y (1993) Thapsigargin, a Ca^{2+}-ATPase inhibitor, depletes the intracellular Ca^{2+} pool and induces apoptosis in human hepatoma cells. Cell Biol Intern 17:969–970
97. Uchino H, Elmér E, Uchino K, Lindvall O, Siesjö BK (1995) Cyclosporin A dramatically ameliorates CA1 hippocampal damage following transient forebrain ischaemia in the rat. Acta Physiol Scand 155:469–471
98. Uchino H, Elmer E, Uchino K, Li PA, He QP, Smith ML, Siesjö BK (1998) Amelioration by cyclosporin A of brain damage in transient forebrain ischemia in the rat. Brain Res 812:216–226
99. Verma A, Ross CA, Verma D, Supattapone S, Snyder SH (1990) Rat brain endoplasmic reticulum calcium pools are anatomically and functionally segregated. Cell Regul 1:781–790
100. Wang S, Longo FM, Chen J, Butman M, Graham SH, Haglid KG, Sharp FR (1993) Induction of glucose regulated protein (grp78) and inducible heat shock protein (hsp70) mRNAs in rat brain after kainic acid seizures and focal cerebral ischemia. Neurochem Int 23:575–582
101. Waring P, Beaver J (1996) Cyclosporin A rescues thymocytes from apoptosis induced by very low concentrations of thapsigargin: effects on mitochondrial function. Exp Cell Res 227:264–276
102. Wei HF, Perry DC (1996) Dantrolene is cytoprotective in two models of neuronal cell death. J Neurochem 67:2390–2398
103. Wei HF, Wei WL, Bredesen DE, Perry DC (1998) Bcl-2 protects against apoptosis in neuronal cell line caused by thapsigargin-induced depletion of intracellular calcium stores. J Neurochem 70:2305–2314
104. Weidemann A, Paliga K, Dürrwang U, Czech C, Evin G, Master CL, Beyreuther K (1997) Formation of stable complexes between two Alzheimer's disease gene products: presenilin-2 and β-amyloid precursor protein. Nature Med 3:328–332
105. Wiessner C, Neumann-Haefelin T, Brink I, Vogel P, Back T, Hossmann K-A (1994) The genomic response of the rat brain following cerebral ischemia: generalized versus cell and region specific responses. In: Pharmacology of Cerebral Ischemia (Kriegelstein J, Oberpichler-Schwenk H, eds.), Stuttgart, Wissenschaftliche Verlagsgesellschaft, pp 455–465
106. Widmann R, Kuroiwa T, Bonnekoh P, Hossmann K-A (1991) [^{14}C] Leucine incorporation into brain proteins in gerbils after transient ischemia: Relationship to selective vulnerability of hippocampus. J Neurochem 56:789–796
107. Widmann R, Miyazawa T, Hossmann K-A (1993) Protective effect of hypothermia on hippocampal injury after 30 min forebrain ischemia in rats is mediated by postischemic recovery of protein synthesis. J Neurochem 61:200–209

108. Willmott NJ, Galione A, Smith PA (1995) Nitric oxide induces intracellular calcium mobilization and increases secretion of incorporated 5-hydroxytryptamine in rat pancreatic β-cells. FEBS Lett 371:99–104
109. Wong WL, Brostrom MA, Brostrom CO (1991) Effects of Ca^{2+} and ionophore A23187 on protein synthesis in intact rabbit reticulocytes. Int J Biochem 23:605–608
110. Wong WL, Brostrom MA, Kuznetsov G, Gmitter-Yellen D, Brostrom CO (1993) Inhibition of protein synthesis and early protein processing by thapsigargin in cultured cells. Biochem J 289:71–79
111. Xie Y, Seo K, Hossmann KA (1989) Effect of barbiturate treatment on post-ischemic protein biosynthesis in gerbil brain. J Neurol Sci 92:317–328
112. Yoshimoto T, Siesjö BK (1999) Posttreatment with the immunosuppressant cyclosporin A in transient focal ischemia. Brain Res 839:283–291
113. Younkin SG (1995) Evidence that Aβ42 is the real culprit in Alzheimer's Disease. Ann Neurol 37:287–288
114. Yu ZF, Luo H, Fu WM, Mattson MP (1999) The endoplasmic reticulum stress-responsive protein GRP78 protects neurons against excitotoxicity and apoptosis: Suppression of oxidative stress and stabilization of calcium homeostasis. Exp Neurol 155:302–314
115. Zhang L, Andou Y, Masuda S, Mitani A, Kataoka K (1993) Dantrolene protects against ischemic, delayed neuronal death in gerbil brain. Neurosci Lett 158:105–108
116. Zhou Y-P, Teng D, Dralyuk F, Ostrega D, Roe MW, Philipson L, Polonsky KS (1998) Apoptosis in insulin-secreting cells. Evidence for the role of intracellular Ca^{2+} stores and arachidonic acid metabolism. J Clin Invest 101:1623–1632
117. Zhu L, Ling S, Yu XD, Venkatesh LK, Subramanian T, Chinnadurai G, Kuo TH (1999) Modulation of mitochondrial Ca^{2+} homeostasis by Bcl-2. J Biol Chem 274:33267–33273

Role of mitochondria in neuronal cell death

The role of mitochondrial dysfunction in reperfusion damage in the brain

B. K. Siesjö[1], T. Kristián[1], F. Shibasaki[2], H. Uchino[1,3]

Abstract

Several lines of evidence suggest the involvement of mitochondrial dysfunction in reperfusion damage in the brain. It has been commonly assumed that mitochondrial damage may be a delayed event, which is caused by oxidative stress and/or secondary calcium accumulation. This is traditionally believed to be mediated by peroxidation of membrane lipids, or oxidation of proteins such as those constituting the respiratory complexes. However, much interest has recently been focussed on the assembly of a mitochondrial permeability transition (MPT) pore, a large conductance channel which short-circuits the inner mitochondrial membrane to H^+, thereby causing cessation of ATP synthesis and a burst of production of reactive oxygen species.

The MPT pore assembly is an adverse event, which is triggered by depolarization of mitochondrial membranes by calcium accumulation, and by oxidative stress. Pore opening is more or less specifically blocked by Cycloporin A (CsA) which has proved to ameliorate ischemic brain damage in both forebrain and focal ischemia, provided that it can be made to pass the blood-brain barrier. In transient focal ischemia, the effect of post-treatment (1 h) of CsA is shared by FK506, an immunosuppressant that does not inhibit the MPT *in vitro*. However, an MPT seems to play a decisive role in global ischemia and when given after only 5 min of recirculation, following 2 h of focal ischemia, CsA has a more pronounced effect than FK506. Available data thus suggests that an MPT plays a pathogenetic role in the immediate recirculation period. In that period, pore formation is promoted by reoxidation of redox couples, by mitochondrial calcium accumulation, and by low pH. When delayed mitochondrial dysfunction occurs after many hours, or days, other mechanisms may come into play.

Introduction

Reperfusion damage in the brain is the result of events occurring in three different phases: (a) the period of ischemia *per se*, (b) a maturation

Keywords: Reperfusion after forebrain and focal ischemia. Mitochondrial dysfunction. Assembly of a mitochondrial transition pore. Effects of Cyclosporin A and of FK506.

[1]Center for the Study of Neurological Disease, The Queen's Medical Center, 1356 Lusitana Street, 8th Floor, Honolulu, Hawaii 96813; [2]Department of Molecular Cell Physiology, The Tokyo Metropolitan Institute of Medical Science, 3-18-22 Honkomagome, Bunkyo-ku, Tokyo 113-8613, Japan; [3]Department of Anesthesiology, Tokyo Medical University, 6-7-1 Nishishinjuku, Shinjuku-ku, Tokyo, 160-0023, Japan
e-mail address: bsiesjo@cns.queens.org.

period during which cells may resume various functions, and in which light microscopical evidence of impending cell damage is usually absent, and (c) a delayed series of catabolic events which leads to the demise of cells.

In this article, we propose that mitochondrial dysfunction developing during the maturation period is the cause of cell demise in the final phase of the death cascade, both because the mitochondria are the targets of a cascade of events that encompass a pathological calcium load, and enhanced formation of free radicals, and because they may release substances which trigger (apoptotic or necrotic) cell death.

1. Events leading to cell death in ischemia – reperfusion

a. The period of ischemia

Ischemia results whenever blood flow decreases, locally or globally, to values that are insufficient for maintaining normal mitochondrial functions (Siesjö 1992). These functions encompass the sequential oxidation of pyruvate and other substrates to CO_2 and water, during which sufficient energy is tapped off to generate ATP from ADP and inorganic phosphate (P_i). Ischemia is a mitochondrial disease since it leads to unsaturation of cyt a-a_3 with oxygen and, thereby, to a critical decrease in the generation of ATP by the mitochondrial respiratory chain (Fig. 1). Secondary to this there is reduction of pyruvate to lactate, which accumulates together with a stoichiometrical amount of H^+, yielding lactic acidosis, and a breakdown of ion homeostasis, encompassing the entry of calcium into cells. The principal events can be broken down as follows.

Energy is generated by the mitochondria in the form of ATP according to the general reaction energy + ADP + P_i → ATP. Under aerobic conditions, only about 6% of the ATP is formed by glycolysis, i.e. by the anaerobic conversion of glucose (or glycogen) to pyruvate (Siesjö 1978). The remainder is formed in the electron transport chain. Under anaerobic conditions, the rate of glycolysis can be increased 6-7-fold (Siesjö 1978). This would significantly enhance ATP production, but there are two problems: the production is not sufficient to sustain energy metabolism of mature tissues, and it occurs at the cost of a potentially harmful lactic acidosis.

Ischemia, particularly if dense, leads to the rapid hydrolysis of ATP according to the reaction ATP + HOH → ADP_f + P_i + energy where ADP_f is the free ADP concentration. Since ADP_f is only about 10% of the total ADP concentration, and about 1% of the ATP concentration, it would tend to rise precipitously whenever ATP is hydrolyzed (Lawson and Veech 1979; Erecinska and Silver 1989; Ekholm et al. 1992). However, a shift in the creatine kinase reaction to the right, as written below:

$$PCr + ADP_f + H^+ \Leftrightarrow Cr + ATP$$

can retard the rise in ADP_f and replenish some ATP. Nonetheless, ADP_f rises steeply during ischemia, and there is a rapid fall in the ATP/ADP_f ratio (Ekholm et al. 1992, see Fig. 2). This means that reactions that depend on the phosphorylation potential, i.e. on ATP • ADP_f^{-1} • P_i^{-1}, may come to a halt long before ATP concentrations are approaching zero.

Since ion transport is driven by ATP energy, a fall in phosphorylation potential leads to arrest of active $3Na^+/2K^+$ exchange, as well as of $Ca^{2+}/3Na^+$ exchange, the result being depolarization and passive release of K^+ from cells, and their uptake of Ca^{2+}, Na^+, and Cl^- (Siesjö 1981; Hansen 1985). Such a collapse of ion gradients occurs quite precipitously, probably because cessation of ion transport is coupled to activation of ion gates by depolarization and by the release of excitatory amino acids, notably glutamate (Benveniste et al. 1984). When released, glutamate stimulates both ionotropic and metabotropic receptors. They first activate ion channels that provide major entry pathways for calcium, while the latter trigger a cascade of reactions that are normally involved in signal transduction between the environment and the cell interior. Since Ca^{2+} is an important second messenger in signal transduction, a cascade of potentially harmful reactions is triggered, encompassing enhanced lipolysis and proteolysis, as well as changes in protein phosphoryla-

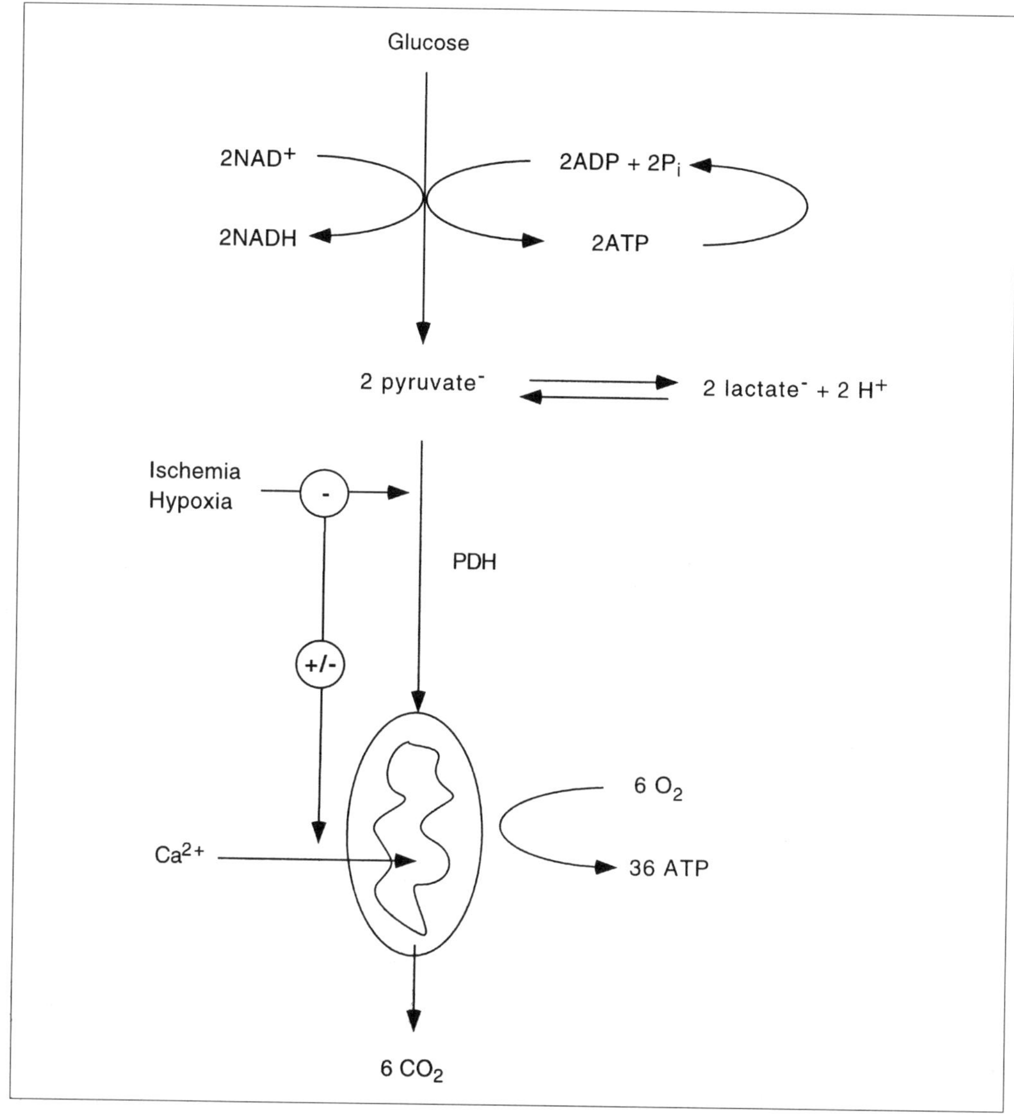

Fig. 1. Schematic diagram illustrating how the glycolytic generation of pyruvate, and the oxidation of the latter by the mitochondria, lead to production of ATP from ADP and P_i. During hypoxia/ischemia, ATP production is reduced, or ceases. This causes reduction of pyruvate to lactate plus H^+, yielding lactic acidosis, and loss of ion homeostasis with influx of calcium into the cell. Slightly modified after Siesjö 1992.

tion and in gene expression (Siesjö 1992; Choi 1995; Tymianski and Tator 1996). Some of these reactions are elicited by the ischemic transient, but others become manifest first during recirculation (see below).

Recirculation, which restores O_2 transport to tissues and mitochondria, leads to resumption of oxidative phosphorylation, and to generation of ATP. If the ischemia is of brief to moderate duration, and under optimal conditions of re-

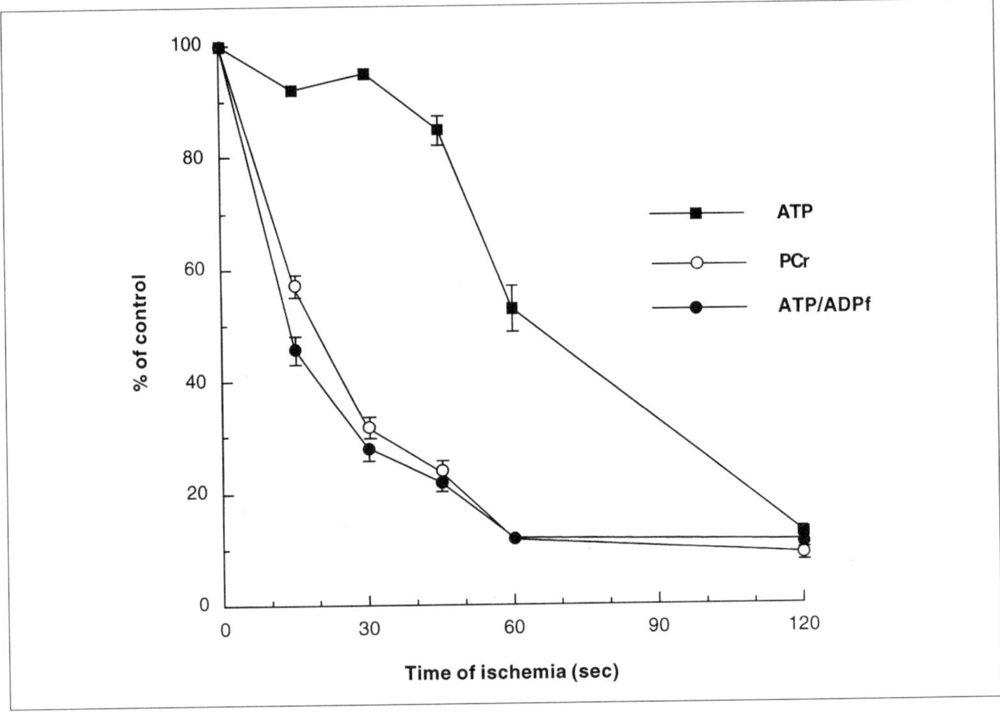

Fig. 2. Changes in the ATP and phosphocreatine (Pcr) concentrations, as well as in the ATP/free ADP ratio, during the first 120 sec of complete ischemia. The values pertain to the neocortex of rats. Data from Ekholm et al. (1992).

flow, the PCr concentration and the phosphorylation potential are restored to normal within 2–3 min while the lactic acidosis is resolved more slowly, particularly in hyperglycemic animals (Ljunggren et al. 1974; see also Hillered et al. 1985; Smith et al. 1986). At the same time, K^+ is accumulated by cells, and Ca^{2+} is extruded (Siemkowicz and Hansen 1981; Katsura et al. 1992, Ekholm et al. 1992). This shows that mitochondrial function is adequately restored.

The situation is different if the ischemia is of long duration, as in middle cerebral artery (MCA) occlusion of 2 h duration. Then, recirculation may fail to completely restore ATP concentration and the phosphorylation potential (Folbergrová et al. 1995). At least in part, this is because ATP is broken down to ADP and AMP, the latter being deaminated and dephosphorylated to nucleosides and bases; thus, the sustained part of the reduction in ATP reflects degradation of the adenine nucleotide pool (Σ ATP + ADP + AMP) (see Kleihues et al. 1974; Chapman et al. 1981). However, a lingering reduction in mitochondrial function is reflected in the persisting increase in lactate content, and mitochondrial dysfunction probably explains the inadequate extrusion of Ca^{2+} from cells to extracellular fluids (Kristián et al. 1998).

b. The maturation period

The concept of maturation of an ischemic lesion, coined by Ito et al. (1975), predicts that the length of the maturation period is inversely proportional to the duration of the ischemia. Thus, a brief ischemic period may be followed by neuronal damage which is delayed by many hours, or by days (Kirino 1982; Pulsinelli et al.

1982a), while ischemia of long duration can trigger damage that develops as soon as recirculation is induced (e.g. Kalimo et al. 1981).

If ischemia is of the global (or forebrain) type the rate of maturation varies between different neuronal populations, some showing signs of cell death within a few hours of the ischemic insult, while others contain cells that survive for days of recirculation (Pulsinelli et al. 1982a; Smith et al. 1988). A comparable situation probably exists in transient focal ischemia, e.g. that caused by middle cerebral artery (MCA) occlusion. However, it should be recalled that MCA occlusion primarily affects cells in the caudoputamen and the neocortex, i.e. regions that either show a rapid or an intermediate rate of maturation in experiments on forebrain ischemia (Pulsinelli et al. 1982a). This means that, even if an MCA occlusion is of brief duration, one cannot expect to see very slowly developing lesions, as is observed in the CA1 sector of the hippocampus in forebrain ischemia.

During the maturation period, cell death seems to be absent and cells may resume certain function, e.g. those underlying EEG and evoked potentials (Hossmann and Kleihues 1973). Nonetheless, pathological events occur, or those of a physiological nature may be distorted or exaggerated. For example, areas containing cells which are destined to die show a persisting reduction in overall protein synthesis (Thilmann et al. 1989; Hossmann 1985), and previously ischemic tissues may be underperfused and hypometabolic for sustained periods (Pulsinelli et al. 1982b; Kozuka et al. 1989). Furthermore, heat shock and stress proteins are expressed (Nowak et al. 1993) and so are many genes. Some of the latter encompass the immediate early genes of the *fos*, *jun*, and *krox* families (Kiessling et al. 1993; Kamme et al. 1995), while others code for enzymes that are potentially harmful in the sense that they give rise to a delayed inflammatory and immunological response. Examples of the latter are the inducible forms of nitric oxide synthase (iNOS) and of cyclooxygenase 2 (COX-2) (Bazan 1997; Vane et al. 1998). It is now widely held that stimulation of surface receptors for glutamate and neurotrophic factors, influx of calcium, or production of reactive oxygen species (ROS), trigger death or survival pathways by activating a web of kinases, phosphatases, and transcription factors. In the present context, though, our interest will be focussed on the role of mitochondria in mediating delayed cell death.

c. The death effector phase

At the end of the maturation period, i.e. after hours or days of recirculation, cells die, as evidenced by plasma and mitochondrial membrane breaks in light and electron microscopical specimens, and by assays demonstrating fragmentation of DNA. Evidence available from experiments on forebrain ischemia suggests that the mechanisms leading to cell death involve bioenergetic failure and mitochondrial dysfunction (Pulsinelli and Duffy 1983; Sims and Pulsinelli 1987). The evidence suggests that the primary event is mitochondrial dysfunction with bioenergetic failure being the secondary one, but the casual relationship has not been established (Sims 1990). The results nonetheless put the mitochondria in the focus of interest. The question arises whether mitochondrial dysfunction develops gradually during the maturation period and if such dysfunction, when sufficiently pronounced, elicits cell death. If this is the case, one has to probe into the mechanisms of mitochondrial dysfunction.

2. Mitochondria as generators of ATP, as targets of adverse stimuli, and as mediators of cell death

According to the chemiosmotic theory of Mitchell (1966) H^+ is extruded from the mitochondria at three sites of the respiratory chain, creating a large electrochemical gradient for H^+ ($\Delta\mu_{H}{}^{+}$). The back flow of H^+ through the ATPase (complex V) is what allows ATP to be generated.

It is possible to envisage two major ways in which postischemic conditions may disturb oxidative phosphorylation. One would be peroxidation of lipid components of mitochondrial membranes by phospholipase A_2 activity, secondarily affecting electron flow through the respiratory complexes (Nakamura et al. 1992; Sun and Gilboe 1994). The second one would be direct oxidation of proteins in these complexes by free radicals (Wagner et al. 1990; Almeida et al. 1995). However, more recent results suggest a third possibility. This is the assembly of a mitochondrial permeability transition (MPT) pore, i.e. a voltage-sensitive and Ca^{2+}-activated channel in the inner mitochondrial membrane which is indiscriminately permeable to solutes with a molecular mass < 1500 Daltons (Zoratti and Szabó 1995; Bernardi et al. 1999; Kroemer and Reed 2000). Since the pore is permeable to all physiological ions, the electrochemical potential for H^+ collapses, and ATP production ceases; in fact, reversal of the ATPase reaction leads to consumption of available ATP stores. This sequence of events is potentially detrimental, particularly since it encompasses enhanced formation of ROS. It has also been emphasized that an MPT could constitute one important factor in reperfusion injury in heart and liver ischemia (see Halestrap et al. 1998, Lemasters et al. 1998).

The concept of an MPT pore as a major pathogenetic factor in brain ischemia has received considerable, albeit indirect support. The evidence is, to a large extent, based on the well-known fact that, *in vitro*, the immunosuppressant cyclosporin A (CsA) is a more or less specific blocker of the pore. However, since CsA poorly penetrates the blood-brain barrier (BBB), probably because of counter-transport by the P-glycoprotein system, this fact remained unrecognized until it was found that, following opening of the blood-brain barrier (BBB) by a unilateral needle lesion, CsA given systemically in a dose of 10 mg • kg^{-1} virtually eliminated CA1 cell damage caused by 7 or 10 min of forebrain ischemia in rats (Uchino et al.1995, 1998). In these studies, it was found that CsA was equally affective when given as pretreatment or when it was given 30 min after the start of reperfusion. These results were confirmed by Friberg et al. (1998), who also reported that when CsA was given 2 h after the ischemic transient, its neuroprotective effect was gone.

It has remained unclarified if an MPT is assembled *in vivo* under conditions of ischemia and reperfusion, and it has been difficult to unequivocally demonstrate under what conditions it occurs *in vitro*, either in isolated mitochondria (Andreyev and Fiskum 1999) or in cultured cells (Kristal and Dubinsky 1997). As Figure 3a shows, heart mitochondria buffer a few calcium loads and then release the calcium; this release is accompanied by mitochondrial swelling and can be prevented by CsA (Fontaine et al. 1998; Kristián et al. 2000a). Brain mitochondria behave differently since, at least with complex 1 substrates, saturation of calcium uptake does not lead to calcium release, but a moderate release is observed after the first calcium pulse (Fig. 3b), which is blocked by CsA. Furthermore, only about a third of the nonsynaptic mitochondria studied showed swelling when loaded with calcium, while virtually all mitochondria swelled in response to alamethacin (see Kristián et al. 2000a). Clearly, it appears highly justified to explore if the mitochondrial population gives an inhomogenous swelling response *in vivo* and, if that is the case, to find out what cells and what cellular compartments are affected.

CsA has three major effects: (a) it modulates protein folding by influencing peptidyl-prolyl-cis-trans-isomerase activity, (b) it reacts with several immunophilins, such as cyclophilin D, thereby reducing the phosphatase activity of calcineurin, and (c) it blocks the MPT pore. The first two of these effects are shared by FK506, an immunosuppressant that binds to a different class of immunophilins, the FK-binding proteins (Snyder et al. 1998); however, FK506 does not block the MPT pore (Friberg et al. 1998).

In view of these facts, it is of interest that FK506 seems to have a less robust effect on brain damage caused by forebrain ischemia than CsA (Drake et al. 1996; Ide et al. 1996), particularly if it is given during reperfusion (Friberg et al. 2000). It is also of note that CsA, but not FK506, ameliorates damage due to hypoglycemic coma (Friberg et al. 1998). These results suggest that an MPT plays a dominating role in the pathogenesis of hypoglycemic brain dam-

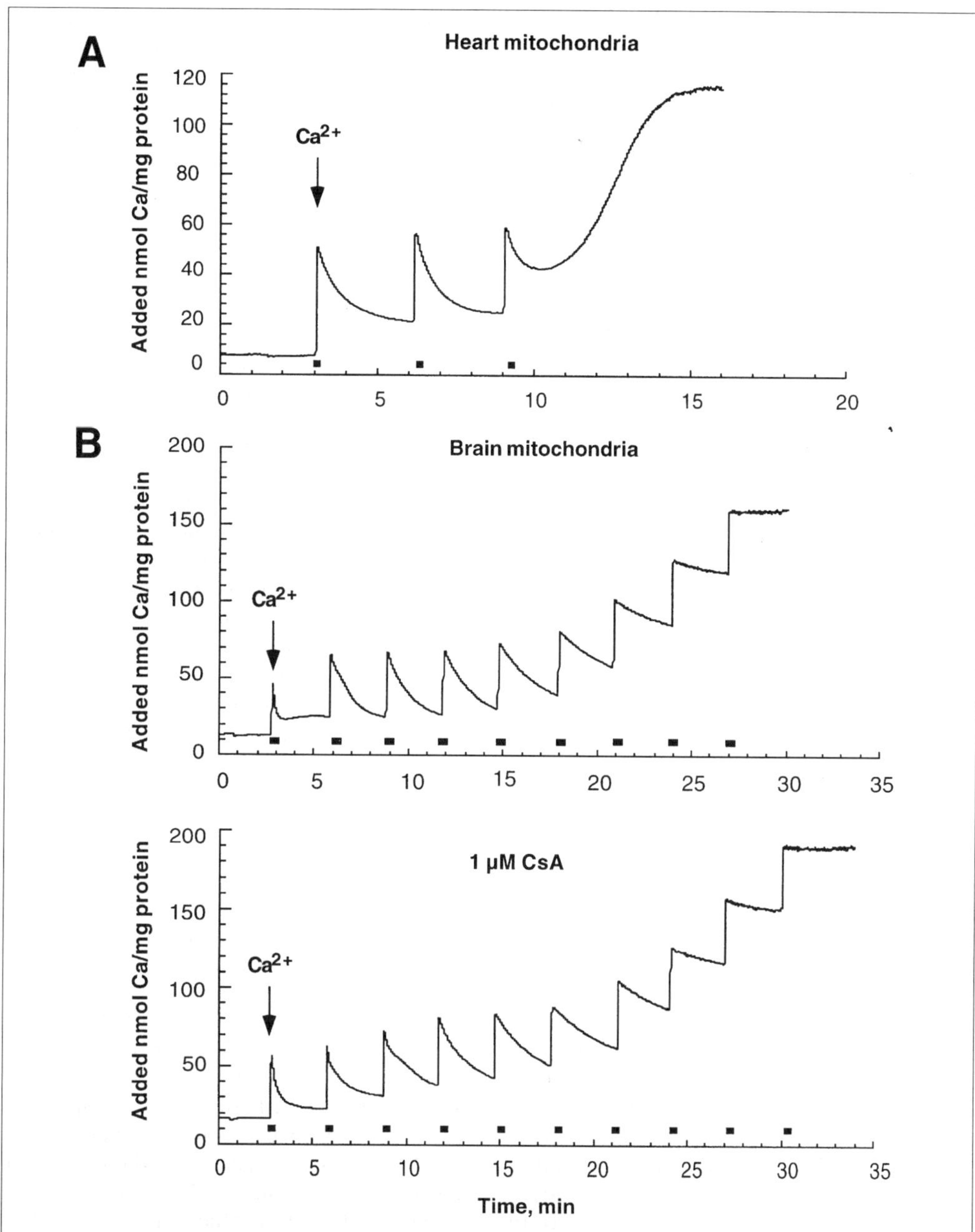

Fig. 3. Measurement of calcium uptake by heart and brain mitochondria. The calcium uptake by isolated mitochondria (0.25 mg protein • ml^{-1}) energized by malate and glutamate was measured in the presence of calcium indicator Calcium Green-5N. Equivalent pulses of $CaCl_2$ (40 nmol • mg^{-1} proteins, 10 µM) were added to mitochondria every 3 min. *Panel A* represents the typical recording when heart mitochondria were exposed to calcium pulses, and *Panel B* shows the calcium uptake and release by non-synaptic brain mitochondria under the same experimental conditions, and also the effect of CsA (1 µM). The small horizontal bars represent the time points when the calcium pulses were added to the medium.

age, and that it contributes to the damage caused by brief periods of forebrain ischemia. Clearly, although several mechanisms could contribute to cause delayed mitochondrial dysfunction (damage to lipid or protein components of mitochondrial membranes, the assembly of an MPT), it is less evident how such dysfunction could cause cell death. The simplest explanation would be failure of ATP synthesis, with cell demise being the result of bioenergetic failure. However, it is now generally considered that dysfunctional mitochondria can mediate cell death by releasing proteins such as apoptosis-inducing factor (AIF) and cytochrome c (cyt c). When cyt c is released from mitochondria to cytosol, it binds to an apoptosis-activating factor (Apaf-1); this, in turn, binds to pro-caspase 9, resulting in the proteolytic processing and activation of the caspase. The result is activation of caspase-3, a serine-threonine protease which is considered the executioner of cell death since it activates CAD, fodrin, poly (ADP-ribose) polymerase (PARP) and other enzymes which degrade cell structure (Reed 1997; Green and Reed 1998; Susin et al. 1999). By long tradition, such cell death has been considered to be of the apoptotic type; however, it is now realized that necrosis could be the end result of an apoptotic program. If this is the case, one could explain why caspase-3 inhibitors ameliorate damage (Chen et al. 1998) in settings in which cell injury has the morphological characteristics of necrosis (Desphande et al. 1992; Petito et al. 1997; Colbourne et al. 1999).

Pathways of mitochondrial-triggered cell death are schematically illustrated in Fig. 4. The figure makes the point that mitochondrial depolarization can lead to an MPT, to collapse of the electrochemical potential for H^+, to ROS production, and necrotic cell death. Possibly, necrosis results when large amounts of cyt c and other essential mitochondrial constituents are lost, or large amounts of ROS are formed. At least *in vitro*, rapidly developing necrotic cell death results when the insult is severe and/or prolonged, while apoptosis, which develops more slowly, is the result of mild insults (Ankarcrona et al. 1995). However, apoptotic cells are believed to undergo secondary necrosis, possibly because caspases activated by cyt c aggravate the mitochondrial damage; alternatively, activated caspases may degrade ATP-extruding enzymes localized to the plasma membrane (Nicotera, this volume). Apoptotic cell death is believed to be triggered by cyt c release, but such release can occur either with or without a preceding depolarization, or an MPT. Since cyt c is bound to the outer face of the inner mitochondrial membrane, its release from the mitochondria requires that the outer membrane develops breaks, or that pores are formed allowing cyt c to pass. Since an MPT is associated with swelling, overstretching of the outer membrane could be what increases its permeability.

For the sake of simplicity, we will confine the discussion to cell death (apoptotic or necrotic) which is triggered by mitochondrial membrane depolarization, assuming that an MPT is involved. We will also use the terms pro- and anti-apoptotic without reference to the mode of cell death. As shown in the upper part of Fig. 4 Ca^{2+} accumulation and redox stress are proapoptotic while CsA has the opposite effect. Most importantly, the Bcl-2 family of proteins modulate mitochondrial membranes, with Bcl-2 and Bcl-x_L being anti- and Bax, Bic, and Bad proapoptotic (Reed 1997; Green and Reed 1998). Clearly, a change in gene expression with upregulation of Bax, Bic, or Bad, or downregulation of Bcl_2 or Bcl-x_L, could significantly shift the balance between life and death in a proapoptotic direction.

The figure gives the impression that CsA and the proto-oncogene products are mechanistically different. In reality, this may not be so. As already mentioned, CsA and FK506 bind to immunophilins, thereby preventing activation of calcineurin, a serine-threonine phosphatase which is the only one activated by calcium. One can then envisage a scenario where calcium enters cells, combines with calmodulin, and activates calcineurin which acts on its substrates that include nuclear factor of activated T cells (NF-AT), nitric oxide synthases, the NMDA receptor, and others (Asai et al. 1999). However, calcineurin *per se* is proapoptotic, and its activation may trigger cell death; in fact, it has been speculated that certain neuronal

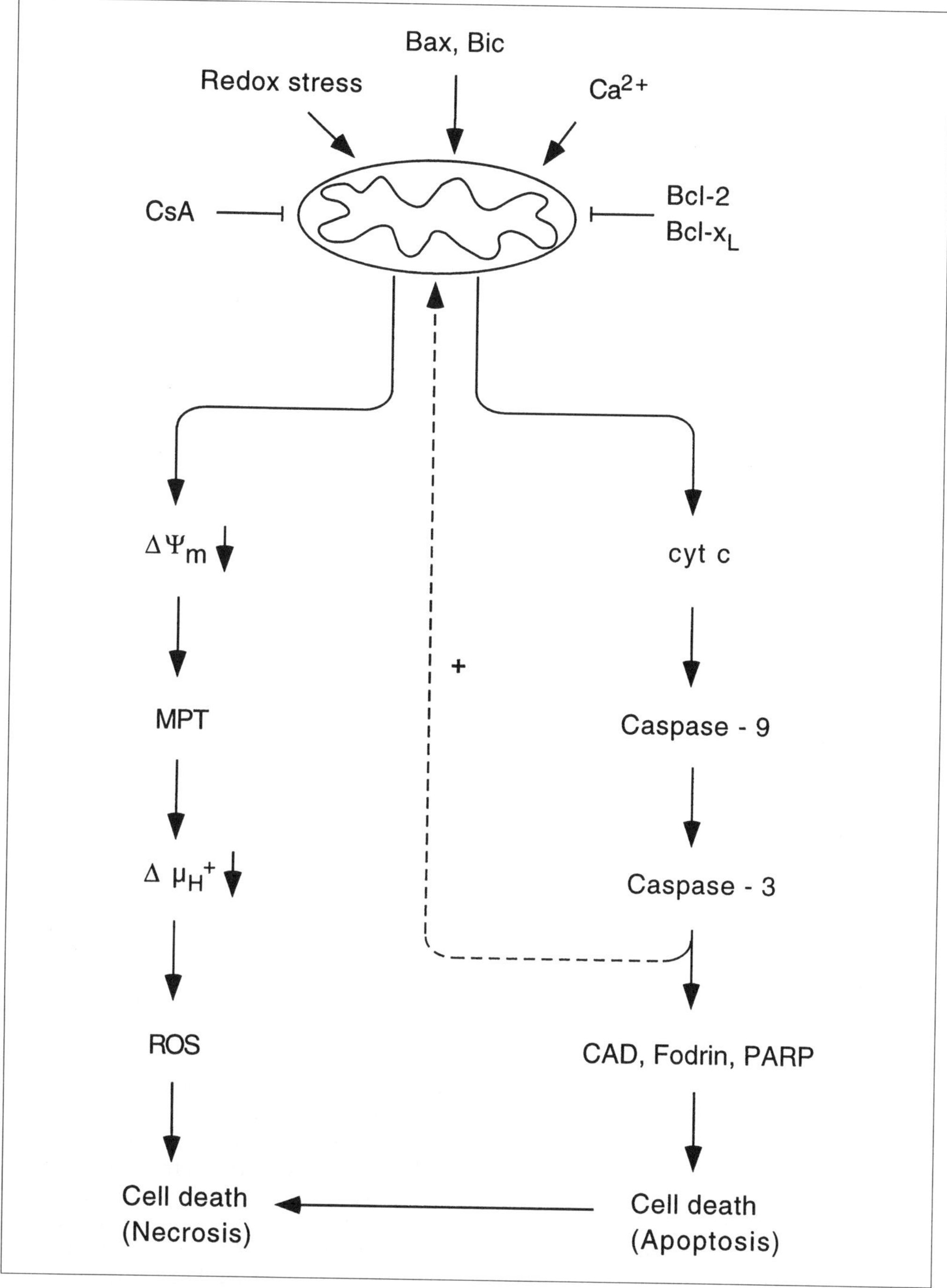

Fig. 4. Schematic diagram illustrating some of the reactions leading to mitochondria – mediated necrotic and apoptotic cell death. For explanation of symbols, and further details, see text.

populations are vulnerable to various insults because they constitutively contain a high calcineurin concentration (Asai et al. 1999).

A coupling seems to exist between calcineurin and the Bcl-2 family of proteins. Thus, Bcl-2 has been found to form a tight complex with calcineurin, resulting in the targeting of calcineurin to Bcl-2 sites on cytoplasmic membranes (Shibasaki et al. 1997). When calcineurin is bound to Bcl-2 it is unable to promote the nuclear translocation of NF-AT, and Bcl-2 blocks the cell death resulting from calcineurin overexpression. Interestingly, the pro-apoptotic Bax interferes with interactions between calcineurin and Bcl-2.

A subsequent article (Wang et al. 1999) reported that calcineurin was found to dephosphorylate Bad, thus enhancing Bad heterodimerization with Bcl-x_L and promoting apoptosis. Many of the experiments quoted were obtained on non-neuronal cells, and the triggers of apoptosis may have been remote from what elicits cell death due to ischemia. However, Wang et al. (1999) reported that glutamate-induced Ca^{2+} influx caused calcineurin activation in hippocampal neurons, triggering mitochondrial targeting of Bad and apoptosis. Both could be suppressed by a dominant-inhibitory mutant of calcineurin, or by pharmacological inhibition of calcineurin.

3. The anti-ischemic effects of CsA and FK506: What mechanisms are involved?

As already mentioned, CsA seems to have a more robust effect on FK506 in forebrain ischemia, suggesting that an MPT plays a relatively dominant role. However, if this is the case, the results indicate that the MPT pore must be assembled during the first 30–60 min of reperfusion. It also remains unexplained why FK506 does not ameliorate ischemic damage when given in the late recirculation period following 10 min of forebrain ischemia. For these reasons, it seems justified to put scrutiny on experiments on focal ischemia.

An anti-ischemic effect of CsA in focal ischemia was first suggested by Shiga et al. (1992), who occluded the MCA in rats for 90 min, using an intraluminal filament technique. Later, Sharkey and Butcher (1994) found a robust effect of FK506 in MCA occlusion induced by endothelin injection. Subsequent results have given information that is pertinent to the following questions. First, is there a difference between the anti-ischemic effects of CsA and FK506? Second, what is the therapeutic window of opportunity for CsA and FK506? Third, if a difference is found between the two immunosuppressants, what is the molecular explanation?

Thirty min of MCA occlusion gives a lesion, primarily in the form of selective neuronal necrosis (SNN), which is restricted to the dorsolateral caudoputamen, but when the occlusion is performed in hyperglycemic animals, the lesion takes on the characteristics of pannecrosis, and extends into neocortical areas (Nedergaard 1987; Gisselsson et al. 1999). When this model was adopted, pretreatment with CsA and FK506 equally reduced the damage, most of the FK506-injected animals having virtually no lesions in TTC-stained sections (Kuroda et al. 1999).

Results obtained in rats, subjected to 90–120 min of MCA occlusion, demonstrate that CsA and FK506 are equally efficacious when given 1 to 3 h after the start of recirculation, infarct volume being reduced to 35–40% of control (Yoshimoto and Siesjö 1999; Yoshimoto et al 2000). In these experiments, the low rate of penetration of CsA across the BBB was circumvented by an increase in the systemically administered dose (Matsumoto et al. 1999), or by direct intracarotid infusion (Yoshimoto and Siesjö 1999). In the experiments of Matsumoto et al. 1999, the CsA analogue Me ValCsA had an effect similar to that of CsA. Since this analogue blocks the MPT pore *in vitro*, but has only a weak immunosuppressive effect, the authors suggested that CsA and its analogues work by preventing the opening of an MPT pore. However, what speaks against this possibility is the fact that FK506 and CsA were equally efficacious when given 1 or 3 h after the start of recirculation (Yoshimoto and Siesjö 1999). It is also of note that both FK506 and CsA prevented apoptosis (and necrosis) in cerebellar granule cells subjected to glutamate exposure *in vitro* (Ankarcrona et al. 1995).

Results obtained with intracarotid infusion of CsA nonetheless suggest that an MPT pore opening plays a role in the pathophysiology of focal ischemic damage. Thus, when CsA was infused 5 min after the start of recirculation, following 2 h of MCA occlusion, the size of the infarct was reduced to 5–10% of control (Yoshimoto and Siesjö 1999). Since this additional effect was not observed when FK506 was given at the same time point, the results suggest that a CsA-sensitive MPT pore is assembled in the immediate recirculation period. However, the opening of an MPT pore in this *in vivo* situation remains to be directly demonstrated and, in view of the *in vitro* results discussed above, it seems highly justified to explore if a population of mitochondria swell within the first 5–15 min of recirculation. Furthermore, the results do not only raise the question about the molecular mechanisms of the additional effect of CsA, when given after 5 min of recirculation, but also about the mechanisms underlying the shared effects of CsA and FK506.

At the present time, therefore, experiments on both forebrain and focal ischemia suggest that CsA has an anti-ischemic effect which is not shared by FK506. This effect becomes prominent if CsA is given either before, or just after recirculation, suggesting that an MPT pore is opened in this period.

It has previously been concluded that an MPT is not likely to occur during ischemia when pore opening is inhibited by the reduction of NAD^+ and $NADP^+$; besides, low pH was assumed to prevent the assembly of an MPT pore (Halestrap 1991; Bernardi et al. 1992). However, these results were obtained in de-energized mitochondria in the absence of inorganic phosphate (P_i). When experiments on brain and heart mitochondria were conducted on energized mitochondria in the presence of P_i, i.e. under conditions more close to those prevailing *in vivo* during recirculation, low pH was shown to promote the assembly of an MPT pore, an effect which seemed related to an increased influx of P_i into mitochondria (Kristián et al. 2000b). This makes it likely that an MPT pore can be opened in the immediate recirculation period when redox systems quickly get oxidized, and pH is low. One may even speculate that preischemic hyperglycemia aggravates damage by exaggerating and prolonging the acidotic transient, thereby promoting pore opening.

References

1. Almeida A, Allen K, Bates T, Clark J (1995) Effects of reperfusion following cerebral ischaemia on the activity of the mitochondrial respiratory-chain in the gerbil brain. J Neurochem 65:1698–1703
2. Andreyev A, Fiskum G (1999) Calcium induced release of mitochondrial cytochrome c by different mechanisms selective for brain versus liver. Cell Death Differ 6:825–832
3. Ankarcrona M, Dypbukt J, Boncoffo E, Zhivotovsky B, Orrenius S, Lipton S, Nicotera P (1995) Glutamate-induced neuronal death: A succession of necrosis or apoptosis depending on mitochondrial function. Neuron 15:961–973
4. Asai A, Qiu J, Narita Y, Chi S, Saito N, Shinoura N, Hamada H, Kuchino Y, Kirino T (1999) High level calcineurin activity predisposes neuronal cells to apoptosis. J Biol Chem 274:34450–34458
5. Benveniste H, Drejer J, Schousboe A, Diemer NH (1984) Elevation of the extracellular concentrations of glutamate and aspartate in rat hippocampus during transient cerebral ischemia monitored by intracerebral microdialysis. J Neurochem 43:1369–1374
6. Bernardi P, Vassanelli S, Veronese P, Colonna R, Szabo I, Zoratti M (1992) Modulation of the mitochondrial permeability transition pore. Effect of protons and divalent cations. J Biol Chem 267:2934–2939
7. Bernardi P, Scorrano L, Colonna R, Petronilli V, Di Lisa F (1999) Mitochondria and cell death. Mechanistic aspects and methodological issues. Eur J Biochem 264:687–701
8. Chapman A, Westerberg E, Siesjö B (1981) The metabolism of purine and pyrimidine nucleotides in rat cortex during insulin-induced hypoglycemia and recovery. J Neurochem 36:179–189
9. Chen J, Nagayama T, Jin K, Stetler RA, Zhu RL, Graham SH, Simon RP (1998) Induction of caspase-3-like protease may mediate delayed neuronal death in the hippocampus after transient cerebral ischemia. J Neurosci 18:4914–4928
10. Choi D (1995) Calcium: still center-stage in hypoxic-ischemic neuronal death. TINS 18:58–60
11. Colbourne F, Sutherland G, Auer R (1999) Electron microscopic evidence against apoptosis as the mechanism of neuronal death in global ischemia. J Neurosci 19:4200–4210
12. Connern CP, Halestrap AP (1992) Purification and N-terminal sequencing of peptidyl-prolyl cis-trans-isomerase from rat liver mitochondrial matrix reveals the existence of a distinct mitochondrial cyclophilin. Biochem J 284:381–385
13. Desphande J, Bergstedt K, Lindén T, Kalimo H, Wieloch T (1992) Ultrastructural changes in the hippocampal CA1 region following transient cerebral ischemia:evidence against programmed cell death. Exp Brain Res 88:91–105
14. Drake M, Friberg H, Boris-Möller F, Sakata K, Wieloch T (1996) The immunosuppressant FK506 ameliorates ischemic damage in the rat brain. Acta Physiol Scand 158:155–159

15. Ekholm A, Asplund B, Siesjö BK (1992) Perturbation of cellular energy state in complete ischemia: relationship to dissipative ion fluxes. Exp Brain Research 90:47–53
16. Erecinska M, Silver I (1989) ATP and brain function. J Cereb Blood Flow Metab 9:2–19
17. Folbergrová J, Zhao Q, Katsura K, Siesjö B (1995) N-tert-butyl-a-phenylnitrone improves recovery of brain energy state in the rats following transient focal ischemia. Proc Nat Acad Sci, USA 92:5057–5061
18. Fontaine E, Ichas F, Bernardi P (1998) A ubiquinone-binding site regulates the mitochondrial permeability transition pore. J Biol Chem 273:25734–25740
19. Friberg H, Elmér E, Wieloch T (2000) Effects of cyclosporin A and FK506 on brain damage when administered after transient forebrain ischemia in the rat. Submitted
20. Friberg H, Ferrand-Drake M, Bengtsson F, Halestrap AP, Wieloch T (1998) Cyclosporin A, but not FK 506, protects mitochondria and neurons against hypoglycemic damage and implicates the mitochondrial permeability transition in cell death. J Neurosci 18:5151–5159
21. Gisselsson L, Smith M-L, Siesjö B (1999) Hyperglycemia and focal brain ischemia. The influence of hyperglycemia on brain damage and blood flow in focal ischemia. Journal of Cerebral Blood Flow and Metabolism 19:288–297
22. Green DR, Reed JC (1998) Mitochondria and apoptosis. Science 281:1309–1312
23. Halestrap AP (1991) Calcium-dependent opening of a non-specific pore in the mitochondrial inner membrane is inhibited at pH values below 7. Implications for the protective effect of low pH against chemical and hypoxic cell damage. Biochem J 278:715–719
24. Halestrap A, Kerr P, Javadov S, Woodfield K-Y (1998) Elucidating the molecular mechanism of the permeability transition pore and its role in reperfusion injury of the heart. Biochimica et Biophysica Acta 1366:79–94
25. Hansen AJ (1985) Effects of anoxia on ion distribution in the brain. Physiol Rev 65(1):101–148
26. Hillered L, Smith M, Siesjö B (1985) Lactic acidosis and recovery of mitochondrial function following forebrain ischemia in the rat. J Cereb Blood Flow Metab 5:259–266
27. Hossmann K-A (1985) Post-ischemic resuscitation of the brain: selective vulnerability versus global resistance. Progr Brain Res 63:3–17
28. Hossmann K-A, Kleihues P (1973) Reversibility of ischemic brain damage. Arch Neurol (Chic) 29:375–382
29. Ide T, Morikawa E, Kirino T (1996) An immunosuppressant, FK506, protects hippocampal neurons from forebrain ischemia in the mongolian gerbil. Neurosci Lett 204:157–160
30. Ito U, Spatz M, Walker JT, Klatzo I (1975) Experimental cerebral ischemia in mongolian gerbils. I. Light microscopic observations. Acta Neuropathol (Berl) 32:209–223
31. Kalimo H, Rehncrona S, Soderfeldt B, Olsson Y, Siesjö B (1981) Brain lactic acidosis and ischemic cell damage: 2. Histopathology. J Cereb Blood Flow Metab 1:313–327
32. Kamme F, Campbell K, Wieloch T (1995) Biphasic expression of the fos and jun families of transcription factors following transient forebrain ischemia in the rat. Effect of hypothermia. Eur J Neurosci 7:2007–2016
33. Katsura K, Ekholm A, Siesjö BK (1992) Coupling among changes in energy metabolism, acidbase homestasis and ion fluxes in ischemia. Can J Physiol Pharmacol 70:S170–S175
34. Kiessling M, Stumm G, Xie Y, Herdegen T, Aguzzi A, Bravo R, Gass P (1993) Differential transcription and translation of immediate early genes in the gerbil hippocampus after transient global ischemia. J Cereb Blood Flow Metab 13:914–924
35. Kirino T (1982) Delayed neuronal death in the gerbil hippocampus following transient ischemia. Brain Res 239:57–69
36. Kleihues P, Kobayashi K, Hossman K-A (1974) Purine nucleotide metabolism in the cat brain after one hour of complete ischemia. J Neurochem 23:417–425
37. Kozuka M, Smith M-L, Siesjö B (1989) Preischemic hyperglycemia enhances postischemic depression of cerebral metabolic rate. J Cereb Blood Flow Metab 9:478–490
38. Kristal BS, Dubinsky JM (1997) Mitochondrial permeability transition in the central nervous system: induction by calcium cycling-dependent and -independent pathways. J Neurochem 69:524–538
39. Kristián T, Gertsch J, Bates T, Siesjö BK (2000a) Characteristics of the calcium-triggered mitochondrial permeability transition in nonsynaptic brain mitochondria: effect of cyclosporin A and ubiquinone O. J Neurochem 74:1999–2009
40. Kristián T, Bernardi P, Siesjö BK (2000b) Acidosis promotes the permeability transition in energized mitochondria: Implications for reperfusion injury. Submitted for publication
41. Kristián T, Gido G, Kuroda S, Schutz A, Siesjo BK (1998) Calcium metabolism of focal and penumbral tissues in rats subjected to transient middle cerebral artery occlusion. Exp Brain Res 120:503–509
42. Kroemer G, Reed JC (2000) Mitochondrial control of cell death [In Process Citation]. Nat Med 6:513–519
43. Kuroda S, Janelidze S, Siesjo BK (1999) The immunosuppressants cyclosporin A and FK506 equally ameliorate brain damage due to 30-min middle cerebral artery occlusion in hyperglycemic rats. Brain Res 835:148–153
44. Lawson JW, Veech RL (1979) Effects of pH and free Mg^{2+} on the Keq of the creatine kinase reaction and other phosphate hydrolyses and phophate transfer reactions. J Biol Chem 254:6528–6537
45. Lemasters J, Nieminen A-L, Qian T, Trost L, Elmore S, Nishimura Y, Crowe R, Cascio W, Bradham C, Brenner D, Herman B (1998) The mitochondrial permeability transition in cell death: a common mechanism in necrosis, apoptosis and autophagy. Biochimica et Biophysica Acta 1366:177–196
46. Ljunggren B, Ratcheson RA, Siesjö BK (1974) Cerebral metabolic state following complete compression ischemia. Brain Research 73:291–307
47. Matsumoto S, Friberg H, Ferrand-Drake M, Wieloch T (1999) Blockade of the mitochondrial permeability transition pore diminishes infarct size in the rat after transient middle cerebral artery occlusion. J Cereb Blood Flow & Metab 19:736–741
48. Mitchell P (1966) Chemiosmotic coupling in oxidative and photosynthetic phosphorylation. Biol Rev 41:445–502
49. Nedergaard M (1987) Transient focal ischemia in hyperglycemic rats is associated with increased cerebral infarction. Brain Res 408:79–85
50. Nowak TS, Osborne OC, Suga S (1993) Stress protein and proto-oncogene expression as indicators of neuronal pathophysiology after ischemia. In: Neurobiology of ischemic brain damage., (K Kogure, K-A Hossmann, BK Siesjös, eds), Amsterdam, Elsevier Science; pp 195–208
51. Petito CK, Torres-Munoz J, Roberts B, Olarte JP, Nowak TS, Jr., Pulsinelli WA (1997) DNA fragmentation follows delayed neuronal death in CA1 neurons exposed to transient global ischemia in the rat. J Cereb Blood Flow Metab 17:967–976
52. Pulsinelli W, Jacewicz M, Buchan A (1992) Antagonists of excitatory amino acid neurotransmitters: A comparison of their effects on global vesus focal ischemia. Drug Research related to neuroactive amino acids. Copenhagen, Munksgaard
53. Pulsinelli W, Levy D, Duffy T (1982b) Regional cerebral blood flow and glucose metabolism following transient forebrain ischemia. Ann Neurol 11:499–509
54. Pulsinelli WA, Brierley JB, Plum F (1982a) Temporal profile of neuronal damage in a model of transient forebrain ischemia. Ann Neurol 11:491–498

55. Pulsinelli WA, Duffy TE (1983) Regional energy balance in rat brain after transient forebrain ischemia. J Neurochem 40:1500–1503
56. Reed J (1997) Cytochrome c: Can't Live with It-Can't Live without It. Cell 91:559–562
57. Sharkey J, Butcher SP (1994) Immunophilins mediate the neuroprotective effects of FK506 in focal cerebral ischaemia. Nature 371:336–339
58. Shibasaki F, Kondo E, Akagi T, McKeon F (1997) Suppression of signalling through transcription factor NF-AT by interactions between calcineurin and Bcl-2. Nature 386:728–731
59. Shiga Y, Onodera H, Matsuo Y, Kogure K (1992) Cyclosporin A protects against ischemia-reperfusion injury in the brain. Brain Res 595:145–148
60. Siemkowicz E, Hansen AJ (1981) Brain extracellular ion composition and EEG activity following 10 minutes ischemia in normo- and hyperglycemic rats. Stroke 12:236–240
61. Siesjö BK (1981) Cell damage in the brain: A speculative synthesis. J Cereb Blood Flow Metab 1:155–185
62. Siesjö BK (1992) Pathophysiology and treatment of focal cerebral ischemia. I. Pathophysiology. J Neurosurg 77:169–184
63. Sims N (1990) Rapid isolation of metabolically active mitochondria from rat bain and subregions using Percoll density gradient centrifugation. J Neurochem 55:698–707
64. Sims N, Pulsinelli W (1987) Altered mitochondrial respiration in selectively vulnerable brain subregions following transient forebrain ischemia in the rat. J Neurochem 49:1367–1374
65. Smith M, von Hanwehr R, Siesjö B (1986) Changes in extra- and intracellular pH in the brain during and following ischemia in hyperglycemic and in moderately hypoglycemic rats. J Cereb Blood Flow Metab 6:574–583
66. Smith M-L, Kalimo H, Warner DS, Siesjö BK (1988) Morphological lesions in the brain preceding the development of postischemic seizures. Acta Neuropathol (Berl) 76:253–264
67. Susin SA, Lorenzo HK, Zamzami N, Marzo I, Snow BE, Brothers GM, Mangion J, Jacotot E, Costantini P, Loeffler M, Larochette N, Goodlett DR, Aebersold R, Siderovski DP, Penninger JM, Kroemer G (1999) Molecular characterization of mitochondrial apoptosis-inducing factor [see comments]. Nature 397:441–446
68. Thilmann R, Xie Y, Kleihues P, Kiessling M (1989) Persistent inhibition of protein synthesis precedes delayed neuronal death in post-ischemic gerbil hippocampus. Acta Neuropathol 71:88–93
69. Tymianski M, Tator CH (1996) Normal and abnormal calcium homeostasis in neurons: a basis for the pathophysiology of traumatic and ischemic central nervous system injury. Neurosurgery 38:1176–1195
70. Uchino H, Elmér E, Uchino K, Li P-A, He Q-P, Smith M-L, Siesjö B (1998) Amelioration by cyclosporin A of brain damage in transient forebrain ischemia in the rat. Brain Res 812:216–226
71. Uchino H, Elmér E, Uchino K, Lindvall O, Siesjö B (1995) Cyclosporin A dramatically ameliorates CA1 hippocampal damage following transient forebrain ischemia in the rat. Acta Physiol Scand 155:469–471
72. Wagner K, Kleinholz M, Myers R (1990) Delayed decrease in specific brain mitochondrial electron transfer complex activities and cytochrome concentrations following anoxia/ischemia. J Neurosurg Sci 100:142–151
73. Wang HG, Pathan N, Ethell IM, Krajewski S, Yamaguchi Y, Shibasaki F, McKeon F, Bobo T, Franke TF, Reed JC (1999) Ca^{2+}-induced apoptosis through calcineurin dephosphorylation of BAD. Science 284:339–343
74. Yoshimoto T, Siesjö B (1999) Posttreatment with the immunosuppressant cyclosporin A in transient focal ischemia. Brain Research 839:283–291
75. Yoshimoto T, Kristián T, Hu B, Ouyang Y-B, Siesjö BK (2000) Cyclosporin A and NXY-059 ameliorate secondary deterioration of mitochondrial function following focal ischemia. Submitted for publication
76. Zoratti M, Szabó I (1995) The mitochondrial permeability transition. Biochimica et Biophysica Acta 1241:139–176

Mitochondria as targets of neuroprotection by Bcl-2 family proteins

G. Fiskum[1], B. M. Polster[1,2], A. J. Kowaltowski[3]

Abstract

Neural cell death that accompanies cerebral ischemia/reperfusion is mediated in part by mitochondrial alterations caused by elevated intracellular Ca^{2+}, oxidative stress, and redistribution or activation of pro-apoptotic proteins, e.g., Bax and Bid. Bcl-2 is membrane protein localized primarily to mitochondria that protects against ischemic brain injury, hypoxic neural cell death, oxidative stress, and mitochondrial respiratory dysfunction caused by exposure to elevated Ca^{2+}. Bcl-2 also protects against the release of cytochrome *c* and other pro-apoptotic mitochondrial proteins evoked by either Ca^{2+} or by peptides that contain a BH3 cell death domain. This report summarizes experiments performed with permeabilized cells where mitochondrial cytochrome *c* release and mitochondrial membrane potential were monitored in response to the addition of either Ca^{2+} plus pro-oxidants, e.g., t-butyl hydroperoxide, or a synthetic peptide containing the BH3 domain of Bax. The results support the hypotheses that: 1. Bcl-2 inhibits the Ca^{2+}-stimulated mitochondrial permeability transition and associated cytochrome *c* release by increasing mitochondrial resistance to pyridine nucleotide oxidation and; 2. Bcl-2 inhibits cytochrome *c* release elicited by the Bax-BH3 peptide by a different mechanism that is independent of the mitochondrial pyridine nucleotide redox state.

Introduction

Mitochondria are primary targets of ischemia/reperfusion brain injury (Lipton 1999; Fiskum et al. 1999) and of neuronal excitotoxicity (Nicholls and Budd 1998; Reynolds 1999). The mechanisms by which excitotoxic and ischemic mitochondrial injury result in cell death are far from resolved. In addition to inhibition of oxidative phosphorylation and subsequent metabolic failure, increased generation of reactive oxygen species (ROS) and release of apoptosis promoting factors such as cytochrome *c* have been strongly implicated as mechanisms by which injury results in death (Fig. 1). The extent to which each of these mechanisms contributes to neural cell death in both *in vitro* and *in vivo* paradigms has, however, not been determined.

Keywords: Apoptosis, bcl-2, calcium, pyridine nucleotides, Bax, cytochrome *c*

[1]Department of Anesthesiology and [2]Program in Neuroscience, The University of Maryland Baltimore School of Medicine, Baltimore, MD, 21201 USA and [3]Cicade Universitaria, San Palo, Brazil 05513-970
e-mail: gfiskum@anesthlab.ummc.umaryland.edu

J. Krieglstein, S. Klumpp (Eds.) Pharmacology of Cerebral Ischemia 2000

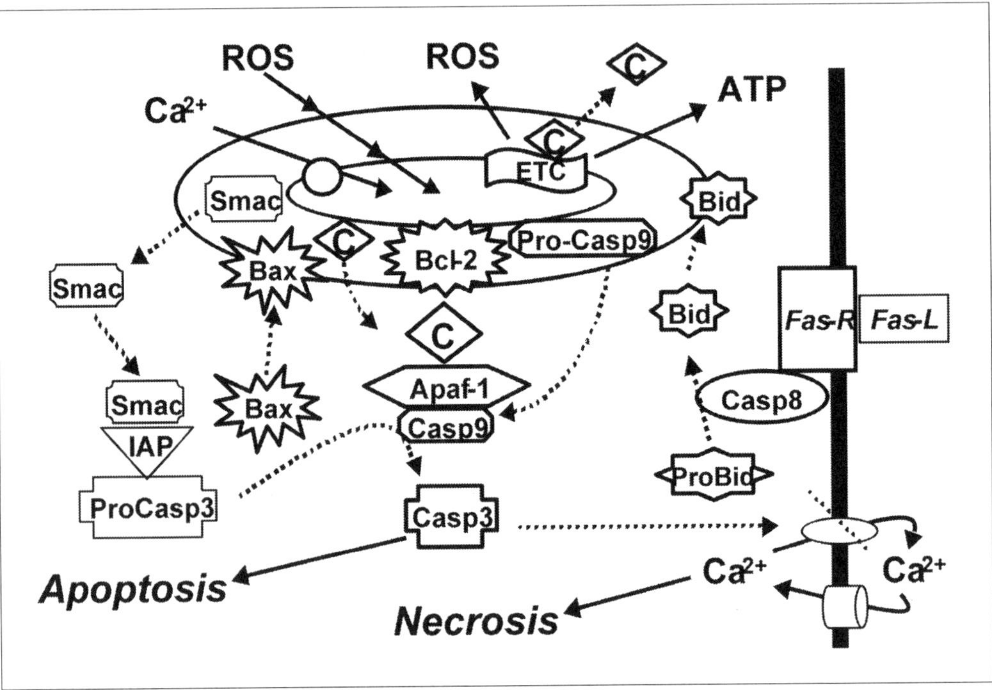

Fig. 1. Mitochondria as targets and mediators of cell death signals. Ca^{2+}, reactive oxygen species (ROS) and pro-apoptotic proteins, e.g., Bax and Bid, all can cause the release of other apoptotic proteins from the mitochondrial intermembrane space into the cytosol. The macromolecular apoptosome, consisting of cytochrome *c*, apoptosis activating factor 1 (Apaf-1) and caspase 9, is capable of proteolytically activating other caspases, e.g., caspase 3, that mediate the later stages of apoptosis. Mitochondria also release at least one factor (Smac) that binds to inhibitor of apoptosis proteins (IAP), relieving their inhibition and allowing pro-caspases, e.g., pro-caspase 3 to be activated by the apoptosome. Although the Fas ligand (Fas-L), Fas receptor (Fas-R) system can trigger apoptosis through caspase 8-mediated activation of Bid, caspase 8 can also bypass the mitochondrial pathway by directly activating caspase 3 (not shown). Necrotic cell death can also be mediated by some of the same events that elicit apoptosis. For example, the plasma membrane Ca^{2+} ATPase pump is susceptible to inactivation by caspase 3, leading to an enormous net influx of Ca^{2+}, followed by autolysis and necrosis. Also, release of cytochrome *c* from mitochondria will ultimately inhibit respiration and oxidative phosphorylation, leading to a net decline in cellular ATP, loss of ionic homeostasis, cell swelling and disruption. Moreover, loss of cytochrome *c* can increase the leakage of electrons from upstream sites of the electron transport chain to O_2 forming superoxide anion radical. Superoxide and its reaction products, e.g., H_2O_2 and peroxynitrite, can cause oxidative damage to mitochondrial proteins and lipids, and oxidative stress that will compromise normal bioenergetic activities and promote membrane permeability alterations that potentiate further release of cytochrome *c* and other proteins.

It appears that relatively mild mitochondrial injury where the process of oxidative phosphorylation is preserved leads primarily to apoptosis, whereas more extensive injury accompanied by metabolic failure leads primarily to necrosis (Ankarcrona et al. 1995; Nicotera et al. 1998; Kruman and Mattson 1999).

Factors that contribute to mitochondrial functional alterations during ischemia/reperfusion include the accumulation of abnormally high amounts of Ca^{2+}, exposure to substantially elevated levels of ROS, and the activation and mitochondrial redistribution of a variety of pro-apoptotic proteins, e.g., Bax, Bid, and Bad (Fiskum et al. 1999). The molecular events that transpire in response to these factors vary. Supranormal mitochondrial accumulation of Ca^{2+}, particularly during oxidative stress, and exposure to pro-apoptotic proteins both share the common effect of releasing cytochrome *c* and other apoptotic signaling proteins into the cytosol from their normal location between the outer and inner mitochondrial membranes (Kroemer et al. 1998). In addition to activating the cascade of caspase activities that mediate apoptosis, release of cytochrome *c* can both inhibit electron transport and oxidative phosphorylation and result in elevated production of superoxide anion and its metabolites from sites in the electron transport chain proximal to cytochrome *c* (Cai et al. 1998).

The Bcl-2 gene codes for an approximately 26 kDa protein that is located primarily on the membranes of mitochondria, endoplasmic reticulum and the nucleus (Krajewski et al. 1993; Gotow et al. 2000). When overexpressed, this gene product is capable of inhibiting the death of a wide variety of cells in response to a wide variety of insults. For example, cultured neural cells overexpressing Bcl-2 are resistant to death caused by the metabolic challenge and oxidative stress of exposure to glucose deprivation in the presence of the respiratory poison cyanide (Myers et al. 1995). More importantly, Bcl-2 overexpressing transgenic mice are resistant to cell death and brain injury caused by both focal and global cerebral ischemia (Martinou et al. 1994; Kitagawa et al. 1998). Preconditioning paradigms have also associated cell-selective induction of Bcl-2 expression with cell-selective resistance to death following cerebral ischemia (Shimazaki et al. 1994). Thus, understanding the mechanisms of cytoprotection by Bcl-2 is an extremely important goal as it could lead to the development of neuroprotective interventions that act either via the stimulation of Bcl-2 activities or by simulation of the modes by which Bcl-2 exerts its effects.

Much of the research on Bcl-2 has focused on its influence over mitochondrial activities and sensitivity of mitochondria to alterations associated with the pathogenesis of both necrotic and apoptotic cell death. Bcl-2 possesses the remarkable ability to protect even isolated mitochondria from dysfunction caused by Ca^{2+}, ROS, or pro-apoptotic proteins, e.g., Bax (Murphy et al. 1996; Kowaltowski et al. 2000; Brenner et al. 2000). It is therefore possible that each of these stimuli act upon mitochondria by a common mechanism sensitive to inhibition by Bcl-2 or that these stimuli act by several mechanisms each independently inhibited by Bcl-2. A common mechanism of action that has been proposed by Kroemer and others is the activation of the mitochondrial permeability transition (Jacotot et al. 1999). This mechanism could certainly explain the ability of each of these stimuli to induce the release of inter-membrane proteins, e.g., cytochrome *c*, as the permeability transition causes non-selective release through osmotic lysis. The permeability transition would also be consistent with observations in many apoptotic cell death paradigms indicating an early loss of mitochondrial membrane potential. There are, however, reports of cytochrome *c* release with isolated mitochondria and in cells undergoing apoptosis in the absence of a loss of membrane potential or in the absence of other markers of the permeability transition, e.g., mitochondrial swelling or sensitivity to the permeability transition inhibitor cyclosporin A (Kluck et al. 1999). The following experiments represent examples of studies in progress in our laboratory directed at determining the mechanism or mechanisms of action of Bcl-2 specifically related to its ability to block cytochrome *c* release by either Ca^{2+} plus chemical pro-oxidants or by a peptide representing a portion of the Bax molecule that contains the BH3 cell death domain.

Methods and materials

GT1-7 Neural Cell Cultures

Immortalized hypothalamic PC-12 and GT1-7 neural cell lines transfected with the *bcl-2* gene (Bcl-2(+)) or with a control retroviral construct (Bcl-2(–)) were kindly provided by Dr. Dale Bredesen (Buck Center for Research on Aging, Novato, CA) and maintained as described previously (Murphy et al. 1996). Prior to the experiments, the cells were trypsinized and suspended in growth media supplemented with 5 mM EGTA. Stock suspensions of cells were kept at room temperature for up to 5 hours. Cell viability, as assessed by a cell count in Trypan Blue, was > 90% during this period. Immediately prior to the experiments, aliquots of the stock cell suspensions were centrifuged and resuspended in standard reaction medium consisting of 130 mM KCl, HEPES (pH 7.0) and other components as indicated in the Figure legends.

Mitochondrial Membrane Potential (ΔΨ) Determinations

Mitochondrial ΔΨ was monitored by measuring the fluorescence changes of safranine O (5 μM) recorded on a Perkin-Elmer LS-3 fluorescence spectrophotometer equipped with continuous stirring, operating at excitation and emission wavelengths of 485 and 586 nm, respectively (Akerman and Wikstrom 1976). The fluorescence of safranine in cell or mitochondrial suspensions decreases as ΔΨ increases, due to quenching as it accumulates within the mitochondria. The fluorescent recordings are presented in the figures so that an increase in the signal corresponds to an increase in ΔΨ.

Measurements of Cytochrome *C* Release

Aliquots of the digitonin-permeabilized cell suspensions were centrifuged at 10,000 x g for 2 min. The supernatants were collected and used for cytochrome *c* immunoblots, performed with 7H8 mouse anti-cytochrome *c* antibodies (PharMingen), as described previously (Andreyev et al. 1998).

Determination of NAD(P) Redox State

The redox state of pyridine nucleotides in digitonin-permeabilized cells was followed fluorometrically at 352 nm excitation and 464 nm emission wavelengths. Extent of pyridine nucleotide oxidation was calculated as a percentage of the oxidation induced by the respiratory uncoupler FCCP. Statistical difference between oxidation for Bcl-2(–) and (+) cells was tested using Student's *t* test.

Materials

Tert-butyl hydroperoxide (*t*-bOOH), phenylarsine oxide (PhAsO), safranine O, rotenone, succinate, malate, glutamate, digitonin, carbonyl cyanide p-trifluoromethoxyphenylhydrazone (FCCP) and alamethicin were purchased from Sigma Chemical Co. Cyclosporin A was purchased from Alexis Corporation. The Bax-BH3 peptide had the sequence of DASTKKLSE-CLKRIGDELDSNMELQRMIAAVDTD and was the generous gift of Dr. Kathleen Kinnally (New York University, NY, NY).

Results and Discussion

Bcl-2 Inhibits Hydroperoxide-Induced Mitochondrial Permeability Transition (MPT) and Cytochrome *C* Release by Inhibiting Oxidation of Pyridine Nucleotides

In this work, we studied the MPT as assessed by the decline in mitochondrial ΔΨ measured by changes in safranine O fluorescence within suspensions of digitonin-permeabilized Bcl-2 non-expressing and Bcl-2 overexpressing PC-12 neural cells. At the concentration of digitonin used in these experiments, membrane cholesterol and other β-hydroxysterols bind to digitonin in a manner where the plasma membrane becomes freely permeable to solutes and molecules without affecting the structure or permeability of mitochondrial membranes (Fiskum et al. 1980).

The experiments shown in Figure 2 measuring changes in ΔΨ were performed to test the hypothesis that Bcl-2 confers resistance against the MPT induced by a pro-oxidant that works via oxidation of pyridine nucleotides but does not inhibit the MPT induced by an agent that directly oxidizes protein sulfhydryl groups. Tert-butyl hydroperoxide (*t*-bOOH) is generally thought to induce the MPT indirectly, through its metabolism by glutathione peroxidase and reductase leading to net oxidation of glutathione and pyridine nucleotides (Castilho et al. 1995). This shift in redox state promotes the MPT by allowing for oxidation of protein sulfhydryls that regulate permeability transition

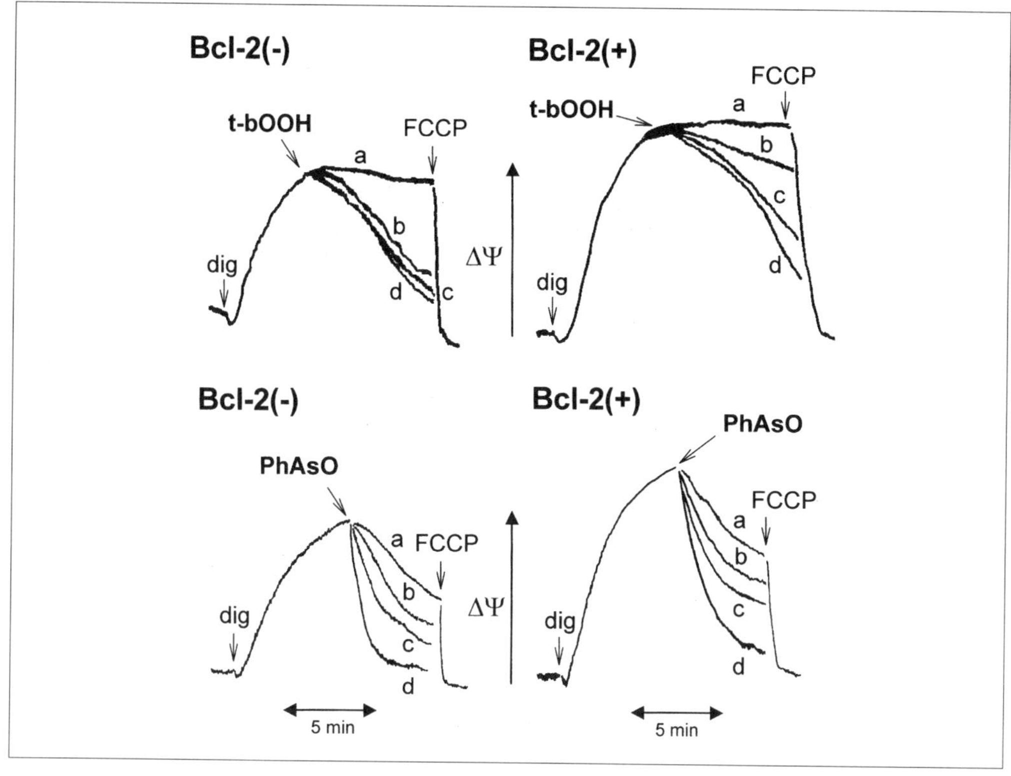

Fig. 2. Bcl-2 inhibition of PC12 neural cell mitochondrial permeability transition induced by *t*-butyl hydroperoxide but not phenylarsine oxide. Bcl-2(–) or (+) PC12 cells (2×10^7/ml) were incubated in standard reaction medium containing 5 mM malate plus 5 mM glutamate as oxidizable substrates, 8 µM Ca^{2+}, and 5 µM safranine O for fluorescent measurement of mitochondrial ΔΨ. Digitonin (dig) was added at 0.01% w/v to permeabilize the plasma membrane of the cells in suspension. In the upper panels, *t*-bOOH was added at a concentration of either 200 µM (line b), 400 µM (line c), or 800 µM (lines a and d). In line a, cyclosporin A was present at 1 µM. In the lower panels, PhAsO was added at a concentration of 2 µM (line a), 5 µM (line b), 10 µM (line c), or 15 µM (line d). The fluorescent detection of changes in ΔΨ was confirmed by the addition of 1 µM FCCP. Modified from Kowaltowski et al. 2000.

pore opening. In contrast, phenylarsine oxide (PhAsO) is a dithiol reagent that reacts directly with membrane protein thiols, promoting MPT independently of ROS or pyridine nucleotide oxidation (Vercesi et al. 1997). In the upper panels of Figure 2, increasing concentrations of *t*-bOOH were added to both Bcl-2(–) and Bcl-2(+) PC12 cells. As the MPT is generally dependent on the presence of Ca^{2+}, a small concentration of Ca^{2+} (8 µM) that was not in itself sufficient to induce the MPT was present to allow for induction by pro-oxidants. Addition of *t*-bOOH to Bcl-2(–) cells at concentrations of 200 µM (line b), 400 µM (line c) or 800 µM (line d) *t*-bOOH promoted essentially identical rates and extents of decline in ΔΨ. However, in Bcl-2(+) cells, a *t*-bOOH dose-dependent loss of ΔΨ was apparent with maximal loss occurring at 800 µM *t*-bOOH (compare lines b-d). For both Bcl-2(–) and (+) cells the drop in ΔΨ was fully inhibited by the classical MPT inhibitor cyclosporin A at all *t*-bOOH concentrations (lines a), confirming that changes in ΔΨ reflect MPT activity.

These comparisons therefore indicate that the MPT can be observed with Bcl-2 overexpressing cells if sufficient levels of *t*-bOOH are added, suggesting that higher levels of *t*-bOOH are necessary in Bcl-2(+) cells to promote extensive pyridine nucleotide oxidation. In contrast to the different dose-response relationships for *t*-bOOH induced MPT with Bcl-2(–) and Bcl-2(+) cells, similar dose-response relationships were observed for 2–15 μM PhAsO (Fig. 2, lower traces). This result indicates that when MPT is triggered by a direct oxidant of protein sulfydryl groups, Bcl-2 is ineffective at inhibiting this phenomenon.

Fluorescent measurements were made of the reduced pyridine nucleotide species (NAD(P)H) in suspensions of the permeabilized cells to confirm that the reason a greater concentration of *t*-bOOH is necessary for induction of the MPT in Bcl-2(+) cells than in Bcl-2(–) cells is due to the resistance of Bcl-2(+) cells to oxidation. As shown in Figure 3, addition of 200 or 800 μM *t*-bOOH to digitonin-permeabilized Bcl-2(–) PC12 cells resulted in rapid and extensive pyridine nucleotide oxidation that approached the degree of oxidation that can be elicited by maximizing respiration-dependent NAD(P)H oxidation by the addition of a respiratory uncoupler. Exposure of Bcl-2(+) cells to 200 μM *t*-bOOH resulted in only partial pyridine nucleotide oxidation whereas the presence of 800 μM *t*-bOOH elicited almost complete oxidation. Figure 3 provides a quantitative comparison of pyridine nucleotide oxidation by *t*-bOOH for Bcl-2(–) versus (+) cells. At 200 μM *t*-bOOH, the extent of oxidation, expressed as a percentage of that obtained with uncoupler, was significantly less in Bcl-2(+) compared to Bcl-2(–) cells ($p < 0.05$, $n = 6$). Other experiments performed either in the presence of cyclosporin A or in the absence of Ca^{2+} to inhibit the MPT yielded similar differences in pyridine nucleotide oxidation (not shown), indicating that differential susceptibility to oxidation is the cause rather than the result of disparate MPT activities. These results obtained *in vitro* with mitochondria present within digitonin-permeabilized cells are consistent with those of Ellerby et al. showing that Bcl-2 shifts the redox potential of several cell types to a reduced state (Ellerby et al. 1996) and with those of Esposti et al., who determined that Bcl-2 overexpressing mitochondria exhibit an increased amount of NAD(P)H and are resistant to increases in cellular ROS generation induced by tumor necrosis factor (Esposti et al. 1999).

In a variety of experimental conditions, large amplitude mitochondrial swelling associated with MPT is followed by the release of cytochrome *c* from the mitochondrial intermembrane space into the cytosol, an event that can trigger apoptotic cells death through caspase activation (Green and Reed 1998). Figure 4 depicts immunoblots used to detect cytochrome *c* in the supernatants obtained following centrifugation of cell suspensions incubated under conditions similar to those used in the experiments described by Figures 2 and 3. In all cell suspensions treated with PhAsO, cytochrome *c* was released into the media, but only Bcl-2(–) cells released cytochrome *c* upon the addition of 200 μM *t*-bOOH. Release of cytochrome *c* under these conditions often approached the extent obtained in the presence of alamethicin, an artificial, non-specific pore former that induces massive mitochondrial swelling. Consistent with the effects on mitochondrial membrane potential, cyclosporin A eliminated cytochrome *c* release elicited by Ca^{2+} and *t*-bOOH and partially blocked the release induced by Ca^{2+} and PhAsO. Ultrastructural analysis of the mitochondria present within the permeabilized cells following treatment with *t*-bOOH confirmed the relationship between mitochondrial swelling and cytochrome *c* release and further established the relative resistance of Bcl-2(+) cell mitochondria to the MPT induced by *t*-bOOH (Kowaltowski et al. 2000).

In our experiments, cytochrome *c* release was elicited in a manner directly related to MPT and mitochondrial swelling. In cytochrome *c*-induced cell death, cytochrome *c* release may occur by both MPT-dependent and independent mechanisms (Lemasters et al. 1998; Kluck et al. 1997). However, studies have shown that MPT and cytochrome *c* release are early events in several models of apoptosis (Kroemer et al. 1998). Thus, our observations concerning the mechanisms of inhibition of MPT by Bcl-2 provide a plausible explanation for the preven-

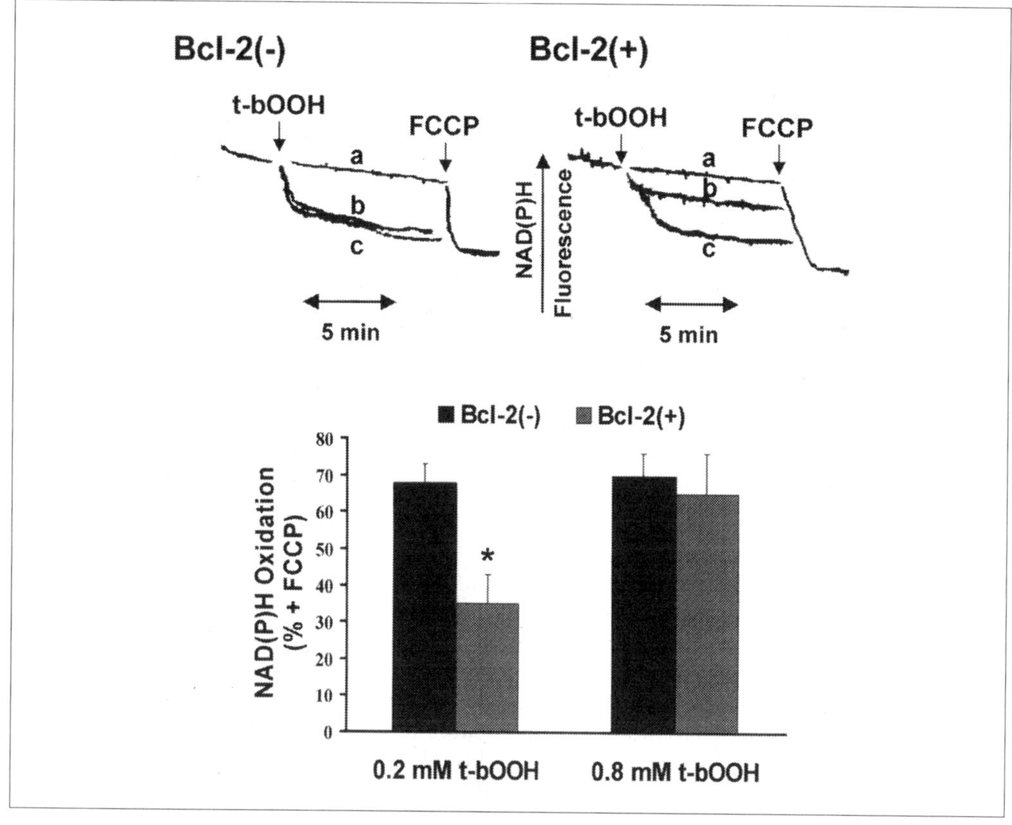

Fig. 3. Bcl-2 inhibition of pyridine nucleotide oxidation caused by *t*-butyl hydroperoxide in PC12 neural cells. PC12 cells (2 x 10^7/ml) were incubated in standard reaction medium containing malate, glutamate, Ca^{2+}, and digitonin. The top panels are representative examples of the autofluorescence emitted by reduced pyridine nucleotides (NAD(P)H) at 352 nm excitation and 464 nm emission wavelengths. In the absence (line a) or presence of either 200 μM *t*-bOOH (line b) or 800 μM *t*-bOOH (line c). 1 μM FCCP was added to induce complete pyridine nucleotide oxidation. The bottom panel describes the means ± s.e. (n = 6) for the pyridine nucleotide oxidation expressed as a percentage of that observed upon addition of FCCP. Modified from Kowaltowski et al. 2000.

tion of cytochrome *c* release promoted by Bcl-2 in many situations, and particularly under conditions that favor oxidative stress. This postulate is supported by the observation that Bcl-2 prevention of apoptosis can be overcome by glutathione depletion of these cells (Wright et al. 1998) and that Bcl-2 protection against mitochondrial injury and cell death can be mimicked by N-acetylcysteine, an antioxidant and precursor of glutathione (Murphy et al. 1996; Ferrari et al. 1995).

Bcl-2 Inhibits Cytochrome *C* Release Evoked by a Bax-BH3 Peptide by a Mechanism Different from that Responsible for Inhibition of the Mitochondrial Permeability Transition

Although Ca^{2+} and oxidative stress may be particularly important in triggering mitochondrial alterations, including cytochrome *c* release, during acute excitotoxicity and during cerebral ischemia/reperfusion, the actions of pro-apoptotic proteins, e.g., Bax and Bid, may

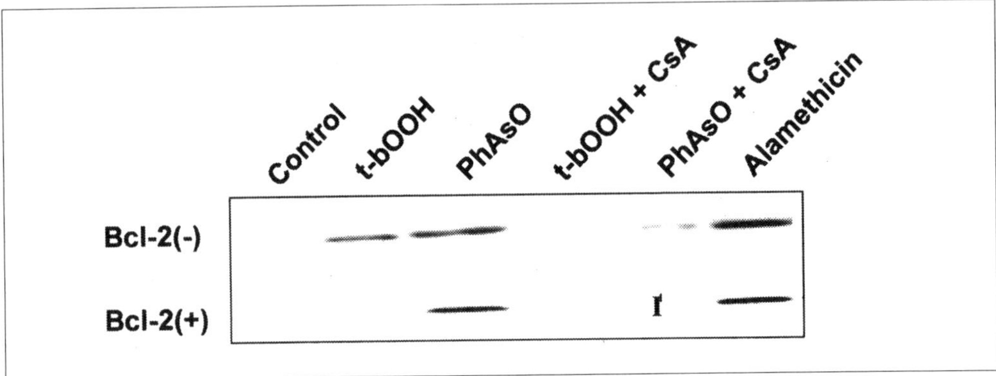

Fig. 4. Inhibition by Bcl-2 and cyclosporin A of pro-oxidant induced release of cytochrome *c* from mitochondria within PC12 neural cells. Supernatants obtained following centrifugation of digitonin-permeabilized cell suspensions (1.6 x 10^8/ml) incubated under the conditions described for Figure 2 were used for immunoblot detection of cytochrome *c* (see Methods and Materials). Modified from Kowaltowski et al. 2000.

be just as important (Krajewski et al. 1999; Crompton 2000). The mechanism by which these proteins release cytochrome *c* and other pro-apoptotic factors from mitochondrial is highly controversial. While some evidence suggests that the MPT is directly involved (Brenner et al. 2000), several studies indicate that these proteins affect the permeability of the mitochondrial outer membrane without influencing the permeability characteristics of the inner membrane (Eskes et al. 1998; Shimizu et al. 1999). Bcl-2 inhibits the actions of these proteins on mitochondria; however, it is not clear whether the mechanism of inhibition is the same or distinctly different from that responsible for inhibition of the MPT by Bcl-2. The following few experiments represent those in progress in our lab designed to answer these questions.

In our experiments a Bax-BH3 peptide was used as a model of proteins that contain the BH3 death domain that are capable of acting on mitochondria to initiate the process of apoptosis. This peptide contains the amino acids 53–86 of 192 residues present in the Bax protein (see Methods and Materials). The cytochrome *c* immunoblot results of Figure 5 were obtained from an experiment where GT1-7 neural cells were suspended in a KCl-based medium in the presence of digitonin to permeabilize the plasma membranes. In these suspensions, no Ca^{2+} was added and EGTA was present to chelate contaminating Ca^{2+}. Physiological concentrations of Mg^{2+} and ATP were also included. The immunoblot of cytochrome *c* present in the supernatants obtained following centrifugation of the cell suspensions demonstrates a dose-dependent release of cytochrome *c* by the Bax-BH3 peptide. Comparison between Bcl-2(–) and (+) cells indicates that Bcl-2 overexpression inhibits the ability of this peptide to release cytochrome *c*. Other results indicate that release under these conditions is not affected by the MPT inhibitor cyclosporin A (not shown).

Confirmation that MPT activity was not associated with the release of cytochrome *c* by Bax-BH3 peptide came from fluorescent measurements of mitochondrial $\Delta\Psi$ in the suspensions of permeabilized GT1-7 cells. In Figure 6, concentrations of Bax-BH3 that elicited a robust release of cytochrome *c* in Bcl-2(–) cells produced only a very modest decline in $\Delta\Psi$. Other experiments indicate that this small decline in $\Delta\Psi$ is due to respiratory inhibition caused by cytochrome *c* release and can be reversed by the addition of exogenous cytochrome *c* to the suspension (not shown). Little if any change in $\Delta\Psi$ was observed with Bcl-2(+) cells, consistent with the loss of much less cytochrome *c* from Bcl-2(+) mitochondria.

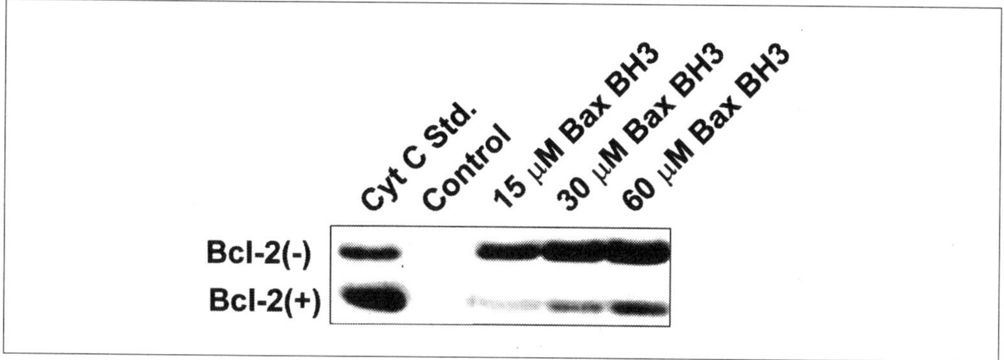

Fig. 5. Bcl-2 inhibition of cytochrome *c* release from GT1-7 neural cell mitochondria evoked by Bax-BH3 peptide. GT1-7 cells (3 x 10^7/ml) were incubated at 30° in standard reaction medium containing 5 mM succinate, 2 µM rotenone, 2 mM KH_2PO_4, 4 mM ATP, 3 mM $MgCl_2$ and 0.25 mM EGTA in the presence of 0.005% digitonin. Following 5 min of incubation in the absence and presence of different concentrations of Bax-BH3 peptide, the permeabilized cell suspension were centrifuged and the supernatants were used for immunoblot detection of cytochrome *c* (see Methods and Materials).

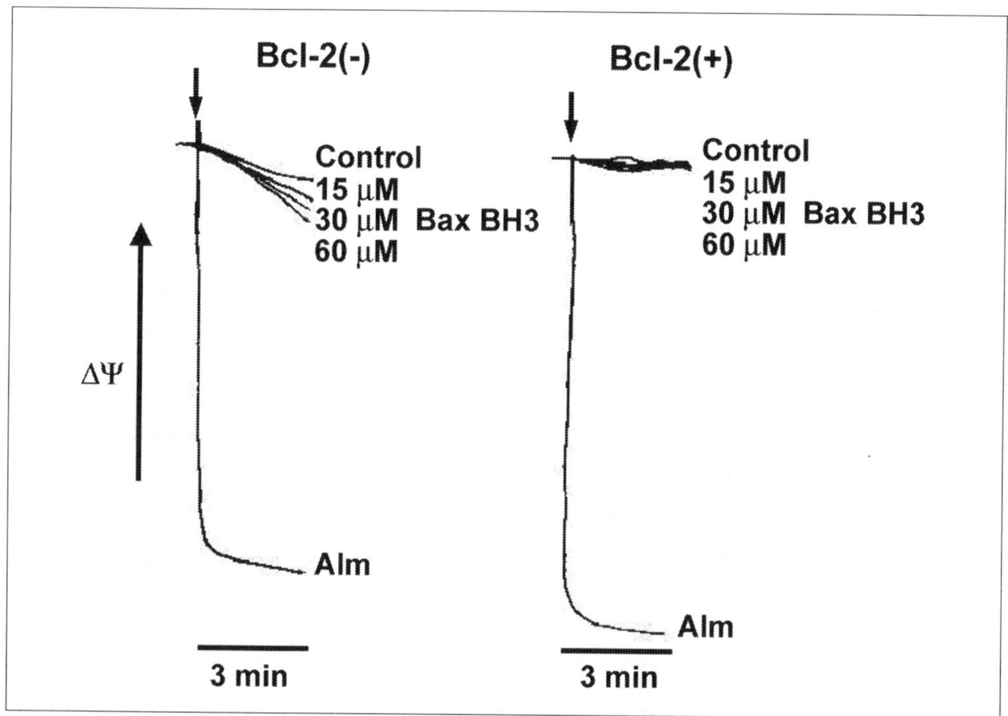

Fig. 6. Maintenance of mitochondrial membrane potential (ΔΨ) during cytochrome *c* release from GT1-7 neural cell mitochondria evoked by Bax-BH3 peptide. GT1-7 cells (3 x 10^7/ml) were incubated at 30° in standard reaction medium containing 5 mM succinate, 2 µM rotenone, 2 mM KH_2PO_4, 4 mM ATP, 3 mM $MgCl_s$, 0.25 mM EGTA, 0.005% digitonin, and 5 µM safranine O for fluorescent measurement of mitochondrial ΔΨ. The arrow indicates when either Bax-BH3 peptide, or alamethicin (8 µg/ml) were added.

Despite the evidence that the MPT is not involved in cytochrome *c* release evoked by the Bax-BH3 peptide, it is possible that the influence of Bcl-2 on mitochondrial redox state could mediate its inhibitory effects on cytochrome *c* release evoked by both pro-oxidants plus Ca^{2+} and by Bax-BH3 peptide. The experiment described in Figure 7 was designed to test the effects of mitochondrial pyridine nucleotide redox state on cytochrome *c* release from permeabilized GT1-7 Bcl-2(+) cells by Bax-BH3. In Figure 7A, redox state was monitored by continuously measuring the autofluorescence of NAD(P)H. When the electron transport chain complex I inhibitor rotenone was added, the redox state shifted rapidly to a completely reduced level, due to inhibition of NADH oxidation by respiratory inhibition. When the respiratory uncoupler FCCP was added, the redox state shifted to the maximally oxidized level, due to stimulation of NADH oxidation by accelerated electron transport. The subsequent addition of Bax-BH3 peptide in the presence or absence of rotenone or FCCP had little effect on redox state. Although the addition of Bax-BH3 might be expected to cause a reduction of NAD(P) due to cytochrome *c* release and respiratory inhibition, the concentration of peptide used with the Bcl-2(+) cells caused an incomplete release of cytochrome *c* that was insufficient to impair respiration. The release of cytochrome *c* into the suspension medium is described by the immunoblot shown in Figure 7B. No cytochrome *c* was released in the absence of

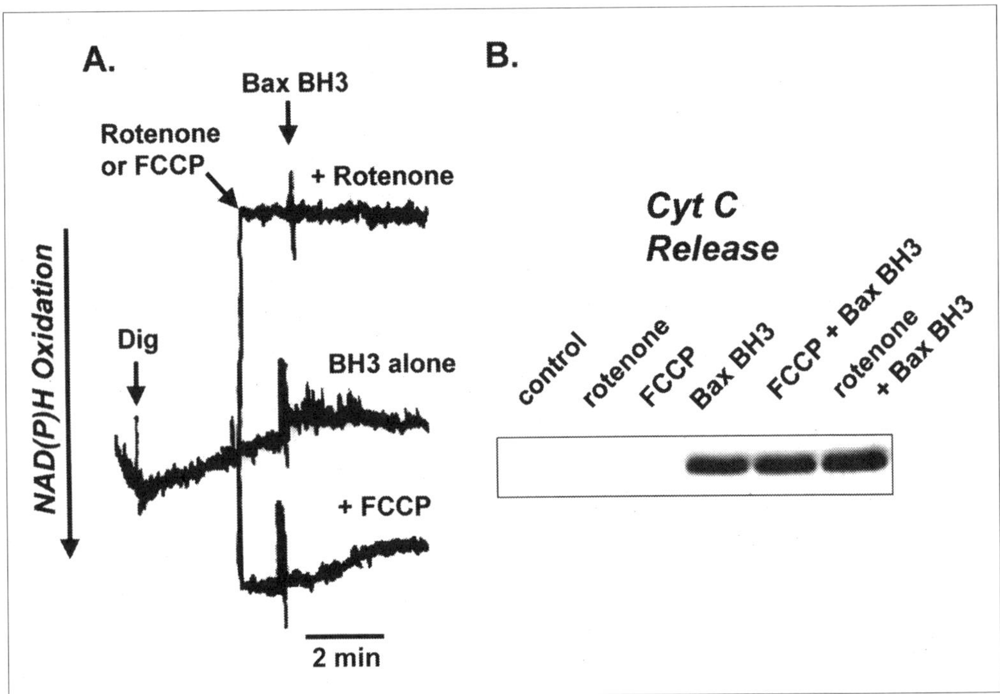

Fig. 7. Pyridine nucleotide (NAD(P)H) redox state does not affect cytochrome *c* release from GT1-7 neural cell mitochondria evoked by Bax-BH3 peptide. GT1-7 cells (3 x 10^7/ml) were incubated at 30° in standard reaction medium containing 5 mM malate, 5 mM glutamate, 2 mM KH_2PO_4, 4 mM ATP, 3 mM $MgCl_s$, 0.25 mM EGTA, and 0.005% digitonin. **A.** Autofluorescence emitted by reduced pyridine nucleotides (NAD(P)H) was measured at 352 nm excitation and 464 nm emission wavelengths. Additions were Bax-BH3 peptide (60 μM), rotenone (2 μM), and FCCP (1 μM). **B.** Following 6 min of incubation in the absence and presence of Bax-BH3 peptide, the permeabilized cell suspensions were centrifuged and the supernatants were used for immunoblot detection of cytochrome *c* (see Methods and Materials).

Bax-BH3 either in the absence or presence of FCCP or rotenone. Release induced by Bax-BH3 was unaffected by the presence of FCCP or rotenone. We therefore conclude that mitochondrial redox state has no effect on the release of cytochrome *c* by Bax-BH3 and that the ability of Bcl-2 to inhibit this phenomenon is unrelated to its influence over mitochondrial redox state.

Recent research has underscored the importance of the BH3 death domain in MPT-independent cytochrome *c* release and apoptosis (Lutz 2000). It has been suggested that BH3-only pro-apoptotic proteins function either by promoting the oligomerization and insertion of other pro-apoptotic proteins, e.g. Bax and Bak (Wei et al. 2000) or by inhibiting the function of anti-apoptotic proteins, e.g. Bcl-X_L (Zha et al. 1997; Kelekar et al. 1997). Specifically, the BH3 domain of the BH3-only pro-apoptotic protein Bid was necessary for Bid to trigger the cyclosporin A-independent release of cytochrome *c* release following cleavage by caspase-8 and the BH3 death domain was also required for dephosphorylated Bad to heterodimerize with Bcl-X_L and initiate apoptosis. The data presented here are consistent with a model whereby Bcl-2 inhibits BH3 peptide-induced cytochrome *c* release by a mechanism independent of the MPT and involving the modulation of the interaction of the BH3 death domain with its protein targets.

Summary

In the quest for developing safe neuroprotective interventions aimed at reducing the mortality and morbidity associated with global and focal cerebral ischemia and traumatic brain injury, a thorough analysis of endogenous mechanisms of neuroprotection should be performed. Bcl-2 and other family members, e.g., Bcl-X_L, are well-documented examples of native proteins that posses the ability to protect against ischemic, hypoxic, and excitotoxic neural cell death. Their mechanism of action appears closely linked with their ability to protect mitochondria against several forms of injury, including that mediated by exposure to excessive Ca^{2+}, oxidative stress, and pro-apoptotic proteins. The results presented here support the hypothesis that there is more than one mechanism of protection by Bcl-2 against these mediators of mitochondrial and cellular injury. Much more needs to be understood about the molecular and bioenergetic explanations for the abilities of Bcl-2 to inhibit both MPT-dependent and independent modes of cytochrome *c* release and the mitochondrial functional alterations associated with these membrane permeability changes.

Acknowledgements

This work was supported by NIH grant NS34152 to G. F. and a FAPESP grant to A.J.K.

References

1. Akerman KE, Wikstrom MK (1976) Safranine as a probe of the mitochondrial membrane potential. FEBS Lett 68:191–197
2. Andreyev AY, Fahy B, Fiskum G (1998) Cytochrome *c* release from brain mitochondria is independent of the mitochondrial permeability transition. FEBS Lett 439:373–376
3. Ankarcrona M, Dypbukt JM, Bonfoco E, Zhivotovsky B, Orrenius S, Lipton SA, Nicotera P (1995) Glutamate-induced neuronal death: a succession of necrosis or apoptosis depending on mitochondrial function. Neuron 15:961–973
4. Brenner C, Cadiou H, Vieira HL, Zamzami N, Marzo I, Xie Z, Leber B, Andrews D, Duclohier H, Reed JC, Kroemer G (2000) Bcl-2 and Bax regulate the channel activity of the mitochondrial adenine nucleotide translocator. Oncogene 19:329–336
5. Cai J, Yang J, Jones DP (1998) Mitochondrial control of apoptosis: the role of cytochrome *c*. Biochim Biophys Acta 1366:139–149
6. Castilho RF, Kowaltowski AJ, Meinicke AR, Bechara EJ, Vercesi AE (1995) Permeabilization of the inner mitochondrial membrane by Ca^{2+} ions is stimulated by *t*-butyl hydroperoxide and mediated by reactive oxygen species generated by mitochondria. Free Radic Biol Med 18:479–486
7. Crompton M (2000) Bax, Bid and the permeabilization of the mitochondrial outer membrane in apoptosis. Curr Opin Cell Biol 12:414–419
8. Ellerby LM, Ellerby HM, Park SM, Holleran AL, Murphy AN, Fiskum G, Kane DJ, Testa MP, Kayalar C, Bredesen DE (1996) Shift of the cellular oxidation-reduction potential in neural cells expressing Bcl-2. J Neurochem 67:1259–1267
9. Eskes R, Antonsson B, Osen-Sand A, Montessuit S, Richter C, Sadoul R, Mazzei G, Nichols A, Martinou JC (1998) Bax-induced cytochrome *C* release from mitochondria is independent of the permeability transition pore but highly dependent on Mg^{2+} ions. J Cell Biol 143:217–224
10. Esposti MD, Hatzinisiriou I, McLennan H, Ralph S (1999) Bcl-2 and mitochondrial oxygen radicals. New approaches with reactive oxygen species-sensitive probes. J Biol Chem 274:29831–29837

11. Ferrari G, Yan CY, Greene LA (1995) N-acetylcysteine (D- and L-stereoisomers) prevents apoptotic death of neuronal cells. J Neurosci 15:2857–2866
12. Fiskum G, Craig SW, Decker GL, Lehninger AL (1980) The cytoskeleton of digitonin-treated rat hepatocytes. Proc Natl Acad Sci USA 77:3430–3434
13. Fiskum G, Murphy AN, Beal MF (1999) Mitochondria in neurodegeneration: acute ischemia and chronic neurodegenerative diseases. J Cereb Blood Flow Metab 19:351–369
14. Gotow T, Shibata M, Kanamori S, Tokuno O, Ohsawa Y, Sato N, Isahara K, Yayoi Y, Watanabe T, Leterrier JF, Linden M, Kominami E, Uchiyama Y (2000) Selective localization of Bcl-2 to the inner mitochondrial and smooth endoplasmic reticulum membranes in mammalian cells. Cell Death Differ 7:666–674
15. Green DR, Reed JC (1998) Mitochondria and apoptosis. Science 281:1309–1312
16. Jacotot E, Costantini P, Laboureau E, Zamzami N, Susin SA, Kroemer G (1999) Mitochondrial membrane permeabilization during the apoptotic process. Ann NY Acad Sci 887:18–30
17. Kelekar A, Chang BS, Harlan JE, Fesik SW, Thompson CB (1997) Bad is a BH3 domain-containing protein that forms an inactivating dimer with Bcl-XL. Mol Cell Biol 17:7040–7046
18. Kitagawa K, Matsumoto M, Tsujimoto Y, Ohtsuki T, Kuwabara K, Matsushita K, Yang G, Tanabe H, Martinou JC, Hori M, Yanagihara T (1998) Amelioration of hippocampal neuronal damage after global ischemia by neuronal overexpression of BCL-2 in transgenic mice [see comments]. Stroke 29:2616–2621
19. Kluck RM, Bossy-Wetzel E, Green DR, Newmeyer DD (1997) The release of cytochrome *c* from mitochondria: a primary site for Bcl-2 regulation of apoptosis [see comments]. Science 275:1132–1136
20. Kluck RM, Esposti MD, Perkins G, Renken C, Kuwana T, Bossy-Wetzel E, Goldberg M, Allen T, Barber MJ, Green DR, Newmeyer DD (1999) The pro-apoptotic proteins, Bid and Bax, cause a limited permeabilization of the mitochondrial outer membrane that is enhanced by cytosol. J Cell Biol 147:809–822
21. Kowaltowski AJ, Vercesi AE, Fiskum G (2000) Bcl-2 prevents mitochondrial permeability transition and cytochrome c release via maintenance of reduced pyridine nucleotides. Cell Death Differ
22. Krajewski S, Krajewska M, Ellerby LM, Welsh K, Xie Z, Deveraux QL, Salvesen GS, Bredesen DE, Rosenthal RE, Fiskum G, Reed JC (1999) Release of caspase-9 from mitochondria during neuronal apoptosis and cerebral ischemia. Proc Natl Acad Sci USA 96:5752–5757
23. Krajewski S, Tanaka S, Takayama S, Schibler MJ, Fenton W, Reed JC (1993) Investigation of the subcellular distribution of the bcl-2 oncoprotein: residence in the nuclear envelope, endoplasmic reticulum, and outer mitochondrial membranes. Cancer Res 53:4701–4714
24. Kroemer G, Dallaporta B, Resche-Rigon M (1998) The mitochondrial death/life regulator in apoptosis and necrosis. Annu Rev Physiol 60: 619–642
25. Kruman II, Mattson MP (1999) Pivotal role of mitochondrial calcium uptake in neural cell apoptosis and necrosis. J Neurochem 72:529–540
26. Lemasters JJ, Nieminen AL, Qian T, Trost LC, Elmore SP, Nishimura Y, Crowe RA, Cascio WE, Bradham CA, Brenner DA, Herman B (1998) The mitochondrial permeability transition in cell death: a common mechanism in necrosis, apoptosis and autophagy. Biochim Biophys Acta 1366:177–196
27. Lipton P (1999) Ischemic cell death in brain neurons. Physiol Rev 79:1431–1568
28. Lutz RJ (2000) Role of the BH3 (Bcl-2 homology 3) domain in the regulation of apoptosis and Bcl-2-related proteins. Biochem Soc Trans 28:51–56
29. Martinou JC, Dubois-Dauphin M, Staple JK, Rodriguez I, Frankowski H, Missotten M, Albertini P, Talabot D, Catsicas S, Pietra C (1994) Overexpression of BCL-2 in transgenic mice protects neurons from naturally occurring cell death and experimental ischemia. Neuron 13:1017–1030
30. Murphy AN, Bredesen DE, Cortopassi G, Wang E, Fiskum G (1996) Bcl-2 potentiates the maximal calcium uptake capacity of neural cell mitochondria. Proc Natl Acad Sci USA 93:9893–9898
31. Murphy AN, Myers KM, Fiskum G (1996) Bcl-2 and N-acetylcysteine inhibition of mitochondrial respiratory impairment following exposure of neural cells to chemical hypoxia/aglycemia. In: Pharmacology of Cerebral Ischemia, edited by J. Krieglstein. Stuttgart, Germany: Wissenschaftliche Verlagsgesellschaft, p 163–172
32. Myers KM, Fiskum G, Liu Y, Simmens SJ, Bredesen DE, Murphy AN (1995) Bcl-2 protects neural cells from cyanide/aglycemia-induced lipid oxidation, mitochondrial injury, and loss of viability. J Neurochem 65:2432–2440
33. Nicholls DG, Budd SL (1998) Neuronal excitotoxicity: the role of mitochondria. Biofactors 8:287–299
34. Nicotera P, Leist M, Ferrando-May E (1998) Intracellular ATP, a switch in the decision between apoptosis and necrosis. Toxicol Lett 102–103:139–142
35. Reynolds IJ (1999) Mitochondrial membrane potential and the permeability transition in excitotoxicity. Ann NY Acad Sci 893:33–41
36. Shimazaki K, Ishida A, Kawai N (1994) Increase in bcl-2 oncoprotein and the tolerance to ischemia-induced neuronal death in the gerbil hippocampus. Neurosci Res 20:95–99
37. Shimizu S, Narita M, Tsujimoto Y (1999) Bcl-2 family proteins regulate the release of apoptogenic cytochrome *c* by the mitochondrial channel VDAC [see comments]. Nature 399:483–487
38. Vercesi AE, Kowaltowski AJ, Grijalba MT, Meinicke AR, Castilho RF (1997) The role of reactive oxygen species in mitochondrial permeability transition. Biosci Rep 17:43–52
39. Wei MC, Lindsten T, Mootha VK, Weiler S, Gross A, Ashiya M, Thompson CB, Korsmeyer SJ (2000) tBID, a membrane-targeted death ligand, oligomerizes BAK to release cytochrome c. Genes Dev 14:2060–2071
40. Wright SC, Wang H, Wei QS, Kinder DH, Larrick JW (1998) Bcl-2-mediated resistance to apoptosis is associated with glutathione-induced inhibition of AP24 activation of nuclear DNA fragmentation. Cancer Res 58:5570–5576
41. Zha J, Harada H, Osipov K, Jockel J, Waksman G, Korsmeyer SJ (1997) BH3 domain of BAD is required for heterodimerization with BCL-XL and pro-apoptotic activity. J Biol Chem 272:24101–24104

Regulation of active cell death in ischemic brain injury: the role of Bax and the mitochondrial pathway

J. Chen[1], X.-M. Yin[2]

Abstract

Recent work has implied a central role of activation of caspases, especially caspase-3, in mediating neuronal apoptosis resulting from ischemic brain injury. Caspase activation in neuronal apoptosis may involve both extrinsic (cell membrane-bound death receptor-mediated) and intrinsic (mitochondrial damage-mediated) pathways, although the precise mechanism in ischemic cell death is unclear. The Bcl-2 family member protein Bax is a potent pro-apoptotic molecule which triggers the activation of effector caspases by damaging mitochondria and releasing cytochrome c. Previous studies demonstrated that Bax is overexpressed in selective ischemic neurons that destine to die, thus Bax may be involved in the cascade of ischemic cell death. Here we further provide evidence suggesting that Bax may play a key role in mediating ischemic cell death via the intrinsic pathway of caspase activation. The evidence includes that Bax is translocated from the cytoplasm to the mitochondria in neurons at time points preceding or coinciding with cell death after transient focal ischemia in rat brain, that following ischemia there is an enhanced heterodimeric binding of Bax to the anti-apoptotic protein Bcl-xl and the mitochondrial permeability transition pore proteins VDAC and ANT that are implicated in the process of cytochrome c release, and that Bax-deficient mice show increased resistance to transient ischemia-induced cell death, release of cytochrome c and activation of caspase-3. Further work elucidating the mechanisms through which Bax is translocated after ischemia and the precise molecular process of Bax-mitochondria interactions is pending.

Introduction

Brain injury resulting from cerebral ischemia may involve mixed types of cell death. While ischemic neurons often die from necrosis, a significant number of neurons exhibit a type of active cell death reminiscent of apoptosis, in which a tightly controlled genetic program of apoptosis is activated (for reviews see Lipton 1999; Schulz et al. 1999). Strongly supporting a role of active cell death in ischemic brain injury, several biochemical features of apoptosis are reproducibly detected in ischemic brain (Linnik et al. 1993; MacManus et al. 1993; Li et al. 1995) and a number of apoptosis-regulatory genes are found to be activated in neurons after ischemia (Krajewski et al. 1995; Chen et al. 1996, 1998; Namura et al. 1998).

Recent studies on basic biology of apoptosis have established a paradigm in which a group of

Departments of Neurology[1] and Pathology[2] University of Pittsburgh School of Medicine, Pittsburgh, PA 15213, USA.
e-mail: jun@med.pitt.edu

J. Krieglstein, S. Klumpp (Eds.) Pharmacology of Cerebral Ischemia 2000

cysteine proteases, known as caspases, play a central role in the execution of active cell death (for review see Thornberry and Lazebnik 1998). Based on the relative substrate specificity, the structure and the function in the caspase cascade, caspases may be categorized into three subgroups (Garcia-Calvo et al. 1998; Thornberry 1998). Group I caspases, such as caspases 1, 4, and 5, are mainly involved in inflammation response, while group II and III are mostly linked with apoptosis see in general. Group III caspases are upstream initiator caspases, such as caspases 8 and 9, and serve mainly to activate downstream group II effector casapses, such as caspase 3 or 7. Effector caspases cleave a variety of cytoplasmic and nuclear substrates, such as ICAD (inhibitor of caspase activated DNAase), PARP (poly(ADP-ribose)polymerase), lamin B among others, ensuring the inevitability of cell death (Liu et al. 1997; Enari et al. 1998; Sakahira et al. 1998; Thornberry 1998).

Caspase-3 appears to be the central executioner of active cell death in ischemic injury. Gene expression and protease activity of caspase-3 are upregulated in injured neurons after ischemia (Chen et al. 1998; Namura et al. 1998; Ni et al. 1998). Caspase-3-mediated cleavage of cell death substrates such as PARP and DNA-dependent protein kinase is detected in ischemic brain (Chen et al. 1998; Shackelford et al. 1999). Furthermore, pharmacological inhibition of caspase-3 activity significantly decreases infarct size (Hara et al. 1997; Namura et al. 1998) or attenuates the loss of hippocampal CA1 neurons following transient cerebral ischemia (Chen et al. 1998). These observations strongly suggest a pivotal role of caspase-3 in ischemic neuronal death, however, the precise mechanism through which caspase-3 is activated in ischemic neurons is poorly understood.

The Bcl-2 family proteins are important endogenous regulators of downstream caspases (Adams and Cory 1998). Recent studies confirm that several members of the bcl-2 family mediate apoptosis via the mitochondrial pathway, also called the intrinsic pathway, by promoting cytochrome c release and subsequently activating death-effector caspases. The induction of these death signals is prevented by death suppressors, BCL-2, BCL-X_L etc., but is promoted by death effectors such as Bax or BID (for review see Green and Reed 1998). Bax is a stress-inducible protein that is overexpressed in selective neurons destined to die after transient cerebral ischemia (Krajewski et al. 1995; Chen et al. 1996; Gillardon et al. 1996). Thus, Bax could serve as a cell death trigger in ischemic neurons by provoking caspase activation through the mitochondrial pathway. The recent findings that caspase-activating factors such as cytochrome c and caspase-9 are released from mitochondria in ischemic neurons strongly suggest that caspase activation after ischemia involves a mitochondrial mechanism (Fujimura et al. 1998, 1999; Krajewski et al. 1999). Accordingly, we investigated the potential role of Bax in cytochrome c release, caspase-3 activation and consequent neuronal death in a model of transient focal cerebral ischemia. Here, we provide evidence, which support such a role for Bax.

Experimental Procedures

Animal model of transient focal ischemia

Transient focal ischemia (30 min) was induced in isoflurane-anesthetized male adult Sprague-Dawley rats or C57BL/6 mice using the intraluminal vascular occlusion of the middle cerebral artery (MCA). Physiological variables were monitored and maintained in the normal range throughout the experiments. Temporalis muscle and rectal temperature were maintained in the range of 36.5–37.5 °C using a heating pad and a temperature-regulated heating lamp. Cortical blood flow was monitored before, during and after MCA occlusion using laser Doppler flowmetry. A sham operation was performed in additional animals using the same anesthesia and surgical procedures except that the intraluminal suture was not inserted; these brains served as nonischemic controls.

Mitochondrial and cytosolic protein isolation

Animals were killed at 1, 3, 6, or 24 h after 30 min of ischemia or 24 h after sham operation. The caudate-putamen, which is affected by MCA occlusion, was dissected from the brain. All procedures for mitochondria and protein isolation were carried out at 4 °C using the protocol described previously (Yan et al. 2000). In brief, brain tissues were homogenized using a Dounce homogenizer in hypotonic buffer containing freshly prepared protease inhibitors. After lysis for 30 min on ice, unbroken cells and nuclei were pelleted at 1200 xg. The supernatant, containing the mitochondria, was centrifuged at 10000 xg for 15 min to pellet the mitochondria, and the resulting supernatant (cytosolic fraction) was removed. To further isolate mitochondrial protein, the pellet was resuspended in a solution containing 3% Ficoll 400, 0.12 M manitol, 0.03 M sucrose, and 25 μM EDTA (pH 7.4), and gently layered twice in 6% Ficoll 400 solution to produce a discontinuous density gradient. After centrifugation at 10,400 xg for 25 min, the sediment was resuspended in the lysis buffer containing 10 mM Hepes (pH 7.4), 142.5 mM KCl, 5 mM $MgCl_2$, 1 mM EGTA, 0.5% NP-40, 0.5 mM PMSF, 10 μg/ml aprotinin, and 1 μg/ml each of leupeptin, chymostatin, antipain, and pepstatin (Narita et al. 1998), followed by sonication. The lysate was centrifuged at 130,000 xg for 1 h, concentrated to 5–10 mg/ml protein, and stored at –80 °C in aliquots.

Western blot analysis

For the detection of Bax and cytochrome c in subcellular fractions, mitochondrial or cytosolic proteins were denatured in SDS-loading buffer (100 mM Tris-HCl, 200 mM dithiothreitol, 4% SDS, 0.2% bromophenol blue, and 20% glycerol) at 100 °C for 6 min and then separated on 12% SDS-polyacrylamide gels (40 μg per lane). Immunoblotting was performed as described previously (Chen et al. 1996), using a chemiluminescent detection system (Clontech, Palo Alto, CA). The working dilution for Bax and cytochrome c antibodies in the present study was 1:500 and 1:3000, respectively. To control for equal sample loading in each subcellular fraction, immunoblotting was performed using antibodies against the mitochondrial marker cytochrome c oxidase IV and the cytosolic marker α-tubulin respectively.

Immunoprecipitation

Immunoprecipitation was performed to examine protein-protein interaction in mitochondria. Mitochondrial lysates (200 μg protein per sample) were incubated with 1 μg of the primary antibody and the mixture was incubated for 2 h at 4 °C. The samples were then transferred to Eppendorf tubes containing 20 μl of Protein A/G PLUS-Agarose beads and incubated overnight at 4 °C. The beads were collected by centrifugation and washed four times with the lysis buffer containing 10 mM Hepes (pH 7.4), 142.5 mM KCl, 5 mM $MgCl_2$, 1 mM EGTA, 0.5% Nonidet P-40, 0.5 mM PMSF, 10 μg/ml aprotinin and 1 μg/ml each of leupeptin, chymostatin, antipain and pepstatin. After the final wash, the beads were resuspended in 40 μl of SDS-PAGE sample buffer, boiled for 5 min and centrifuged. The supernatant was then subjected to electrophoresis and immunoblotting.

Immunohistochemistry

Animals were anesthetized with 8% chloral hydrate at 6, 24 or 72 h after 30 min of ischemia or 24 h after sham operation (n = 4 per time point). Their brains were rapidly removed, frozen in 2-methylbutane at –30 °C, covered with mounting medium and stored at –80 °C. Coronal sections (15-μm thick) were cut on a cryostat at –20 °C. Sections at the level of midcaudate (anteroposterior, +0.2 mm from the bregma) were selected and processed for immunohistochemical staining. The sections were fixed with 4% paraformaldehyde in 0.1 M PBS (pH 7.4) for 15 min followed by three washes in PBS. After being preblocked using 2% normal goat serum in PBS for 20 min, the sections were incubated for 2 h at 37 °C in the primary antibody diluted (1:250 for Bax) in PBS, pH 7.4, containing 2% goat serum, 0.2% Triton X-100, 0.5% bovine serum albumin, and 0.2% glycine. After washes, the sections were incubated for 1.5 h at room temperature at a 1:2500 dilution with goat anti-rabbit Cy3.18. All steps were performed in the dark. A Zeiss light microscope equipped for epifluorescent illumination was used for observations.

For the detection of co-localization of Bax with the mitochondrial marker cytochrome c oxidase IV, double-label immunohistochemistry was performed on sections obtained at 6 h after ischemia. Sections were first processed for Bax immunohistochemical staining as described above, and then incubated in the anti-cytochrome c oxidase IV antibody (1:2000) for 2 h at 37 °C followed by PBS washes and incubation with horse anti-mouse Cy2 immunoconjugate. The rest of the procedures were the same as described above.

Detection of DNA damage

In situ detection of DNA fragmentation in brain cells after ischemia or sham operation was performed using the method previously described (Chen et al. 1998). In brief, coronal sections obtained from mice killed at 72 h after 30 min of ischemia were fixed with 4% paraformaldehyde in PBS for 15 min. After the sections were permeabilized with 1% triton X-100 in PBS for 30 min, they were incubated in a moist-air chamber at 37 °C for 1 h in a reaction mixture containing: 5 mM $MgCl_2$, 5 mM 2-mercaptoethanol, 10 μM each of dGTP, dCTP, dTTP, biotinylated dATP and 30 U/ml Klenow fragment of DNA polymerase I (Sigma) in PBS (pH 7.4). The reaction was terminated by three washes in PBS for 10 min each. The sections were then incubated at room temperature for 15 min in flurescein-avidin D (cell-sorting grade; Vector Laboratories, Burlingame, CA) diluted at 7.5 μg/ml. After four PBS washes of 10 min each, the sections were counterstained with Hoechst 33258 and then coverslipped for fluorescence microscopy examinations. The percentages of DNA-damaged cells in the caudate were quantified.

Measurement of caspase activities

Measurement of caspase-3-like protease activity in brain cell extracts was performed as described (Chen et al. 1998). The animals were anesthetized using 8% chloral hydrate and decapitated at 24 h after ischemia or sham operation (n = 4 per experimental condition). Brains were quickly removed and tissues were dissected from the caudate-putamen. Protein extracts were prepared on ice by Dounce homogenization of tissues in the lysis buffer (Chen et al. 1998). Cell lysate was centrifuged at 14,000 rpm for 30 min (4 °C), and the supernatant was used for the enzymatic assay. Fifty micrograms of protein were incubated for 1 h at 37 °C with the reaction buffer containing 25 mM HEPES (pH 7.5), 10% sucrose, 0.1% 3-[(3-cholamidopropyl)dimethylammonio]-1-propane sulfonate, 5 mM DTT, and 5 mM EDTA in a total volume of 100 μl. The reaction mixture contained 25 μM of the peptide cleavage substrate (Ac-DEVD-AMC, Biomol).

Data analysis

All data are presented as means ± SEM. Comparisons of caspase activities, Bax protein expression, cytochrome c release, infarct size, cell survival or DNA-damaged cells after ischemia versus sham controls were made using ANOVA and *post hoc* Fisher's PLSD tests. A level of $p < 0.05$ was considered statistically significant.

Results

Overexpression and mitochondrial translocation of Bax after ischemia

In this study, we examined Bax protein expression in normal and ischemic brains, focusing on the caudate-putamen (Cpu), a region affected by transient focal ischemia (30 min). In particular, the changes in subcellular distribution of Bax after ischemia were studied at the cellular levels using indirect immunoflurescence and at the tissue levels using Western blotting.

As shown in Figure 1, the cellular distribution of Bax immunoreactivity was examined using immunofluorescence in non-ischemic brains and in brains 6 or 24 h after ischemia (representatives of 4 brains per time point). In non-ischemic Cpu (A), Bax immunoreactivity was faint and diffusely distributed in the cytosol (arrows) and generally difficult to be distinguished from the background. At 6 h after ischemia, increased Bax immunoreactivity was detected in many medium-sized neurons and showed a punctate pattern (B). This punctate pattern of Bax immunostaining was consistent with a mitochondrial localization as previously described in cell culture studies (Rosse et al. 1998; Saikumar et al. 1998; Desagher et al. 1999). At 24 h after ischemia, Bax immunoreactivity was further increased in neurons, exhibiting a mixture of diffusive and punctate patterns suggestive of both cytosol- and mitochondria-associated distributions (C).

To confirm the mitochondrial localization of Bax after ischemia, double-label immunofluorescence was performed to co-localize Bax and the mitochondria marker cytochrome c oxidase IV. As shown in Figure 2, the punctual Bax immunoreactivity was largely overlapping that

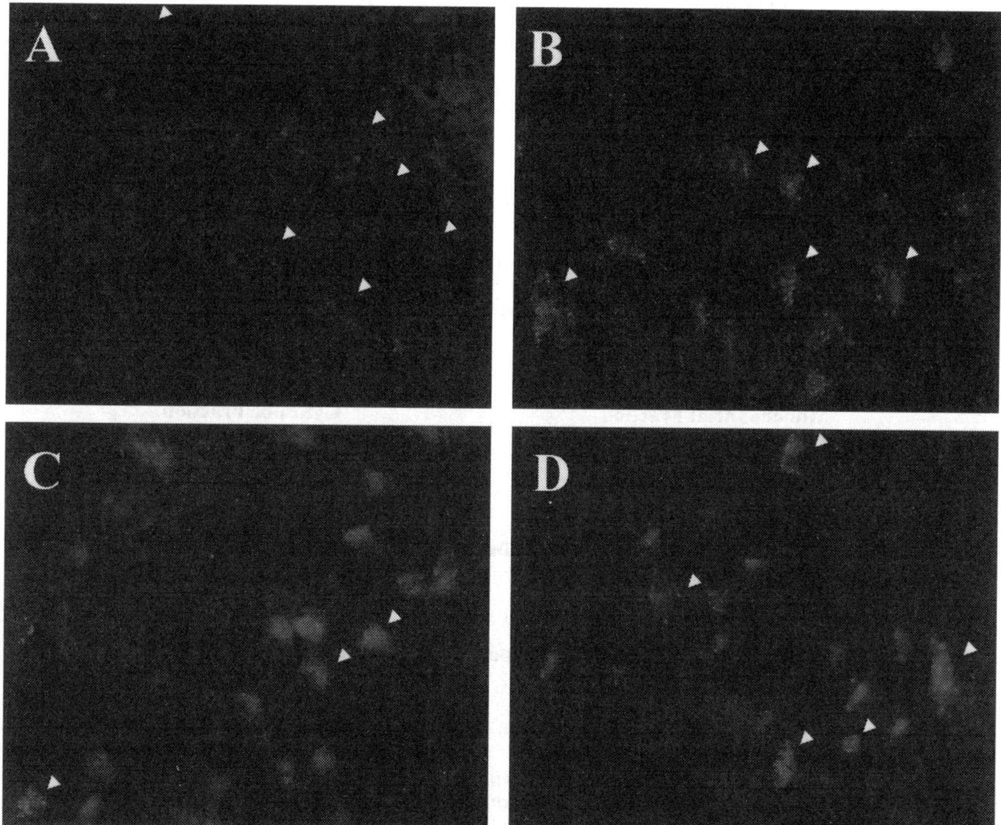

Fig. 1. Representative micrographs showing Bax immunoreactivity in the caudate-putamen at 24 h after sham operation (A) or 6 (B), 24 (C), or 72 h (D) after 30 min of MCA occlusion. Note that, as compared to the sham-control brain, Bax immunoreactivity was increased and showed a punctate pattern in ischemic neurons.

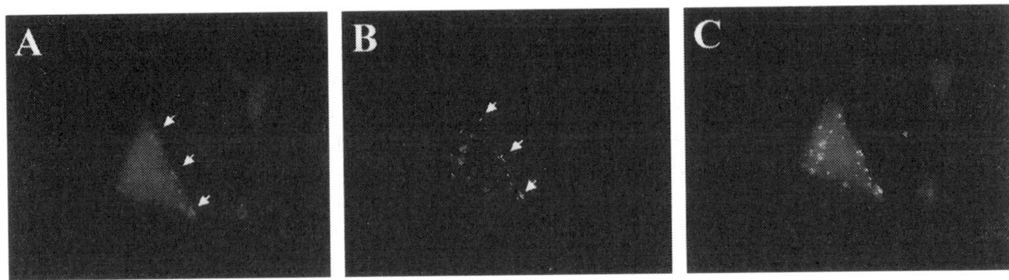

Fig. 2. Representative double-label immunofluorescent images of Bax (*A*) and cytochrome c oxidase IV (*B*) in caudate neurons at 6 hours after ischemia. The overlapping images of *A* and *B* are shown in *C*. Note that Bax is at least partially co-localized with cytochrome c oxidase IV (yellow puncta in *C*). Magnification X 1000.

of the mitochondrial marker in the ischemic brain.

To examine the subcellular distribution of Bax after ischemia, Western blotting was performed after protein fractionation (Fig. 3). In non-ischemic brains, Bax immunoreactivity was readily detected in the cytosol and, to a lesser extent, in the mitochondria. Bax immunoreactivity began to be increased in the mitochondrial fraction at 3–6 h and peaked at 24 h after ischemia. In the cytosolic fraction, Bax immunoreactivity was unchanged (1–3 h) or slightly decreased (6 h) at earlier time points but increased at 24 h after ischemia. These results are consistent with the overexpression and mitochondrial translocation of Bax after ischemia.

Enhanced Bax-mitochondria interactions after ischemia

To study the potential interaction of Bax with mitochondria-associated proteins, mitochondria were isolated from the CPu of sham-operated brains and CPu at 6 or 24 h after ischemia. The mitochondrial lysates were subjected to immu-

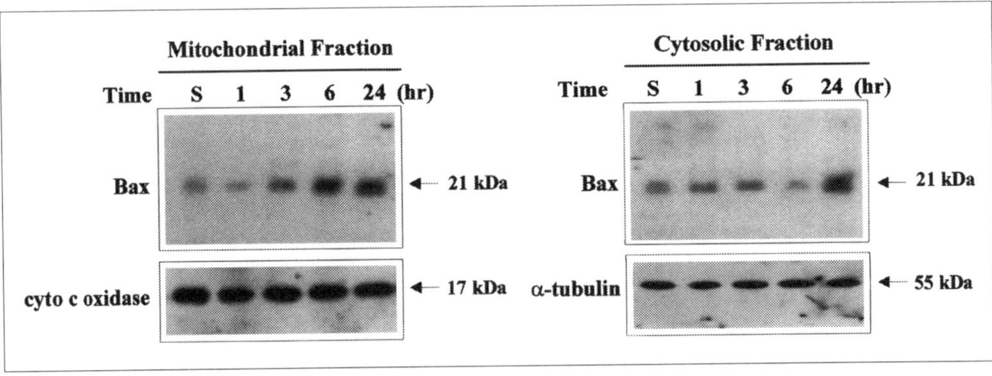

Fig. 3. Representative Western blots showing changes in Bax immunoreactivity in the mitochondrial and cytosolic fractions after ischemia. Mitochondrial or cytosolic protein was purified from the caudate-putamen at 1, 3, 6, or 24 hours after ischemia or 24 hours after sham operation and subjected to Western blot analysis. Note that Bax immunoreactivity was increased in the mitochondria at 3 h after ischemia and thereafter, while it was increased in the cytosol only at 24 h postischemia. Control Western blots (for protein loading) show that the purified mitochondrial and cytosolic fractions are enriched in the mitochondrial membrane-bound protein cytochrome c oxidase IV (COX-IV) and the cytosolic protein α-tubulin respectively.

noprecipitation with monoclonal anti-Bax antibody and the resulting immune complexes analyzed by Western blotting using antibodies against the mitochondrial permeability transition pore proteins VDAC (voltage-dependent anion channel) and ANT (adenine nucleotide translocator) or the Bcl-2 family members Bid, Bad, Bak, bcl-2, bcl-w, bcl-xl or Bax, respectively. As shown in Figure 4, endogenous Bax was coimmunoprecipitated with VDAC, ANT and bcl-xl. These immune complexes were detected in non-ischemic samples as well as in ischemic samples. However, the amounts of VDAC-Bax and ANT-Bax immune complexes were elevated in ischemic samples. Furthermore, increases in the Bax immune complexes following ischemia were coincidence with the increase in the amount of Bax protein in the mitochondrial lysates, suggesting that a large portion of the complexes resulted from Bax that translocates to the mitochondria after ischemia. In contrast, Bax coimmunoprecipitation with other proteins was not detected (not shown).

Additional immunoprecipitation experiments were performed using anti-VDAC and anti-ANT antibodies respectively. The immune complexes were subjected to Western blotting using the anti-Bax antibody. The results were consistent with the interactions of Bax with the two pore proteins. While the levels of neither VDAC nor ANT were changed in the mitochondrial lysates following ischemia, immunoprecipitate of ANT and VDAC contained increased amount of Bax in ischemic samples (Fig. 4).

Bax-null mice are resistant to ischemic brain injury

Bax-null male mice (Bax–/–) and wild type littermates with body weight of 25–30 grams were subjected to 30 min of MCA occlusion. Cortical blood flow was dropped to approximately 15% of baseline values during ischemia and returned to about 85% of baseline once the reperfusion was established; no statistic significance was detected between the two groups ($p > 0.05$). Blood pressure, blood pH, arterial O_2 and CO_2 were maintained during and after ischemia.

Histology and *in situ* DNA fragmentation were performed at 72 h after MCA occlusion, focusing on the caudate-putamen. Neuronal cell death in the caudate was significantly reduced in Bax-null mice as compared to the heterozygous (Bax+/–) and wild type mice ($n = 6$ per group, Fig. 5A).

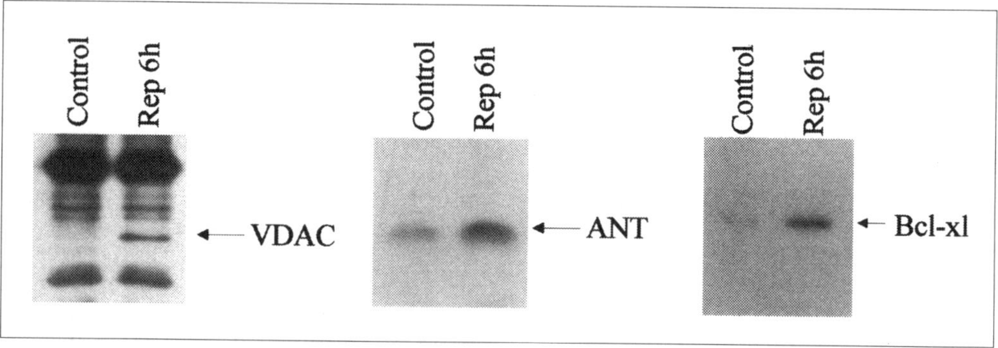

Fig. 4. Western blots showing co-immunoprecipitation of Bax and the mitochondrial permeability transition pore complex proteins VDAC and ANT and the antiapoptotic Bcl-2 family member Bcl-xl after ischemia. Mitochondrial protein was purified from the caudate cell extracts after sham operation (control) or 6 h after 30 min of MCA occlusion and subjected to immunoprecipitation using the anti-Bax monoclonal antibody. The resulting immune complex was then analyzed by Western blotting using antibodies against VDAC, ANT or Bcl-xl. Note that the heterodimerization between Bax and all three proteins was increased in ischemic samples. The blots are representatives of 3 independent experiments with similar results.

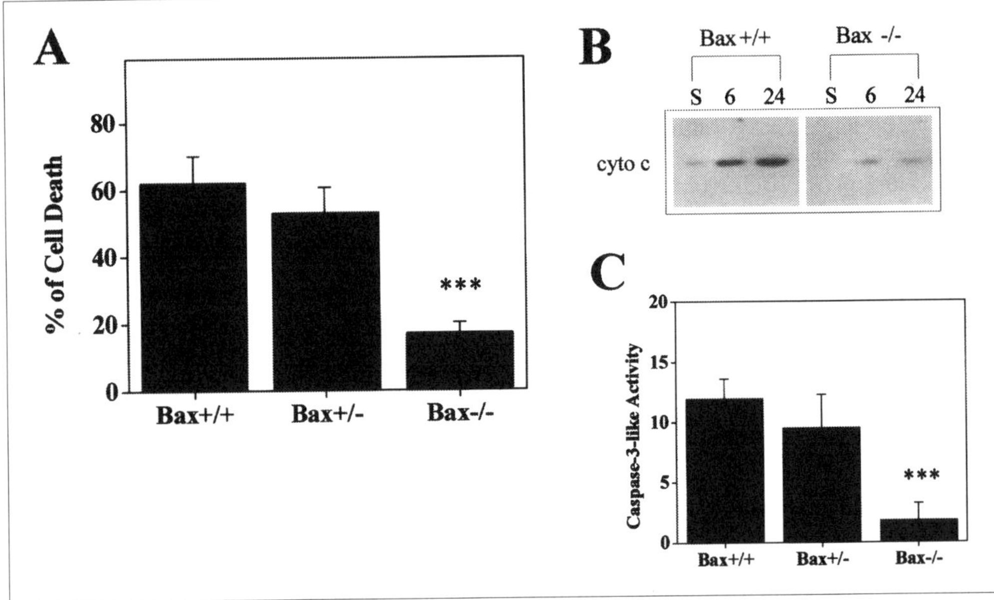

Fig. 5. Bax-null mice are resistant to ischemic brain injury. (A) Bax-null (Bax–/–) or Bax heterozygous (Bax+/–) mice or their wild-type littermates (Bax+/+) were subjected to 30 min of MCA occlusion. Brains were removed at 72 h after ischemia; coronal sections were subjected to TUNEL staining and counterstained with the DNA dye Hoechst 33258 and the percentage of TUNEL-positive cells versus total cell accounts in the caudate was quantified. Note that Bax–/– mice showed significantly less amounts of cell death. Data are mean ± SEM, n = 6 per group. ***$p < 0.001$ versus the wild-type littermates (ANOVA and post hoc PLSD tests). (B) Representative Western blots showing decreased cytochrome c release in Bax–/– mice at 6 and 24 h following transient focal ischemia. (C) Caspase-3-like proteolytic activity was significantly decreased in Bax–/– mice at 24 h following transient focal ischemia. *** $p < 0.001$ versus the wild-type littermates (n = 4 per group, ANOVA and post hoc PLSD tests).

Additional Bax-null and wild type mice were subjected to 30 min of MCA occlusion and the brains were removed at 6 or 24 h after ischemia for cytochrome c release analysis (n = 3 per group) and at 24 h after ischemia for caspase-3 activity measurement (n = 4 per group). Cytochrome c release and caspase-3 activation were reduced in Bax-null mice (Fig. 5B-C).

Discussion

Recent evidence suggests that mitochondria play a crucial role in apoptosis by releasing apoptogenic factors such as cytochrome c and apoptosis-inducing factor from the intermembrane space into the cytoplasm (Liu et al. 1996; Kluck et al. 1997; Yang et al. 1997; Marzo et al. 1998). Cytochrome c release activates caspase-9, in concert with the cytosolic molecules Apaf-1 and dATP, and subsequently activates caspase-3. Although the apoptotic signal-transduction pathway downstream from the mitochondria is relatively clear, the precise mechanism by which the cell death signals are transmitted to the mitochondria during apoptosis are poorly understood. However, it has been postulated that the BH3 domain-containing death agonist Bax may be an important apoptosis signal transducer linking the upstream apoptotic cascade and mitochondria. Bax is a soluble protein that is mainly localized in the cytoplasm but it translocates to the mitochondria at the early stage of apoptosis (Wolter et al. 1997). Bax is an extremely potent inducer for cytochrome c release in isolated mitochondria, including those of the brain origin (Yan et al. 2000).

Two mechanisms by which Bax targets mitochondria and promotes cell death have been hypothesized (for review see Adams 1998). One is through competitive heterodimerization with anti-apoptotic family members such as Bcl-2 and Bcl-xl and, therefore, to block their anti-apoptotic functions (Oltvai et al. 1993; Yin et al. 1994). Deletion analysis has indicated that the BH3 domain of Bax is required for it to heterodimerize with Bcl-2 or Bcl-xl and to promote cell death. The second mode in which Bax triggers apoptosis is through enhanced mitochondrial membrane permeability, which leads to the release of cytochrome c (Wolter et al. 1997; Jurgensmeier et al. 1998; Pastorino et al. 1998; Rosse et al. 1998). The latter mechanism requires interactions between Bax and the mitochondrial membrane permeability transition pore complex which includes VDAC, ANT, creatine kinase (CK), and the peripheral benzodiazepine receptor (PBR) (Beutner et al. 1998; Marzo et al. 1998; Narita et al. 1998; Shimizu et al. 1999). However, alternative mechanisms by which Bax increases mitochondrial membrane permeability that are independent of protein-protein heterodimerization may also exist. One such mechanism that has been proposed is the channel-forming activity of Bax, which has been shown *in vitro* in lipid membrane (Antonsson et al. 1997; Schlesinger et al. 1997). It may be hypothesized that the channel activity created by Bax may affect mitochondrial permeability and thus regulate either the release of cytochrome c or other mitochondrial functions that are associated with caspase-independent apoptosis.

The present study provides strong evidence that Bax may be an important cell death agonist in the brain after transient cerebral ischemia. The expression of Bax protein was found to be upregulated and translocated to the mitochondria during early stage of ischemic brain injury. Furthermore, the data show that Bax formed heterodimetric complexes with the permeability transition pore proteins VDAC and ANT and the anti-apoptotic protein Bcl-xl in mitochondria of the ischemic brain. Finally, the Bax-deficient mice showed significantly decreased ischemic cell death and caspase-3 activity compared to the wild type littermates. These results thus suggest an important role of Bax in apoptotic signal transduction in ischemic brain injury by an enhanced interaction with mitochondrial proteins.

What remains to be elucidated is how the postulated mechanisms discussed above contribute to the cell death-agonizing effect of Bax in ischemic neurons. Also, it is important to determine whether the effect by Bax on mitochondria requires the synergic actions of other proapoptotic Bcl-2 family members, as a recent study suggests that Bid-induced conformational changes of Bax may be essential for Bax-induced cytochrome c release (Desagher et al. 1999). Further investigation thus is warranted to address these issues.

References

1. Adams JM, Cory S (1998) The Bcl-2 protein family: arbiters of cell survival. Science 281:1322–1326
2. Antonsson B, Conti F, Ciavatta A, Montessuit S, Lewis S, Martinou I, Bernasconi L, Bernard A, Mermod JJ, Mazzei G, Maundrell K, Gambale F, Sadoul R, Martinou JC (1997) Inhibition of Bax channel-forming activity by Bcl-2. Science 277:370–372
3. Beutner G, Ruck A, Riede B, Brdiczka D (1998) Complexes between porin, hexokinase, mitochondrial creatine kinase and adenylate translocator display properties of the permeability transition pore. Implication for regulation of permeability transition by the kinases. Biochim Biophys Acta 1368:7–18
4. Chen J, Nagayama T, Jin K, Stetler RA, Zhu RL, Graham SH, Simon RP (1998) Induction of caspase-3-like protease may mediate delayed neuronal death in the hippocampus after transient cerebral ischemia. J Neurosci 18:4914–4928
5. Chen J, Zhu RL, Nakayama M, Kawaguchi K, Jin K, Stetler RA, Simon RP, Graham SH (1996) Expression of the apoptosis-effector gene, Bax, is up-regulated in vulnerable hippocampal CA1 neurons following global ischemia. J Neurochem 67:64–71
6. Desagher S, Osen-Sand A, Nichols A, Eskes R, Montessuit S, Lauper S, Maundrell K, Antonsson B, Martinou JC (1999) Bid-induced conformational change of Bax is responsible for mitochondrial cytochrome c release during apoptosis. J Cell Biol 144:891–901
7. Enari M, Sakahira H, Yokoyama H, Okawa K, Iwamatsu A, Nagata S (1998) A caspase-activated DNase that degrades DNA during apoptosis, and its inhibitor ICAD [see comments] [published erratum appears in Nature 1998 May 28;393(6683):396]. Nature 391:43–50
8. Fujimura M, Morita-Fujimura Y, Murakami K, Kawase M, Chan PH (1998) Cytosolic redistribution of cytochrome c after transient focal cerebral ischemia in rats. J Cereb Blood Flow Metab 18:1239–1247

9. Fujimura M, Morita-Fujimura Y, Kawase M, Copin JC, Calagui B, Epstein CJ, Chan PH (1999) Manganese superoxide dismutase mediates the early release of mitochondrial cytochrome C and subsequent DNA fragmentation after permanent focal cerebral ischemia in mice. J Neurosci 19:3414–3422
10. Garcia-Calvo M, Peterson EP, Leiting B, Ruel R, Nicholson DW, Thornberry NA (1998) Inhibition of human caspases by peptide-based and macromolecular inhibitors. J Biol Chem 273:32608–32613
11. Gillardon F, Lenz C, Waschke KF, Krajewski S, Reed JC, Zimmermann M, Kuschinsky W (1996) Altered expression of Bcl-2, Bcl-X, Bax, and c-Fos colocalizes with DNA fragmentation and ischemic cell damage following middle cerebral artery occlusion in rats. Brain Res Mol Brain Res 40:254–260
12. Green DR, Reed JC (1998) Mitochondria and apoptosis. Science 281:1309–1312
13. Hara H, Friedlander RM, Gagliardini V, Ayata C, Fink K, Huang Z, Shimizu-Sasamata M, Yuan J, Moskowitz MA (1997) Inhibition of interleukin 1beta converting enzyme family proteases reduces ischemic and excitotoxic neuronal damage. Proc Natl Acad Sci U S A 94:2007–2012
14. Jurgensmeier JM, Xie Z, Deveraux Q, Ellerby L, Bredesen D, Reed JC (1998) Bax directly induces release of cytochrome c from isolated mitochondria. Proc Natl Acad Sci USA 95:4997–5002
15. Kluck RM, Bossy-Wetzel E, Green DR, Newmeyer DD (1997) The release of cytochrome c from mitochondria: a primary site for Bcl-2 regulation of apoptosis [see comments]. Science 275:1132–1136
16. Krajewski S, Mai JK, Krajewska M, Sikorska M, Mossakowski MJ, Reed JC (1995) Upregulation of bax protein levels in neurons following cerebral ischemia. J Neurosci 15:6364–6376
17. Krajewski S, Krajewska M, Ellerby LM, Welsh K, Xie Z, Deveraux QL, Salvesen GS, Bredesen DE, Rosenthal RE, Fiskum G, Reed JC (1999) Release of caspase-9 from mitochondria during neuronal apoptosis and cerebral ischemia. Proc Natl Acad Sci USA 96:5752–5757
18. Li Y, Chopp M, Jiang N, Yao F, Zaloga C (1995) Temporal profile of in situ DNA fragmentation after transient middle cerebral artery occlusion in the rat. J Cereb Blood Flow Metab 15:389–397
19. Linnik MD, Zobrist RH, Hatfield MD (1993) Evidence supporting a role for programmed cell death in focal cerebral ischemia in rats. Stroke 24:2002–2008; discussion 2008–2009
20. Lipton P (1999) Ischemic cell death in brain neurons. Physiol Rev 79:1431–1568
21. Liu X, Zou H, Slaughter C, Wang X (1997) DFF, a heterodimeric protein that functions downstream of caspase-3 to trigger DNA fragmentation during apoptosis. Cell 89:175–184
22. Liu X, Kim CN, Yang J, Jemmerson R, Wang X (1996) Induction of apoptotic program in cell-free extracts: requirement for dATP and cytochrome c. Cell 86:147–157
23. MacManus JP, Buchan AM, Hill IE, Rasquinha I, Preston E (1993) Global ischemia can cause DNA fragmentation indicative of apoptosis in rat brain. Neurosci Lett 164:89–92
24. Marzo I, Brenner C, Zamzami N, Jurgensmeier JM, Susin SA, Vieira HL, Prevost MC, Xie Z, Matsuyama S, Reed JC, Kroemer G (1998) Bax and adenine nucleotide translocator cooperate in the mitochondrial control of apoptosis. Science 281:2027–2031
25. Namura S, Zhu J, Fink K, Endres M, Srinivasan A, Tomaselli KJ, Yuan J, Moskowitz MA (1998) Activation and cleavage of caspase-3 in apoptosis induced by experimental cerebral ischemia. J Neurosci 18:3659–3668
26. Narita M, Shimizu S, Ito T, Chittenden T, Lutz RJ, Matsuda H, Tsujimoto Y (1998) Bax interacts with the permeability transition pore to induce permeability transition and cytochrome c release in isolated mitochondria. Proc Natl Acad Sci USA 95:14681–14686
27. Ni B, Wu X, Su Y, Stephenson D, Smalstig EB, Clemens J, Paul SM (1998) Transient global forebrain ischemia induces a prolonged expression of the caspase-3 mRNA in rat hippocampal CA1 pyramidal neurons. J Cereb Blood Flow Metab 18:248–256
28. Oltvai ZN, Milliman CL, Korsmeyer SJ (1993) Bcl-2 heterodimerizes in vivo with a conserved homolog, Bax, that accelerates programmed cell death. Cell 74:609–619
29. Pastorino JG, Chen ST, Tafani M, Snyder JW, Farber JL (1998) The overexpression of Bax produces cell death upon induction of the mitochondrial permeability transition. J Biol Chem 273:7770–7775
30. Rosse T, Olivier R, Monney L, Rager M, Conus S, Fellay I, Jansen B, Borner C (1998) Bcl-2 prolongs cell survival after Bax-induced release of cytochrome c [see comments]. Nature 391:496–499
31. Saikumar P, Dong Z, Patel Y, Hall K, Hopfer U, Weinberg JM, Venkatachalam MA (1998) Role of hypoxia-induced Bax translocation and cytochrome c release in reoxygenation injury. Oncogene 17:3401–3415
32. Sakahira H, Enari M, Nagata S (1998) Cleavage of CAD inhibitor in CAD activation and DNA degradation during apoptosis [see comments]. Nature 391:96–99
33. Schlesinger PH, Gross A, Yin XM, Yamamoto K, Saito M, Waksman G, Korsmeyer SJ (1997) Comparison of the ion channel characteristics of proapoptotic BAX and antiapoptotic BCL-2. Proc Natl Acad Sci USA 94:11357–11362
34. Schulz JB, Weller M, Moskowitz MA (1999) Caspases as treatment targets in stroke and neurodegenerative diseases. Ann Neurol 45:421–429
35. Shackelford DA, Tobaru T, Zhang S, Zivin JA (1999) Changes in expression of the DNA repair protein complex DNA-dependent protein kinase after ischemia and reperfusion. J Neurosci 19:4727–4738
36. Shimizu S, Narita M, Tsujimoto Y (1999) Bcl-2 family proteins regulate the release of apoptogenic cytochrome c by the mitochondrial channel VDAC [see comments]. Nature 399:483–487
37. Thornberry NA (1998) Caspases: key mediators of apoptosis. Chem Biol 5:R97–103
38. Thornberry NA, Lazebnik Y (1998) Caspases: enemies within. Science 281:1312–1316
39. Wolter KG, Hsu YT, Smith CL, Nechushtan A, Xi XG, Youle RJ (1997) Movement of Bax from the cytosol to mitochondria during apoptosis. J Cell Biol 139:1281–1292
40. Yan C, Chen J, Chen D, Minami M, Pei W, Yin XM, Simon RP (2000) Overexpression of the cell death suppressor Bcl-w in ischemic brain: implications for a neuroprotective role via the mitochondrial pathway. J Cereb Blood Flow Metab 20:620–630
41. Yang J, Liu X, Bhalla K, Kim CN, Ibrado AM, Cai J, Peng TI, Jones DP, Wang X (1997) Prevention of apoptosis by Bcl-2: release of cytochrome c from mitochondria blocked [see comments]. Science 275:1129–1132
42. Yin XM, Oltvai ZN, Korsmeyer SJ (1994) BH1 and BH2 domains of Bcl-2 are required for inhibition of apoptosis and heterodimerization with Bax [see comments]. Nature 369:321–323

The effect of pH on state 3 and state 4 brain mitochondrial metabolism

D. B. Kintner, K. A. Sailor, D. D. Gilboe

Abstract

We have measured the effect of decreasing the pH of a sucrose-based media over the range of 7.4 to 5.6 on the pyruvate/malate supported respiration, membrane potential and ΔpH of mitochondria isolated from the rat forebrain. At the lowest pH level in this study, State 4 respiration increased by 400%, State 3 respiration decreased by 34% and RCR decreased by 83%. We monitored mitochondrial membrane potential with the fluorescent probe tetramethylrhodamine methyl ester (TMRM) and ΔpH with the fluorescent probe 2',7'-bis-(2-carboxyethyl)-5(6)-carboxyfluorescein (BCECF). The decrease in membrane potential is best described by a sigmoid curve which covered the range from 165 mV to 115 mV as reaction media pH decreased. The decrease in membrane potential was partially compensated by a concurrent increase in ΔpH from 4.4 mV to 33 mV. The time required to reestablish the membrane potential following ADP-stimulated State 3 respiration increased from 34 s to 101 s as pH decreased from 7.4 to 5.6. In mitochondria exposed to acidosis, the calculated membrane conductance during State 4 respiration increased by 472%, indicating a significant proton leak. Attempts to pharmacologically block the effects of acidosis on mitochondria with cyclosporin A, 6-ketocholestanol or the spin-trap agent PNM were unsuccessful.

Introduction

Elevated pre-ischemic blood glucose levels coincide with changes in brain histology, metabolism, and functional recovery following temporary global cerebral ischemia. Several studies have shown that hyperglycemic ischemia accelerates the onset of delayed brain damage, disrupts the blood-brain barrier, facilitates development of infarctions and triggers post-ischemic seizures (Siesjö et al. 1996; Li and Siesjö 1997). The increased brain lactate levels following hyperglycemic ischemia suggest the possibility that ischemic brain damage might be associated with acidosis. The extracellular pH (pH_e) and intracellular pH (pH_i) have been determined using both glass electrodes and ^{31}P-NMR. Both pH values varied linearly with the amount of lactate formed during ischemia (Combs et al. 1990; Katsura et al. 1991). Nevertheless, the precise mechanism(s) by which

Keywords: Mitochondrial respiration, Acidosis, Protonmotive force, Membrane conductance, Free radicals

University of Wisconsin Medical School, Department of Neurological Surgery, 1300 University Ave., 4630 MSC, Madison, WI 53706-1532, U.S.A.
e-mail: ddgilboe@facstaff.wisc.edu

increased [H^+] contributed to increased post-ischemic brain damage remain unclear.

It has been suggested that a lower pH_i might alter the charge, and consequently the function of critical intracellular proteins (Maruki et al. 1995). However, severe non-ischemic hypercapnia in rats decreases pH_i to a level similar to that in normoglycemic or mildly hyperglycemic brains during ischemia, but fails to disrupt energy metabolism, cause histological damage, or affect subsequent neurological recovery (Cohen et al. 1990; Xu et al. 1991). Thus, it appears that pH-induced changes in protein function *per se* are insufficient to cause irreversible brain damage.

By inducing hypercapnia prior to the insult (Katsura et al. 1994), it is possible to decrease pH_e during normoglycemic ischemia to values seen during hyperglycemic ischemia. The result is exaggerated histologic damage compared to that observed during normocapnic ischemia and damage comparable to that seen with hyperglycemic ischemia. Although this suggests that the detrimental effect of hyperglycemic ischemia is the result of acidosis, the increased acidity apparently acts in conjunction with one or more pathologic processes initiated by energy failure.

Surprisingly, it appears that some of the values improve as a result of the decreased pH_i resulting from ischemia. *In vitro* studies have shown a decrease in cell death consequent to both glutamate exposure and anoxia when pH_e is reduced from 7.4 to 6.5 (Giffard et al. 1990; Tombaugh 1994). During ischemia, the hyperglycemic brain produces additional ATP to fuel membrane pumps, which may delay cell depolarization and calcium influx (Gisselsson et al. 1999). The increase in $[H^+]_i$ during ischemia may also decrease mitochondrial membrane permeability transition, thereby delaying the influx of calcium into the mitochondria and the resultant collapse of the electrochemical H^+ gradient.

Data from a variety of tissues suggest that decreases in pH_i coincide with reductions in the respiratory function of mitochondria (Mitchelson and Hird 1973; Mukherjee et al. 1979; Hillered et al. 1984a; Duerr and Hillman 1993). Impaired mitochondrial function has been linked to both necrotic and apoptotic cell death, consequently mitochondrial function may provide some insight into the relation between [H^+] and brain damage. In brain, Hillered et al. (1984a) reported systematic decreases in both State 3 and ADP/O ratios as mitochondria were exposed to buffers in which pH was decreased from pH 7.1 to 6.1 by either addition of lactic acid or hypercapnia. Few if any studies have followed up on these results and attempted to identify the underlying mechanism behind the pH induced impairment of mitochondrial respiration.

In this study, we measured mitochondrial respiration, membrane potential, membrane pH gradient and the recovery of membrane potential following ADP stimulation as buffer pH was varied from 5.6 to 7.4. We attempted to inhibit the reduction of mitochondrial respiratory function caused by increased H^+ concentration either by blocking free radical damage (spin trap reagent PBN), activation of the membrane permeability transition (cyclosporin A) and activation of uncoupler proteins (6-ketocholestanol).

Methods

Isolation of brain mitochondria

Rat brain mitochondria were isolated using a minor modification of the method described by Lee et al. (1993). Male Sprague-Dawley rats (300–350 g) were decapitated and the forebrain immediately removed and placed into 10 mL of ice-cold isotonic sucrose medium (SM) containing 150 mM sucrose, 10 mM N-[2-hydroxyethyl] piperazine-N'-[2-ethanesulfonic acid] (HEPES), 1 mg/mL bovine serum albumin (BSA), 0.5 mM ethylendiamine tetraacetic acid (EDTA) and 0.5 mM ethyleneglycol-bis-(β-amino-ethyl ether) N, N'-tetraacetic acid (EGTA) at pH 7.4. The forebrains were minced with scissors, decanted and rinsed with another 10 mL aliquot of SM. The minced tissue was then incubated with gentle stirring for 2 min in 10 mL of SM containing 2.5 mg/mL nagarse.

An additional 10 mL SM was then added and the tissue homogenized with three up and down strokes in a Dounce glass homogenizer with a 50.8 μm clearance pestle. The homogenate is immediately placed in two 12 mL tubes and centrifuged at 2,000 g for 3 min. The supernatants were decanted and centrifuged at 12,000 g for 8 min. The resulting pellets were resuspended in 10 mL of SM and centrifuged at 12,000 g for 8 min. The supernatants were decanted, the pellets were combined and suspended in 10 mL of 0.25 M sucrose and centrifuged at 12,000 g for 10 min. The resulting pellets were combined in 0.8 mL 0.25 M sucrose. All operations were carried out at 4° centigrade.

Respiratory activities

The respiratory activity of the rat brain mitochondrial preparations was determined polarographically using a Clark-type oxygen electrode fitted into a thermostated polycarbonate chamber with a capacity of 1 mL (Yellow Springs, Yellow Springs. OH USA). The reaction mixture (RM) consisted of 150 mM sucrose, 25 mM tris(hyroxymethyl)aminomethane hydrochloride (Tris-HCl), 10 mM KH_2PO_4, 1 mM EDTA, 1 mg/ml BSA and 0.5 mg of mitochondrial protein maintained at 30 °C. Pyruvate (4 mM) and malate (4 mM) were added and the rate of oxygen consumption determined (State 4 respiration). State 3 respiration was determined in a similar manner following addition of 0.5 μmoles ADP. Reaction mixture pH (RM_{pH}) was adjusted to pH values ranging from 5.6 to 7.4 as appropriate prior to State 4 determination by addition of concentrated HCl or KOH.

In some experiments mitochondrial respiration was determined at pH 7.4 and pH 6.0 in the presence of either 2 μM cyclosporin A (CsA) to block activation of permeability transition, 80 μM 6-ketocholestanol (kCh) to block activation of uncoupler proteins, or 5 mM of the spin-trap agent N-t-butyl-α-phenylnitrone (PBN) to scavenge free radicals.

Mitochondrial membrane potential

The rhodamine derivative, tetramethylrhodamine methyl ester (TMRM), was used to determine the membrane potential of mitochondria ($\Delta\psi$) as described by Scaduto and Grotyohann (1999). Rat brain mitochondria (0.5 mg protein/mL) were incubated in 1 mL of RM along with 4 mM pyruvate/malate and 0.2 μM TMRM. Ratiometric determinations were made at an emission of 590 nm after excitation at both 545 nm and 573 nm using a PTI DeltaScan D-140 ratio spectrofluorometer (Photon Technology International, Monmouth Junction, NJ, USA) with 2 nm bandwidth monochromometers and a water-jacketed cuvette holder that was maintained at 30 °C. Instrument control and data analyses were accomplished with FeliX™ software (PTI, Monmouth Junction, NJ, USA). The partition coefficients for the mitochondrial binding of TMRM were determined (Scaduto and Grotyohann 1999). The matrix concentration of free dye was calculated from the difference between total dye concentration and the media concentration at equilibrium. A calibration curve was then constructed between the shift in the ratio of fluorescence excitation energy and $\Delta\psi$.

Mitochondrial $\Delta\psi$ was determined during State 4 respiration at a RM_{pH} of 7.4, 7.1, 6.8, 6.4, 6.0, or 5.6. The rate at which mitochondrial $\Delta\psi$ was reestablished during State 3 respiration was determined by the addition of 0.5 mM ADP to the initial solution.

pH gradient (ΔpH)

ΔpH was determined in isolated mitochondria using the fluorescent pH indicator 2',7'-bis-(2-carboxyethyl)-5(6)-carboxyfluorescein (BCECF) as described by Czyz et al. (1995). Mitochondria were loaded with the membrane-permeant acetoxymethyl ester of BCECF (BCECF-AM) by incubation in a solution containing 0.25 M sucrose and 10 μM BCECF-AM for 10 min at 20 °C. Mitochondria were subsequently washed twice with 0.25 M sucrose. BCECF loaded rat brain mitochondria (0.5 mg protein/mL) were incubated in 1 mL of RM along with 4 mM pyruvate and 4 mM malate. The ratios of the emissions at 530 nm after excitation at both 440 nm and 490 nm ($R_{490/440}$) were measured using a PTI DeltaScan D-140 ratio spectrofluorometer in a manner similar to the $\Delta\psi$ determinations. Mitochondrial matrix pH was determined at a RM_{pH} of 7.4, 7.1, 6.8, 6.4, 6.0, or 5.6. The system was calibrated by clamping internal pH with RM_{pH} by the addition of 5 μM nigerician and 0.5 μM carbonyl cyanide 4-trifluoromethoxyphenylhydrazone (FCCP) and constructing a standard curve of RM_{pH} versus $R_{490/440}$.

Lipid peroxidation

In some experiments the RM was assayed for the production of thiobarbituric acid reactive substances (TBAR) using the method of Erdahl et al. (1991). One-tenth of a milliliter of RM was mixed with 2 mL of a solution containing 0.395% (wt/vol) 2-thiobarbituric acid, 15% (wt/vol) trichloracetic acid in a 0.25 M aqueous HCl solution containing 0.2% BHT. Color was developed by heating the tube to 80 °C for 15 min. After cooling the tubes were centrifuged to remove turbidity. The absorbance at 600 nm was subtracted from the absorbance at 532 nm and TBAR calculated from a standard curve.

Results

Mitochondrial respiration

Figure 1 shows the effect of RM_{pH} on State 4 respiratory rates in isolated brain mitochondria. As [H^+] increases in the absence of ADP there is a corresponding increase in the oxygen consumed by nonphosphorylating mitochondria. State 4 respiration increases to three times the

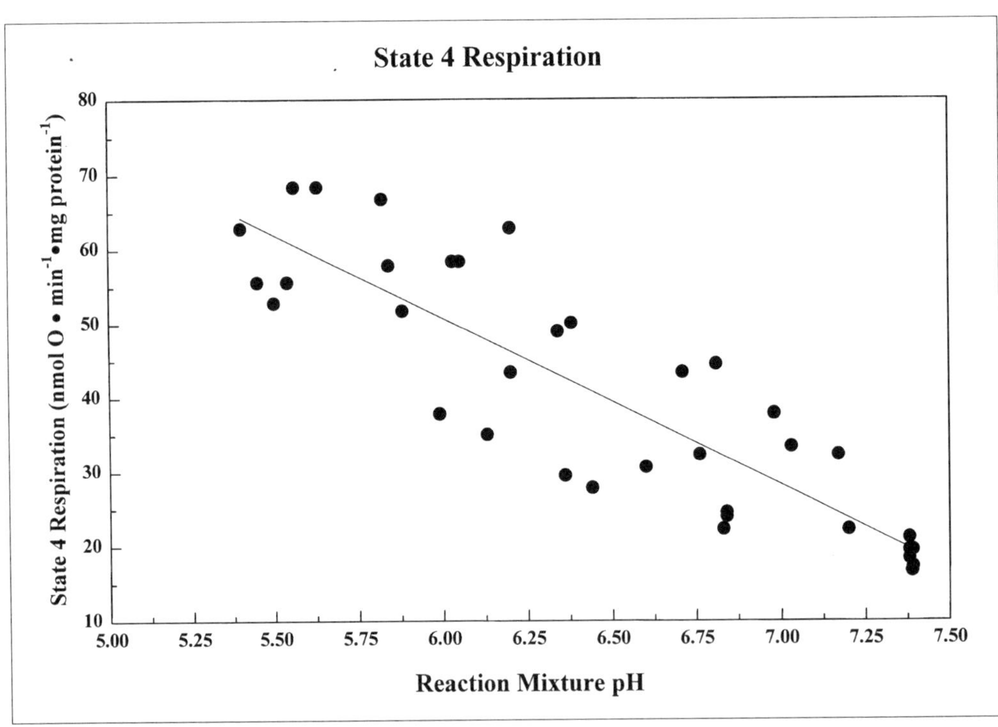

Fig. 1. State 4 respiration was initiated by the adding 4 μmol pyruvate/malate to a reaction chamber containing 0.5 mg/ml mitochondria in RM with a pH that varied from 5.4 to 7.4 ($n = 7$). Data were fitted by linear regression, $r = 0.88$, $p < 0.02$.

control rate when RM_{pH} reaches ~5.37. This suggests that an increase in $[H^+]$ results in a significant increase in the proton leak across the mitochondrial innermembrane.

Figure 2 shows the effect of RM_{pH} when pyruvate/malate supported respiration is associated with ADP phosphorylation (State 3) in isolated mitochondria. Although there is considerable scatter in the data, State 3 respiration does appear to slow as $[H^+]$ increases. At a pH of 5.6, State 3 respiration decreases to about 66% of the control rate. The effect of RM_{pH} on the respiratory control ratio (RCR) is shown in Figure 3. An increase in $[H^+]$ results in a profound loss of calculated respiratory control, which decreases to 20% of control levels at the acidic extreme. Most of the change in RCR can be attributed to the increase in State 4 respiratory rate.

There is some evidence that an increase in free radical production following hyperglycemic ischemia may result in peroxidative damage to brain mitochondrial lipids. We hypothesized that the $[H^+]$ stimulation of State 4 respiratory rate might be the result of leaky membranes caused by their exposure to free radicals. Table 1 shows that even when the concentration of a known free radical scavenger, the spin-trap reagent PBN, was increased to 10 mM, State 4 respiration continued to be stimulated by an increased level of $[H^+]$. The permeability transition inhibitor cyclosporin A has been shown to prevent mitochondrial damage induced by free radicals. However, in our system, CsA failed to prevent the $[H^+]$ stimulation of State 4 respiratory rate (Table 1). To further confirm these results we measured the level of TBAR in the RM after 10 min of State 4 respiratory activity when RM_{pH} was varied. Table 2 demonstrates that there is no measurable increase in the by-products of lipid peroxidation in these mitochondria. Taken together these data sug-

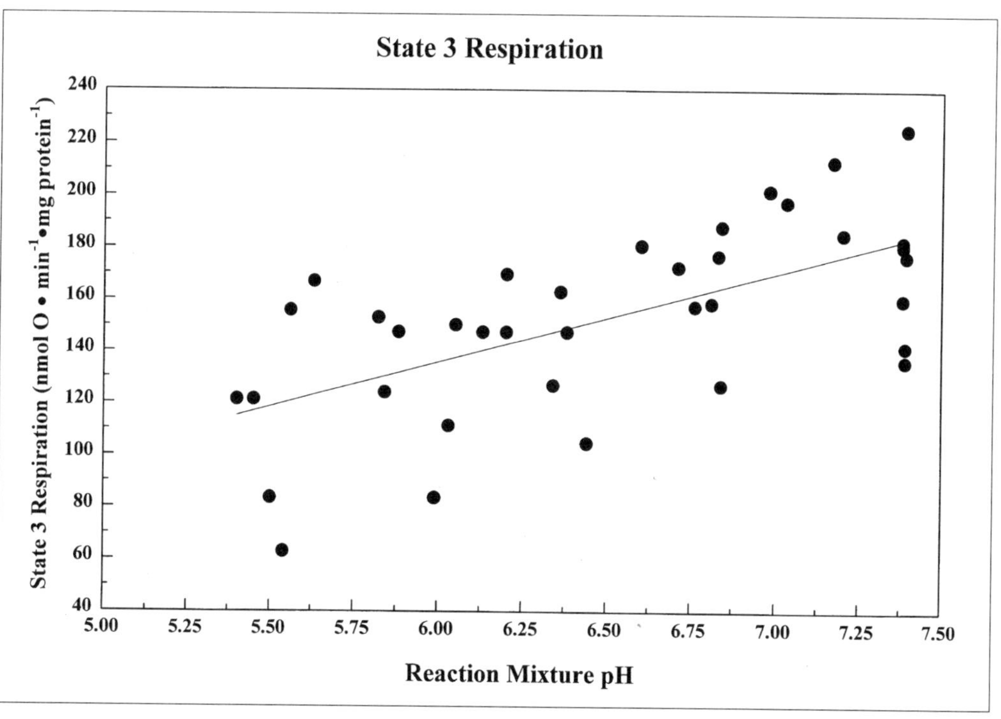

Fig. 2. State 3 respiration was initiated by the addition 0.25 μmol ADP to a reaction chamber containing 4 μmol pyruvate/malate and 0.5 mg/ml mitochondria in RM with a pH that varied from 5.4 to 7.4 (n = 7). Data were fitted by linear regression, r = 0.63, p < 0.10.

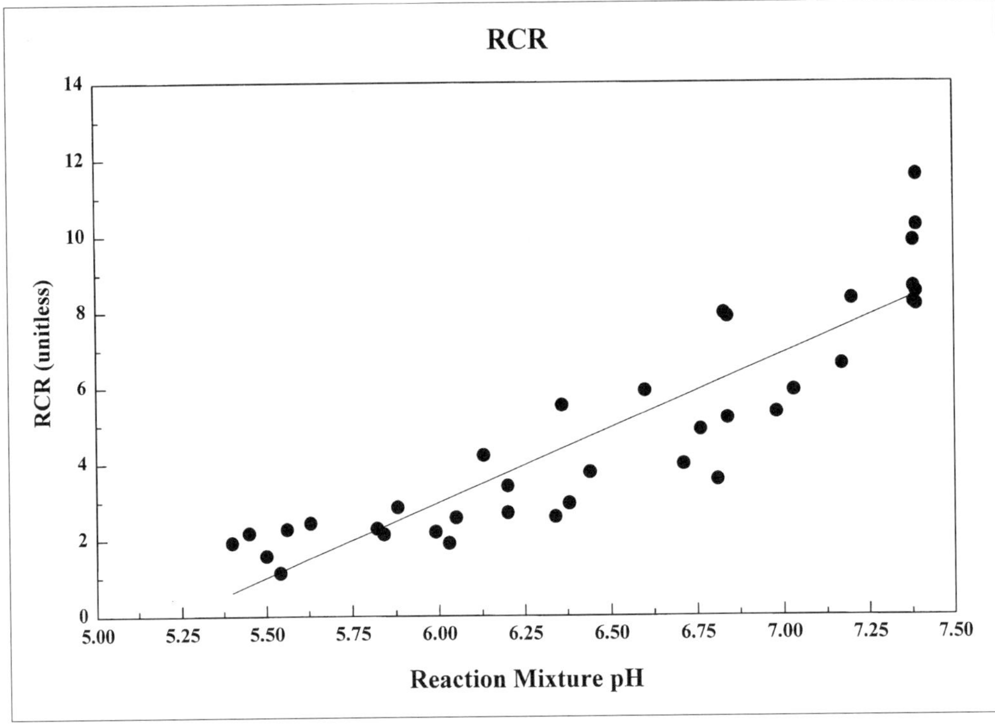

Fig. 3. State 3 and State 4 data (n = 7) from Figures 1 and 2 expressed as RCR (State 3/State 4). Data were fitted by linear regression, $r = 0.90$, $p < 0.01$.

Table 1.

	RM_{pH}	State 4 nmol O/min/g	State 3 nmol O/min/g	RCR
Control	7.4	18 ± 1	179 ± 7	10.2 ± 0.3
Control	6.0	89 ± 13	202 ± 12	2.3 ± 0.4
0.5 mM PBN	6.0	78 ± 18	188 ± 10	2.5 ± 0.7
1.0 mM PBN	6.0	76 ± 17	193 ± 10	2.6 ± 0.5
5.0 mM PBN	6.0	68 ± 19	186 ± 13	2.9 ± 0.7
10 mM PBN	6.0	77 ± 17	193 ± 12	2.6 ± 0.7
2 µM CsA	7.4	20 ± 2	184 ± 6	9.2 ± 0.6
2 µM CsA	6.0	84 ± 15	176 ± 13	2.1 ± 0.8

State 4 and State 3 respiration was determined by the addition of 4 µmol pyruvate/malate and 0.25 µmol ADP respectively to 0.5 mg/ml mitochondria in RM_{pH} of either 7.4 or 6.0. PBN was added to $RM_{pH} = 6.0$ at concentrations varying from 0.5 mM to 10 mM before determination of respiratory parameters. Data are expressed as mean ± SD, n = 3. In separate experiments, the respiratory parameters were determined in RM containing 2 µM CsA at a pH of 7.4 or 6.0. Data expressed as mean ± SD, n = 3

Table 2.

RM_{pH}	TBAR nmol/mg	State 4 nmol 0/min/mg
7.4	1.36 ± 0.39	15.1 ± 3.8
7.1	3.82 ± 4.00	25.5 ± 7.0
6.8	4.02 ± 5.71	35.4 ± 5.4*
6.4	4.07 ± 6.21	51.0 ± 7.0*
6.0	2.91 ± 4.05	60.0 ± 12.1*
5.6	1.98 ± 3.43	63.9 ± 11.0*

State 4 respiration was initiated by the addition of 4 mM pyruvate/malate to 0.5 mg/ml mitochondria in RM with a pH that varied from 5.6 to 7.4. After 5 min, an aliquot of the reaction chamber contents were assayed for TBAR; data expressed as mean ± SD, n = 3, * $p < 0.02$ compared to pH = 7.4, paired t-test.

gest that the stimulation of State 4 respiration is not the result of free radical induced oxidative damage to the innermembrane of mitochondria.

Protonmotive force

Membrane protonmotive force (Δp) is the electrochemical potential resulting from combining the electrical gradient ($\Delta\psi$), which occurs when charged species are separated by a membrane, and the chemical gradient (ΔpH), which occurs when species exist at different concentrations on either side of a membrane. Figure 4 shows the effect of decreasing RM_{pH} on mitochondrial $\Delta\psi$, ΔpH and Δp. $\Delta\psi$ decreases with decreases in RM_{pH} falling to 70% of control

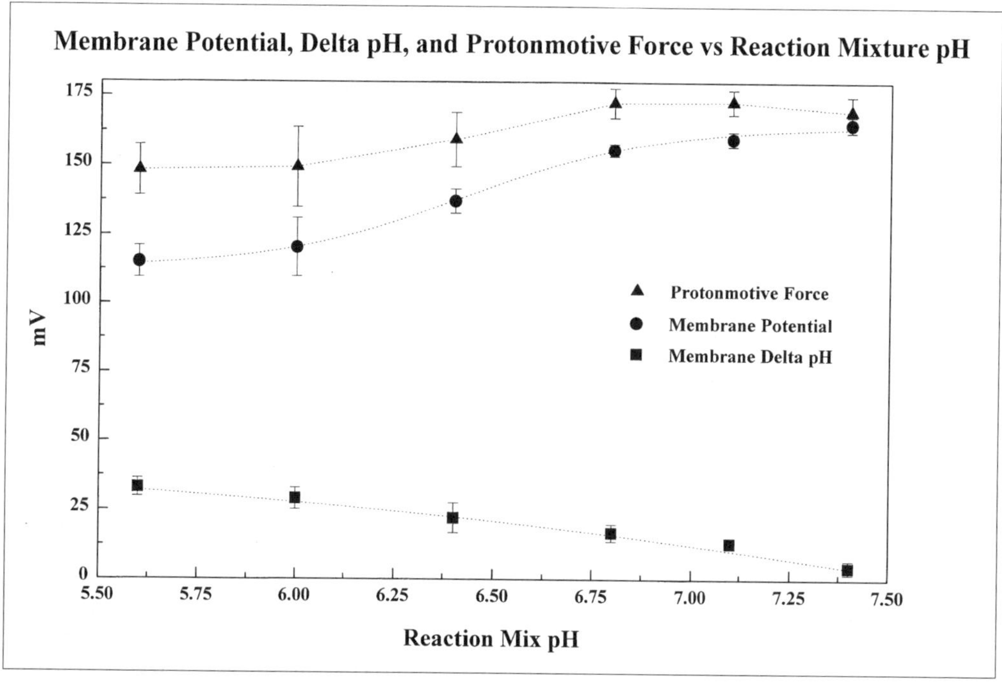

Fig. 4. The changes in mitochondrial Ψ (●), Δ pH (■) and Δ p (▲) were determined at RM_{pH} of 7.4, 7.1, 6.8, 6.4, 6.0 and 5.6. Ψ was determined by incubating mitochondria (0.5 mg/mL) with 4 mM pyruvate/malate and measuring the ratio of the emissions at 590 nm of 0.2 μM TMRM when excited at 545 nm and 573. For details see Methods. Data are expressed as mean ± SD and fit with a sigmoid curve, n = 4). Δ pH was determined by loading mitochondria with BCECF-AM and subsequently incubating the mitochondria (0.5 mg/mL) with 4 mM pyruvate/malate and determining the ratio of the emissions at 530 nm when excited at 440 nm and 490 nm. For details see Methods. Data are expressed at mean ± SD and fitted with a sigmoid curve, n = 4. Δ p was calculated from the equation $\Delta p = \Delta\Psi - Z\Delta pH$, where $Z = 2.3\ RT/F = 59$ mV using the data for ΔΨ and ΔpH from above.

when RM_{pH} reaches 5.6. A decrease in State 4 mitochondrial $\Delta\psi$ implies a change in the equilibrium between the rate that protons are pumped out by the electron transport chain and the rate at which protons reenter the matrix without the production of ATP. The points are well fit by a sigmoid curve which is typical of receptor binding kinetics. The half-maximal response occurs at a RM_{pH} of 6.45. An explanation for this relationship might be found in the proposal of Starkov (1997) who recently suggested that protonated superoxide ($HO_2^{\bullet}$) serves as an endogenous factor controlling the degree of coupling in mitochondria by effecting proteins that regulate the proton permeability of the inner mitochondrial membrane. To test this hypothesis, we measured the effect of 80 μM 6-ketocholestanol, a compound that increases the membrane dipole potential and modulates the [H^+] stimulation of State 4 respiration by both artificial and endogenous protonophores. In one experiment, however, we found that kCh failed to prevent the increase in State 4 respiration or the depression of State 3 respiration as RM_{pH} increased (data not shown).

At RM_{pH} of 7.4, the ΔpH of the mitochondria membrane in a sucrose-based low-potassium RM is very low (Fig. 4). This agrees with the studies of Czyz et al. (1995) who demonstrated that it is the electrophoretic K^+ fluxes which compensate for the electric charge transfer produced by the electron transport chain pumps and results in the formation of ΔpH in isolated mitochondria. When RM_{pH} is decreased, Δ pH increases by nearly 7.5 times (Fig. 4) and serves to partially compensate for the decrease in $\Delta\psi$. However, there is some evidence that $\Delta\psi$ and ΔpH are not thermodynamically equivalent since only the $\Delta\psi$ induces the rotary torque capable of driving ATP synthase (Dimroth et al. 2000).

$\Delta\psi$ and State 3 respiration

In a series of experiments, $\Delta\psi$ was monitored during ADP-stimulated State 3 respiration under identical conditions to our mitochondrial respiration studies (Fig. 5). $\Delta\psi$ fell immediately on addition of ADP, then it recovered slowly as ADP was phosphorylated. Typically, the $\Delta\psi$ plateaued at a level slightly higher than the initial value. The time between the lowest value of $\Delta\psi$ and the new plateau was plotted as a function of RM_{pH} (Fig. 6). When the RM_{pH} decreased from 7.4 to 5.6 there was nearly a 3-fold decrease in the rate of mitochondrial phosphorylation of ADP. The points were well fit with a straight line ($r = 0.98$). This result supports our observations that State 3 respiration and protonmotive force are depressed as RM_{pH} decreases and suggests that ATP synthase is slowed by acidosis.

Discussion

Reaction mixtures

There have been several *in-vitro* studies reporting the effect of various RM_{pH} on respiration of isolated mitochondria. The results of the studies do not clearly implicate a specific mechanism that may be responsible for the effect of RM_{pH} on mitochondrial function (Tonkonogi and Sahlin 1999). In some studies State 3 respiration decreased significantly when RM_{pH} was decreased (Fry et al. 1980; Hillered et al. 1984b; Duerr and Hillman 1993), but in other studies there was no significant response of mitochondrial function to RM acidification (Tobin et al. 1972; Senger 1975; Sitaramam and Rao 1991). These disparate findings may result from differences in experimental conditions, such as different composition of the RM. For example, Devin et al. (1997) have reported that State 3 respiration is stimulated in ionic media, yet Rolfe et al. (1994) reported that the RCR of mitochondria was decreased in ionic media. Typically, mitochondria from muscle, liver or kidney were used with a sucrose-based RM. An exception is the study of Hillered et al. (1984b), who used mitochondria from rat brain and a RM with an elevated KCl. As in our study, Hillered et al. (1984b) demonstrated that State 3 respiration slowed as RM_{pH} decreased. However, in contrast to our study, they did not observe an increase in State 4 respiration. A possible explanation for this discrepancy may be the differ-

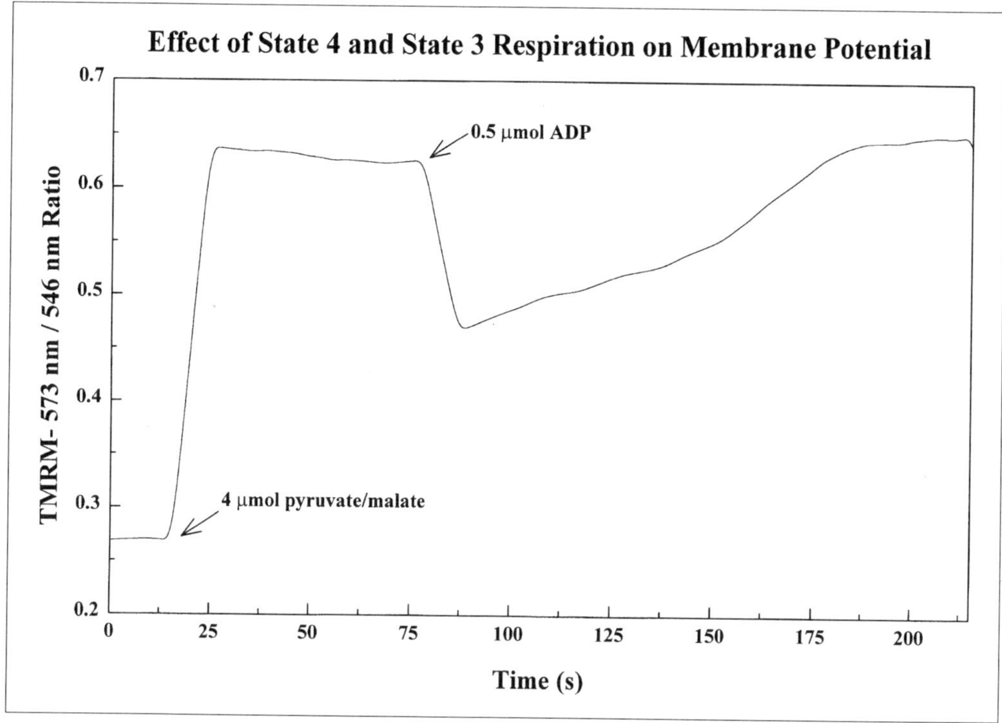

Fig. 5. A representative recording of the monitoring of 573/546 fluorescence ratio after the addition of 4 µmol pyruvate/malate to 0.5 mg/ml mitochondria. State 3 respiration was initiated by the addition of 0.5 µmol ADP. The time between when 573/546 reached its lowest value after addition of ADP and when 573/546 returned to its pre-addition value was determined. Data shown were subjected to a Lowess (locally weighted regression scatter plot smoothing) 5% smoothing using Peakfit® (SPSS Science, Chicago, IL, USA) software to reduced the noise. There was no difference in the time for restoration of $\Delta\Psi$ when determined using either raw or smoothed data.

ence in the composition of the RM used in the various studies. The RM used by Hillered et al. (1984b) was 10 mM $NaHCO_3$ in isotonic KCl equilibration with 5% CO_2. RM_{pH} was adjusted by varying both lactate and RM PCO_2. Although this RM more closely resembles cerebral intracellular fluid and would appear more appropriate, it should be noted that the buffer capacity of the RM is decreased compared to the cytosol or the RM used by other investigators. Our results are more in agreement with the study of Tonkonogi and Sahlin (1999) who observed an increase in State 4 respiration and a decrease in State 3 respiration of rat skeletal muscle mitochondria when non-ionic RM_{pH} was decreased with lactic acid.

Recently, the use of ionic media in studies of isolated mitochondria has been called into question. Devin et al. (1997) observed a 20% increase in matrix volume of liver mitochondria in ionic RM as compared to sucrose RM. These workers also observed a left shift in the relationship between State 3-respiration rate and $\Delta\psi$ in liver mitochondria in ionic RM. This suggested the possibility of an increase in inner-membrane permeability to protons. They hypothesize that the increased permeability may be due to an ionic media induced activation of the ADP/ATP translocase, which can function as a H^+-specific conductor. Alternately, the use of ionic medium may cause the activation of various transmembrane cation pathways which

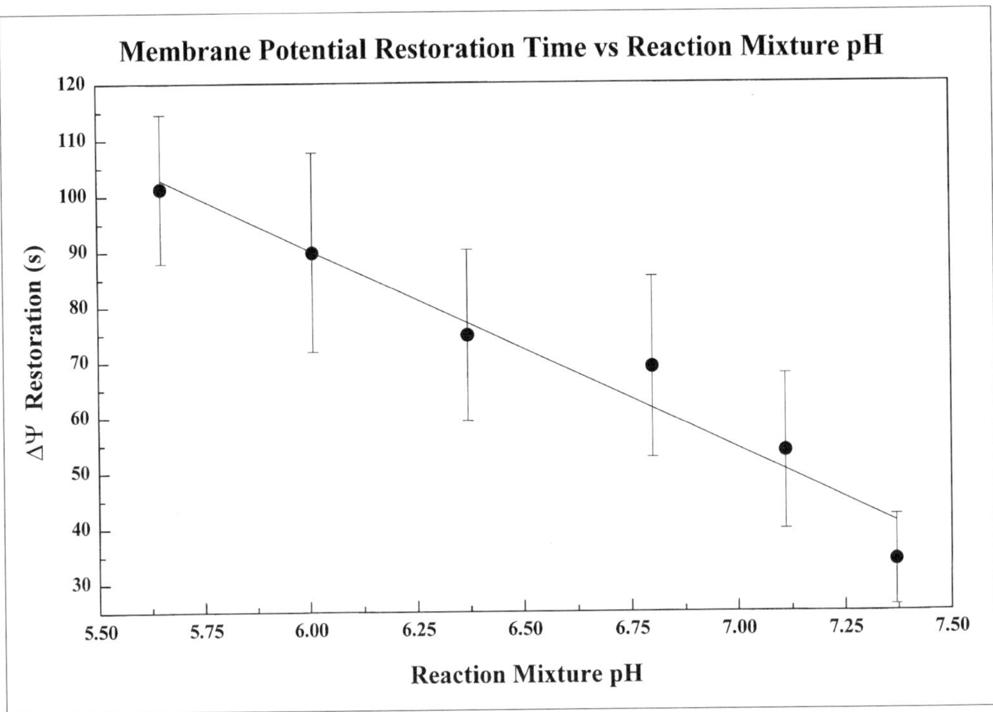

Fig. 6. Mitochondria (0.5 mg/ml) were incubated with 4 μmol pyruvate/malate in RM_{pH} at 7.4, 7.1, 6.8, 6.4, 6.0 or 5.6. State 3 respiration was initiated by the addition of 0.5 μmol ADP and the time between when ΔΨ reached its lowest value and its return to the pre-addition value. Data were expressed as mean ± SD and fit to a straight line using linear regression, n = 4, r = 0.99, $p < 0.01$.

have been described, including electroneutral cation/H^+ exchangers and electrogenic cation uniports, which can lead to dissipation of the free energy stored in protonmotive force as heat. As with all *in-vitro* studies, investigators should interpret their results cautiously and in the light of the specific experimental conditions.

Acidosis and mitochondrial function

As electrons are passed along the electron transport chain, oxygen is consumed and protons are translocated from the mitochondrial matrix to the inter-membrane space. The energy stored in this electrochemical gradient is then used by ATP synthase ($[F_0F_1]$-ATPase) to generate ATP from ADP and P_i. The production of ATP is not, however, the only route by which the electrochemical proton gradient can be dissipated. The flux through other nonproductive proton conductance pathways has been termed "proton leak". State 4 respiration is a measure of the energy required to maintain protonmotive force, which would counter this proton leak. In early work, State 4 proton conductance was considered an artifact due to damage of mitochondrial membranes sustained during the isolation procedure. However, Nobes et al. (1990) have shown that State 4 proton conductance was at least as great in mitochondria functioning in rat hepatocytes as in isolated mitochondria. This suggests that basal State 4 proton conductance across mitochondrial membranes is a normal physiological feature of undamaged mitochondria. In fact, studies have indicated that the contribution of proton leak to the standard metabolic rate of the rat is the largest single component of cellular energy metabolism and is at least 20% of the total (Brand et al. 1999).

Nicholls (1997) has proposed the concept of a proton circuit in which the transmembrane current of protons is considered to be the current and the Δp the voltage in an equivalent electrical circuit. Assuming a relationship that obeys Ohms law and a ratio of H^+/O that is invariant (Stuart et al. 1999), we calculated proton conductance during State 4 respiration as a function of RM_{pH} (Fig. 7). Acidosis increased nonproductive proton conductance across brain mitochondria membrane in a linear fashion. There are several possible mechanisms which may explain this relationship.

The mitochondrial respiratory chain produces 95% of all *in vivo* superoxide radicals ($O^{\bullet}{}_2^-$) via oxidative metabolism. During State 4 respiration, a small number a of oxygen molecules can accept a single electron to form $O^{\bullet}{}_2^-$ (Liu 1999). Other reactive oxygen species (ROS) can also be formed from $O^{\bullet}{}_2^-$. However, the activity of Mn^{2+}-superoxide dismutase and other scavenging enzymes in the mitochondria metabolize $O^{\bullet}{}_2^-$ and maintain physiological levels that are extremely low. Siesjö et al. (1985) demonstrated that acidosis promotes brain lipid peroxidation *in vitro* via increased production of ROS. ROS production has also been shown to directly result in proton leak (Mason et al. 1997; Brookes 1998) as well as result in the production of free fatty acids which are known uncouplers of oxidative phosphorylation (Wojtczak and Wieckowski 1999). However, we were unable to block the acidosis-induced increase in State 4-proton conductance with a spin-trap agent nor were we able to measure significant increases in TBAR levels. These results argue against a role for increased levels

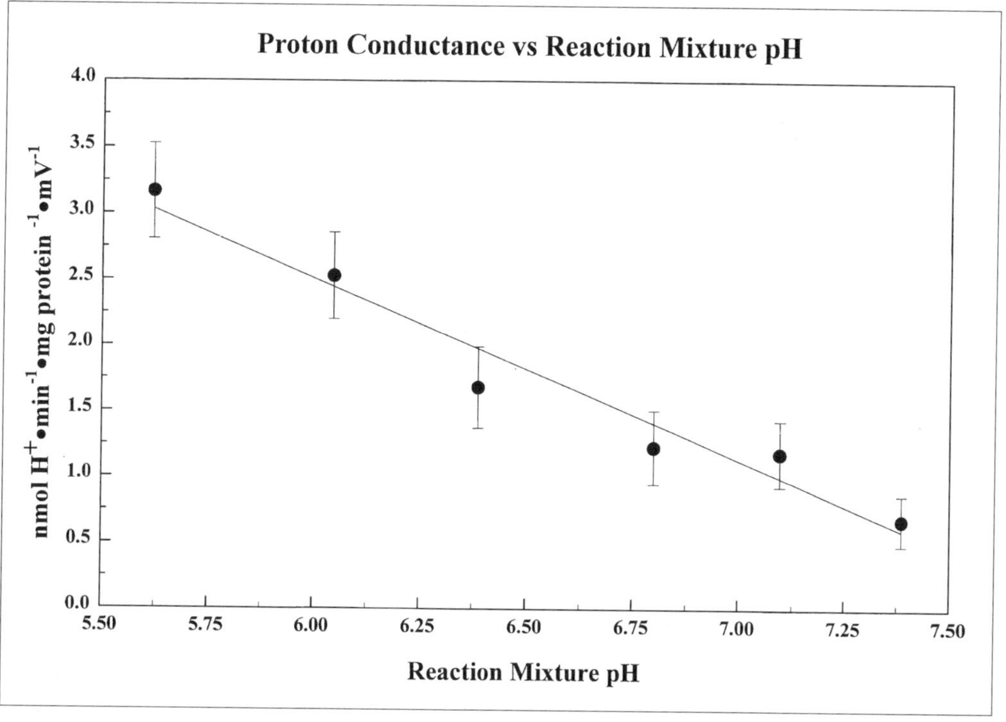

Fig. 7. The data from Figure 4 were used to calculate proton conductance (C_mH^+) using the following equation: $C_mH^+ = (JO * H/O)/\Delta p$), where JO is State 4 respiration and the H/O for NADH substrates is assumed to be 6. Data are expressed as mean ± SD and fitted with a linear regression, $n = 4$, $r = 0.96$, $p < 0.01$.

of ROS or free fatty acids in acidosis-induced increase in proton conductance.

It has been proposed that a non-productive dissipation of the proton gradient can result from the activation of a futile cycle involving K^+/H^+ antiporters and electrogenic K^+ uniporters (Belyaeva and Wojtczak 1994). However, given that we used a low-K^+ RM and the fact that most membrane ion channels are slowed by acidosis, this mechanism appears unlikely to play a role in acidosis-induced increases in State 4 proton conductance. Recently, Sanchis et al. (1998) have reported the expression of a mouse and human brain mitochondrial carrier protein (BMCP1) and shown that it uncouples respiration when cloned in yeast spheroplasts. However, there is no evidence to suggest an up-regulation of BMCP1 with a decrease in pH. This, together with the fact that kCh failed to block the acidosis-induced increase in State 4 respiration, suggests that the involvement of uncoupling protein is highly speculative; however, it is worthy of further investigation.

Finally, it has been documented that, under certain conditions, proton leakage can occur during State 4 respiration through either ADP/ATP translocase or F_0F_1-ATPase (Tonkonogi and Sahlin 1999). We plan future experiments using the specific ADP/ATP translocase blocker atractyloside and the ATP synthase blocker oligomycin to investigate the roles these enzymes might play in the acidosis-induced increase in proton conductance that we observe.

Acidosis, mitochondria and ischemic brain damage

There is no doubt that the level of acidosis during global brain ischemia negatively influences subsequent recovery; however, the precise mechanisms involved in this pathology remain unclear (Siesjö et al. 1996). It is doubtful that the acidosis-induced damage which occurs either during the insult or the initial stages of reoxygenation is only manifested hours or even days following the insult. Thus, we are confronted with envisioning mechanisms that would explain how damage related to acidosis "matures" over a period of time. Such mechanisms might include depression of mitochondrial bioenergetics, activation of DNAses, or enhancement of free radical damage (Li and Siesjö 1997).

The principle finding of our study is that acidosis increased mitochondrial State 4 proton conductance and depressed State 3 respiration in low-KCl RM. These results appear to contradict our findings that mitochondria isolated from rats following 30 min of global hyperglycemic ischemia had significantly higher RCR values at the end of ischemia and following 60 min of reoxygenation than normoglycemic rats (Kintner et al. 1997). There was no change in State 4 respiration at the end of ischemia or following reoxygenation in either normo- or hyperglycemic rats (unreported results). Wagner and Myers (1986) have reported similar findings using mitochondria isolated from the brains of normo- and hyperglycemic cats subjected to 8 min of anoxia. However, both of these studies used high-KCl RM to determined mitochondrial respiratory indexes and the question remains as to how mitochondria that have been made ischemic would respond when the RM_{pH} is decreased *in vitro*.

We have used high field strength ^{31}P-NMR to determine brain pH_e and pH_i during 12 min of normoglycemic (blood glucose = 5.5 mM) and hyperglycemic ischemia (blood glucose = 15 mM) in the intact rat (data not shown). After 5.5 min of normoglycemic ischemia, pH reached a plateau of 6.4 for both pH_i and pH_e. In contrast, the pH_i and pH_e of hyperglycemic rats decreased significantly further (pH = 5.8) and took considerably longer (8.5 min) to plateau. Our data would suggest that upon reoxygenation the rate to ATP restoration should be significantly depressed in hyperglycemic rats (Fig. 6) and that the mitochondrial membrane proton conductance would be enhanced (Fig. 7). It is not clear, however, how these factors would negatively impact post-ischemic recovery. Hurn et al. (1991) have proposed a pH_i of 5.5–5.7 as an apparent endpoint for the recovery of high-energy metabolites in the ischemic dog brain. In our study, this level of RM_{pH} would be expected to result in a profound inhibition of ADP phosphorylation (Fig. 6). On the other hand, the acidosis-induced decrease of mitochondrial $\Delta\psi$ at a pH_i of 5.5–5.7 would tend to decrease the rate of ROS production by the electron transport chain (Liu 1999), although it should be noted that Siesjö et al. (1985) have proposed a theoretical connection between acidosis and free radical production through the release of iron from transferrin-like proteins.

It is far from clear what the effect of acidosis is on brain mitochondria both during and following ischemia and what further investigation is warranted. In particular, it is important to learn how mitochondria, which have been subjected to ischemia prior to isolation, perform in a RM that is similar in pH to that in cytosol found from either normo- or hyperglycemic brains subjected to ischemia.

Acknowledgement

The authors thank Donna Brackett for her skillful preparation of this manuscript and Dr. Jeff Walker for the use of the spectrofluorometer. This research was supported by University of Wisconsin Department of Neurological Surgery Research and Development Funds.

References

1. Belyaeva EA, Wojtczak L (1994) An attempt to quantify K^+ fluxes in rat liver mitochondria. Biochem Mol Biol Int 33:165–175
2. Brand MD, Brindle KM, Buckingham JA, Harper JA, Rolfe DF, Stuart JA (1999) The significance and mechanism of mitochondrial proton conductance. Int J Obes Relat Metab Disord 23(Suppl 6):S4–S11
3. Brookes PS (1998) Mitochondrial proton leak and superoxide generation: an hypothesis. Biochem Soc Trans 26:S331
4. Cohen Y, Chang LH, Litt L, Kim F, Severinghaus JW, Weinstein PR, Davis RL, Germano I, James TL (1990) Stability of brain intracellular lactate and ^{31}P-metabolite levels at reduced intracellular pH during prolonged hypercapnia in rats. J Cereb Blood Flow Metab 10:277–284
5. Combs DJ, Dempsey RJ, Maley M, Donaldson D, Smith C (1990) Relationship between plasma glucose, brain lactate, and intracellular pH during cerebral ischemia in gerbils. Stroke 21:936–942
6. Czyz A, Szewczyk A, Nalecz MJ, Wojtczak L (1995) The role of mitochondrial potassium fluxes in controlling the protonmotive force in energized mitochondria. Biochem Biophys Res Commun 210:98–104
7. Devin A, Guerin B, Rigoulet M (1997) Control of oxidative phosphorylation in rat liver mitochondria: effect of ionic media. Biochim Biophys Acta 1319:293–300
8. Dimroth P, Kaim G, Matthey U (2000) Crucial role of the membrane potential for ATP synthesis by F(1)F(o) ATP synthases. J Exp Biol 203:t-9
9. Duerr JM, Hillman SS (1993) An analysis of pH tolerance and substrate preference of isolated skeletal muscle mitochondria from Bufo marinus and Rana catesbeiana. Comp Biochem Physiol [B] 106:889–893
10. Erdahl WL, Krebsbach RJ, Pfeiffer DR (1991) A comparison of phospholipid degradation by oxidation and hydrolysis during the mitochondrial permeability transition. Arch Biochem Biophys 285:252–260
11. Fry DE, Ratcliffe DJ, Yates JR (1980) The effects of acidosis on canine hepatic and renal oxidative phosphorylation. Surgery 88:269–273
12. Giffard RG, Monyer H, Christine CW, Choi DW (1990) Acidosis reduces NMDA receptor activation, glutamate neurotoxicity, and oxygen-glucose deprivation neuronal injury in cortical cultures. Brain Res 506:339–342
13. Gisselsson L, Smith ML, Siesjo BK (1999) Hyperglycemia and focal brain ischemia. J Cereb Blood Flow Metab 19:288–297
14. Hillered L, Ernster L, Siesjö BK (1984b) Influence of *in vitro* lactic acidosis and hypercapnia on respiratory activity of isolated rat brain mitochondria. J Cereb Blood Flow Metab 4:430–437
15. Hillered L, Siesjö BK, Arfors KE (1984a) Mitochondrial response to transient forebrain ischemia and recirculation in the rat. J Cereb Blood Flow Metab 4:438–446
16. Hurn PD, Koehler RC, Norris SE, Blizzard KK, Traystman RJ (1991) Dependence of cerebral energy phosphate and evoked potential recovery on end-ischemic pH. Am J Physiol 260:Pt 2):H532–541
17. Katsura K, Ekholm A, Asplund B, Siesjö BK (1991) Extracellular pH in the brain during ischemia: relationship to the severity of lactic acidosis. J Cereb Blood Flow Metab 11:597–599
18. Katsura K, Kristian T, Smith ML, Siesjö BK (1994) Acidosis induced by hypercapnia exaggerates ischemic brain damage. J Cereb Blood Flow Metab 14:243–250
19. Kintner DB, Fitzpatrick JH, Jr., Gilboe DD (1997) Hyperglycemic damage to mitochondrial membranes during cerebral ischemia: Amelioration by PAF antagonist BN 50739. J Neurochem 69:1219–1227
20. Lee CP, Sciamanna MA, Peterson PL (1993) Intact Rat Brain Mitochondria from a Single Animal: Prepartion and Properties. In: Methods in Toxicology, vol 2 Academic Press, pp 41–50
21. Li PA, Siesjö BK (1997) Role of hyperglycaemia-related acidosis in ischaemic brain damage. Acta Physiol Scand 161:567–580
22. Liu SS (1999) Cooperation of a "reactive oxygen cycle" with the Q cycle and the proton cycle in the respiratory chain-superoxide generating and cycling mechanisms in mitochondria. J Bioenerg Biomembr 31:367–376
23. Maruki Y, Koehler RC, Kirsch JR, Blizzard KK, Traystman RJ (1995) Tirilazad pretreatment improves early cerebral metabolic and blood flow recovery from hyperglycemic ischemia. J Cereb Blood Flow Metab 15:88–96
24. Mason RP, Walter MF, Mason PE (1997) Effect of oxidative stress on membrane structure: small-angle X-ray diffraction analysis. Free Radic Biol Med 23:4–25
25. Mitchelson KR, Hird FJ (1973) Effect of pH and halothane on muscle and liver mitochondria. Am J Physiol 225:1393–1398
26. Mukherjee A, Wong TM, Templeton G, Buja LM, Willerson JT (1979) Influence of volume dilution, lactate, phosphate, and calcium on mitochondrial functions. Am J Physiol 237:H224–H238
27. Nicholls DG (1997) The non-Ohmic proton leak – 25 years on. Biosci Rep 17:251–257

28. Nobes CD, Brown GC, Olive PN, Brand MD (1990) Non-ohmic proton conductance of the mitochondrial inner membrane in hepatocytes. J Biol Chem 265:12903–12909
29. Rolfe DF, Hulbert AJ, Brand MD (1994) Characteristics of mitochondrial proton leak and control of oxidative phosphorylation in the major oxygen-consuming tissues of the rat. Biochim Biophys Acta 1188:405–416
30. Sanchis D, Fleury C, Chomiki N, Goubern M, Huang Q, Neverova M, Gregoire F, Easlick J, Raimbault S, Levi-Meyrueis C, Miroux B, Collins S, Seldin M, Richard D, Warden C, Bouillaud F, Ricquier D (1998) BMCP1, a novel mitochondrial carrier with high expression in the central nervous system of humans and rodents, and respiration uncoupling activity in recombinant yeast. J Biol Chem 273:34611–34615
31. Scaduto RCJ, Grotyohann LW (1999) Measurement of mitochondrial membrane potential using fluorescent rhodamine derivatives. Biophys J 76:t-77
32. Senger H (1975) Changes of the oxidative phosphorylation in mitchondria of rat skeletal muscle following strenous exercise. Acta Biol Med Ger 34:181–188
33. Siesjö BK, Bendek G, Koide T, Westerberg E, Wieloch T (1985) Influence of acidosis on lipid peroxidation in brain tissues *in vitro*. J Cereb Blood Flow Metab 5:253–258
34. Siesjö BK, Katsura KI, Kristian T, Li PA, Siesjö P (1996) Molecular mechanisms of acidosis-mediated damage. Acta Neurochir Suppl (Wien) 66:8–14
35. Sitaramam V, Rao NM (1991) Oxidative phosphorylation in rat liver mitochondria: influence of physical parameters. Indian J Biochem Biophys 28:401–407
36. Starkov AA (1997) "Mild" uncoupling of mitochondria. Biosci Rep 17:273–279
37. Stuart JA, Brindle KM, Harper JA, Brand MD (1999) Mitochondrial proton leak and the uncoupling proteins. J Bioenerg Biomembr 31:517–525
38. Tobin RB, Mackerer CR, Mehlman MA (1972) pH effects on oxidative phosphorylation of rat liver mitochondria. Am J Physiol 223:83–88
39. Tombaugh GC (1994) Mild acidosis delays hypoxic spreading depression and improves neuronal recovery in hippocampal slices. J Neurosci 14:5635–5643
40. Tonkonogi M, Sahlin K (1999) Actively phosphorylating mitochondria are more resistant to lactic acidosis than inactive mitochondria. Am J Physiol 277:t-93
41. Wagner KR, Myers RE (1986) Hyperglycemia preserves brain mitochondrial respiration during anoxia. J Neurochem 47:1620–1626
42. Wojtczak L, Wieckowski MR (1999) The mechanisms of fatty acid-induced proton permeability of the inner mitochondrial membrane. J Bioenerg Biomembr 31:447–455
43. Xu Y, Cohen Y, Litt L, Chang LH, James TL (1991) Tolerance of low cerebral intracellular pH in rats during hyperbaric hypercapnia. Stroke 22:1303–1308

Cytochrome c release in apoptotic and excitotoxic neuron death

J. H. M. Prehn, N. T. Bui, A. J. Krohn, C. M. Luetjens, M. Poppe, C. Reimertz

Abstract

Apoptotic and excitotoxic mechanisms have been implicated in neuron death after cerebral ischemia. Evidence is accumulating that mitochondria play an important role in both types of cell death by increasing the production of reactive oxygen species and by releasing pro-apoptotic factors into the cytosol. Excitotoxic neuron death was induced in cultured rat hippocampal neurons by a brief exposure to the glutamate receptor agonist N-methyl-D-aspartate. Apoptotic neuron death was induced by an exposure to the protein kinase inhibitor staurosporine. During excitotoxic neuron death, mitochondria depolarized, increased the production of reactive oxygen species, and released cytochrome c. During apoptotic neuron death, mitochondria also released cytochrome c, but remained polarized until apoptosis was maximally activated. Staurosporine-induced cytochrome c release and apoptosis were insensitive to inhibitors of the permeability transition pore (PTP). Moreover, the selective PTP inhibitor N-methylvaline-4-cyclosporin did not alter the kinetics of staurosporine-induced cytochrome c release monitored confocally in MCF-7 cells stably overexpressing green fluorescent protein-tagged cytochrome c. Treatment with N-methylvaline-4-cyclosporin also failed to inhibit cytochrome c release during excitotoxic neuron death. Our data suggest that excitotoxic and apoptotic neuronal injury trigger the mitochondrial release of cytochrome c, but question the role of the PTP in these events.

Introduction

Apoptotic cell death is required for the development of the nervous system (Li and Yuan 1999). Evidence is growing that apoptotic mechanisms are also involved in neuron death after cerebral ischemia (Dirnagl et al. 1999). Most of the morphological and biochemical changes during neuronal apoptosis are caused by the activation of a family of cytosolic cysteine proteases, the caspases (Li and Yuan 1999; Porter and Jänicke 1999). Release of cytochrome c from the mitochondrial intercristal space into the cytosol triggers caspase activation during apoptosis (Liu et al. 1996; Kroemer and Reed 2000). Cytoplasmic cytochrome c induces a caspase-3 activating complex, composed of cytochrome

Keywords: Mitochondrial membrane potential; Permeability transition pore; Cytochrome c; Reactive oxygen species; Apoptosis; Excitotoxicity

Interdisciplinary Center for Clinical Research (IZKF), University of Münster, Röntgenstr. 21, D-48149 Münster, Germany.
e-mail: prehn@uni-muenster.de

c, Apaf-1, dATP and procaspase-9 (Li et al. 1997; Zou et al. 1997). In the so-called extrinsic pathway, ligand binding to death receptors triggers the caspase-8-mediated cleavage of Bid, a BH3 domain-containing pro-apoptotic Bcl-2 family member (Li et al. 1998; Luo et al. 1998). The truncated form tBid triggers cytochrome c release from mitochondria and thereby amplifies the apoptotic caspase cascade (Li et al. 1998; Luo et al. 1998). In the so-called intrinsic pathway, release of cytochrome c occurs independently of upstream caspases (Bossy-Wetzel et al. 1998) and is tightly controlled by the activity of pro- and anti-apoptotic Bcl-2 family members (Kluck et al. 1997; Yang et al. 1997; Kroemer and Reed 2000).

The release of cytochrome c from the intracristal space requires a reversible or irrevserible permeability increase of the outer mitochondrial membrane. The precise release mechanisms in apoptosis are still controversial (Kroemer and Reed 2000), with several theories arguing for selective opening (of pores) of the outer mitochondrial membrane (Van der Heiden et al. 1997; Eskes et al. 1998; Kluck et al. 1999; Shimizu et al. 1999; Shimizu and Tsujimoto 2000), and another theory arguing for opening of the inner and outer mitochondrial membranes after the induction of the permeability transition pore (PTP) (Bernardi and Petronilli 1996; Beutner et al. 1996; Marchetti et al. 1996; Nicolli et al. 1996; Marzo et al. 1998). The PTP is induced by an increase in matrix Ca^{2+}, prooxidants, mitochondrial depolarization, and results in ATP depletion and matrix swelling (Zoratti and Szabo 1995). The PTP allows the non-specific permeability of solutes under 1.5 kDa. Since cytochrome c has a molecular weight of 12.5 kDa, the PTP could trigger cytochrome c release by inducing mitochondrial swelling and a rupture of the outer mitochondrial membrane. Because PTP opening results in inner membrane permeability to protons, it is associated with a reversible or irreversible decrease in mitochondrial transmembrane potential ($\Delta\Psi m$) (Zoratti and Szabo 1995; Bernardi and Petronilli 1996). Interestingly, mitochondrial depolarization has been shown to be an early signal specific for another form of neuronal injury, excitotoxic neuron death (White and Reynolds 1996). In light of the increasing evidence that both excitotoxic and apoptotic mechanisms are involved in ischemic neuron death, we investigated the role of cytochrome c release and $\Delta\Psi m$ in both types of neuronal injury.

Release of cytochrome c in excitotoxic neuron death is accompanied by mitochondrial depolarization

We investigated the role of mitochondrial depolarization and cytochrome c release in Ca^{2+}-dependent excitotoxic neuron death of cultured rat hippocampal neurons. A 5-min exposure to the selective glutamate receptor agonist N-methyl-D-aspartate (NMDA; 300 μM) induced a delayed cell death in approx. 40% of the hippocampal neurons assessed 24 h after the exposure (Sengpiel et al. 1998; Luetjens et al. 2000). The percentage of damaged neurons did not increase up to 4–8 h after termination of the NMDA exposure (Lankiewicz et al. 2000; Luetjens et al. 2000). To investigate changes in $\Delta\Psi m$ during and after the 5-min NMDA exposure, we determined the uptake of rhodamine-123 (R-123), a voltage-sensitive probe that detects changes in $\Delta\Psi m$ (Emaus et al. 1986), using confocal laser scanning microscopy. Cells were exposed to NMDA or Hepes-buffered saline (sham exposure) and loaded with R-123 (30 nM). Mitochondrial R-123 uptake was indistinguishable from that of sham-exposed controls immediately as well as 2 h after the 5-min NMDA exposure. However, a significant decline in mitochondrial R-123 uptake was observed 6 h after the NMDA exposure, suggesting a delayed mitochondrial depolarization (Fig. 1).

We next investigated changes in cytochrome c distribution by immunofluorescence analysis. In sham-exposed controls, cytochrome c immunoreactivity was intense, distributed in a rod-like pattern, and co-localized with Mitotracker Green FM, a potential-insensitive mitochondrial marker (Krohn et al. 1999) (Fig. 1). Two h after the NMDA exposure, cytochrome c immunoreactivity was comparable to that of sham-exposed controls. By 8 h, many hippocampal

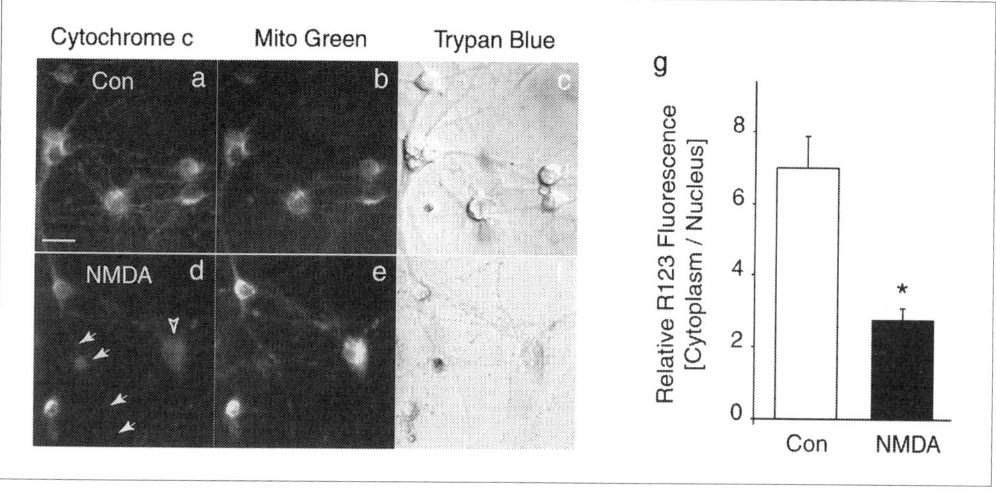

Fig. 1. NMDA-induced cytochrome c release is accompanied by mitochondrial depolarization. Loss of mitochondrial cytochrome c after NMDA receptor overactivation. **a.–c.** Control culture 8 h after sham-exposure (Con), showing a rod-like cytochrome c immunofluorescence that colocalizes with Mitotracker Green FM fluorescence. **d.–f.** Hippocampal neurons 8 h after a 5-min NMDA exposure (300 µM). Note the loss of cytochrome c immunofluorescence in the neuron indicated by an open arrowhead. Mitochondria could still be labeled with the potential-insensitive marker Mitotracker Green FM (Mito Green). Trypan blue was excluded from the cell. Loss of cytochrome c immumofluorescence was particularly pronounced along neurites of individual hippocampal neurons (arrows). Scale bar = 25 µm. **g.** Mitochondrial depolarization after NMDA receptor overactivation. Confocal imaging of R-123 uptake was performed in hippocampal neurons 6 h after a 5-min exposure to NMDA (300 µM) or Mg^{2+}-free Hepes-buffered saline (Con). Fluorescence data in the histogram are given as the ratio between the average pixel intensity of the neuronal soma and the nucleus according to Wadia et al. (1998) to compensate for background differences and unequal R-123 loading. Data are means ± SEM from n = 60 and 64 neurons, respectively, in n = 3 separate cultures per treatment. Difference between NMDA- and sham-exposed cells: * $p < 0.05$ (t-test).

neurons showed a reduced, diffuse cytochrome c immunofluorescence in their neuronal soma, as well as a significant loss of cytochrome c immunofluorescence along their neurites (Fig. 1). Of note, mitochondria could still be labeled with Mitotracker Green FM. Similar results were obtained by double-staining with an antibody recognizing the mitochondrial matrix protein superoxide dismutase-2 (Luetjens et al. 2000). After 8 h, approx. 54% of the hippocampal neurons that excluded trypan-blue lost their cytochrome c immunoreactivity, but were still positive for mitochondrial markers. These data indicate that delayed mitochondrial depolarization during excitotoxic neuron death is accompanied by mitochondrial cytochrome c release.

To investigate the invovement of the PTP in NMDA-induced cytochrome c release, we treated cultured rat hippocampal neurons with N-methylvaline-4-cyclosporin (1.6 µM). This drug inhibits the opening of the mitochondrial PTP by binding to the matrix protein cyclophilin D (Nicolli et al. 1996). Hippocampal neurons pretreated for 30 min with N-methylvaline-4-cyclosporin released their cytochrome c to the same extent as NMDA-exposed cultures treated with the vehicle (Table 1).

Mitochondrial superoxide production – an event downstream of mitochondrial cytochrome c release

While many studies have focused on the role of cytochrome c release to activate the caspase cascade (Liu et al. 1996; Li et al. 1997), loss of cytochrome c may also affect mitochondrial electron transport and mitochondrial free radical

Table 1. The PTP inhibitor N-methylvaline-4-cyclosporin does not alter NMDA-induced cytochrome c release.

Exposure	Treatment	Loss of Cytochrome C (% Cells)
Sham	Vehicle	6.7 ± 3.6
Sham	SDZ, 1.6 µM	9.6 ± 2.0
NMDA	Vehicle	49.7 ± 7.8
NMDA	SDZ, 1.6 µM	50.1 ± 8.8

Cultured rat hippocampal neurons were exposed to 300 µM NMDA or Mg^{2+}-free Hepes-buffered saline (Sham) for 5 min, washed and returned to the original culture medium. Cultures were pretreated for 30 min with N-methylvaline-4-cyclosporin (SDZ) or vehicle. The drug was present in the cultures during and after the NMDA exposure. After 8 h, cultures were fixed and cytochrome c distribution was determined by immunofluorescence analysis using a mouse monoclonal antibody. Data are means ± SD from n = 3 independent experiments. There was no statistically significant difference between the respective vehicle- and drug-treated cultures.

production (Krippner et al. 1996; Cai and Jones 1998). Cytochrome c transports electrons between complexes III and IV of the mitochondrial respiratory chain. A pronounced loss of cytochrome c could cause a disruption of the mitochondrial electron transport, leading to an accumulation of reducing equivalents. As a consequence, complex I and the ubiquinone at complex II will maintain in their reduced state. This condition is known to increase 1-electron reduction of molecular oxygen, presumably due to autooxidation of complex I and ubiquinone, and will lead to an enhanced superoxide formation (Boveris et al. 1976; Turrens and Boveris 1980). We were therefore interested to quantify superoxide production in the hippocampal neuron cultures after the NMDA-induced release of cytochrome c using the oxidation-sensitive probe hydroethidine. Hydroethidine is oxidized by superoxide to its fluorescent product, ethidium (Bindokas et al. 1996). Cultures exposed to NMDA for 5 min and allowed to recover for 8 h indeed showed an increased superoxide production compared to sham-exposed controls (Fig. 2). Increased superoxide production was also observed in cultures treated with the mitochondrial complex III inhibitor antimycin A (10 µM) (Fig. 2).

A previous study provided evidence that the loss of cytochrome c could be related to the increased superoxide production during apoptosis (Cai and Jones 1998). If electron flow through complex III was already inhibited by a treatment with antimycin A, NMDA should fail to stimulate a further increase in superoxide production. Quantification of hydroethidine oxidation in rat hippocampal neurons 8 h after the exposure revealed that NMDA indeed failed to increase superoxide production in the presence of antimycin A (Fig. 2). In contrast, NMDA-exposed neurons increased their superoxide production in the presence of paraquat (100 µM), an agent that increases superoxide inde-

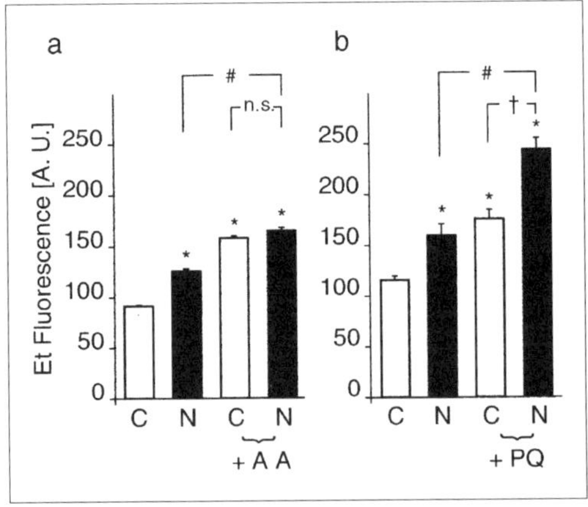

Fig. 2. Delayed superoxide production in NMDA-exposed neuron cultures: effect of antimycin A and paraquat. Cultured rat hippocampal neurons were exposed to 300 µM NMDA (N) or Mg^{2+}-free Hepes-buffered saline (C) for 5 min, washed and returned to the original culture medium. After 8 h, cultures were incubated at 37 °C in Hepes buffer supplemented with 2 µg/ml hydroethidine plus 1 µM of the NMDA antagonist dizocilpine, and either 10 µM antimycin A (AA) (**a.**), 100 µM paraquat (PQ) (**b.**), or respective vehicle. Ethidium (Et) production of individual hippocampal neurons was quantified by fluorescence microscopy. Data are means ± SEM from n = 174–373 neurons in two separate experiments per treatment. * $P < 0.05$: Different from sham-exposed controls. # $P < 0.05$: Different from NMDA-exposed controls. † $P < 0.05$: Different from respective drug-treated control. n.s., not statistically significant (ANOVA and Tukey test). A.U., arbitrary fluorescence units. Data from Luetjens et al. (2000).

pendently of the activity of the mitochondrial respiratory chain (Smith et al. 1978).

Superoxide production and cytochrome c release have also been observed during nerve growth factor withdrawal- and staurosporine (STS)-induced neuronal apoptosis at similar time points in the death cascade (Greenlund et al. 1995; Deshmukh and Johnson 1998; Krohn et al. 1998, 1999). We investigated the relationship between cytochrome c release and superoxide production in human D283 medulloblastoma cells deficient in mitochondrial respiration (ρ^- cells). Treatment with the apoptosis-inducing protein kinase inhibitor STS (Falcieri et al. 1993) induced mitochondrial release of cytochrome c, caspase activation and apoptotic cell death both in control and ρ^- cells (Luetjens et al. 2000). Only in control cells, however, loss of cytochrome c was accompanied by an increased superoxide production. It is therefore conceivable that loss of cytochrome c triggers an increased mitochondrial superoxide production via a defect in mitochondrial electron transport.

Staurosporine-induced neuronal apoptosis does not require mitochondrial depolarization

Exposure of rat hippocampal neurons to STS has been shown to trigger neuronal apoptosis (Prehn et al. 1997; Krohn et al. 1998, 1999). We investigated changes in $\Delta\Psi_m$ during STS-induced neuronal apoptosis. To determine a time-course of caspase activation in this model, hippocampal neuron cultures were exposed to 300 nM STS. Caspase-3-like activity was determined by quantifying the cleavage of the fluorogenic caspase-3 substrate acetyl-DEVD-aminomethylcoumarin (Ac-DEVD-AMC) by extracts from STS-treated neurons (Krohn et al. 1999). By 2 h of STS exposure, cleavage activity had already increased 5- to 7-fold compared to controls. By 8 h, caspase-3-like activity reached its maximum (Fig. 3). Tetramethylrhodamine ethyl ester (TMRE), a cationic, lipophilic dye was used for the estimation of

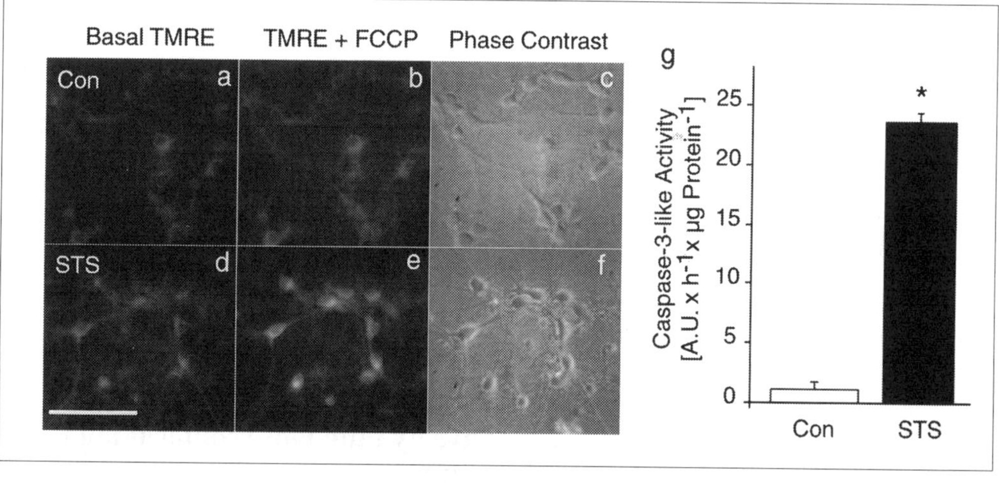

Fig. 3. Mitochondria do not depolarize during staurosporine-induced neuronal apoptosis. Representative TMRE images from vehicle- and 300 nM staurosporine (STS)-treated rat hippocampal neurons. **a.** Control cultures exposed for 8 h to vehicle (dimethylsulfoxide). Baseline TMRE fluorescence image was taken after loading cells with 100 nM TMRE. **b.** Peak TMRE fluorescence after treatment with 0.1 µM FCCP. **c.** Phase contrast image. **d.** and **e.** Basal and FCCP fluorescence of cultures exposed for 8 h to 300 nM STS. Note that cells take up TMRE and respond to FCCP-induced mitochondrial depolarization. The higher fluorescence of STS-treated cells is clearly visible. **f.** Phase contrast image. Bar = 50 µm. **f.** Detection of caspase 3-like protease activity in cultures treated for 8 h with vehicle (Con) or 300 nM STS. Caspase-3-like protease activity was measured by cleavage of the fluorogenic substrate Ac-DEVD-AMC (10 µM). Activities are represented as increase in AMC fluorescence (in arbitrary fluorescence units) over 60 min per µg protein. Data are means ± SEM from n = 6 cultures. Different from controls * $p < 0.05$ (t-test).

$\Delta\Psi_m$ during STS-induced apoptosis. In this set of experiments, TMRE uptake was quantified by digital video microscopy. Cultures treated with 300 nM STS were loaded with 100 nM TMRE in a Hepes-buffered salt solution. TMRE remained present in the buffer solution during the entire course of the data collection. In comparison to controls exposed to the vehicle dimethylsulfoxide, there was no decrease in mitochondrial TMRE uptake, indicative of mitochondrial depolarization, during the STS exposure (Fig. 3). On the contrary, STS-treated cells showed increased TMRE fluorescence values, which was already significant at 2 h and became more pronounced during the course of STS treatment (Krohn et al. 1998, 1999). Neuron size remained unchanged up to 12 h after addition of STS, suggesting that cell shrinkage occured only later (Krohn et al. 1999).

We also proved that STS-treated cells were able to functionally respond to a pharmacological manipulation of $\Delta\Psi_m$ by examining the reaction of TMRE-loaded neurons to the protonophore carbonyl cyanide *p*-trifluoromethoxy-phenylhydrazone (FCCP; 0.1 μM) (Fig. 3; Krohn et al. 1999). FCCP depolarizes mitochondria, releasing TMRE into the cytoplasm. At the TMRE concentration used here, the release of TMRE is accompanied by a transient increase in fluorescence ("unquenching"; Duchen and Biscoe 1992; Prehn et al. 1994). Of note, the mitochondria of STS-treated hippocampal neurons could still be depolarized with FCCP up to 12 h after onset of the STS exposure. Fluorescence values after the 5-min exposure to FCCP showed the same trend as the basal values, i.e. a gradual increase in TMRE fluorescence (Krohn et al. 1999). These results indicate that the increased basal TMRE fluorescence values were not a result of TMRE release from the mitochondria through depolarization. The Nernstian behavior of this cationic probe would predict a concomittant increase in uptake as either mitochondrial or plasma potential increases (Ehrenberg et al. 1988). Incubation in high K^+ buffer, which decreases plasma membrane potential and resulted in lower TMRE uptake in control cells, prevented the increase in TMRE uptake observed after the STS treatment (Krohn et al. 1999).

We also examined mitochondrial release of cytochrome c in conjunction with monitoring of $\Delta\Psi_m$ using the potential-sensitive probe Mitotracker Red (CMXRos). Unlike TMRE, CMXRos forms stable thiol conjugates with mitochondrial proteins. This inhibits the release of CMXRos once the dye is taken up by mitochondria, and also allows fixation and double-labeling of cells with an antibody to cytochrome c. Examination of cells with a 100X oil objective allowed the resolution of individual mitochondria and mitochondria-rich regions (Fig. 4). Comparable to the results seen with TMRE, we saw no decrease in neuronal CMXRos uptake during the STS treatment, but rather an increase by 8 h. In contrast, cytochrome c staining of STS-exposed cells was clearly lower than that of the respective controls by this time.

We also investigated the invovement of the PTP in STS-induced cytochrome c release. Hippocampal neurons pre-treated for 1 h with cyclosporin A (CsA; 10 μM) released their cytochrome c to the same extent as cultures exposed to STS only (Fig. 4). We also investigated the effects of CsA (10 μM) and another inhibitor of the PTP, bongkrekic acid (50 μM), on STS-induced cell death. Bongkrekic acid inhibits PTP opening by binding to the adenine nucleotide translocator (Marzo et al. 1998). After 24 h of exposure, we assessed apoptotic nuclear morphology (Hoechst staining of nuclear chromatin) or the extent of secondary necrosis (trypan-blue staining). Neither PTP inhibitor reduced the level of STS-induced apoptosis or secondary necrosis (Krohn et al. 1999).

Cytochrome c release monitored live by time-lapse confocal microscopy

In intact cells, cytochrome c release can only be indirectly monitored by using potential-sensitive dyes. Moreover, as demonstrated above, the release of cytochrome c may also occur independently of changes in $\Delta\Psi m$ (Bossy-Wetzel et al. 1998; Krohn et al. 1998, 1999). On the other hand, immunocytochemistry and

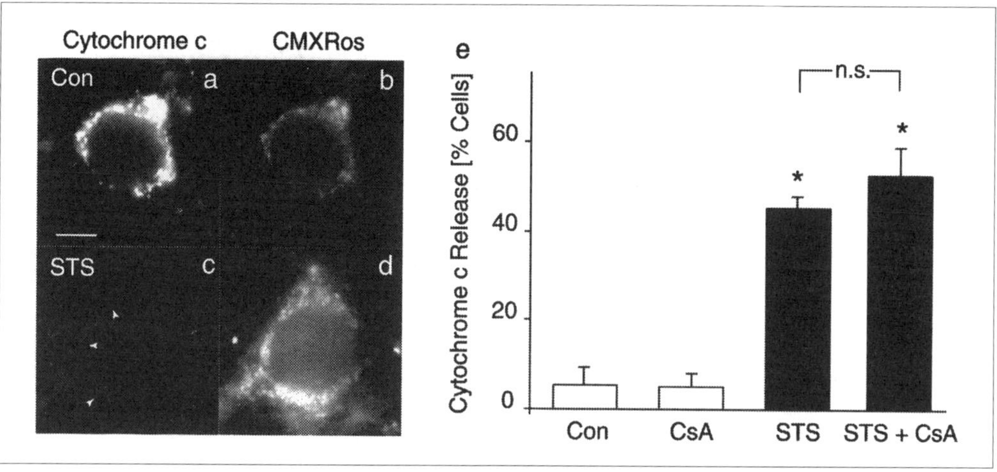

Fig. 4. Cytochrome c release during STS-induced neuronal apoptosis. High resolution of cytochrome c immunofluorescence in cultures treated for 8 h with vehicle (Con; **a.** and **b.**) or 300 nM STS (**c.** and **d.**). Cytochrome c immunofluorescence (**a.** and **c.**) and CMXRos uptake (**b.** and **d.**) were observed with a 100X oil objective. Mitochondria from control cells show a high level of staining for cytochrome c. In comparison, mitochondria from STS-treated cells show extensive loss of cytochrome c. Mitochondria from STS-treated cells show no loss of CMXRos uptake 8 h after addition of STS. Bar = 10 µm. **e.** Quantification of hippocampal neurons exhibiting cytochrome c release in control cultures and cultures exposed for 8 h to 300 nM STS. Cultures were pre-treated for one hour with vehicle (saline) or the PTP inhibitor cyclosporin A (CsA; 10 µM) and analyzed by immunofluorescence microscopy. Data are means ± SEM from n = 4 cultures. Different from respective controls * $p < 0.05$ (ANOVA and Tukey test).

subcellular fractionation experiments fail to enlighten the actual translocation of mitochondrial proteins, and do not reveal the kinetics of this event. To directly monitor the release of cytochrome c, we have generated a breast carcinoma cell line (MCF-7/Casp-3) that overexpresses enhanced green fluorescent protein (EGFP)-tagged cytochrome c. Previous studies have shown that cytochrome c-GFP distributes into the cytosol and nucleus during apoptosis and co-localizes with endogenous cytochrome c after its release (Heiskanen et al. 1999; Goldstein et al. 2000). We analyzed cytochrome c release kinetics in the MCF-7/Casp-3/Cytochrome c-EGFP cells during the exposure to STS, both in the presence and absence of the selective PTP inhibitor N-methylvaline-4-cyclosporin. Exposure of cytochrome c-EGFP-transfected MCF-7/Casp-3 cells to 3 µM STS induced morphological changes characteristic of apoptosis. After 6 to 8 h of treatment, caspase-3-like protease activity determined with the Ac-DEVD-AMC cleavage assay increased significantly. Epifluorescence microscopy revealed that the cytochrome c-EGFP signal was diffuse in STS-treated cells and distributed into the entire cytoplasm. However, a transition from a mitochondrial EGFP-signal to a diffuse cytoplasmic distribution state could be rarely detected. To determine the kinetic of the cytochrome c release, cytochrome c-EGFP-transfected MCF-7/Casp-3 cells were monitored with a time-lapse confocal laserscan microscope. Incubation with STS induced a rapid redistribution of the cytochrome c-EGFP signal (Fig. 5). All mitochondria from a STS-treated MCF-7/Casp-3 cytochrome c-EGFP cell started releasing large quantities of cytochrome c-EGFP into the cytoplasm within minutes. A distinct starting point within the cell could not be detected. However, the release event was not synchronized among neighbouring cells. STS-induced cytochrome c release of individual cells was completed in less than 30 min. After 30 min, the

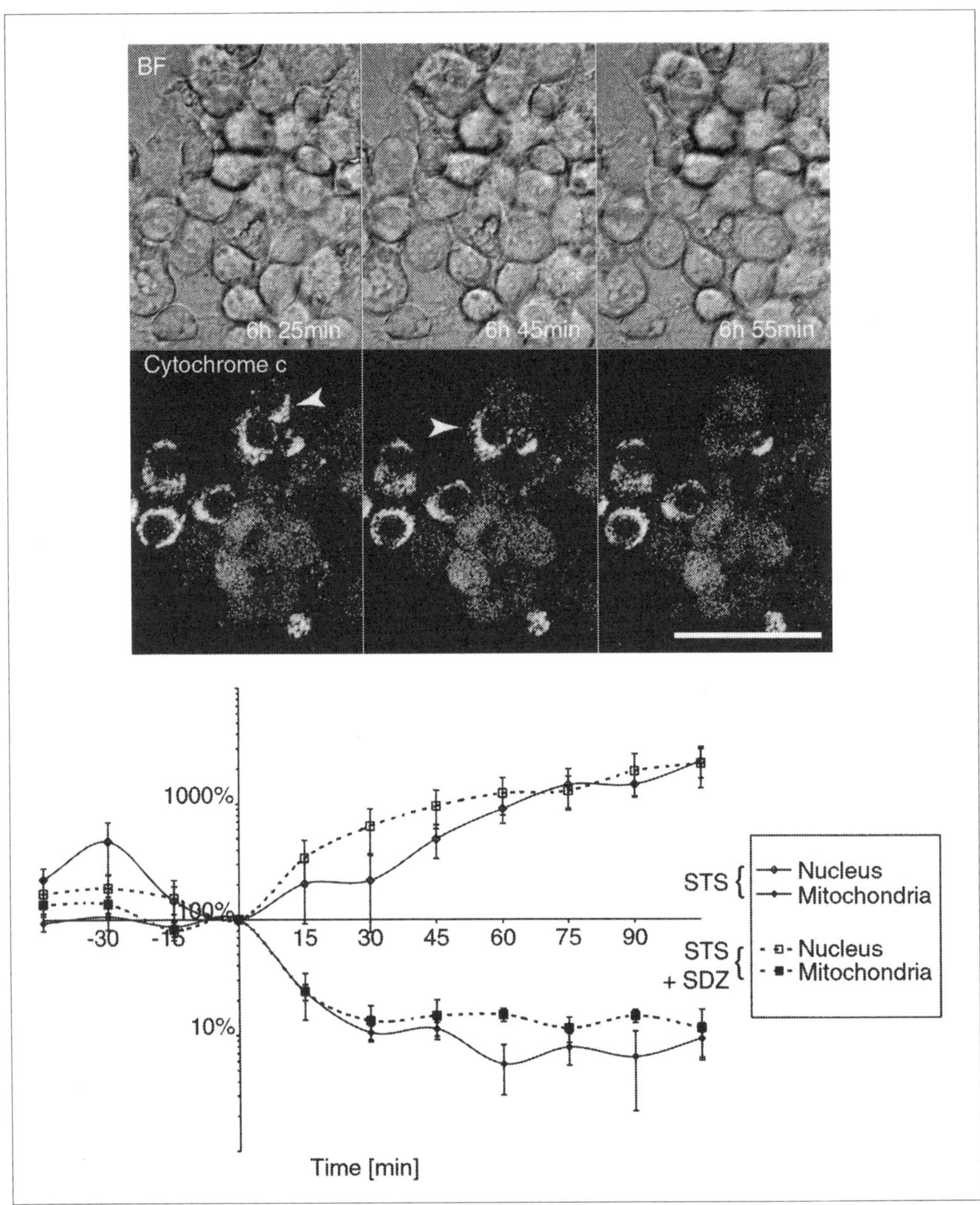

Fig. 5. Cytochrome c release monitored live by confocal laser scanning microscopy. MCF-7/Casp-3 cytochrome c-EGFP cells release cytochrome c within minutes during an exposure to 3 μM STS. **Upper Panel:** Bright field (BF) images. **Middel Panel:** Three confocal images of an 8 h time-lapse experiment demonstrating the release event of individual cells. Arrows indicate cells which will have released cytochrome c-EGFP in the following image. Scale bar = 50 μm. **Lower Panel:** Standardized graph showing relative fluorescence at different time points before and after the release event for mitochondrial rich regions and nuclei in cultures exposed to 3 μM STS, either in the absence or presence of the PTP inhibitor N-methylvaline-4-cyclosporin (SDZ; 1.6 μM). Mean release kinetics were determined from n = 8 and 6 cells in a typical experiment. Eleven time points per release event have been considered. Note the semi-logarithmic scale.

fluorescence signal appeared also in the nuclei and became later equally distributed throughout the entire cell compartments. Treatment with the PTP inhibitor N-methylvaline-4-cyclosporin (1.6 μM) did not alter the kinetics of STS-induced cytochrome c release (Fig. 5).

Discussion

An increased permeability of the outer mitochondrial membrane and a subsequent loss of the pro-apoptotic factor cytochrome c may occur in both excitotoxic and apoptotic neuron death (Figs. 1 and 4; Deshmukh and Johnson 1998; Krohn et al. 1999; Budd et al. 2000; Luetjens et al. 2000). Excitotoxic neuron death caused by NMDA receptor overactivation is a Ca^{2+}-dependent cell death. Mitochondrial Ca^{2+} overloading is known to occur in excitotoxic neuron death (White and Reynolds 1995; Peng and Greenamyre 1998; Stout et al. 1998) and could trigger PTP opening. However, although the NMDA-induced loss of cytochrome c was accompanied by mitochondrial depolarization (Fig. 1; Luetjens et al. 2000), it was insensitive to the selective and potent PTP inhibitor N-methylvaline-4-cyclosporin. In this context, it has recently been demonstrated that Ca^{2+}-induced cytochrome c release from isolated brain mitochondria may also occur via PTP-independent pathways (Andreyev et al. 1998).

In contrast to NMDA, the STS-induced cytochrome c release proceeded while mitochondria remained polarized (Figs. 3 and 4; Krohn et al. 1999). Interestingly, cellular and mitochondrial Ca^{2+} overloading have also been observed during STS-induced neuronal apoptosis (Kruman and Mattson 1999). In line with these findings, we have previously demonstrated that STS-induced apoptosis of hippocampal neurons is inhibited in cells overexpressing the Ca^{2+} binding protein calbindin D_{28k} (Prehn et al. 1997). Of note, various PTP inhibitors failed to inhibit STS-induced cytochrome c release and apoptosis activation (Figs. 4 and 5; Krohn et al. 1999; see also Budd et al. 2000).

Many studies have focused on the role of cytochrome c release to activate the caspase cascade (Liu et al. 1996; Li et al. 1997). Activation of caspases is a well established process in neuronal apoptosis (Schulz et al. 1996; Stefanis et al. 1996; Armstrong et al. 1997; Krohn et al. 1998). On the other hand, previous studies have found little evidence for a prominent activation of executioner caspases after glutamate receptor overactivation, despite the mitochondrial release of cytochrome c (Armstrong et al. 1997; Yu et al. 1999; Budd et al. 2000; Lankiewicz et al. 2000). We have recently demonstrated that this apparent discrepancy could be due to a Ca^{2+}- and calpain-dependent suppression of the caspase cascade (Lankiewicz et al. 2000). However, loss of cytochrome c may also affect mitochondrial respiration, and hence mitochondrial ATP and free radical production (Krippner et al. 1996; Cai and Jones 1998). Energy depletion has been shown to occur when glutamate receptors are overactivated for a longer period of time, and is generally associated with necrotic cell death (Ankarcrona et al. 1995). It remains to be shown whether loss of cytochrome c plays a role in ATP depletion during excitotoxic neuron death. On the other hand, our data indicate that loss of cytochrome c may also cause a delayed increase in mitochondrial superoxide production, both in excitotoxicity and in neuronal apoptosis (Krohn et al. 1998, 1999; Luetjens et al. 2000; see also Greenlund et al. 1995). Moreover, inhibition of superoxide formation has been shown to reduce both excitotoxic and apoptotic neuron death (Chan et al. 1990; Greenlund et al. 1995; Jordan et al. 1995; Patel et al. 1996; Krohn et al. 1998; Luetjens et al. 2000). It is conceivable that mitochondrial superoxide production secondary to a significant loss of cytochrome c is an important downstream cell death effector in both types of neuron death.

Acknowledgements

This research was funded by grants from IZKF Universität Münster (BMBF 01 KS 9604/0), DFG (Pr 338/8-1 and 9-1), Alzheimer Forschung Initiative e.V. and Stiftung VERUM to J.H.M.P.

References

1. Andreyev AY, Fahy B, Fiskum G (1998) Cytochrome c release from brain mitochondria is independent of the mitochondrial permeability transition. FEBS Lett 20:373–376
2. Ankarcrona M, Dypbukt JM, Bonfoco E, Zhivotovsky B, Orrenius S, Lipton SA, Nicotera P (1995) Glutamate-induced neuronal death: a succession of necrosis or apoptosis depending on mitochondrial function. Neuron 15:961–973
3. Armstrong RC, Aja TJ, Hoang KD, Gaur S, Bai X, Alnemri ES, Litwack G, Karanewsky DS, Fritz LC, Tomaselli KJ (1997) Activation of the CED3/ICE-related protease CPP32 in cerebellar granule neurons undergoing apoptosis but not necrosis. J Neurosci 15:553–562
4. Bernardi P, Petronilli V (1996) The permeability transition pore as a mitochondrial calcium release channel: a critical appraisal. J Bioenerg Biomembr 28:131–138
5. Beutner G, Ruck A, Riede B, Welte W, Brdiczka D (1996) Complexes between kinases, mitochondrial porin and adenylate translocator in rat brain resemble the permeability transition pore. FEBS Lett 396:189–195
6. Bindokas VP, Jordan J, Lee CC, Miller RJ (1996) Superoxide production in rat hippocampal neurons: sensitive imaging with ethidine. J Neurosci 16:1,324–1,336
7. Bossy-Wetzel E, Newmeyer DD, Green DR (1998) Mitochondrial cytochrome c release in apoptosis occurs upstream of DEVD-specific caspase activation and independently of mitochondrial transmembrane depolarization. EMBO J 17:37–49
8. Boveris A, Cadenas E, Stoppani AOM (1976) Role of ubiquinone in the mitochondrial generation of hydrogen peroxide. Biochem J 156:435–444
9. Budd SL, Tenneti L, Lishnak T, Lipton SA (2000) Mitochondrial and extramitochondrial apoptotic signaling pathways in cerebrocortical neurons. Proc Natl Acad Sci USA 97:6,161–6,166
10. Cai JY, Jones DP (1998) Superoxide in apoptosis – mitochondrial generation triggered by cytochrome c loss. J Biol Chem 273:11,401–11,404
11. Chan PH, Chu L, Chen SF, Carlson EJ, Epstein C (1990) Attenuation of glutamate-induced neuronal swelling and toxicity in transgenic mice overexpressing human CuZn-superoxide dismutase. Acta Neurochir 51:245–247
12. Deshmukh M, Johnson Jr EM (1998) Evidence of a novel event during neuronal death: development of competence-to-die in response to cytoplasmic cytochrome c. Neuron 21:695–705
13. Dirnagl U, Iadecola C, Moskowitz MA (1999) Pathobiology of ischaemic stroke: an integrated view. Trends Neurosci 22:391–397
14. Duchen MR, Biscoe TJ (1992) Relative mitochondrial membrane potential and $[Ca^{2+}]$ in type I cells isolated from the rabbit carotid body. J Physiol 450:33–61
15. Ehrenberg B, Montana V, Wie MD, Wuskell JP, Loew LM (1988) Membrane potential can be determined in individual cells from the nernstian distribution of cationic dyes. Biophys J 53:785–794
16. Emaus RK, Grunwald R, Lemasters JJ (1986) Rhodamine 123 as a probe of transmembrane potential in isolated rat liver mitochondria: spectral and metabolic properties. Biochem Biophys Acta 850:436–448
17. Eskes R, Antonsson B, Osen-Sand A, Montessuit S, Richter C, Sadoul R, Mazzei G, Nichols A, Martinou JC (1998) Bax-induced cytochrome C release from mitochondria is independent of the permeability transition pore but highly dependent on Mg^{2+} ions. J Cell Biol 143:217–224
18. Falcieri E, Martelli AM, Bareggi R, Cataldi A, Cocco L. (1993) The protein kinase inhibitor staurosporine induces morphological changes typical of apoptosis in MOLT-4 cells without concomitant DNA fragmentation. Biochem Biophys Res Commun 193:19–25
19. Goldstein JC, Waterhouse NJ, Juin P, Evan GI, Green DR (2000) The coordinate release of cytochrome c during apoptosis is rapid, complete and kinetically invariant. Nat Cell Biol 2:156–162
20. Greenlund LJS, Deckwerth TL, Johnson Jr EM (1995) Superoxide dismutase delays neuronal apoptosis: a role for reactive oxygen species in programmed cell death. Neuron 14:303–315
21. Heiskanen KM, Bhat MB, Wang HW, Ma J, Nieminen AL (1999) Mitochondrial depolarization accompanies cytochrome c release during apoptosis in PC6 cells. J Biol Chem 274:5,654–5,658
22. Jordan J, Ghadge GD, Prehn JHM, Toth P, Roos RP, Miller RJ (1995) Expression of human Cu/Zn superoxide dismutase inhibits the death of sympathetic neurons caused by withdrawal of nerve growth factor. Mol Pharmacol 47:1,095–1,100
23. Kluck RM, Bossy-Wetzel E, Green DR, Newmeyer DD (1997) The release of cytochrome c from mitochondria: a primary site for Bcl-2 regulation of apoptosis. Science 275:1,132–1,136
24. Kluck RM, Esposti MD, Perkins G, Renken C, Kuwana T, Bossy-Wetzel E, Goldberg M, Allen T, Barber MJ, Green DR, Newmeyer DD (1999) The pro-apoptotic proteins, Bid and Bax, cause a limited permeabilization of the mitochondrial outer membrane that is enhanced by cytosol. J Cell Biol 147:809–822
25. Krippner A, Matsuno-Yagi A, Gottlieb RA, Babior BM (1996) Loss of function of cytochrome c in Jurkat cells undergoing Fas-mediated apoptosis. J Biol Chem 271:21,629–21,636
26. Kroemer G, Reed JC (2000) Mitochondrial control of cell death. Nat Med 6:513–519
27. Krohn AJ, Preis E, Prehn JHM (1998) Staurosporine-induced apoptosis of cultured rat hippocampal neurons involves caspase-1-like proteases as upstream initiators and increased production of superoxide as a main downstream effector. J Neurosci 18:8,186–8,197
28. Krohn AJ, Wahlbrink T, Prehn JHM (1999) Mitochondrial depolarization is not required for neuronal apoptosis. J Neurosci 19:7,394–7,404
29. Kruman II, Mattson MP (1999) Pivotal role of mitochondrial calcium uptake in neural cell apoptosis and necrosis. J Neurochem 72:529–540
30. Lankiewicz S, Luetjens CM, Bui NT, Krohn AJ, Poppe M, Cole GM, Saido TC, Prehn JHM (2000) Activation of calpain I converts excitotoxic neuron death into a caspase-independent cell death. J Biol Chem 275:17,064–17,071
31. Li H, Yuan J (1999) Deciphering the pathways of life and death. Curr Op Cell Biol 11:261–266
32. Li H, Zhu H, Xu CJ, Yuan J (1998) Cleavage of BID by caspase 8 mediates the mitochondrial damage in the Fas pathway of apoptosis. Cell 94:491–501
33. Li P, Nijhawan D, Budihardjo I, Srinivasula SM, Ahmad M, Alnemri ES, Wang X (1997) Cytochrome c and dATP-dependent formation of Apaf-1/caspase-9 complex initiates an apoptotic protease cascade. Cell 91:479–489
34. Liu X, Kim CN, Yang J, Jemmerson R, Wang X (1996) Induction of apoptotic program in cell-free extracts: requirement for dATP and cytochrome c. Cell 86:147–157
35. Luetjens CM, Bui NT, Sengpiel B, Münstermann G, Poppe M, Krohn AJ, Bauerbach E, Krieglstein J, Prehn JHM (2000) Delayed mitochondrial dysfunction in excitotoxic neuron death: cytochrome c release and a secondary increase in superoxide production. J Neurosci 20:5715–5723
36. Luo X, Budihardjo I, Zou H, Slaughter C, Wang, X. (1998) Bid, a Bcl2 interacting protein, mediates cytochrome c release from mitochondria in response to activation of cell surface death receptors. Cell 94:481–490

37. Marchetti P, Castedo M, Susin SA, Zamzami N, Hirsch T, Macho A, Haeffner A, Hirsch F, Geuskens M, Kroemer G (1996) Mitochondrial permeability transition is a central coordinating event of apoptosis. J Exp Med 184:1,155–1,160
38. Marzo I, Brenner C, Zamzami N, Jürgensmeier JM, Susin SA Vieira HLA, Prévost MC, Xie Y, Matsuyama S, Reed JC, Kroemer G (1998) Bax and adenine nucleotide translocator cooperate in the mitochondrial control of apoptosis. Science 281:2,027–2,031
39. Nicolli A, Basso E, Petronilli V, Wenger RM, Bernardi P (1996) Interactions of cyclophilin with the mitochondrial inner membrane and regulation of the permeability transition pore, and cyclosporin A-sensitive channel. J Biol Chem 271:2,185–2,192
40. Patel M, Day BJ, Crapo JD, Fridovich I, McNamara JO (1996) Requirement for superoxide in excitotoxic cell death. Neuron 16:345–355
41. Peng TI, Greenamyre JT (1998) Priviliged access to mitochondria of calcium influx through N-methyl-D-aspartate receptors. Mol Pharmacol 53:974–980
42. Porter AG, Janicke RU (1999) Emerging roles of caspase-3 in apoptosis. Cell Death Differ 6: 99–104
43. Prehn JHM, Bindokas VP, Marcuccilli CJ, Krajewski S, Reed JC, Miller RJ (1994) Regulation of neuronal Bcl2 protein expression and calcium homeostasis by transforming growth factor type β confers wide-ranging protection on rat hippocampal neurons. Proc Natl Acad Sci USA 91:12,599–12,603
44. Prehn JHM, Jordan J, Ghadge GD, Preis E, Galindo MF, Roos RP, Krieglstein J, Miller RJ (1997) Ca^{2+} and reactive oxygen species in staurosporine-induced neuronal apoptosis. J Neurochem 68:1,679–1,685
45. Schulz JB, Weller M, Klockgether T (1996) Potassium deprivation-induced apoptosis of cerebellar granule neurons: a sequential requirement for new mRNA and protein synthesis, ICE-like protease activity, and reactive oxygen species. J Neurosci 16:4,696–4,706
46. Sengpiel B, Preis E, Krieglstein J, Prehn JHM (1998) NMDA-induced superoxide production and neurotoxicity in cultured rat hippocampal neurons: role of mitochondria. Eur J Neurosci 10:1,903–1,910
47. Shimizu S, Narita M, Tsujimoto Y (1999) Bcl-2 family proteins regulate the release of apoptogenic cytochrome c by the mitochondrial channel VDAC. Nature 399:483–487
48. Shimizu S, Tsujimoto Y (2000) Proapoptotic BH3-only Bcl-2 family members induce cytochrome c release, but not mitochondrial membrane potential loss, and do not directly modulate voltage-dependent anion channel activity. Proc Natl Acad Sci USA 97:577–582
49. Smith LL, Rose MS, Wyatt I (1978) The pathology and biochemistry of paraquat. Ciba Found Symp 65:321–341
50. Stefanis L, Park DS, Yun C, Yan I, Farinelli SE, Troy CM, Shelanski ML, Greene LA (1996) Induction of CPP32-like activity in PC12 cells by withdrawal of trophic support. J Biol Chem 271:30,663–30,671
51. Stout AK, Raphael HM, Kanterewicz BI, Klann E, Reynolds IJ (1998) Glutamate-induced neuron death requires mitochondrial calcium uptake. Nat Neurosci 1:366–373
52. Turrens JF, Boveris A (1980) Generation of superoxide anion by the NADH dehydrogenase of bovine heart mitochondria. Biochem J 191:421–427
53. Van der Heiden MG, Chandel NS, Williamson EK, Schumaker PT, Thompson CB (1997) Bcl-xL regulates the membrane potential and volume homeostasis of mitochondria. Cell 91:627–637
54. Wadia JS, Chalmers-Redman RME, Ju WJH, Carlile GW, Phillips JL, Fraser AD, Tatton WG (1998) Mitochondrial membrane potential and nuclear changes in apoptosis caused by serum and nerve growth factor withdrawal: time course and modification by (–)-deprenyl. J Neurosci 18:932–947
55. White RJ, Reynolds IJ (1995) Mitochondria and Na^+/Ca^{2+} exchange buffer glutamate-induced calcium in cultured cortical neurons. J Neurosci 15:1,318–1,328
56. White RJ, Reynolds IJ (1996) Mitochondrial depolarization in glutamate-stimulated neurons: an early signal specific to excitotoxin exposure. J Neurosci 16:5,688–5,697
57. Yang J, Liu X, Bhalla K, Kim CN, Ibrado AM, Cai J, Peng TI, Jones DP, Wang X (1997) Prevention of apoptosis by Bcl-2: release of cytochrome c from mitochondria blocked. Science 275:1,129–1,132
58. Yu SP, Yeh C-H, Strasser U, Tian M, Choi DW (1999) NMDA receptor-mediated K^+ efflux and neuronal apoptosis. Science 284:336–339
59. Zoratti M, Szabo I (1995) The mitochondrial permeability transition. Biochim Biophys Acta 1241:139–176
60. Zou H, Henzel WJ, Liu X, Lutschg A, Wang X (1997) Apaf-1, a human protein homologous to C. elegans CED-4, participates in cytochrome c-dependent activation of caspase-3. Cell 90:405–413

Regulation of the mitochondrial permeability transition pore by ubiquinone analogs

P. Bernardi[1], E. Fontaine[2]

Summary

We briefly review the properties and consequences of the mitochondrial permeability transition in the context of ischemic brain damage. Pharmacological evidence supports the notion that onset of the permeability transition plays a causative role in ischemic injury. We report here on the discovery of the modulatory properties of quinones on this process, and of a study where we correlate some quinone structure features with their effects on the permeability transition.

Regulation of ion fluxes across the inner mitochondrial membrane is essential both for metabolic regulation and for energy conservation. The inner membrane possesses an intrinsically low permeability to ions and solutes, which allows energy conservation in the form of a proton electrochemical potential difference (Mitchell 1979). Yet, mitochondria *in vitro* can easily undergo a permeability increase to solutes with molecular masses of about 1,500 Da or lower, which is followed by deenergization, disruption of ionic homeostasis and swelling, the "permeability transition" (PT) (see Bernardi 1999a for review). Recent years have witnessed an exponential increase of the interest in the PT as a potential mediator of cell death both in the context of necrosis and of apoptosis (see Bernardi et al. 1999b for review). The PT could play a role by causing ATP depletion and dysregulation of Ca^{2+} homeostasis, and by contributing (through matrix swelling and outer membrane rupture) to the release of cytochrome *c* (Liu et al. 1996) and smac/diablo (Du et al. 2000; Ekert et al. 2000), which cooperate in the activation of cytosolic procaspase 9. It is widely assumed that the PT is due to opening of a proteinaceous pore, the PTP, whose molecular identity remains debated (Bernardi 1999a).

The discovery of the effects of Cyclosporin A (CsA), which in isolated mitochondria inhibits the PT with a Ki of about 10 nM (e.g. Nicolli et al. 1996), prompted extensive investigations in cell, organ as well as animal models of disease. These studies tried to assess whether the PT represents a potential factor for mitochondrial dysfunction, and the results are particularly convincing in the context of brain injury. Increasing evidence indeed indicates that PTP opening is a key event in the damage to the nervous tissue that follows forebrain ischemia (Uchino et al. 1995, 1998), hypergly-

Keywords: mitochondria; quinones; permeability transition; ischemia; brain

[1]Consiglio Nazionale delle Ricerche Unit for the Study of Biomembranes and Department of Biomedical Sciences, University of Padova Medical School, I-35121 Padova, Italy (e-mail: bernardi@civ.bio.unipd.it) and [2]Laboratoire de Bioénergétique Fondamentale et Appliquée, Université Joseph Fourier, F-38041 Grenoble-cedex 09, France
e-mail: eric.fontaine@ujf-grenoble.fr

J. Krieglstein, S. Klumpp (Eds.) Pharmacology of Cerebral Ischemia 2000

cemia (Li et al. 1997), and hypoglycemic coma (Friberg et al. 1998; Ferrand-Drake et al. 1999); that CsA displays a dramatic protective effect in all these models (Uchino et al. 1995, 1998; Li et al. 1997; Friberg et al. 1998; Ferrand-Drake et al. 1999); and that the PT represents a viable target for pharmacological intervention.

CsA has multiple effects on cells, particularly in relation to inhibition of the cytosolic phosphatase calcineurin, which is involved in nuclear translocation of NF-AT and is responsible for the immunosuppressive effects of this drug (Crabtree 1999). Even if derivatives devoid of effects on calcineurin but still active on the PT have been described, such as MeVal-4-cyclosporin (Nicolli et al. 1996), all cellular cyclophilins are inhibited by this drug (Nicolli et al. 1996). Furthermore, CsA does not readily cross the blood-brain barrier, which would limit its usefulness in a clinical setting.

We have long been involved in the study and characterization of PTP inducers and inhibitors, with the long-term goals of defining the PTP regulatory features and molecular nature, and of developing better drugs for its modulation *in vivo*. In a series of recent studies we have shown that the PTP is modulated by electron flux through respiratory Complex I (Fontaine et al. 1998a), which led to the discovery that the PT is inhibited by Q0 and decylubiquinone (Fontaine et al. 1998b). Inhibition by these quinones could be specifically relieved by Q1, which is inactive *per se*, suggesting that quinones could be competing for a common binding site (see Fontaine and Bernardi 1999 for review). To identify the structural features required for regulation of the PTP by ubiquinone analogs, we have carried out a detailed analysis with several structural variants. We show that three quinone functional classes can be defined: (i) PTP inhibitors [Q0; decylubiquinone; Q2; 2,3-dimethyl-6-decyl-1,4-benzoquinone; 2,3,5-trimethyl-6-geranyl-1,4-benzoquinone]; (ii) PTP inducers [2,3-dimethoxy-5-methyl-6-(10-hydroxydecyl)-1,4-benzoquinone; 2,5-dihydroxy-6-undecyl-1,4-benzoquinone]; and (iii) PTP-inactive quinones that compete with both inhibitors and inducers [Q1; 2,3,5-trimethyl-6-(3-hydroxyisoamyl)-1,4-benzoquinone]. The structure-function correlation indicates that minor modifications in the isoprenoid side chain can turn an inhibitor into an activator, and that the methoxy groups are not essential for the effects of quinones on the PTP. Since the analogs used in this study have a similar midpoint potential and decrease production of mitochondrial reactive oxygen species to the same extent, we favor the idea that quinones modulate the PTP through a common binding site rather than through oxidation-reduction reactions. Occupancy of this site could modulate the PTP open-closed transitions, possibly through secondary changes of the Ca^{2+}-binding affinity (Walter et al. 2000).

References

1. Bernardi P (1999a) Mitochondrial transport of cations: Channels, exchangers and permeability transition. Physiol Rev 79:1127–1155
2. Bernardi P, Scorrano L, Colonna R, Petronilli V, Di Lisa F (1999b) Mitochondria and cell death. Mechanistic aspects and methodological issues. Eur J Biochem 264:687–701
3. Crabtree GR (1999) Generic signals and specific outcomes: Signaling through Ca^{2+}, calcineurin and NF-AT. Cell 96:611–614
4. Du C, Fang M, Li Y, Li L, Wang X (2000) Smac, a Mitochondrial Protein that Promotes Cytochrome c-Dependent Caspase Activation by Eliminating IAP Inhibition. Cell 102:33–42
5. Ekert PG, Silke J, Connolly LM, Reid GE, Moritz RL, Vaux DL (2000) Identification of DIABLO, a Mammalian Protein that Promotes Apoptosis by Binding to and Antagonizing IAP Proteins. Cell 102:43–53
6. Ferrand-Drake M, Friberg H, Wieloch T (1999) Mitochondrial permeability transition induced DNA-fragmentation in the rat hippocampus following hypoglycemia. Neuroscience 90:1325–1338
7. Fontaine E, Bernardi P (1999) Progress on the Mitochondrial Permeability Transition Pore. Regulation by Complex I and Ubiquinone Analogs. J Bioenerg Biomembr 31:335–345
8. Fontaine E, Eriksson O, Ichas F, Bernardi P (1998a) Regulation of the permeability transition pore in skeletal muscle mitochondria. Modulation by electron flow through the respiratory chain complex I. J Biol Chem 273:12662–12668
9. Fontaine E, Ichas F, Bernardi P (1998b) A ubiquinone-binding site regulates the mitochondrial permeability transition pore. J Biol Chem 273:25734–25740
10. Friberg H, Ferrand-Drake M, Bengtsson F, Halestrap AP, Wieloch T (1998) Cyclosporin A, but not FK 506, protects mitochondria and neurons against hypoglycemic damage and implicates the mitochondrial permeability transition in cell death. J Neurosci 18:5151–5159
11. Li PA, Uchino H, Elmer E, Siesjo BK (1997) Amelioration by cyclosporin A of brain damage following 5 or 10 min of ischemia in rats subjected to preischemic hyperglycemia. Brain Res 753:133–140
12. Liu X, Kim CN, Yang J, Jemmerson R, Wang X (1996) Induction of apoptotic program in cell-free extracts: requirement for dATP and cytochrome c. Cell 86:147–157

13. Mitchell P (1979) Keilin's respiratory chain concept and its chemiosmotic consequences. Science 206:1148–1159
14. Nicolli A, Basso E, Petronilli V, Wenger RM, Bernardi P (1996) Interactions of cyclophilin with the mitochondrial inner membrane and regulation of the permeability transition pore, a cyclosporin A-sensitive channel. J Biol Chem 271:2185–2192
15. Uchino H, Elmer E, Uchino K, Li PA, He QP, Smith ML, Siesjo BK (1998) Amelioration by cyclosporin A of brain damage in transient forebrain ischemia in the rat. Brain Res 812:216–226
16. Uchino H, Elmer E, Uchino K, Siesjo BK (1995) Cyclosporin A dramatically ameliorates CA1 hippocampal damage following transient forebrain ischemia in the rat. Acta Physiol Scand 155:469–471
17. Walter L, Nogueira V, Leverve X, Bernardi P, Fontaine E (2000) Three Classes of Ubiquinone Analogs Regulate the Mitochondrial Permeability Transition Pore through a Common Site. J Biol Chem 275:29521–29527

Inflammation and neuronal cell death

Do caspase and proteasome inhibitors influence the delayed maturation of cortical infarction by preventing apoptosis or neuroinflammation?

A. M. Buchan

Abstract

Transient cortical ischemia ultimately results in cerebral infarction which is an energetically active process characterized in death by morphological pan-necrosis. The many biochemical features, however, suggest at least a component of the apoptotic pathway. With brief ischemia there is a slow maturation of injury, endonuclease dependant DNA laddering, end labelling or tunel staining of the dying neurones, mitochondrial release of cytochrome c, and activation of a series of caspases and proteins influenced by the activation of NF-κB. Spontaneously hypertensive rats were subjected to 30, 45, 60, 90, or 120 minutes of middle cerebral artery occlusion followed by reperfusion. Volumes of cerebral infarction were calculated with an image analyzing system. Animals were treated with a variety of caspase inhibitors including ICV-Z.VAD.FMK, ICV-Z.DEVD.FMK and an IV caspase inhibitor, the Cytovia compound, CV1013. Animals were also treated with two proteasome inhibitors IV-CVT-634 and IV-PS-519 to inhibit the activation of the transcription factor NF-κB. No infarction was detected following 30 minutes of ischemia although selective neuronal injury was observed after seven days. With 45 and 60 minutes of ischemia, less than 50% of the maturing infarct was seen at 24 hours, but this then evolved, in a delayed fashion over a period of 7–14 days, to the full infarct (20% of hemisphere). With 90 minutes of ischemia, 85% of the infarct was apparent at 24 hours with further maturation to a complete infarct at 7 days. Durations of ischemia of 120 minutes or 3 or 4 hours demonstrate a complete infarct within 24 hours of the onset of reperfusion.

Both ICV and IV caspase inhibition achieved a 30% infarct volume reduction following 90 minutes of ischemia. Both novel proteasome inhibitors which prevent the activation of NF-κB, PS-519 and CVT-634, achieved approximately 40% infarct volume reductions at 24 hours. These drugs reduce a number of inflammatory events including the migration of polymorphs. In a comparative study, neither caspase nor NF-κB inhibition prevented CA_1 injury following global ischemia using the 4-vessel occlusion model, which induces little in the way of inflammation.

Brief periods of ischemia give rise to a slowly maturing infarct which can be inhibited by either caspase or NF-κB inhibitors. These disease modifiers protect through anti-inflammatory, rather than anti-apoptotic mechanisms.

Keywords: Selective neuronal death, cortical infarction, apoptosis, caspases, proteasomes, inflammation

University of Calgary/Foothills Medical Centre, Room 1162, 1403–29th Street N.W., Calgary, Alberta, Canada, T2N 2T9
e-Mail: abuchan@ucalgary.ca

J. Krieglstein, S. Klumpp (Eds.) Pharmacology of Cerebral Ischemia 2000

Introduction

The delayed maturation of cell death following global ischemia is clearly demonstrated by the temporal pattern of selective loss of CA_1 neurons (Ito et al. 1975). While no observable injury is seen at 24 hours, after a latency of greater than 48 hours there is a progressive loss of cells moving in a medial to lateral direction (Pulsinelli et al. 1982; Kirino 1982). We have recently shown that, although briefer durations of ischemia appear to produce less initial injury, once a critical ischemic duration (ie. 5 minutes) is exceeded, simply takes longer for the expression of injury. Despite briefer ischemia, the same percentage of CA_1 cell death results, ie. the briefer the duration of ischemia the longer the necessary maturation period (Colbourne et al. 1999a). We now describe a maturation phenomena following transient focal ischemia which suggests that once a critical duration of focal ischemia is exceeded, although briefer durations appear to produce less injury, this is an illusion. In reality the cortical infarct is simply maturing more slowly. Although much of the injury is delayed, the same volume of injury results. Longer periods of reperfusion are required to realize the full extent of the pathology.

In terms of the putative mechanism of this maturation of focal infarction, we studied the injury which evolved out from the core lesion (ie. that seen at 24 hours) and looked at the role of both caspase and NF-κB activation, and the effects of inhibitors. We speculate that these neuroprotective effects may be mediated by anti-inflammatory mechanisms.

Methods

Focal ischemia

Male spontaneously hypertensive rats (SHR) weighing 200–250 grams were subjected to transient middle cerebral artery occlusion (MCA). The detailed methods have previously been described (Buchan et al. 1992). Briefly, animals are anesthetized with a mixture of 70% N_2, 28% O_2, and 2% halothane. The right common carotid artery is exposed and a loose ligature placed around it. The temporalis muscle is dissected and a 1 mm burr hole drilled 2–3 mm rostral to the point of fusion of the zygomatic arch with the temporal bone, exposing the right MCA. Regional cerebral blood flow (rCBF) is recorded in two locations using laser doppler flowmetry, the first 3 mm dorsal to the exposure for the MCA (to measure core ischemic blood flow) and the second 3 mm posterior and 5 mm lateral to bregma to measure the penumbral blood flow. Blood flow is recorded as a percentage of pre-occlusion baseline flows. A microaneurysm clip is placed on the MCA proximal to the point where it crosses the inferior cerebral vein in the rhinal fissure, and the right common carotid artery (CCA) is permanently occluded. Post-occlusion cerebral blood flow is measured prior to closing the wound. At the end of ischemia, the animals are briefly anesthetized, rCBF is measured, and the MCA clip removed. Body temperatures are maintained at 37.5±0.5 °C throughout ischemia and reperfusion. At the time of sacrifice, animals are anesthetized and blood flow is measured. Brains are then removed and frozen in –80 °C isopentane, and 20 μm thick sections are taken at 500 μm intervals throughout the entire area of ischemic-injured cortex and stained with hematoxylin and eosin. Areas outside the infarct are examined for selective cortical neuronal death. In the infarcted area, ipsi-lateral and contra-lateral hemispheres are traced and the infarctions expressed as percentage of the contra-lateral hemisphere. The infarct volume as a percentage of the hemisphere is calculated for each brain. Neutrophil counts were made in the area of infarction and selective neuronal injury.

Maturation phenomena

To study the influence of increasing durations of transient focal ischemia, animals were subjected to 30 (n = 20), 45 (n = 20), 60 (n = 15), 90 (n = 18) and 120 minutes of ischemia (n = 17).

Following ischemia animals were allowed to survive for one, seven, fourteen and twenty-one

Table 1. Cortical Infarct Volumes for Differing Ischemic Durations and Periods of Reperfusion

Ischemic Duration (Min)	Cortical Infarction % ± SD (n)			
	Reperfusion Period			
	1 Day	7 Days	14 Days	21 Days
30	0 ± 0% (5)	0 ± 0% (5)	1 ± 1% (5)	2 ± 1% (5)
45	3 ± 2% (5)	3 ± 1% (5)	4 ± 2% (5)	3 ± 2% (5)
60	10 ± 3% (5)	17 ± 2% (5)	21 ± 3% (5)	N/A
90	19 ± 3% (7)	20 ± 4% (6)	22 ± 2% (5)	N/A
120	21 ± 3% (5)	22 ± 3% (7)	23 ± 3% (5)	N/A

days. The number of rats included in each reperfusion period is presented in Table 1.

Experiments with inhibitors of caspase

Animals exposed to 90 minutes of ischemia were infused ICV with DMSO, Z.VAD, or Z.DEVD. In a further experiment animals were randomized to receive an IV infusion of either placebo or the caspase inhibitor CV-1013. The number of animals and drug dosages for each group are demonstrated in Table 2.

Experiments with inhibitors of NF-κB

Following 90 minutes of transient focal ischemia animals were treated IV with either a placebo or the proteasome inhibitor CVT-634 and allowed to survive for one or seven days. Neutrophil counts were made in CVT-634 treated and placebo treated rats. In addition animals were treated IV with either placebo or the proteasome inhibitor PS-519. The number of animals, dosages, and outcomes are detailed in Table 3.

Table 2. Cortical Infarct Volumes and the Effects of ICV Caspase Inhibitors (z-VAD, z-DEVD) and IV Caspase Inhibitors, Following 90 Minutes Ischemia and 24 Hours Reperfusion

Caspase Inhibitor	Cortical Infarction % ± SD (n)	
DMSO Control	13 ± 5% (7)	
z-VAD (2 μl ICV)	14 ± 3% (7)	
z-DEVD ((2 μl ICV)	18 ± 4% (7)	
DMSO Control	25 ± 6% (8)	
z-VAD (1 μl ICV x 3)	21 ± 7% (7)	
z-DEVD (1 μl ICV x 3)	22 ± 9% (9)	
DMSO Control	27 ± 6% (7)	
z-VAD (1 μl ICV x 4)	17 ± 6% (6)	$p < 0.05$
z-DEVD (1 μl ICV x 4)	20 ± 8% (6)	$p < 0.05$
Tris-Base Control	24 ± 7% (7)	
CV-1013 (20 mg/kg IV + 5 mg/kg/hr IV infusion x 6 hrs)	13 ± 6% (7)	$p < 0.01$

Table 3. Percentage of Cortical Infarction Following Infusion with Proteasome Inhibitors CVT-634 and PS-519 (90 Minutes of Focal Ischemia With Reperfusion for 24 Hours or 7 Days)

Proteasome Inhibitor	Cortical Infarction % ± SD (n)	
24 Hours Reperfusion		
Control	23 ± 4% (10)	
PS-519 (1 mg/kg)	16 ± 2% (10)	$p < 0.003$
Saline Control	21 ± 3% (8)	
DMSO Control	21 ± 3% (8)	
CVT-634 (50 mg/kg)	14 ± 3% (7)	$p < 0.002$
7 Days Reperfusion		
Saline Control	19 ± 4% (8)	
DMSO Control	21 ± 3% (8)	
CVT-634 (50 mg/kg x 3)	15 ± 3% (8)	$p < 0.024$
CVT-634 (50 mg/kg x 7)	12 ± 2% (7)	$p < 0.001$

Results

There were no significant differences in regional cerebral blood flow among the different groups in the maturation experiment and in those experiments in which either caspase or NF-κB inhibitors were used. Similarly, arterial blood gases, arterial pressure, glucose and hematocrit were also similar among the groups. Cortical cerebral blood flow dropped to 10–15% of baseline throughout ischemia and recovered upon reperfusion. Histological results are expressed as percentage infarct volume (mean ± standard deviation) in Figure 1 and Tables 1, 2, and 3. Neutrophil counts are demonstrated in Figures 2 and 3.

Maturation experiment

The rate of maturation of extension of cortical infarction relates to the duration of ischemia, as illustrated in Figure 1. In those animals exposed to 30 minutes of ischemia there was no injury following one day of reperfusion. There were scant selective neuronal eosinophilia which appeared in the cortex in animals at seven days of survival. Small, but well demarcated, volumes of cortical infarction occurred by fourteen days. With 45 minutes of ischemia, similar small cortical infarcts (3–4% of hemisphere) were evident at 24 hours, although there was no subsequent recruitment. In animals exposed to 60 and 90 minutes of ischemia there was significantly more injury in the groups allowed to survive for seven and fourteen days, as compared to one day. After 60 minutes of ischemia, 50% of the eventual infarct was seen at 24 hours, which progressed to 75% at seven days, and 100% was achieved by fourteen days. Following 90 minutes of ischemia, 85% of the resulting infarct was seen at 24 hours, which reached 100% by seven days. Following 120 minutes, a full infarct (100% infarct or 25% by hemispheric volume) was seen at 24 hours with no subsequent interval increase over four-

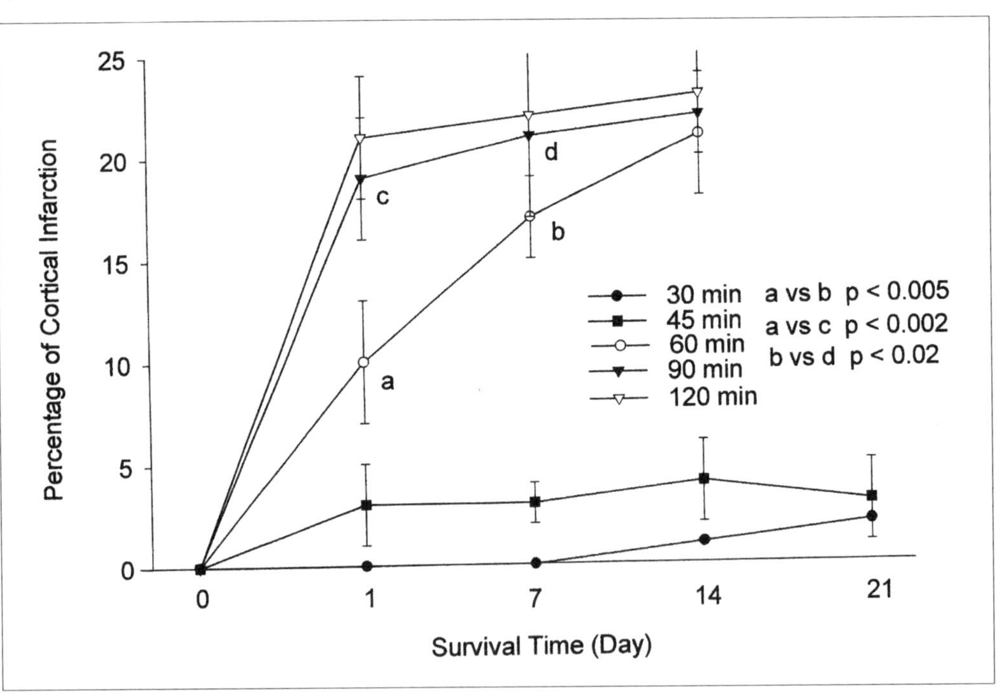

Fig. 1. The maturation of cortical infarction following 30, 45, 60, 90, and 120 minutes of ischemia with survival times ranging from 1–21 days. The maturation of ischemic injury was dependent on the duration of ischemia.

teen days. The progressive influence of neutrophil invasion is seen in Figure 2.

Influence of caspase inhibitors

Following ICV injection with Z.DEVD and Z.VAD, there were reductions in the volume of focal infarction by approximately 30%–40% less than control. Although injections of Z.DEVD appeared to increase temperature, controlling for temperature did not produce a greater degree of protection (Li et al. 2000a). Volumes of infarction were also reduced almost 50% by the systemic administration of an IV caspase inhibitor. The effect of caspase inhibitors on infarct volumes is demonstrated in Table 2.

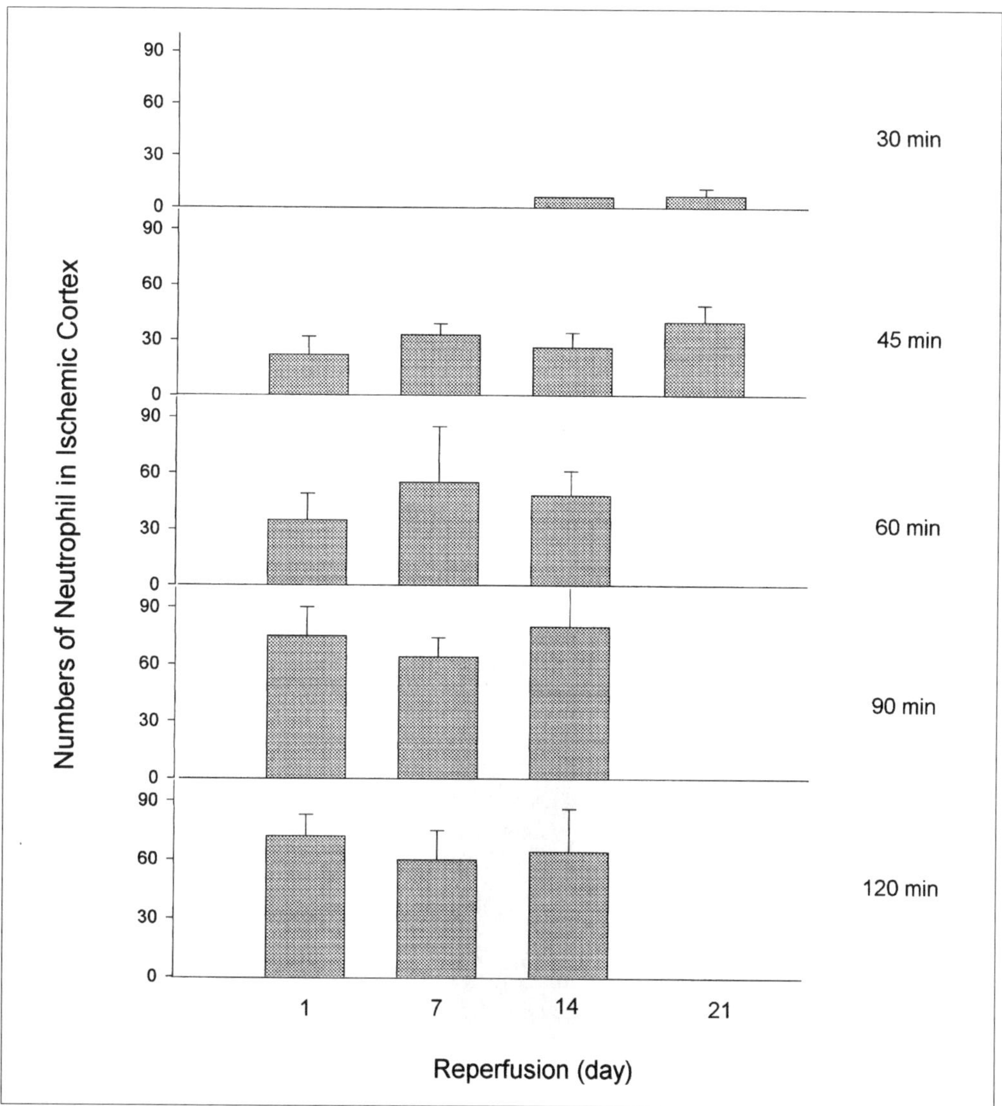

Fig. 2. Number of neutrophils in infarcted cortex following 30, 45, 60, 90 and 120 minutes of ischemia with survival times ranging from 1–21 days.

Influence of proteasome inhibitors

The effect of both proteasome inhibitors was to reduce infarct volumes by approximately 30–40% with no evidence for subsequent maturation of the injury in the following seven days. The reduction of infarction for both CVT-634 and PS-519 are demonstrated in Table 3. A striking reduction in the number of polymorphs was seen for those animals treated with CVT-634 (Fig. 3).

Discussion

We have previously shown that the maturation rate of CA_1 death is not static; it depends on the duration of ischemia. In this study we have demonstrated that there is an analogous slow maturation of cortical infarction whose rate is also dependent on the duration of ischemia. With briefer periods of ischemia, the rate of infarction is not static, but is fully dependent on the duration of reperfusion once a critical ischemic temporal threshold is exceeded. After a brief insult (60 minutes), at 24 hours there is a core of ischemic injury, which is followed by slow maturation of injury. There is a 50% infarct at 24 hours, maturing to 75% at seven days, and reaching 100% of the infarction at fourteen days. With 90 minutes of ischemia, 80–90% of the infarct is seen at 24 hours, with subsequent maturation by seven days, while with 120 minutes of ischemia, a full infarct is seen, with no subsequent interval increase, at 24 hours. The volume of injury is therefore not simply a function of the duration of ischemia. Once the critical ischemic duration is exceeded,

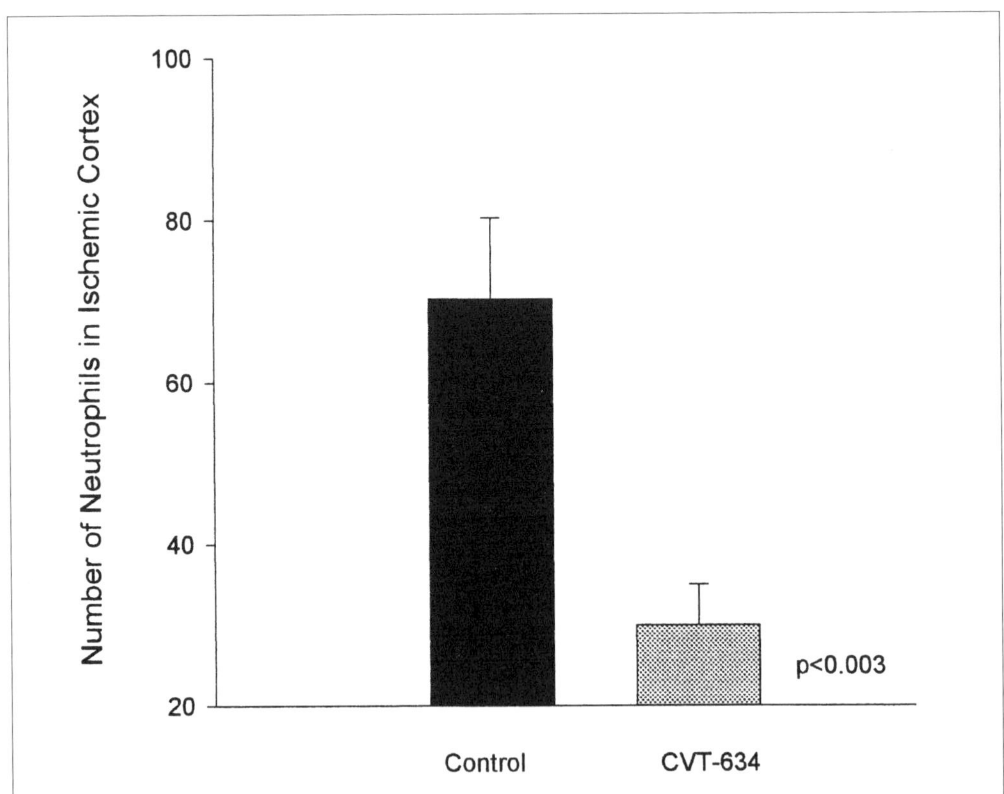

Fig. 3. Number of neutrophils observed in the ischemic cortex of the control versus the CVT-634-treated group.

there is a direct correlation between the duration of ischemia and the rate of maturation of injury.

This previously witnessed slowly evolving injury had implied a role for apoptosis in the progression of cerebral infarction (Du et al. 1996). The morphology in this study, however, was strongly suggestive of necrosis, in agreement with the observations of van Lookeren Campagne et al. (1996) with no evidence for membrane delineated cellular injury (Colbourne et al. 1999a, 1999c).

There are, however, many biochemical features that suggest an active process such as apoptosis during reperfusion following a transient focal ischemic event. These include the activation of the pro-apoptotic Bax (Krajewski et al. 1995) and the observation that supplementation with anti-apoptotic BCl-2 reduces injury (Martinou et al. 1994). To explore this we used inhibitors of caspase to limit or reduce the amount of cortical infarction. Previous experiments have shown that inhibiting interleukin-converting enzyme reduces both ischemic and excito-toxic injury, and that transgenic mice expressing a mutant ICE inhibitory protein also have an attenuation of cortical injury (Hara et al. 1997a, 1997b). In our experiments we were able to demonstrate that caspase inhibitors reduce neuronal injury following focal, but not global, cerebral ischemia (Li et al. 2000a). We were able to confirm the effects of an ICV injection using a systemically (IV) administered caspase inhibitor (Li et al. 2000b). Previous reports had suggested that caspase inhibitors would inhibit the injury to CA_1 cells, but we were unable to confirm this, and speculate that the contradictory data of Chen et al (1998) resulted from premature examination of the pathology. These authors looked at injury within three days of reperfusion. Had they looked at later time points, we speculate that they would have discovered that caspase inhibition was postponing CA_1 injury (Colbourne et al. 1999a) rather than achieving indefatigable cell survival (Colbourne et al 1999b).

In our experiments with focal ischemia, we have been able to achieve neuroprotection with two proteasome inhibitors, which prevent the activation of NF-κB and, therefore, the downstream effects of NF-κB-mediated transcription products. With the CVT-634 compound we were able to demonstrate that the abrogation of injury persisted and there was evidence of sustained protection with an absence of the subsequent delayed maturation of the injury (Buchan et al. 2000). In addition, there was a reduction in the inflammatory component of the injury. With the PS-519 compound, a lactacystin derived proteasome inhibitor (Fenteany et al. 1995), we demonstrated once again a reduction in focal infarction in contrast to a lack of neuroprotection for CA_1 cells following global ischemia (Li et al. 2000c).

NF-κB is a crucial transcription factor and, once activated, promotes cell death following focal cerebral ischemia (Schneider et al. 1999). It appears to be a central mediator of gene expression induced in cells by both ischemia (Clemens et al. 1997) and inflammatory cytokines (Rothwell et al. 1997). While genes transcribed by the activation of NF-κB may be either anti-apoptotic (Mattsan et al. 1997) or pro-apoptotic (Clemens et al. 1998), it is known that injurious cytokines are strong activators of NF-κB (Schneider et al. 1999; Mattsan et al. 1997). Neuroprotection has been achieved with Aspirin, which acts as an inhibitor of NF-κB (Grilli et al. 1996), and with the proteasome inhibitors (Buchan et al. 2000; Li et al. 2000c; Elliott et al. 1999) presented here.

In our observations with PS-519 we also demonstrated that this NF-κB inhibitor had efficacy in an *in vivo* T-lymphocyte-dependent contact sensitivity model in the mouse and reduced inflammation in an ischemia-reperfusion injury model in the rabbit. Both of these observations suggested that its actions have anti-inflammatory components. Further evidence for this comes from the fact that, following focal ischemia and the infusion of both PS-519 and CVT-634, there are fewer inflammatory cells (polymorphs and lymphocytes) in the ischemic vascular bed (Elliott et al. 1999; Li et al. 2000c; Buchan et al. 2000).

In global ischemia, following reperfusion, evidence for apoptosis is dependent on the detection of DNA ladders and the activation of pro-apoptotic enzymes. Morphologically, CA_1 cells appear to die via necrosis (Colbourne et al. 1999a, 1999c) and it appears that the DNA ladders have sticky ends rather than the flush or blunt ends seen in archetypal apoptosis (MacManus et al. 1999). The evidence presented here suggests that neither caspase inhibition nor NF-κB inhibition reduce CA_1 injury.

In conclusion, we present data that suggest that focal infarction, like CA_1 injury, progresses following a latency (Du et al. 1996) and with a maturation rate which is proportional to the ischemic duration (Li and Buchan, 2000). Both caspase and NF-κB inhibition prevent the evolution of this slow injury. Neither caspase nor proteasome inhibitors prevented CA_1 cell death. We speculate that this difference is because the drugs are blocking neuro-inflammation, rather than preventing the activation of an apoptotic cascade. Neuro-inflammation may be more important in post-focal, compared to post-global, maturation of injury.

Acknowledgements

This work was supported by grants from the Heart and Stroke Foundation of Canada, the Medical Research Council of Canada, and the Alberta Heritage Foundation for Medical Research.

References

1. Buchan AM, Xue D, Slivka A (1992) A new model of temporary focal neocortical ischemia in the rat. Stroke 23:273–279
2. Buchan AM, Li H, Blackburn B (2000) Neuroprotection achieved with a novel proteasome inhibitor which blocks NF-κB activation. NeuroReport 11:427–430
3. Chen J, Nagayama T, Jin K, Stetler RA, Zhu RL, Graham SH, Simon RP (1998) Induction of caspase-3-like protease may mediate delayed neuronal death in the hippocampus after transient cerebral ischemia. J Neurosci 18:4914–4928
4. Clemens JA, Stephenson DT, Smalstig EB, Dixon EP, Little SP (1997) Global ischemia activates nuclear-factor-κB in forebrain neurons of rats. Stroke 28:1073–1081
5. Clemens JA, Stephenson DT, Yin T, Smalstig EB, Panetta JA, Little SP (1998) Drug-induced neuroprotection from global ischemia is associated with prevention of persistent but not transient activation of nuclear factor-κB in rats. Stroke 29:677–682
6. Colbourne F, Li H, Buchan AM (1999a) Continuing postischemic neuronal death in CA_1: influence of ischemic duration and cytoprotective doses of NBQX and SNX-111 in rats. Stroke 30:662–668
7. Colbourne F, et al. Li H, Buchan AM, (1999b) Indefatigable CA_1 sector neuroprotection with mild hypothermia induced 6 hours after severe forebrain ischemia in rats. J Cereb Blood Flow Metab 19:742–749
8. Colbourne F, Sutherland GR, Auer RN (1999c) Electron microscope evidence against apoptosis as the mechanism of neuronal death in global ischemia. J Neurosci 19:4200–4210
9. Du C, Hu R, Csernansky CA, Hsu CY, Choi DW (1996) Very delayed infarction after mild focal cerebral ischemia: a role for apoptosis? J Cereb Blood Flow Metab 16:195–201
10. Elliott PJ, Pien CS, McCormack TA, Chapman ID, Adams J (1999) Proteasome inhibition: a novel mechanism to combat asthma. J Allergy Clin Immun 104:294–300
11. Fenteany G, Standaert RF, Lane WS, Choi S, Corey EJ, Schreiber SL (1995) Inhibition of proteasome activities and subunit-specific amino-terminal threonine modification by lactacystin. Science 268:726–731
12. Grilli M, Pizzi M, Memo M, Spano PF (1996) Neuroprotection by aspirin and sodium salicylate through blockade of NF-κB activation. Science 274:1383–1385
13. Hara H, Fink K, Endres M, Friedlander RM, Gagliardini V, Yuan J, Moskowitz MA (1997a) Attenuation of transient focal cerebral ischemic injury in transgenic mice expressing a mutant ICE inhibitory protein. J Cereb Blood Flow Metab 17:370–375
14. Hara H, Friedlander RM, Gagliardini V, Ayata C, Fink K, Huang Z, Shimizu-Sasamata M, Yuan J, Moskiwitz MA (1997b) Inhibition of interleukin 1β converting enzyne family proteases reduces ischemic and excitotoxic neuronal damage. Proc Natl Acad Sci USA 94:2007–2012
15. Ito U, Spatz M, Walker Jt Jr, Klatzo I (1975) Experimental cerebral ischemia in mongolian gerbils. I. Light microscope observations. Acta Neuropathol (Berl) 32:209–223
16. Kirino T (1982) Delayed neuronal death in the gerbil hippocampus following ischemia. Brain Res 239:57–69
17. Krajewski S, Mai JK, Krajewska M, Sikorska M, Mossakowski MJ, Reed JC (1995) Upregulation of Bax protein levels in neurons following cerebral ischemia. J Neurosci 15:6364–6376
18. Li H, Buchan AM (2000) Delayed maturation of cortical infarction: the influence of ischemic duration. (Abstract) Stroke, 31,345
19. Li H, Colbourne F, Sun P, Zhao Z, Buchan AM (2000a) Caspase inhibitors reduce neuronal injury after focal but not global cerebral ischemia in rats. Stroke 31:176–182
20. Li H, van Bruggen N, Cai SX, Buchan AM (2000b) Intravenous administration of a novel caspase inhibitor affords neuroprotection following focal ichemia in rats. Canadian Journal Neurological Science, S16
21. Li H, Zhao Z, Sun P, Elliott P, Buchan AM (2000c) "Proscript 519, Proteasome Inhibitor, Reduces Cortical Neuronal Injury Following Focal Ischemia in Rats" Stroke, 31:277
22. MacManus JP, Fliss H, Preston E, Rasquinha I, and Preston E (1999) Cerebral ischemia produces laddered DNA fragments distinct from cardiac ischemia and archetypal apoptosis. J Cereb Blood Flow Metab 19:502–510
23. Martinou JC, Dubois-Dauphin M, Staple JK, Rodriguez I, Frankowski H, Missotten M, Albertini P, Talabot D, Catsicas S, Pietra C, Huarte J (1994) Overexpression of BCL-2 in transgenic mice protects neurons from naturally occurring cell death and experimental ischemia. Neurol 13:1017–1030
24. Mattsan MP, Goodman Y, Luo H, Fu W, Furukawa K (1997) Activation of NF-κB protects hippocampal neurons against oxidative stress-induced apoptosis: evidence for induction of manganese superoxide dismutase and suppression of peroxynitrite production and protein tyrosine nitration. J Neurosci Res 49:681–697

25. Pulsinelli WA, Brierley JB, Plum F (1982) Temoral profile of neuronal damage in a model of transient forebrain ischemia. Ann Neurol 11:491–498
26. Rothwell N, Allan S, Toulmond S (1997) The role of interleukin 1 in acute neurodegeneration and stroke: pathophysiological and therapeutic implications. J Clin Invest 100:2648–2652
27. Schneider A, Martin Villalba A, Weih F, Vogel J, Wirth T, Schwaninger M (1999) NF-κB is activated and promotes cell death in focal cerebral ischemia. Nature Med 5:554–559
28. van Lookeren Campagne M, Gill R (1996) Ultrastructural morphological changes are not characteristic of apoptotic cell death following focal cerebral ischemia in the rat. Neurosci Lett 213:111–114

Inflammation-related genes and ischemic brain injury

C. Iadecola[1], M. Alexander[1], S. Nogawa[2], E. Araki[1], M. E. Ross[1]

1.1 Introduction

Focal cerebral ischemia results from a permanent or transient reduction in cerebral blood flow that is restricted to the territory of a major cerebral artery, most frequently, the middle cerebral artery (MCA). In the center of the ischemic territory, or ischemic core, the flow reduction is most marked and the tissue undergoes irreversible damage within a few hours. At the periphery of ischemic territory, however, the reduction in blood flow is less marked and neurons survive for many hours, perhaps, even days (Baird et al. 1997; Dereski et al. 1993; Garcia et al. 1993; Marchal et al. 1996; Touzani et al. 1995). The size of the brain infarct depends, ultimately, on the fate of this peripheral region, commonly referred to as "ischemic penumbra". Studies in experimental models of cerebral ischemia and in human stroke indicate that inflammatory mechanisms play an important role in the delayed progression of brain injury in the ischemic penumbra. Thus, interventions aimed at decreasing the inflammatory reaction of the post-ischemic brain offer an attractive therapeutic strategy in human stroke because of their potentially-wide therapeutic window. In this chapter the experimental evidence that inflammation contributes to ischemic injury will be reviewed with emphasis on the role of inflammation-related genes and transcription factors.

1.2 Cerebral ischemia and inflammation

Studies in animal models of focal cerebral ischemia and in human stroke have demonstrated accumulation of neutrophils and monocytes in the infarct territory. In a primate model of focal cerebral ischemia produced by MCA occlusion, the accumulation of neutrophils is maximal at 48–72 hours, and it is followed by accumulation of macrophages 7–16 days after occlusion (Garcia and Kamijyo 1974). In rodents, the neutrophilic infiltration begins a few hours after arterial occlusion and peaks 12–24 hours depending on the model (Barone et al. 1991; Clark et al. 1993; Garcia et al. 1994). In vivo studies of human cerebral ischemia, in which circulating leukocytes were labeled with Indium-111, showed delayed leukocyte accumulation 2–14 days after the onset of symptoms (Pozzilli et al. 1985). The inflammatory reaction that involves the ischemic brain is driven by activation of a complex array of genes, the expression of which is triggered by the ischem-

[1]Center for Clinical and Molecular Neurobiology, Department of Neurology, University of Minnesota School of Medicine, Box 295 UMHC, 420 Delaware street S.E., Minneapolis, MN 55455, USA
email: iadec001@tc.umn.edu
[2]Department of Neurology, Keio University, Tokyo, Japan

J. Krieglstein, S. Klumpp (Eds.) Pharmacology of Cerebral Ischemia 2000

ic event. Ischemia induces expression of inflammatory cytokines, including tumor necrosis factor-α (TNF-α) and interleukin-1β (IL-1β), which, in turn, lead to expression of adhesion molecules on endothelial cells and leukocytes (see Feuerstein et al. 1998 for a review). The adhesion molecules-mediated interactions between leukocytes and endothelial cells ultimately result in migration of blood borne leukocytes across the vascular wall and into the ischemic brain parenchyma. Other pro-inflammatory molecules termed chemokines, such as interleukin-8, monocyte chemoattractant protein-1 and macrophage inflammatory protein-1, are produced by the injured brain and guide the migration of blood borne inflammatory cells towards their target in the ischemic territory (Kim et al. 1996).

Several lines of evidence suggest that post-ischemic inflammation has a deleterious effect on the outcome of the ischemic tissue. First, interventions aimed at reducing the number of circulating neutrophils improve the outcome of cerebral ischemia. Thus, treatments that induce neutropenia reduce infarct volume and improve functional outcome (Table 1). Second, antibodies blocking the action of adhesion molecules reduce the influx of neutrophils and improve tissue outcome (Table 2). Third, null mice lacking the adhesion molecules ICAM-1 or P-selectin are less susceptible to ischemic damage (Table 2). Fourth, intervention blocking the action of cytokines reduces ischemic damage (Table 3).

The mechanisms whereby inflammation contributes to cerebral ischemic damage are not well understood. Several hypotheses have been put forward (see Feuerstein et al. 1998 for a review). Although leukocyte adhesion to the microvascular endothelium could produce microvascular plugging and worsen the ischemia (Del Zoppo et al. 1991), the pathogenic significance of this process remains controversial (Dirnagl et al. 1994). Toxic substances could also be released by injured or dying cells in response to the inflammatory reaction that involves the brain. Certain cytokines produced during ischemia, such as IL-1β and TNF-α, can produce neuronal damage directly (Rothwell and Hopkins 1995). However, there are instances in which TNF-α can ameliorate neuronal injury. For example, TNF-α receptor-null mice have an increased susceptibility to ischemic damage (Bruce et al. 1996; Gary et al. 1998), and TNF-α can induce protection from subsequent ischemic injury (ischemic pre-conditioning) (Liu et al. 2000). Thus, in some conditions, this cytokine can be protective, an effect thought to be mediated by NFkB-induced expression of the free radical-scavenging enzyme superoxide dismutase (see Shohami et al. 1999 and Mattson et al. 2000 for a review). On the other hand, inflammatory cells could contribute to neuronal damage by producing oxygen free radicals and other inflammation-related products, that are toxic to neurons (Iadecola et al. 1995b; Ward 1991).

Over the past several years we have been investigating the mechanisms by which post-

Table 1. Effect of systemic leukocyte depletion on the outcome of focal cerebral ischemia

Intervention	Outcome	Selected references
Mechlorethamine and vinblastine	Improved histological or functional outcome in dog, rabbit and rat models of focal ischemia	Dutka et al. 1989 Heinel et al. 1994 Helps and Gorman 1991
Anti-neutrophilic antibodies	Reduction in infarct size or edema in rabbit and rat models of focal cerebral ischemia	Bednar et al. 1991 Shiga et al. 1991 Matsuo et al. 1994
Neutrophil inhibitory factor	Reduction in infarct size in rats with transient MCAO	Jiang et al. 1995

Abbreviations: MCAO, middle cerebral artery occlusion.

Table 2. Effect of inhibition of adhesion molecules on the outcome of focal cerebral ischemia

Intervention	Outcome	Selected references
Anti-ICAM-1 antibodies	Reduction in infarct size in rats with transient MCAO	Zhang et al. 1994
ICAM-1 null mice	Reduction in infarct size in transient and permanent MCAO	Soriano et al. 1996 Connolly et al. 1996 Kitagawa et al. 1998
Anti-CD18 monoclonal antibodies	Increased reflow in microvessels of different sizes in primates	Mori et al. 1992
Anti-CD11b monoclonal antibody	Reduction in infarct size in rats with transient MCAO	Chen et al. 1994
Mac-1 (CD11b/CD18) null mice	Reduction in infarct size in rats with transient MCAO	Soriano et al. 1999
CY-1503, analog of sialyl-Lewis (x)	Reduction in infarct size in rats with transient MCAO	Zhang et al. 1996
Synthetic oligopeptide corresponding to the lectin domain of selectins	Reduction in infarct size in rats with transient MCAO	Morikawa et al. 1996
P-selectin null mice	Reduction in infarct size in rats with transient MCAO	Connolly et al. 1997
Anti-P-selectin monoclonal antibody	Reduction in infarct size in rats with transient or permanent MCAO	Goussev et al. 1998 Suzuki et al. 1999

Abbreviations: MCAO, middle cerebral artery occlusion; ICAM-1, intercellular adhesion molecule-1; Mac-1, macrophage-1 antigen complex.

ischemic inflammation contributes to cerebral ischemic injury. Evidence will be presented that expression of iNOS, COX-2 and related transcription factors are important pathogenic factors in the progression of cerebral ischemic damage.

1.3 iNOS

Nitric oxide (NO) is a free radical that can act both as a signaling molecule and a neurotoxin (Iadecola 1999). NO is synthesized from L-arginine by the enzyme nitric oxide synthase (NOS). There are three isoforms of NOS: neuronal NOS (nNOS), endothelial NOS (eNOS), and inducible or immunological NOS (iNOS) (Marletta 1994). nNOS and eNOS are expressed constitutively in a selected group of neurons and in endothelial cells, respectively, and their activity is regulated by intracellular calcium (Garthwaite and Boulton 1995). iNOS is normally not present in most cells and its expression is induced in many cell types during inflammation and injury (Nathan 1995). iNOS activity is independent of intracellular calcium, and generates toxic levels of NO, which are thought to contribute to the tissue damage associated with inflammation (Gross and Wolin 1995).

In brain, iNOS is induced in the setting of post-ischemic inflammation. Following transient or permanent MCA occlusion in rodents, iNOS mRNA is upregulated and peaks 12–48 h after ischemia (Grandati et al. 1997; Iadecola et al. 1996, 1995b). iNOS is induced in neutrophils infiltrating the injured brain and in cerebral blood vessels in the ischemic territory. A recent study using immunohistochemistry showed that iNOS is also expressed in the

Table 3. Effect of inhibition of cytokines on the outcome of focal cerebral ischemia

Intervention	Outcome	Selected references
TNFα soluble receptor type 1	Reduction in infarct size in rat and mouse with permanent MCAO	Dawson et al. 1996 Nawashiro et al. 1997
Anti-TNF-α monoclonal antibody	Reduction in infarct size in rat and mouse with MCAO	Barone et al. 1997 Yang et al. 1998
IL-1β administration	Increase in infarct size in rat with transient MCAO	Yamasaki et al. 1995
IL-1β receptor antagonist	Reduction in infarct size in rat and mouse with MCAO	Betz et al. 1995 Loddick and Rothwell 1996 Relton et al. 1996 Yang et al. 1997
IL-6 administration	Reduction in infarct size in rat with permanent MCAO	Loddick et al. 1998
Anti-IL-8 monoclonal antibody	Reduction in infarct size in rabbits with transient ischemia	Matsumoto et al. 1997
Anti-CINC antibody	Reduction in infarct size in rat with transient MCAO	Yamasaki et al. 1997

Abbreviations: MCAO, middle cerebral artery occlusion; IL-, interleukin-, CINC, cytokine-induced neutrophil chemoattractant; TNF-α, tumor necrosis factor-α.

human brain following ischemic stroke (Forster et al. 1999). As in rodents, iNOS immunoreactivity is observed in neutrophils and blood vessels within the ischemic territory. Immunoreactivity for nitrotyrosine, a relatively-specific marker of NO-derived peroxynitrite, is observed in infiltrating neutrophils, suggesting that iNOS is catalytically active also in the post-ischemic human brain (Forster et al. 1999).

Several lines of evidence suggest that iNOS contributes to ischemic injury (Table 4). First, administration of the iNOS inhibitor aminoguanidine, starting 6 or 24 hours after MCA occlusion, attenuates post-ischemic iNOS activity and reduces the volume of the infarct by 30–40% (Table 4) (Iadecola et al. 1996; Iadecola et al. 1995a). The reduction in histological damage is associated with improvement in neurological deficits (Nagayama et al. 1998). Aminoguanidine does not influence cerebral blood flow, indicating that its protective effect is not related to preservation of post-ischemic blood flow (Iadecola et al. 1995a). Second, delayed administration of the iNOS inhibitor 1400W, an agent structurally distinct from aminoguanidine, reduces infarct volume in rats after MCA occlusion (Parmentier et al. 1999). Third, iNOS deficient mice have smaller infarcts following MCA occlusion and a better neurological outcome than wild-type controls (Table 4). The reduction in infarct volume is more pronounced in homozygous (–/–) than in heterozygous (+/–) null mice (Zhao et al. 2000). The reduction in CBF produced by MCA occlusion and the degree of neutrophilic infiltration and astrocytic activation is comparable in iNOS knockout mice and wild-type controls (Iadecola et al. 1997). Therefore, the protection cannot be attributed to cerebrovascular effects related to iNOS deletion or to differences in the cellular reaction to ischemia. It must be noted, however, that in models of brain trauma iNOS expression is beneficial to the injured brain (Sinz et al. 1999). Therefore, the deleterious effects of iNOS in cerebral ischemia do not apply to other modalities of brain injury.

Table 4. Role of iNOS, COX-2, NFkB and IRF-1 in animal models of focal cerebral ischemia

Intervention	Outcome	Selected references
iNOS inhibition/deletion		
Aminoguanidine 1400W	Reduction in infarct size in rats with transient and permanent MCAO	Iadecola et al. 1995a Iadecola et al. 1996 Nagayama et al. 1998 Parmentier et al. 1999
iNOS knockout mice	Reduction in infarct size in permanent MCAO	Iadecola et al. 1997 Nagayama et al. 1999a Zhao et al. 2000
COX-2 inhibitors		
NS 398	Reduction in infarct size in rat and mouse with MCAO	Nogawa et al. 1997 Nagayama et al. 1999b
NFkB inhibition/deletion		
N-acetylcysteine CVT-634	Reduction in infarct size in rats with transient MCAO	Carroll et al. 1998 Buchan et al. 2000
Mice lacking p50 subunit	Reduction in infarct size in transient MCAO	Schneider et al. 1999
IRF-1 deletion		
IRF-1 knockout mouse	Reduction in infarct size in permanent MCAO	Iadecola et al. 1999b

Abbreviations: COX-2, cyclooxygenase-2; iNOS, inducible nitric oxide synthase; IRF-1, interferon regulatory factor-1; MCAO, middle cerebral artery occlusion; NFkB, nuclear factor-kappa B.

The mechanisms by which NO and its derived chemical species exert their cytotoxic effect are multiple and include inhibition of ATP-producing enzymes (Gross and Wolin 1995), DNA damage (Szabo and Ohshima 1997), and oxidative damage produced by peroxynitrite, a highly reactive chemical specie formed by the reaction of NO with superoxide (Beckman et al. 1990).

1.4 COX-2

Cyclooxygenase (COX) is a rate-limiting enzyme in the synthesis of prostaglandins and thromboxanes. Two isoforms have been described: COX-1 and COX-2. COX-1 is constitutively expressed in many cells, where it produces prostanoids that are involved in normal cellular function (Vane et al. 1998). COX-2 is normally not expressed, except at low levels in some cells, such as neurons (Breder et al. 1995; Yamagata et al. 1993). However, in many cells COX-2 is upregulated in response to mitogens, inflammatory mediators, and hormones (see Wu 1995 for a review). In models of inflammation, COX-2 is upregulated and contributes to tissue damage through the production of reactive oxygen species and toxic prostanoids (Seibert et al. 1995). The catalytic activity of COX-2 is associated with production of reactive oxygen species (Armstead et al. 1988; Kontos et al. 1980; Smith and DeWitt 1995). Superoxide produced by COX-2 could react with NO to form peroxynitrite, a highly reactive oxidant that mediates many of the toxic effects of NO (e.g., Szabo and Ohshima 1997).

There is evidence that COX-2 participates in the mechanisms of cerebral ischemia (Table 4). COX-2 mRNA and protein expression are upregulated 12–24 h after cerebral ischemia in rodents (Miettinen et al. 1997; Nogawa et al. 1998, 1997; Planas et al. 1995). COX-2 expression in rodents is observed in neurons at the periphery of the infarct, in vascular cells and, possibly, microglia (Miettinen et al. 1997;

Nogawa et al. 1997). Recently, COX-2 has been found to be expressed also in human brain after ischemic stroke (Iadecola et al. 1999a; Sairanen et al. 1998). As in rodents, COX-2 immunoreactivity is observed in ischemic neurons at the border of ischemic territory, and in neutrophils and vascular cells. The upregulation in COX-2 immunoreactivity is confined to the area of damage (Iadecola et al. 1999a). Administration of NS398, a relatively selective COX-2 inhibitor, 6 hours after ischemia, reduces the infarct volume by 20–30% in a model of focal ischemia in rats (Table 4). COX-2 inhibition also reduces CA1 hippocampal neuronal damage in a model of global cerebral ischemia (Nakayama et al. 1998). The observation that delayed administration of NS398 reduces infarct volume supports the hypothesis that COX-2 is involved in the late stages of ischemic injury. The deleterious role that COX-2 plays in cerebral ischemia, however, cannot be generalized, because in models of kainate-induced seizures NS398 aggravates hippocampal damage (Baik et al. 1999).

1.5 Interaction between iNOS and COX-2

COX-2 and iNOS are upregulated with a similar time course and in cells that are in close proximity to each other (Nogawa et al. 1998). The spatial and temporal proximity between iNOS and COX-2 raises the possibility that, in the post-ischemic brain as in other organs during inflammation, NO produced by iNOS activates COX-2 and enhances the toxic output of the enzyme (Salvemini et al. 1994). Recent experimental evidence supports this view. After MCA occlusion, inhibition of iNOS by aminoguanidine attenuates COX-2 reaction products only in the ischemic region (Nogawa et al. 1998). Furthermore, post-ischemic prostaglandin production is reduced in iNOS null mice, despite normal COX-2 mRNA and protein expression (Nogawa et al. 1998). These findings are consistent with the hypothesis that, in the post-ischemic brain, iNOS-derived NO activates COX-2.

The interaction between iNOS-derived NO and COX-2 raises the possibility that some of the deleterious effects of iNOS expression induced by cerebral ischemia are mediated through COX-2 reaction products. This hypothesis is supported by a recent study in which the COX-2 inhibitor NS398 was found to attenuate ischemic brain damage in wild-type mice, but not in iNOS deficient mice (Nagayama et al. 1999b). Thus, inhibition of COX-2 in iNOS deficient mice did not confer protection greater than that attained by iNOS deletion alone. In contrast, administration of the nNOS inhibitor 7-nitroindazole reduced infarct volume in iNOS null mice (Nagayama et al. 1999b). Thus, the failure of NS398 to ameliorate the injury is not due to the fact that iNOS null mice are maximally protected. The data support the hypothesis that COX-2 activation is an important factor in the damage produced by iNOS-derived NO, and that iNOS-derived NO is required for the full expression of COX-2 neurotoxicity.

iNOS and COX-2 are expressed in the human brain in the acute stage of focal cerebral ischemia (Forster et al. 1999; Iadecola et al. 1999a). While it remains to be established whether iNOS-derived NO and COX-2 reaction products contribute to the pathogenesis of human stroke, the similarity in the timing and cellular localization of iNOS and COX-2 between rodents and humans, suggests that the interaction between iNOS-derived NO and COX-2 reported in rodents may also occur in the human brain.

1.6 Inflammation-related transcription factors and cerebral ischemic injury

The molecular mechanisms of iNOS and COX-2 gene expression are not fully understood. Gene expression is controlled by transcription factors, DNA-binding proteins that initiate mRNA transcription. Transcription factors that are important in the expression of inflammation-related genes, such as iNOS and COX-2, include nuclear factor kappa B (NFkB) and interferon regulatory factor-1 (IRF-1) (see Baeuerle and Baltimore 1996 and Nguyen et al. 1997 for review).

NFkB activates transcription of a wide variety of genes, including those encoding for adhesion molecules, chemokines, iNOS and COX-2 (Mattson et al. 2000). In resting cells, the two subunits of NFkB, p65 and p50, are bound to the inhibitory factor IkB and the complex is sequestered in the cytoplasm. Cell stimulation leads to degradation of IkB in the proteosome, unmasking a nuclear localization signaling sequence that allows NFkB to be translocated to the nucleus. NFkB then binds to cognate DNA sequences and activates gene transcription (see Baeuerle and Baltimore 1996 for a review). Ischemia-reperfusion, physical stress and reactive oxygen species are potent stimuli for NFkB activation (Mattson et al. 2000).

Cerebral ischemia activates NFkB (Salminen et al. 1995; see Carroll et al. 2000 for a review). After transient focal ischemia in rat, increased immunoreactivity of p65 is found in neurons at the periphery of the infarct, in reactive glia, and in inflammatory cells (Gabriel et al. 1999; Stephenson et al. 2000). NFkB activation is observed 6–96 hours after ischemia, depending on model and specie (Gabriel et al. 1999; Schneider et al. 1999; Stephenson et al. 2000). Immunoreactivity for NFkB is also observed in glial cells of human infarcts, particularly at the border zone between ischemic and non-ischemic areas (Terai et al. 1996). NFkB activation occurs also in vulnerable hippocampal neurons after global ischemia (Clemens et al. 1997).

Several studies have investigated the role of NFkB in ischemic brain injury. NFkB transcription factor decoys, oligonucleotides that compete with NFkB for promoter binding sites, were used in cultured endothelial cells. NFkB decoys block the increase in ICAM-1 mRNA levels and the upregulation of surface ICAM-1 following exposure to TNF-α or hypoxia-reoxygenation (Hess et al. 2000). Administration of the NFkB activation inhibitor N-acetylcysteine to rats with transient focal ischemia reduces infarct volume (Carroll et al. 1998). Similarly, blockade of NFkB activation by treatment with the proteosome inhibitor CVT-634 reduces infarct volume in a rat model of transient focal ischemia (Buchan et al. 2000). Furthermore, null mice lacking the p50 subunits of NFkB are more resistant to focal cerebral ischemia (Schneider et al. 1999). On the other hand, in some models of brain injury NFkB plays a protective role (Mattson et al. 2000). For example, p50 null-mice are more susceptible to hippocampal damage produced by kainate administration (Yu et al. 1999). Furthermore, administration of NFkB decoys to wild-type mice worsens such injury (Yu et al. 1999). Therefore, the role of NFkB in neuronal damage is complex and model dependent.

IRF-1 is a transcription factor involved in multiple functions, including cell growth, differentiation, and cytokine signaling (Mamane et al. 1999). Recent evidence suggests that this transcription factor is also involved in cerebral ischemic injury. Interferon-γ and other cytokines bind to cell surface receptors that carry JAK/STAT proteins (Janus kinases and signal transduction and activator of transcription). The resulting activation of JAK/STAT results in the expression of many genes including the IRF-1 gene. IRF-1 protein binds to DNA promoter elements shared by many pro-inflammatory genes, such as iNOS and COX-2 (Blanco et al. 2000; Kamijo et al. 1994) and activates their expression.

IRF-1 mRNA is upregulated after focal cerebral ischemia (Iadecola et al. 1999b). The increase begins at 12 hours after ischemia, is maximal at 4 days, and subsides at 7 days (Iadecola et al. 1999b). Immunocytochemical studies revealed that IRF-1 expression occurs in cerebral endothelial cells and in cells with the morphological characteristics of neurons, both at the center and periphery of the ischemic territory (M. Alexander, C. Forster, K. Sugimoto and C. Iadecola, unpublished observations). Furthermore, gel-shift assay experiments demonstrated that IRF-1 binding activity is enhanced after focal ischemia (Fig. 1), suggesting that the upregulation in IRF-1 protein is functionally significant. The role of IRF-1 in focal cerebral ischemia was studied in IRF-1-null mice subjected to MCA occlusion. It was found that IRF-1 –/– mice do not express IRF-1 after cerebral ischemia and have smaller infarct compared to wild-type mice (Table 4). The reduc-

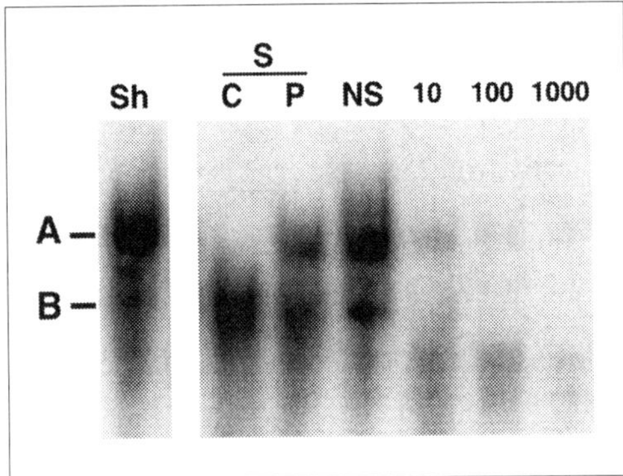

Fig. 1. Gel mobility-shift assay was used to determine whether IRF-1 binding activity is increased following cerebral ischemia. The assay was performed on nuclear extracts from brains of mice sacrificed 24 hours after MCA occlusion. Sham-operated mice served as controls. Two complexes, A and B, were found in sham-operated mice (Sh) (cf. Martin et al. 1994). Complex B was upregulated following cerebral ischemia. The upregulation was more marked in samples taken from the center of the ischemic territory (C) than from the periphery (P). In contrast, complex A disappeared in the ischemic core and was attenuated in the periphery. The complexes observed in the non-ischemic side of the brain (NS) were similar to those observed in sham-operated animals. Complexes A and B were progressively attenuated by incubation with increasing concentrations of cold probe (10, 100, 1000 fold excess). These data suggest that complex B represents IRF-1 binding activity is increased in the post-ischemic brain.

tion in infarct volume was greater in IRF-1 –/– (≈ 46%) mice than in IRF-1 +/– mice (≈ 23%), and was associated with improvement in the neurological deficits produced by cerebral ischemia (Iadecola et al. 1999b). These studies demonstrate that IRF-1-dependent genes contribute to the late stages of cerebral ischemia. Further studies are necessary to identify the gene products involved, and to determine whether IRF-1 expression is also relevant to human stroke.

1.7 Summary and Conclusions

We have presented evidence that post-ischemic expression of iNOS and COX-2 contributes to the delayed progression of the brain damage produced by cerebral ischemia. iNOS and COX-2 are expressed in the setting of a massive genomic response driven by ischemia-induced activation of transcription factors. In particular, IRF-1 and NFkB are activated after cerebral ischemia and play a major role in gene expression in the late stages of ischemic brain injury. Although the evidence indicates that in focal cerebral ischemia iNOS and COX-2 contribute to tissue damage, in other models of brain injury these gene products seem to be protective. Similarly, the cytokine TNF-α and the transcription factor NFkB promote cell death in some settings, but act as neuroprotectants in others. Therefore, the conclusions reached on the basis of data in models of cerebral ischemia cannot be generalized to other brain pathologies. In addition, studies of post-ischemic inflammation have, thus far, focused on the participation of the inflammatory process in the mechanisms of tissue damage. The role of inflammation in tissue repair and remodeling after stroke, and the effects of anti-inflammatory interventions on these processes remain to be investigated. Nevertheless, the evidence thus far accumulated provides a strong rationale for exploring further the therapeutic potential of interventions aimed at modulating post-ischemic inflammation.

Acknowledgments

The studies summarized in this chapter were supported by grants from the National Institutes of Health (NS34179 and NS35806). C.I. is the recipient of a Javits Award from NINDS. We wish to thank Mr. Tim Murphy for editorial assistance.

References

1. Armstead WM, Mirro R, Busija DW, Leffler CW (1988) Postischemic generation of superoxide anion by newborn pig brain. Am J Physiol 255:H401–403
2. Baeuerle PA, Baltimore D (1996) NF-kappa B: ten years after. Cell 87:13–20
3. Baik EJ, Kim EJ, Lee SH, Moon C (1999) Cyclooxygenase-2 selective inhibitors aggravate kainic acid induced seizure and neuronal cell death in the hippocampus. Brain Res 843:118–129

4. Baird AE, Benfield A, Schlaug G, Siewert B, Lövblad K-O, Edelman RR, Warach S (1997) Enlargement of human cerebral ischemic lesion volumes measured by diffusion-weighted magnetic resonance imaging. Ann Neurol 41:581–589
5. Barone FC, Arvin B, White RF, Miller A, Webb CL, Willette RN, Lysko PG, Feuerstein GZ (1997) Tumor necrosis factor-alpha. A mediator of focal ischemic brain injury. Stroke 28:1233–1244
6. Barone FC, Hillegass LM, Price WJ, White RF, Lee EV, Feuerstein GZ, Sarau HM, Clark RK, Griswold DE (1991) Polymorphonuclear leukocyte infiltration into cerebral focal ischemic tissue: myeloperoxidase activity assay and histologic verification. J Neurosci Res 29:336–345
7. Beckman JS, Beckman TW, Chen J, Marshall PA, Freeman BA (1990) Apparent hydroxyl radical production by peroxynitrite: implications for endothelial injury from nitric oxide and superoxide. Proc Natl Acad Sci USA 87:1620–1624
8. Bednar MM, Raymond S, McAuliffe T, Lodge PA, Gross CG (1991) The role of neutrophils and platelets in a rabbit model of thromboembolic stroke. Stroke 22:44–50
9. Betz AL, Yang GY, Davidson BL (1995) Attenuation of stroke size in rats using an adenoviral vector to induce overexpression of interleukin-1 receptor antagonist in brain. J Cereb Blood Flow Metab 15:547–551
10. Blanco JC, Contursi C, Salkowski CA, DeWitt DL, Ozato K, Vogel SN (2000) Interferon regulatory factor (IRF)-1 and IRF-2 regulate interferon gamma-dependent cyclooxygenase 2 expression. J Exp Med 191:2131–2144
11. Breder CD, Dewitt D, Kraig RP (1995) Characterization of inducible cyclooxygenase in rat brain. J. Comp. Neurol. 355:296–315
12. Bruce AJ, Boling W, Kindy MS, Peschon J, Kraemer PJ, Carpenter MK, Holtsberg FW, Mattson MP (1996) Altered neuronal and microglial responses to excitotoxic and ischemic brain injury in mice lacking TNF receptors. Nat Med 2:788–794
13. Buchan AM, Li H, Blackburn B (2000) Neuroprotection achieved with a novel proteasome inhibitor which blocks NF-kappaB activation. Neuroreport 11:427–430
14. Carroll JE, Hess DC, Howard EF, Hill WD (2000) Is nuclear factor-kappaB a good treatment target in brain ischemia/reperfusion injury? Neuroreport 11:R1–4
15. Carroll JE, Howard EF, Hess DC, Wakade CG, Chen Q, Cheng C (1998) Nuclear factor-kappa B activation during cerebral reperfusion: effect of attenuation with N-acetylcysteine treatment. Brain Res Mol Brain Res 56:186–191
16. Chen H, Chopp M, Zhang RL, Bodzin G, Chen Q, Rusche JR, Todd RFIII (1994) Anti-CD11b monoclonal antibody reduces ischemic cell damage after transient focal cerebral ischemia in rat. Ann Neurol 35:458–463
17. Clark RK, Lee EV, Fish CJ, White RF, Price WJ, Jonak ZL, Feuerstein GZ (1993) Development of tissue damage, inflammation and resolution following stroke: an immunohistochemical and quantitative planimetric study. Brain Res. Bull 31:565–572
18. Clemens JA, Stephenson DT, Smalstig EB, Dixon EP, Little SP (1997) Global ischemia activates nuclear factor-kappa B in forebrain neurons of rats. Stroke 28:1073–1080
19. Connolly ES, Jr., Winfree CJ, Prestigiacomo CJ, Kim SC, Choudhri TF, Hoh BL, Naka Y, Solomon RA, Pinsky DJ (1997) Exacerbation of cerebral injury in mice that express the P-selectin gene: identification of P-selectin blockade as a new target for the treatment of stroke. Circ Res 81:304–310
20. Connolly ES, Jr., Winfree CJ, Springer TA, Naka Y, Liao H, Yan SD, Stern DM, Solomon RA, Gutierrez-Ramos JC, Pinsky DJ (1996) Cerebral protection in homozygous null ICAM-1 mice after middle cerebral artery occlusion. Role of neutrophil adhesion in the pathogenesis of stroke. J. Clin. Invest. 97:209–216
21. Dawson DA, Martin D, Hallenbeck JM (1996) Inhibition of tumor necrosis factor-alpha reduces focal cerebral ischemic injury in the spontaneously hypertensive rat. Neurosci Lett 218:41–44
22. Del Zoppo GJ, Schmid-Schonbein GW, Mori E, Copeland BR, Chang CM (1991) Polymorphonuclear leukocytes occlude capillaries following middle cerebral artery occlusion and reperfusion in baboons. Stroke 22:1276–1283
23. Dereski MO, Chopp M, Knight RA, Rodolosi LC, Garcia JH (1993) The heterogeneous temporal evolution of focal ischemic neuronal damage in the rat. Acta Neuropathol 85:327–333
24. Dirnagl U, Niwa K, Sixt G, Villringer A (1994) Cortical hypoperfusion after global forebrain ischemia in rats is not caused by microvascular leukocyte plugging. Stroke 25:1028–1038
25. Dutka AJ, Kochanek PM, Hallenbeck JM (1989) Influence of granulocytopenia on canine cerebral ischemia induced by air embolism. Stroke 20:390–395
26. Feuerstein GZ, Wang X, Barone FC (1998) Inflammatory mediators and brain injury: The role of cytokines and chemokines in stroke and CNS diseases. In: Cerebrovascular Diseases (M. D. Ginsberg and J. Bogousslavsky, eds), Cambridge, MA, Blackwell Science, pp 507–531
27. Forster C, Clark HB, Ross ME, Iadecola C (1999) Inducible nitric oxide synthase expression in human cerebral infarcts. Acta Neuropathol (Berl) 97:215–220
28. Gabriel C, Justicia C, Camins A, Planas AM (1999) Activation of nuclear factor-kappaB in the rat brain after transient focal ischemia. Brain Res Mol Brain Res 65:61–69
29. Garcia JH, Kamijyo Y (1974) Cerebral infarction. Evolution of histopathological changes after occlusion of a middle cerebral artery in primates. J Neuropathol Exp Neurol 33:408–421
30. Garcia JH, Liu KF, Yoshida Y, Lian J, Chen S, del Zoppo GJ (1994) Influx of leukocytes and platelets in an evolving brain infarct. Am J. Pathol 144:188–199
31. Garcia JH, Yoshida Y, Chen H, Li Y, Zhang ZG, Lian J, Chen S, Chopp M (1993) Progression from ischemic injury to infarct following middle cerebral artery occlusion in the rat. Am J Pathol 142:623–635
32. Garthwaite J, Boulton CL (1995) Nitric oxide signaling in the central nervous system. Ann Rev Physiol 57:683–706
33. Gary DS, Bruce-Keller AJ, Kindy MS, Mattson MP (1998) Ischemic and excitotoxic brain injury is enhanced in mice lacking the p55 tumor necrosis factor receptor. J Cereb Blood Flow Metab 18:1283–1287
34. Goussev AV, Zhang Z, Anderson DC, Chopp M (1998) P-selectin antibody reduces hemorrhage and infarct volume resulting from MCA occlusion in the rat. J Neurol Sci 161:16–22
35. Grandati M, Verrecchia C, Revaud ML, Allix M, Boulu RG, Plotkine M (1997) Calcium-independent NO-synthase activity and nitrites/nitrates production in transient focal cerebral ischaemia in mice. Br J Pharmacol 122:625–630
36. Gross SS, Wolin MS (1995) Nitric oxide: pathophysiological mechanisms. Ann Rev Physiol 57:737–769
37. Heinel LA, Rubin S, Rosenwasser RH, Vasthare US, Tuma RF (1994) Leukocyte involvement in cerebral infarct generation after ischemia and reperfusion. Brain Res Bull 34:137–141
38. Helps SC, Gorman DF (1991) Air embolism of the brain in rabbits pretreated with mechlorethamine. Stroke 22:351–354
39. Hess DC, Howard E, Cheng C, Carroll J, Hill WD, Hsu CY (2000) Hypertonic mannitol loading of NF-kappaB transcription factor decoys in human brain microvascular endothelial cells blocks upregulation of ICAM-1. Stroke 31:1179–1186
40. Iadecola C (1999) The role of NO in cerebrovascular regulation and stroke. In: (R. T. Mathie and T. M. Griffith, eds), London, Imperial College Press, pp 202–225
41. Iadecola C, Forster C, Nogawa S, Clark HB, Ross ME (1999a)

Cyclooxygenase immunoreactivity in the human brain following cerebral ischemia. Acta Neuropathologica 98:9–14
42. Iadecola C, Salkowski CA, Zhang F, Aber T, Nagayama M, Vogel SN, Ross ME (1999b) The Transcription Factor Interferon Regulatory Factor 1 Is Expressed after Cerebral Ischemia and Contributes to Ischemic Brain Injury. J Exp Med 189:719–727
43. Iadecola C, Zhang F, Casey R, Clark HB, Ross ME (1996) Inducible nitric oxide synthase gene expression in vascular cells after transient focal cerebral ischemia. Stroke 27:1373–1380
44. Iadecola C, Zhang F, Casey R, Nagayama M, Ross ME (1997) Delayed reduction in ischemic brain injury and neurological deficits in mice lacking the inducible nitric oxide synthase gene. J. Neurosci. 17:9157–9164
45. Iadecola C, Zhang F, Xu X (1995a) Inhibition of inducible nitric oxide synthase ameliorates cerebral ischemic damage. Am J. Physiol 268:R286–R292
46. Iadecola C, Zhang F, Xu X, Casey R, Ross ME (1995b) Inducible nitric oxide synthase gene expression in brain following cerebral ischemia. J. Cereb. Blood Flow Metab. 15:378–384
47. Jiang N, Moyle M, Soule HR, Rote WE, Chopp M (1995) Neutrophil inhibitory factor is neuroprotective after focal ischemia in rats. Ann Neurol 38:935–942
48. Kamijo R, Harada H, Matsuyama T, Bosland M, Gerecitano J, Shapiro D, Le J, Koh SI, Kimura T, Green SJ, Mak TW, Taniguchi T, Vilcek J (1994) Requirement for transcription factor IRF-1 in NO synthase induction in macrophages. Science 263:1612–1615
49. Kim Y, Busto R, Dietrich WD, Kraydieh S, Ginsberg MD (1996) Delayed postischemic hyperthermia in awake rats worsens the histopathological outcome of transient focal cerebral ischemia. Stroke 27:2274–2280
50. Kitagawa K, Matsumoto M, Mabuchi T, Yagita Y, Ohtsuki T, Hori M, Yanagihara T (1998) Deficiency of intercellular adhesion molecule 1 attenuates microcirculatory disturbance and infarction size in focal cerebral ischemia. J Cereb Blood Flow Metab 18:1336–1345
51. Kontos HA, Wei EP, Povlishock JT, Dietrich WD, Magiera CJ, Ellis EF (1980) Cerebral arteriolar damage by arachidonic acid and prostaglandin G2. Science 209:1242–1245
52. Liu J, Ginis I, Spatz M, Hallenbeck JM (2000) Hypoxic preconditioning protects cultured neurons against hypoxic stress via TNF-alpha and ceramide. Am J Physiol Cell Physiol 278:C144–153
53. Loddick SA, Rothwell NJ (1996) Neuroprotective effects of human recombinant interleukin-1 receptor antagonist in focal cerebral ischemia in the rat. J. Cereb. Blood Flow Metab. 16:932–940
54. Loddick SA, Turnbull AV, Rothwell NJ (1998) Cerebral interleukin-6 is neuroprotective during permanent focal cerebral ischemia in the rat. J Cereb Blood Flow Metab 18:176–179
55. Mamane Y, Heylbroeck C, Genin P, Algarte M, Servant MJ, LePage C, DeLuca C, Kwon H, Lin R, Hiscott J (1999) Interferon regulatory factors: the next generation. Gene 237:1–14
56. Marchal G, Beaudouin V, Rioux P, de la Sayette V, Le Doze F, Viader F, Derlon J-M, Baron J-C (1996) Prolonged persistence of substantial volumes of potentially viable brain tissue after stroke. Stroke 27:599–606
57. Marletta MA (1994) Nitric oxide synthase: aspects concerning structure and catalysis. Cell 78:927–930
58. Martin E, Nathan C, Xie QW (1994) Role of interferon regulatory factor 1 in induction of nitric oxide synthase. J. Exp Med 180:977–984
59. Matsumoto T, Ikeda K, Mukaida N, Harada A, Matsumoto Y, Yamashita J, Matsushima K (1997) Prevention of cerebral edema and infarct in cerebral reperfusion injury by an antibody to interleukin-8. Lab Invest 77:119–125
60. Matsuo Y, Onodera H, Shiga Y, Nakamura M, Ninomiya M, Kihara T, Kogure K (1994) Correlation between myeloperoxidase-quantified neutrophil accumulation and ischemia brain injury in the rat. Stroke 25:1469–1475
61. Mattson MP, Culmsee C, Yu Z, Camandola S (2000) Roles of nuclear factor kappaB in neuronal survival and plasticity. J Neurochem 74:443–456
62. Miettinen S, Fusco FR, Yrjanheikki J, Keinanen R, Hirvonen T, Roivainen R, Narhi M, Hokfelt T, Koistinaho J (1997) Spreading depression and focal brain ischemia induce cyclooxygenase-2 in cortical neurons through N-methyl-D-aspartic acid-receptors and phospholipase A2. Proc Natl Acad Sci USA 94:6500–6505
63. Mori E, del Zoppo GJ, Chambers JD, Copeland BR, Arfors KE (1992) Inhibition of polymorphonuclear leukocyte adherence suppresses no-reflow after focal cerebral ischemia in baboons. Stroke 23:712–718
64. Morikawa E, Zhang SM, Seko Y, Toyoda T, Kirino T (1996) Treatment of focal cerebral ischemia with synthetic oligopeptide corresponding to lectin domain of selectin. Stroke 27:951–955
65. Nagayama M, Aber T, Nagayama T, Ross ME, Iadecola C (1999a) Age-dependent increase in ischemic brain injury in wild-type mice and in mice lacking the inducible nitric oxide synthase gene. J Cereb Blood Flow Metab 19:661–666
66. Nagayama M, Niwa K, Nagayama T, Ross ME, Iadecola C (1999b) The cyclooxygenase-2 inhibitor NS-398 ameliorates cerebral ischemic injury in wild-type mice but not in mice with deletion of the inducible nitric oxide synthase gene. J Cereb Blood Flow Metab 19:1213–1219
67. Nagayama M, Zhang F, Iadecola C (1998) Delayed treatment with aminoguanidine decreases focal cerebral ischemic damage and enhances neurologic recovery in rats. J Cereb Blood Flow Metab 18:1107–1113
68. Nakayama M, Uchimura K, Zhu RL, Nagayama T, Rose ME, Stetler RA, Isakson PC, Chen J, Graham SH (1998) Cyclooxygenase-2 inhibition prevents delayed death of CA1 hippocampal neurons following global ischemia. Proc Natl Acad Sci USA 95:10954–10959
69. Nathan C (1995) Inducible nitric oxide synthase: regulation subserves function. Current Topics in Microbiology & Immunology 196:1–4
70. Nawashiro H, Martin D, Hallenbeck JM (1997) Neuroprotective effects of TNF binding protein in focal cerebral ischemia. Brain Res 778:265–271
71. Nguyen H, Hiscott J, Pitha PM (1997) The growing family of interferon regulatory factors. Cytokine Growth Factor Rev 8:293–312
72. Nogawa S, Forster C, Zhang F, Nagayama M, Ross ME, Iadecola C (1998) Interaction between inducible nitric oxide synthase and cyclooxygenase-2 after cerebral ischemia. Proc Natl Acad Sci USA 95:10966–10971
73. Nogawa S, Zhang F, Ross ME, Iadecola C (1997) Cyclooxygenase-2 gene expression in neurons contributes to ischemic brain damage. J. Neurosci. 17:2746–2755
74. Parmentier S, Bohme GA, Lerouet D, Damour D, Stutzmann JM, Margaill I, Plotkine M (1999) Selective inhibition of inducible nitric oxide synthase prevents ischaemic brain injury. Br J Pharmacol 127:546–552
75. Planas AM, Soriano MA, Rodriguez-Farre E, Ferrer I (1995) Induction of cyclooxygenase-2 mRNA and protein following transient focal ischemia in the rat brain. Neurosci Lett 200:187–190
76. Pozzilli C, Lenzi GL, Argentino C, Carolei A, Rasura M, Signore A, Bozzao L, Pozzilli P (1985) Imaging of leukocytic infiltration in human cerebral infarcts. Stroke 16:251–255
77. Relton JK, Martin D, Thompson RC, Russell DA (1996) Peripheral administration of Interleukin-1 Receptor antagonist

inhibits brain damage after focal cerebral ischemia in the rat. Exp Neurol 138:206–213

78. Rothwell NJ, Hopkins SJ (1995) Cytokines and the nervous system II: Actions and mechanisms of action. Trends Neurosci 18:130–136
79. Sairanen T, Ristimaki A, Karjalainen-Lindsberg ML, Paetau A, Kaste M, Lindsberg PJ (1998) Cyclooxygenase-2 is induced globally in infarcted human brain. Ann Neurol 43:738–747
80. Salminen A, Liu PK, Hsu CY (1995) Alteration of transcription factor binding activities in the ischemic rat brain. Biochemical & Biophysical Research Communications 212:939–944
81. Salvemini D, Seibert K, Masferrer JL, Misko TP, Currie MG, Needleman P (1994) Endogenous nitric oxide enhances prostaglandin production in a model of renal inflammation. J. Clin. Invest. 93:1940–1947
82. Schneider A, Martin-Villalba A, Weih F, Vogel J, Wirth T, Schwaninger M (1999) NF-kappaB is activated and promotes cell death in focal cerebral ischemia. Nat Med 5:554–559
83. Seibert K, Masferrer J, Zhang Y, Gregory S, Olson G, Hauser S, Leahy K, Perkins W, Isakson P (1995) Mediation of inflammation by cyclooxygenase-2. Agents & Actions Suppl. 46:41–50
84. Shiga Y, Onodera H, Kogure K, Yamasaki Y, Yashima Y, Syozuhara H, Sendo F (1991) Neutrophil as a mediator of ischemic edema formation in the brain. Neurosci Lett 125:110–112
85. Shohami E, Ginis I, Hallenbeck JM (1999) Dual role of tumor necrosis factor alpha in brain injury. Cytokine Growth Factor Rev 10:119–130
86. Sinz EH, Kochanek PM, Dixon CE, Clark RS, Carcillo JA, Schiding JK, Chen M, Wisniewski SR, Carlos TM, Williams D, DeKosky ST, Watkins SC, Marion DW, Billiar TR (1999) Inducible nitric oxide synthase is an endogenous neuroprotectant after traumatic brain injury in rats and mice. J Clin Invest 104:647–656
87. Smith WL, DeWitt DL (1995) Biochemistry of prostaglandin endoperoxide H synthase-1 and synthase-2 and their differential susceptibility to nonsteroidal anti-inflammatory drugs. Sem. Nephrol. 15:179–194
88. Soriano SG, Coxon A, Wang YF, Frosch MP, Lipton SA, Hickey PR, Mayadas TN (1999) Mice deficient in Mac-1 (CD11b/CD18) are less susceptible to cerebral ischemia/reperfusion injury. Stroke 30:134–139
89. Soriano SG, Lipton SA, Wang YF, Xiao M, Springer TA, Gutierrez-Ramos JC, Hickey PR (1996) Intercellular adhesion molecule-1-deficient mice are less susceptible to cerebral ischemia-reperfusion injury. Ann Neurol 39:618–624
90. Stephenson D, Yin T, Smalstig EB, Hsu MA, Panetta J, Little S, Clemens J (2000) Transcription factor nuclear factor-kappa B is activated in neurons after focal cerebral ischemia. J Cereb Blood Flow Metab 20:592–603
91. Suzuki H, Hayashi T, Tojo SJ, Kitagawa H, Kimura K, Mizugaki M, Itoyama Y, Abe K (1999) Anti-P-selectin antibody attenuates rat brain ischemic injury. Neurosci Lett 265:163–166
92. Szabo C, Ohshima H (1997) DNA damage induced by peroxynitrite: subsequent biological effects. Nitric Oxide 1:373–385
93. Terai K, Matsuo A, McGeer EG, McGeer PL (1996) Enhancement of immunoreactivity for NF-kappa B in human cerebral infarctions. Brain Res 739:343–349
94. Touzani O, Young AR, Derlon J-M, Beaudouin V, Marchal G, Rioux P, Mezenge F, Baron J-C, MacKenzie ET (1995) Sequential studies of severely hypometabolic tissue volumes after permanent middle cerebral artery occlusion: A positron emission tomographic investigation in anesthetized baboons. Stroke 26:2112–2119
95. Vane JR, Bakhle YS, Botting RM (1998) Cyclooxygenases 1 and 2. Annu Rev Pharmacol Toxicol 38:97–120
96. Ward PA (1991) Mechanisms of endothelial cell killing by H2O2 or products of activated neutrophils. Am J Med 91:89–94
97. Wu KK (1995) Inducible cyclooxygenase and nitric oxide synthase. Adv Pharmacol 33:179–207
98. Yamagata K, Andreasson KI, Kaufmann WE, Barnes CA, Worley PF (1993) Expression of a mitogen-inducible cyclooxygenase in brain neurons: regulation by synaptic activity and glucocorticoids. Neuron 11:371–386
99. Yamasaki Y, Matsuo Y, Zagorski J, Matsuura N, Onodera H, Itoyama Y, Kogure K (1997) New therapeutic possibility of blocking cytokine-induced neutrophil chemoattractant on transient ischemic brain damage in rats. Brain Res 759:103–111
100. Yamasaki Y, Matsuura N, Shozuhara H, Onodera H, Itoyama Y, Kogure K (1995) Interleukin-1 as a pathogenetic mediator of ischemic brain damage in rats. Stroke 26:676–680
101. Yang GY, Gong C, Qin Z, Ye W, Mao Y, Betz AL (1998) Inhibition of TNFalpha attenuates infarct volume and ICAM-1 expression in ischemic mouse brain. Neuroreport 9:2131–2134
102. Yang GY, Zhao YJ, Davidson BL, Betz AL (1997) Overexpression of interleukin-1 receptor antagonist in the mouse brain reduces ischemic brain injury. Brain Res 751:181–188
103. Yu Z, Zhou D, Bruce-Keller AJ, Kindy MS, Mattson MP (1999) Lack of the p50 subunit of nuclear factor-kappaB increases the vulnerability of hippocampal neurons to excitotoxic injury. J Neurosci 19:8856–8865
104. Zhang RL, Chopp M, Li Y, Zaloga C, Jiang N, Jones ML, Miyasaka M, Ward PA (1994) Anti-ICAM-1 antibody reduces ischemic cell damage after transient middle cerebral artery occlusion in the rat. Neurology 44:1747–1751
105. Zhang RL, Chopp M, Zhang ZG, Phillips ML, Rosenbloom CL, Cruz R, Manning A (1996) E-selectin in focal cerebral ischemia and reperfusion in the rat. J Cereb Blood Flow Metab 16:1126–1136
106. Zhao X, Haensel C, Ross ME, Iadecola C (2000) Gene-dosing effect and persistence of reduction in ischemic brain injury in mice lacking inducible nitric oxide synthase. Brain Res in press

Metalloproteinase generation and matrix injury during focal cerebral ischemia

G. J. del Zoppo, J. Lucero, N. Hosomi, J. H. Heo

1.0 Introduction

Middle cerebral artery occlusion (MCA:O) promotes rapid (del Zoppo et al. 1991; del Zoppo 1994; Haring et al. 1996b; Little et al. 1975, 1976; Mori et al. 1992; Okada et al. 1994; Thomas et al. 1993) changes in microvascular integrity and permeability (del Zoppo et al. 1986; Haring et al. 1996a), loss of basal lamina matrix as well as endothelial cell and astrocyte integrin antigens (del Zoppo et al. 1996; Hamann et al. 1995, 1996; Wagner et al. 1997), the appearance of select microvascular activation antigens (Abumiya et al. 1999), and changes in astrocyte ultrastructure (del Zoppo et al. 1991; Garcia et al. 1983). These occur in temporal and topographical association with neuron injury. Importantly, the alterations in microvascular extracellular matrix (ECM), predominantly the basal lamina, are related to the appearance of localized hemorrhage (Hamann et al. 1995, 1996). The changes observed in the microvascular ECM are consistent with a role for localized specialized protease activity initiated during focal cerebral ischemia. Work in several laboratories, including our own, has pursued the potential that matrixins, matrix-degrading enzymes, and plasminogen activators participate in cerebral tissue injury following blood flow cessation in vulnerable regions of the brain. During the early moments following MCA:O, subtle changes in endothelial cell ultrastructure and increases in endothelial permeability coincide with swelling of astrocyte end-foot processes and astrocyte cytoplasmic reorganization. The rapidity of these changes, together with the onset of neurological symptoms, the loss of integrin receptor antigens on endothelial cells and astrocytes, and coincident appearance of metalloproteinases (MMPs) and plasminogen activators (PAs) with neuron injury suggest the hypothesis that microvascular and neuron injury are related. In this context the effects of MMPs and PAs on matrix integrity must be examined together (Fig. 1).

1.1 The microvascular basal lamina and extracellular matrix

The ECM within microvessels comprises a fabric of laminins, type IV collagen, fibronectin, and heparan sulfates containing varying amounts of entactin, thrombospondin, and ni-

The work described in this manuscript is supported in part by grants RO1 NS 26945 and NS 38710 of the National Institutes of Neurological Disorders and Stroke. This is manuscript 13475-MEM of The Scripps Research Institute

Department of Molecular and Experimental Medicine, The Scripps Research Institute, 10550 North Torrey Pines Road, MEM 132, La Jolla, CA 92037
e-mail: grgdlzop@hermes.scripps.edu

J. Krieglstein, S. Klumpp (Eds.) Pharmacology of Cerebral Ischemia 2000

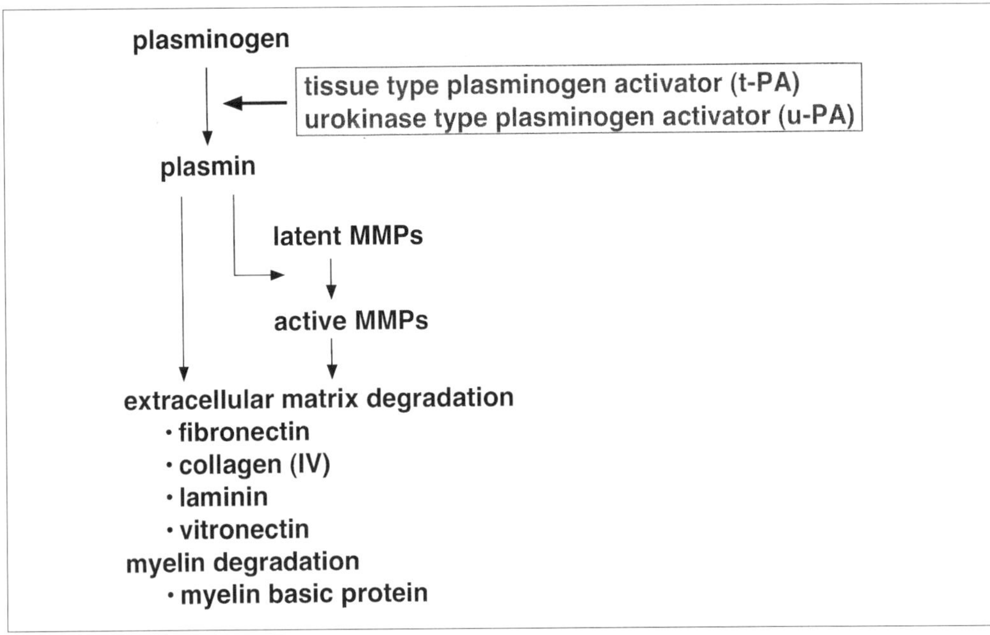

Fig. 1. General relationship of matrix protein degradation to the interaction of metalloproteinases (MMPs) and plasminogen activator (PA) systems (selected elements).

dogen (Yurchenko and Schittny 1986). Although less well appreciated, selected proteoglycans have been identified between neurons and neighboring cells (Carlson and Hockfield 1996). Generated by endothelial cells and astrocytes in concert during development, the basal lamina forms a biologically active connection between these two cell compartments. Organotypic tissue cultures have shown that intact basal lamina requires the juxtaposition of microvascular endothelium and astrocytes (Bernstein et al. 1985; Kusaka et al. 1985). Microvascular endothelial cells and astrocytes play reciprocal roles in the generation of matrix proteins. In culture, astrocytes secrete laminin, fibronectin, and chondroitin sulfate proteoglycan, while collagens stimulate astrocyte-induced endothelial cell maturation (Ard and Faissner 1991; Tagami et al. 1992; Webersinke et al. 1992). Conversely, endothelial cell-derived ECM components stimulate astrocyte growth and function (Kozlova et al. 1993; Nagano et al. 1993). The blood-brain barrier also relies upon the interdependence of endothelial cells and astrocytes. This has been elegantly shown in chick-quail adrenal vascular tissue/brain tissue xenograft (Janzer and Raff 1987) and fetal-adult hippocampal/neocortex allograft preparations (Hurwitz et al. 1993). Soluble factor(s) generated by astrocytes are necessary to maintain endothelial blood-brain barrier characteristics including the induction of tight-junctions, transendothelial resistance, and glucose/amino acid transport polarity (Estrada et al. 1990; Hurwitz et al. 1993; Minakawa et al. 1991). The basal lamina and blood-brain barriers, then, depend exquisitely upon cooperation between these two unrelated cell types.

1.2 Endothelial cell-astrocyte-neuron interrelationships

The proximity of the endothelium to neighboring astrocytes in cerebral capillaries and post-capillary venules suggests a close functional relationship for communication and nutrient supply. Adhesion receptors on endothelial cells and on astrocyte end-feet are presumed to maintain close cell-cell apposition (del Zoppo et al. 1996; Haring et al. 1996a; Wagner et al. 1997). The association of astrocytes with neurons suggests the presence of direct interactions between cerebral microvessels and the neurons they serve.

The endothelium and astrocyte end-feet attach to matrix laminins and collagen IV by integrin receptors. Integrins are $\alpha\beta$ heterodimeric transmembrane glycoproteins which participate in vascular development, structural integrity, and intercellular communication (Albelda and Buck 1990; Luscinskas and Lawler 1994; Ruoslahti 1991). The matrix attachments of individual cells occur at focal contact points (Pasqualini and Hemler 1994). In one formulation, when cells attach to matrix via integrin receptors, respective MMP(s) is (are) not secreted; but with cell detachment, the MMP is secreted and the receptor is not expressed at the contact point (Chintala et al. 1996; Partridge et al. 1997). It might be predicted that in cerebral microvessels where the endothelium and astrocyte end-feet detach from the matrix, connections with neurons may be lost.

1.3 Cell-specific generation of proteases

Proteases which degrade matrix constituents can be generated by cellular constituents of microvessels, neurons and non-neuronal cells of brain tissue, and activated cells of the circulation (e.g., leukocytes). For instance, MMP expression has been associated with endothelial cells and astrocytes, microglia, and oligodendrocytes under specific conditions of culture (Cross and Woodroofe 1999; Gottschall and Deb 1996; Gottschall et al. 1995; Pagenstecher et al. 1998; Uhm et al. 1998; Wells et al. 1996). Both gelatinases A and B, MMP-2 and MMP-9, are synthesized by leukocytes, and secreted upon activation of the cells (Anthony et al. 1997; Hibbs et al. 1985). Synthesis of plasminogen activators (e.g., urokinase (u-PA)) has been attributed to a number of cell-types within the central nervous system (CNS), including endothelial cells, neurons, astrocytes, and microglia *in vivo* and *in vitro* (Masos and Miskin 1996; Nakajima et al. 1992; Tranque et al. 1994; van Hinsbergh et al. 1990). The reactions of these cell-types to ischemia within the CNS, their ability to generate MMPs or PAs, potential effects on microvascular matrix, and their impact on neuron integrity have not been detailed.

This loss of microvascular basal lamina during ischemia is greatest in the region where neuron injury is maximal (Hamann et al. 1995; Wagner et al. 1997). The disappearance of matrix antigens may be due to proteolysis, blockade of transcription, inhibition of translation, protein folding, or a combination of these. Remodelling of the microvascular basal lamina occurs when secreted proteases such as MMPs and PAs, which are associated with the cerebral microvasculature, degrade laminin, collagen, or fibronectin (Krane 1994; Levin and del Zoppo 1994). Activated serine proteases generated during ischemia may augment these processes. Among serine proteases, thrombin is interesting because it has multiple actions and targets. For instance, thrombin stimulates MMP-2 and MMP-9 secretion by vascular smooth muscle cells (Fabunmi et al. 1996; Galis et al. 1997). Also, PMN leukocyte granule enzymes, including collagenase (MMP-8), gelatinase B (MMP-9), elastase, and cathepsin G are released during the inflammatory phase following ischemia and degrade laminins and collagens (Heck et al. 1990; Krane 1994; Murphy et al. 1987; Pike et al. 1989; Watanabe et al. 1990). However, the appearance of PMN leukocytes does not uniformly coincide with initial evidence of laminin degradation within the primate (Abumiya et al. 1999; del Zoppo et al. 1991; Hamann et al. 1995, 1996).

1.4 Microvascular basal lamina and focal cerebral ischemia

During focal cerebral ischemia, microvascular basal lamina antigens are lost. The ECM components of the basal lamina (e.g.laminin-1, laminin-5, collagen IV, and fibronectin) disappear together during MCA:O in the primate (Hamann et al. 1995, 1996; Wagner et al. 1997). These changes are most prominent in the region of most severe ischemic neuron injury (Ic), and may be detectable as early as 2 hours after MCA:O (e.g., laminin-5) (Wagner et al. 1997).

When viewed from the perspective of functional activity microvascular basal lamina may serve as i) a physical barrier to extravasation of circulating cells (e.g., erythrocytes, leukocytes), ii) as a stabilizer of endothelial cell and astrocyte viability, and iii) a scaffolding to maintain the proximity of the endothelial and astrocyte compartment in the CNS. Implications of these assertions are that degradation of microvascular matrix may allow cellular extravasation from the circulation, resulting in detectable hemorrhage. A second consequence of disruption of endothelial cell-astrocyte proximity is acceleration of neurodegeneration under conditions of tissue injury. This latter notion may be restated as the hypothesis that neuron viability requires integrity of microvascular matrix and endothelial cell-astrocyte proximity. Both concepts are testable.

2.0 Metalloproteinases

Focal cerebral ischemia stimulates the generation of a number of proteases which include MMPs, select PAs, and other serine proteases, together with activated enzymes of the coagulation cascade and the immune system. MMPs are Ca^{2+} dependent Zn^{2+} containing endopeptidases which cleave ligands in the ECM. More than twenty distinct members of the matrixin family have been identified (Woessner Jr. 1994). All members of this family share common structural domains which include (NH_2- to COOH-terminal) a signal peptide, a pro-domain, a Zn^{2+} containing catalytic site, and one or more hemapexin-like domains. Secreted in latent form as proenzymes, pro-MMP-2 and pro-MMP-9 are activated to their respective 72 kDa and 92 kDa enzymes by separate mechanisms. Latent MMP-2 is activated on cellular membrane surfaces by MT1-MMP (MMP-14) or MT3-MMP (MMP-16), while latent MMP-9 is activated by plasmin (generated by PAs), select serine proteases, and specific MMPs including MMP-1, MMP-2, MMP-3, and MMP-8.

Latent MMP-2 is expressed in constitutive fashion by a number of cell types. MMP-2 participates in cellular responses including adhesion, proliferation, and migration. Vascular endothelial cells secrete pro-MMP-2, contributing to detectable levels in plasma. Pro-MMP-2 and MMP-9 are associated with PMN leukocytes, macrophages, and platelets in the circulation. Non-vascular parenchymal cells of the CNS also have the capacity to generate MMPs (Cross and Woodroofe 1999; Gottschall and Deb 1996; Gottschall et al. 1995; Pagenstecher et al. 1998; Uhm et al. 1998; Wells et al. 1996). Activities of MMP-2 and MMP-9 are modulated by the specific inhibitors TIMP-2 and TIMP-1, respectively, which are themselves under regulation. The intermolecular interactions of the MMPs and their inhibitors is understood in large part (Bode et al. 1999). For instance, pro-MMP-2 and MMP-2 have homologous binding sites for TIMP-2. MMP-2, in addition, exposes the Zn^{2+}-containing active site which offers a second binding site for inhibition by TIMP. The participation of latent MMPs, their activators, and their active products in the CNS, however, are not yet understood. Interest in the generation of MMPs in the CNS derives from the loss of microvascular matrix following MCA:O, activation of hypoxic microvessels, the coincidence of hemorrhage with focal cerebral ischemia, and the evolution of neuron injury.

2.1 Targets of MMP activity in the CNS

Constitutive generation of pro-MMP-2 activity has been noted in uninjured basal ganglia and cortex of non-human primates and rodents (Heo et al. 1999), the purposes of which remain uncertain. The laminins and collagen IV which comprise microvascular basal lamina within the CNS are appropriate substrates for MMP-2 and MMP-9. The presence of these substrates in the extracellular space within the neuropil has not yet been reported, but detection methods may be inadequate.

2.2 Responses of MMPs to MCA:O

Anthony et al. have reported the marked increased expression of latent MMP-9 by PMN leukocytes in human brain within one week of ischemic stroke, and the association of MMP-2 with macrophages accumulated in ischemic tissue thereafter (Anthony et al. 1997). No explanation was provided for the initial appearance of MMP-2 immune reactivity in neurons in nonischemic brain and its subsequent disappearance after stroke. In anesthetized Wistar-Kyoto and spontaneously hypertensive (SHR) rats, Rosenberg et al. showed that pro-MMP-9 increased by 12–24 hours and pro-MMP-2 by 5 days after MCA:O in isolated brain tissues (Rosenberg et al. 1996). Those findings have been variably corroborated by others (Table 1) (Clark et al. 1997; Fujimura et al. 1999; Gasche et al. 1999). In aggregate, the results suggest that in rodents subject to MCA:O increased pro-MMP-9 expression precedes that of pro-MMP-2. Variability in the timing of the appearance of pro-MMP activity in rodents is most probably due to technical differences in MMP extraction and tissue handling (see below).

2.3 Relationship of MMP expression to neuron injury

In contrast, a significant rapid increase in the expression of the latent form of MMP-2 occurs 1–2 hours after MCA:O in buffer perfused ischemic basal ganglia of the nonhuman primate, which correlates significantly with the size of the Ic region (Heo et al. 1999) (Fig. 2). Those findings suggest that MMP-2 secretion may be directly related to early neuron injury. Moreover, *in situ* hybridization experiments have demonstrated the appearance of MMP-2 mRNA transcripts in both microvessels and nonvascular non-neuronal cell nuclei in the Ic region by 2 hours MCA:O (unpublished). Furthermore, evidence of coexpression of two activators of latent MMP-2 has been obtained. Hence, MMP-2 may be synthesized *de novo* by microvascular cells in direct association with neuron injury, in the same time and location as microvascular matrix and integrin loss. Finally, activated MMP-2 accounted for < 2% of total MMP-2 activity at any time following MCA:O (Heo et al. 1999).

2.4 MMP expression and hemorrhagic transformation

pro-MMP-9 activity increases in the ischemic regions of those primate subjects displaying he-

Table 1. Matrix Metalloproteinases-2 and -9 in Response to Focal Cerebral Ischemia (see legend Table 2)

authors	date	species	ischemia	assay	MMP-2	MMP-9	TIMP-1
Rosenberg	1996	SHR	MCA:O	zymo	↑ 120 hr	↑ 12–120 hr	
Anthony	1997	human	stroke	IH	↑ > 7d	↑ < 7d	
Clark	1997	human	stroke	zymo	↑ 4–84 mo	↑ 48–96 hr	
Romanic	1998	SHR	MCA:O	zymo, IH	↑ > 120 hr	↑ 6–120 hr	~
Heo	1999	primate	MCA:O/R	zymo	↑ 1–2 hr	**hemorrhage**	
Fujimura	1999	m	MCA:O/R	zymo zymo(r)	↑ 23 hr	↑ 1–23 hr	~
Gauche	1999	m	MCA:O	zymo zymo(r)	↑ 4–24 hr	↑ 2–24 hr	~

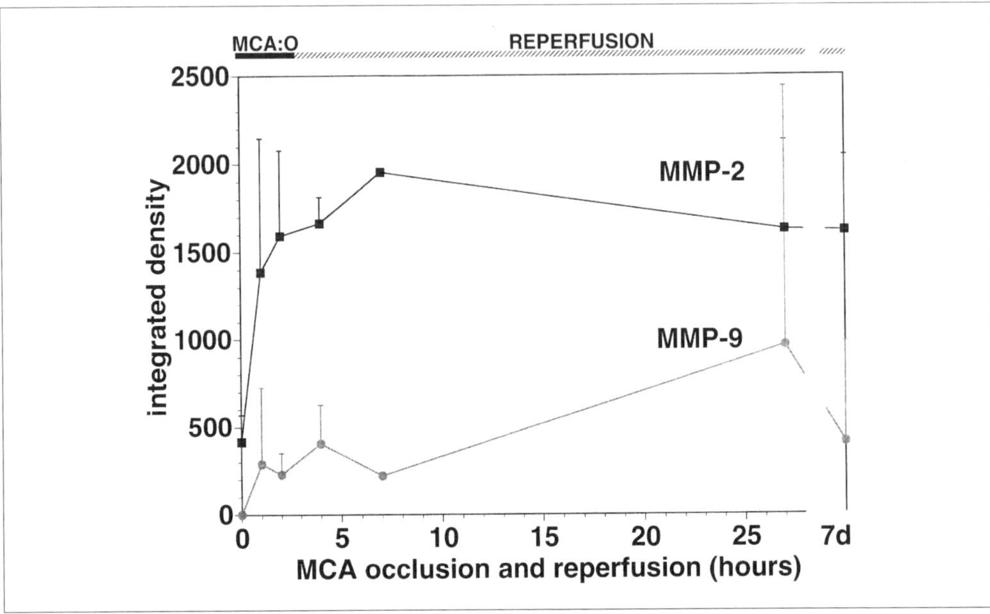

Fig. 2. Response of latent MMP-2 and MMP-9 activities to focal cerebral ischemia in the basal ganglia initiated by MCA:O. Note the constitutive generation of pro-MMP-2 activity, and its rapid increase following MCA:O. Activity normalized for Ic region, and derived by zymography from 10 μm frozen sections. All data represents mean ± S.D.

morrhagic transformation compared to those without hemorrhage (2 p = 0.018) (Fig. 3) (Heo et al. 1999). No relationship to duration of ischemia or neuron injury was observed. Hence, a clear dichotomy between the expression of pro-MMP-2 and pro-MMP-9 has been seen following MCA:O in the primate, which was differentially related to neuron injury, and in rodent experimental models. It should be noted that primate tissues were perfused of blood elements.

3.0 Plasminogen Activators

Plasminogen activators, serine proteases which convert plasminogen to plasmin within the circulation and on the surface of forming thrombi, may also affect MMP activities between and among cells of the cerebral microvessels and the neuropil. Their generation and secretion under conditions of focal cerebral ischemia may contribute to the evolving injury.

3.1 Components of the endogenous fibrinolytic system

The fibrinolytic system within the vascular circulation is responsible for thrombus dissolution. This (*endogenous*) system consists of plasminogen, plasmingen activators, and inhibitors of fibrinolysis. Plasmin formation occurs in the plasma, where it can cleave circulating fibrin(ogen), and on reactive surfaces (e.g., thrombi or cells). The fibrin network offers a site for plasminogen activation, while various cells, including PMN leukocytes, platelets, and endothelial cells, express receptors for plasminogen binding (Plow et al. 1991). Specific cellular receptors also concentrate specific PAs (e.g., urokinase plasminogen activator receptor (u-PAR) for u-PA) to enhance local plasmin production. Plasmin can also mediate the proteolytic cleavage of matrix substrates, including the laminins, collagens, and fibronectin which comprise basement membranes and vascular

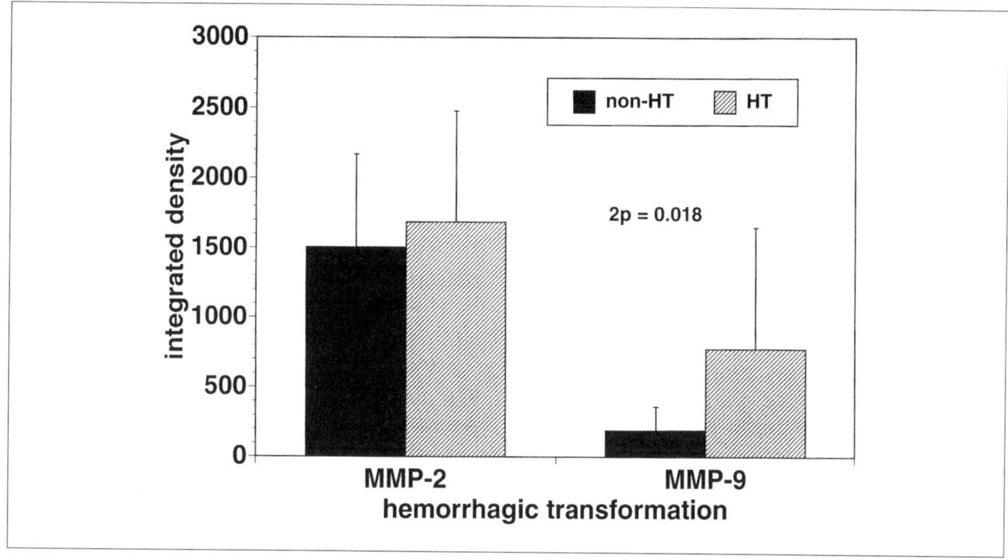

Fig. 3. Association of latent MMP-9 activity (per zymography) with detectable hemorrhagic transformation following MCA:O.

basal lamina. Plasmin has been shown to degrade myelin basic protein.

Plasmin is derived from the zymogen, plasminogen, a single-chain 92 kDa glycosylated serine protease containing 5 kringle structures (Bachmann 1994; Forsgren et al. 1987; Peterson and Serenson 1990; Tran-Thong et al. 1986). Plasminogen is present in two forms: glu-plasminogen (with an NH_2-terminal glutamic acid), and lys-plasminogen (lacking an NH_2-terminal 8 kDa peptide). Plasmin cleavage of the NH_2-terminal fragment converts glu-plasminogen to lys-plasminogen (Holvoet et al. 1985; Wallen and Wiman 1973). The primary contributor to plasminogen activation within the circulation appears to be t-PA which is secreted from the endothelium and other cellular sources. Thrombin, activated protein C (APC), and histamine stimulate t-PA secretion from endothelial stores (Gelehrter and Sznycer-Laszuk 1986; Hanss and Collen 1987; Levin et al. 1984, 1986; Sakata et al. 1985). Within the circulation t-PA and several serine proteases, including Factor IX, Factor X, prothrombin (Factor II), protein C, chymotrypsin and trypsin, various elastases (of leukocyte origin), and plasmin itself can convert plasminogen to plasmin by cleaving the arg^{560}-val^{561} bond (Bachmann 1994; Robbins et al. 1967; Robbins 1995).

t-PA is a 70 kDa single-chain glycosylated serine protease (Rijken 1988; Robbins et al. 1967), with four distinct domains which include a finger (F-) domain, a growth factor (E-) domain, two kringle regions (K_1 and K_2), and a serine protease domain (Pennica et al. 1983). The finger domain is responsible for fibrin-affinity, while the growth factor domain (residues 50–87) is homologous with epidermal growth factor (EDF). The single-chain form is converted to the two-chain form by plasmin cleavage of the arg^{275}-$isoleu^{276}$ bond.

Single-chain urokinase plasminogen activator (scu-PA) is a 54 kDa glycoprotein synthesized by endothelial cells (renal cells and certain malignant cells) (Plow et al. 1991). Cleavage or removal of lys^{158} from scu-PA by plasmin produces the high molecular weight (54 kDa) two-chain u-PA which has a disulfide bridge at cys^{148} and cys^{279} between the A-chain and the glycosylated B-chain. Further cleavages at lys^{135} and arg^{156} produce the low molecular weight 31 kDa u-PA (Rijken 1988). The two forms of u-PA exhibit measurable fibrinolytic and fibrinogenolytic activities *in vitro* and *in vivo* (Fletcher et al. 1965; Kakkar and Scully 1978; Stump and Mann 1988; White et al. 1966).

In hemostasis, t-PA and u-PA differ primarily in the domain organization of their noncatalytic regions, which differentially regulate their function as plasminogen activators. Therefore, although both PAs can generate plasmin, t-PA may be primarily involved in the maintenance of hemostasis through the dissolution of fibrin, while u-PA may be involved in generating pericellular proteolytic activity in relation to cells expressing its receptor u-PAR, needed for degradation of extracellular matrix.

In the circulation fibrin(ogen)olysis is regulated by specific inhibitors. Plasmin binds rapidly to the inhibitor α_2-antiplasmin and is thereby inactivated. Excess plasmin is inactivated by covalent binding to α_2-macroglobulin. Thrombospondin interferes with fibrin-associated plasminogen activation by t-PA (Bachmann 1987). Inhibitors of the contact activation system and complement (C1 inhibitor) have an indirect effect on fibrinolysis, and histidine-rich glycoprotein (HRG) is a competitive inhibitor of plasminogen. Plasminogen activator inhibitor-1 (PAI-1) is the principal plasma inhibitor of t-PA and u-PA, deriving from the endothelial cell and plasma compartment (Loskutoff et al. 1983; Philips et al. 1984; Thorsen et al. 1988). PAI-1 is also an acute phase reactant (Juhan-Vague et al. 1984).

3.2 Plasminogen activators in cerebral tissue

PAs may be involved in cell migration, development, vascular remodeling, and neuron viability in the CNS. Resident nonvascular cells of the CNS have been reported to variously express t-PA, u-PA, or PAI-1. t-PA and u-PA have been reported to be secreted by endothelial cells, neurons, astrocytes, and microglia *in vivo* or *in vitro* (Krystosek and Seeds 1986; Levin and del Zoppo 1994; Masos and Miskin 1996; Nakajima et al. 1992; Pittman 1985; Toshniwal et al. 1987; Tranque et al. 1994; Tsirka et al. 1997; Vincent et al. 1998). In normal cerebral tissue t-PA antigen is associated with microvessels of a size similar to those of the vasa-vasorum of the aorta (Levin and del Zoppo 1994). Expression of PA activity has been reported in nonischemic cerebral tissues of mouse, spontaneously hypertensive rats, and primates (Danglet et al. 1986; Levin and del Zoppo 1994; Matsuo et al. 1992). The roles of the principal t-PA inhibitor, PAI-1, in the neuropil are uncertain.

u-PA mRNA is expressed in neurons and oligodendrocytes during process outgrowth in rodent brain (Dent et al. 1993). t-PA is expressed by neurons in many brain regions, but extracellular proteolysis seems confined to specific discrete brain regions (Sappino et al. 1993). Recent studies suggesting that t-PA may mediate hippocampal neurodegeneration during excitotoxicity or following focal cerebral ischemia (Wang et al. 1998), have opened a discussion that PAs may play roles in cellular viability outside the *endogenous* fibrinolytic system. However, at this writing conflicting evidence of increasing injury by t-PA has been balanced against credible reports of no effect or reduction in infarct volume in rodent focal cerebral ischemia models. The potential roles of PAs in the CNS have not been clarified by murine knockout preparations. For instance, plasminogen$^{(-/-)}$ constructs subject to MCA:O display larger regions of injury than (strain-specific) wild-type, while t-PA$^{(-/-)}$ constructs have smaller injury regions (Nagai et al. 1999).

3.3 PAs and matrix degradation

Plasmin is capable of degrading selected matrix proteins of the basal lamina, elastin, and myelin basic protein either directly or through the activation of latent MMPs (Mackay et al. 1990; McGuire and Seeds 1989; Norton et al. 1978; Saksela and Rifkin 1988; Vassalli et al. 1991). There is no zymographic evidence of free plasmin in normal brain issue (Sappino et al. 1993). The roles of PAs in altering matrix integrity in response to focal cerebral ischemia have not yet been clearly defined (Chen and Strickland 1997; Tsirka et al. 1997), but they may facilitate degradation of basal lamina via several paths. Plasmin and u-PA, but not t-PA, can activate latent MMP-1, MMP-3, and MMP-9, or in the case of pro-MMP-2 through the proteolytic activation of MT1-MMP (He et al. 1989; Kazes et al. 1998; Mackay et al. 1990; Mazzieri et al. 1997; Vassalli et al. 1991). Similarly, other serine proteases can also activate latent MMP-9. The roles of these proteases, including plasmin and PAs, in the CNS have not been clearly defined.

3.4 Responses of PAs to MCA:O

A limited number of recently reported studies have focused on responses of PAs, derived from CNS tissues, to focal ischemia in rodents (Table 2). Rosenberg et al. first described increased u-PA-like proteinase activity and decreased t-PA-like proteinase activity by 12–24 hours after permanent MCA:O in anesthetized Wistar-Kyoto rats SHRs (Rosenberg et al. 1996). Ahn et al. (1999) reported an increase in u-PA-like proteinase activity and no change in t-PA-like proteinase activity in bilateral cerebral tissues following MCA:O in C57BL/6J mice. Pfefferkorn et al. also observed an increase in PA activity within the caudate putamen by 9 hours following MCA:O in Wistar rats, although the exact PA was not defined (Pfefferkorn et al. 2000). In contrast, Wang et al. suggested that increases in t-PA-like proteinase activity following MCA:O contribute to neurodegeneration within the ischemic zone (Wang et al. 1998), while in separate experiments neuron injury in the hippocampus was thought to be laminin-dependent (Chen and Strickland 1997; Tsirka et al. 1997). t-PA, but not u-PA, has been assigned a role in neuron injury within the murine hippocampus (Tsirka et al. 1997; Wang et al. 1998). In short, no consensus in the response of t-PA in these species was possible. PAI-1 antigen was reported to be increased after 4 hours following MCA:O in Wistar rats (Zhang et al. 1999). However, no relation of PAI-1 with u-PA and t-PA activity in cerebral ischemia has been reported.

By contrast, rapid and persistent increase in gelatin-proteolytic activity due mainly to significantly increased u-PA in the Ic regions of ischemic basal ganglia occurred following MCA:O in the nonhuman primate (Hosomi et al. 2000). A transient decrease in t-PA activity 2 hours after MCA:O coincided with a significant persistent increase in PAI-1 antigen, producing an increase in t-PA·PAI-1 complex, although total t-PA antigen was unchanged. The significant increase in u-PA within the ischemic basal ganglia coincides with pro-MMP-2 generation, but was not related to neuron injury following MCA:O in that model. Immunohistochemical localization of these antigens is in progress.

Table 2. Responses of Plasminogen Activators to Focal Cerebral Ischemia

Authors	date	species	ischemia	assay	u-PA	t-PA	PAI-1
Rosenberg	1996	SHR	MCA:O	zymo	↑ 12–240 hr	↓ 12–24 hr	
Wang	1998	m	MCA:O/R	zymo IS		↑ 24 hr	
Ahn	1999	m	MCA:O	zymo	↑ 4–24 hr	~	
Zhang	1999	Wistar	MCA:O	IH, ISH			↑ 4 hr
Docagne	1999	m	MCA:O	RT PCR		~	↑ 24–72 hr

IH immunohistochemistry
ISH *in situ* hybridization
RT PCR reverse transcriptase-PCR
zymo zymography
zymo(r) reverse zymograpy
zymo IS *in situ* zymography
MCA:O middle cerebral artery occlusion
MCA:O/R middle cerebral artery occlusion and reperfusion
SHR spontaneously hypertensive rat
m mouse

4.0 Technical Issues

The differences in timing and behavior of MMP and PA responses to MCA:O requires explanation. Technical differences among the reported experiences with MMP-2 and MMP-9 expression exist. Tissue sampling (Rosenberg et al. 1996), the use of extraction procedures (Fujimura et al. 1999; Gasche et al. 1999), and the lack of cerebrovascular perfusion of blood elements (Ahn et al. 1999; Rosenberg et al. 1996), can each lead to differences in activity levels. Specific details of the zymographic technologies used, most of which employ substrates for the human enzymes, suggest that none have been optimized. Importantly, there appears to be a substantial difference in the responses of MMP-2 and MMP-9 according to species, with substantial contributions from circulating leukocyte subpopulations possible (Anthony et al. 1997). These issues make comparison across experiments difficult, but must be resolved for firm conclusions regarding mechanism to be drawn.

5.0 Conclusion

The evolution of ischemic injury to the final pathology of cerebral tissues following occlusion of a brain-supplying artery involves the generation of several families of proteases. Among these, select MMPs have been identified with the focal ischemic lesion in both rodent and primate species including man. Although the time course and order of expression vary, dependent in part upon technical and tissue-handling issues. In the non-human primate basal ganglia, latent MMP-2 expression is immediately upregulated following MCA:O. While latent MMP-9 expression is associated with hemorrhagic transformation. The latter may be explained in part by the known effects of MMP-9 on microvascular matrix, although other explanations are sought. PAs, through the actions of plasmin, may degrade matrix proteins directly and activate certain latent MMPs. PA activity also increases rapidly following MCA:O. The precise targets and effects of these proteases, generated by cerebral tissues, are not completely understood. However, the concident appearance with neuron injury of selected MMPs and PAs, both topographically and temporarily, suggests a neurodegenerative effect. Future studies will further address this hypothesis.

References

1. Abumiya T, Lucero J, Heo JH, Tagaya M, Koziol JA, Copeland BR, del Zoppo GJ (1999) Activated microvessels express vascular endothelial growth factor and integrin $\alpha_v\beta_3$ during focal cerebral ischemia. J Cereb Blood Flow Metab 19:1038–1050
2. Ahn MY, Zhang ZG, Tsang W, Chopp M (1999) Endogeneous plasminogen activator expression after embolic focal cerebral ischemia in mice. Brain Res 837:169–176
3. Albelda SM, Buck CA (1990) Integrins and other cell adhesion molecules. FASEB J 4:2868–2880
4. Anthony DC, Ferguson B, Matyzak MK, Miller KM, Esiri MM, Perry VH (1997) Differential matrix metalloproteinase expression in cases of multiple sclerosis and stroke. Neuropathol Appl Neurobiol 23:406–415
5. Ard MD, Faissner A (1991) Components of astrocytic extracellular matrix are regulated by contact with axons. Ann N Y Acad Sci 633:566–569
6. Bachmann F (1987) Fibrinolysis. In:Thrombosis and Haemostasis (Verstraete M, Vermylen J, Lijnen HR, Arnout J, eds), Leuven, ISTH/University of Leuven Press, pp 227–265
7. Bachmann F (1994) Molecular aspects of plasminogen, plasminogen activators and plasmin. In: Haemostasis and Thrombosis (Bloom AL, Forbes CD, Thomas DP, Tuddneham EGD, eds), Edinburgh, Churchill Livingstone, pp 575–613
8. Bernstein JJ, Getz R, Jefferson M, Kelemen M (1985) Astrocytes secrete basal lamina after hemisection of rat spinal cord. Brain Res 327:135–141
9. Bode IO, Fernandez-Catalan C, Grans F, Gomis-Rüth F-X, Nagase H, Tschesche H, Maskos K, Greenwold RA, Zucker S, Golub LM (1999) Insight into MMP-TIMP Interactions In Inhibition of Matrix Metalloproteinases. Ann NY Acad Sciences 878:73–91
10. Carlson SS and Hockfield S (1996) Central nervous system. In:Extracellular Matrix, Volume 1 (Comper WD, eds), Melbourne, Harwood Academic Publishers, pp 1–23
11. Chen ZL, Strickland S (1997) Neuronal death in the hippocampus is promoted by plasmincatalyzed degradation of laminin. Cell 91:917–925
12. Chintala SK, Sawaya R, Gokaslan ZL, Rao JS (1996) Modulation of matrix metalloprotease-2 and invasion in human glioma cells by $\alpha_3\beta_1$ integrin. Cancer Lett 103:201–208
13. Clark AW, Krekoski CA, Bou Shao-Sun, Chapman KR, Edwards DR (1997) Increased gelatinase A (MMP-2) and gelatinase B (MMP-9) activities in human brain after focal ischemia. Neurosci Lett 238:53–56
14. Cross AK, Woodroofe MN (1999) Chemokine modulation of matrix metalloproteinase and TIMP production in adult rat brain microglia and a human microglial cell line *in vitro*. GLIA 28(3):183–189
15. Danglet G, Vinson D, Chapeville F (1986) Qualitative and quantitative distribution of plasminogen activators in organs from healthy adult mice. FEBS Lett 194:96–100

16. del Zoppo GJ (1994) Microvascular changes during cerebral ischaemia and reperfusion. Cerebrovasc Brain Metab Rev 6:47–96
17. del Zoppo GJ, Copeland BR, Harker LA, Waltz TA, Zyroff J, Hanson SR, Battenberg E (1986) Experimental acute thrombotic stroke in baboons. Stroke 17:1254–1265
18. del Zoppo GJ, Haring H-P, Tagaya M, Wagner S, Akamine P, Hamann GF (1996) Loss of $\alpha_1\beta_1$ integrin immunoreactivity on cerebral microvessels and astrocytes following focal cerebral ischemia/reperfusion. Cerebrovasc Dis 6:9
19. del Zoppo GJ, Schmid-Schönbein GW, Mori E, Copeland BR, Chang C-M (1991) Polymorphonuclear leukocytes occlude capillaries following middle cerebral artery occlusion and reperfusion in baboons. Stroke 22:1276–1283
20. Dent MA, Sumi Y, Morris RJ, Seeley PJ (1993) Urokinase-type plasminogen activator expression by neurons and oligodendrocytes during process outgrowth in developing rat brain. Eur J Neurosci 5:633–647
21. Estrada C, Bready JV, Berliner JA, Pardridge WM, Cancilla PA (1990) Astrocyte growth stimulation by a soluble factor produced by cerebral endothelial cells *in vitro*. J Neuropathol Exp Neurol 49:539–549
22. Fabunmi RP, Baker AH, Murray EJ, Booth RFG, Newby AC (1996) Divergent regulation by growth factors and cytokines of 95 kDa and 72 kDa gelatinases and tissue inhibitors of metalloproteinases-1, -2, and -3 in rabbit aortic smooth muscle cells. Biochem J 315:335–342
23. Fletcher AP, Alkjaersig N, Sherry S, Genton E, Hirsh J, Bachmann F (1965) The development of urokinase as a thrombolytic agent. Maintenance of a sustained thrombolytic state in man by its intravenous infusion. J Lab Clin Med 65:713–731
24. Forsgren M, Raden B, Israelsson M, Larsson K, Heden LO (1987) Molecular cloning and characterization of a full-length cDNA clone for human plasminogen. FEBS Lett 213:254–260
25. Fujimura M, Gasche Y, Morita-Fujimura Y, Massengale J, Kawase M, Chan PH (1999) Early appearance of activated matrix metalloproteinase-9 and blood-brain barrier disruption in mice after focal cerebral ischemia and reperfusion. Brain Res 842:92–100
26. Galis ZS, Kranzhöfer R, Fenton JWII, Libby P (1997) Thrombin promotes activation of matrix metalloproteinase-2 produced by cultured vascular smooth muscle cells. Arterioscler Thromb Vasc Biol 17:483–489
27. Garcia JH, Mitchem HL, Briggs L, Morawetz R, Hudetz AG, Hazelrig JB, Halsey JH, Jr., Conger KA (1983) Transient focal ischemia in subhuman primates: Neuronal injury as a function of local cerebral blood flow. J Neuropathol Exp Neurol 42:44–60
28. Gasche Y, Fujimura M, Morita-Fujimura Y, Copin JC, Kawase M, Massengale J, Chan PH (1999) Early appearance of activated matrix metalloproteinase-9 after focal cerebral ischemia in mice: a possible role in blood-brain barrier dysfunction. J Cereb Blood Flow Metab 19:1020–1028
29. Gelehrter TD, Sznycer-Laszuk R (1986) Thrombin induction of plasminogen activator-inhibitor in cultured human endothelial cells. J Clin Invest 77:165–169
30. Gottschall PE, Deb S (1996) Regulation of matrix metalloproteinase expressions in astrocytes, microglia and neurons. Neuroimmunomodulation 3(2–3):69–75
31. Gottschall PE, Yu X, Bing B (1995) Increased production of gelatinase B (matrix metalloproteinase-9) and interleukin-6 by activated rat microglia in culture. J Neurosci Res 42(3):335–342
32. Hamann GF, Okada Y, del Zoppo GJ (1996) Hemorrhagic transformation and microvascular integrity during focal cerebral ischemia/reperfusion. J Cereb Blood Flow Metab 16:1373–1378
33. Hamann GF, Okada Y, Fitridge R, del Zoppo GJ (1995) Microvascular basal lamina antigens disappear during cerebral ischemia and reperfusion. Stroke 26:2120–2126
34. Hanss M, Collen D (1987) Secretion of tissue-type plasminogen activator and plasminogen activator inhibitor by cultured human endothelial cells: Modulation by thrombin endotoxin and histamine. J Lab Clin Med 109:97–104
35. Haring H-P, Akamine P, Habermann R, Koziol JA, del Zoppo GJ (1996a) Distribution of the integrin-like immunoreactivity on primate brain microvasculature. J Neuropathol Exp Neurol 55:236–245
36. Haring H-P, Berg EL, Tsurushita N, Tagaya M, del Zoppo GJ (1996b) E-selectin appears in non-ischemic tissue during experimental focal cerebral ischemia. Stroke 27:1386–1392
37. He CS, Wilhelm SM, Pentland AP, Marmer BL, Grant GA, Eisen AZ, Goldberg GI (1989) Tissue cooperation in a proteolytic cascade activating human interstitial collagenase. Proc Natl Acad Sci USA 86:2632–2636
38. Heck LW, Blackburn WD, Irwin MH, Abrahamson DR (1990) Degradation of basement membrane laminin by human neutrophil elastase and cathepsin G. Am J Pathol 136:1267–1274
39. Heo JH, Lucero J, Abumiya T, Koziol JA, Copeland BR, del Zoppo GJ (1999) Matrix metalloproteinases increase very early during experimental focal cerebral ischemia. J Cereb Blood Flow Metab 19:624–633
40. Hibbs MS, Hasty KA, Seyer JM, Kang AH, Mainardi CL (1985) Biochemical and immunological characterization of the secreted forms of human neutrophil gelatinase. J Biol Chem 260:2493–2500
41. Holvoet P, Lijnen HR, Collen D (1985) A monoclonal antibody specific for lys-plasminogen. Application to the study of the activation pathways of plasminogen *in vivo*. J Biol Chem 260:12106–12111
42. Hosomi N, Lucero J, Copeland BR, del Zoppo GJ (2000) Rapid endogenous urokinase (u-PA), but not t-PA, expression by ischemic brain tissue during acuto middle cerebral artery occlusion. Stroke 31:281
43. Hurwitz AA, Berman JW, Rashbaum WK, Lyman WD (1993) Human fetal astrocytes induce the expression of blood-brain barrier specific proteins by autologous endothelial cells. Brain Res 625:238–243
44. Janzer RC, Raff MC (1987) Astrocytes induce blood-brain barrier properties in endothelial cells (Letter). Nature 325:353–355
45. Juhan-Vague I, Moerman B, de Cock F, Aillaud MF, Collen D (1984) Plasma levels of a specific inhibitor of tissue-type plasminogen activator (and urokinase) in normal and pathological conditions. Thromb Res 33:523–530
46. Kakkar VV, Scully MF (1978) Thrombolytic therapy. Br Med Bull 34:191–199
47. Kazes I, Delarue F, Hagege J, Bouzhir-Sima L, Rondeau E, Sraer JD, Nguyen G (1998) Soluble latent membrane-type 1 matrix metalloprotease secreted by human mesangial cells is activated by urokinase. Kidney Int 54:1976–1984
48. Kozlova M, Kentroti S, Vernadakis A (1993) Influence of culture substrata on the differentiation of advanced passage glial cells in cultures from aged mouse cerebral hemispheres. Int J Dev Neurosci 11:513–519
49. Krane SM (1994) Clinical importance of metalloproteinases and their inhibitors. In: Inhibition of Matrix Metalloproteinases: Therapeutic Potential (Eds. R.A. Greenwald, L.M. Golub). Ann N Y Acad Sci 732:1–10
50. Krystosek A, Seeds NW (1986) Normal and malignant cells, including neurons, deposit plasminogen activator on growth substrata. Exp Cell Res 166:31–46
51. Kusaka H, Hirano A, Bornstein MB, Raine CS (1985) Basal lamina formation by astrocytes in organotypic cultures of

mouse spinal cord tissue. J Neuropathol Exp Neurol 44:295–303
52. Levin EG, del Zoppo GJ (1994) Localization of tissue plasminogen activator in the endothelium of a limited number of vessels. Am J Pathol 144:855–861
53. Levin EG, Marzec U, Anderson J, Harker LA (1984) Thrombin stimulates tissue plasminogen activator release from cultured human endothelial cells. J Clin Invest 74:1988–1995
54. Levin EG, Stern DM, Nawrath PP, Marlar RA, Fair DS, Fenton II JW, Harker LA (1986) Specificity of the thrombin-induced release of tissue plasminogen activator from cultured human endothelial cells. Thromb Haemost 56:115–119
55. Little JR, Kerr FWL, Sundt TM, Jr. (1975) Microcirculatory obstruction in focal cerebral ischemia. Relationship to neuronal alterations. Mayo Clin Proc 50:264–270
56. Little JR, Kerr FWL, Sundt TM, Jr. (1976) Microcirculatory obstruction in focal cerebral ischemia: An electron microscopic investigation in monkeys. Stroke 7:25–30
57. Loskutoff DJ, van Mourik JA, Erickson LA, Lawrence DA (1983) Detection of an unusually stable fibrinolytic inhibitor produced by bovine endothelial cells. Proc Natl Acad Sci USA 80:2956–2960
58. Luscinskas FW, Lawler J (1994) Integrins as dynamic regulators of vascular function. FASEB J 8:929–938
59. Mackay AR, Corbitt RH, Hartzler JL, Thorgeirsson UP (1990) Basement membrane type IV collagen degradation: evidence for the involvement of a proteolytic cascade independent of metalloproteinases. Cancer Res 50:5997–6001
60. Masos T, Miskin R (1996) Localization of urokinase-type plasminogen activator mRNA in the adult mouse brain. Brain Res Mol Brain Res 35:139–148
61. Matsuo O, Okada K, Fukao H, Suzuki A, Ueshima S (1992) Cerebral plasminogen activator activity in spontaneously hypertensive stroke-prone rats. Stroke 23:995–999
62. Mazzieri R, Masiero L, Zanetta L, Monea S, Onisto M, Garbisa S, Mignatti P (1997) Control of type IV collagenase activity by components of the urokinase-plasmin system: a regulatory mechanism with cell-bound reactants. EMBO J 16:2319–2332
63. McGuire PG, Seeds NW (1989) The interaction of plasminogen activator with a reconstituted basement membrane matrix and extracellular macromolecules produced by cultured epithelial cells. J Cell Biochem 40:215–227
64. Minakawa T, Bready J, Berliner J, Fisher M, Cancilla PA (1991) *In vitro* interaction of astrocytes and pericyte with capillary-like structures of brain microvessel endothelium. Lab Invest 65:32–40
65. Mori E, Chambers JD, Copeland BR, Arfors K-E, del Zoppo GJ (1992) Inhibition of polymorphonuclear leukocyte adherence suppresses no-reflow after focal cerebral ischemia. Stroke 23:712–718
66. Murphy G, Reynolds JJ, Bretz U, Baggiolini M (1987) Collagenase is a component of the specific granules of human neutrophil leukocytes. Biochem J 162:195–197
67. Nagai N, De Mol M, Lijnen HR, Carmeliet P, Collen D (1999) Role of plasminogen system components in focal cerebral ischemic infarction: a gene targeting and gene transfer study in mice. Circulation 99:2440–2444
68. Nagano N, Aoyagi M, Hirakawa K (1993) Extracellular matrix modulates the proliferation of rat astrocytes in serum-free culture. GLIA 8:71–76
69. Nakajima K, Tsuzaki N, Shimojo M, Hamanoue M, Kohsaka S (1992) Microglia isolated from rat brain secrete a urokinase-type plasminogen activator. Brain Res 577:285–292
70. Norton WT, Cammer W, Bloom BR, Gordon S (1978) Neutral proteinases secreted by macrophages degrade basic protein: a possible mechanism of inflammatory demyelination. Adv Exp Med Biol 100:365–381
71. Okada Y, Copeland BR, Mori E, Tung M-M, Thomas WS, del Zoppo GJ (1994) P-selectin and intercellular adhesion molecule-1 expression after focal brain ischemia and reperfusion. Stroke 25:202–211
72. Pagenstecher A, Stalder AK, Kincaid CL, Shapiro SD, Campbell IL (1998) Differential expression of matrix metalloproteinase and tissue inhibitor of matrix metalloproteinase genes in the mouse central nervous system in normal and inflammatory states. American Journalof Pathology 152(3):729–741
73. Partridge CA, Phillips PG, Niedbala MJ, Jeffrey JJ (1997) Localization and activation of type IV collagenase/gelatinase at endothelial focal contacts. Lung Cell Mol Physiol 16:L813–L822
74. Pasqualini R, Hemler ME (1994) Contrasting roles for integrin β_1 and β_5 cytoplasmic domains in subcellular localization, cell proliferation, and cell migration. J Cell Biol 125:447–460
75. Pennica D, Holmes WE, Kohr WJ, Harkins RN, Vehar GA, Ward CA, Bennett WF, Yelverton E, Seeburg PH, Heyneker HL, Goeddel DV, Collen D (1983) Cloning and expression of human tissue-type plasminogen activator cDNA in *E. coli.* Nature 301:214–221
76. Peterson LC, Serenson E (1990) Effect of plasminogen and tissue-type plasminogen activator on fibrin gel structure. Fibrinolysis 5:51–59
77. Pfefferkorn T, Staufer B, Liebetrau M, Bultemeier G, Vosko MR, Zimmermann C, Hamann GF (2000) Plasminogen activation in focal cerebral ischemia and reperfusion. J Cereb Blood Flow Metab 20:337–342
78. Philips M, Juul AG, Thorsen S (1984) Human endothelial cells produce a plasminogen activator inhibitor and a tissue-type plasminogen activator-inhibitor complex. Biochim Biophys Acta 802:99–110
79. Pike MC, Wicha MS, Yoon P, Mayo L, Boxer LA (1989) Laminin promotes the oxidative burst in human neutrophils via increased chemoattractant receptor expression. J Immunol 142:2004–2011
80. Pittman RN (1985) Release of plasminogen activator and a calcium-dependent metalloprotease from cultured sympathetic and sensory neurons. Dev Biol 110:91–101
81. Plow EF, Felez J, Miles LA (1991) Cellular regulation of fibrinolysis. Thromb Haemost 66:132–136
82. Rijken DC (1988) Structure/function relationships of t-PA. In: Tissue Type Plasminogen Activator (t-PA): Physiological and Clinical Aspects. Volume 1 (Kluft C, eds), Boca Raton, CRC Press, pp 101–122
83. Robbins KC (1995) The plasminogen-plasmin system. In: Thrombolytic Therapy for Peripheral Vascular Disease (Comerota AJ, eds), Philadelphia, J.B. Lippincott, pp 41–65
84. Robbins KC, Summaria L, Hsieh B, Shah RJ (1967) The peptide chains of human plasmin. J Biochem 242:2333–2342
85. Rosenberg GA, Navratil M, Barone F, Feuerstein G (1996) Proteolytic cascade enzymes increase in focal cerebral ischemia in rat. J Cereb Blood Flow Metab 16:360–366
86. Ruoslahti E (1991) Integrins. J Clin Invest 87:1–5
87. Sakata Y, Curriden S, Lawrence D, et al. (1985) Activated protein C stimulates the fibrinolytic activity of cultured endothelial cells and decreases antiactivator activity. Proc Natl Acad Sci USA 82:1121–1125
88. Saksela O, Rifkin DB (1988) Cell-associated plasminogen activation: regulation and physiological functions. Annu Rev Cell Biol 4:93–126
89. Sappino A-P, Madani R, Huarte J, Belin D, Kiss JZ, Wohlwend A, Vassalli J-D (1993) Extracellular proteolysis in the adult murine brain. J Clin Invest 92:679–685
90. Stump DC, Mann KH (1988) Mechanisms of thrombus formation and lysis. Ann Emerg Med 17:1138–1147
91. Tagami M, Yamagata K, Fujino H, Kubota A, Nara Y, Yamori Y (1992) Morphological differentiation of endothelial cells co-

cultured with astrocytes on type-I or type-IV collagen. Cell Tissue Res 268:225–232

92. Thomas WS, Mori E, Copeland BR, Yu J-Q, Morrissey JH, del Zoppo GJ (1993) Tissue factor contributes to microvascular defects following cerebral ischemia. Stroke 24:847–853
93. Thorsen S, Philips M, Selmer J, Lecander I, Astedt B (1988) Kinetics of inhibition of tissue-type and urokinase-type plasminogen activator by plasminogen-activator inhibitor type 1 and type 2. Eur J Biochem 175:33–39
94. Toshniwal PK, Firestone SL, Barlow GH, Tiku ML (1987) Characterization of astrocyte plasminogen activator. J Neurol Sci 80:277–287
95. Tran-Thong C, Kruithof EKO, Atkinson J, Bachmann F (1986) High-affinity binding sites for human glu-plasminogen unveiled by limited plasmic degradation of human fibrin. Eur J Biochem 160:559–604
96. Tranque P, Naftolin F, Robbins R (1994) Differential regulation of astrocyte plasminogen activators by insulin-like growth factor-I and epidermal growth factor. Endocrinology 134:2606–2613
97. Tsirka SE, Rogove AD, Bugge TH, Degen JL, Strickland S (1997) An extracellular proteolytic cascade promotes neuronal degeneration in the mouse hippocampus. J Neurosci 17:543–552
98. Uhm JH, Dooley NP, Oh LY, Yong VW (1998) Oligodendrocytes utilize a matrix metalloproteinase, MMP-9, to extend processes along an astrocyte extracellular matrix. GLIA 22(1):53–63
99. van Hinsbergh VW, van den Berg EA, Fiers W, Dooijewaard G (1990) Tumor necrosis factor induces the production of urokinase-type plasminogen activator by human endothelial cells. Blood 75:1991–1998
100. Vassalli JD, Sappino AP, Belin D (1991) The plasminogen activator/plasmin system. J Clin Invest 88:1067–1072
101. Vincent VA, Lowik CW, Verheijen JH, de Bart AC, Tilders FJ, Van Dam AM (1998) Role of astrocyte-derived tissue-type plasminogen activator in the regulation of endotoxin-stimulated nitric oxide production by microglial cells. GLIA 22:130–137
102. Wagner S, Tagaya M, Koziol JA, Quaranta V, del Zoppo GJ (1997) Rapid disruption of an astrocyte interaction with the extracellular matrix mediated by $\alpha_6\beta_4$ during focal cerebral ischemia/reperfusion. Stroke 28:858–865
103. Wallen P, Wiman B (1973) Characterization of human plasminogen. II. Separation and partial characterization of different molecular forms of human plasminogen. Biochim Biophys Acta 257:122–134
104. Wang YF, Tsirka SE, Strickland S, Stieg PE, Soriano SG, Lipton SA (1998) Tissue plasminogen activator (tPA) increases neuronal damage after focal cerebral ischemia in wild-type and tPA-deficient mice. Nature Medicine 4:228–231
105. Watanabe H, Hattori S, Katsuda S, Nakanishi I, Nagai Y (1990) Human neutrophil elastase: Degradation of basement membrane components and immunolocalization in the tissue. J Biochem 108:753–759
106. Webersinke G, Bauer H, Amberger A, Zach O, Bauer HC (1992) Comparison of gene expression of extracellular matrix molecules in brain microvascular endothelial cells and astrocytes. Biochem Biophys Res Commun 189:877–884
107. Wells GM, Catlin G, Cossins JA, Mangan M, Ward GA, Miller KM, Clements JM (1996) Quantitation of matrix metalloproteinases in cultured rat astrocytes using the polymerase chain reaction with a multi-competitor cDNA standard. GLIA 18(4):332–340
108. White FW, Barlow GH, Mozen MM (1966) The isolation and characterization of plasminogen activators (urokinase) from human urine. Biochemistry 5:2160–2169
109. Woessner JF, Jr. (1994) The family of matrix metalloproteinases. Ann N Y Acad Sci 732:11–21
110. Yurchenko PD, Schittny JC (1986) Molecular architecture of basement membranes. J Biol Chem 261:1577–1590
111. Zhang GZ, Chopp M, Goussev A, Lu D, Morris D, Tsang W, Powers C, Ho K-L (1999) Cerebral microvascular obstruction by fibrin is associated with upregulation of PAI-1 acutely after onset of focal embolic ischemia in rats. J Neurosci 19:10898–10907

Inhibition of inflammation and neuroprotection by tetracyclines

J. Yrjänheikki*, T. Tikka*, G. Goldsteins*, M. Koistinaho*, R. Keinänen*, P. H. Chan‡, J. Koistinaho*†

Abstract

Minocycline and doxycycline are safe semisynthetic tetracycline derivates, which have multiple anti-inflammatory effects unrelated to their antimicrobial action. Because inflammation is an important component of ischemic neuronal death, we studied whether these tetracyclines protect against brain ischemia in vivo and against excitotoxicity in vitro. In gerbil global ischemia minocycline increased the survival of CA1 pyramidal neurons from 10.5% to 77% when the treatment was started 12 h before ischemia and to 71% when the treatment was started 30 min after ischemia. The survival with pre- and post-treatment with doxycycline was 57% and 47%, respectively. In transient focal brain ischemia of the rat, minocycline reduced cortical infarction volume by 76% when the treatment was started 12 h before ischemia and by 63% when started even 4 h after the onset of ischemia. The treatment inhibited activation of microglia and induction of IL-1β-converting enzyme, reduced cyclooxygenase-2 expression and prostaglandin E_2 production, and slightly down-regulated induction of inducible nitric oxide synthase. Minocycline had no effect on astrogliosis or spreading depression. In cell cultures minocycline inhibited microglial proliferation and salvaged primary neurons from glutamate and kainate toxicity. These findings indicate that the activation of microglia contributes to ischemic neuronal death, which is inhibited by minocycline, an antibiotic used in severe human infections.

J. Krieglstein, S. Klumpp (Eds.) Pharmacology of Cerebral Ischemia 2000

Tetracyclines are well-known broad-spectrum antibiotics (Sande and Mandell 1995). The second-generation tetracyclines, doxycycline and minocycline were synthetized about 30 years ago (Fig. 1). These semi-synthetic antibiotics are very lipophilic, are absorbed rapidly and completely even in aged population (Barza et al. 1975; Kramer et al. 1978; Cunha et al. 1982; Klein and Cunha 1995), and compared to many other antibiotics, they penetrate well into the brain and cerebrospinal fluid (Aronson 1980; Klein and Cunha 1995). A special feature of doxycycline and minocycline is that they exert biological effects that are completely separate and distinct from their antimicrobial action. These

Keywords: Inflammation; cytokines; microglia; nitric oxide; focal ischemia; global ischemia; glutamate

*A.I. Virtanen Institute for Molecular Sciences, University of Kuopio, P.O. Box 1627, †Department of Neurology, Kuopio University Hospital, P.O. Box 1627, FIN-70211 Kuopio, Finland, ‡Neurosurgical Laboratories, Department of Neurosurgery, Department of Neurology and Neurobiological Sciences, Program in Neurosciences, Stanford University School of Medicine, 701B Welch Road #148, Palo Alto, CA 94304, USA.
e-mail: jari.koistinaho@uku.fi

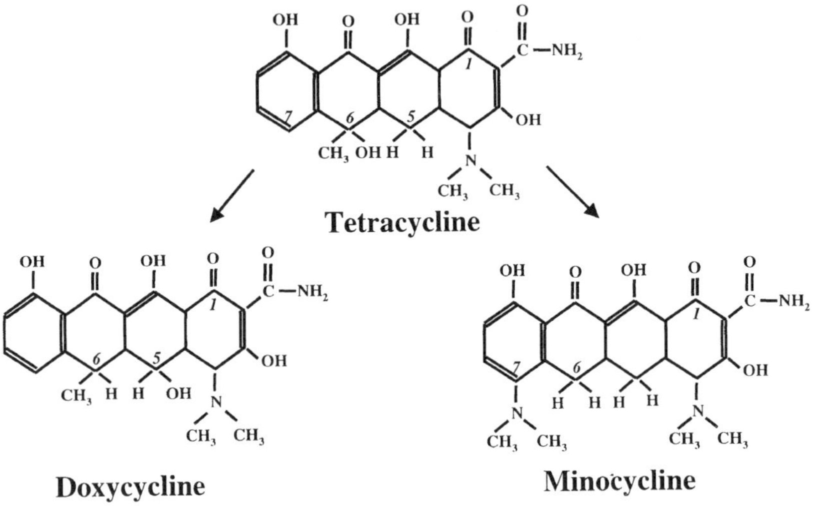

Fig. 1. Structure of tetracycline, doxycycline and minocycline. Doxycycline differs from tetracycline by substitutions of the fifth and sixth position and minocycline by substitutions on the sixth and seventh position on the basic structure.

effects include inhibition of matrix metalloproteases (Golub et al. 1991), modulation of cyclooxygenase-2 activity (Patel et al. 1999), depression of oxygen radical release from polymorphonuclear neutrophils (Gabler and Creamer 1991), inhibition of inducible nitric oxide synthase (iNOS) (Amin et al. 1996, 1997), and inhibition of protein tyrosine nitration by scavenging peroxynitrite (Whiteman and Halliwell 1997). Both experimental and clinical studies indicate that minocycline and doxycycline may be beneficial in treatment of peripheral inflammatory diseases (Greenwald et al. 1992; Furst 1998; Nordstrom et al. 1998) The drugs are clinically well tolerated and minocycline has been considered for treatment of rheumatoid arthritis, a severe inflammatory human disease (Furst 1998).

Inflammation, which involves non-neuronal cells, has an important role in pathogenesis of stroke (Rothwell et al. 1997; Barone and Feuerstein 1999; Dirnagl et al. 1999; Lee et al. 1999; del Zoppo et al. 2000). In global ischemia hippocampal CA1 pyramidal neurons die as late as 3 to 5 days after the insult (Siesjö 1978), indicating that hippocampal ischemic cell death involves slowly developing mechanisms. Moreover, focal ischemia caused by occlusion of the middle cerebral artery (MCA) involves secondary inflammation that significantly contributes to the outcome after ischemic insult (Nogawa et al. 1997; DeGraba 1998; Sairanen et al. 1998; Barone and Feuerstein 1999; Dirnagl et al. 1999; Lee et al. 1999; del Zoppo et al. 2000). Several genes or mediators that promote inflammation, such as inducible nitric oxide synthase (iNOS), cyclooxygenase-2 (COX-2), and cytokines, are strongly expressed in the ischemic brain (Nogawa et al. 1997; Dirnagl et al. 1999; del Zoppo et al. 2000). Inflammation is now regarded as an attractive pharmacologic target, because it progresses over several days after acute brain injury, and intervention with inflammatory mechanisms, which are not fundamental for physiological brain functions, may not result in intolerable side effects (Barone and Feuerstein 1999), as the wide clinical use of non-steroidal anti-inflammatory drugs (NSAIDs) demonstrates. We therefore studied, whether minocycline and doxicycline reduce ischemic brain damage caused by global or transient focal ischemia. We studied the effect of minocycline also in primary neuronal cultures, because neurotoxicity of excitatory amino acids, e.g. glutamate, is a major contributing factor in acute stroke. We chose to use mixed spinal cord cultures, because cultured spinal cord neurons maturate fast and express functional glutamate receptors after 7 days in vitro.

Studies on global ischemia model

Using global gerbil ischemia as a model, we first screened the effect of the following antibiotics: erythromycin, tetracycline, doxycycline, minocycline and cefritriaxone, a third generation cephalosporine. The antibiotics were administered intraperitoneally twice a day starting 24 h before ischemia and the treatment was continued until the day the animals were sacrificed (Yrjänheikki et al. 1998). The screening studies indicated neuroprotective potential of doxycycline and minocycline, which together with tetracycline were studied more in detail in the same gerbil model. We used the dose of 180–90 mg/kg per day because the treatment did not result in severe side effects and the maximal penetration of the drugs to the brain was desired. Twelve hours before ischemia, gerbils were injected with 45 mg/kg of minocycline, doxycycline or tetracycline hydrochloride. Thereafter, the animals were injected twice a day, at a dose of 90 mg/kg during the first day after ischemia and 45 mg/kg starting 36 h after ischemia. The postischemic treatment was started 30 min after ischemia with 90 mg/kg. Both minocycline and doxycycline treatments increased significantly the number of surviving neurons (Fig. 2). Six days after ischemia the minocycline-pretreated gerbils had 76.7%, minocycline-postreated gerbils had 71.4%, doxycycline-pretreated gerbils had 57.2%, and doxycycline-postreated gerbils had 47.1% of the neuron profiles left in the CA1 pyramidal cell layer, whereas in untreated gerbils 10.5% of the CA1 neurons were left. The neuroprotection was statistically significant in every animal group. Tetracycline did not provide any protection. Minocycline and doxycycline did not reduce the postoperative body temperatures.

To determine whether neuroprotection by minocycline is associated with activation of

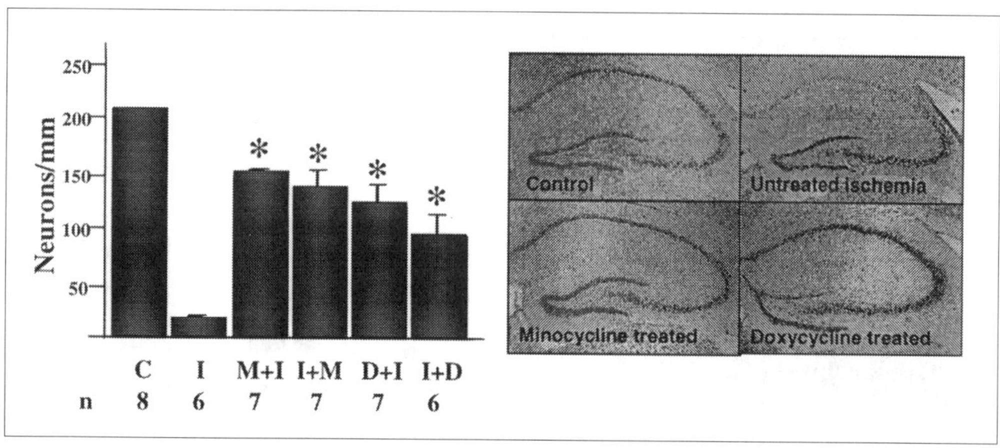

Fig. 2. Effect of minocycline and doxycycline treatment on the CA1 pyramidal neurons after global brain ischemia. The graph summarizes the quantitative results of CA1 neuronal counts: C, sham-operated; I, saline-treated; M+I/D+I, minocycline/doxycycline treatment started before ischemia; I+M/I+D, minocycline/doxycycline treatment started after ischemia. *, $P < 0.05$, when compared with saline-treated ischemic (I) gerbils. n, number of animals. On the left panel, the hippocampus is shown in a cresyl violet-stained section from a sham-operated gerbil (control), from a ischemia-operated gerbils treated with saline (untreated ischemia), and from a minocycline and doxycycline-treated sgerbil. Modified from a figure in Yrjänheikki et al. 1998.

nonneuronal cells, we studied GFAP expression, a marker of astrogliosis, and phosphotyrosine immunoreactivity and isolectin B4 binding, which are markers of activated microglia. The results showed that expression of GFAP mRNA in the hippocampus was increased to the same extent in saline- and minocycline-treated gerbils and that immunoreactivity for GFAP was similar in these two groups. Instead, microglial activation appeared to be significantly reduced in minocycline-treated gerbils (Fig. 3A). We therefore next studied whether induction of interleukin-1β converting enzyme (ICE), an apoptosis-promoting gene that is strongly induced in microglia after global ischemia, or iNOS, an enzyme suggested to produce toxic concentration of nitric oxide in nonneuronal cells after global brain ischemia (Endoh et al. 1994), are affected by neuroprotective minocycline treatment. The semiquantitative RT-PCR showed that 4 days after ischemia, expression of ICE mRNA was attenuated by approximately 70% and expression of iNOS mRNA by 30% in the hippocampus of minocycline-treated gerbils (Fig. 3B). In addition, 6 days after ischemia, NADPH-diaphorase-reactive cells were seen in the hippocampi of saline-treated, but not in minocycline-treated, ischemic gerbils. Most of the NADPH-diaphorase-reactive cells resembling microglia were located in the pyramidal cell layer of the CA1 subfield and some NADPH-diaphorase-reactive cells with the morphology typical of astrocytes were detected in the stratum radiatum. Therefore, minocycline inhibited NOS activity also in astrocytes, even though it did not block astrogliosis.

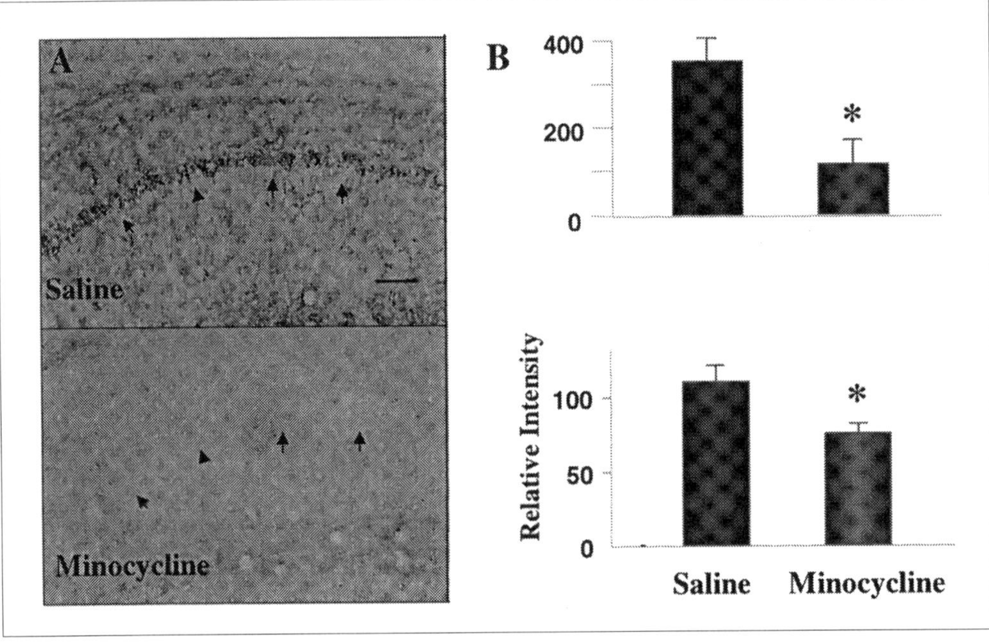

Fig. 3. Activation of microglial cells (A) in the CA1 hippocampus six days after global brain ischemia and induction of ICE (B, upper panel) and iNOS (B, lower panel) mRNA four days after ischemia is prevented by minocycline. (A) Microglia was detected by phosphotyrosine immunoreactivity, which was particularly intense in the pyramidal cell layer (arrows) of saline-treated gerbils. Bar = 250 μM. (B) Semiquantitative results of RT-PCR analysis of ICE and iNOS mRNA induction. The amplification products (n = 4 in each group) were analyzed with a Bio-Rad Imaging Densitometer using RT-PCR of glyceraldehydes-3-phosphate dehydrogenase as a reference. *$p < 0.05$, one-way ANOVA.
Modified from figures in Yrjänheikki et al.1998.

Studies on focal ischemia model

Because minocycline was more neuroprotective than doxycycline in global brain ischemia, we decided to continue with minocycline in focal brain ischemia model of the rat (Yrjänheikki et al. 1999). Treatment with minocycline (45 mg/kg i.p. twice a day for the first day; 22.5 mg/kg for the subsequent 2 days) did not affect rectal temperature, arterial blood pressure, plasma glucose, or arterial blood gases. However, the treatment started 12 h before ischemia reduced the size of the infarct in the cerebral cortex by 76% and in the striatum by 39%. Starting the minocycline treatment 2 h after the onset of ischemia resulted in a reduction in the size of cortical (by 65%) and striatal (by 42%) infarct, a reduction similar to the one obtained with pretreatment. The cortical infarct size was reduced by 63% even when the treatment was started 4 h after the onset of ischemia (Fig. 4).

Because cortical spreading depression (SD), an energy-consuming wave of transient depolarizations of astrocytes and neurons, contributes to the evolution of ischemia to infarction in focal ischemia (Mies et al. 1993; Back et al. 1996; Busch et al. 1996; Rawanduzy et al. 1997), we tested whether minocycline provides protection by inhibiting cortical SD. In a separate set of rats that were not subjected to MCA occlusion, minocycline did not alter the number, duration, or amplitude of direct current potentials induced by a 60-min exposure to topical 3 M KCl, whereas MK-801, an NMDA receptor antagonist known to reduce partially ischemic damage by blocking cortical SD, completely prevented KCl-induced direct current potentials.

As nonneuronal cells are characteristically activated in the brain in response to injury (Banati et al. 1993; Giulian and Corpuz 1993; McGeer and McGeer 1995), and minocycline was found to reduce microglial activation in global ischemia model, we studied astrogliosis and microglial activation in focal ischemia model. At 24 h after 90 min of ischemia, a

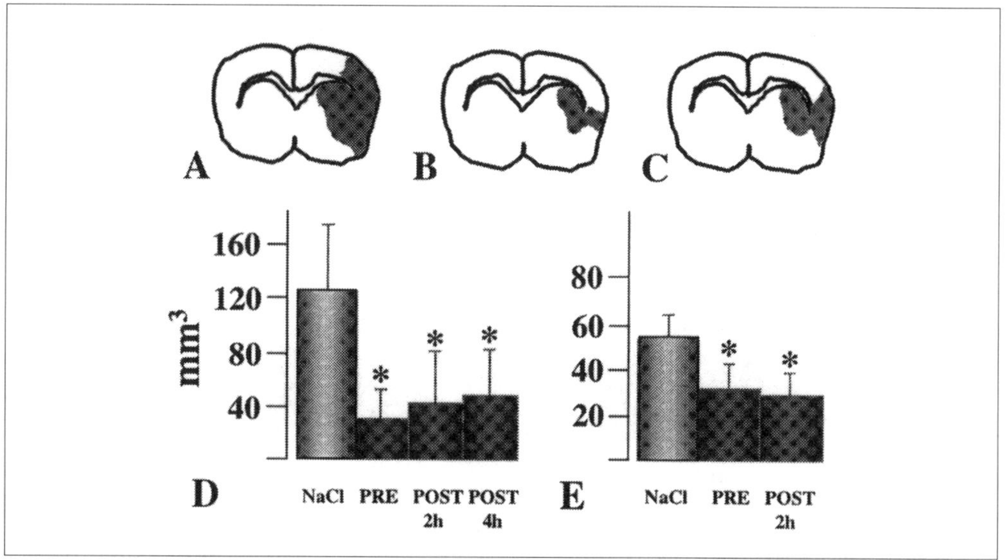

Fig. 4. Minocycline treatment started 12 h before the onset of ischemia (B) and two hours after the onset of ischemia (C) reduces the infarction area (seen in gray in the figure) detected in triphenyltetrazolium chloride-stained brain slices 3 days after ischemia.. The infarction area is significantly reduced in the cortex (D) and striatum (E) compared with saline (NaCl)-treated animals when the minocycline treatment is started 12 hours before ischemia (PRE, n = 10), 2 hours after the onset of ischemia (POST 2 h, n = 10), or 4 hours after the onset of ischemia (POST 4 h, n = 12). *p < 0.01 (one-way ANOVA followed by the Bonferoni's test). Modified from a figure in Yrjänheikki et al. 1999.

strong induction of CD11b immunoreactivity was observed around and inside the infarction core in untreated rats. The immunoreactive cells had an amoeboid shape in the penumbra zone. Minocycline treatment started 12 h before ischemia decreased the number of CD11b-immunoreactive cells and prevented the appearance of the amoeboid-shaped microglia adjacent to the infarction core (Fig. 5A, B). Instead, GFAP-immunoreactivity in the ischemic hemispheres of untreated and minocycline-treated animals was similarly increased. Similar to global ischemia studies, pretreatment with minocycline decreased also the induced ICE mRNA levels by 83% in the penumbra (Fig. 5C), indicating that minocycline treatment inhibits expression of the enzyme needed for IL-1β activation in microglia.

COX-2 is highly expressed in the brain after global and focal brain ischemia and produces superoxides and proinflammatory prostaglandins such as PGE_2 (Sairanen et al. 1998; Nogawa et al. 1997; Miettinen et al. 1997; Koistinaho et al. 1999). In general, expression of COX-2 is reduced by antiinflammatories and can be induced by cytokines, including IL-1β. Because minocycline treatment inhibited microglial activation, we studied whether the treatment also affects COX-2. In global brain ischemia of gerbil, we studied the hippocampal expression of COX-2 mRNA and found that minocycline down-regulated the expression by 30–40%. The protein levels and activity of COX-2 was studied in focal brain ischemia model. In untreated rats, the PGE_2 concentration was increased 5-fold in the ischemic penumbra and was preced-

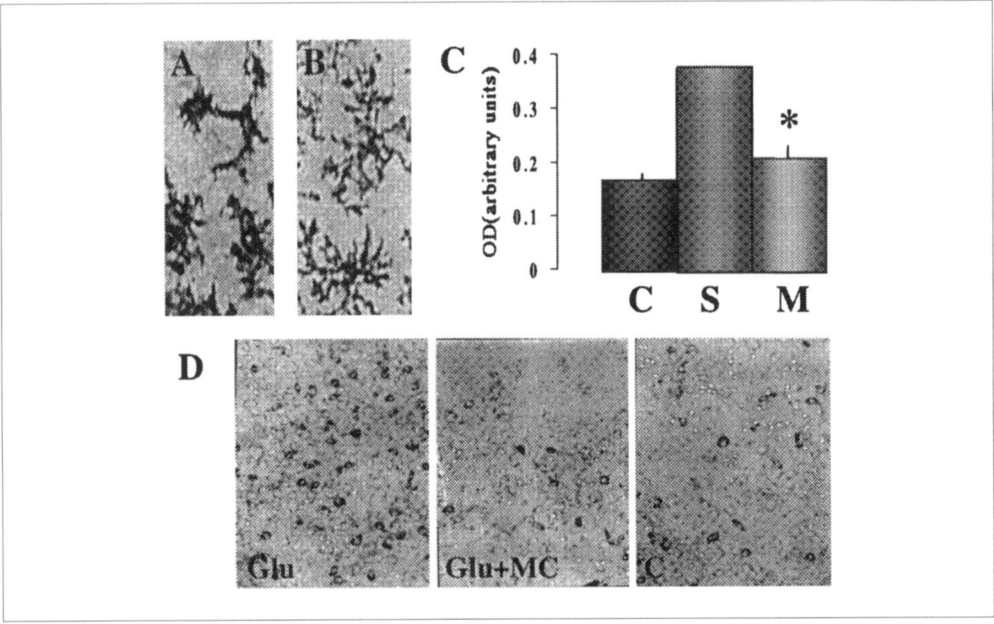

Fig. 5. Minocycline treatment inhibits ischemia and excitotoxin-induced activation of microglia and reduces ischemia-induced induction of ICE mRNA in penumbra. Twentyfour hours after focal brain ischemia ameboid-shaped CD-11b (OX-42)-immunoreactive cells are seen around infarction core in saline-treated (A), but not in minocycline-treated (B) animals. (C) RT-PCR analysis of ICE mRNA levels revealed a significant increase 12 h after the onset of ischemia in penumbra of saline-treated animals (S) compared to control samples (C). Minocycline treatment (M) reduced the induction ($p < 0.01$, one-way ANOVA followed by Bonferroni's test, n = 4 in each group). (D) Minocycline inhibits excitotoxin-induced proliferation of OX-42 positive microglial cells in mixed spinal cord cultures. The number of immunoreactive microglial cells (identified by dark staining) is significantly increased after a 24-h exposure to 500 μM glutamate (Glu) compared to untreated (C) cultures. Minocycline pretreatment completely prevents the microglial proliferation.

ed by the induction of COX-2 immunoreactive neurons. Pretreatment with minocycline reduced the PGE_2 concentration in the penumbra by 55% and almost completely prevented the appearance of COX-2 immunoreactivity at 24 h.

Studies on Cell Culture Model

Tetracyclines, including minocycline, reduce efficiently inflammation in the peripheral sysmtem, for example by inhibiting the function of polymorphonuclear neutrophils (Gabler and Creamer 1991; Gabler et al. 1992). To find out, whether minocycline has direct effects on the brain cells, we studied minocycline in primary neuronal cultures. Mixed spinal cord cultures that consist of neurons (70%), astrocytes (24%), and microglia (6%) and that are devoid of endothelial cells and peripheral cells, were used. When the cultures were treated with 0.02 μM minocycline, the lactate dehydrogenase release induced by 500 μM glutamate or 100 μM kainate, a major mediator of neuronal death in the brain, was decreased by 50–85%. We also found that glutamate and kainate treatment increase the number of OX-42 positive cells in mixed spinal cord cultures and that this increase is inhibited by 0.02 μM minocycline (Fig. 5D). Therefore, we concluded that minocycline provides major neuroprotection against excitotoxicity in mixed brain cell cultures by a mechanism that is independent of peripheral systems. Instead, minocycline inhibits microglial proliferation. Because microglial cells have been reported to enhance excitotoxicity (Rogove and Tsirka 1998), it is possible that the beneficial effect of minocycline is at least partially based on inhibited release of microglial toxins, such as tumor necrosis factor alpha, interleukin-1β, nitric oxide and extracellular proteases.

Minocycline and doxycycline are widely used antibiotics with proven safety. It is possible that even high doses of these antibiotics may not provide sufficient protection against human brain ischemia. However, minocycline and doxycycline may represent lead molecules for development of novel derivatives with potent anti-inflammatory effects for stroke therapy.

Acknowledgements

The study was supported by the Sigrid Juselius Foundation (J.K., T.T., J.Y.), the Saastamoinen Foundation (T.T.), the North Savo Fund of the Finnish Cultural Foundation (T.T.), and The Finnish Cultural Foundation (J.Y).

References

1. Amin AR, Attur MG, Thakker GD, et al (1996) A novel mechanism of action of tetracyclines: effects on nitric oxide synthases. Proc Natl Acad Sci USA 93:14014–14019
2. Amin AR, Patel RN, Thakker GD, et al (1997) Post-transcriptional regulation of inducible nitric oxide synthase mRNA in murine macrophages by doxycycline and chemically modified tetracyclines. FEBS Lett 410:259–264
3. Aronson AL (1980) Pharmacotherapeutics of the newer tetracyclines. J Am Vet Med Assoc 176:1061–1068
4. Back T, Ginsberg MD, Dietrich WD, et al (1996) Induction of spreading depression in the ischemic hemisphere following experimental middle cerebral artery occlusion: Effect on infarct morphology. J Cereb Blood Flow Metab 16:202–213
5. Banati RB, Gehrmann J, Schubert P, et al (1993) Cytotoxicity of microglia. Glia 7:111–118
6. Barone, FC, Feuerstein GZ (1999) Inflammatory mediators and stroke: new opportunities for novel therapeutics. J Cereb Blood Flow Metab 19:819–834
7. Barza M, Brown RB, Shanks C, et al (1975) Relation between lipophilicity and pharmacological behavior of minocycline, doxycycline, tetracycline, and oxytetracycline in dogs. Antimicrobiol Agents Chemother 8:713–720
8. Busch E, Gyngell ML, Eis M, et al (1996) Potassium-induced cortical spreading depressions during focal cerebral ischemia in rats: contribution to lesion growth assessed by diffusion-weighted NMR and biochemical imaging. J Cereb Blood Flow Metab 16:1090–1099
9. Cunha BA, Sibley C, Ristuccia PA (1982) Doxycycline. Ther Drug Monit 4:115–130
10. DeGraba TJ (1998) The role of inflammation after acute stroke: utility of pursuing anti-adhesion molecule therapy, Neurology 51, Suppl. 3, S62–S68
11. Dirnagl U, Iadecola C, Moskowitz MA (1999) Pathobiology of ischaemic stroke: an integrated view. Trends Neurosci 22:391–397
12. Endoh M, Maiese K, Wagner J (1994) Expression of the inducible form of nitric oxide synthase by reactive astrocytes after transient global ischemia. Brain Res 651:92–100
13. Furst DE (1998) Update on clinical trials in the rheumatic diseases. Cur Opin Rheumatol 10:123–128
14. Gabler W, Creamer H (1991) Suppression of human neutrophil functions by Tetracyclines. J Periodontal Res 26: 52–58.
15. Gabler W, Smith J, Tsukuda N (1992) Comparison of doxycycline and a chemically modified tetracycline inhibition of leukocyte functions. Res Commun Chem Pathol Pharmacol 8:151–160
16. Giulian D, Corpuz M (1993) Microglial secretion products and their impact on the nervous system. Adv Neurol 59:315–320
17. Golub LM, Ramamurthy NS, McNamara TF (1991) Tetracyclines inhibit connective tissue breakdown: new therapeutic implications for an old family of drugs. Crit RevOral Biol Med 2:297–322

18. Greenwald RA, Moak SA, Ramamurthy NS et al (1992) Tetracyclines suppress matrix metalloproteinase activity in adjuvant arthritis and in combination with flurbiprofen, ameliorate bone damage. J Rheumatol 19:927–938
19. Klein NC, Cunha BA (1995) Tetracyclines. Med Clin North Amer 79:789–801
20. Koistinaho J, Pasonen S, Chan PH (1999) Expression of cyclooxygenase-2 mRNA after global ischemia is regulated by AMPA receptors and glucocorticoids. Stroke 30:1900–1905
21. Kramer PA, Chapron DJ, Benson J, Mercik SA (1978) Tetracycline absorption in elderly patients with achlorhydria. Clin Pharmacol Ther 23:467–472
22. Lee JM, Zipfel G, Choi DW (1999) The changing landscape of ischaemic brain injury mechanisms. Nature 399:6738 Suppl:A7–14
23. McGeer PL, McGeer EG (1995) The inflammatory response system of brain: implications for therapy of Alzheimer and other neurodegenerative diseases. Brain Res Rev 21:195–218
24. Mies G, Iijima T, Hossmann KA (1993) Correlation between peri-infarct DC shifts and ischaemic neuronal damage in rat. Neuroreport 4:709–711
25. Miettinen S, Fusco FR, Yrjänheikki J, et al (1997) Spreading depression and focal brain ischemia induce cyclooxygenase-2 in cortical neurons through N-methyl-D-aspartic acid-receptors and phospholipase A2. Proc Natl Acad Sci USA 94:6500–6505
26. Nogawa S, Zhang F, Ross ME, et al (1997) Cyclo-oxygenase-2 gene expression in neurons contributes to ischemic brain damage. J Neurosci 17:2746–2755
27. Nordstrom D, Lindy O, Lauhio A, et al (1998) Anti-collagenolytic mechanism of action of doxycycline treatment in rheumatoid arthritis. Rheumatol Int 17:175–180
28. Patel RN, Attur MG, Dave MN, et al (1999) A novel mechanism of action of chemically modified tetracyclines: inhibition of COX-2-mediated prostaglandin E2 production. J Immunol 163:3459–3467
29. Rawanduzy A, Hansen A, Hansen TW, et al (1997) Effective reduction of infarct volume by gap junction blockade in a rodent model of stroke. J Neurosurg 87:916–920
30. Rogove AD, Tsirka SE (1998) Neurotoxic responses by microglia elicited by excitotoxic injury in the mouse hippocampus. Curr Biol 8:19–25
31. Rothwell NJ, Loddick SA, Stroemer P (1997) Interleukins and cerebral ischaemia. Int Rev Neurobiol 40:281–298
32. Sairanen T, Ristimaki A, Karjalainen-Lindsberg ML, et al (1998) Cyclooxygenase-2 is induced globally in infarcted human brain. Ann Neurol 43:738–747
33. Sande MA, Mandell GL (1985) in The Pharmacological Basis of Therapeutics (Goodman LS, Gilman A, eds) Macmillan, New York, pp. 1170–1192
34. Siesjö BK (1978) Brain Energy Metabolism (Wiley, New York)
35. Whiteman M, Halliwell B (1997) Prevention of peroxynitrite-dependent tyrosine nitration and inactivation of alpha1-antiproteinase by antibiotics. Free Rad Res 26:49–56
36. Yrjänheikki J, Keinänen R, Pellikka M, et al (1998) Tetracyclines inhibit microglial activation and are neuroprotective in global brain ischemia. Proc Natl Acad Sci USA 95:15769–15774.
37. Yrjänheikki J, Tikka T, Keinänen R, et al (1999) A tetracycline derivative, minocycline, reduces inflammation and protects against focal cerebral ischemia with a wide therapeutic window. Proc Natl Acad Sci USA 96:13496–13500
38. del Zoppo G, Ginis I, Hallenbeck JM, et al. (2000) Inflammation and stroke: putative role for cytokines, adhesion molecules and iNOS in brain response to ischemia. Brain Pathol 10:95–112

Non-neuronal cells in the injured brain: Cellular pathology and molecular activation signals

G. Raivich

Summary

Brain damage regularly results in cellular changes not only in the injured neurons but also in the adjacent glial cells. Frequently, it is also accompanied by changes in the vasculature und recruitment of blood-borne cells that belong to the immune system. Overall, this neuroglial activation is a common and routine hallmark in the injured brain and occurs in almost all forms of brain pathology. Recent work in mice that are genetically deficient for different cytokines (M-CSF, IL-6, IL1, TNFα, or TGF-β1) has begun to shed light on the molecular signals that regulate this cellular response. Here, the availability of cytokine-deficient animals with reduced or abolished neuroglial activation provides a direct approach to determine the function of the different components of the cellular response, leading to repair and regeneration following neural trauma.

Introduction

Acute injury to the nervous system results in the triggering of a large network of morphologic and metabolic changes which appear to play a role in enabling repair and regeneration (for reviews see Raivich et al. 1995; Kreutzberg and Raivich 2000; Barron 1983; Grafstein and McQuarrie 1978). The injured neurons assume a state of emergency, rapidly changing their gene expression and stimulating nearby microglia and astrocytes for support. These glial changes form a stereotypic cellular response, particularly well described for astrocytes and microglia. Almost all forms of pathology lead to the activation of microglia and astrocytes. Even slight or indirect injury will lead to rapid glial activation, as shown by the retrograde response to a peripheral injury in the axotomized facial motor nucleus. This activation of glial cells is a very graded response and their level depends on the extent of damage to neural parenchyma. The following text will summarize these changes and then focus on the molecules responsible for this cellular reaction.

Microglial activation

On the morphological level, injury-activated microglia increase in cell body size, decrease in ramification and form stout, proximal processes (for a review see Raivich et al. 1999). The extent of these changes and the accompanying molecular events form a highly graded response.

Keywords: microglia, astrocyte, immune system, trauma, regeneration

Department of Neuromorphology, Max-Planck Institute for Neurobiology, Am Klopferspitz 18A, D-82152 Martinsried, Germany.

J. Krieglstein, S. Klumpp (Eds.) Pharmacology of Cerebral Ischemia 2000

In the mildest form, microglia will simply increase in the expression of early adhesion molecules (aMb2, ICAM1, thrombospondin, IgG receptors) and reduce peripheral branching, an alert response or phase 1 (Werner et al. 1998; Kloss et al. 1999). In the second phase (2), these microglia will express mid-phase adhesion molecules (α5β1, α6β1 integrin), the major histocompatibility complex antigens and high levels of the MCSF receptor, and will home onto the damage cellular structures (Raivich et al. 1998a; Kloss et al. 1999; Raivich and Kreutzberg 2000). Axotomized neurons, degenerating neurite terminals or terminally affected oligodendrocytes are common targets. In the case of living neurons, the adhering microglia will move in-between the neuronal surface and the neurite terminals, a phenomenon called "synaptic stripping" (Blinzinger and Kreutzberg 1968). Microglial proliferation starts between phase 1 and phase 2, leading to an overall 4–6 fold increase in microglial cell number within 3–7 days of the initial injury (Kreutzberg 1966; Sjöstrand 1966; Raivich et al. 1994; Klein et al. 1997). The following changes depend on the consequences of injury. If no additional insults occur and the neurons recover, the microglia will return gradually, over the following weeks, to their resting state (Jones et al. 1997).

Neuronal cell death, however, will lead to further transformation of microglia into amoeboid, phagocytotic macrophages that remove neural debris or phase 3a (Streit et al. 1988; Angelov et al. 1995; Möller et al. 1996). They express very high levels of the major histocompatibility complex (MHC), costimulatory factors and proteases (Werner et al. 1998; Bohatschek et al. 1999). This points to a role as a competent, antigen presenting cells, a suggestion is supported by their frequent interaction with T-lymphocytes that enter injured brain (Raivich et al. 1998b; Werner et al. 1998). Interestingly, phagocytotic macrophages will also elicit an activation of the neighboring cells (bystander activation), including the adjacent, non-phagocytotic microglia (phase 3b), suggesting a production of stimulatory, and possibly cytotoxic factors (Raivich et al. 1999). Finally, microglia will also respond to infection and autoimmune disease with a very strong upregulation of MHC2, costimulatory factors, and iNOS (phase 4), exceeding the response apparent in all the previous stages (Schluter et al. 1998; Wong et al. 1984).

Astrocyte reaction

As in microglia, the astrocyte response to injury proceeds through several stages and depends on the extent of trauma. In the protoplasmic astrocytes predominant in the CNS gray matter, activation begins with a rapid induction of GFAP, CD44 and other reactive astrocyte markers on the mRNA and protein level (Graeber et al. 1986; Eddleston and Mucke 1993; Ridet et al. 1997; Raivich et al. 1999; Jones et al. 2000). This early molecular response is followed, in the second phase, by the reorganization of cytoskeleton-associated molecules, such as GFAP to the perinuclear cytoplasm and the main astrocyte branches. It also leads to the appearance of stellar, GFAP-positive astrocytes, a stellarization phenomenon that depends on the presence of IL6 after injury (Klein et al. 1997; Raivich et al. 1999) and is inhibited by endogenous TGFβ1 in the uninjured tissue (Jones et al. 1998a). This reorganization of de novo synthesized GFAP and vimentin appears to contribute to tissue rigidity and the stability of newly formed vessels (Pekny et al. 1999).

The creation of physical barriers between damaged and healthy tissue appears to be the main function of reactive astrocytes. Although the extent of scarring depends on the severity of brain damage and injury site (Alonso and Privat 1993), a rudimentary response around affected neurons is already observed in the mild, indirect trauma due to axomoty (Graeber et al. 1988). This response is rather slow. Beginning 2 weeks after injury, the reactive astrocytes enwrap injured neurons with thin and flat cytoplasmic processes. These processes form a multilayered stack of astrocyte lamellae surrounding the axotomized neuron, which could act a small glial scar. Successful regeneration leads to a partial retraction of these astrocyte processes and the repopulation of the neuronal surface with synaptic terminals (Guntinas-Lichius et al. 1997). Thus, synaptic stripping is basically a reversible process.

Direct physical trauma, ischemia and inflammation will lead to a much stronger response, with astrocyte proliferation and the formation of massive scars. There is also a recruitment of NG2+ astrocyte/oligodendrocyte precursors that will proliferate, and later differentiate into additional mature astrocytes (Stallcup and Beasley 1987; Levine 1994). Disruption of the blood brain barrier, collateral activation of resident microglia and the influx of blood borne leukocytes, and their synthesis of proinflammatory cytokines, all appear to play a role in the regulation of this process (Giulian and Lachman 1985; Lindholm et al. 1992; Balasingham et al. 1994). The glial scars are composed of a dense network of hypertrophied astrocytes, with thick, interdigitating processes and associated extracellular matrix. They inhibit neurite outgrowth, a phenomenon attributed both to the molecules on the cell surface of reactive astrocytes and their precursors, and components of the extracellular matrix including chrondroitin sulfate proteoglycans such as NG2, collagen IV and tenascin (Giftochristos and David 1988; McKeon et al. 1991; Laywell et al. 1992; Brodkey et al. 1995; Stichel et al. 1999; Moon et al. 2000). Both pro- and anti-inflammatory cytokines regulate glial scar formation, and the inhibitory properties of this structure are an interesting target for pharmacological intervention.

Vascular changes and leukocyte recruitment

Changes in blood vessels and the entry of leukocytes into the damaged brain are among the first hallmarks of the celluar response to neural injury. This leukocyte recruitment is again a graded phenomenon, described in detail in a previous review (Raivich et al. 1999). In the indirect trauma associated with retrograde response (grade 1), the recruitment is limited to lymphocytes. Extensive neuronal cell death (grade 2) will greatly enhance this entry of T-cells, but not the recruitment of other leukocyte subtypes. The entry of granulocytes and macrophages is limited to direct trauma (grade 3) and immune response in infection and autoimmune disease (grade 4). All 3 cell types are present in grades 3 and 4, but the lymphocytes are more abundant in pathology associated with active immune response. Leukocyte entry in the injured spinal cord confers with this general picture, although the absolute number of recruited macrophages and granulocytes is considerably higher than that in the more rostral parts of the CNS such as the cerebral cortex (Schnell et al. 1999). Thus, injured spinal cord could be particularly susceptible to a cytotoxic effect of these leukocytes. The reduction of spinal cord tissue loss and axonal degeneration in macrophage-depleted animals clearly supports such a cytotoxic effect (Popovich et al. 1999).

In addition to the graded response there are also differences in the distribution pattern and time course in specified pathology such as spinal cord or cerebral cortex injury, where all three cell-types are recruited. Lymphocytes are found even very far, up to 5 mm from the site of trauma, and appear to avoid the direct injury zone. Blood-borne macrophages appear restricted to the lesion site. The granulocytes tend to take an intermediate distribution pattern (Raivich et al. 1999; Schnell et al. 1999; Jones et al. in press). In addition, there are differences in the temporal pattern. The granulocytes peak within 24 hours after injury (Streit et al. 1998), the lymphocytes plateau between day 1 and day 4 (Raivich et al. 1998b; Schnell et al. 1999), a macrophages reach a maximum at day 4–7 (Schnell et al. 1999; Popovich et al. 1999). Although attractive, the differences in time course do not allow a simple conclusion with respect to cellular hierarchy such as granulocytes → lymphocytes → macrophages, and the resulting signaling cascade. Thus, depletion of macrophages with liposome encapsulated clodronate strongly inhibits granulocyte recruitment in a rabbit model of bacterial meningitis (Zysk et al. 1997). Intracisternal application of clodronate and the elimination of local microglia/macrophages has no effect, pointing to a crucial role of the circulating monocytes (Trostdorf et al. 1999).

Studies on the expression of adhesion molecules on the luminal side of brain vascular endothelium have begun to unveil the chemical signals involved in this rather complicated and graded pattern of leukocyte recruitment. Indirect trauma associated with neuronal cell death and strong, selective recruitment of lymphocytes (grade 2) leads to an upregulation of the endothelial α5β1 and α6β1 integrins (Kloss et al. 1999) but leave the levels of ICAM1 and VCAM1 unchanged (Werner et al. 1998). More severe pathology (grade 3, 4) will lead to endothelial increase in ICAM1, VCAM1, but also in P- and E-selectin (Bo et al. 1996; Jander et al. 1996; Lou et al. 1997; Suzuki et al. 1997; Zhang et al. 1998). In the in vitro models, these molecules are involved in different stages of leukocyte adhesion and extravasation. In vivo, genetic ablation of ICAM1, E-selectin or P-selectin greatly inhibits neutrophil extravasation, disturbance of blood brain barrier and loss of tissue in the stroke, meningitis and sepsis models (Connoly et al. 1996, 1997; Soriano et al. 1996; Bohatschek and Raivich, unpublished observations). Combined deletion of several adhesion molecules is particularly effective (Tang et al. 1996), pointing to a certain level of redundancy for each individual endothelial cell surface component. This redundancy can be an important problem in evaluating a specific deletion, and needs to be considered in designing experimental or pharmacological trials.

Cytokine pyramid

The activation of microglial cells, astrocytes and the recruitment of leukocytes appear closely related with the local synthesis of inflammation-associated cytokines, which is a highly graded response, forming a "cytokine pyramid". Moderate levels of MCSF and TGFβ1 are already present in the normal brain. Slight or indirect injury leads to increased synthesis of TGFβ1, and the induction of IL6 and the receptor for MCSF. Neural cell death is associated with high levels of two additional cytokines, IL1β and TNFα. High levels of IFNγ are restricted to conditions with florid immune response, in infection and in autoimmune disease. Recent studies using cytokine-deficient mice have begun to unveil the molecular cascades involved in microglial activation (for a review see Raivich et al. 1999). As one would expect, they differ with the grade of the response and the extent of pathology in the affected brain. The early cytokines, MCSF, IL6 and TGFβ1 play a key role in the early phases of microglial activation (stages 1, 2); TNF and TNF receptor type 1 are involved in the bystander activation (Bohatschek et al. 1999) and IFNγ for the immune-mediated response (Deckert-Schlueter et al. 1996). Interestingly, constitutive levels of TGFβ1, and to lesser extent, MCSF, are already needed to maintain normal microglial biology even in the normal, uninjured brain (Raivich et al. 1994; Jones et al. 1998a).

Macrophage colony stimulating factor (MCSF)

MCSF is a homodimeric, 45–90 kD glycoprotein that is a potent mitogen for monocyte precursors (Roth and Stanley 1992) and related cell types including brain-derived amoeboid macrophages (Giulian and Ingeman 1998; Hao et al. 1990; Sawada et al. 1990) and ramified microglia (Kloss et al. 1997). MCSF is constitutively expressed during brain development and in the adult central nervous system (Théry et al. 1990; Chang et al. 1994). Although there are mixed reports on the further MCSF increase in response to injury (Du Yan et al. 1997; Hulkower et al. 1993; Raivich et al. 1998a), all brain pathologies studied so far have shown a strong and selective induction of MCSF receptors on activated, postmitotic microglia (Raivich et al. 1991; Hulkower et al. 1993; Akiyama et al. 1994; Raivich and Kreutzberg 2000).

New insights into the function of MCSF and its receptor have come from *osteopetrotic* mice which carry a natural, frameshift mutation in the coding region for MCSF (Yoshida et al. 1990). In the homozygous animals (*op/op*) this mutation leads to a complete absence in the biological activity for this hematopoetic molecule (Wiktor-Jedrzejczak et al. 1990). In the facial axotomy, there is a 70–80% reduction in microglial proliferation in the MCSF-deficient, homozygous mice, compared with phenotypically normal, heterozygous littermates. This is accompanied by a strong inhibition of microglial activation markers (thrombospondin, αMβ2-integrin, MCSF receptor), suggesting a severe defect in the overall microglial activation (Raivich et al. 1996). Absence of MCSF does not affect posttraumatic changes in the adjacent motoneurons or astrocytes. This is in line with the selective expression of MCSF receptors on the activated microglia and not on neurons or astrocytes (Raivich et al. 1991; Raivich et al. 1998a). Interestingly however, the absence of MCSF does enhance neuronal cell death in a cerebral ischemia model (Berezovskaya et al. 1995). This effect could be abolished by transplantation of MCSF-secreting cells, pointing to the importance of MCSF-dependent microglial activation in promoting recovery in severely damaged neural tissue.

Tumor necrosis factor-α (TNFα)

TNFα is a proinflammatory cytokine which is strongly induced following trauma, ischemia, infection or excitotoxic injury (Bruce et al. 1996; Seilhean et al. 1997; Uno et al. 1997). Interestingly, it is absent though during the early stage of indirect injury to the brain, like for example, the axotomized facial nerve model (Kiefer et al. 1993; Raivich et al. 1998b). This suggests that the function of TNFα is restricted to the more severe forms of brain pathology. Thus, deletion of TNFR1 strongly inhibits the bystander activation in the response to neuronal cell death and microglial phagocytosis (Bohatschek et al. 1999). In vitro, TNFα is a pleiotrophic molecule with direct effects on neurons, oligodendrocytes, astrocytes and microglia. Two different TNF receptor types, p55 and p75, have been identified, which are both expressed on neurons and glial cells. Combined transgenic deletion of both TNF receptors led to severe changes in the cellular response to injury. The absence of the TNF-receptors exacerbated neuronal damage following focal cerebral ischemia and epileptic seizures and reduced microglial isolectin B4 immunoreactivity, but did not affect the adjacent astrocytes (Bruce et al. 1996). Since the TNFα-immunoreactivity was localized to the activated microglia, these data suggest an important neuroprotective function for this microglial cytokine. Moreover, the direct neuronal effects of TNFα also suggest that the neuroprotective action of MCSF following cerebral ischemia (see above) could be due to this microglial synthesis of TNFα.

Interleukin-6 (IL6)

IL6 is a 28 kD proinflammatory cytokine which belongs to a family of neurokines that also includes Leukemia inhibitory factor (LIF), Oncostatin-M, growth promoting activity (GPA), interleukin-11 (IL11) and cardiotrophin-1/CT1 (Patterson and Nawa 1993; Pennica et al. 1995). It is a multifunctional cytokine that plays an important role in promoting hematopoiesis, immune response, bacterial phagocytosis by the reticuloendothelial system and the associated acute phase reaction. It is also a potent neurotrophic factor and enhances astrocyte activation (Patterson and Nawa 1993; Balasingham et al. 1994; Fattori et al. 1995). These trophic effects are dosage-dependent. Strong overexpression of IL6 under the control of the GFAP promotor leads to a disruption of the blood brain barrier, reactive gliosis and protracted neuronal cell death in the particularly affected cerebellum (Campbell et al. 1993).

The induction of IL6 is an early and almost ubiquitous marker of tissue damage in brain pathology. It occurs following direct trauma, ischemia, infection, in neurodegeneration (Alzheimer, Parkinson), in autoimmune disease or following indirect injury (for reviews see Hopkins and Rothwell 1995; Raivich et al. 1996). The receptors for IL6 are localized on neurons and astrocytes, but not on microglia, and this expression pattern does not change after injury (Klein et al. 1997). The absence of IL6 following transgenic deletion leads to striking changes in the pattern of neuroglial activation. In the axotomized facial motor nucleus model, all three major cell types, neurons, astrocytes and microglia, are affected. Compared to normal, wildtype control mice, the IL6-deficient animals show a much smaller, and sometimes completely absent, posttraumatic induction of GFAP-positive astrocytes. Similar, but more moderate effects are also observed on microglial proliferation. The injured neurons however, respond with a strong, late increase of galanin, a neuropeptide expressed during motoneuron regeneration (Raivich et al. 1995).

The current data suggest a hierarchy in the cellular action of IL6, with reactive astrocytes being the primary target. Astrocytes express high levels of IL6 receptors and are particularly affected by IL6-deficiency. The effects on astrocytes also closely follow the onset of IL6 expression following injury. The absence of microglial receptors clearly suggests that the IL6 action on microglia is indirect. The late onset in the neuronal expression of Galanin could also point to an indirect effect, emphasizing the role of reactive astrocytes in the overall orchestration of the cellular response in the injured nervous system.

Transforming growth factor-beta 1 (TGFβ1)

Unlike MCSF, TNFα or IL6, TGFβ1 is an anti-inflammatory cytokine. It is a homodimeric protein that belongs to a family of pleiotrophic cytokines with potent neutrophic and immunosuppressive properties. TGFβ1 is already present at low levels in the normal central nervous system (Kiefer et al. 1993) and is strongly upregulated in almost all forms of brain pathology, which is quite similar to the regulation of the MCSF receptor and of IL6 (Morgan et al. 1993; Kiefer et al. 1995). Although TGFβ receptors are present on many different cultured cell types, their expression in the brain appears to be restricted to neurons (Unsicker et al. 1996). Transection of the facial nerve led to a selective upregulation of the TGFβ receptor II (TR2) on axotomized motoneurons but not on the adjacent astrocytes or microglia (Jones and Raivich 1998a). This selective neuronal expression could be one explanation for the striking differences in the glial response in cell culture and in vivo following transgenic deletion of TGFβ1: in vitro the effects of TGFβ1 are direct; in vivo they are probably mediated by the TGFβ1-responsive, TR2-positive neurons.

On cultured astrocytes, TGFβ1 leads to a strong increase in their synthesis of the cytoskeletal protein GFAP and extracellular matrix (laminin, fibronectin), but inhibits their proliferation, the γ-interferon-induced expression of MHC2 and the associated antigen presentation. TGFβ1 also inhibits the proliferation of brain-derived amoeboid macrophages (Suzumura et al. 1993) and of the ramified microglia (Jones et al. 1998b). TGFβ deprivation using neutralizing antibodies has a reverse effect and enhances microglial proliferation. In vivo however, the absence of TGFβ1 leads to a completely different response. The microglia of TGFβ1-deficient animals exhibit a severe decrease in their normal cell density, their ability to proliferate in the axotomized facial motor nucleus model, the diminished expression of activation markers αMβ2-integrin and ICAM-1, and a striking reduction of their normally ramified morphology (Jones and Raivich 1998a). These TGFβ1-deficient microglia also constitutively express CD44, a cell adhesion molecule which normally is only induced on microglia following direct trauma. This aberrant microglial response is accompanied by a strong increase of CD44- and GFAP-positive, activated astrocytes in the uninjured brain. The absence of TGFβ1 also leads to an overall increase in the astrocyte activation following facial axotomy.

These effects of TGFβ1 on the astrocytes are apparently dosage-dependent. The abnormal neuroglial response in the TGFβ1-deficient animals may reflect the moderate concentrations of the cytokine following axotomy (Kiefer et al. 1993), which are mediated indirectly by the highly TGFβ1-sensitive, TR2-positive neurons. On the other hand, high concentrations of TGFβ1 could have a direct effect on the TR2-negative, but TR1-expressing glial cells (Ata et al. 1997). Thus, high levels of exogenous TGFβ1 have been shown to enhance glial scarring and extracellular matrix deposition following direct cerebral trauma (Logan et al. 1994). Strong overexpression of TGFβ1 under the control of the GFAP promoter also induces severe reactive astrogliosis and abundant production of extracellular matrix in the transgenic animals (Wyss-Coray et al. 1995).

Conclusion

Recent studies on pro- and anti-inflammatory cytokines have begun to uncover the molecular mechanisms that underlie posttraumatic cellular activation responses in the injured brain. Although the data on the molecular mechanisms are not complete, they do point to a set of substances including MCSF, IL6, TNFα and TGFβ1, which are strongly induced after tissue damage and exert different, cell-specific actions in the overall glial response. Relatively little is known however about the molecules that regulate neuronal activation. Their elucidation will greatly enhance our insight into the cellular and molecular activation cascade in the injured neural tissue.

References

1. Akiyama H, Nishimura T, Kondo H, Ikeda K, Hayashi Y, McGeer PL (1994) Expression of the receptor for macrophage colony stimulating factor by brain microglia and its upregulation in brains of patients with Alzheimer's disease and amyotrophic lateral sclerosis. Brain Res 639:171–174
2. Angelov DN, Gunkel A, Stennert E, Neiss WF (1995) Phagocytic microglia during delayed neuronal loss in the facial nucleus of the rat – time course of the neuronofugal migration of brain macrophages. GLIA 13:113–129
3. Ata AK, Funa K, Olsson Y (1997) Expression of various TGF-beta isoforms and type I receptor in necrotizing human brain lesions. Acta Neuropathol 93:326–333
4. Alonso G, Privat A (1993) Reactive astrocytes involved in the formation of lesional scars differ in the mediobasal hypothalamus and in other forebrain regions. J Neurosci Res 34:523–538
5. Balasingham V, Tejada-Berges T, Wright E, Bouckova R, Yong VW (1994) Reactive astrogliosis in the neonatal mouse brain and its modulation by cytokines. J Neurosci 14:846–856
6. Barron KD (1983) Comparative observations on the cytologic reactions of central and peripheral nerve cells to axotomy. in: Kao CC, Bunge RP, Reier PJ, eds, Spinal Cord Reconstruction. New York, Raven Press, pp 7–40
7. Berezovskaya O, Maysinger D, Fedoroff S (1995) The hematopoietic cytokine, colony-stimulating factor 1, is also a growth factor in the CNS: congenital absence of CSF-1 in mice results in abnormal microglial response and increased neuron vulnerability to injury. Int J Dev Neurosci 13:285–299
8. Blinzinger K, Kreutzberg GW (1968) Displacement of synaptic terminals from regenerating motoneurons by microglial cells. Z Zellforsch 85:145–157
9. Bo L, Peterson JW, Mork S, Hoffman PA, Gallatin WM, Ransohoff RM, Trapp BD (1996) Distribution of immunoglobulin superfamily members ICAM-1, -2, -3 and the beta 2 integrin LFA-1 in multiple sclerosis lesions. J Neuropathol Exp Neurol 55: 1060–1072
10. Bohatschek M, Gschwendtner A, von Malzan X, Kloss CUA, Pfeffer K, Labow M, Bluthmann H, Kreutzberg GW, Raivich G (1999) Cytokine-mediated regulation of MHC1, MHC2 and B7.2 in the axotomized facial motor nucleus. Soc Neurosci Abstr 29:610.7
11. Brodkey JA, Laywell ED, O'Brien TF, Faissner A, Stefansson K, Doerries HU, Schachner M, Steindler DA (1995) Focal brain injury and upregulation of a developmentally regulated extracellular matrix protein. J Neurosurg 82:106–112
12. Bruche AJ, Boling W, Kindy MS, Peschon J, Kraemer PJ, Carpenter MK, Holtsberg FW, Mattson MP (1996) Altered neuronal and microglial responses to excitotoxic and ischemic brain injury in mice lacking TNF receptors. Nature Med 2:788–794
13. Campbell L, Abraham CR, Masliah E, Kemper P, Inglis JD, Oldstone MB, Mucke L (1993) Neurologic disease induced in transgenic mice by cerebral overexpression of interleukin 6. Proc Natl Acad Sci USA, 90:10061–10065
14. Chang Y, Albright S, Lee F (1994) Cytokines in the central nervous system: expression of macrophage colony stimulating factor and its receptor during development. J Neuroimmunol 52:9–17
15. Connolly ES Jr, Winfree CJ, Springer TA, Naka Y, Liao H, Yan SD, Stern DM, Solomon RA, Gutierrez-Ramos JC, Pinsky DJ (1996) Cerebral protection in homozygous null ICAM-1 mice after middle cerebral artery occlusion. Role of neutrophil adhesion in the pathogenesis of stroke. J Clin Invest 97:209–216
16. Connolly ES Jr, Winfree CJ, Prestigiacomo CJ, Kim SC, Choudhri TF, Hoh BL, Naka Y, Solomon RA, Pinsky DJ (1997) Exacerbation of cerebral injury in mice that express the P-selectin gene: identification of P-selectin blockade as a new target for the treatment of stroke. Circulation Res 81:304–310
17. Deckert-Schlueter M, Rang A, Weiner D, Huang S, Wiestler OD, Hof H, Schlueter D (1996) Interferon-gamma receptor-deficiency renders mice highly susceptible to toxoplasmosis by decreased macrophage activation. Lab Invest 75:827–841
18. Du Yan S, Zhu H, Fu J, Yan SF, Roher A, Tourtellotte WW, Rajavashisth T, Chen X, Godman GC, Stern D, Schmidt AM (1997) Amyloid-beta peptide-receptor for advanced glycation endproduct interaction elicits neuronal expression of macrophage-colony stimulating factor: a proinflammatory pathway in Alzheimer disease. Proc Natl Acad Sci USA 94:5296–5301
19. Eddleston M, Mucke L (1993) Molecular profile of reactive astrocytes. Neurosci 54:15–36
20. Fattori E, Lazzaro D, Musiani P, Modesti A, Alonzi T, Cilberto G (1995) IL-6 expression in neurons of transgenic mice causes reactive astrocytosis and increase in ramified microglial cells but no neuronal damage. Eur J Neurosci 7:2441–2449
21. Giftochristos N, David S (1988) Laminin and heparan sulfate proteoglycan in the lesioned adult mammalian central nervous system and their possible relationship to axonal sprouting. J Neurocytol 17:385–398
22. Giulian D, Lachman LB (1985) Interleukin-1 stimulation of astrocyte proliferation after brain injury. Science 228:497–499
23. Giulian D, Ingeman JE (1988) Colony stimulating factors as promoters of ameboid microglia. J Neurosci 8:4707–4717
24. Graeber MB, Kreutzberg GW (1988) Delayed astrocyte reaction following facial nerve axotomy. J Neurocytol 17:209–220

25. Graeber MB, Kreutzberg GW (1986) Astrocytes increase in glial fibrillary acidic protein during retrograde changes of facial motor neurons. J Neurocytol 15:363–374
26. Graeber MB, Streit WJ, Kreutzberg GW (1988) The microglial cytoskeleton vimentin is localized with activated cells in situ. J Neurocytol 17:573–580
27. Grafstein B, McQuarrie IG (1978) Role of the nerve cell body in axonal regeneration. In: Cotman CW, ed, Neuronal Plasticity. New York, Raven Press, pp 155–195
28. Guntinas-Lichius O, Martinez-Portillo F, Lebek J, Angelov DN, Stennert E, Neiss WF (1997) Nimodipine maintains in vivo the increase in GFAP and enhances the astroglial ensheathment of surviving motoneurons in the rat following permanent target deprivation. J Neurocytol 26:241–248
29. Hao C, Guilbert LJ, Fedoroff S (1990) Production of colony-stimulating factor-1 (CSF-1) by mouse astroglia *in vitro*. J Neurosci Res 27:314–323
30. Hol EM, Schwaiger FW, Werner A, Schmitt A, Raivich G, Kreutzberg GW (1999) Regulation of the LIM-type homeobox gene islet-1 during neuronal regeneration. Neurosci 88:917–925
31. Hopkins SJ, Rothwell NJ (1995) Cytokines and the nervous system: expression and recognition. Trends Neurosci 18:83–88
32. Hulkower K, Brosnan CF, Aquino DA, Cammer W, Kulshrestha S, Guida MP, Rapoport DA, Berman JW (1993) Expression of CSF-1, c-fms, and MCP-1 in the central nervous system of rats with experimental allergic encephalomyelitis. J Immunol 150:2525–2533
33. Jander S, Pohl J, Gillen C, Schroeter M, Stoll G (1996) Vascular cell adhesion molecule-1 mRNA is expressed in immune-mediated and ischemic injury of the rat nervous system. J Neuroimmunol 70:75–80
34. Jones LL, Banati R, Graeber MB, Bonfanti L, Raivich G, Kreutzberg GW (1997) Population control of microglia: does apoptosis play a role? J Neurocytol 26:755–770
35. Jones LL, Shen J, Kreutzberg GW, Raivich G (1998a) Neuroglial activation in the injured central nervous system: role of transforming growth factor β1. Soc Neurosci Abstr 28:710.2
36. Jones LL, Kreutzberg GW, Raivich G (1998b) Transforming growth factor β's 1, 2 and 3 inhibit proliferation of ramified microglia on an astrocyte monolayer. Brain Res 795:301–306
37. Jones LL, Liu ZQ, Shen J, Werner A, Kreutzberg GW, Raivich G (2000) Regulation of the cell adhesion molecule CD44 after nerve transection and direct trauma to the mouse brain. J Comp Neurol, in press
38. Kiefer R, Lindholm D, Kreutzberg GW (1993) Interleukin-6 and transforming growth factor-beta-1 mRNAs are induced in rat facial nucleus following mononeuron axotomy. Eur J Neurosci 5:775–781
39. Kiefer R, Streit WJ, Toyka KV, Kreutzberg GW, Hartung H (1995) Transforming growth factor-beta-1: A lesion-associated cytokine of the nervous system. Int J Dev Neurosci 13:331–339
40. Klein MA, Möller JC, Jones LL, Bluethmann H, Kreutzberg GW, Raivich G (1997) Impaired neuroglial activation in Interleukin-6 deficient mice. GLIA 19:227–233
41. Kloss CUA, Kreutzberg GW, Raivich G (1997) Proliferation of ramified microglia on an astrocyte Monolayer: characterization of stimulatory and inhibitory cytokines. J Neurosci Res 49:248–254
42. Kloss CUA, Werner A, Shen J, Klein MA, Kreutzberg GW, Raivich G (1999) The integrin family of cell adhesion molecules in the injured brain: regulation and cellular localization in the normal and regenerating mouse facial nucleus. J Comp Neurol 441:162–178
43. Kreutzberg GW (1966) Autoradiographische Untersuchungen über die Beteiligung von Gliazellen an der axonalen Reaktion im Fazialiskern der Ratte. Acta Neuropathol 7:149–161
44. Kreutzberg GW, Raivich G (2000) Neurbiology of regeneration and degeneration. In: The Facial Nerve (May M, Ed). Thieme, New York, 2nd edition, pp 67–79
45. Laywell ED, Dorries U, Bartsch U, Faissner A, Schachner M, Steindler DA (1992) Enhanced expression of the developmentally regulated extracellular matrix molecule tenascin following adult brain injury. Proc Natl Acad Sci USA 89:2634–2638
46. Lindholm D, Castren E, Kiefer R, Zafra F, Thoenen H (1992) Transforming growth factor-β1 in the rat brain: Increase after injury and inhibition of astrocyte proliferation. C Cell Biol 117:395–400
47. Levine JM (1994) Increased expression of the NG2 chondroitin-sulfate proteoglycan after brain injury. J Neurosci 14:4716–4730
48. Logan A, Berry M, Gonzalez AM, Frautschy SA, Sporn MB, Baird A (1994) Effects of transforming growth factor beta 1 on scar production in the injured central nervous system of the rat. Eur J Neurosci 6:355–363
49. Lou J, Chofflon M, Juillard C, Donati Y, Mili N, Siegrist CA, Grau GE (1997) Brain microvascular endothelial cells and leukocytes derived from patients with multiple sclerosis exhibit increased adhesion capacity. NeuroReport 8:629–633
50. McKeon RJ, Schreiber RC, Rudge JS, Silver J (1991) Reduction of neurite outgrowth in a model of glial scarring following CNS injury in correlated with the expression of inhibitory molecules on reactive astrocytes. J Neurosci 11:3398–3411
51. Möller JC, Klein MA, Haas S, Jones LL, Kreutzberg GW, Raivich G (1996) Regulation of thrombospondin in the regenerating mouse facial nucleus. Glia 17:121–132
52. Moon LD, Brecknell JE, Franklin RJ, Dunnett SB, Fawcett JW (2000) Robust regeneration of CNS axons through a track depleted of CNS glia. Exp Neurol 161:49–66
53. Morgan TE, Nichols NR, Pasinetti GM, Finch CE (1993) TGF beta-1 mRNA increases in macrophage-microglial cells of the hippocampus in response to deafferentation and kainic acid-induced neurodegeneration. Exp Neurol 120:291–301
54. Patterson PH, Nawa H (1993) Neuronal differentiation factors, cytokines and synaptic plasticity. Neuron 10:123–137
55. Pekny M, Johansson CB, Eliasson C, Stakeberg J, Wallen A, Perlmann T, Lendahl U, Betsholtz C, Berthold CH, Frisen J (1999) Abnormal reaction to central nervous system injury in mice lacking glial fibrillary acidic protein and vimentin. J Cell Biol 145:503–514
56. Pennica D, King KL, Shaw KJ, Luis E, Rullamas J, Luoh S, Darbonmne WC, Knutzon DS, Yen R, Chien KR, Baker JB, Wood WI: Expression cloning of cardiotrophin 1, a cytokine that induces cardiac myocyte hypertrophy. Proc Natl Acad Sci USA 92:1142–1146
57. Popovich PG, Guan Z, Wei P, Huitinga I, van Rooijen N, Stokes BT (1999) Depletion of hematogenous macrophages promotes partial hindlimb recovery and neuroanatomical repair after experimental spinal cord injury. Exp Neurol 158:351–365
58. Raivich G, Gehrmann J, Kreutzberg GW (1991): Increase of macrophage colony-stimulating factor and granulocyte-macrophage colony stimulating factor receptors in the regenerating rat facial nucleus. J Neurosci Res 30:682–686
59. Raivich G, Moreno-Flores MT, Möller JC, Kreutzberg GW (1994) Inhibition of posttraumatic microglial proliferation in a genetic model of macrophage colony-stimulating factor deficiency in the mouse. Eur J Neurosci 6:1615–1618
60. Raivich G, Reddington M, Haas CA, Kreutzberg GW (1995) Peptides in motoneurons. Prog Brain Res 104:3–20
61. Raivich G, Bluethmann H, Kreutzberg GW (1996) Signaling molecules and neuroglial activation in the injured central nervous system. Keio J Med 45:239–247
62. Raivich G, Haas S, Werner S, Klein MA, Kloss CUA, Kreutzberg GW (1998a) Regulation of MCSF receptors on microglia

in the normal and injured central nervous system: A quantitative immunofluorescence study using confocal laser microscopy. J Comp Neurol 395:342–358
63. Raivich G, Jones LL, Kloss CUA, Werner A, Neumann H, Kreutzberg GW (1998b) Immune surveillance in the injured nervous system: T-lymphocytes invade the axotomized mouse facial motor nucleus and aggregate around sites of neuronal degeneration. J Neurosci 18:5804–5816
64. Raivich G, Bohatschek M, Kloss CUA, Werner A, Jones LL, Kreutzberg GW (1999) Neuroglial activation in the injured brain: graded response, molecular mechanisms and cues to physiological function. Brain Res Rev 30:77–105
65. Raivich G, Kreutzberg GW (2000) Inflammatory response following nerve injury. In: Neural Regeneration (Ingoglia N, Murray M, Eds). Marcel Decker, New York, pp 287–314
66. Ridet JL, Malhotra SK, Privat A, Gage FH (1997) Reactive astrocytes: cellular and molecular cues to biological function. Trends Neurosci 20:570–577
67. Rieske E, Graeber MB, Tetzlaff W, Czlonkowska A, Streit WJ, Kreutzberg GW (1989) Microglia and microglia-derived brain macrophages in culture: Generation from axotomized rat facial nuclei, identification and characterization in vitro. Brain Res 492:1–14
68. Roth P, Stanley E (1992) The biology of CSF-1 and its receptor. Curr. Topics Microbiol Immunol 181:141–167
69. Sawada M, Suzumura A, Yamamoto H, Marunouchi T (1990) Activation and proliferation of the isolated microglia by colony stimulating factor-1 and possible involvement of protein kinase C. Brain Res 509:119–124
70. Schluter D, Bertsch D, Frei K, Hubers SB, Wiestler OD, Hof H, Fontana A, Deckert-Schluter M (1998) Interferon-gamma antagonizes transforming growth factor-beta2-mediated immunosuppression in murine Toxoplasma encephalitis. J Neuroimmunol 81:38–48
71. Schnell L, Schneider R, Berman MA, Perry VH, Schwab ME (1997) Lymphocyte recruitment following spinal cord injury in mice is altered by prior viral exposure. Eur J Neurosci 9:1000–1007
72. Schnell L, Fearn S, Klassen H, Schwab ME, Perry VH (1999) Acute inflammatory responses to mechanical lesions in the CNS: differences between brain and spinal cord. European Journal of Neuroscience 11:3648–3658
73. Seilhean D, Kobayashi K, He Y, Uchihara T, Rosenblum O, Katlama C, Bricaire F, Duyckaerts C, Hauw JJ (1997) Tumor necrosis factor-alpha, microglia and astrocytes in AIDS dementia complex. Acta Neuropath 93:508–517
74. Sjöstrand J (1966) Studies on glial cells in the hypoglossal nucleus of the rabbit during nerve regeneration. Acta Physiologica Scandinavica 67 (Suppl 270), 1–17
75. Soriano SG, Lipton SA, Wang YF, Xiao M, Springer TA, Gutierrez-Ramos JC, Hickey PR (1996) Intercellular adhesion molecule-1-deficient mice are less susceptible to cerebral ischemia-reperfusion injury. Ann Neurol 39:618–624
76. Stallcup WB, Beasley L (1987) Bipotential glial precursor cells of the optic nerve express the NG2 proteoglycan. J Neurosci 7:2737–2744
77. Stichel CC, Hermanns S, Luhmann HJ, Lausberg F, Niermann H, D'Urso D, Servos G, Hartwig HG, Muller HW (1999) Inhibition of collagen IV deposition promotes regeneration of injured CNS axons. Eur J Neurosci 11:632–646
78. Streit WJ, Graeber MB, Kreutzberg GW (1988) Functional plasticity of microglia: a review. Glia 1:301–307
79. Streit WJ, Semple-Rowland SL, Hurley SD, Miller RC, Popovich PG, Stokes BT (1998) Cytokine mRNA profiles in contused spinal cord and axotomized facial nucleus suggest a beneficial role for inflammation and gliosis. Exp Neurol 152:74–87
80. Suzuki H, Abe K, Tojo S, Morooka S, Kimura K, Mizugaki M, Itoyama Y (1997) Expressions of P-selectin- and HSP72-like immunoreactivities in rat brain after transient middle cerebral artery occlusion. Brain Res 759:321–329
81. Suzumura A, Sawada M, Yamamoto H, Marunouchi T (1993) Transforming growth factor-beta suppresses activation and proliferation of microglia in vitro. J Immunol 151:2150–2158
82. Tang T, Frenette PS, Hynes RO, Wagner DD, Mayadas TN (1996) Cytokine-induced meningitis is dramatically attenuated in mice deficient in endothelial selectins. J Clin Invest 97:2485–2490
83. Théry C, Hétier E, Evrard C, Mallat M (1990) Expression of macrophage colony-stimulating factor gene in the mouse brain during development. J Neurosci Res 26:129–133
84. Trostdorf F, Bruck W, Schmitz-Salue M, Stuertz K, Hopkins SJ, van Rooijen N, Huitinga I, Nau R (1999) Reduction of meningeal macrophages does not decrease migration of granulocytes into the CSF and brain parenchyma in experimental pneumococcal meningitis. J Neuroimmunol 99:205–210
85. Uno H, Matsuyama T, Akita H, Nishimura H, Sugita M (1997) Induction of tumor necrosis factor-alpha in the mouse hippocampus following transient forebrain ischemia. J Cereb Blood Flow Metabol 17:491–499
86. Unsicker K, Meier C, Krieglstein K, Sartor MB, Flanders KC (1996) Expression, localization and function of transforming growth factor-beta s in embryonic chick spinal cord, hindbrain and dorsal root ganglia. J Neurobiol 29:262–276
87. Werner A, Kloss CUA, Walter J, Kreutzberg GW, Raivich G (1998) Intercellular adhesion molecule-1 (ICAM1) in the regenerating mouse facial motor nucleus. J Neurocytol 27:219–232
88. Wiktor-Jedrzejczak W, Bartocci A, Ferrante W, Ahmed-Ansari A, Sell KW, Pollard JW, Stanlay ER (1990) Total absence of colony-stimulating factor 1 in the macrophage-deficient osteopetrotic (op/op) mouse. Proc Natl Acad Sci USA 87:4828–4832
89. Wong GH, Bartlett PF, Clark-Lewis I, Battye F, Schrader JW (1984) Inducible expression of H-2 and la antigens on brain cells. Nature 310:688–691
90. Wyss-Coray T, Feng L, Masliah E, Ruppe MD, Lee HS, Toggas SM, Rockenstein EM, Mucke L (1995) Increased central nervous system production of extracellular matrix components and development of hydrocephalus in transgenic mice overexpressing transforming growth factor-beta 1. Am J Pathology 147:53–67
91. Yoshida H, Hayashi SI, Kunisasa Z, Ogaea M, Nishikawa S, Okamura H, Sudo T, Shultz LD, Nishikawa SI (1990) The murine mutation osteopetrosis is in the coding region of the macrophages colony stimulating factor gene. Nature 345:442–444
92. Zhang R, Chopp M, Zhang Z, Jiang N, Powers C (1998) The expression of P- and E-selectins in three models of middle cerebral artery occlusion. Brain Res 785:207–214
93. Zysk G, Bruck W, Huitinga I, Fischer FR, Flachsbarth F, van Rooijen N, Nau R (1997) Elimination of blood-derived macrophages inhibits the release of interleukin-1 and the entry of leukocytes into the cerebrospinal fluid in experimental pneumococcal meningits. J Neuroimmunol 73:77–80

Ultrastructural behavior of astrocytes to singly dying cortical neurons

U. Ito[1,3,5], T. Kuroiwa[2], S. Hanyu[3], Y. Hakamata[3], S. Ito[4], I. Nakano[3], K. Oyanagai[5]

Abstract

We investigated the temporal profile of astrocytic behaviors and isolated neuronal death in the cerebral cortex after an under threshold ischemic insult to induce infarction. In this cortex, dying neuron with disseminated selective neuronal necrosis (DSNN) without infarction increased in number, slowly until 4 days after the ischemic insult. The cell body, processes and end-feet of neighboring astrocytes were swollen, with an increase in both number and volume of mitochondria and accumulated glycogen granules. The DSNN of a neuron almost always started and progressed with homogeneous condensation of isolated neuronal cytosol and organelles with small loosely aggregated chromatin condensations in the nuclear matrix and margin. These neurons were surrounded by swollen astrocytic cell processes in which astrocytic mitochondria and glycogen granules were increased in number. Finally, the isolated neuron became completely shrunken, resulting in intensely high electron density of the entire cell, and surrounded by remarkably swollen astrocytic cell processes. The shrunken neuron was fragmented by astrocytic cell processes and phagocytized by them. Activity of macrophages and other inflammatory cells did not become conspicuous until 4 days after the ischemic insult. These processes of neuronal death are discussed with respect to ischemic cell necrosis versus apoptosis.

Introduction

Following a large ischemic insult, cerebral infarction develops rapidly. We slowed down the process of the maturation phenomenon (Ito et al. 1975) of ischemic injuries in the cerebral cortex by giving a threshold amount of ischemic insults to induce cerebral infarction (Hanyu et al. 1995; Ito et al. 1997b). Thus, the temporal profile of the histopathology revealed that only disseminated selective neuronal necrosis (DSNN) develops in the cerebral cortex after an ischemic insult given just under the threshold to induce infarction. Following ischemic insult at the threshold, DSNN develops first and focal infarction appears later and enlarges in size in

Keywords: disseminated selective neuronal necrosis, astrocyte, ischemic neuronal change, dark neuron

[1]Department of Neurosurgery, Musashino Red Cross Hospital, 4-22-24, Zenpukuji, Suginami-ku, Tokyo 167-0041, Japan, [2]Department of Neuropathology, Medical Research Institute, Tokyo Medical and Dental University, Tokyo, [3]Department of Neurology, Jichi Medical School, Tochigi, [4]Department of Neurosurgery, School of Medicine, University of Chiba, Chiba, [5]Tokyo Metropolitan Institute of Neuroscience, Tokyo

J. Krieglstein, S. Klumpp (Eds.) Pharmacology of Cerebral Ischemia 2000

the cerebral cortex in which DSNN is still progressing (Ito et al. 1975; Marcoux et al. 1982; Ito et al. 1999a). Using this model, we have studied urtrastructural temporal profile of progressing DSNN, with special attention to the behavior of astrocytes surrounding the isolated dying neuron.

Materials and methods

Under 2% halothane and 70% nitrous oxide and 30% oxygen anesthesia, the left carotid artery of adult Mongolian gerbils was twice occluded for 10 minutes, with a 5 h interval between the two occlusions (Hanyu et al. 1997). After each cervical surgery, the animals soon recovered from the anesthesia and moved spontaneously. Ischemia-positive animals were selected based on the stroke index score determined after the first occlusion (Ohno et al. 1984).

The gerbils were sacrificed at 15 min, at 5, 12, 24 h, and at 4 days following the second ischemic insult by intracardiac perfusion with glutaraldehyde fixative for electron microscopy and phosphate-buffered formaldehyde fixative for light microscopy.

Ultrathin sections including the 3rd~5th cortical layers were prepared from the left ischemic cerebral hemisphere at the mid-point between the interhemispheric and rhinal fissures at the coronal level of chiasma (face A) and infundibulum (face B). Alternative sections were double stained by uranyl acetate and lead solution, and observed under an electron microscope.

Paraffin sections were stained with hematolxylin-eosin (HE) and peroxide fuchsin Shiff (PAS), and for glial fibril acidic protein (GFAP).

Results

We investigated the temporal profile of astrocytic behavior in the post ischemic cerebral cortex after a just under threshold ischemic insult to induce infarction (Ito et al. 1996, 1997a). In this cortex, disseminated selective neuronal necrosis (DSNN) without infarction progressed slowly until 4 days after the ischemic insult, with an increase in number of electron-dense dark neurons. These necrotic neurons were compatible with the ischemic neuronal changes visualized by light microscopy, which produced a homogeneous eosinophilic cell body containing a pycnotic and/or karyorrhectic nucleus (Ito et al. 1999a).

Swelling of astrocytic cell processes, perivascular end-feet, and cell body had started already 15 min after the ischemic insult, without accumulation of glycogen granules (Ito et al. 1999b). At this stage, isolated dark neurons with a diffuse increase in electron density appeared disseminated among the almost normal looking neurons, some of which showed slight disorganization of their rough endoplasmic reticulum and slight swelling of the Golgi apparatus. These dark neurons with increased electron density were surrounded by swollen astrocytic cell processes without glycogen granules. Small dots of chromatin condensation were scattered in the nuclear matrix as well as along the nuclear margin of these neurons. However, no swelling was observed in their mitochondria or other cytosolic organelles. These dark neurons were never found in the control animals after the same processes of fixation and preparation as those applied for the postischemic animals.

From 5 to 24 hours, isolated dark neurons with different grades of high electron density (Fig. 1) increased in number among the almost normal looking neurons, some of which still showed slight disorganization of their rough endoplasmic reticulum and slight swelling of the Golgi apparatus. In the astrocytic cell processes, enlarged mitochondria with slightly swollen cristae and boosted electron density of the matrices were increased in number; and there was an increased accumulation of glycogen granules (Ito et al. 1999b, 2000). These dark neurons were surrounded by remarkably swollen astrocytic cell processes in which glycogen granules and mitochondria were increased in number. These swollen astrocytic processes were especially prominent nearby the dendritic synapses. Later than 12 h after the ischemic insult, some mitochondria of these dark neurons showed partial swelling of the matrices,

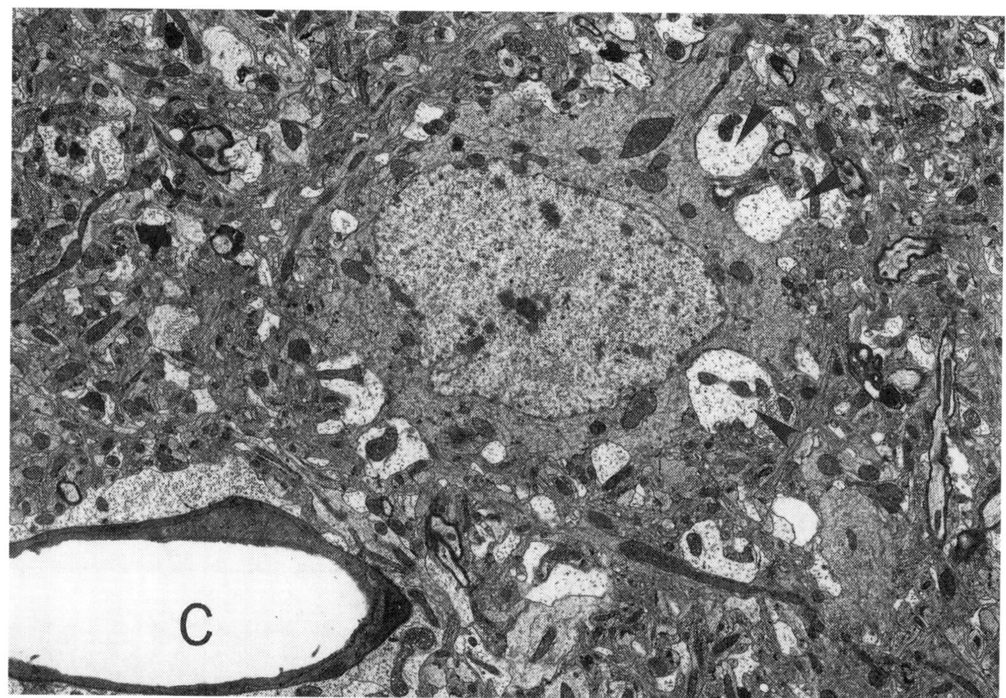

Fig. 1. Electron dense dark neuron, 5 h after the ischemic insult. Diffuse concentration of the cytosol without swelling of organelles, and of the nucleus with dotted chromatin condensations scattered in the nucleus and along the margin. Astrocytic cell processes are swollen accumulating glycogen granules, especially around the dark neuron adjacent to the dendritic synapses, (arrows) and inside the endfeet around the capillary (C). x 2,500

along with disintegration of cristae with wooly densities (Fig. 2).

Among these dark neurons, completely shrunken neurons with intensely high electron density of the entire cell increased in number from 5 to 24 hours after the ischemic insult. These shrunken neurons often contained mitochondria with swollen matrices having woolly densities and were surrounded by remarkably swollen astrocytic cell processes (Fig. 3).

At 4 days after the ischemic insult, these shrunken neurons became fragmented by astrocytic cell processes and phagocytized by them. Up to this stage no inflammatory wandering cells appeared in this lesion. Phagocytic activity of the perivascular microglia was also observed.

Discussion

In this model, post ischemic injuries mature slowly in the cerebral cortex. Only DSNN progressed slowly in the face B coronally cut at the infundibulum. In face A, coronally cut at the chiasma, first DSNN progressed followed by focal infarction 12 hours after the ischemic insult. In the focal infarcts, all neurons and astrocytes showed massive necrosis with marked swelling and destruction of the entire membranous system of these cells (Ito et al. 1996, 1999a). In order to study ultrastructural temporal profile of DSNN, in the present study we investigated face B (Ito et al. 1997a).

The DSNN appeared from the early post ischemic stage, and under the electronmicroscopic observation, it manifested as an isolated dark neuron with a diffuse increase in electron

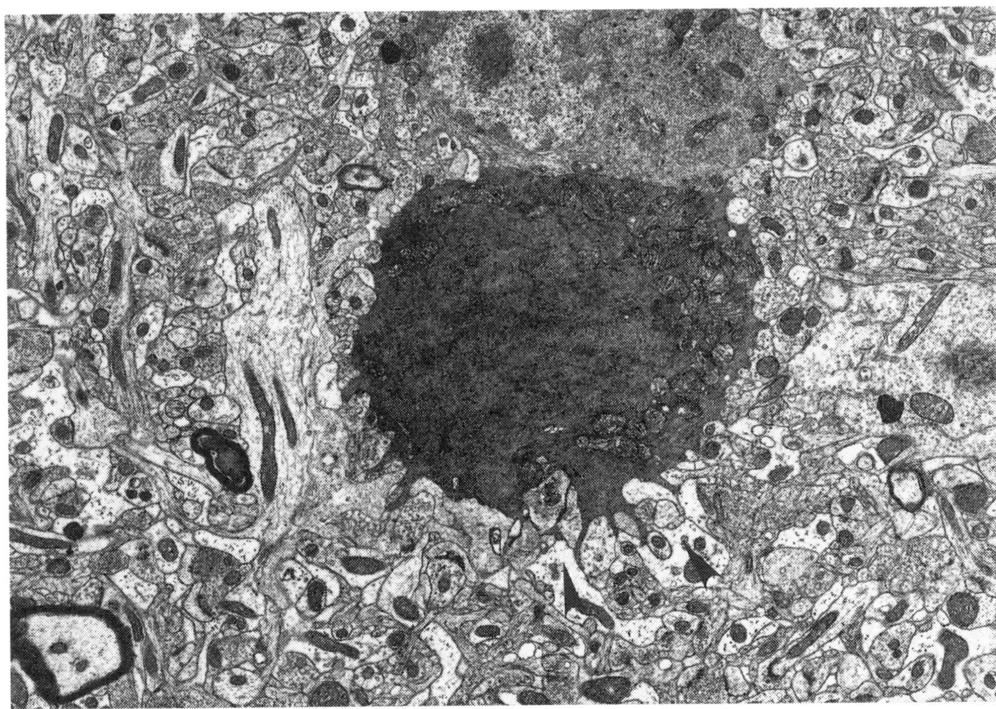

Fig. 2. Electron dense dark neuron, 12 h after the ischemic insult. Diffuse condensation of the entire cell is more advanced than that observed in Figure 1. It contains mitochondria showing slight swelling of the matrices along with disintegration of cristae with wooly densities in some of them. The dark neuron is surrounded by remarkably swollen astrocytic cell processes (arrows) in which glycogen granules and mitochondria were increased in number. x 4,000

density of its cytosol and nucleus. No swelling of mitochondria and other cytosolic organelles was observed except in the completely shrunken neurons with intensely high electron density of the entire cell, which increased in number from 5 to 24 hours after the ischemic insult. As the dark neuron showed small loosely aggregated chromatin condensations scattered in the nuclear matrix as well as along the nuclear margin, cellular activity seemed to be decreased (Ghdially 1997). These isolated dark neurons increased in number from 15 min to 24 h, and were still observed until 4 days after the ischemic insult.

These dark neurons were surrounded by swollen astrocytic cell processes in which the mitochondria had increased in number and size: however, no accumulation of glycogen granules was observed at 15 min after the ischemic insult (Ito et al. 1999b). These astrocytic cell processes were remarkably swollen, especially nearby the dendritic synapses (von-Lubitz et al. 1983), and showed increases in number and size of mitochondria and accumulating glycogen granules from 5 to 24 h after the ischemic insult. These astrocytic mitochondria showed moderately swollen cristae and increased electron densities in matrices (Ito et al. 1999b, 2000). These findings strongly suggest activated astrocytic energy metabolism, generating lactate as a neuronal fuel (Hamprecht and Dringen 1995; Coles 1995), and scavenging potassium (Newman 1995), neurotransmitters (Martin 1995; Levi and Gallo 1995) and other metabolites from the neuron and dendritic synapses, and promoting survival of the astrocytes themselves (Kraig et al. 1995). As this fuel does not transfer smoothly to neurons due to de-

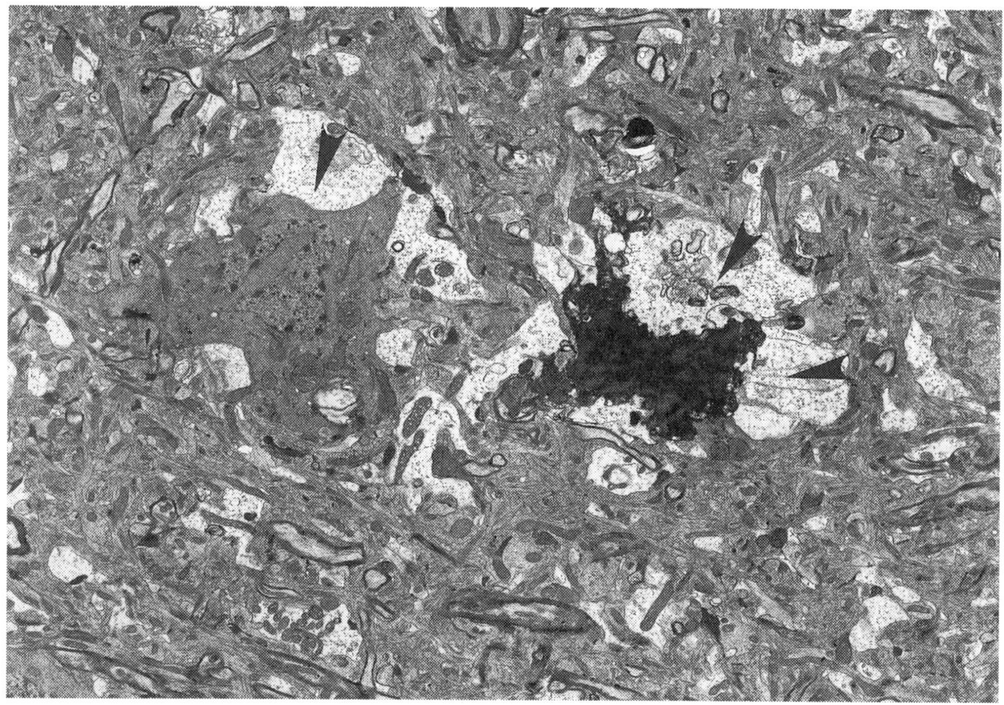

Fig. 3. Completely shrunken neurons with intensely high electron density of the entire cell, among the dark neurons, 12 hours after the ischemic insult. The shrunken neuron contains mitochondria with swollen matrices having woolly densities, and is surrounded by remarkably swollen astrocytic cell processes with accumulation of glycogen granules (arrows). x 2,000

ranged neuronal energy metabolism, glycogen accumulates in the astrocytic cell processes via glycogeno-neogenesis from lactate (Hamprecht and Dringen 1995; Dringen et al. 1993; Sokoloff 1992; Sokoloff et al. 1996; Swanson and Choi 1993).

Among the dark neurons with increased electron density, completely shrunken neurons with intensively high electron density of the entire cell increased in number from 5 to 24 hours after the ischemic insult. These dead neurons were fragmented by astrocytic cell processes and phagocytized by them 4 days after the ischemic insult. No inflammatory cells or phagocytes were noted in this study. Only perivascularly located microglia showed slight phagocytic activities. Later than 12 h after the ischemic insult, some mitochondria of the isolated dark neurons showed partial swelling of the matrices and disintegration of the cristae with wooly densities. Many of the mitochondria in the shrunken neurons also showed swollen matrices with occasional wooly densities and disintegrated cristae, and these had been considered to be an irreversive damage leading to cell death (Ghdially 1997). From these findings, not every dark neuron dies, becoming a shrunken neuron; rather some of them survive. Further quantitative study of the fate of these isolated dark neurons is necessary.

The present study suggests that the astrocytic cell processes around the dark neuron rescue the injured neuron by scavenging neuronal and synaptic metabolites (Kimelberg et al. 1995; Kempski and Volk 1996; Levi and Gallo 1995; Martin 1995; Newman 1995; Rosenberg and Aizeman 1989), and also dispose these dead neurons by shrinking, smashing and phagocytosis. Further study is necessary to elucidate the turning point from the living to the dying dark neuron.

Necrosis versus apoptosis, both resulting in cell death, has been controversial. In the present study, the morphological findings on the dark neuron suggested necrosis, i.e., eosinophilic ghosting of cells in histology and the presence of small loose aggregates of nuclear chromatin in the nuclear matrix and margin seen by EM, instead of the marginal condensed coarse granular aggregates of the nuclear chromatin and apoptotic bodies seen in apoptosis. However, they also suggested apoptosis in term of the scattered individual affected cells observed histologically (shrinkage necrosis), the lack of exudative inflammation, and the condensation of the cytosol with structurally intact mitochondria and other organelles, instead of swelling of all cell components followed by rupture of cell membrane and destruction of cytosolic organelles seen in necrosis (Wyllie et al. 1980; Majno and Joris 1995). Farber (1994) pointed out "there is no field of basic cell biology and cell pathology that is more confusing and more unintelligible than the area of apoptosis versus necrosis. It is easy to see, single cell necrosis indistinguishable from so-called apoptosis, in many tissue in which necrosis has been induced by toxic and ischemic and other environmental perturbations." (Farber 1994). All one can say is that sometimes dead cells are swollen and sometimes they are shrunken depending on the cell's environment (Ghdially 1997). Therefore, swollen perineuronal astrocytes may act to cause condensation, resulting in shrinkage, in DSNN. While, when astrocytes die in infarction, all neurons and astrocytes swell; and all of their membrane systems rupture. Further investigation is necessary to determine what ultrastructure corresponds to the positive TUNEL staining of fragmented DNA (Wijsman et al. 1993).

Acknowledgment

The authors wish to thank Ms. Emiko Kawakami for electronmicroscopical preparations.

References

1. Coles JA (1995) Glial cells and the supply of substrates of energy metabolism to neurons. Neuroglia (Kettenmann H, Ransom B, eds) New York Oxford, Oxford University Press. pp 793–804
2. Dringen R, Schmoll D, Cesar M, Hamprecht B (1993) Incorporation of radioactivity from [14C]lactate into the glycogen of cultured mouse astroglial cells. Evidence for glyconeogenesis in brain cells. Biol Chem Hoppe Seyler 374(5):343–347
3. Farber E (1994) Ideas in pathology. Programmed cell death: Necrosis versus apoptosis. Mod Pathol 7:605–612
4. Ghdially FN (1997) Ultrastructural Pathology of the Cell and Matrix. vol. 1, Butterworth-Heinemann pp 18–29, 246–258
5. Hamprecht B, Dringen R (1995) Energy metabolism. In: Neuroglia (Kettenmann H, Ransom B, eds) New York Oxford, Oxford University Press. pp 473–487
6. Hanyu S, Ito U, Hakamata Y, Yoshida M (1995) Transition from ischemic neuronal necrosis to infarction in repeated ischemia. Brain Res 686:44–48
7. Hanyu S, Ito U, Hakamata Y, Nakano I (1997) Topographical analysis of cortical neuronal loss associated with disseminated selective neuronal necrosis and infarction after repeated ischemia. Brain Res 767(1):154–157
8. Ito U, Spatz M, Walker J Jr, Klatzo I (1975) Experimental cerebral ischemia in mongolian gerbils. I. Light microscopic observations. Acta Neuropathol Berl 32(3):209–223
9. Ito U, Hanyu S, Hakamata Y, Nakamura M, Arima K (1996) Ultrastructure of astrocytes associated with progressing selective neuronal death or impending infarction after repeated ischemia. In: Pharmacology of Cerebral Ischemia (Krieglstein J, ed), Stuttgart, Medpharm Scientific Publ pp 385–392
10. Ito U, Hanyu S, Hakamata Y, Nakamura M, Arima K (1997a) Ultrastructure of astrocytes associated with selective neuronal death of cerebral cortex after repeated ischemia. Acta Neurochir Suppl Wien 70:46–49
11. Ito U, Hanyu S, Hakamata Y, Kuroiwa T, Yoshida M (1997b) Features and threshold of infarct development in ischemic maturation phenomenon. In: Maturation Phenomenon in Cerebral Ischemia II (Ito U, Kirino T, Kuroiwa T, Klatzo I, eds). Berlin, Heidelberg, Springer-Verlag. pp 115–121
12. Ito U, Hanyu S, Hakamata Y, Arima K, Oyanagi K, Kuroiwa T, Nakano I (1999a) Temporal profile of cortical injury following ischemic insult just-below and at the threshold level for induction of infarction-light and electron microscopic study. In: Maturation Phenomenon in Cerebral Ischemia III (Ito U, Orzi F, Kuroiwa T, Fieschi C, Klatzo I, eds), Springer-Verlag
13. Ito U, Kuroiwa T, Hanyu S, Hakamata Y, Arima K, Nakano I, Oyanagi K (1999 b) Ultrastructural features of astroglial mitochondria following temporary ischemia of threshold level needed to induce infarction. In: Pharmacology of cerebral ischemia (Krieglstein, ed), Medpharm Science Publication, Stuttgart, pp 113–117
14. Ito U, Kuroiwa T, Hanyu S, Hakamata Y, Arima K, Nakano I, Oyanagi K (2000) Ultrastructure and morphometry of astroglial mitochondria following temporary threshold ischemia to induce focal infarction. In: Maturation Phenomenon in Cerebral Ischemia IV (Bazan NG, Ito U, Kuroiwa T, Klatzo I, eds) Springer-Verlag, Berlin, Heidelberg, (to be published)
15. Kempski O, Volk C (1996) Glial protection against neuronal damage. In: Maturation Phenomenon in Cerebral Ischemia II (Ito U, Kirino T, Kuroiwa T, Klatzo I, eds) Berlin, Heidelberg, Springer-Verlag. pp 115–121
16. Kimelberg HK, Rutledge E, Goderie S, Charniga C (1995) Astrocytic swelling due to hypotonic or high K+ medium causes inhibition of glutamate and aspartate uptake and increases their release. J Cereb Blood Flow Metab 15(3):409–416

17. Kraig RP, Lascola CD, Caggiano A (1995) Glial response to brain ischemia. Neuroglia (Kettenmann H, Ransom B, eds) New York Oxford, Oxford University Press. pp 964–976
18. Levi G, Gallo V (1995) Release of neuroactive amino acids from glia. Neuroglia (Kettenmann H, Ransom B, eds), New York Oxford, Oxford University Press. pp 815–826
19. Majno G, Joris I (1995) Apoptosis, oncosis and necrosis: an overview of cell death. Am J Pathol 146:143–115
20. Marcoux FW, Morawetz RB, Crowell RM, DeGirolami U, Halsey J, Jr (1982) Differential regional vulnerability in transient focal cerebral ischemia. Stroke 13(3):339–346
21. Martin DL (1995) The role of glia in the inactivation of neurotransmitters. Neuroglia (Kettenmann H, Ransom B, eds) New York Oxford, University Press. pp 732–745
22. Newman EA (1995) Glial cell regulation of extracellular potassium. In: Neuroglia (Kettenmann H, Ransom B, eds) New York Oxford, Oxford University Press. pp 717–731
23. Ohno K, Ito U, Inaba Y (1984) Regional cerebral blood flow and stroke index after left carotid artery ligation in the conscious gerbil. Brain Res 297(1):151–157
24. Rosenberg GA, Aizeman E (1989) Hundred-fold increase in neuronal vulnerability to glutamate toxicity in astrocyte-poor cultures of rat cerebral cortex. Neuroscience letters 103:162–168
25. Sokoloff L (1992) Energy metabolism and effects of energy depletion or exposure to glutamate. Can J Physiol Pharmacol 70(12):S107–112
26. Sokoloff L, Gotoh J, Law MJ, Takahashi S (1996) Functional activation of energy metbolism in nervous tissue: Roles of neurons and astroglia. In: Pharmacology of cerebral ischemia (Krieglstein J, ed), Stuttgart, Medpharm Scientific Publ. pp 259–270
27. Swanson RA, Choi DW (1993) Glial glycogen stores affect neuronal survival during glucose deprivation in vitro. J Cereb Blood Flow Metab 13(1):162–169
28. von-Lubitz DK, Diemer NH (1983) Cerebral ischemia in the rat: ultrastructural and morphometric analysis of synapses in stratum radiatum of the hippocampal CA-1 region. Acta Neuropathol Berl 61(1):52–60
29. Wijsman JH, Jonker RR, Keijr R et al. (1993) A new method to detect apoptosis in paraffin sections: in situ end-labelling of fragmentation DNA. J Histochem Cytochem 41:47–12
30. Wyllie AH, Kerr JFR, Currie AR (1980) Cell death: the significance of apoptosis. Int Rev Cytol 68:251–301

Circulation

Dynamic investigation of the rat cortical microcirculation using confocal videomicroscopy in transient focal ischemia and related penumbral depolarizations

H. Nallet*, S. Roussel*, O. Issertial, E. T. Mac Kenzie*, J. Seylaz, E. Pinard[1]

Abstract

The aim of the study was to directly assess the influence of recurrent penumbral depolarizations on surface arteriole diameter and velocity of erythrocytes through parenchymal capillaries.

Cortical microcirculation was explored in halothane-anesthetized rats for 3 min every 20 min during 2-hour MCA occlusion and 1-hour reperfusion, using in vivo confocal fluorescence microscopy. In rats made ischemic under the microscope by an intraluminal remotely controlled method (n = 6), both arteriolar constrictions and dilatations occurred, but the mean arteriole diameter did not change significantly. The mean velocity of capillary erythrocytes was depressed by 35%. Under SD-like depolarizations, a significant increase in diameter occurred, while capillary erythrocyte velocity was further depressed by 15%. This decrease in velocity was more pronounced (25%) when the depolarizations were associated with inversions of blood flow directions in arterioles. Following reperfusion, all microvascular variables returned to baseline. No clear sign of BBB permeability changes were observed, neither were present thrombi, although blood seemed extremely viscous in venules. A displacement of the capillary network with respect to surface microvessels suggested brain edema. All rats exhibited infarcts 24 hours after the occlusion.

It is concluded that, even in moderately ischemic tissue, SD-like depolarizations have an adverse influence on penumbral microcirculation, ie a reduction in capillary perfusion by erythrocytes.

Introduction

A variety of noxious stimuli induce a transient functional disturbance of cerebral cortex, characterized by a shift of the cortical steady potential and a reversible silence of electrocorticographic activity. This phenomenon is caused by neuronal depolarization, propagating like a wave across the cerebral cortex or other grey matter regions. It was first described by Leao (1944) and called spreading depression (SD). It has been shown that SD propagation involves high extracellular K^+ (Gardner-Medwin 1981; Hansen and Zeuten 1981) and Ca^{++} influx through NMDA receptors (Lauritzen and Hansen 1992; Nellgard and Wieloch 1992), and causes the activation of the sodium/potassium-

Keywords: Focal ischemia, Microcirculation, Penumbra, Spreading depression, in vivo confocal microscopy

[1]Laboratoire de Recherches Cérébrovasculaires, CNRS UPR 646, Université Paris 7, IFR 6, 10 Avenue de Verdun, 75010 Paris, France.
e-mail: pinard@ext.jussieu.fr
*CNRS UMR 6551, Université de Caen

stimulated ATPase and other energy-dependent ion exchange pumps, resulting in an increase in glucose and oxygen consumption (Shinohara et al. 1979; Mayevski and Weiss 1991).

In healthy tissue, repeated SDs do not produce neuronal damage since there is no mismatch between the local increased energy demand and blood flow. The rise in metabolic activity due to mitochondrial calcium loading (Erecinska et al. 1991) is coupled to a parallel increase in blood flow to ensure adequate oxygen delivery (Mayevsky and Weiss 1991). Interestingly, cortical SD induces a widespread expression of immediate early genes (Herdegen et al. 1993), followed by an upregulation of trophic factors, and an activation of glial cells (Matsushima et al. 1998).

Transient cortical depolarizations following focal ischemia were first described by Nedergaard and Astrup (1986) who used intracortical microelectrodes for the recording of the direct current (DC) potential. Such periinfarct current shifts are prevented by either NMDA (Gill et al. 1992; Iijima et al. 1992) or AMPA receptor antagonists (Mies et al. 1994). In addition, these spontaneous waves of neuronal depolarizations were shown to participate in the extent of the ischemic damage (Back et al. 1996; Gill et al. 1992; Mies et al. 1993), indicating a difference in vulnerability to spreading depression in intact and ischemic brains. This difference has been postulated to be due to the fact that the increased oxygen demand of the repolarizing tissue is not coupled to an adequate increase in blood flow in the ischemic penumbra, further enhancing the mismatch between energy requirement and availability.

In areas with moderate reduction in blood flow, a transient increase in local blood supply following the onset of the DC shift has been measured by laser-Doppler flowmetry (Iijima et al. 1992; Nallet et al. 2000). In contrast, in severely ischemic areas, LDF did not reveal any blood flow changes during transient depolarisations, while tissue PO2 was decreased (Back and Hossman 1994). However, in these conditions, regional tissue perfusion reflected by LDF may have been dissociated from cerebral capillary perfusion, as shown by Hudetz et al. (1998) with a different experimental protocol. Some microvascular phenomena may be not fully reflected by a change in regional CBF, especially because LDF does not distinguish between capillary flow and shunt flow.

In the present study, we have reevaluated the issue of tissue perfusion under periinfarct depolarizations, using an original method that we have recently developed. This method is based on the combined use of laser-scanning confocal fluorescence microscopy and of fluorescently labeled erythrocytes and plasma. Such an approach allows the dynamic on-line visualization of both the erythrocytes flowing through parenchymal capillaries and the pial microvascular network (Seylaz et al. 1999; Pinard et al. 1998). The aims of our work were: 1) to directly assess the dynamic microcirculatory changes induced by focal ischemia and reperfusion in the penumbral zone, 2) to determine the influence of spontaneous depolarizations on the penumbral microcirculation, and 3) to address the questions of capillary recruitment within the penumbra, of thrombus formation in microvessels and indirectly of blood-brain barrier permeability.

Materials and methods

All experimental procedures were carried out in accordance with the National Institute of Health guidelines for the care and use of laboratory animals. Experiments were performed under permit No 02934 from the French Ministry of Agriculture.

Surgery protocol

The experiments were performed on nine adult male Sprague-Dawley rats weighing 270–320 grams (R. Janvier Breeding Center, France). Anaesthesia was induced with halothane 4% in O_2:N_2O (30:70) and animals were intubated and artificially ventilated. Anaesthesia was maintained during the surgery with halothane 1.5–2% in O_2:N_2O (30:70). A femoral artery was cannulated for continuous blood pressure recording and to obtain arterial samples for blood gas and pH analysis. A catheter was placed in the femoral vein to administer the fluorescent tracers. Rectal temperature was kept close to 37.5 °C throughout the experiment with a feed-back controlled heating pad connected to a rectal probe.

A cranial window was performed on the right fronto-parietal cortex. The dura mater was removed over an area of 4 mm^2 and a 150 μm thick quartz microscope coverglass was sealed to the bone with dental cement (Palaferm, Kuzler) to make the preparation waterproof.

In addition, a right frontal craniotomy (diameter 2 mm) was performed 2 mm rostral to the bregma and 2 mm lateral to the sagittal suture. The dura mater was kept intact. One Ag/AgCl wire (diameter 0.07 mm, uncoated tip 1.5 mm) was placed between the calvarium and the meningeal surface to record the DC potential and the electrocorticogram (ECoG). An Ag/AgCl disk electrode was inserted under the skin of the neck as a reference electrode.

Finally, after isolation of the right carotid arterial tree, a cylinder of melt adhesive (2 mm long, diameter 0.38 mm) attached to a nylon thread (0.22 mm in diameter) was advanced from the lumen of the external carotid artery (ECA), into the internal carotid artery 5 mm after the external skull base. The portion of the thread remaining outside the ECA stump was inserted into a catheter and secured with a suture. Such a surgical preparation enabled us to induce reversible focal cerebral ischemia under the confocal microscope by a remote controlled method of intraluminal middle cerebral artery occlusion (MCAo) (Roussel et al. 1994).

Confocal microscopy protocol

The rat was placed under the confocal microscope and its head was secured in a custom-built stereotaxic device closely fitting the confocal microscope stage. A BioRad Viewscan confocal laser-scanning unit, attached to a Nikon Optiphot-2 microscope was used. The scanning unit scanned 50 fields per second. A detailed description of the apparatus has been published (Seylaz et al. 1999). The light source was an argon-krypton laser ($\lambda = 488$, 568 and 647nm). An appropriate filter was used for fluorescence microscopy of fluorescein.

Electrodes were connected to a polygraph (Gould) for continuous DC potential and ECoG recording. The arterial catheter was connected to a pressure transducer (Statham). Arterial blood was regularly sampled to check blood gases and pH (Corning). The hematocrit was measured before and at different times after injecting the tracers.

Fluorescein-isothiocyanate (FITC)-Dextran (molecular weight = 70,000) diluted in 0.9% NaCl (2.5 mg/ml) was injected (0.5 ml) into the blood circulation to visualize microvessels and delineate their internal walls. FITC-labeled erythrocytes (previously prepared *in vitro*) were injected via the same route at a tracer dose (< 2%). The whole cranial window was systematically explored with a 10x objective. The most appropriate area of investigation (presence of at least one pial arteriole and a dense capillary network) was then chosen with 20x objective lens (Fig. 1). This 20x objective lens was used for the whole experiment. Intraparenchymal capillaries were visualized by changing the focus from the pial arterioles to a depth of 200 μm beneath the surface of the brain. Images were recorded at video speed (50 frames per second) with a SIT camera (Hamamatsu) and a PAL-VHS video recorder (Panasonic).

Limited sequences of videorecording (approximately 3 min each, with a focus on arterioles for about 1 min and on capillaries for about 2 min) were used to avoid continuous laser illumination, which could have damaged the tissue. These recording sequences were performed every 15–20 min during a control period, during MCAO (initiated by further advancing the nylon thread by 4 mm) and during reperfusion. Additional sequences of images were also recorded following the start of each neuronal depolarization.

At the end of the experiment, the frontal craniotomy and the closed cranial window were covered with pieces of silicone rubber, the scalp was sutured, the femoral catheters were re-

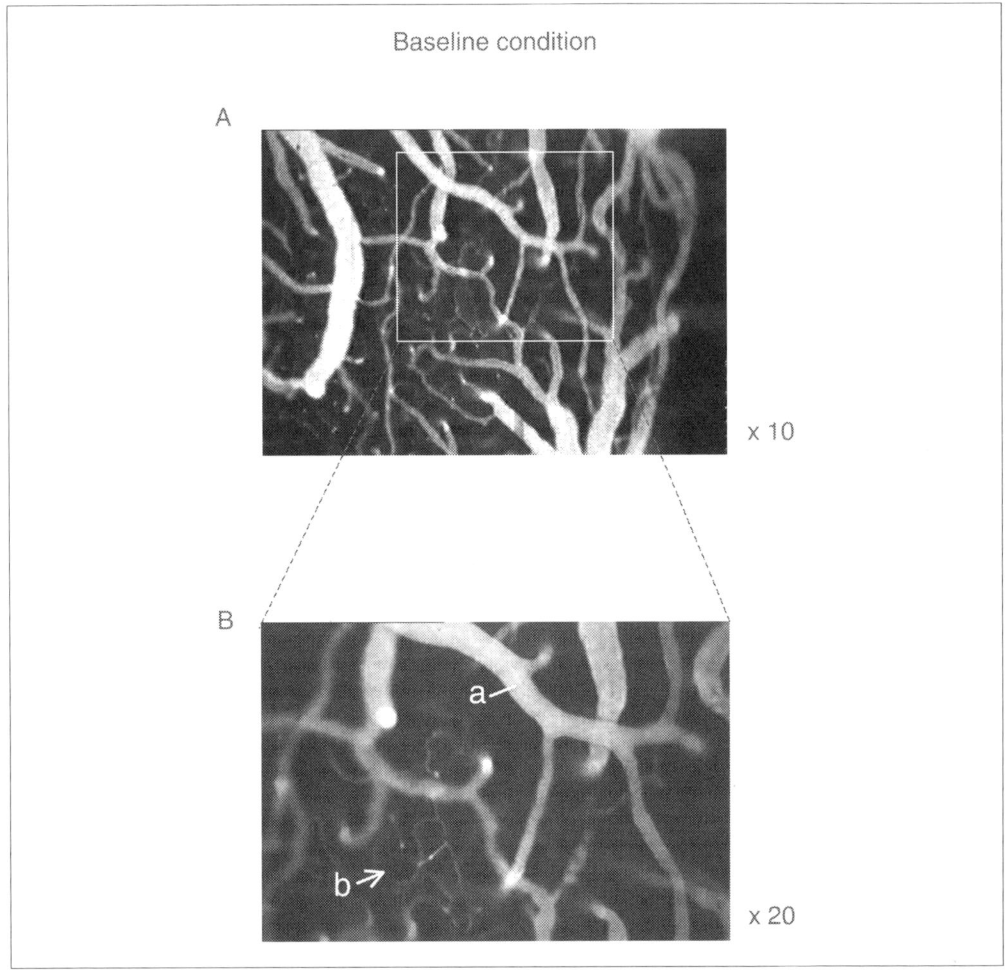

Fig. 1. A. Example of a rat microvascular network through a closed cranial window visualised under baseline conditions by fluorescence confocal microscopy with a 10x objective lens. **B.** Area (20x objective lens) corresponding to the box in A, which was selected as the region of interest for the whole experiment on the basis of the presence of at least one pial arteriole -a- and a dense capillary -b- network. The white dots in the capillary network are FITC-labelled erythrocytes.

moved and the animal was extubated. An intraperitoneal injection of physiological saline (5 ml) was performed before awakening and return to the animal house.

Histopathological evaluation

Twenty four hours after ischemia, animals were anaesthetized with halothane 5% in O_2:N_2O (30:70), decapitated and the brain was removed. The brain was frozen during 1 minute in isopentane –40 °C and stored at –80 °C. The brains were cut coronally with a cryostat into 15 µm slices at 500 µm intervals. These sections were stained with cresyl violet. An image analysis system (BIOCOM) was used to measure the surface of cortical and striatal infarcted and non-infarcted tissues. The volume of the infarct was then calculated, corrected from edema.

Materials

FITC-Dextran (molecular weight 70,000) and FITC Isomer I were purchased from Sigma Chemical Co.

Data and statistical analyses

Images were digitized and analyzed off-line to determine the arteriolar diameter and the velocity of fluorescently-labeled erythrocytes through capillaries.

Two to four arteriolar segments from one arteriole per rat were selected. Their internal diameter was automatically measured on digitized images using a custom-built Optimas software procedure at each period of interest. Measures from all segments of the same arteriole at the same time were averaged, since changes in diameter were similar in all parts of the same arteriole.

The erythrocyte velocity was measured through 3–5 capillaries per rat at approximately the same time periods than arteriole diameters. The velocity was measured over capillary segments of about 70–130 μm long.

For both arteriolar diameter and erythrocyte velocity in capillaries, we calculated the average value over each recording sequence in each rat. The recording sequences were classified by categories as baseline (before MCAo), MCAo (during MCAo excepted during a transient SD-like depolarization), SD (during MCAo while a SD-like depolarization occurred) and reperfusion, and these categories were used as "sequence category" factor levels in ANOVAs.

Mean arteriolar diameter for each recording sequence was expressed either as % of the baseline value or as % of the mean MCAo value. Mean erythrocyte velocity through capillaries was expressed either as absolute value (mm/s) or as % of the mean MCAo value.

In addition, each sequence was carefully examined visually to detect the presence of at least one inversion or arrest of arteriolar blood flow. When such a change in blood flow was detected, the sequence was classified as "with perturbation". The other sequences were classified as "without perturbation".

Statistical analyses were performed by ANOVA using Statview software (Abacus Concepts, USA), followed, when appropriate, by Fisher PLSD post-hoc tests. Values are given as means ± standard deviation and $p < 0.05$ was accepted as significant.

Results

Physiological parameters

In both experimental groups (sham: n = 3, ischemia: n = 6), physiological variables were within the expected ranges for halothane-anesthetized artificially ventilated rats ($PaO_2 = 140 \pm 40$ mmHg; $PaCO_2 = 37.4 \pm 6.2$ mmHg; pHa $= 7.45 \pm 0.05$; mean arterial pressure $= 72 \pm 9$ mmHg; rectal temperature $= 36.8 \pm 1.1$ °C). Hematocrit ($39.2 \pm 1.9\%$) was not significantly modified by the injection of FITC-labelled erythrocytes.

Microcirculation during basal conditions and following MCA occlusion

In basal conditions, the mean arteriolar diameter was 33 ± 12 μm and the mean velocity of labelled erythrocytes through capillaries was 0.51 ± 0.19 mm/sec. No significant change in microvascular variables was measured at any time of the experiment in sham rats (n = 3).

In the other rats (n = 6), the advancement of the thread up to the MCA branching induced either dilatations (up to 140% of baseline diameter) or constrictions (down to 80% of baseline diameter) of arterioles or both. On average, however, only a small non-significant increase in arteriole diameter was obtained ($107 \pm 18\%$ of baseline; one-way ANOVA for sequence category effect, $p < 0.029$; post-hoc test: $p > 0.47$). Following MCAo, a significant slowering of the erythrocyte velocity through capillaries was observed (0.33 ± 0.14 mm/sec during MCAo vs 0.51 ± 0.19 mm/sec during baseline conditions; one-way ANOVA for sequence category effect, $p < 0.0001$; post-hoc test: $p = 0.0001$). No significant correlation was obtained between the changes in diameter and the changes in erythrocyte velocity.

Both arteriolar and venular circulations were visibly reduced, often exhibiting viscous blood and sluggish blood flow. No circulating thrombus was observed, but stops in blood flow and reversions of the blood flow direction were sometimes detected in arterioles (such perturbations were observed in 15% of the MCAo recording sequences and never in baseline sequences). A transient opening of the blood-brain barrier, objectivated by fluorescein leakage across the arteriolar wall, was observed in only one rat, during the period of ischemia. A marked displacement of the capillary bed with respect to the surface vessels was also observed, at the end of the ischemia period as compared to the baseline period.

Microcirculation under penumbral depolarization

No neuronal depolarizations occurred in sham rats. Transient ischemic depolarizations occurred in all MCA-occluded rats, with a mean number of 4.5 ± 3.0 over the 2 hours of ischemia and a mean duration of 1.99 ± 1.06 min.

Transient ischemic depolarizations induced a significant transient increase in arteriolar diameter ($119 \pm 23\%$ of baseline; Fig. 2) as compared to baseline or MCAo ($107 \pm 18\%$ of baseline) (one-way ANOVA for sequence category effect, $p < 0.029$; post-hoc test SD vs baseline: $p < 0.048$; post-hoc test SD vs MCAo: $p < 0.015$).

Blood flow arrests and inversions in arterioles (Fig. 3) were frequent during ischemic depolarizations (these perturbations were observed in 41% of the SD recording sequences). The proportion of sequences "with" and "without perturbations" is significantly dependent on the sequence category (chi-square test: $p < 0.022$).

To correct inter-animal differences in absolute velocity of labelled erythrocytes and arteriolar diameters following MCAo, we analyzed the influence of transient ischemic depolarizations and arteriolar blood flow perturbations on these hemodynamic parameters in percentages of mean MCAo values. One-way ANOVAs were then used with the following factor levels: MCAo without perturbations, MCAo with perturbations, SD without perturbations and SD with perturbations.

The mean changes in arteriolar diameter during ischemia are presented in Figure 4 and those of velocity of labelled erythrocytes through capillaries in Figure 5. Arteriolar diameter was significantly increased during SD-like depolarizations without perturbations as compared to MCAo (with or without perturbations). The velocity of labelled erythrocytes through capillaries was significantly reduced during SD-like depolarizations with perturbations as compared to SD-like depolarizations without perturbations or MCAo without perturbations.

Finally, we compared the capillary erythrocytes velocities during MCAo and SD-like depolarizations, independently of the presence or absence of perturbations (data correponding to "with" and "without perturbations" pooled). The average velocity of erythrocytes was significantly decreased during SD-like depolarizations as compared to MCAo (Student's t test, $p < 0.031$).

Microcirculation under reperfusion

When the thread was removed, there was no significant change in mean arteriolar diameter ($104 \pm 26\%$ of baseline; one-way ANOVA for sequence category effect, $p < 0.029$; post-hoc test reperfusion vs baseline: $p > 0.67$; post-hoc test vs MCAo: $p > 0.58$), but the arteriolar blood flow was visibly increased. The velocity of labelled erythrocytes through capillaries returned to its baseline value attaining 0.50 ± 0.24 mm/sec. No capillary recruitment (i.e. newly perfused capillaries) was observed. Sluggish blood flow persisted in some venules, and many round black masses, possibly activated monocytes, were rolling and fixing.

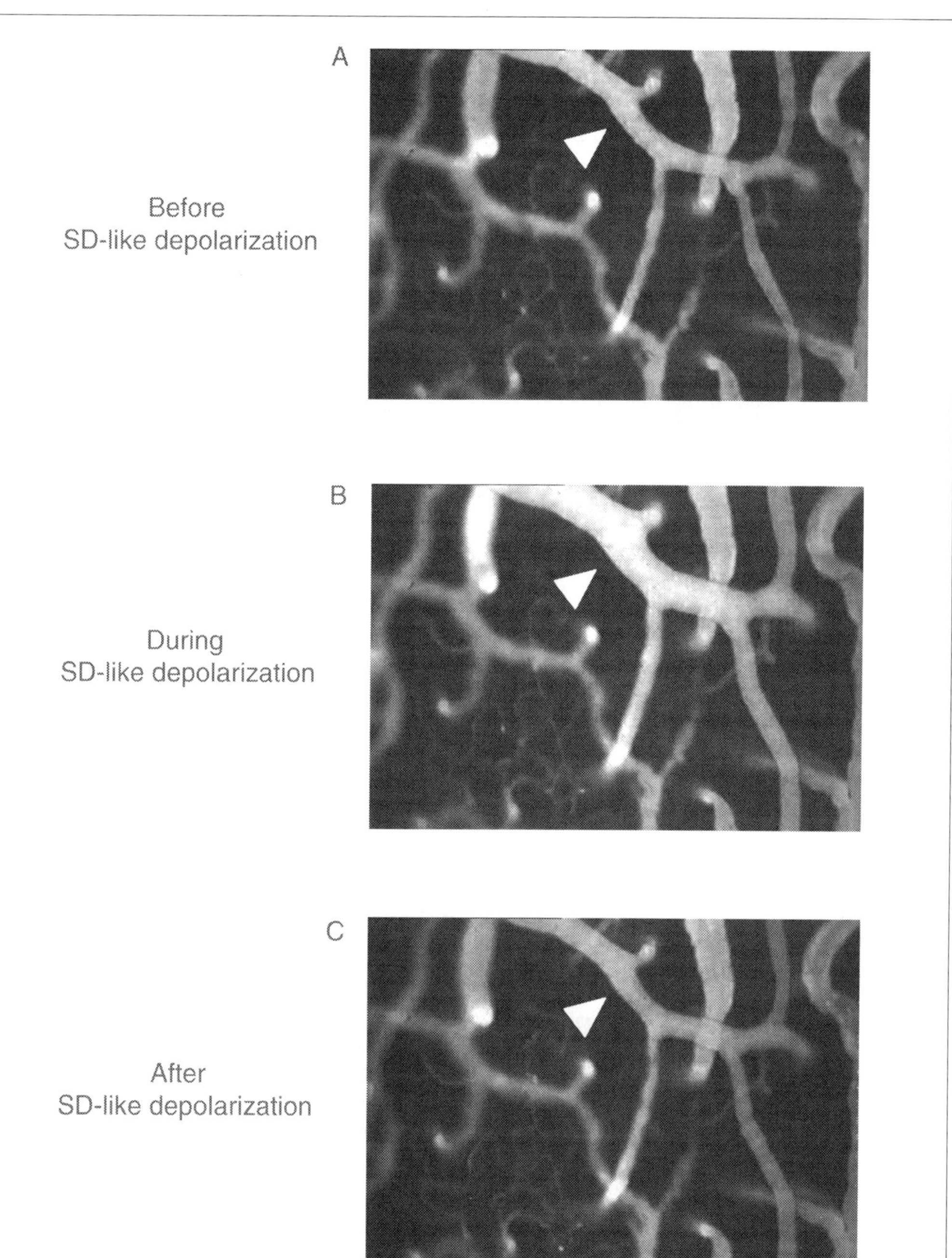

Fig. 2. Example of a change in arteriolar diameter associated with SD-like depolarization. **A.** Before SD-like depolarization; **B.** Dilation during SD-like depolarization; **C.** After the wave of SD-like depolarization, return of the arteriolar diameter to the pre-event state.

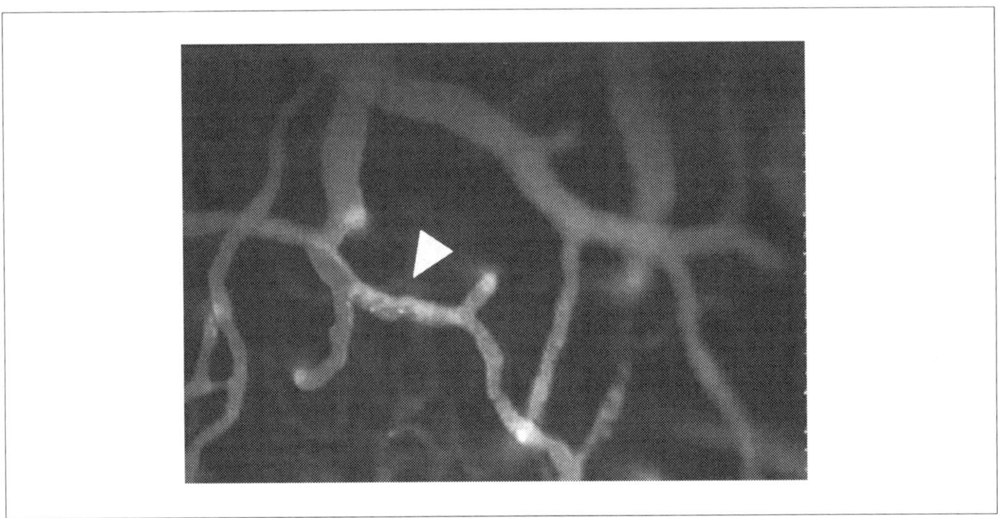

Fig. 3. Example of arteriolar blood flow arrest (arrow) during a SD-like depolarization.

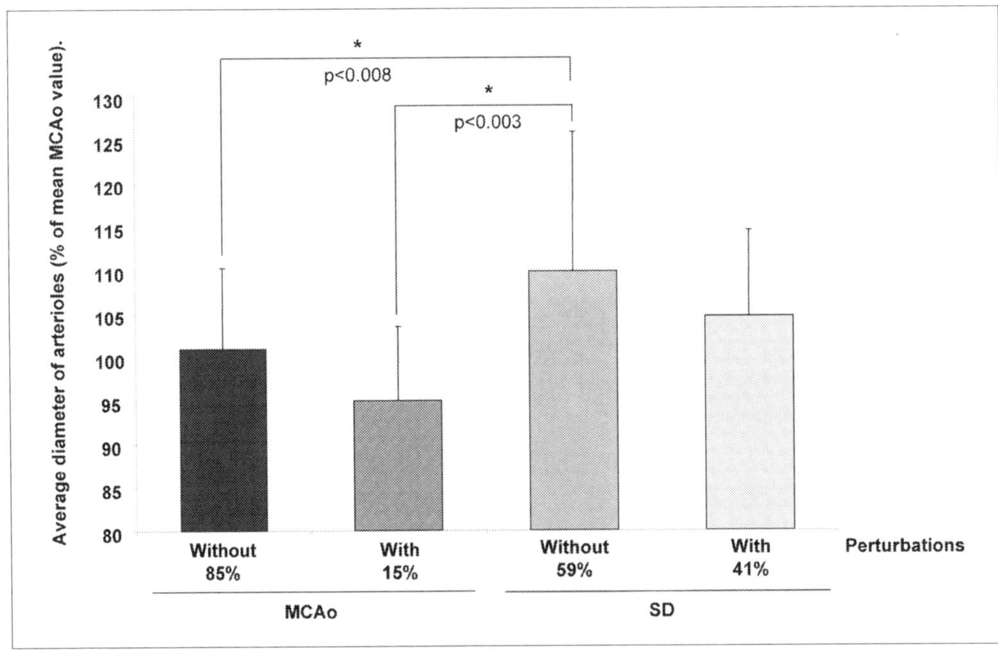

Fig. 4. Average diameter of arterioles during MCAo and SD-like depolarization as a function of the presence or absence of arteriolar flow perturbation (inversion or arrest). The values are expressed as percentage from the mean MCAo value (obtained by pooling "with" and "without perturbation" measures). The percentages of sequences "with" and "without perturbations" for each sequence type (MCAo or SD) are indicated.
*: Significant Fischer-PLSD post-hoc test following a significant one-way ANOVA ($p < 0.011$).

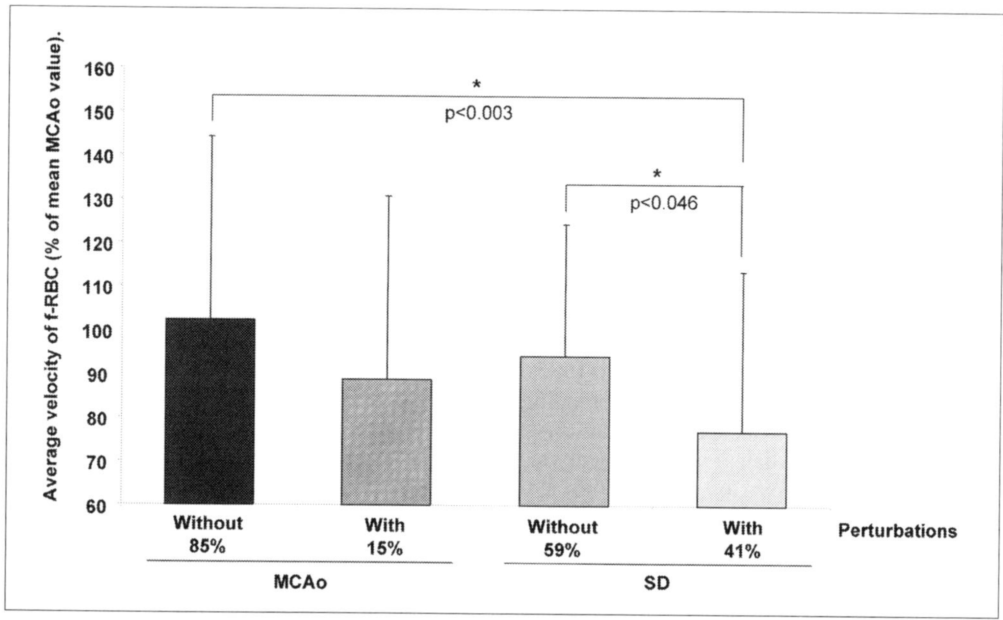

Fig. 5. Average velocity of FITC-labelled erythrocytes during MCAo and SD-like depolarization as a function of the presence or absence of arteriolar flow perturbation (inversion or arrest). The values are expressed as percentage from the mean MCAo value (obtained by pooling "with" and "without perturbation" measures). The percentages of sequences "with" and "without perturbations" for each sequence type (MCAo or SD) are indicated.
*: Significant Fischer-PLSD post-hoc test following a significant one-way ANOVA ($p < 0.021$).

Histopathology

Sham rats ($n = 3$) did not exhibit any brain lesion, contrarily to MCA-occluded rats ($n = 6$). The occlusion induced infarction in both cortex and subcortex in 4 rats, and in subcortex only in 2 rats. The mean total infarct volumes were respectively 127.0 ± 14.3 mm^3 (cortex 107.5 ± 11.3 mm^3, subcortex 19.5 ± 7.7 mm^3) and 18.9 ± 1.3 mm^3.

Discussion

This is the first study reporting direct visualization in real-time of plasma and erythrocytes flowing through pial microvessels and intraparenchymal capillaries within the penumbral zone following MCA occlusion and reperfusion. Such data were lacking, as underlined by Del Zoppo (1994), and they should contribute to draw the picture of the dynamic microvascular consequences of focal cerebral ischemia.

The decrease in erythrocyte capillary perfusion under focal ischemia was unassociated with changes in mean arteriolar diameter and followed by an increase in blood viscosity. The spontaneous transient waves of neuronal depolarizations induced a further decrease in erythrocyte capillary perfusion, associated with an arteriolar dilatation and with frequent local inversions of blood flow direction in arterioles. All microvascular variables returned to pre-ischemic basal levels at reperfusion.

Capillary recruitment, in terms of both plasma flow and erythrocyte flow, did not occur at any time of the reperfusion period, as we previously found following global ischemia (Pinard et al. 2000).

No clear sign of vascular permeability to FITC-Dextran was observed, indicating no major increase in BBB permeability for large molecular weight proteins, contrarily to what we observed in global ischemia (ibid). In contrast, a geometrical rearrangement of the parenchymal capillary network with respect to the pial arteriole and venule pattern was striking, indicating changes in parenchymal volume due to transient focal ischemic conditions. Such a rearrangement was suggestive of marked tissue edema. Such indications of no early increase in permeability to proteins and of early brain edema following occlusion of the MCA in the rat are in good agreement with data on the time course of these parameters (Gotoh et al. 1985).

The phenomenon of periinfarct spreading depressions and the concept of ischemic penumbra have been exhaustively and nicely reviewed respectively by Hossmann (1996) and by Obrenovitch (1995). The following discussion will thus concentrate on the present data.

In the present investigation of the penumbral zone, the anastomoses of arteriolar circulation were functional in ischemic conditions, with blood flowing in either direction, but they were not sufficient to prevent a decrease in parenchymal capillary perfusion. In addition to decreased perfusion pressure, mechanical factors such as astrocytic endfeet swelling and/or venous thrombosis, may be partly responsible for the reduction in erythrocyte flow through capillaries. Polymorphonuclear leukocytes may have also restricted transit through capillary portions of microvascular beds (Del Zoppo 1994).

The decrease in capillary erythrocyte velocity measured in the present study indicates the penumbral localization of the field we explored by confocal fluorescence microscopy. Furthermore, since the duration of transient depolarizations has been reported to be inversely proportional to the residual blood flow (Mies 1997), the duration we measured (about 2 min) was also indicative of a moderate reduction of perfusion. In such an ischemic state, a transient moderate or no increase in blood flow during the depolarizations is expected, as previously shown by laser-Doppler flowmetry (Iijima 1992; Nallet et al. 2000). This contrasts with the present finding of a reduction in erythrocyte velocity through capillaries. Not only the LDF method may not reflect the actual tissue perfusion, as shown by Hudetz et al. (1998), but the penumbra may comprise subareas with differential fates, as suggested by the diversity of penumbral pH changes (Back et al. 2000) and the microcirculatory abnormalities revealed by capillary filling at the borderline between normal and ischemic tissue (Vogel et al. 1999).

The arteriolar dilatation occurring during the passage of SD-like depolarizations has been suggested to be due to many factors, notably to nitric oxide (NO) released by neurons. Ohta et al. (1997) have measured a significant increase in NO concentration in ischemic regions exhibiting anoxic depolarizations. Mutant mice with disrupted type 1 NO synthase gene showed fewer SD-like events after focal ischemia than wild type mice (Shimizu-Sasamata et al. 1998). However, no direct demonstration of the vasodilatatory role of NO released from neurons under transient ischemic depolarizations has been provided. The fact that the vasodilatation can also be transmitted upstream and downstream, and that propagated vasodilatation in arterioles may occur independently of changes in blood flow has to be taken into consideration (Segal et al. 1989), as well as autoregulatory mechanisms which are still efficient in this moderately ischemic area. Another possible explanation is a vasodilatatory effect of extracellular K^+, whose increase in concentration during transient depolarizations may remain in the range of smooth muscle relaxation (<30 mmol) at the pial level, as shown by Strong et al. (1983). Conversely, the enhancement of depressed capillary perfusion by erythrocytes under SD-like depolarizations could be due to a constriction of intraparenchymal precapillary arterioles in contact with the highest increase in K^+ concentration, ie in the range of its vasoconstrictory effect (about 60 mM) (Nedergaard and Hansen 1993). Capillary compression due to further astrocytic endfeet swelling during transient depolarizations may also contribute to the capillary perfusion impairment.

An alternative hypothesis which may explain the simultaneous pial arteriolar dilatation and the decrease in parenchymal perfusion is the occurrence of a steal phenomenon. The vasodilatation would improve the perfusion of a tissue located outside the area of investigation at the expense of the tissue under investigation. Such a steal phenomenon has been described in case of vasodilatatory drugs administered to ischemic brains. More recently, a paradoxical response of cerebral collateral vessels, which provide blood flow to the surrounding ischemic penumbra, has been reported under selective inhibition of NOS and attributed to a vascular steal phenomenon through collaterals (Muhonen et al. 1994). The hypothesis of a steal phenomenon in the present experiments is supported by the numerous changes in blood direction through arterioles occurring during the propagation of neuronal depolarizations. They probably reflect focal changes in arteriolar resistance due to constiction or dilatation and associated with a reduction of capillary perfusion in the area of investigation.

In conclusion, the present investigation confirms that the penumbra is a highly dynamic and heterogeneous structure. The present data suggest that the propagation of transient neuronal depolarizations plays a deleterious role in the extent of the infarct at least in part via a decrease in tissue perfusion and is a key pathological event for the evolution of hemodynamics in focal ischemia, even in moderately ischemic tissue with efficient arteriolar anastomoses.

References

1. Back T, Hossmann KA (1994) Cortical negative DC deflections following middle cerebral artery occlusion and KCl-induced spreading depression: effect on blood flow, tissue oxygenation, and electroencephalogram. J Cereb Blood Flow Metab 14:12–19
2. Back T, Ginsberg MD, Dietrich WD, Watson BD (1996) Induction of spreading depression in the ischemic hemisphere following experimental middle cerebral artery occlusion: effect on infarct morphology. J Cereb Blood Flow Metab 16:202–213
3. Back T, Hoehn M, Mies G, Busch E, Schmitz B, Kohno K, Hosmann KA (2000) Penumbral tissue alkalosis in focal cerebral ischemia: relationship to energy metabolism, blood flow, and steady potential. Ann Neurol 47:485–492
4. Del Zoppo GJ (1994) Microvascular changes during cerebral ischemia and reperfusion. Cereb Brain Metab Rev 6:47–96
5. Erecinska M, Delson D, Chance B (1991) Depolarization-induced changes in cellular energy production. Proc Natl Acad Sci USA 88:7600–7604
6. Gardner-Medwin AR (1981) Possible roles of vertebrate neuroglia in potassium dynamics, spreading depression and migraine. J Exp Biol 95:111–127
7. Gill R, Andiné P, Hillered L, Persson L, Hagberg H (1992) The effect of MK-801 on cortical spreading depression in penumbral zone following focal ischaemia in the rat. J Cereb Blood Flow Metab 12:371–379
8. Gotoh O, Asano T, Koide T, Takakura K (1985) Ischemic brain edema following occlusion of the MCA in the rat. I: The time courses of the brain water, sodium and potassium contents and blood-brain barrier permeability to ^{125}I-albumin. Stroke 16:101–109
9. Hansen AJ, Zeuthen T (1981) Extracellular ion concentrations during spreading depression and ischemia in the rat brain cortex. Acta Physiol Scand 113:437–445
10. Herdegen T, Sandkühler J, Gass P, Kiessling M, Bravo R, Zimmermann M (1993) JUN, FOS, KROX, and CREB transcription factor proteins in the rat cortex: basal expression and induction by spreading depression and epileptic seizures. J Comp Neurol 333:271–288
11. Hossmann KA (1996) Periinfarct depolarizations. Cereb Brain Metab Rev 8:195–208
12. Hudetz AG, Shen H, Kampine JP (1998) Nitric oxide from neuronal NOS plays critical role in cerebral capillary flow response to hypoxia. Am J Physiol 43:H982–H989
13. Iijima T, Mies G, Hossmann KA (1992) Repeated negative DC deflections in rat cortex following middle cerebral artery occlusion are abolished by MK-801: effect on volume of ischemic injury J Cereb Blood Flow Metab 12:727–733
14. Lauritzen M, Hansen AJ (1992) The effects of glutamate receptor blockade on anoxic depolarization and cortical spreading depression. J Cereb Blood Flow Metab 12:223–229
15. Leao AP (1944) Spreading depression of activity in the cerebral cortex. J Neurophysiol 7:359–390
16. Matsushima K, Schmidt-Kastner R, Hogan MJ, Hakim AM (1998) Cortical spreading depression activates trophic factor expression in neurons and astrocytes and protects against subsequent focal brain ischemia. Brain Res 807:47–60
17. Mayevsky A, Weiss HR (1991) Cerebral blood flow and oxygen consumption in cortical spreading depression. J Cereb Blood Flow Metab 11:829–836
18. Mies G, Iijima T, Hossmann KA (1993) Correlation between peri-infarct DC shifts and ischaemic neuronal damage in rat. NeuroReport 4:709–711
19. Mies G, Kohno K, Hossmann KA (1994) Prevention of periinfarct direct current shifts with glutamate antagonist NBQX following occlusion of the middle cerebral artery in the rat. J Cereb Blood Flow Metab 14:802–807
20. Mies G (1997) Blood flow dependent duration of cortical depolarizations in the periphery of focal ischemia of rat brain. Neurosci Lett 221:165–168
21. Muhonen MG, Heistad DD, Faraci FM, Loftus CM (1994) Augmentation of blood flow through cerebral collaterals by inhibition of nitric oxide synthase. J Cereb Blood Flow Metab 14:704–714
22. Nallet H, MacKenzie ET, Roussel S (2000) Blood Flow changes associated with transient penumbral depolarizations following focal cerebral ischaemia in the rat. Brain Res (in press)
23. Nedergaard M, Astrup J (1986) Infarct rim: effect of hyperglycemia on direct current potential and [^{14}C]2-deoxyglucose phosphorylation. J Cereb Blood Flow Metab 6:607–615
24. Nedergaard M, Hansen AJ (1993) Characterization of cortical depolarizations evoked in focal cerebral ischemia. J Cereb Blood Flow Metab 13:568–574
25. Nellgard B, Wieloch T (1992) NMDA-receptor blockers but not NBQX, an AMPA-receptor antagonist, inhibit spreading depression in the rat-brain. Acta Physiol Scand 146:497–503
26. Obrenovitch TP (1995) The ischaemic prenumbra: twenty years on. Cereb Brain Metab Rev 7:297–323
27. Ohta K, Graf R, Heiss WD (1997) Profiles of cortical tissue depolarization in cat focal cerebral ischemia in relation to calcium ion homeostasis and nitric oxide production. J Cereb Blood Flow Metab 17:1170–1181

28. Pinard E, Engrand N, Von Euw D, Charbonne R, Nanri K, Borredon J, Meric P, Seylaz J (1998) *In vivo* confocal microscopy investigation of rat cerebral circulation in ischemic conditions. In: Pharmacology of Cerebral Ischemia (Krieglstein J, ed), Stuttgart, Medpharm, pp 43–50
29. Pinard E, Engrand N, Seylaz J (2000) Dynamic cerebral microcirculatory changes in transient forebrain ischemia in rats: involvement of nitric oxide from neurons. J Cereb Blood Flow Metab, in press
30. Roussel SA, Van Bruggen N, King MD, Houseman J, Williams SR, Gadian DG (1994) Monitoring the initial expansion of focal ischaemia changes by diffusion-weighted MRI using a remote controlled method of occlusion. NMR Biomed 7:21–28
31. Segal SS, Damon DN, Duling BR (1989) Propagation of vasomotor responses coordinates arteriolar resistances. Am J Physiol 256:H832–H837
32. Seylaz J, Charbonne R, Nanri K, Von Euw D, Borredon J, Kacem K, Meric P, Pinard E (1999) Dynamic *in vivo* measurement of erythrocyte velocity and flow in capillaries and of microvessel diameter in the rat brain by confocal laser microscopy. J Cereb Blood Flow Metab 19:863–870
33. Shimizu-Sasamata M, Bosque-Hamilton P, Huang PL, Moskowitz MA, Lo EH (1998) Attenuated neurotransmitter release and spreading depression-like depolarizations after focal ischemia in mutant mice with disrupted type I nitric oxide synthase gene. J Neurosci 18:9564–9571
34. Shinohara M, Dollinger B, Brown G, Rapoport S, Sokoloff L (1979) Cerebral glucose utilization: local changes during and after recovery from spreading cortical depression. Science 203:188–190
35. Strong AJ, Venables GS, Gibson G (1983) The cortical ischaemic penumbra associated with occlusion of the middle cerebral artery in the cat: 1. Topography of changes in blood flow, potassium ion activity, and EEG. J Cereb Blood Flow Metab 3:86–96
36. Vogel J, Hermes A, Kuschinski W (1999) Capillary perfusion in ischemic rat brain. J Cereb Blood Flow Metab 19:S718

Cerebral vasospasm of penetrating arteries in brain stem

A. Y. Zubkov, J. H. Zhang

Abstract

Cerebral vasospasm is defined as a prolonged contraction of major cerebral arteries after subarachnoid hemorrhage (SAH). However, the possible vasospasm in penetrating arteries that could be affected easily by blood clot or other spasmogens, due to a thinner vessel wall, remain undetermined. Vasospasm of penetrating arteries may affect the survival of neurons and may be equally important as vasospasm in major arteries. This study was undertaken to examine the occurrence of penetrating vasospasm using a dog double hemorrhage model.

Forty-seven mongrel dogs were divided into nine groups of 4–6 each. In SAH groups, dogs were undergone angiography and then autologous arterial blood injection, after withdrawn equal amount of CSF, into cisterna magna on day 0. The same injection was repeated on day 2. The dogs were sacrificed on day 3, 5 or 7. In control group, no surgery was conducted. In the treatment group, dogs were treated from day 3–6 either with mitogen-activated protein kinase (MAPK) inhibitor PD98059 or U0126, or with caspase II or III inhibitors. Vehicle treatment (DMSO) was served in 4 dogs. The dogs were angiogramed and sacrificed on day 7. Penetrating arteries from brain stem were collected and fixed for transmission electron microscopy.

Mild vasospasm of basilar artery was observed on day 3 and severe vasospasm on day 5 and 7 in angiography. Penetrating arteries were removed and found spastic on days 3, 5 and 7, but not in control group. Endothelial dystrophy and partial desquamation were recorded in all dogs sacrificed on day 5 and 7. Condensation of chromatin, blebbing of membrane, condensation of cytoplasm were identified in many endothelial cells, features consistent with apoptosis. PD98059 prevented vasospasm in both major (angiographic) and penetrating arteries. U0126 failed to prevent angiographic vasospasm but prevented penetrating vasospasm. Both caspase inhibitors failed to prevent angiographic vasospasm but prevented to a mild degree of penetrating vasospasm. Vehicle treatment failed to prevent either angiographic or penetrating vasospasm.

Penetrating vasospasm occurs at a similar time course of angiographic vasospasm. The severe penetrating vasospasm on day 5 and 7 will drastically reduce the blood supply to the brain tissue. MAPK activation may be involved in penetrating vasospasm, since MAPK inhibitors prevented vasospasm. Apoptosis in endothelial cells was observed that might be resulted from severe vasoconstriction since apop-

Keyword: Penetrating arteries, apoptosis, vasospasm, subarachnoid hemorrhage

Department of Neurosurgery, University of Mississippi Medical Center, 2500 North State Street, Jackson, MS, 39216-4505, USA
e-mail: jzhang@neurosurgery.umsmed.edu

J. Krieglstein, S. Klumpp (Eds.) Pharmacology of Cerebral Ischemia 2000

tosis was not observed in penetrating arteries in dogs treated with MAPK inhibitors. Caspase inhibitors, at a low concentration, failed to prevent angiographic vasospasm, and reduced slightly penetrating vasospasm. Penetrating vasospasm may contribute to the neurological deficits of cerebral ischemia and treatment of penetration vasospasm may be a new strategy for the future studies.

Introduction

Cerebral vasospasm is considered a delayed and prolonged contraction of *major* cerebral arteries to a subarachnoid blood clot (Weir 1995). However, there are two clinical discrepancies that can not be explained by vasospasm in the major cerebral arteries. First, some patients have severe angiographic vasospasm without clinical symptoms or have clinical vasospasm with less angiographic vasospasm (Mayberg 1998). Second, vasoactive drugs, such as nimodipine, fail to prevent or reverse angiographic vasospasm but improve the clinical outcome of patients (Mayberg 1998), and some therapies, such as angioplasty, reverse angiographic vasospasm but sometimes fail to improve the neurological deficit (Zubkov et al. 1999).

These discrepancies led us to hypothesize that the clinical presentation of cerebral vasospasm reflexes not only vasospasm in the major arteries, but also in the *penetrating arteries*. Similarly, the effectiveness of treatments depends not only on the reversal of vasospasm in the major cerebral arteries but also in the penetrating arteries. In this study, we, first, investigated the morphology of penetrating arteries during vasospasm in a dog model of SAH. The vasospastic changes in penetrating arteries were correlated with angiographic vasospasm. Second, we tested if penetrating vasospasm can be reversed by vasodilators such as the inhibitors for the mitogen activated protein kinase (MAPK). Third, we examined if apoptosis occurred in penetrating arteries and if inhibitors of apoptosis will reduce vasospasm.

Materials and methods

Dog double hemorrhage model

Fourty-seven mongrel dogs of either sex, weighing 17–25 kg, were used for the dog double hemorrhage model. The dogs were anesthetized with thiopental (10 mg/kg) and mechanically ventilated during the experiments. The body temperature was kept at 37 °C with a heating blanket, and mean arterial blood pressure and blood gases were monitored through a 4F catheter inserted into the femoral artery and were maintained in normal range. Experimental subarachnoid hemorrhage was induced according to the method of Varsos et al. (1983). Cerebral angiography was performed on Exposcop 7000 (Ziehm International Medical Systems, Riverside, CA). One of the vertebral arteries was catheterized with a 4F catheter via the femoral artery, and the baseline vertebrobasilar angiogram was obtained. The cisterna magna was punctured transcutaneously, and 0.4 ml/kg of cerebrospinal fluid (CSF) was withdrawn. An equivalent amount of arterial blood was withdrawn from the femoral artery and immediately injected into the cisterna magna. The first injection was considered to be day 0 subarachnoid hemorrhage. On day 2, the same blood injection procedure was repeated without angiography.

The dogs were divided randomly into nine groups include a control (without blood injection, N = 4) group, and three hemorrhage groups to be sacrificed on days 3 (N = 4), 5 (N = 5), and 7 (N = 4). In another five groups, dogs were treated on day 3–6 with either vehicle (DMSO, N = 6), MAPK inhibitors PD98059 (N = 6), U0126 (N = 6), or caspase II (N = 6) and caspase III (N = 6) inhibitors.

Angiograph was repeated in all groups on the day of sacrifice, and the dogs were euthanized by an overdose of pentobarbital (120 mg/kg). This protocol was evaluated and approved by the University of Mississippi Medical Center Animal Care and Use Committee.

Measurements of arterial diameter

The diameters of the basilar arteries were measured in a double-blinded fashion from magnified angiograms. In order to eliminate differences in the magnification, a penny was placed on each dog's chin during the angiography run. The coin was used as a standard, and all values of the arterial diameter were relatively adjusted to the size of the coin. Two researchers independently measured the arterial diameters on the magnified angiograms at three points: distal, central, and proximal parts of the basilar artery. The mean of the three measurements was taken for the arterial diameter. The mean of all measurements of both studies was taken as a final diameter.

Morphological studies

The brain was immediately removed within 10 minutes after euthanasia and the basilar artery with the penetrating arteries were perfused with 2% glutaraldehyde solution. Under the guidance of a surgical microscope, the brain stem penetrating arteries (paramedian and short circumferential branches of the basilar artery) were isolated and kept in 2% glutaraldehyde. At least 6 penetrating arteries were studies from each dog. The penetrating arteries were post-fixed with osmium tetroxide, dehydrated in a graded series of acetone, embedded in epon-araldite epoxy resin, sectioned at 60 Å, and examined with a LEO 906 (Leo, Thoenwood, NY) transmission electron microscope (TEM).

Inhibitors

Two selective MAPK inhibitors were chosen for the study: PD98059 (BIOMOL Research Laboratories, Inc., Plymouth Meeting, PA) and U0126 (Promega, Madison, WI). Both drugs were diluted in dimethyl sulfoxide (DMSO) to 10 mM. Two selective antagonists for caspase-2 (Z-VDVAD-FMK) and caspase-3 (Z-DEVD-FMK) were purchased from R & D Systems Inc., Minneapolis, MN. Both drugs were diluted in dimethyl sulfoxide (DMSO) to 20 mM.

The doses of antagonists were calculated for each dog to reach the same drug levels in the dogs' cerebrospinal fluid (CSF), taking into account the relative size of the CSF space. MAPK inhibitors (~ 40 μl) or caspase inhibitors (~ 20 μl) were mixed with 1 ml of CSF and injected intracisternally to obtain a final concentration in CSF of 10 μM, assuming that the canine CSF volume is 2.0 ml/kg (Zoghbi et al. 1985).

Data analysis

Data are expressed as the mean ± the standard error of the mean. Statistical differences between angiographic values in the control and other groups were compared using one-way analysis of variance (ANOVA) and, then, a Tukey-Kramer multiple comparison procedure if significant variance was found. The clinical scores were compared by a Kruskal-Wallis One Way ANOVA on Ranks, followed by Dunn's multiple comparison procedure if the significant differences were found by ANOVA on Ranks analysis. A value of $P < 0.05$ was considered statistically significant.

Results

Angiographic vasospasm

The residual diameter of the basilar artery, which was compared with day 0 angiogram, decreased gradually in a time-dependent manner from day 3 (80%), day 5 (68%) through day 7 (53.5%). MAPK inhibitor PD98059, but not U0126, significantly reversed vasospasm and increased residual diameter to 79.0% on day 7. Caspase III, but not caspase II inhibitor, partially reversed ($P < 0.058$) angiographic cerebral vasospasm.

Morphology of normal penetrating arteries

The endothelial cells form a continuous monolayer overlying the internal elastic lamina (IEL). The endothelial cells have tight junctions between each other and with the basal membrane. No corrugation is observed in the IEL. Smooth muscle cells (1–4 layers) lie under the IEL, surrounded by the collagen matrix and are elongated in shape. The adventitial layer consists of fibroblast cells surrounded by connective tissue (Fig. 1A).

The normal endothelial cells have an ovoid and elongated shape. All organelles are clearly present in the cytoplasm. Normal peripheral heterochromatin is present in all cells without any condensation of chromatin. No blebbing or vacuolization of cytoplasm is noticed. The tight junctions between the cells and contact between the cells and the basal membrane are well preserved (Fig. 1B).

Morphology of penetrating arteries after SAH

Beginning on the third day, vasospasm developed in the penetrating arteries (Fig. 1C). A morphological review showed that the arteries appeared contracted with a corrugation of the IEL. The smooth muscle cells were contracted in a round shape although to necrotic changes were visible. The endothelial cells were shortened and slightly protruding into the lumen. Dystrophy of the endothelial cells was observed (Fig. 1D). The apoptosis-like changes characterized by the chromatin condensation appeared in some of the endothelial cells and blebbing of the cytoplasmic membrane. There was no marked desquamation of the endothelial cells from the basal membrane. There were no changes noted on the adventitial side of the vessel.

On day 5, severe vasoconstriction was noticed (Fig. 2A). Excessive corrugation of the IEL accompanied by partial endothelial desquamation, disruption of the tight junctions between the endothelial cells, and protruding of the remaining endothelial cells into the lumen were the most striking features. The smooth muscle cells were shortened, and no morphological alterations were noticed in the smooth muscle cells or in the adventitia. The apoptotic-like changes in endothelial cells were characterized by chromatin condensation, blebbing, condensation of cytoplasm, vacuolization of cytoplasm, and on occurrence of apoptotic bodies (Fig. 2B).

Similar morphological changes were observed in sample from day 7 dogs. The corrugation of the IEL, contraction of the smooth muscle cells (Fig. 2C) and protruding of the endothelial cells were all noticed. The chromatin condensation, dystrophy of the endothelial cytoplasm, and vacuolization of cytoplasm occurred (Fig. 2D).

Morphology of penetrating arteries after treatment

(1) Vehicle group

The penetrating arteries were severely contracted with a corrugation of the IEL, partial desquamation of the endothelial cells, and dystrophic changes in the endothelial cells. The smooth muscle cells appeared to be contracted without any dystrophic changes (Fig. 3A).

(2) PD98059 Group

No severe morphological vasospasm in the penetrating arteries was noted. The penetrating arteries had a slight corrugation of the IEL and a slight contraction of smooth muscle cells, but the endothelial and smooth muscle cells had not dystrophic changes as noted on transmission microscopy study (Fig. 3B).

(3) U0126 Group

The penetrating arteries did not develop morphological vasospasm. The endothelial cells preserved their tight junctions and their attachment to the basal membrane. No dystrophic changes

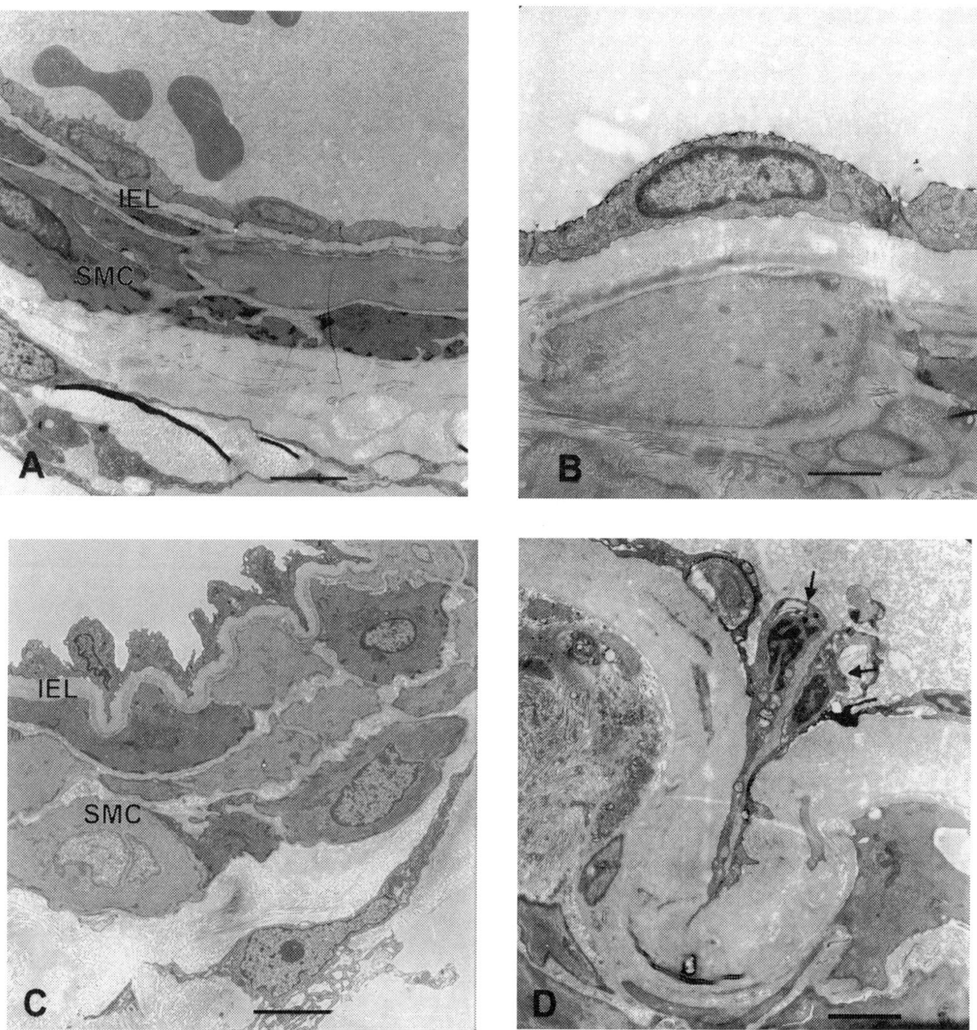

Fig. 1. Normal penetrating arteries (**A**) consist of three layers: endothelial, smooth muscle, and adventitial layers. The endothelial layer is a monolayer of ovoid endothelial cells connected by tight junctions. The internal elastic lamina (IEL) consists of elastic fibers, lies smoothly under the endothelial cells, and is not corrugated. The smooth muscle layer (SMC) includes 1–3 layers of smooth muscle cells surrounded by connective tissue, consisting predominantly of collagen fibers. The adventitial layer is a connective tissue consisting predominantly of fibroblasts and collagen.
Normal endothelial cells (**B**) are ovoid shaped, connected tightly with neighboring endothelial cells, and underlying the basal lamina. The nucleus is ovoid shaped and possesses euchromatin and peripheral heterochromatin. No condensation of chromatin, no blebbing of the membrane, and no vacuolization were observed. All intracellular organelles have normal appearance.
The penetrating arteries from day-3 dogs after SAH (**C**) appears contracted with corrugation of the IEL. The smooth muscle cells are rounded up and shortened. No necrosis is observed in either the smooth muscle cells or in the adventitial layer. The endothelial cells (**D**) are dystrophic with blebbing of the membrane and condensation of chromatin under larger magnifications. No endothelial detachment from the basal lamina is noted.
Bars: ***A****. 3.36 μm,* ***B****. 1.56 μm,* ***C****. 4.34 μm,* ***D****. 2.01 μm.*

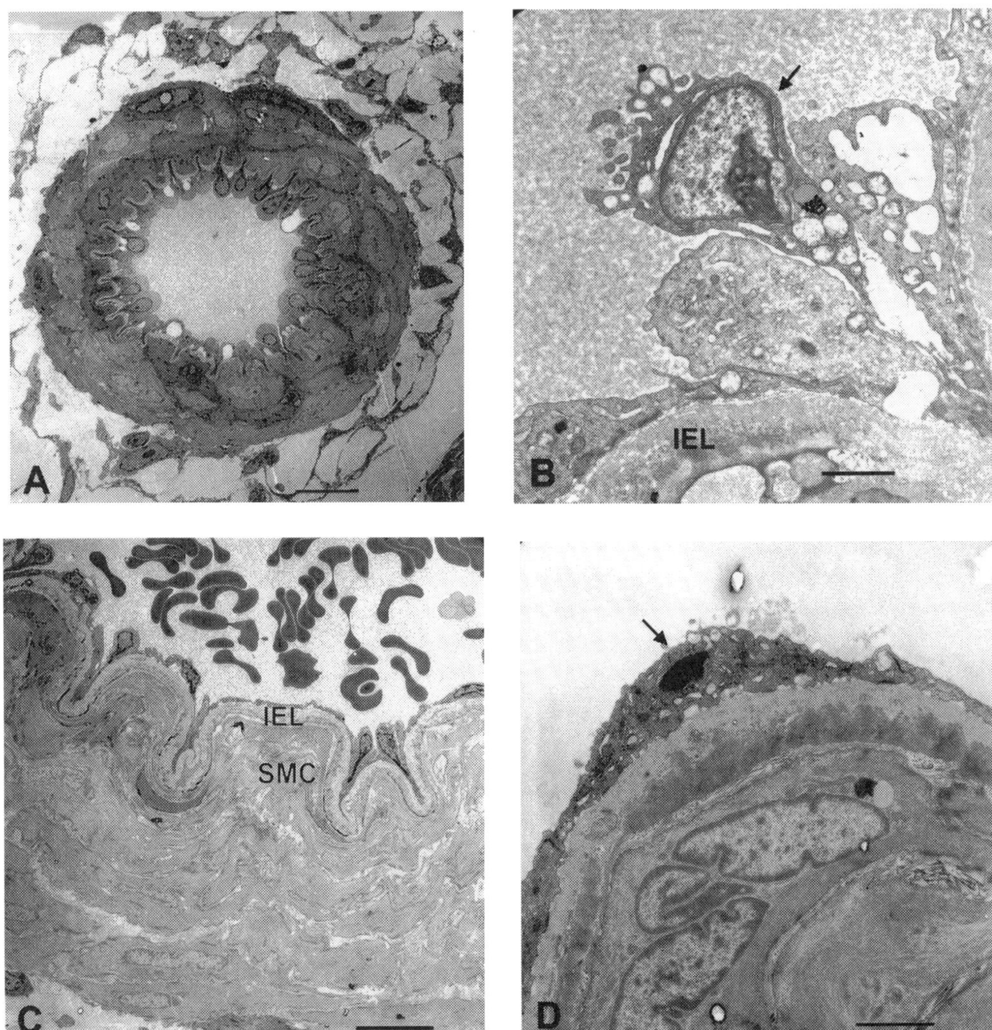

Fig. 2. The penetrating arteries from day-5 dogs after SAH are contracted (**A**) with excessive corrugation of the IEL and rounding of smooth muscle cells. No necrotic changes are noted in the smooth muscle cells. Partial desquamation of endothelial cells is visible in some areas of the vessels (**B**). Condensation of chromatin, vacuolization, condensation of cytoplasm, and blebbing of the membrane are recorded in the endothelial cells under larger magnifications.
The penetrating arteries from day-7 dogs after SAH (**C**) are contracted with excessive corrugation of the IEL and rounding of the smooth muscle cells. No necrotic cells are noted in the smooth muscle layer. Disrupted tight junctions between the endothelial cells and detachment of the endothelial cells from the basal lamina are recorded (**D**). Vacuolization in cytoplasm, blebbing of membrane, and condensation of chromatin in the endothelial cells are noted to be more wide spread than the penetrating arteries from the day-3 dogs (arrow).
Bars: ***A.*** *15.6 μm,* ***B.*** *2.01 μm,* ***C.*** *9.3 μm,* ***D.*** *2.01 μm.*

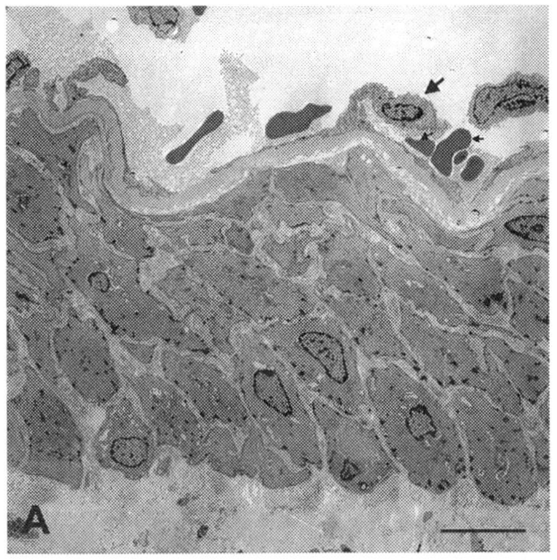

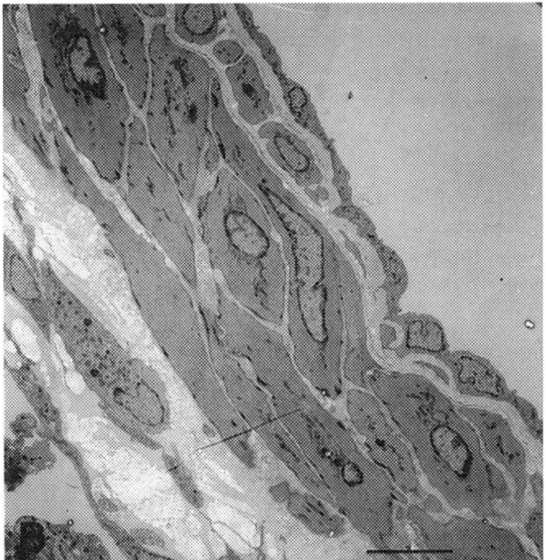

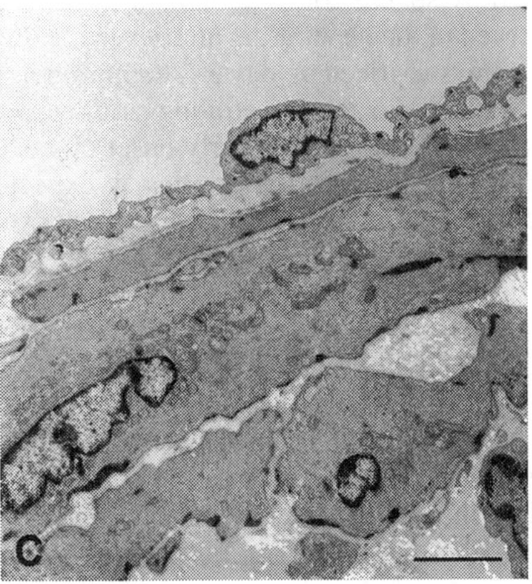

were noted in the endothelial and smooth muscle cells. The IEL was not corrugated (Fig. 3C).

(4) Caspase-2 inhibitor group

The penetrating arteries were moderately contracted, demonstrated by corrugation of IEL, some endothelial cells had apoptosis-like changes, such as peripheral condensation of chromatin (Fig. 4A).

(5) Caspase-3 inhibitor group

The morphological picture of vasospasm in the penetrating arteries resembled the picture in the SAH and DMSO groups: the vessels were contracted with corrugation of the IEL, contraction of the smooth muscle cells, and dystrophic changes in endothelial cells. Tight junctions between the endothelial cells were disrupted. Some endothelial cells demonstrated condensation of chromatin, condensation of cytoplasm, vacuolization of cytoplasm, and blebbing of the cytoplasmic membrane (Fig. 4B).

Fig. 3. Morphological findings in the penetrating arteries in the SAH with vehicle treatment group (**A**). The penetrating arteries appeared to be significantly contracted. IEL was severely corrugated. The endothelial cells (EC) were dystrophic with an occasional disruption of the tight junctions (C. arrow). The smooth muscle cells (SMC) were contracted and dystrophic. All five dogs developed severe vasospasm in the large arteries (not shown).
Morphological changes in the SAH with PD98059 treatment group (**B**). The IEL was less corrugated in comparison to the control and DMSO-treated groups. The endothelial cells (EC) and smooth muscle cells (SMC) did not have any dystrophic changes. The smooth muscle cells appeared to be more elongated and less contracted.
Morphological changes in SAH with the U0126 treatment group (**C**). Severe vasospasm, of a comparable degree with vasospasm in the control and vehicle-treated groups, developed in the basilar arteries of all four dogs. However, an injection of U0126 completely abolished the occurrence of vasospasm in the penetrating arteries. No corrugation IEL was detected. The endothelial cells (EC) maintained potent tight junction and were not dystrophic. The smooth muscle cells (SMC) did not have any dystrophic changes and were not contracted.
Bars: A. – 7.2 μm, B. – 7.2 μm, C. – 2.6 μm.

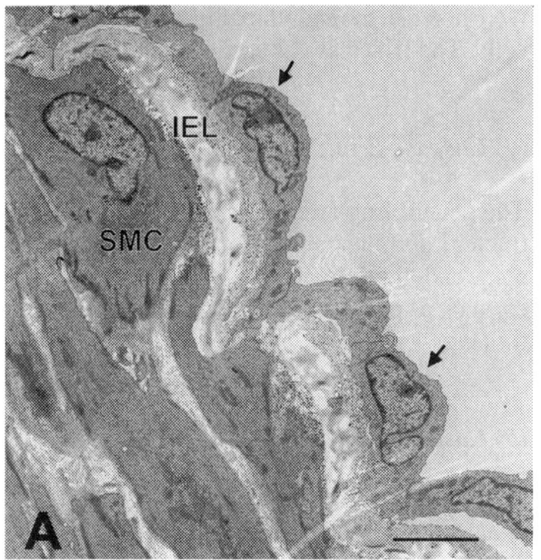

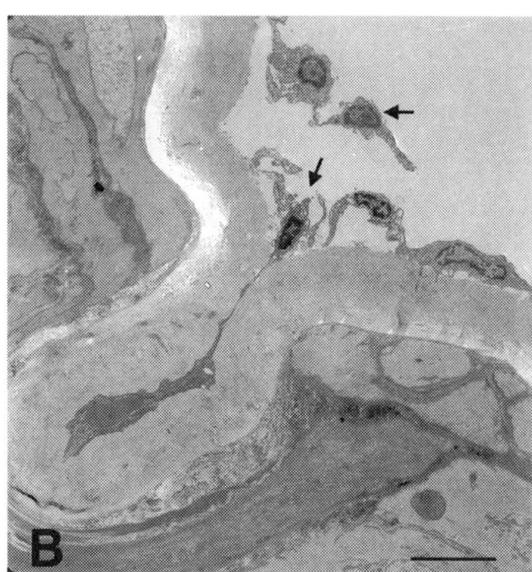

Fig. 4. Morphological presentation of penetrating arteries in caspase-2-treated group (**A**). The penetrating arteries were morphologically contracted, with corrugation of the IEL, and contraction of the smooth muscle cells. In some cell, condensation of chromatin was detected (arrows), but overall there were less dystrophic changes than in the SAH and DMSO groups.
Morphological presentation of brainstem penetrating arteries in caspase-3-treated group (**B**). Penetrating arteries were morphologically contracted, demonstrated by severe corrugation of the IEL, and contraction of the smooth muscle cells. The endothelial cells were dystrophic, with partial loss of morphological integrity of the tight junctions between cells and with basal lamina. Some cells had apoptosis-like changes as demonstrated by the condensation of the peripheral chromatin, electron condensation of the cytoplasm (arrows).
Bars: A. – 3.4 μm, B. – 5.6 μm.

Discussion

Penetrating vasospasm

Several attempts were made to describe morphological changes in the penetrating arteries prior to the study. Hughes et al. (Hughes and Schianchi 1978) demonstrated by light microscopy in an autopsy series of patients who died from SAH that the intima was lifted with exudate in addition to corrugation of the IEL in the small cerebral arteries. Okhuma et al. (1997) demonstrated the constriction of the intraparenchymal arterioles that occurred after SAH in a double-hemorrhage dog model. In contrast, Nihei et al. (1991) failed to demonstrate any significant vasospasm in the small pial arteries of the brain stem in a *rabbit* double hemorrhage model and concluded that the larger arteries were affected by vasospasm after SAH more readily than the smaller arteries. In the current study, severe microscopic vasospasm, demonstrated by severe corrugation of the IEL, was observed in the penetrating arteries in the dogs that were sacrificed on day 3. The morphological changes in the penetrating arteries progressed up to day 7. The early onset of vasospasm in the penetrating arteries is expected since the penetrating arteries have thinner vessel walls than the large arteries and are more likely to be affected by blood clot components, which are a proposed causative agent for vasospasm (Macdonald et al. 1991), from the adventitial side. The discrepancy between our study and Nihei et al. (1991) may be due to differences in the species.

The alteration of endothelial cells is a major part of the morphological presentation of vasospasm in the major arteries. In the recent past, these changes were attributed to apoptosis by Ogihara et al. (1999). The authors found that oxyhemoglobin caused cell death in cultured endothelial cells. The cells exposed to oxyhemoglobin for 24 hours demonstrated DNA ladders and apoptotic morphological changes. Zubkov et al. (2000) described the apoptotic changes in endothelial cells of a patient, who died from vasospasm. In the current study, morphological changes in the penetrating arteries after SAH in a dog double-hemorrhage model revealed that apoptosis of endothelial cells developed on Day 3 after SAH and persisted at least until Day 7. The same pattern of apoptotic changes was observed in the major cerebral arteries (Zubkov, unpublished data).

Role of apoptosis in penetrating vasospasm

Although the presented data suggests on occurrence of apoptosis in the endothelial cells of vasospastic penetrating arteries, the role of apoptosis in the pathogenesis of prolonged vessel contraction remained unknown. Apoptosis of endothelial cells will cause cell death and the detachment of endothelial cells, expose IEL and collagen to the blood flow, activate platelets and form thrombus. All these might lead to narrowing of the lumen diameter. Thus, apoptosis might be one of the causes of vasospasm. On the contrary, apoptosis might be a consequence of vasospasm due to the severe and prolonged contraction of cerebral arteries. However, regardless the cause or consequence of vasospasm, apoptosis certainly promotes and maintains vasoconstriction, and enhances cerebral ischemia. In this study, we hypothesized that apoptosis might be important for vasospasm and apoptosis inhibitors might reduce vasospasm.

However, caspase II and III inhibitors failed to reverse either angiographic or penetrating vasospasm in this dog model study. Furthermore, both caspase inhibitors failed to prevent apoptosis in endothelial cells. Even though caspase inhibitors did not prevent vasospasm in this study, the role of apoptosis in cerebral vasospasm cannot be excluded for the following reasons. First, we used a low concentration of caspase inhibitors (10 μM) in this study. High concentration of caspase inhibitors (100 μM) were used in the prevention of apoptosis in other disorders (Liu et al. 1998), and caspase inhibitors prevented apoptosis in neurons (Wiessner et al. 2000), myocardium (Weiland et al. 2000), and vascular endothelial cells (Farber et al. 1999; He et al. 2000). Thus, higher doses of the drugs may be required to have a therapeutic effect. Second, caspase inhibitors were injected into the cisterna magna and need to penetrate all layers of the vascular wall to reach endothelial cells. The information regarding the permeability of caspase inhibitors 2 or 3 through the vessel wall are not available. Third, the signal transduction in apoptosis is complex. Caspase-2 or -3 may not be involved in the endothelial apoptosis in the dog model of vasospasm, or inhibitors of caspase-2 or -3 may not prevent all the signals for apoptosis. Other caspases such as caspase 4, 6, 7 or 9 are all involved in apoptosis in different tissues (Cohen 1997). On the contrary, it may be possible that apoptosis is a parallel entity in the pathogenesis of vasospasm and might be a contributing factor, but not a primary cause, of vasospasm. However, apoptosis may not only occur in the major or penetrating arteries but may be also in the smaller arterioles and neuronal tissue. Thus, the possible protective effect of apoptosis inhibitors in neurons need to be studied in the future.

Role of MAPK in penetrating vasospasm

Several studies reported an important role of MAPK in cerebral vasospasm. The MAPK activation started on day 2 in the dog double-hemorrhage model and was still above baseline on day 7 (Fujikawa et al. 1999). Hemolysate-induced stimulation of MAPK started within 3 minutes and lasted up to 120 minutes. PD98059 effectively blocked the hemolysate-induced contraction of the rabbit basilar artery and hemolysate-induced enhancement of MAPK immunoprecipitation (Zubkov et al. 1999). In another study, the effects of PD98059 and U0126 on an endothelin-1-induced contraction of the rabbit basilar artery were examined. Both drugs significantly inhibited the contraction induced by endothelin-1 (Zubkov et al. 2000). In this study, PD98059 reduced vasospasm in major and penetrating arteries. Although U0126 failed to prevent angiographic vasospasm, U0126 reduced vasospasm of the penetrating arteries. The failure of U0126 in reversing angiographic vasospasm may be explained by its poor stability and penetrating ability in major arteries. The MAPK inhibitors were administered starting on day 3 after experimental SAH, rather than beginning treatment immediately after or prior to SAH, to reflect clinical practice. The concentration of MAPK inhibitors was the same or lower than the concentration used in isolated arteries (Zubkov et al. 1999). This study demonstrated that MAPK is involved in vasospasm in the major arteries as well as the penetrating arteries.

Conclusions

This study demonstrated cerebral vasospasm in the penetrating arteries. The time course of vasospasm is consistent between major and penetrating arteries. The contraction of the penetrating arteries is attributed, at least in part, to the activation of MAPK. Apoptosis of the endothelial cells in the penetrating arteries coincide with the onset of the vasospasm. The role of apoptosis in penetrating vasospasm is unclear and requires further investigation.

Acknowledgment

This work was partially supported by a grant-in-aid to J.H.Z. from the American Heart Association and by a NIH grant 1S10RR11321-01A1 to the Department of Anatomy. The authors thank Glenn Hoskins for assistance with transmission electron microscopy.

References

1. Cohen GM (1997) Caspases: the executioners of apoptosis. Biochem J 326:1–16
2. Farber A, Kitzmiller T, Morganelli PM et al. (1999) A caspase inhibitor decreases oxidized low-density lipoprotein-induced apoptosis in bovine endothelial cells. J Surg Res 85:323–330
3. Fujikawa H, Tani E, Yamaura I et al. (1999) Activation of protein kinases in canine basilar artery in vasospasm. J Cereb Blood Flow Metab 19:44–52
4. He J, Xiao Y, Zhang L (2000) Cocaine induces apoptosis in human coronary artery endothelial cells [In Process Citation]. J Cardiovasc Pharmacol 35:572–580
5. Hughes JT, Schianchi PM (1978) Cerebral artery spasm. A histological study at necropsy of the blood vessels in cases of subarachnoid hemorrhage. J Neurosurg 48:515–525
6. Liu W, Staecker H, Stupak H et al. (1998) Caspase inhibitors prevent cisplatin-induced apoptosis of auditory sensory cells. Neuroreport 9:2609–2614
7. Macdonald RL, Weir BK, Runzer TD et al. (1991) Etiology of cerebral vasospasm in primates. J Neurosurg 75:415–424
8. Mayberg MR (1998) Cerebral vasospasm. Neurosurg Clin N Am 9:615–627
9. Nihei H, Kassell NF, Dougherty DA et al. (1991) Does vasospasm occur in small pial arteries and arterioles of rabbits? Stroke 22:1419–1425
10. Ogihara K, Zubkov AY, Bernanke DH et al. (1999) Oxyhemoglobin Induces Apoptosis in Cultured Endothelial Cells. J Neurosurg 91:459–465
11. Ohkuma H, Itoh K, Shibata S et al. (1997) Morphological changes of intraparenchymal arterioles after experimental subarachnoid hermorrhage in dogs. Neurosurgery 41:230–235
12. Varsos VG, Liszczak TM, Han DH et al. (1983) Delayed cerebral vasospasm is not reversible by aminophylline, nifedipine, or papaverine in a "two-hemorrhage" canine model. J Neurosurg 58:11–17
13. Weiland U, Haendeler J, Ihling C et al. (2000) Inhibition of endogenous nitric oxide synthase potentiates ischemia-reperfusion-induced myocardial apoptosis via a caspase-3 dependent pathway. Cardiovasc Res 45:671–678
14. Weir B (1995) The pathophysiology of cerebral vasospasm. Br J Neurosurg 9:375–390
15. Wiessner C, Sauer D, Alaimo D et al. (2000) Protective effect of a caspase inhibitor in models for cerebral ischemia in vitro and in vivo. Cell Mol Biol 46:53–62
16. Zoghbi HY, Okumura S, Laurent JP et al. (1985) Acute effect of glycerol on net cerebrospinal fluid production in dogs. J Neurosurg 63:759–762
17. Zubkov AY, Ogihara K, Bernanke DH et al. (2000a) Apoptosis of endothelial cells in vessels affected by cerebral vasospasm. Surg Neurol 53:260–266
18. Zubkov A, Lewis AI, Scalzo D et al. (1999a) Morphological Changes after Percutaneous Transluminal Angioplasty. Surg Neurol 51:399–403
19. Zubkov A, Rollins K, Parent A et al. (2000b) Mechanism of endothelin-1-induced contraction in rabbit basilar artery. Stroke 31:526–533
20. Zubkov AY, Ogihara K, Tumu P et al. (1999b) Mitogen-activated protein kinase mediates hemolysate-induced contraction in rabbit basilar artery. J Neurosurg 90:1091–1097

Repair, recovery and neuroprotection

DNA damage and repair in the setting of mild injury

H.-M. Lee, G. H. Greeley, Jr., E. W. Englander

Abstract

Reactive oxygen species (ROS) generated in the course of hypoxia/ischemia and reperfusion damage lipids, proteins and DNA. We measured the formation of oxidative DNA damage and the extent of DNA repair in the rat brain after hypoxia using the Quantitative Polymerase Chain Reaction (QPCR) methodology. The principle of this detection method is that many types of DNA damage block thermostable polymerase-mediated DNA amplification. This results in a decrease in amplification product amounts since only intact DNA templates can be amplified. Hence, with this assay, amplification is a measure of DNA templates without damage. We employed two QPCR-based assays; one to measure the integrity of the entire mitochondrial genome and the other the integrity of transcribed regions in nuclear DNA. The later is a novel assay, which utilizes the Short Interspersed DNA Elements (SINEs) residing in high copy numbers in mammalian genomes. Using these assays, we found that hypoxia injures both, mitochondrial and nuclear DNA in the rat brain and that subsequently the DNA repair process is activated. The activation of DNA repair under these conditions was further substantiated in an increase in immunoreactivity of DNA repair enzymes involved in the repair of oxidative DNA damage, polymerase β and AP endonuclease.

Introduction

The roles of DNA damage and DNA repair processes are being increasingly recognized in neurodegenerative disorders (Citterio et al. 2000; Hermon et al. 1998; Lovell et al. 2000; Mandir et al. 1999), in aging (Atamna et al. 2000; Feuers 1998; Michikawa et al. 1999; Schmitz et al. 1999), in multiple brain injuries including, ischemia (Chen et al. 1997; Hayashi et al. 1999; Jin et al. 1999; Tobita et al. 1995), cold injury (Morita-Fujimura et al. 1999), trauma (Kaya et al. 1999) and most recently in seizures induced by systemic kainic acid (Lan et al. 2000). Impaired cerebral energy metabolism during hypoxia/ischemia has been decisively linked to excessive generation of reactive oxygen species (ROS) that damage macromolecules, ie, lipids, proteins and DNA (Cao et al. 1988; Chopp et al. 1996; Facchinetti et al. 1998;

Keywords: hypoxia, oxidative DNA damage, DNA repair, rat, DNA polymerase β, AP endonuclease

Department of Surgery and Shriners Hospitals for Children, The University of Texas Medical Branch, 815 Market Street, Galveston, Texas 77550
e-mail: elenglan@utmb.edu

Hayashi et al. 1999; Hou et al. 1997; Jin et al. 1996; Liu et al. 1996; Mehmet et al. 1998; Ozawa 1997; Piantadosi and Zhang 1996; Piantadosi, Zhang and Demchenko 1997; Ratan 1994; Sakhi et al. 1994; Tan et al. 1999). Furthermore, a definitive correlation of an ischemic insult with direct oxidative DNA damage and activation of DNA repair in the mouse brain has been recently established (Liu et al. 1996). In that study, eight different types of oxidative DNA lesions consistent with induction by free radicals were detected in total cellular DNA. Interestingly, partial removal of damage was observed within 4–6 hours of reperfusion, yet, the subsequent appearance of nuclei with DNA fragmentation and morphological changes suggestive of cell death were also observed. Oxidative DNA damage is considered particularly injurious to mtDNA because mitochondria are the primary sites of oxygen metabolism, and their genomes, unprotected by chromatin proteins, are located close to the inner membrane, the site of electron transport and generation of free radicals (Fujimura et al. 1998; Murakami et al. 1998; Suzuki et al. 1998). Hence, accumulation of DNA damage and resultant mitochondrial deletions have been strongly implicated in the etiology of brain dysfunction, aging and neurodegenerative disease (Ames et al. 1995; Croteau and Bohr 1997; Druzhyna et al. 1998; Fujimura et al. 1998; Murakami et al. 1998; Schapira 1996; Suzuki et al. 1998; Wei 1998). Interestingly, in the human brain, an increased frequency of mtDNA deletions has been correlated with a condition of chronic hypoxia and linked to impaired energy metabolism suggesting that chronic hypoxia should be more closely examined in the pathophysiology of central nervous system diseases (Merril et al. 1996).

To assess the formation of oxidative DNA damage in the rat brain in our experimental model where hypoxia is produced by exposure of rats to reduced respiratory oxygen we used the quantitative PCR (QPCR)-based approach. This approach is based on the fact that many types of DNA lesions form blocks to thermostable polymerase-mediated DNA synthesis (Fig. 1). This results in decreased amplification since only intact DNA templates are amplified (Govan et al. 1990; Kalinowski 1992; Yakes and van Houten 1997b). Since current technologies support amplification of long segments of

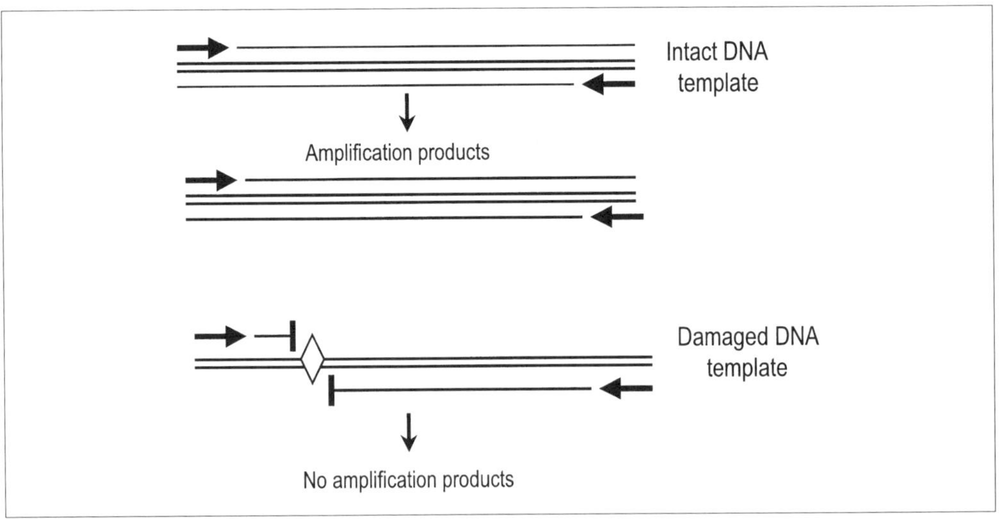

Fig. 1. Schematic representation of the application of Quantitative Polymerase Chain Reaction (QPCR) for detection of DNA damage. With this assay only intact DNA, free of lesions can be duplicated and serve as template for subsequent rounds of amplification. A DNA lesion, which blocks the thermostable polymerase-mediated DNA synthesis and abolishes amplification, is depicted. Thus, amplification is a measure of intact templates without lesions.

DNA (> 10 kb) the assay provides adequate sensitivity for detection of physiologically relevant levels of damage. Lesion frequency is calculated assuming random distribution of lesions and using the Poisson equation [$f(x) = e^{-\lambda} \lambda/x!$]. *The frequency* of lesions is then expressed as $\lambda = -\ln A_D/A_C$, where A_D is amount amplification from damaged and A_C from intact control templates (Yakes and van Houten 1997b). In our studies, two sensitive QPCR-based assays are employed; one measures the integrity of the complete mitochondrial genome (Yakes and van Houten 1997a), and the other monitors the overall integrity of genomic DNA. To accomplish the latter, we utilize the *S*hort *In*terspersed repetitive DNA *E*lements (SINEs) which reside in high copy numbers in transcribed regions of mammalian genomes (Dieninger 1989). We use PCR primers complementary to the SINE consensus sequence, to simultaneously amplify long, random segments of DNA abutted by pairs of SINEs and thus, obtain information on the overall integrity of the genome (Englander et al. 1999; Englander and Howard 1997; Wang et al. 1999a; Wang et al. 1999b; Wang et al. 2000). We found that in the hippocampus and cortex, damage is formed in mitochondrial and nuclear DNA and that this damage is partially repaired in the course of a recovery period in ambient air.

Oxidative DNA lesions which include oxidized bases, abasic sites and DNA strand breaks with non-ligatable ends, are thought to be repaired by the base excision repair (BER) pathway (Mitra et al. 1997). Of primary interest to us therefore, were DNA repair enzymes which are involved in BER pathway, and are expressed in the rat brain. Specifically, we focused on the AP-endonuclease (APE) (Edwards et al. 1998a; Edwards et al. 1998b; Ramana et al. 1998; Walker et al. 1994; Xu et al. 1998) and DNA polymerase β (Srivastava et al. 1998; Zucconi et al. 1992) and found that immunoreactivity of these repair enzymes increased in the brain following a hypoxic episode.

Methods

Model of Brain Hypoxia in the Rat

We have used a brain hypoxia model in which conscious rats are exposed to 4% oxygen/nitrogen mixtures for 30 min (Marti and Risau 1998; Semenza et al. 1991; Wiener et al. 1996). Following administration of hypoxia, rats were sacrificed or allowed to recover in ambient air for three hours (Englander et al. 1999). The number of animals in each test group was eight. Sacrifice was by decapitation. Harvested brains were immediately dissected on ice. Brain regions (cortex, and hippocampus) were collected and snap frozen in liquid nitrogen. The dissection of each brain and tissue collection was carried out within 2–2.5 minutes. Additional rats were used for collecting brains for histology and immunohistochemistry.

Detection of DNA Damage

High molecular weight DNA was purified from hippocampus and cortex of control and test animals. Typically, 25 mg aliquots of tissue were homogenized on ice and processed using QIAamp Tissue Kit (Qiagen, CA). The quality of DNA was verified by electrophoresis in agarose gels and EtBr staining. DNA was quantified by ethidium bromide fluorescence with an A4-filter fluorometer (Optical Technology Devices, Elmsford, NY) according to the manufacturer. Quantitative PCR for nuclear DNA was carried out using the Expand 20 Kb^{plus} PCR System (Boehringer Mannheim), with primers corresponding to the consensus sequence of the rat SINE, ID (sense:5'-GGCTGGGGATTTAG-3' and antisense 5'-TTCGGAGCTGGGGA-3'). Total DNA, 15 ng, was amplified by 8 cycles (10 seconds at 94 °C, 30 seconds at 52 °C, 3 minutes at 72 °C), with 0.75 μCi of 3000 Ci/mM [α-^{32}P]dCTP, 350 μM dNTPs, 300 nmoles primer and 2.5 u enzyme. Amplification products were resolved in 7 M urea, 6% polyacrylamide gels and quantified using the ImageQuant software on a phosphoimager (Molecular Dynamics). Amplification counts obtained with damaged DNA were divided by counts obtained with control templates, to express the relative amount of intact DNA templates present in the reaction.

For detection of damage in mitochondrial DNA, the QPCR assay was conducted as described previously (Yakes and van Houten 1997) with some modifications. The primers for amplification of complete rat mitochondrial genome (sense 5'-CCTCCCATTCATTATCG-CCGCCCTTGC-3' and antisense primer: 5'-GATGGGGCCGGTAGGTCGATAAAG-GAG-3') were designed by Dr. Bennett van Houten. Briefly, PCR reaction was initiated by addition of enzyme during a hot-start at 70 °C, 15 ng total DNA was amplified by 27 cycles (15 seconds at 94 °C, 12 minutes at 68 °C), with 0.75 µCi of 3000 Ci/mM [α-^{32}P]dCTP, 350 µM dNTPs, 300 nmoles primer and 2.5 u enzyme using the Expand 20 Kb^{plus} PCR System (Boehringer Mannheim). Amplification products were resolved in native 4% polyacrylamide gels. The incorporated label was quantified and the ratio of non-damaged templates was calculated as described above for nuclear DNA.

Histological and Immunohistochemical Examination of the Rat Brain

The brains were removed, postfixed in neutral-buffered formalin overnight at 4 °C and paraffin embedded. 3 µm coronal brain sections were stained by standard procedures; immunohistochemical staining: Antibodies for pol-β were a kind gift from Dr. S. Wilson and for APE from Santa Cruz (Santa Cruz, CA). Specificity of staining was verified by substitution of primary antisera with nonimmune serum. Immunocytochemistry was performed using the avidin/biotin/peroxidase procedure (Vector Laboratories, Burlingame, CA) according to the manufacturer, after staining, sections were lightly counterstained with hematoxylin.

Results

Detection of DNA Damage

Rats were exposed to 4% O_2 for 30 min. Control group and two test groups were examined; hypoxia alone (4% O_2 for 30 min) and hypoxia followed by a 3-hour recovery (n = 8 rats/group). Following treatment, DNA was purified and examined for formation of DNA damage. QPCR with primers that amplify the complete mitochondrial genome was carried out. Radiolabeled amplification products were resolved in native polyacrylamide gels and quantified. A reduction in amplification product amounts, which is indicative of DNA damage, was observed with DNA isolated after hypoxia from both the hippocampus and cortex (Fig. 2, arrowheads). In the hippocampus (Fig. 2, left panel), a substantial DNA damage was detected in mitochondrial DNA, followed by some restoration of amplification signal indicating partial removal of damage after the 3-hour recovery period. Interestingly, recent findings by others show that a capacity for repair of oxidative DNA damage exists in mitochondria (Croteau and Bohr 1997; Cullinane and Bohr 1998; Dianov et al. 1998). The damage detected in mitochondrial DNA from the cortex (Fig. 2, right panel) persisted and no significant removal of lesions was noted during the 3-hour recovery period. The ratio between damaged and intact DNA was calculated by dividing counts obtained with DNA from either test group by counts obtained from the control group. The relative amplification for each group is shown as bar graphs (Fig. 2, bottom) and represents the ratio between intact DNA templates present in reactions assembled for each treatment and those present in the control group.

The same DNA samples from hippocampus and cortex of control and hypoxic rat brains were examined also for nuclear DNA damage. QPCR assays with primers complementary to the consensus sequence of the rat SINE, ID were conducted to assess the overall integrity of genomic DNA. Radiolabeled amplification products were resolved on denaturing polyacrylamide gels, visualized and quantified. A re-

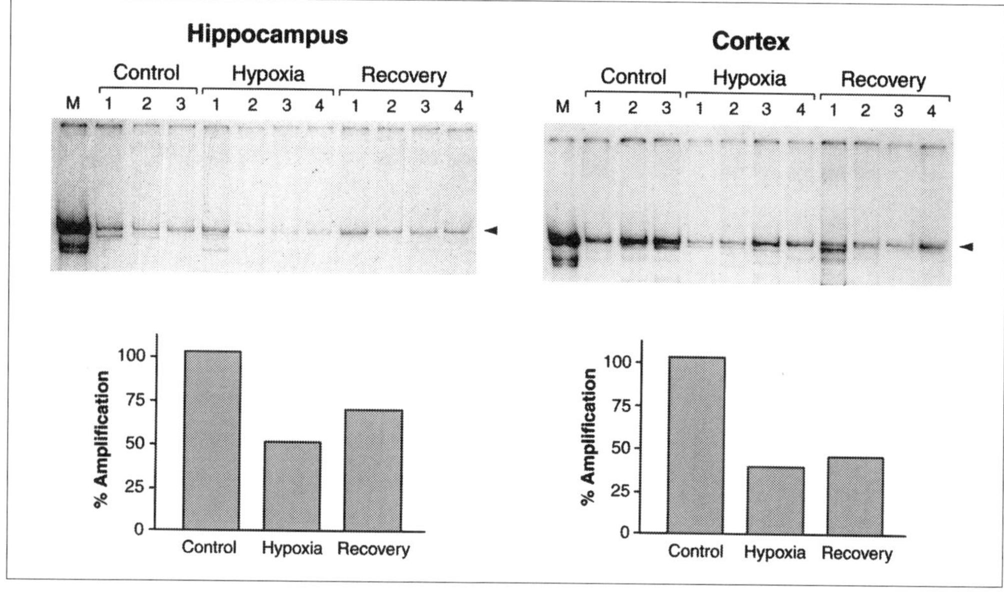

Fig. 2. Hypoxia-induced mitochondrial DNA damage in rat hippocampus and cortex. A representative autoradiogram shows a substantial reduction in amplification products (arrowheads) in the hippocampus and cortex. Samples collected from 8 rats per group were analyzed, of which 4 samples for each group are shown (control, hypoxia, hypoxia and recovery). A substantial decrease in amplification is observed in the hippocampus and cortex after hypoxia. In the hippocampus an increase in amplification is seen after a subsequent 3-hour recovery in ambient air. No significant increase in amplification is observed at that time in the cortex. Label incorporated into individual bands was quantified as integrated volume using a phosphoimager (Molecular Dynamics) with ImageQuant software. Each DNA sample was analyzed by three PCR reactions. Values recorded for each group (n = 8) in 3 independent PCR reactions were averaged to generate the relative amplification signal for each experimental group. Amplification signal obtained with control group were assigned the value of 100%. Lane 1 is molecular size marker, λ/Hind3. Bottom panel shows graphic representation of inhibition of amplification with treatment.

duction in amplification product amounts was observed with DNA isolated after hypoxia from both the hippocampus and cortex (Fig. 3, arrowheads). Following a three-hour recovery after hypoxia, the repair of nuclear DNA was evidenced in a substantial restoration of amplification signal. The ratio between damaged and intact DNA templates was calculated as described for mitochondrial DNA and the relative resultant amplification for each group is shown as bar graphs (Fig. 3, bottom).

Immunohistochemical Analysis for DNA Polymerase β (pol-β) and Apurinic/Apyrimidinic Endonuclease (APE)

The levels and distribution of two enzymes involved in the repair of oxidative DNA damage (pol-β and APE) were visualized in the brain by immunohistochemical analysis. Brain sections from control and hypoxic rats (4% O_2 for 30 min followed by a 3-hour recovery in ambient air) were prepared. Representative regions from control and treatment brains stained with either polymerase-β or AP endonuclease antibody are shown by light microscopy (Figs. 4–5). A specific spatial and intercellular compartmentalization pattern of immunoreactivity was detected for protein. The pattern and inten-

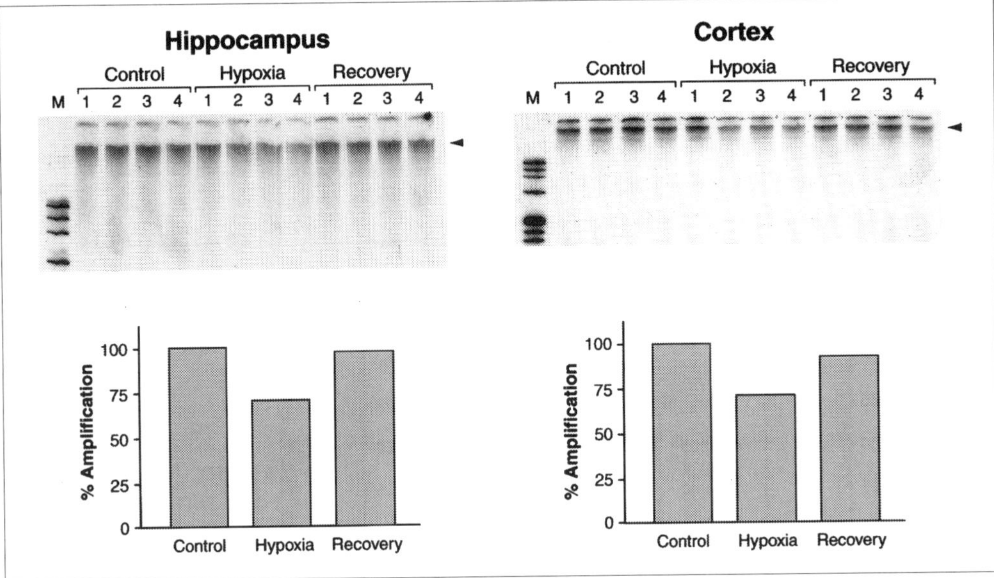

Fig. 3. Hypoxia-induced DNA damage in nuclear DNA in hippocampus and cortex detected by SINE-mediated QPCR assay. Amplification products (arrowheads) for 4 rats out of 8 included in each experimental group were resolved in denaturing gels and visualized by autoradiography. Demarcations are as in Figure 2. A representative autoradiogram shows a reduction in amplification products after hypoxia when compared to control rats and, a restoration of amplification signal after a subsequent 3-hour recovery period in ambient air. Amplification products obtained with the control group were assigned the value of 100%. Lane 1 is molecular size marker, phi 174/Hae3. Bottom panel shows graphic representation of inhibition of amplification.

sity of staining were altered by hypoxia treatment. In Fig. 4A, an increased immunoreactivity for pol-β is shown in the hippocampal region. Increased immunoreactivity is detected also in the cortex, in particular in the nuclei of large neuronal cells (Fig. 4B). Similarly, an elevated level of APE protein is detected (Fig. 5). A representative photomicrograph shows intensified staining in the CA3 hippocampal region. Interestingly, in this case strong immunoreactivity appears to be localized in the nucleoli. To quantitatively assess these alterations, non-adjacent brain sections in each group were scored microscopically by counting specifically stained cells with visible nuclei at 2 levels of staining intensity (light, dark). The corresponding cell counts, summarized in Table 1, show that the number of cells expressing basal levels (light) of both proteins is only moderately increased with treatment. However, the number of cells showing strong immunoreactivity (dark) is dramatically elevated after hypoxia. The immunohistochemical analysis therefore, demonstrates that at least two repair enzymes involved in the base excision repair (BER) pathway are elevated in the rat brain in this experimental model. The data show also that the expression patterns of β-pol and APE overlap in part and suggest that these enzymes may cooperate in repair of oxidative DNA damage in the brain.

Discussion

The presence of DNA damage and inadequate DNA repair capacity are being increasingly implicated as contributing factors to neurodegenerative disorders (Citterio et al. 2000; Hermon et al. 1998; Lovell et al. 2000; Mandir et al. 1999), age-associated neurodegeneration (Feu-

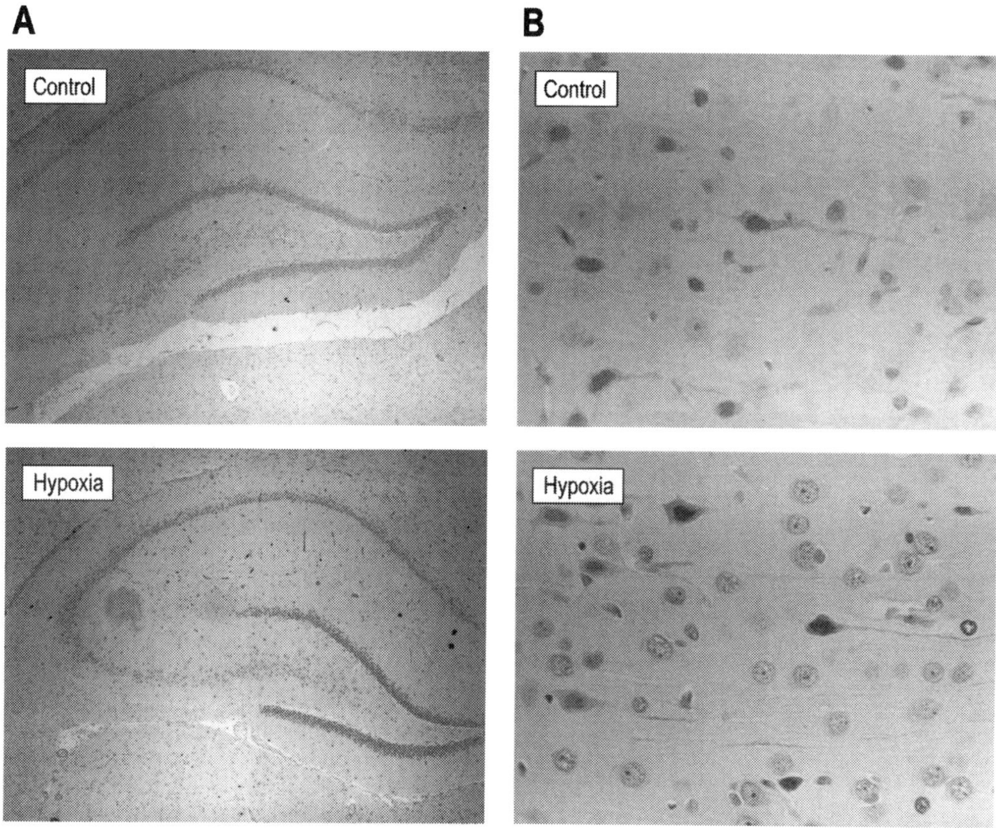

Fig. 4. Immunohistochemical analysis of DNA polymerase β: (A) Representative photomicrographs of the hippocampal region (x4); sections from rats subjected to hypoxia show elevated staining when compared to controls. (B) In the cortex, pol-β staining is markedly increased especially in the nuclear compartment. Note the strongly elevated immunoreactivity in nuclei of large neurons (x100).

ers 1998; Michikawa et al. 1999; Schmitz et al. 1999) and to the adverse outcomes of chronic hypoxia in humans (Love et al. 1998; Love et al. 1999). In experimental models, the formation of DNA damage in the brain was clearly documented in ischemia (Chen et al. 1997; Hayashi et al. 1999; Jin et al. 1999; Tobita et al. 1995), cold injury (Morita-Fujimura et al. 1999), trauma (Kaya et al. 1999) and most recently in seizures induced by systemic kainic acid (Lan et al. 2000). Thus, it is plausible that in humans, genetic or age-related impairments in DNA repair as well as a variety of insults that compromise cerebral energy metabolism (causing excessive generation of ROS) may contribute separately or in combination to a broad spectrum of neuropathologies.

The central nervous system depends on an uninterrupted supply of oxygen in order to maintain its functional and structural integrity. Free radicals generated in the course of hypoxia/ ischemia and reperfusion induce a wide spectrum of DNA lesions, primarily base modifications, base loss and strand breaks (Imlay et al. 1988; Imlay and Linn 1988). Hence, an accurate assessment of the integrity of DNA subsequently to such insults relies on the capacity to detect a broad spectrum of lesions. Notably, many free radical-induced DNA lesions form strong blocks to thermostable polymerase-mediated DNA syn-

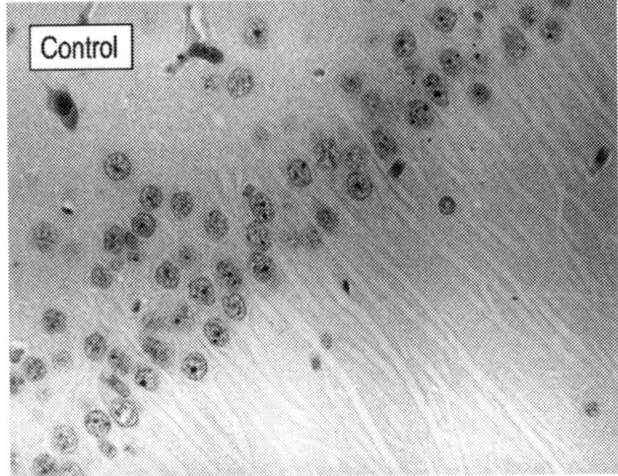

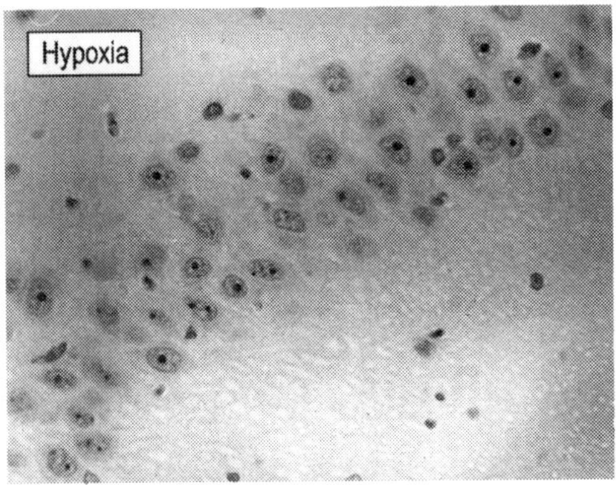

Fig. 5. Immunohistochemical analysis of APE protein: In control sections of the CA3 subregion of the hippocampus, punctate nuclear staining is observed, in sections obtained after hypoxia staining is intensified and localized specifically to the nucleoli (x200).

thesis. These lesions include, in addition to DNA strand breaks, about 35–50% of the approximately 80 different types of free radical-induced adducts (Yakes and van Houten 1997a). By comparison, the canonical adduct, conventionally used for measuring oxidative DNA damage, 8-oxodeoxyguanine, represents only about 10% of oxidative modifications in DNA (Yakes and van Houten 1997). In this study, therefore, we used the QPCR-mediated approach for detection of DNA damage. Two QPCR assays were employed; one to measure the integrity of the entire mitochondrial genome and the other the integrity of nuclear DNA. The latter, SINE-mediated QPCR, is a novel assay which supports simultaneous amplification of long random segments of DNA. This feature offers increased sensitivity and uniformity in detection of DNA damage and eliminates the concern of a potential bias in the distribution of DNA damage as a function of genomic localization or a specialized chromatin structure (Pfeifer 1997; Suquet et al. 1995; Wang et al. 1991).

Table 1. Immunohistochemical Detection – Cell Count

	Light[a]		Dark[b]	
	Control	**Hypoxia**	**Control**	**Hypoxia**
β-pol	35 ± 9	56 ± 15	4 ± 1	71 ± 17*
APE	16 ± 5	40 ± 10	1 ± 1	43 ± 10*

[a]basal level of staining (ie, expression). [b]induced level of staining. *Number of dark cells detected with each antibody that was significantly different in hypoxia brains compared to control brains. Student's t test ($p < 0.001$).

Thus, using this approach, it is possible to detect low levels of DNA damage, which appears to be compatible with cell capacity for DNA repair and with cellular survival. In this system therefore, it is possible to study molecular events invoked by DNA damage, ie, activation of DNA repair processes without activation of pathways leading to cell death. This new capability will now assist in understanding the roles that DNA damage and DNA repair may play in brain pathologies in which the presence of DNA damage in absence of adequate DNA repair capacity exist.

Acknowledgments

This work was supported by a research grant from Shriners Hospitals for Children to E.W.E.

References

1. Ames BN, Shigenaga MK, Hagen TM (1995) Mitochondrial decay in aging. Biochim Biophys Acta 1271:165–170
2. Atamna H, Cheung I, Ames BN (2000) A method for detecting abasic sites in living cells: age-dependent changes in base excision repair. Proc Natl Acad Sci USA 97:686–691

3. Cao W, Carney JM, Duchon A, Floyd RA, Chevion M (1988) Oxygen free radical involvement in ischemia and reperfusion injury to brain. Neurosci Lett 88:233–238
4. Chen J, Jin K, Chen M, Pei W, Kawaguchi K, Greenberg DA, Simon RP (1997) Early detection of DNA strand breaks in the brain after transient focal ischemia: implications for the role of DNA damage in apoptosis and neuronal cell death. J Neurochem 69:232–245
5. Chopp M, Chan PH, Hsu CY, Cheung ME, Jacobs TP (1996) DNA damage and repair in central nervous system injury: National Institute of Neurological Disorders and Stroke Workshop Summary. Stroke 27:363–369
6. Citterio E, Vermeulen W, Hoeijmakers JH (2000) Transcriptional healing. Cell 101:447–450
7. Croteau DL, Bohr VA (1997) Repair of oxidative damage to nuclear and mitochondrial DNA in mammalian cells. J Biol Chem 272:25409–25412
8. Cullinane C, Bohr VA (1998) DNA interstrand cross-links induced by psoralen are not repaired in mammalian mitochondria. Cancer Res 58:1400–1404
9. Dianov G, Bischoff C, Piotrowski J, Bohr VA (1998) Repair pathways for processing of 8-oxoguanine in DNA by mammalian cell extracts. J Biol Chem 273:33811–33816
10. Dieninger P (1989) SINEs: short interspersed repeated DNA elements in higher eucaryotes. In: (Berg DE, Howe MM, eds) Mobile DNA, American Society for Microbiology, Washington DC, pp 619–636
11. Druzhyna N, Nair RG, LeDoux SP, Wilson GL (1998) Defective repair of oxidative damage in mitochondrial DNA in Down's syndrome. Mutat Res 409:81–89
12. Edwards M, Kent TA, Rea HC, Wei J, Quast M, Izumi T, Mitra S, Perez-Polo JR (1998a) APE/Ref-1 responses to ischemia in rat brain. Neuroreport 9:4015–4018
13. Edwards M, Rassin DK, Izumi T, Mitra S, Perez-Polo JR (1998b) APE/Ref-1 responses to oxidative stress in aged rats. J Neurosci Res 54:635–638
14. Englander EW, Greeley GH, Wang G, Perez-Polo JR, Lee HM (1999) Hypoxia-Induced Mitochondrial and Nuclear DNA Damage in the Rat Brain. Journal of Neuroscience Research 58:262–269
15. Englander EW, Howard BH (1997) Alu-mediated detection of DNA damage in the human genome. Mutat Res 385:31–39
16. Facchinetti F, Dawson VL, Dawson TM (1998) Free radicals as mediators of neuronal injury. Cell Mol Neurobiol 18:667–682
17. Feuers RJ (1998) The effects of dietary restriction on mitochondrial dysfunction in aging. Ann NY Acad Sci 854:192–201
18. Fujimura M, Morita-Fujimura Y, Murakami K, Kawase M, Chan PH (1998) Cytosolic redistribution of cytochrome c after transient focal cerebral ischemia in rats. J Cereb Blood Flow Metab 18:1239–1247
19. Govan HLd, Valles-Ayoub Y, Braun J (1990) Fine-mapping of DNA damage and repair in specific genomic segments. Nucleic Acids Res 18:3823–3830
20. Hayashi T, Sakurai M, Itoyama Y, Abe K (1999) Oxidative damage and breakage of DNA in rat brain after transient MCA occlusion. Brain Res 832:159–163
21. Hermon M, Cairns N, Egly JM, Fery A, Labudova O, Lubec G (1998) Expression of DNA excision-repair-cross-complementing proteins p80 and p89 in brain of patients with Down Syndrome and Alzheimer's disease. Neurosci Lett 251:45–48
22. Hou ST, Tu Y, Buchan AM, Huang Z, Preston E, Rasquinha I, Robertson GS, MacManus JP (1997) Increases in DNA lesions and the DNA damage indicator Gadd45 following transient cerebral ischemia. Biochem Cell Biol 75:383–392
23. Imlay JA, Chin SM, Linn S (1988a) Toxic DNA damage by hydrogen peroxide through the Fenton reaction in vivo and in vitro. Science 240:640–642
24. Imlay JA, Linn S (1988) DNA damage and oxygen radical toxicity. Science 240:1302
25. Jin K, Chen J, Kawaguchi K, Zhu RL, Stetler RA, Simon RP, Graham SH (1996) Focal ischemia induces expression of the DNA damage-inducible gene GADD45 in the rat brain. Neuroreport 7:1797–1802
26. Jin K, Chen J, Nagayama T, Chen M, Sinclair J, Graham SH, Simon RP (1999) In situ detection of neuronal DNA strand breaks using the Klenow fragment of DNA polymerase I reveals different mechanisms of neuron death after global cerebral ischemia. J Neurochem 72:1204–1214
27. Kalinowski DP, Illenye S, van Houten B (1992) Analysis of DNA damage and repair in murine leukemia L1210 cells using a quantitative polymerase chain reaction assay. Nucleic Acids Res 20:3485–3494
28. Kaya SS, Mahmood A, Li Y, Yavuz E, Goksel M, Chopp M (1999) Apoptosis and expression of p53 response proteins and cyclin D1 after cortical impact in rat brain. Brain Res 818:23–33
29. Lan J, Henshall DC, Simon RP, Chen J (2000) Formation of the base modification 8-hydroxyl-2'-deoxyguanosine and DNA fragmentation following seizures induced by systemic kainic acid in the rat. J Neurochem 74:302–309
30. Liu PK, Hsu CY, Dizdaroglu M, Floyd RA, Kow YW, Karakaya A, Rabow LE, Cui JK (1996) Damage, repair, and mutagenesis in nuclear genes after mouse forebrain ischemia-reperfusion. J Neurosci 16:6795–6806
31. Love S, Barber R, Wilcock GK (1998) Apoptosis and expression of DNA repair proteins in ischaemic brain injury in man. Neuroreport 9:955–959
32. Love S, Barber R, Wilcock GK (1999) Neuronal accumulation of poly(ADP-ribose) after brain ischaemia. Neuropathol Appl Neurobiol 25:98–103
33. Lovell MA, Xie C, Markesbery WR (2000) Decreased base excision repair and increased helicase activity in Alzheimer's disease brain. Brain Res 855:116–123
34. Mandir AS, Przedborski S, Jackson-Lewis V, Wang ZQ, Simbulan-Rosenthal CM, Smulson ME, Hoffman BE, Guastella DB, Dawson VL, Dawson TM (1999) Poly(ADP-ribose) polymerase activation mediates 1-methyl-4-phenyl-1, 2,3,6-tetrahydropyridine (MPTP)-induced parkinsonism. Proc Natl Acad Sci USA 96:5774–5779
35. Marti HH, Risau W (1998) Systemic hypoxia changes the organ-specific distribution of vascular endothelial growth factor and its receptors. Proc Natl Acad Sci USA 95:15809–15814
36. Mehmet H, Yue X, Penrice J, Cady E, Wyatt JC, Sarraf C, Squier M, Edwards AD (1998) Relation of impaired energy metabolism to apoptosis and necrosis following transient cerebral hypoxia-ischaemia. Cell Death Differ 5:321–329
37. Merril CR, Zullo S, Ghanbari H, Herman MM, Kleinman JE, Bigelow LB, Bartko JJ, Sabourin DJ (1996) Possible relationship between conditions associated with chronic hypoxia and brain mitochondrial DNA deletions. Arch Biochem Biophys 326:172–177
38. Michikawa Y, Mazzucchelli F, Bresolin N, Scarlato G, Attardi G (1999) Aging-dependent large accumulation of point mutations in the human mtDNA control region for replication [see comments]. Science 286:774–779
39. Mitra S, Hazra TK, Roy R, Ikeda S, Biswas T, Lock J, Boldogh I, Izumi T (1997) Complexities of DNA base excision repair in mammalian cells. Mol Cells 7:305–312
40. Morita-Fujimura Y, Fujimura M, Kawase M, Chan PH (1999) Early decrease in apurinic/apyrimidinic endonuclease is followed by DNA fragmentation after cold injury-induced brain trauma in mice. Neuroscience 93:1465–1473
41. Murakami K, Kondo T, Kawase M, Li Y, Sato S, Chen SF, Chan PH (1998) Mitochondrial susceptibility to oxidative stress

exacerbates cerebral infarction that follows permanent focal cerebral ischemia in mutant mice with manganese superoxide dismutase deficiency. J Neurosci 18:205–213
42. Ozawa T (1997) Oxidative damage and fragmentation of mitochondrial DNA in cellular apoptosis. Biosci Rep 17:237–250
43. Pfeifer GP (1997) Formation and processing of UV photoproducts: effects of DNA sequence and chromatin environment. Photochem Photobiol 65:270–283
44. Piantadosi CA, Zhang J (1996) Mitochondrial generation of reactive oxygen species after brain ischemia in the rat. Stroke 27:327–332
45. Piantadosi CA, Zhang J, Demchenko IT (1997) Production of hydroxyl radical in the hippocampus after CO hypoxia or hypoxic hypoxia in the rat. Free Radic Biol Med 22:725–732
46. Ramana CV, Boldogh I, Izumi T, Mitra S (1998) Activation of apurinic/apyrimidinic endonuclease in human cells by reactive oxygen species and its correlation with their adaptive response to genotoxicity of free radicals. Proc Natl Acad Sci USA 95:5061–5066
47. Ratan RR, Murphy TH, Baraban JM (1994) Oxidative stress induces apoptosis in embryonic cortical neurons. J Neurochem 62:376–379
48. Sakhi S, Bruce A, Sun N, Tocco G, Baudry M, Schreiber SS (1994) p53 induction is associated with neuronal damage in the central nervous system. Proc Natl Acad Sci USA 91:7525–7529
49. Schapira AH (1996) Oxidative stress and mitochondrial dysfunction in neurodegeneration. Curr Opin Neurol 9:260–264
50. Schmitz C, Axmacher B, Zunker U, Korr H (1999) Age-related changes of DNA repair and mitochondrial DNA synthesis in the mouse brain. Acta Neuropathol (Berl) 97:71–81
51. Semenza GL, Koury ST, Nejfelt MK, Gearhart JD, Antonarakis SE (1991) Cell-type-specific and hypoxia-inducible expression of the human erythropoietin gene in transgenic mice. Proc Natl Acad Sci USA 88:8725–8729
52. Srivastava DK, Berg BJ, Prasad R, Molina JT, Beard WA, Tomkinson AE, Wilson SH (1998) Mammalian abasic site base excision repair. Identification of the reaction sequence and rate-determining steps. J Biol Chem 273:21203–21209
53. Suquet C, Mitchell DL, Smerdon MJ (1995) Repair of UV-induced (6–4) photoproducts in nucleosome core DNA. J Biol Chem 270:16507–16509
54. Suzuki H, Kumagai T, Goto A, Sugiura T (1998) Increase in intracellular hydrogen peroxide and upregulation of a nuclear respiratory gene evoked by impairment of mitochondrial electron transfer in human cells. Biochem Biophys Res Commun 249:542–545
55. Tan S, Zhou F, Nielsen VG, Wang Z, Gladson CL, Parks DA (1999) Increased injury following intermittent fetal hypoxia-reoxygenation is associated with increased free radical production in fetal rabbit brain. J Neuropathol Exp Neurol 58:972–981
56. Tobita M, Nagano I, Nakamura S, Itoyama Y, Kogure K (1995) DNA single-strand breaks in postischemic gerbil brain detected by in situ nick translation procedure. Neurosci Lett 200:129–132
57. Walker LJ, Craig RB, Harris AL, Hickson ID (1994) A role for the human DNA repair enzyme HAP1 in cellular protection against DNA damaging agents and hypoxic stress. Nucleic Acids Res 22:4884–4889
58. Wang G, Hallberg LM, Englander EW (1999a) Rapid SINE-mediated detection of cisplatin:DNA adduct formation in vitro and in vivo in blood. Mutat Res 434:67–74
59. Wang G, Hallberg LM, Saphier E, Englander EW (1999b) Short interspersed DNA element-mediated detection of UVB-induced DNA damage and repair in the mouse genome, in vitro, and in vivo in skin. Mutat Res 433:147–157
60. Wang G, Hazra TK, Mitra S, Lee HM, Englander EW (2000) Mitochondrial DNA damage and a hypoxic response are induced by CoCl(2) in rat neuronal PC12 cells. Nucleic Acids Res 28:2135–2140
61. Wang ZG, Wu XH, Friedberg EC (1991) Nucleotide excision repair of DNA by human cell extracts is suppressed in reconstituted nucleosomes. J Biol Chem 266:22472–22478
62. Wei YH (1998) Oxidative stress and mitochondrial DNA mutations in human aging. Proc Soc Exp Biol Med 217:53–63
63. Wiener CM, Booth G, Semenza GL (1996) In vivo expression of mRNAs encoding hypoxia-inducible factor 1. Biochem Biophys Res Commun 225:485–488
64. Xu YJ, Kim EY, Demple B (1998) Excision of C-4'-oxidized deoxyribose lesions from double-stranded DNA by human apurinic/apyrimidinic endonuclease (Ape1 protein) and DNA polymerase beta. J Biol Chem 273:28837–28844
65. Yakes FM, van Houten B (1997a) Mitochondrial DNA damage is more extensive and persists longer than nuclear DNA damage in human cells following oxidative stress. Proc Natl Acad Sci USA 94:514–519
66. Yakes FM, van Houten B (1997b) PCR-based assays for the detection and quantitation of DNA damage and repair. In: (GP Preifer ed.): Technologies for Detection of DNA Damage and Mutations, Plenum Press, New York, pp. 171–183
67. Zucconi GG, Carcereri de Prati A, Menegazzi M, Cosi C, Suzuki H (1992) DNA repair enzymes in the brain. DNA polymerase beta and poly (ADP-ribose) polymerase. Ann NY Acad Sci 663:432–435

Functional recovery after brain injury: role of neurotrophic factors and behavior-driven structural events

T. Schallert[1,2], S. T. Bland[2], S. M. Fleming[2]

It is clear from this meeting and its proceedings that enormous progress is being made in preclinical stroke research, but that no single path of investigation can be regarded at this time as the most appropriate. It is nearly impossible for one laboratory to adopt every promising line of inquiry, but attacking the issues from many directions in a joint effort with discussion among many investigators is more likely to provide comprehensive and potentially more effective solutions to enhancing stroke outcome. There are at least five general approaches to reducing behavioral deficits and improving the quality of function in experimental models of ischemic injury. These include preventing initial loss of tissue, preinjury preventive measures, capitalizing on early opportunities for plasticity and repair, avoiding delayed secondary degeneration, and promoting late residual opportunities for deficit compensation. In this paper we focus primarily on the last three approaches, emphasizing use-dependent structural changes that may underlie behavioral deficit compensation and restoration of function.

Limiting tissue loss

The most commonly taken approach has been to limit the extent of the cerebrovascular accident, primarily by using chemical or other treatment interventions during the acute phase to prevent tissue loss. This approach involves, for example, (a) understanding cellular and molecular cascading mechanisms of neuronal death associated with inadequate blood supply or with the toxic effects of reperfusion; and (b) using this information to apply rational therapy to limit the size of the infarct and the extent of acute secondary degeneration.

These are reviewed by investigators writing for the present volume and elsewhere (e.g., Ginsberg and Bogousslavsky 1998; Abe 2000; Cramer and Chopp 2000; Johansson 2000).

Among the most formidable problems that must be addressed with regard to this approach include how to assess neuroprotective treatments effectively and to deal with narrow, ever-changing time windows or multiple interacting cascades of events leading to progressive cell death, which can differ among the models utilized (see Corbett and Nurse 1998; Schallert et al. 2000 for reviews). Moreover, not all ischemic injuries share identical sequelae, particularly within the first few hours, even when the location and extent of primary infarct are similar. Even so, interventions are being developed that appear to have broad protective properties and

[1]Department of Psychology & Center for Human Growth and Development University of Michigan, Ann Arbor, MI.
[2]Department of Psychology & Institute for Neuroscience, Mezes 330, University of Texas, Austin, TX 78712.
e-mail: TSchall@umich.edu

J. Krieglstein, S. Klumpp (Eds.) Pharmacology of Cerebral Ischemia 2000

that can inhibit cell death by rendering tissue less vulnerable to a variety of degenerative pressures.

Although all types of ischemic injury can ultimately lead to cell death, one must recognize that the processes that affect outcome may have unique properties in comparison to other types of brain damage. Nevertheless, preclinical investigations using models of other types of brain injury have benefited greatly from the enormous research effort applied to understanding the acute consequences of ischemia and to minimizing their impact because many of the same neural events and the factors that influence these events are highly informative to non-ischemic injury. This is particularly true for long-term post-injury processes linked to neuroplasticity.

Pre-operative manipulations

A second approach has been to manipulate pre-injury experience in an effort to investigate dietary, genetic, environmental, stroke history (ischemic tolerance) or other factors that might reduce or increase the probability of stroke occurrence, its severity, or how well the brain reacts chronically to the damage (Perez-Pinson, this volume; Chen et al. 1996; Schallert 1989; Kolb 1995; Schallert et al. 2000; Bruce-Keller et al. 1999). For example, restricted feeding or other ingestive regimens before injury can provide functional and neural protection, and pre-operative exposure to a complex environment greatly upregulates trophic factor expression in response to injury (Schallert 1989; Schallert et al. 2000).

Early post-acute neuroplasticity: use-dependency and window of opportunity

Use-dependent events. Research suggests that the first weeks after brain injury represent a special time when trophic factors or other precursors to neuroadaptations are overexpressed such that direct manipulation of motor behavior can enhance functional outcome by shaping mechanisms of neuroplasticity.

It is well established that environmental factors that affect motor behavior can influence neural events (e.g., Schwartz 1964; Black et al. 1975, 1990; Greenough et al. 1976; Withers and Greenough 1989; Rosenzweig 1980; Nudo et al. 1996; Freund 1996; Kaas 1991; Kozlowski et al. 1996a; Karni et al. 1995; Pons et al. 1991; Sanes et al. 1988; Schallert et al. 1980, 1997; Whishaw et al. 1976, 1978, 1982; Johansson 1995, 2000; Whishaw and Schallert 1977).

Interventions that directly affect motor experience after brain injury, including deficit-imposed compensatory behavior, can have significant neural and functional consequences related to plasticity or degeneration. After brain injury, dendritic arborization and synaptogenesis may require new motor learning. These structural changes may be optimal soon after damage because the injured brain might be differentially sensitive to modification at that time.

Motor behavior after brain damage has been examined closely in relation to anatomical changes and then directly manipulated at different post-injury time points (Jones and Schallert 1994; Kozlowski et al. 1996; Schallert et al. 1997; Schallert and Jones 1993; Kolb 1995; Johansson 2000). Damage to the forelimb area of the sensorimotor cortex leaves animals partially hemi-paretic. They are forced by this deficit in the contralateral forelimb to preferentially use the unaffected forelimb for weight shifting and other behaviors. Brain injury may, in certain instances, prime surviving tissue thereby enabling the animal to rely more efficiently on the non-impaired forelimb, using it as a "crutch" to more efficiently negotiate exploration, feeding and social interaction (Jones and Schallert 1992, 1994; Schallert and Jones 1993; Jones et al. 1996; Kolb 1995). Several plasticity-associated events are known to occur as recovery of function progresses, including expression of growth-correlated markers (e.g., FGF-2, Gap-43, synaptophysin), NMDA-dependent hyper-excitability, GABA receptor down-regulation, dendritic arborization, pruning, spine density increases and synaptogenesis (Bury et al. 2000; Jones et al. 1997; Jones and Schallert 1992; Stroemer et al. 1995; Kawamata et al. 1997b; Witte and Stoll 1997; Finklestein 1996; Schallert et al. 1997; Witte 1998). Electron microscopy revealed a large increase in multiple axodendritic synapses and discontinuous expanded postsynaptic receptors in the intact sensorimotor cortex (Jones 1999; Jones et al. 1999). These synapses are similar to those formed after long-term potentiation (LTP) in the hippocampus, an established activity-related model of learning and memory (Harris 1995).

Enhanced dendritic arborization appears to depend on movement because it can be prevented by partially immobilizing the "crutch" forelimb so that it cannot be used for motor function (Jones and Schallert 1994; Schallert and Jones 1993; Schallert et al. 1997; see also Stephan and Frackowiak 1997; Seitz and Freund 1997). Signals from damaged tissue (e.g., diffusable trophic factors) in the injured hemisphere appear to be important as well because immediate aspiration of the debris in the lesion cavity prevents dendritic arborization and greatly prolongs the deficit (Voorhies and Jones 2000).

Nudo et al. (1996) used microstimulation mapping techniques to analyze the functional properties of the motor cortex in squirrel monkeys before and after focal coagulation of blood vessels in the region of the cortical area controlling hand movements. In addition to the primary damage the loss of "hand territorry" gradually extended into healthy cortical tissue. Retraining of hand and wrist food-retrieving skills beginning five days after the injury prevented the extention of tissue loss. Castro-Alamancos et al. (1992, 1995) used movement-contingent reinforcing electrical stimulation to improve functional outcome. Cortical mapping techniques indicated that the region closely adjacent to focal motor cortex injury was reorganized. Thus, rehabilitative training soon after injury can shape functional reorganization in the adjacent intact cortex.

LTP-like neuronal activity or epileptoid bursting in the peri-injury zone may partially underlie the effects of motor interventions on plasticity and behavior (Witte 1998; Johansson 2000; Eysel 1997). The peri-injury zone may extend several millimeters outside the area of damaged tissue and 0.5 to 1 mm outside the "penumbral" tissue in which neural activity is depressed (Eysel 1997). During the first week after focal heat-induced injury to the sensorimotor cortex, in vitro examination of field potentials and single cell electrophysiology suggested that the region outside the penumbra shows increased NMDA-mediated excitatory postsynaptic potentials and reduced GABA-mediated currents. Moreover, the suppressed activity in the penumbral region *in vivo* was not present *in vitro*, suggesting that metabolic, vascular or other deficiencies may have contributed to the penumbral suppression. Normalization of these events occurred after the first week.

Similarly, Witte and his colleagues (e.g., Witte and Stoll 1997; Witte 1998) found that after focal photothrombotic injury, this intermediate peri-penumbral zone is hyperexcitable for several weeks and $GABA_A$ receptors are downregulated. Moreover, in the focal heat injury model the fast $GABA_A$- and the slow $GABA_B$-mediated inhibitory postsynaptic potentials are greatly reduced in vitro (Eysel 1997), which could increase the activation of NMDA receptors (Luhmann and Pronce 1991). Diazepam administered peripherally or GABAergic agonists locally infused into the sensorimotor cortex during the first week after more medially located focal lesions can impair recovery of function chronically, whereas low doses of GABAergic antagonists can improve recovery (Schallert et al. 1986; Schallert and Hernandez 1998; Hernandez and Schallert 1988). Eysel (1997) and Witte and Stoll (1997) suggest that mild LTP-like hyperexcitability of peri-lesional neurons may sometimes favor functional reorganization while neuronal inhibition may impede it, and that early physical therapy or enriched environments may interact in some influential way with these and associated mechanisms (Johansson 2000). The additional role of injury-induced neurotrophic factors in the peri-lesional region is not known, although neurotrophic factors in vitro can enhance synaptic transmission by modulating $GABA_A$ receptors (e.g., Tanaka et al. 1996, 1997).

In the next section, we review evidence suggesting that endogenous or exogenous neurotrophic factors might promote the integrity of perilesional tissue such that neuronal function and plasticity may be enhanced.

FGF-2 and brain injury. Neurotrophic factors are frequently increased after brain injury and it has been argued that they may contribute to neural, glial and other cell survival, maintenance and plasticity (Nieto-Sampedro and Cotman 1985; Riva et al. 1992; Logan et al. 1992; Takami et al. 1992; Speliotes et al. 1996; Thoenen 1995; Mattson and Scheff 1994; Bury et al. 2000; Kolb 1995). Among the most studied of these is basic fibroblast growth factor (FGF-2).

FGF-2 immunoreactivity can be observed in the nuclei of astroglia and neurons all over the brain (Mattson and Scheff 1994; Speliotes et al. 1996). Soon after injury, FGF-2 mRNA expression is found prominently in the nuclei and cell bodies of reactive astrocytes surrounding the damage (Humpel et al. 1994; Finklestein et al. 1988, 1996; Humm et al. 1997; Frautschy et al. 1991). FGF-2 mRNA precedes FGF-2 expression (Speliotes et al. 1996).

Glial, endothelial and neural cells in the brain express high-affinity FGF-2 receptors (Wanaka et al. 1990), and FGF-2 receptor binding on neurons is increased for two weeks after injury (Kato et al. 1992). Binding of FGF-2 to one of its high-affinity receptors initiates an intracellular signal transduction cascade leading to gene expression and protein synthesis (Lee et al. 1989; Dionne et al. 1990; Keegan et al. 1991; Partanen et al. 1991). Even at low concentrations FGF-2 is a potent mitogen, causing cell proliferation and differentiation and causing migration of fibroblasts, endothelial cells, glial cells (especially astrocytes), neuronal precursors, myoblasts and many other cell types (Thomas and Gimenez-Gallego 1986; Thomas 1987; Burgess and Maciag 1989; Walicke 1988; Morrison et al. 1986, 1988; Gritti et al. 1996; Menon and Landerholm 1994; McDermott et al. 1997).

It has been hypothesized that excitatory amino acids or other signals from the injury (e.g., increased free radicals, nitric oxide, heat shock protein induction) may influence FGF-2 and other neurotrophic factor gene expression (Kawamata et al. 1997b; Mattson and Scheff 1994; Sharp et al. 1997). Other events may also play a role, including activation of the polysialic acid-neural cell adhesion molecule (PSA-NCAM), which is increased along with cell mitosis in the forebrain subependyma one week after large frontal cortex suction lesions (Szele and Chesselet 1996), as well as L-1 antigen and other molecules involved in cell proliferation, process outgrowth, and migration (Khoja et al. 1995; Giordana et al. 1994). Interestingly, we have found in the dorsolateral corner of the forebrain subependyma that FGF-2 expression (Humm et al. 1997), as well as cytochrome oxidase activity (Valla et al. 1999), is increased one week after electrolytic or suction lesions of the FLsmc.

Using immunostaining with FGF-2 antisera, Rowntree and Kolb (1997) found that astrocytes expressing FGF-2 were visible in large numbers in the region surrounding a focal suction ablation of the sensorimotor cortex. There was a temporal and spatial increase in FGF-2 immunoreactivity, increasing between Day 2 and Day 7 after injury, and gradually declining (but still readily detectable) by 21 days. The increased expression of FGF-2 in astrocytes may be associated with neuritic outgrowth that occurs later after injury (Nieto-Sampedro and Cotman 1985). Rowntree and Kolb (1997) suggest that the delay in sprouting may be due, at least in part, to the time it takes for locally expressed FGF-2 to be transported retrogradely to neuronal cell bodies (Grothe and Wewetzer 1996).

However, the spatial and temporal aspects of FGF-2 expression are likely to vary to some extent from one lesion model to another, as suggested by the work of Gómez-Pinilla et al. (1992) using entorhinal cortex lesions, and that of Speliotes et al. (1996) using cerebral infarction. Moreover, damage that induces spreading depression or seizures soon after the injury might be expected to have unique FGF-2 onset since these events may contribute to the initiation of FGF-2 and FGF-2 mRNA expression

(Lippoldt et al. 1993; Witte and Stoll 1997; Follesa et al. 1994). It would be important, therefore, to carefully characterize the sequence of specific events for the particular model being adopted and to determine the generalizability of the effects of motor interventions or exogenous FGF-2 manipulations to other models.

Rowntree and Kolb (1997) found that when FGF2-neutralizing antibodies were immediately administered via gelfoam directly into the lesion site, the number of FGF2-positive (but not GFAP-positive) astrocytes was reduced dramatically. Moreover, dendritic arbors and spines in surviving neurons of the same region were greatly reduced, and recovery of movements of the contralateral limb was disrupted severely. Control substances, including saline or biotinylated anti-goat IgG developed in rabbit had no effect on FGF-2 expression, dendritic morphology or motor outcome. FGF-2 antibodies may block the astrocytic expression of FGF-2 by occupying an otherwise active site on the FGF molecule, which prevents the FGF-2 molecule from binding to FGF receptors on cells (Rowntree and Kolb 1997). Thus, FGF-2, a neurotrophic factor that is known to promote neuronal survival and neurite extension (Grothe et al. 1989; Walicke 1988; Anderson et al. 1988; Otto et al. 1989; Sievers et al. 1987), may be necessary for neuronal integrity, neuritic outgrowth (or regrowth) and recovery of function after injury.

Post-injury treatment with exogenous FGF-2. Treatment with exogenous FGF-2 in vivo has been shown to promote survival of neurons and recovery of function after both injury and transplantation (Cummings et al. 1992; Mayer et al. 1993; Sabel et al. 1997; Brecknell et al. 1996). Remarkable neuroprotection has been observed after fluid percussion injury (Dietrich et al. 1996; McDermott et al. 1997), fimbria-fornix transection (Anderson et al. 1988; Cummings et al. 1992; Gómez-Pinilla 1992; Miyamoto et al. 1993; Otto et al. 1989), axon-sparing striatal damage (Frim et al. 1993), neurotoxic damage to nigrostriatal dopaminergic neurons (Otto and Unsicker 1990), vascular injury (Yamada et al. 1991) and kainic acid-induced seizures (Liu et al. 1993).

Finklestein (1996) reported that pretreatment with exogenous FGF-2 prior to unilateral middle cerebral artery occlusion prevented the usual expansion of the infarct into the "penumbral" tissue. Finklestein's group also found that FGF-2 administered intracisternally beginning 24 hours following unilateral middle cerebral artery occlusion, and twice weekly for several weeks thereafter, enhanced recovery of limb-placing function without affecting the size of the infarct detectably (Kawamata et al. 1996).

In collaboration with Finklestein's group, we showed that a similar regimen of intracisternally-infused FGF-2 after injury caused upregulated expression of a growth-associated marker (GAP-43) and facilitated use of the impaired forelimb for simple placing and landing functions that improved interlimb coordination and reduced preferential reliance on the good limb for these movements (Kawamata et al. 1997a). Chronically improved function of the impaired forelimb appears to require as few as two infusions of FGF-2 during the first postoperative week (Finklestein et al., unpublished data, 2000). Whether endogenous expression of FGF-2 is linked directly to cellular changes and recovery of function will require further research, however.

It is possible that FGF-2 influences the expression of other growth factors. For example, FGF-2 increases nerve growth factor (NGF) in astrocytes *in vitro* (Yoshida and Gage 1991) and *in vivo* (Yoshida and Gage 1992). NGF is known to increase dendritic arborization and improve recovery of function after cortical lesions (Kolb et al. 1997; Kolb 1995). Therefore, FGF-2 may interact with NGF to facilitate regeneration which would affect functional outcome after brain injury and if so, the interaction between these two factors might potentially be modulated by motor experience.

Brain injury, of course, directly enhances the expression of a number of other neurotrophic factors (Finklestein 1988; Freund et al. 1997; Johansson 2000, for review). Moreover, epileptoid activity can upregulate mRNA of several neurotrophic factors, including FGF-2 (Gall and Isackson 1989; Enfors et al. 1991; Follesa et al. 1994). This may be significant in view of studies showing that convulsant drugs and electroconvulsant stimulation activates motor behavior violently and can enhance recovery of function after injury, and that anticonvulsant GABAergic agonists can reduce motor behavior, disrupt recovery of function and exaggerate subcortical degeneration associated with anteromedial cortical injury (Hernandez and Schallert 1988; Schallert and Hernandez 1998, for review).

The extent to which neurotrophic factors other than FGF-2 are inhibited by motor disuse after brain injury is unknown. However, considerable evidence indicates that a number of growth factors are highly linked to neurotransmitter release in the intact adult and developing brain and can be modified by decreasing or increasing sensory and motor activity (Lindholm 1997 for review). Indeed, neurotrophin production is thought to be influenced by the balance of excitatory (e.g., glutamatergic) and inhibitory (e.g., GABAergic) neuronal activity (Lindholm 1997). Moreover, as noted above, extracellular glutamate is increased in association with use of the forelimb in FLsmc-related tasks (Bland et al. 1999).

Using a model of the potential dynamics between FGF-2 and glutamatergic mechanisms of neuronal growth and pruning, it has been shown in vitro that FGF-2 (which promotes neurite outgrowth) and glutamate (which can cause dendritic retraction) can offset each other if the doses of each are balanced (Mattson et al. 1993; see Finklestein 1996 and Kozlowski et al. 1994, for review). Without sufficient FGF-2, glutamate can compromise or even kill the cell, and without sufficient glutamate, FGF-2 can produce excessive outgrowth (Mattson et al. 1989, 1993). Cotman et al. (1989) have suggested that growth factors and glutamate interact in a mutually antagonistic way throughout the life span, and may be involved in the production, selection and maintenance of dendritic or axonal processes and synapse formation. Cotman et al. (1989) argued that these interactions are essential not only for normal development, but also for plasticity after brain injury and degenerative disorders, and may be relevant to the erosive process of aging during which growth factors may decline relative to glutamatergic activity (Tropepe et al. 1997).

We have previously reported that animals treated with OP-1 (Osteogenic protein, Creative Biomolecules, Inc.) following permanent middle cerebral artery occlusion (MCAo) showed modest but significantly detectable improvement in limb use asymmetries for combined wall exploration and landing lasting up to 90 days (Schallert et al. 2000). These results are similar to those obtained with FGF-2 in the same stroke model (Kawamata et al. 1997a) and confirm that our battery of tests might be useful in screening potentially beneficial agents for recovery of function after ischemic injury. By 450 days after MCAo, recovery of symmetrical limb use was apparent for both untreated and OP-1 treated animals (see Fig. 1).

Delayed degeneration of tissue: use-dependency and window of vulnerability

A fourth approach is limiting progressive delayed degenerative events in nearby and remote brain sites. Albeit greatly slowed compared to the acute insult, degeneration after brain injury can continue for weeks or months after the primary damage (e.g., Du et al. 1996; Kozlowski et al. 1996; Conti et al. 1998). Chemical and behavioral interventions that slow or exaggerate chronic degeneration of tissue have been documented (Kozlowski et al. 1996).

We have shown that forced overuse, but not disuse, of the affected forelimb via immobilization of the ipsilateral or contralateral limb, respectively, by a unilateral plaster cast for the first 10 days after mild (Bland et al. 1998) and moderate (Bland et al. 2000) distal MCAo using a 3 vessel occlusion model resulted in exacerbation of functional deficits. The distal MCAo model used in those studies resulted in exclusively cortical infarction. As shown in Figure 2, 45 minutes of 3VO resulted in cortical infarction in uncasted and ipsilaterally casted animals, but not in contralaterally casted animals. Note that there was no significant striatal

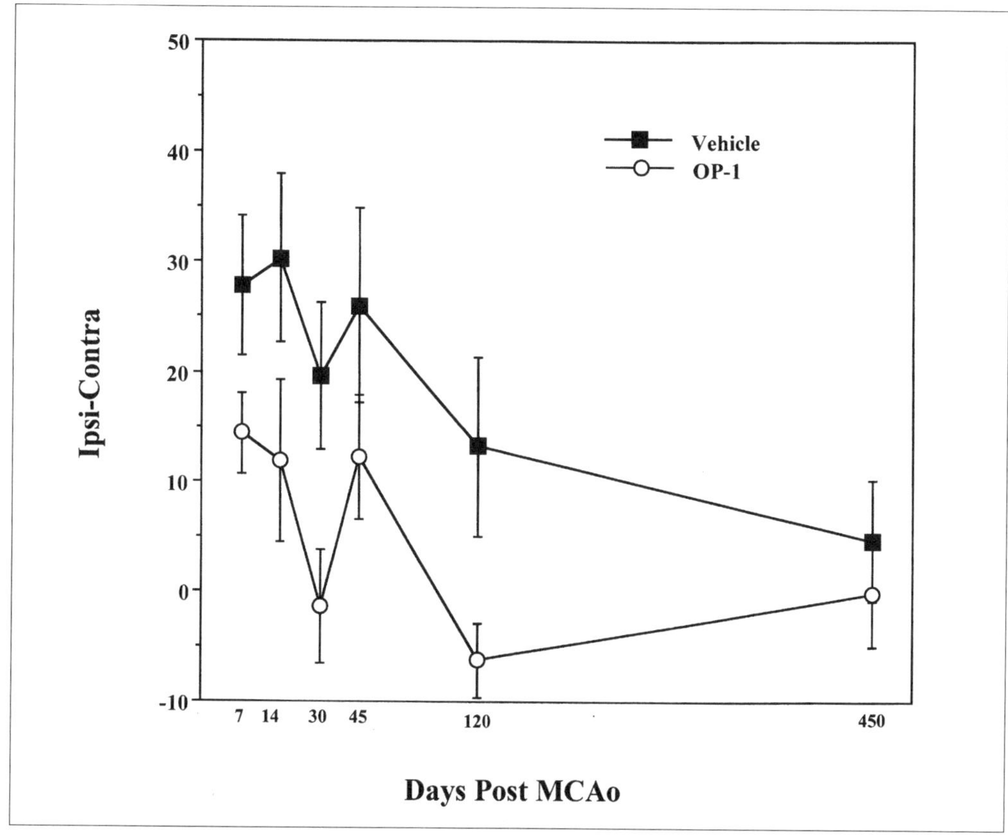

Fig. 1. Instracisternal injections of OP-1 on days one and three after MCAo reduce forelimb use asymmetry during spontaneous movement in a cylinder. Percent ipsilateral minus percent contralateral limb use, with wall and land data pooled, are shown (n = 10 for vehicle group, and n = 9 for OP-1 group).

infarction in any group. The finding of use-dependent exaggeration of functional deficits after cortical infarction is consistent with the work of Kozlowski et al. (1996) who have demonstrated that early forced overuse via ipsilateral forelimb immobilization for the first two weeks after electrolytic lesions of the FLsmc resulted in long-lasting exacerbation of functional deficits.

The detrimental effects of overuse may be site-dependent. Functional outcome is enhanced if overuse of the affected forelimb is forced for one week after unilateral 6-OHDA induced degeneration of ascending nigrostriatal dopamine neurons (Tillerson et al. 2000). We have recently observed that early disuse, rather than overuse, of the affected forelimb worsened functional deficits after 60 minutes of proximal MCAo using the intraluminal suture model (Belayev et al. 1996), which preferentially damages neurons in the striatum (Bland et al., in press). As shown in Figure 3, after 60 minutes of proximal MCAo, all groups had significant striatal infarction, but no groups had cortical infarction. There was no effect of limb use on striatal tissue loss. Figure 4 compares the effects of early disuse and overuse of the affected forelimb on forelimb placing responses after proximal and distal MCAo. When animals were tested 24 days after ischemia and 10 days of

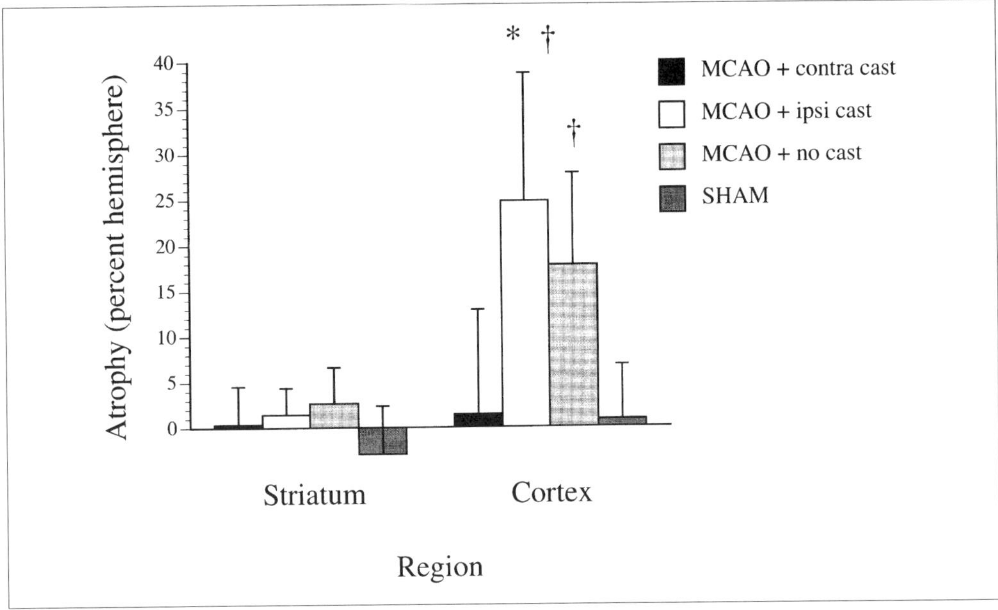

Fig. 2. Mean tissue atrophy in the striatum and cortex after early overuse, disuse, or normal use of the affected forelimb in rats that were subjected to either 45 minute distal MCA occlusion (unilateral MCA and bilateral CCA) or sham surgery. Animals were forced to either overuse (ipsi cast) or disuse (contra cast) the affected forelimb by immobilization of one limb in a plaster cast for 10 days immediately following stroke surgery, or they were uncasted (no cast) to allow normal use of both forelimbs. Atrophy is expressed as a percentage of the contralateral, intact hemisphere. SHAM represents the pooled data of ipsi- contra- and uncasted sham animals.
* $p < .05$, significantly different from SHAM ($p < .05$).
† $p < .05$, significantly different from MCAO + contra.

disuse or overuse of the affected forelimb, forelimb placing is worsened in animals that were forced to *overuse* the affected forelimb after transient *distal* MCAo (Fig. 4 A), but forelimb placing is worsened in animals that were forced to *disuse* the affected forelimb after transient *proximal* MCAo (Fig. 4 B).

Delayed interventions: never too late?

Damage to the motor cortex in humans and other mammals causes transient disruption of function of the contralateral limb. Although gradual recovery of function occurs, if sensitive tests are used, residual impairment can be observed (e.g., Gowland 1987; Schallert et al. 1997, 2000; Whishaw et al. 1991; Fulton and Kennard 1934; Bucy 1944; Barth et al. 1990; Penfield 1954; Passingham et al. 1983; Lashley 1924; Gless and Cole 1950; Twitchell 1951; Travis and Woolsey 1956; Denny-Brown 1960; Lieberman 1986; Kolb 1995; Black et al. 1975).

Taub et al. (1994) suggest that at least some of the residual impairment is due to "learned non-use" of the contralateral forelimb (see also Odin and Franz 1917, cited in Lashley 1924; Denny-Brown 1950; Schallert et al. 1997; Winstein and Pohl 1995). If so, then delayed interventions that target motor learning and motivation should be successful. It is well-known that animals readily learn to adopt alternative motor strategies after injury or drugs in order to compensate for dysfunction (see LeVere 1988; Gentile et al. 1978; Day and Schallert 1996; Schallert 1988, 1989, 1995; Rose et al. 1987;

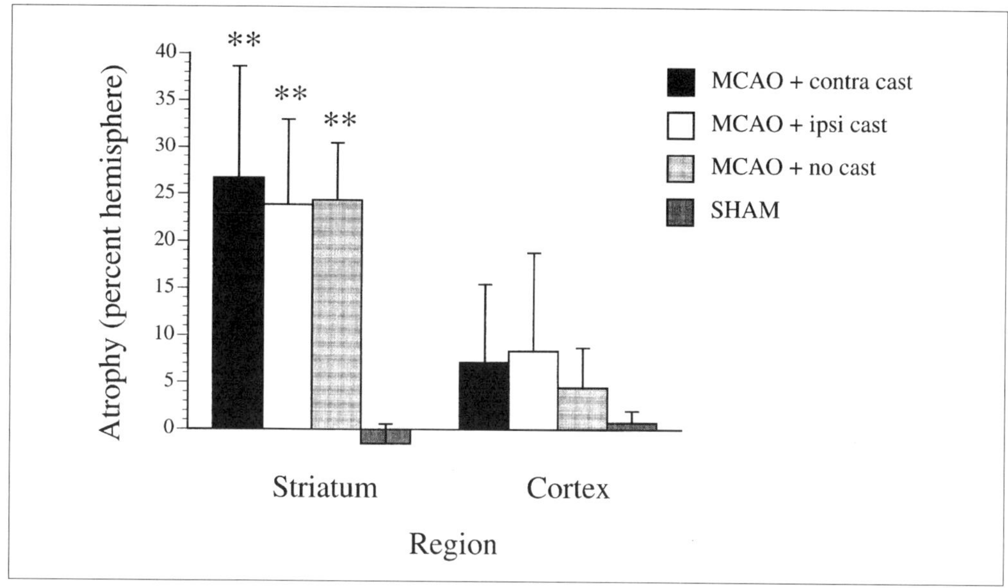

Fig. 3. Mean tissue atrophy in the striatum and cortex after early overuse, disuse, or normal use of the affected forelimb in rats that were subjected to either 60 minute proximal MCA occlusion using the intraluminal suture technique or sham surgery. Animals were forced to either overuse (ipsi cast) or disuse (contra cast) the affected forelimb by immobilization of one limb in a plaster cast for 10 days immediately following stroke surgery, or they were uncasted (no cast) to allow normal use of both forelimbs. Atrophy is expressed as a percentage of the contralateral, intact hemisphere. SHAM represents the pooled data of ipsi- contra- and uncasted sham animals All MCAo groups had significant striatal atrophy. ** $p < .01$, significantly different from SHAM.

Bach-y-rita 1990, 1993; Schallert and Whishaw 1984, 1985; Schallert et al. 1992, 1996, 1997). If these strategies are immediately effective, then the animal may fail to demonstrate its maximum potential for function during a sensitive period soon after injury. Thus, it might be useful to apply moderate rehabilitative pressure that focuses preferentially on the impaired forelimb, which often is *disused* in clinical situations when the patient fails to be self-motivated or when the affected limb is either broken or has been fitted with an intravenous catheter.

Long-standing deficits can show considerable amelioration by repetitive limb-specific training or by preventing use of the unaffected limb (Ostendorff and Wolf 1981; Taub 1980; Liepert et al. 2000; reviewed by Freund 1996). Taub and his colleagues (1993, 1994, 1996; Liepert et al. 2000) showed that months after unilateral stroke, immobilizing the unaffected arm of patients, together with physical rehabilitation of the affected arm, detectably improved the function of the affected arm and was associated with cortical reorganization. The effects were transient following short periods of rehabilitative intervention, but were stable following longer periods of intense motor training.

If one is interested in non-compensation related plasticity that can enhance recovery of function independent of practice, it is important to use tests that are not influenced by repeated testing (reviewed in Schallert et al. 2000; Schallert and Whishaw 1984; Schallert et al. 1986). Interventions that improve performance in these tests are more likely to have an effect on behavior that truly helps to reduce the primary deficit rather than improve motor or other adaptive strategies. Such tests allow long-term assessment of the deficit as well as permit accurate evaluation of the neural plasticity associat-

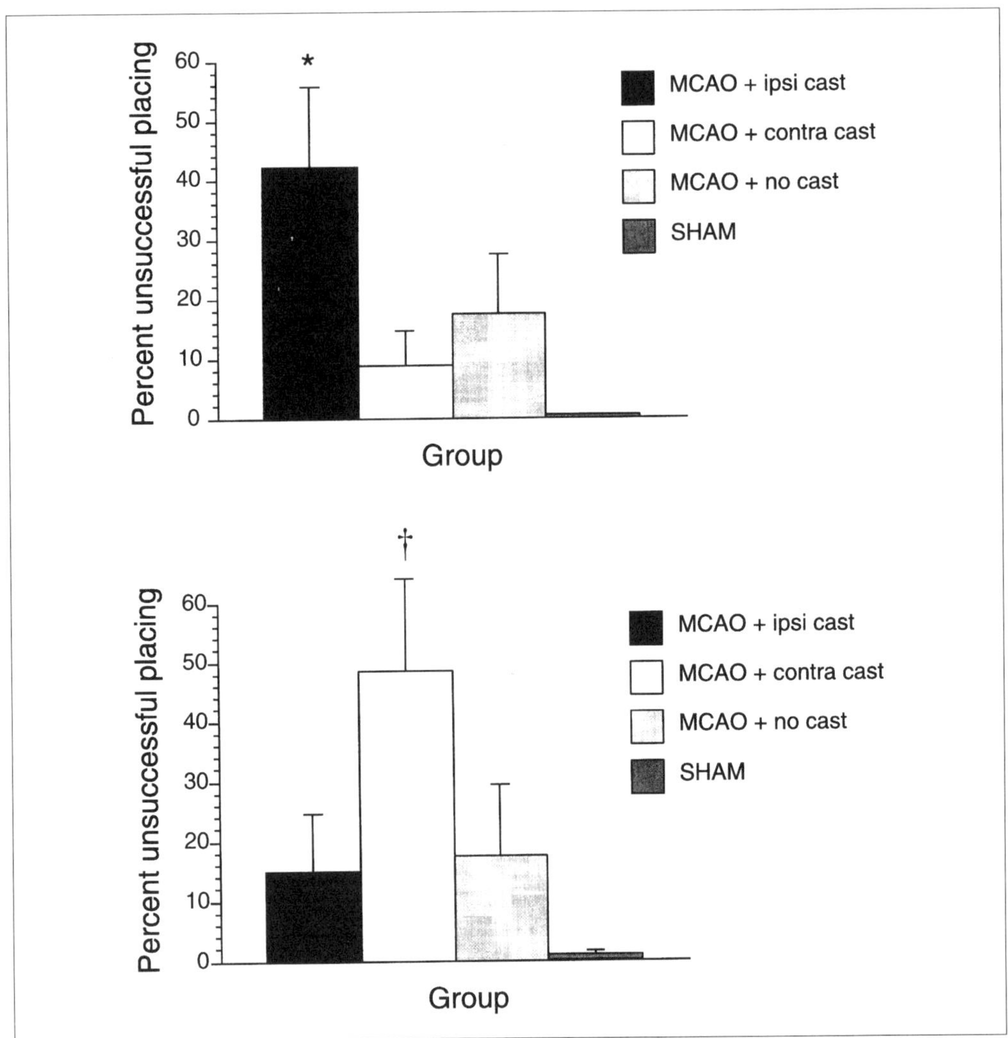

Fig. 4. Early overuse and disuse of the affected forelimb after MCAo differentially affects forelimb placing depending on the stroke model used. Animals were forced to either overuse or disuse the affected forelimb by immobilization of one limb in a plaster cast for 10 days immediately following stroke surgery, or they were uncasted to allow normal use of both forelimbs. Early *overuse* (ipsi cast) worsened the placing deficit after transient *distal* MCAo, but early *disuse* (contra cast) worsened the placing deficit after transient *proximal* MCAo. Placing responses (percent unsuccessful forelimb placing of the affected forelimb) on day 24 are shown after (A) distal MCAo, which preferentially caused cortical damage, and (B) proximal MCAo, which preferentially caused striatal damage. SHAM represents the pooled data of ipsi- contra- and uncasted sham animals.
* p <.05, significantly different from MCAo + contra cast, MCAo + no cast, and SHAM.
† p <.05, significantly different from MCAo + ipsi cast, MCAo + no cast, and SHAM.

ed directly with the damaged brain system rather than neural changes linked to alternative behavioral strategies.

A unique method for evaluating chronic deficits is to provide the animal with a crutch to prevent the need for alternative motor strategies. Recently such a test was developed based on the footfault test (Tim Barth, personal communication). We have extended this and developed a footfault test with random size openings through which an animal can place its fore- or hindlimbs onto a solid surface 1 cm below the grid. Normal animals do not slip their feet through the grid to contact the solid surface, but animals with permanent MCAo do so, primarily with the contralateral limbs (Fig. 5, left panel). The deficit is chronic in this stroke model (which causes damage to both cortex and striatum, Tamura et al. 1981), lasting over a year post-ischemia. Without the solid platform under the grid, footfaults are only transient. We hypothesize that the solid platform allows the impaired limbs to rest directly below the random-grid surface, thus providing a crutch which the animals learn to use on a chronic basis. This technique may reveal the true extent of the injury and deficit because the animals are not forced to compensate.

Extensive rehabilitative training, even long after the injury, can ameliorate the deficit. Animals were housed for 15 says beginning 12 months after MCAo in a cage with a random grid surface with large openings similar to the test apparatus. The animals living in the random grid showed remarkable improvement in performance (Fig. 5, right panel). This method

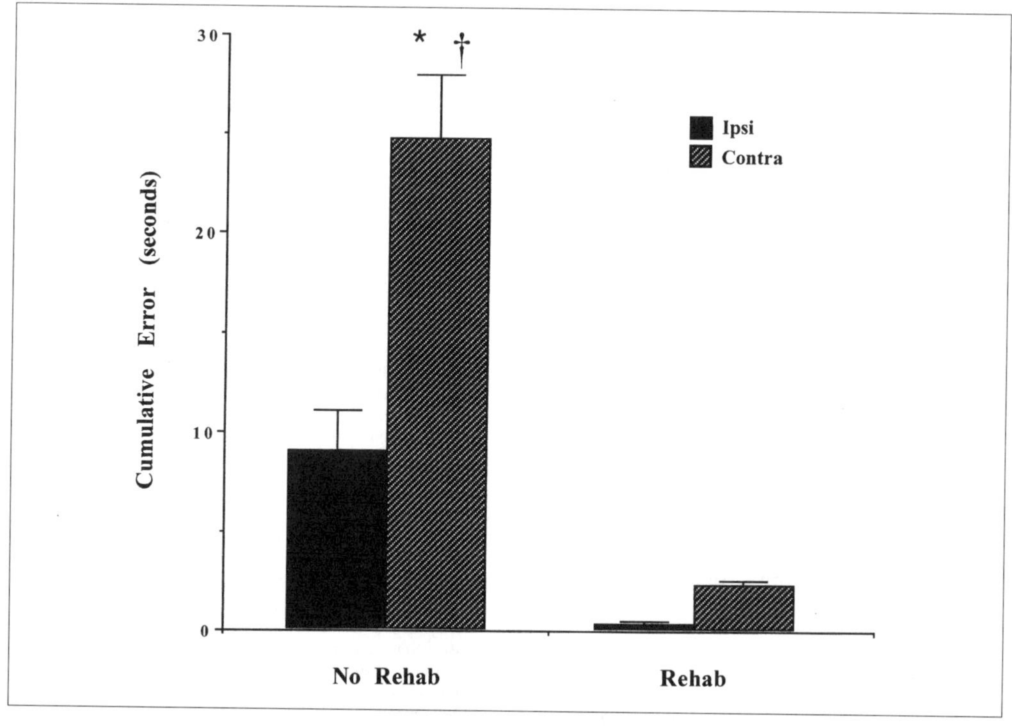

Fig. 5. Twelve months following MCAo animals were housed in cages with random grid floors (Rehab group, n = 10) for 15 days or remained in cages with a sawdust floor (No Rehab group, n = 9). They were then tested on a footfault task with similar random grid openings and a platform 1 cm below the grid. The duration (seconds) of forelimb and hindlimb faults were calculated and combined. Animals in the No Rehab group spent more time faulting with the limb contralateral to the lesion compared to the Rehab group (* = $p < 0.01$) and the No Rehab group faulted more with the contralateral limb compared to the ipsilateral limb († = $p < 0.05$).

may be useful and convenient for rehabilitative training after ischemic or other injury to sensorimotor systems without being too intense. The extent to which this intervention generalizes to other motor test remains to be determined. However, in human stroke patients, the effectiveness of training procedures often are evaluated with tests that match the training goal.

Conclusions

Brain injury causes time-dependent anatomical events in rats that may be altered by behavior. Both plasticity and degenerative events can be modified by manipulating behavioral demand. Early after injury there may be a window of opportunity during which the beneficial effects of motor rehabilitation might be potentiated by endogenous trophic factor expression or by exogenous growth factors. Extreme disuse of the affected forelimb after stroke can impair functional recovery, suggesting that complete motor quiescence during the first week or so after injury may be detrimental. On the other hand, extreme forced overuse of the affected forelimb can exaggerate functional deficits. In stroke models, the extent of the initial infarct and the timing of the intervention can be significant factors in determining whether extreme rehabilitative pressure has an adverse effect on outcome. Use-dependent extracellular glutamate and the NMDA receptor may interact with other factors associated with excessive movement, to degrade peri-lesional tissue, which appears to be vulnerable during the first week or so after injury. Finally, delayed rehabilitation which prevents the use of alternative strategies can be very effective following stroke.

Acknowledgements

This work was supported by NIH NS 23979.

References

1. Abe K (2000) Therapeutic potential of neurotrophic factors and neural stem cells against ischemic brain injury. JCBFM, in press
2. Anderson KJ, Dam D, Lee S, Cotman CW (1988) Basic fibroblast growth factor prevents death of lesioned cholinergic neurons in vivo. Nature 332:360–361
3. Bach-y-Rita P (1990) Brain plasticity as a basis for recovery of function in humans. Neuropsychologia 28(6):547–554
4. Bach-y-Rita P (1993) Recovery from brain damage. Journal of Neurological Rehabilitation 6:191–199
5. Barth TM, Jones TA, Schallert T (1990) Functional subdivisions of the rat somatic sensorimotor cortex. Behavioral Brain Research 39:73–95
6. Belayev L, Alonso OF, Busto R, Zhao W, Ginsberg MD (1996) Middle cerebral artery occlusion in the rat by intraluminal suture. Neurological and pathological evaluation of an improved model. Stroke 27:1616–1622
7. Black JE, Isaacs KR, Anderson BJ, Alcantara AA, Greenough WT (1990) Learning causes synaptogenesis, whereas motor activity causes angiogenesis, in cerebellar cortex of the rat. Proceedings of the National Academy of Sciences 87:5568–5572
8. Black P, Markowitz RS, Cianci SN (1975) Recovery of motor function after lesions in motor cortex in monkeys. In Outcome of Severe Damage to the Central Nervous System (ed. C.E. Symposium), pp 65–70
9. Bland ST, Gonzales RA, Schallert T (1999) Movement related glutamate levels in rat hippocampus, striatum, and sensorimotor cortex. Neuroscience Letters 277:119–122
10. Bland ST, Humm JL, Kozlowski DA, Williams L, Strong R, Aronowski J, Grotta J, Schallert T (1998) Forced overuse of the contralateral forelimb increases infarct volume following a mild, but not a servere, transient cerebral ichemic insult. Soc Neurosci Abstr 24
11. Bland ST, Pillai RN, Aronowski J, Grotta JC, Schallert T (2000) Early overuse and disuse of the affected forelimb after moderately severe intraluminal suture occlusion of the middle cerebral artery in rats. Behavioral Brain Research (in press)
12. Bland ST, Strong R, Aronowski J, Grotta J, Schallert T (2000) Early overuse of the affected forelimb following moderate transient focal ischemia in rats: Functional and anatomical outcome. Stroke 31:1144–1152
13. Brecknell JE, Haque NSK, Du JS, Muir EM, Fidler PS, Hlavin ML, Fawcett JW, Dunnett SB (1996) Functional and anatomical reconstruction of the 6-hydroxydopamine lesioned nigrostriatal system of the adult rat. Neuroscience 71:913–925
14. Bruce-Keller AJ, Umberger G, McFall R, Mattson MP (1999) Food restriction reduces brain damage and improves behavioral outcome following excitotoxic and metabolic insults. Ann Neurol 45:8–15
15. Bucy PC (1944) Effects of extirpation in man. In The precentral motor cortex (Eds) 353–394
16. Burgess W, Maciag T (1989) The heparin-binding (fibroblast) growth factor family of proteins. Annual Review of Biochemistry 58:575–606
17. Bury SD, Eichhorn AC, Kotzer CM, Jones TA (2000) Reactive astrocytic responses to denervation in the motor cortex of adult rats are sensitive to manipulations of behavioral experience. Neuropharmacology 39:743–755
18. Castro-Alamancos MA, Donoghue JP, Connors BW (1995) Different forms of synaptic plasticity in somatosensory and motor areas of the neocortex. Journal of Neuroscience 15:5324–5333
19. Castro-Alamancos MA, Garcia-Segura L, Borrell J (1992) Transfer of function to a specific area of the cortex after induced recovery from brain damage. European Journal of Neuroscience 4:853–863

20. Chen J, Graham SH, Zhu RL, Simon RP (1996) Stress proteins and tolerance to focal cerebral ischemia. J Cereb Blood Flow Metab 16:566–577
21. Conti AC, Raghupathi R, Trojanowski JQ, McIntosh TK (1998) Experimental brain injury induces regionally distinct apoptosis during the acute and delayed post-traumatic period. J Neurosci 18:5663–5672
22. Corbett D, Nurse S (1998) The problem of assessing effective neuroprotection in experimental cerebral ischemia. Progress in Neurobiology 54:531–548
23. Cotman CW, Bridges RJ, Taube JS, Clarke AS, Geddes JW, Monaghan DT (1989) The role of NMDA receptors in central nervous system plasticity and pathology. Journal of WIH Research 1:65–74
24. Cramer S, Chopp M (2000) Recovery recapitulates ontogeny. Trends in Neurosciences 23:265–271
25. Cummings BJ, Yee GJ, Cotman CW (1992) bFGF promotes the survival of entorhinal layer II neurons after perforant path axotomy. Brain Research 591(2):271–276
26. Day LB, Schallert T (1996) Anticholinergic effects on acquisition of place learning in the Morris Water Task: spatial mapping deficit or inability to inhibit nonplace strategies? Behavioral Neuroscience 110:1–8
27. Day LB, Weisand M, Sutherland RJ, Schallert T (1999) The hippocampus is not necessary for a place response but may be necessary for Pliancy. Behavioral Neuroscience 113:914–924
28. Denny-Brown D (1950) Disintegration of motor function resulting from cerebral lesions. Journal of Nervous Mental Disease 112:1–45
29. Denny-Brown D (1960) Motor mechanisms-introduction: the general principles of motor integration. In Handbook of Physiology. Neurophysiology 781–796
30. Dietrich WD, Alonso O, Busto R, Finklestein SP (1996) Posttreatment with intravenous basic fibroblast growth factor reduces histopathological damage following fluid-percussion brain injury in rats. Journal of Neurotrauma 13(6):309–316
31. Dionne CA, Crumley G, Bellot F, Kaplow JM, Searfoss G, Ruta M, Burgess WH, Jaye M, Schlessinger J (1990) Cloning and expression of two distinct high-affinity receptors cross-reacting with acidic and basic fibroblat growth factors. EMBO Journal 9:2685–2692
32. Du C, Hu R, Csernansky CA, Hsu CY, Choi DW (1996) Very delayed infarction after mild focal cerebral ischemia: A role for apoptosis? J Cereb Blood Flow Metab 16:195–201
33. Enfors P, Bengzon J, Kokaia Z, Persson H, Lindvall O (1991) Increased levels of messenger RNAs for neurotrophic factors in the brain during kindling epileptogenesis. Neuron 7:165–176
34. Eysel UT (1997) Perilesional cortical dysfunction and reorganization. In Brain Plasticity, Advances in Neurology, Freund H-J, Sabel BA, Witte OW (Eds), Lippencott-Raven Publishers: Philadelphia
35. Finklestein SP (1996) The potential use of neurotrophic growth factors in the treatment of cerebral ischemia. In Siesjo BK, Wieloch T (Eds), Cellular and Molecular Mechanisms of Ischemic Brain Damage. Raven Press: New York
36. Finklestein SP, Apostolides PJ, Caday CG, Prosser J, Philips MF, Klagsbrun M (1988) Increased basic fibroblast growth factor (bFGF) immunoreactivity at the site of focal brain wounds. Brain Research 460:253–259
37. Follesa P, Gale K, Mocchetti I (1994) Regional and temporal pattern of expression of nerve growth factor and basic fibroblast growth factor mRNA in rat brain following electroconvulsive shock. Experimental Neurology 127:37–44
38. Frautschy SA, Walicke PA, Baird A (1991) Localization of basic fibroblast growth factor and its mRNA after CNS injury. Brain Research 553:291–299
39. Freund HJ (1996) Remapping the brain. Science 272(5269):1754
40. Freund HJ, Sabel BA, Witte OW (1997) Advances in Neurology, Lippincott-Raven Press: New York
41. Frim DM, Uhler TA, Short PM, Ezzedine ZD, Klagsbrun M, Breakfield XO, Isacson O (1993) Effects of biologically-delivered NGF, BDNF and bFGF on striatal excitotoxic lesions. NeuroReport 4:367–370
42. Fulton JF, Kennard MA (1934) A study of flaccid and spastic paralysis produced by lesions of the cerebral cortex in primates. Research Publication of the Association for Mental Disabilities 13:158–210
43. Gall CM, Isackson PI (1989) Limbic seizures increase neuronal production of messenger RNA for nerve growth factor. Science 245:758–761
44. Gentile AM, Green S, Nieburgs A, Schelzer W, Stein DG (1978) Description and recovery of locomotor and manipulatory behavior following cortical lesions in rats. Behavioral Biology 22:417–455
45. Ginsberg MD, Bogousslavsky J (Eds) Cerebrovascular disease. New York: Blackwell Science
46. Giordana MT, Attanasio A, Cavalla P, Migheli A, Vigliani MC, Schiffer D (1994) Reactive cell proliferation and microglia following injury to the rat brain. Neuropathology and Applied Neurobiology 20:163–174
47. Gless P, Cole J (1950) Recovery of skilled motor functions after small repeated lesions in motor cortex in macaque. Journal of Neurophysiology 13:137–148
48. Gómez-Pinilla F, Won-Kyun Lee J, Cotman CW (1992) Basic FGF in adult rat brain: Cellular distribution and response to entorhinal lesion and fimbria-fornix transection. The Journal of Neuroscience 12(1):345–355
49. Gowland C (1987) Management of hemiplegic upper limb. In Stroke Rehabilitation (ed. Brandstater M and Basmajian J), pp 217–245 Baltimore: Williams and Wilkens
50. Greenough WT, Fass B, DeVoogd T (1976) The influence of experience on recovery following brain damage in rodents: Hypotheses based on developmental research. In Environments as Therapy for Brain Dysfunction (ed. Walsh, R and Greenough WT), pp 10–50 New York: Plenum Press
51. Gritti A, Parati EA, Cova L, Froilchsthal P, Galli R, Wanke E, Faravelli L, Morassutti DJ, Roisen F, Nickel DD, Vescovi AL (1996) Multipotential stem cells from the adult mouse brain proliferate and self-renew in response to basic fibroblast growth factor. The Journal of Neuroscience 16(3):1091–1100
52. Grothe C, Wewetzer K (1996) Fibroblast growth factor and its implications for developing and regenerating neurons. International Journal of Developmental Biology 40:403–410
53. Grothe C, Otto D, Frotscher M, Unsicker K (1989) A role of basic fibroblast growth factor for rat septal neurons. EXS 57:251–258
54. Harris KM (1995) How multiple-synapse boutons could preserve input specificity during an interneuronal spread of LTP. Trends in Neuroscience 18:365–369
55. Hernandez TD, Schallert T (1988) Seizures and recovery from experimental brain damage. Experimental Neurology 102:318–324
56. Humm JL, James DC, Gibb R, Kolb B, Schallert T (1997) Forced disuse of the impaired forelimb by restraint after sensorimotor cortical injury inhibits expression of endogenous bFGF in astrocytes and adversely affects behavioral function. Society for Neuroscience Abstracts 23
57. Humpel C, Chadi G, Lippoldt A, Ganten D, Fuxe K, Olson L (1994) Increase of basic fibroblast growth factor (bFGF, FGF-2) messenger RNA and protein following implantation of a microdialysis probe into rat hippocampus. Experimental Brain Research 98:229–237
58. Johansson BB (2000) Brain plasticity and stroke rehabilitation. Stroke 31:223–230

59. Johansson BB (1995) Functional recovery after brain infarction. Cerebrovascular Disorders 5:278–281
60. Jones TA (1999) Motor skills training enhances lesion-induced structural plasticity in the motor cortex of adult rats. Journal of Comparative Neurology 414:57–66
61. Jones TA, Chu CJ, Grande LA, Gregory AD (1999) Motor skills training enhances lesion-induced structural plasticity in the motor cortex of adult rats. Journal of Neuroscience 19:10153–10163
62. Jones TA, Kleim JA, Greenough WT (1996) Synaptogenesis and dendritic growth in the cortex opposite unilateral sensorimotor cortex damage in adult rats: a quantitative electron microscopic examination. Brain Research 733:142–148
63. Jones TA, Klintsova AY, Kilman VL, Sirevaag AM, Greenough WT (1997) Induction of multiple synapses by experience in the visual cortex of adult rats. Neurobiology of Learning and Memory 68:13–20
64. Jones TA, Schallert T (1992) Overgrowth and pruning of dendrites in adult rats recovering from neocortical damage. Brain Research 581:156–160
65. Jones TA, Schallert T (1994) Use-dependent growth of pyramidal neurons after neocortical damage. Journal of Neuroscience 14:2140–2152
66. Kaas JH (1991) Plasticity of sensory and motor maps in adult mammals. Annual Review of Neuroscience 14:137–167
67. Karni A, Meyer G, Jezzard P, Adams MM, Turner R, Ungerleider LG (1995) Functional MRI evidence of adult motor cortex plasticity during motor skill learning. Nature 377:155–158
68. Kato T, Nakano S, Kogure K, Sasaki H, Koiwai K, Yamasaki Y, Katagiri T, Sasaki H (1992) The binding of basic fibroblast growth factor to ischemic neurons in the rat. Neuropathology & Applied Neurobiology 18(3):282–290
69. Kawamata T, Alexis NE, Dietrich WD, Finklestein SP (1996) Intracisternal basic fibroblast growth factor (bFGF) enhances behavioral recovery following focal cerebral infarction in the rat. Journal of Cerebral Blood Flow and Metabolism 16:542–547
70. Kawamata T, Schallert T, Dietrich WD, Benowitz LI, Gotts JE, Cocke RR, Finklestein SP (1997a) Intracisternal basic fibroblast growth factor (bFGF) enhances functional recovery and upregulates the expression of a molecular marker of neuronal sprouting following focal cerebral infarction. Proceedings of the National Academy of Sciences 94:8179–8184
71. Kawamata T, Speliotes EK, Finklestein SP (1997b) The role of polypeptide growth factors in recovery from stroke. In Brain Plasticity, Advances in Neurology, Freund H-J, Sabel BA and Witte OW (Eds), Lippencott-Raven Publishers: Philadelphia
72. Keegan K, Johnson DE, Williams LT, Hayman MJ (1991) Isolation of an additional member of the fibroblast growth factor receptor family, FGFR-3. Proceedings of the National Academy of Sciences 88:1095–1099
73. Khoja I, Herranz AS, Willams JR, Cannon-Spoor HE, Heim RC, Freed WJ, Poltorak M (1995) Localization of gliosis in the corpus striatum of mice following cortical lesion. Restorative Neurology and Neuroscience 9:113–119
74. Kolb B (1995) Brain Plasticity and Behavior. Erlbaum & Associates: New York
75. Kolb B, Cote S, Ribeiro-da-Silva A, Cuello C (1997) NGF treatment prevents dendritic atrophy and promotes recovery of function after cortical injury. Neuroscience 76:1139–1151
76. Kozlowski DA, James DC, Schallert T (1996) Use-dependent exaggeration of neuronal injury following unilateral sensorimotor cortex lesions. Journal of Neuroscience 16:4776–4786
77. Kozlowski DA, Jones TA, Schallert T (1994) Pruning of dendrites and maintenance of function after brain damage: Role of the NMDA receptor. Restorative Neurology and Neuroscience 7:119–126
78. Lashley K (1924) Studies of cerebral function in learning. V. The retention of motor habits after destruction of the so-called motor areas in primates. Archives of Neurological Psychiatry 12:249–276
79. Lee PL, Johnson DE, Cousens LS, Fried VA, Williams LT (1989) Purification and complementary DNA cloning of a receptor for basic fibroblast growth factor. Science 245:57–60
80. LeVere TE (1988) Neural system imbalances and the consequences of large brain injuries. In Finger S, LeVere TE, Almi CR and Stein DG (Eds). Brain Injury and Recovery, Theoretical and Controversial Issues, Plenum Press: New York, pp 15–28
81. Lieberman JS (1986) Hemiplegia: Rehabilitation of the upper extremity. In Stroke Rehabilitation (ed. Kaplan P and Cerullo L), Boston: Butterworths, pp 95–117
82. Liepert J, Bauder H, Miltner WHR, Taub E, Weiller C (2000) Treatment-induced cortical reorganization after stroke in humans. Stroke 31:1210–1216
83. Lindholm D (1997) Neurotrophic factors and neuronal plasticity: Is there a link? In Brain Plasticity, Advances in Neurology, Freund H-J, Sabel BA and Witte OW (Eds), Lippencott-Raven Publishers: Philadelphia
84. Lippoldt A, Andbjer B, Rosen L, Richter E, Ganten D, Cao Y, Pettersson RF, Fuxe K (1993) Photochemically induced focal cerebral ischemia in rat: time dependent and global increase in expression of basic fibroblast growth factor mRNA. Brain Research 625:45–56
85. Liu Z, D'Amore PA, Mikati M, Gatt A, Holmes GL (1993) Neuroprotective effect of chronic infusion of basic fibroblast growth factor on seizure-associated hippocampal damage. Brain Research 626:335–338
86. Logan A, Frautschy SA, Gonzalez AM, Baird, A (1992) A time course for the focal elevation of synthesis of basic fibroblast growth factor and one of its high-affinity receptors (flg) following a localized cortical brain injury. Journal of Neuroscience 12(10):3828–3837
87. Luhmann HJ, Pronce DA (1991) Control of NMDA receptor-mediated activity by GABAergic mechanisms in mature and developing rat neocortex. Developmental Brain Research 54:287–290
88. Mattson MP, Scheff S (1994) Endogenous neuroprotection factors and traumatic brain injury: Mechanisms of action and implications for therapy. Journal of Neurotrauma 11:3–33
89. Mattson MP, Kumar KN, Wang H, Cheng B, Michaelis EK (1993) Basic FGF regulates the expression of a functional 71 kDa NMDA receptor protein that mediates calcium influx and neurotoxicity in hippocampal neurons. Journal of Neuroscience 13: 4575–4588
90. Mattson MP, Murrain M, Guthrie PB, Kater SB (1989) Fibroblast growth factor and glutamate: Opposing roles in the generation and degeneration of hippocampal neuroarchitecture. Journal of Neuroscience 9:3728–3740
91. Mayer E, Dunnett SB, Fawcett JW (1993) Mitogenic effect of basic fibroblast growth factor on embryonic ventral mesencephalic dopaminergic neurone precursors. Developmental Brain Research 72(2):253–258
92. McDermott KL, Raghupathi R, Fernandez SC, Saatman KE, Protter AA, Finklestein SP, Sinson G, Smith DH, McIntosh TK (1997) Delayed administration of basic fibroblast growth factor (bFGF) attenuates cognitive dysfunction following parasagittal fluid percussion brain injury in the rat. Journal of Neurotrauma 14:191–200
93. Menon VK, Landerholm TE (1994) Intralesion injection of basic fibroblast growth factor alters glial reactivity to neural trauma. Experimental Neurology 129:142–154
94. Miyamoto O, Itano T, Fujisawa M, Tokuda M, Matsui H, Nagao S, Hatase O (1993) Exogenous basic fibroblast growth factor and nerve growth factor enhance sprouting of acetylcholineste-

rase positive fibers in denervated rat hippocampus. Acta Medica Okayama 47(3):139–144
95. Morrison RS, Keating RF, Moskal JR (1988) Basic fibroblast growth factor and epidermal growth factor exert differential trophic effects on CNS neurons. Journal of Neuroscience Research 21:71–79
96. Morrison RS, Sharma A, de Vellis J, Bradshaw RA (1986) Basic fibroblast growth factor supports the survival of cerebral cortical neurons in primary culture. Proceedings of the National Academy of Sciences 83:7537–7541
97. Nieto-Sampedro M, Cotman CW (1985) Growth factor induction and temporal order in central nervous system repair. In Cotman CW (ed) Synaptic plasticity, New York: Guilford Press, pp 407–456
98. Nudo RJ, Wise BM, SiFuentes F, Milliken GW (1996) Neural substrates for the effects of rehabilitative training on motor recovery after ischemic infarct. Science 272:1791–1794
99. Ostendorf CG, Wolf SL (1981) Effect of forced use of the upper extremity of a hemiplegic patient on changes in function. Physical Therapy 61:1022–1028
100. Otto D, Unsicker K (1990) Basic FGF reverses chemical and morphological deficits in the nigrostriatal system of MPTP-treated mice. The Journal of Neuroscience 10:1912–1921
101. Otto D, Frotscher M, Unsicker K (1989) Basic fibroblast growth factor and nerve growth factor administered in gel foam rescue medial septal neurons after fimbria fornix transection. Journal of Neuroscience Research 22(1):83–91
102. Partanen J, Mäkelä TP, Eerola E, Korhonen J, Hirvonen H, ClaessonWelsh L, Alitalo K (1991) FGFR-4, a novel acidic fibroblast growth factor receptor with a distinct expression pattern. EMBO Journal 10:1347–1354
103. Passingham RE, Perry VH, Wilkinson F (1983) The long-term effects of removal of sensorimotor cortex in infant and adult rhesus monkeys. Brain 106:675–705
104. Penfield W (1954) Mechanisms of voluntary movement. Brain 77:1–17
105. Pons TP, Garraghty PE, Ommaya K, Kaas JH, Taub E, Mishkin M (1991) Massive cortical reorganization after sensory deafferentation in adult macaques. Science 252:1857–1860
106. Riva MA, Gale K, Mocchetti I (1992) Basic fibroblast growth factor mRNA increases in specific brain regions following convulsive seizures. Molecular Brain Research 15(3–4):311–318
107. Rose FD, Davey MJ, Love S, Dell PA (1987) Environmental enrichment and recovery from contralateral sensory neglect in rats with large unilateral neocortical lesions. Behavioural Brain Research 24:195–202
108. Rosenzweig MR (1980) Animal models for effects of brain lesions and for rehabilitation. In Recovery of Function: Theoretical Considerations For Brain Injury Rehabilitation (ed. Bach-y-Rita P). Baltimore: University Park Press
109. Rowntree S, Kolb B (1997) Blockade of basic fibroblast growth factor retards recovery from motor cortex injury in rats. Eur J Neurosci 9:2432–2441
110. Sabel BA, Kasten E, Kreutz MR (1997) Recovery of vision after partial visual system injury as a model of postlesion plasticity. In Brain Plasticity, Advances in Neurology, Freund H-J, Sabel BA and Witte OW (Eds), Lippencott-Raven Publishers: Philadelphia
111. Sanes JN, Suner S, Lando JF, Donoghue JP (1988) Rapid reorganization of adult rat motor cortex somatic representation patterns after motor nerve injury. Proceedings of the National Academy of Sciences 85(6):2003–2007
112. Schallert T, De Ryck M, Teitelbaum P (1980) Atropine stereotypy as a behavioral trap: A movement subsystem and electroencephalographic analysis. Journal of Comparative and Physiological Psychology 94:1–24
113. Schallert T, Leasure HL, Kolb B (2000) Experience-associated structural events, neuroplasticity and recovery of function following brain injury: a review. J Cereb Blood Flow Metab, in press
114. Schalltert T, Hernandez TD (1998) GABAergic drugs and neuroplasticity after brain injury: Impact on functional recovery. In Restorative Neurology: Advances in the Pharmacotherapy of Recovery after Stroke (Goldstein L, ed), Futura Publishing: Armonk, NY, 91–120
115. Schallert T, Jones TA (1993) "Exuberant" neuronal growth after brain damage in adult rats: The essential role of behavioral experience. Journal of Neural Transplantation Plasticity 4:193–198
116. Schallert T (1988) Aging-dependent emergence of sensorimotor dysfunction in rats recovered from dopamine depletion sustained early in life. In Joseph JA (Ed), Central Determinants of Age-Related Decline in Motor Function, Annals of the New York Academy of Science, 108–120
117. Schallert T (1989) Preoperative intermittent feeding or drinking regimens enhance postlesion sensorimotor function. In Schulkin J (Ed) Preoperative events: Their effects on behavior following brain damage, Lawrence Erlbaum Associates: New Jersey, 1–20
118. Schallert T (1995) Models of neurological defects and defects in neurological models. Brain and Behavioral Sciences 18:68–69
119. Schallert T, Fleming SM, Leasure JL, Tillerson JL, Bland ST (2000) CNS plasticity and assessment of forelimb sensorimotor outcome in unilateral rat models of stroke, cortical ablation, parkinsonism and spinal cord injury. Neuropharmacology 39:777–787
120. Schallert T, Hernandez TD, Barth TM (1986) Recovery of function after brain damage: Severe and chronic disruption by diazepam. Brain Res 379:104–111
121. Schallert T, Jones TA, Weaver MS, Fulton R, Robinson D, Shapiro LE (1992) Pharmacological and anatomical considerations in recovery of function. In Tucker DM (Ed) State of the Art Reviews in Neuropsychology, Hanley & Belfus: Philadelphia
122. Schallert T, Kozlowski DA, Humm JL, Cocke RR (1997) Use-dependent events in recovery of function. In Brain Plasticity, Advances in Neurology 73:229–238
123. Schallert T, Whishaw IQ (1984) Bilateral cutaneous stimulation of the somatosensory system in hemidecorticate rats. Behavioural Neuroscience 98:518–540
124. Schallert T, Whishaw IQ (1985) Neonatal hemidecortication and bilateral cutaneous stimulation in rats. Developmental Psychobiology 18:501–514
125. Schwartz S (1964) Effect of neonatal cortical lesions and early environmental factors on adult rat behavior. Journal of Comparative Physiological Psychology 57:72–77
126. Seitz RJ, Freund H-J (1997) Plasticity of the human motor cortex. In Brain Plasticity, Advances in Neurology 73:321–333
127. Sharp FR, Kinouchi H, Massa SM, Weinstein P, Narasimhan P, Sklar R, Chan P (1997) Stress gene induction in focal ishemia. In Ginsberg MD and Bogousslavsky J (Eds), Cerebrovascular Disease: Pathology, Diagnosis, and Management. Cambridge, MA: Blackwell Science
128. Sievers J, Hausmann B, Unsicker K, Berry M (1987) Fibroblast growth factors promote the survival of adult rat retinal ganglion cells after transection of the optic nerve. Neuroscience Letters 76(2):157–162
129. Speliotes EK, Caday CG, Do T, Weise J, Kowall NNW, Finklestein SP (1996) Increased expression of basic fibroblast growth factor (bFGF) following focal cerebral infarction in the rat. Molecular Brain Research 39:31–42

130. Stephan K-M, Frackowiak RSJ (1997) Recovery from subcortical stroke-PET activation patterns in patients compared with healthy subjects. In Brain Plasticity, Advances in Neurology, Freund H-J, Sabel BA and Witte OW (Eds), Lippencott-Raven Publishers: Philadelphia
131. Stroemer RP, Kent TA, Hulsebosch CE (1995) Neocortical neural sprouting, synaptogenesis, and behavioral recovery after neocortical infarction in rats. Stroke 26:2135–2144
132. Szele FG, Chesselet MF (1996) Cortical lesions induce an increase in cell number and PSA-NCAM expression in the subventricular zone of adult rats. Journal of Comparative Neurology 368(3):439–454
133. Takami K, Iwane M, Kiyota Y, Miyamoto M, Tsukuda R, Shosaka S (1992) Increase of basic fibroblast growth factor immunoreactivity and its mRNA level in rat brain following transient forebrain ischemia. Experimental Brain Research 90:1–10
134. Tamura A, Graham DI, McCulloch T, Teasdale GM (1981) Focal cerebral ischaemia in the rat: 2. Regional cerebral blood flow determined by [^{14}C] iodoantipyrine autoradiography following middle cerebral artery occlusion. J Cereb Blood Flow Metab 1(1):53–60
135. Tanaka T, Saito H, Matsuki N (1996) Basic fibroblast growth factor modulates synaptic transmission in cultured rat hippocampal neurons. Brain Research 723:190–195
136. Tanaka T, Saito H, Matsuki N (1997) Inhibition of GABAA synaptic responses by brain-derived neurotrophic factor (BDNF) in rat hippocampus. Journal of Neuroscience 17:2959–2966
137. Taub E (1980) Somatosensory deafferentation research with monkeys: Implications for rehabilitation medicine. In Ince P (Ed), Behavioral Psychology in Rehabilitation Medicine: Clinical Applications. Williams & Wilkins: New York, 371–401
138. Taub E, Crago JE, Burgio LD, Groomes TE, Cook EW, DeLuca SC, Miller NE (1994) An operant approach to rehabilitation medicine: Overcoming learned non-use by shaping. Journal of the Experimental Analysis of Behavior 61:281–293
139. Taub E, Miller NE, Novack TA, Cook EW, Fleming WC, Nepomuceno CS, Connell JS, Crago JE (1993) Technique to improve chronic motor deficit after stroke. Archives of Physical and Medical Rehabilitation 74:347–354
140. Taub E, Pidikiti D, DeLuca SC, Crago JE (1996) Effects of motor restriction of an unimpaired upper extremity and training on improving functional tasks and altering brain/behaviors. In Imaging in Neurologic Rehabilitation (ed. Toole JF and Good DC) pp 133–154. New York: Demos Vermande
141. Thoenen H (1995) Neurotrophins and neuronal plasticity. Science 170:593–598
142. Thomas KA, Gimenez-Gallego G (1986) Fibroblast growth factors: Broad spectrum mitogens with potent angiogenic activity. Trends in the Biochemical Sciences 11:81–84
143. Thomas KA (1987) Fibroblast growth factors. FASEB Journal 1:434–440
144. Tillerson JL, Castro SL, Zigmond MJ, Schallert T (1998) Motor rehabilitation of forelimb use in a unilateral 6-hydroxydopamine (6-OHDA) rat model of Parkinson's disease. Soc Neurosci Abstr 672.18:1720
145. Tillerson JL, Cohen A, Fleming SM, Castro SC, Philhower J, Miller GW, Zigmond MJ, Schallert T (2000) Effect of physical therapy on the behavioral and neurochemical response to 6-hydroxydopamine. Soc Neurosci Abstr 26:1025
146. Travis AM, Woolsey CN (1956) Motor performance of monkeys after bilateral partial and total cerebral decortication. American Journal of Physiological Medicine 35:273–310
147. Tropepe V, Craig CG, Morshead CM, van der Kooy D (1997) Transforming growth factor – alpha null and sensescent mice show decreased neural progenitor cell proliferation in forebrain subependyma. Journal of Neuroscience 17:7850–7859
148. Twitchell TE (1951) The restoration of motor function following hemiplegia in man. Brain 74:443–480
149. Valla JE, Humm JL, Schallert T, Gonzalez-Lima F (1999) Metabolic activation of the subependymal zone after cortical injury. Neuroreport 10:2731–2734
150. Voorhies AC, Jones TA (2000) Behavioral and structural effects of aspiration of tissue damaged by cortical injury. Society of Neuroscience Abstracts 26:2294
151. Walicke PA (1988) Basic and acidic fibroblast growth factors have trophic effects on neurons from multiple CNS regions. The Journal of Neuroscience 8(7):2618–1627
152. Wanaka A, Johnson EM, Milbrandt J (1990) Localization of FGF receptor mRNA in the adult rat central nervous system by *in situ* hybridization. Neuron 5:267–281
153. Whishaw IQ, Flannigan KP, Schallert T (1982) An assessment of the state hypothesis of animal hypnosis through an analysis of neocortical and hippocampal EEG in spontaneously immobile and hypnotized rabbits. Electroencephalography and Clinical Neurophysiology 54:365–374
154. Whishaw IQ, Schallert T (1977) Hippocampal RSA (theta), apnea, bradycardia and effects of atropine during underwater swimming in the rat. Electro-encephalography and Clinical Neurophysiology 42:389–396
155. Whishaw IQ, Pellis SM, Gorny BP, Pellis VC (1991) The impairments in reaching and the movements of compensation in rats with motor cortex lesions: An endpoint, videorecording, and movement notation analysis. Behavioral Brain Research 42:77–91
156. Whishaw IQ, Robinson TE, Schallert T (1976) Intraventricular anticholinergics do not block cholinergic hippocampal RSA or neocortical desynchronization in the rabbit or rat. Pharmacology, Biochemistry, and Behavior 5:275–283
157. Whishaw IQ, Robinson TE, Schallert T, De Ryck M, Ramirez VD (1978) Electrical activity of the hippocampus and neocortex in rats depleted of brain dopamine and norepinephrine: Relation to behavior and effects of atropine. Experimental Neurology 62:748–767
158. Winstein CJ, Pohl PS (1995) Effects of unilateral brain damage on the control of goal-directed hand movements. Experimental Brain Research 105:163–174
159. Withers GS, Greenough WT (1989) Reach training selectively alters dendritic branching in subpopulations of layer II–III pyramidals in rat motor-somatosensory forelimb cortex. Neuropsychologia 27:61–69
160. Witte O (1998) Lesion-induced plasticity as a potential mechanism for recovery and rehabilitative training. Current Opinion in Neurology 11:655–662
161. Witte OW, Stoll G (1997) Delayed and remote effects of focal cortical infarctions: secondary damage and reactive plasticity. Advances in Neurology 73:207–227
162. Yamada K, Kinoshita A, Kohmura E, Sakaguchi T, Taguchi J, Kataoka K, Hayakawa T (1991) Basic fibroblast growth factor prevents thalamic degeneration after cortical infarction. Journal of Cerebral Blood Flow & Metabolism 11(3):472–478
163. Yoshida K, Gage FH (1992) Cooperative regulation of nerve growth factor synthesis and secretion in fibroblasts and astrocytes by fibroblast growth factor and other cytokines. Brain Research 569(1):14–25
164. Yoshida K, Gage FH (1991) Fibroblast growth factors stimulate nerve growth factor synthesis and secretion by astrocytes. Brain Research 538(1):118–126

Difference in the time windows for the induction of ischemic tolerance: putative mechanisms

M. A. Pérez-Pinzón

Abstract

Animal studies indicate that a mild anoxic/ ischemic or stress insults will promote neuroprotection of the brain against subsequent 'lethal' insults. The main goal in our laboratory is to characterize the mechanisms by which ischemic tolerance is induced. In this manuscript we review the different time windows by which ischemic preconditioning (IPC) promotes neuroprotection and attempt to define common mechanisms of neuroprotection for both IPC windows. Common pathways appear to involve the activation of the adenosine receptor, the ATP sensitive potassium channel, possibly the translocation of PKC isoforms, the induction of neuroprotective genes and changes in the metabolic and antioxidant state of the preconditioned cells.

Introduction

Ischemic preconditioning (IP) refers to the ability of a brief ("sublethal") ischemic episode, followed by a period of reperfusion, to increase an organ's resistance to injury (ischemic tolerance) following a subsequent ischemic event. This induction of tolerance against ischemia resulting from sublethal ischemic or anoxic insults has gained attention as a robust neuroprotective mechanism against conditions of stress such as anoxia/ischemia in heart and brain (Murry et al. 1986; Kato et al. 1992; Lin et al. 1992; Alkhulaifi et al. 1993; Lin et al. 1993; Walker et al. 1993). There are different preconditioning paradigms both in heart and brain. For example, variations in preconditioning paradigms include, the number of preconditioning insults, types of preconditioning insults, and time between preconditioning and the test insults.

In the past, most preconditioning studies in brain have suggested that several hours are required to develop the tolerant state. However, in recent studies we and others suggested that preconditioning with a rapid onset time course, similar to that in heart (within 1 h), can protect synaptic activity after anoxia in brain slices (Schurr et al. 1986; Schurr and Rigor 1987; Pérez-Pinzón et al. 1996; Centeno et al. 1999; Pérez-Pinzón and Born 1999; Pérez-Pinzón et al. 1999a) and reduce histopathology after ischemia in intact brain (Pérez-Pinzón et al. 1997; Pérez-Pinzón et al. 1999b; Stagliano et al. 1999).

This suggested that mechanisms inducing this state of tolerance in heart and brain may be

Key words: ischemia, adenosine, hypoxia, tolerance, hippocampus.

Department of Neurology, University of Miami School of Medicine, P.O. Box 016960, Miami, Fl. 33101, USA
e-mail: perezpinzon@miami.edu

J. Krieglstein, S. Klumpp (Eds.) Pharmacology of Cerebral Ischemia 2000

common to both organs. There are also two windows for the induction of IPC, one with a rapid onset (rapid ischemic preconditioning) and one with a delay onset (delay ischemic preconditioning). However, it is still undefined whether both windows have similar mechanisms of induction. Some recent evidence suggests that this may be the case.

Mechanisms of ischemic preconditioning

Among the suggested mechanisms of IPC are: a) activation of adenosine receptors; b) activation of K^+_{ATP} channels; c) stimulation of PKC; d) increased activation of 5'-nucleotidase; e) effects on cell metabolism; f) antioxidant defense systems; g) expression of neuroprotective genes; and h) others. These putative mechanisms will be considered in the following sections.

a) Activation of adenosine receptors:

Liu et al. (1991) suggested that endogenous adenosine mediates IPC in cardiac muscle (see also Lohse et al. 1987; Yao and Gross 1994). Since adenosine A1 receptor blockers eliminated the protective effect of IPC. Furthermore, acadesine (5-amino-4-imidazolecarboxamide riboside, AICAR), which increases local levels of adenosine (Gruver et al. 1994; Tsuchida et al. 1994; Tsuchida et al. 1994) delayed the natural decay of preconditioning (i.e., IPC protection was prolonged beyond 1 h) (Tsuchida et al. 1994). Acadesine also lowered the threshold for preconditioning (Tsuchida et al. 1993). IPC was also enhanced by dipyridamole, which blocks adenosine uptake (Miura et al. 1992).

Evidence in brain also suggests that adenosine is involved in IPC. For example, when caffeine, an adenosine receptor blocker, was infused during hypoxic preconditioning in neonates, IPC protection was reduced (Fitzgibbons et al. 1994). In contrast, infusion of the adenosine A1 receptor agonist R-(phenylisopropyl)-adenosine (R-PIA) enhanced IPC effects (Fitzgibbons et al. 1994). IPC was also potentiated by blocking adenosine deaminase (which initiates adenosine catabolism) (Gidday et al. 1995). Supporting a role of adenosine also are findings that the nearly complete protection produced by IPC in the CA1 region of rat hippocampus 3 days after 6 min of global cerebral ischemia was abolished by DPCPX (1 mg/kg) (an adenosine A1 receptor antagonist) (Heurteaux et al. 1995). Infusion of cyclopentyl adenosine (CPA) (1 mg/kg) (an adenosine A1 receptor agonist) 15 min prior to ischemia, produced 70% protection of CA1 cells after 3 days of reperfusion. These experiments suggested the role of adenosine in the induction of delay IPC.

We also showed that amplitudes of evoked potentials recovered significantly better after 'test' anoxic insults in preconditioned slices (Pérez-Pinzón et al. 1996). In control slices, transient superfusion with adenosine or an adenosine A1 receptor agonist (2-chloroadenosine) 30 min prior to 'test' anoxia markedly improved evoked potential recovery. Administration of 8-cyclopentyl-1,3-dipropylxanthine, an A1 receptor antagonist, blocked the protection afforded by preconditioning. These data supported the hypothesis that adenosine, probably by its activation of A1 receptors, is involved in the neuroprotection afforded by anoxic preconditioning in hippocampal slices. These experiments suggested the role of adenosine in the induction of rapid IPC.

b) ATP-sensitive potassium channel

Activation of the K^+_{ATP} channel, likely plays a role in at least some of the mechanisms of IPC. This is because blockade of the K^+_{ATP} channel abolished preconditioning and the protection afforded by adenosine and R-PIA (Schulz et al. 1994; Tomai et al. 1994; Van Winkle et al. 1994). In contrast, a K^+_{ATP} channel opener (RP-52891, aprikalim) increased ischemic tolerance (Auchampach et al. 1991; Gross and Auchampach 1992; Auchampach and Gross 1993). Activation of K^+_{ATP} channel with bimakalin (agonist) during a preconditioning ischemic episode reduced the time necessary to produce preconditioning in dogs (Yao and Gross 1994).

Recent evidence in brain also showed that transient infusion of K^+_{ATP} channel antagonist 24 h prior to ischemia (delay IPC) can block IPC protection after forebrain ischemia (Heurteaux et al. 1995). Recently, we have also shown that the K^+_{ATP} channel is involved in APC protection. In control slices, transient superfusion with an ATP-sensitive potassium channel agonist (10 μM pinacidil) 30 min prior to 'test' anoxia markedly improved evoked potential recovery (rapid IPC). Administration of 5 μM of the sulfonylurea tolbutamide, an ATP-sensitive potassium channel antagonist during preconditioning insults, blocked the protection afforded by preconditioning. These data supported the hypothesis that the ATP-sensitive potassium channel is involved in the neuroprotection afforded by anoxic preconditioning in hippocampal slices (Pérez-Pinzón and Born 1999).

Recently, two ATP-sensitive potassium channels have been described. One of these channels resides in the plasmatic membrane; the other resides in the mitochondrial inner membrane. The mtK^+_{ATP} has been suggested to be the key channel involved in ischemic preconditioning, since the $mtK+_{ATP}$ blocker 5HD prevented IPC protection (Auchampach et al. 1992; Schultz et al. 1997). Also, PKC modulates mtK^+_{ATP}. When PMA (an activator of PKC) was superfused on cardiomyocytes, diazoxide (a mtK^+_{ATP} channel opener) induced mtK^+_{ATP} channel opening was increased (Sato et al. 1998). It has been hypothesized that opening of the mtK^+_{ATP} channel may depolarize mitochondrial membrane potential promoting an increase in the electron transport chain rate, and thus increasing ATP production (Inoue et al. 1991).

c) Stimulation of PKC

Stimulation of PKC by the phorbol ester was cardioprotective during ischemia (Ytrehus et al. 1994). This link between PKC activation and cardioprotection is supported by findings that 5 min of ischemia was sufficient to activate PKC and to produce IPC (Strasser et al. 1992). Ytrehus et al. (1994) showed that activation of PKC may be involved in the secondary phase of ischemic preconditioning in rabbit hearts (Downey et al. 1994). In addition, transient activation of adenosine A1 receptors resulted in an upregulation of PKC, which likely reflects its physical translocation into membranes during IPC.

The translocation of cytosolic PKC into membranes may be a key event during IPC in rabbits. Blockade of PKC activity with staurosporine, abolished IPC protection (Liu et al. 1994), while a PKC agonist (1,2-dioctanoyl-sn-glycerol; DOG) provoked IPC (Speechly-Dick et al. 1994). Interestingly, PKC translocation and activation via several mechanisms emulated IPC. For example, alpha-1-adrenergic agonists that activate PKC can similarly emulate IPC, independent of adenosine direct activation of PKC in rabbits (Tsuchida et al. 1994). Thus, IPC was evoked with alpha-adrenoceptor stimulation (Bankwala et al. 1994) or with phenylephrine (and alpha-adrenergic agonist), which can act as a pharmacological preconditioning agent, as did adenosine (Hale and Kloner 1994).

The role of PKC during ischemic preconditioning in the heart has been supported by numerous studies. Downey et al. (1994) proposed the 'translocation theory of ischemic preconditioning' attempting to define the role of PKC during preconditioning. This theory proposed that preconditioning insults would promote activation of the adenosine A1 receptor, which through the production of diacylglycerol (DAG) and inositol trisphosphate, would induce activation of PKC. During a 'test' ischemic insult, PKC in membranes can be rapidly activated upon re-activation of A1 receptors. In this way, proteins responsible for protection against ischemia can be phosphorylated within the first few minutes of 'test' ischemia in preconditioned myocardium. The translocation theory then states that the only difference between a preconditioned heart and a virgin heart is that the former has PKC translocated into its membranes.

In heart, this theory has been supported by numerous studies. In brain however, no evidence for such mechanism has been reported. In a previous study we showed that the role of PKC appears to be negligible in the anoxic preconditioning paradigm used (Pérez-Pinzón and Born 1999). But, it is possible that activation of PKC may be protective in brain under conditions different to those shown in our previous study (Pérez-Pinzón and Born 1999). It is also possible that concentrations for PKC emulation of APC in brain slices are different from those used to normally activate this protein in the CNS.

d) 5'-Nucleotidase

Another proposed mechanism of IPC is activation of the enzyme 5'-nucleotidase, which is involved in dephosphorylation of AMP to adenosine. Kitakaze et al. (1993) showed that IPC increased both, adenosine release and 5'-nucleotidase activity during myocardial ischemia and reperfusion in dogs. IPC was blunted by inhibition of 5'-nucleotidase activity and by attenuation of adenosine release in dog hearts (Kitakaze et al. 1994). IPC increased ectosolic 5'-nucleotidase activity through activation of PKC, and activation of this enzyme contributed to cardioprotection against ischemia (Kitakaze et al. 1994), since this enzyme increases interstitial adenosine levels by dephosphorylation of AMP.

Other factors known to elicit IPC, such as alpha-1-adrenoceptor seemed to do so by increasing ectosolic 5'-nucletidase activity during preconditioning and may contribute to IPC protection in dog hearts (Kitakaze et al. 1994).

e) Metabolism

Another suggested mechanism of IPC is adenosine stimulation of glucose transport that may increase the capacity for anaerobic energy production (Wyatt et al. 1989). This is consistent with findings that IPC stimulated anaerobic glycolysis in the isolated rabbit heart (Janier et al. 1994), and better preserved ATP levels in rat heart (Kaplan et al. 1994). IPC also reduced the energy imbalance during subsequent myocardial ischemia and maintained the rate of net adenine nucleotide degradation and production of purine metabolites and lactate in dog hearts (Van Wylen 1994).

However, there has not been any reports suggesting a change in the energy charge following either window of IPC in the brain.

f) Antioxidants

IPC also affected the antioxidant defense system. For example, malondialdehyde formation (an indirect marker of free radical formation) was decreased after the second ischemic insult in rat hearts (Tosaki et al. 1994). This is likely due to IPC effects on free radical generating and scavenging systems. IPC enhanced manganese-superoxide dismutase (SOD) catalase, and glutathione-peroxidase activities, whereas it reduced glutathione reductase activity (Das et al. 1992; Hoshida et al. 1993). In brain, the role of superoxide dismutase on IPC has been suggested (Ohtsuki et al. 1992; Kato et al. 1995).

g) Gene expression

A protective effect of IPC may be modulated in part by low molecular weight stress proteins. An important role of stress proteins such as heat shock proteins (HSP) and ubiquitin has been suggested (Kirino et al. 1991; Aoki et al. 1993; Kato et al. 1993; Liu et al 1993; Nishi et al. 1993). Expression of HSP70 seems essential in ischemic tolerance since tolerance disappeared by procedures, which counteracted HSP70 (Liu et al. 1992; Aoki et al. 1993; Nakata et al. 1993; Kato et al. 1994). Interestingly, expression of heat shock proteins in heart due to hyperthermia resulted in a preconditioning effect (Liu et al. 1992), in which antioxidant activity and cell metabolism were improved leading to tolerance against ischemia and reperfusion injury.

Recently, the role of the proto-oncogene bcl-2 on IPC was suggested. First, it was shown that bcl-2 is expressed in neurons that survive focal ischemia in rats (Chen et al. 1995). Shimazaki et al. (1994) showed that ischemic preconditioning promoted increased bcl-2 immunoreactivity. This evidence led to the suggestion that both anti-apoptotic genes, bcl-2 and bcl-x_L are increased in tolerant brain (Chen and Simon 1997).

h) Others

1) Depolarization: Several studies have demonstrated that depolarization of brain cells lead to the induction of tolerance. Previous studies demonstrated that cortical spreading depression (CSD) induced tolerance against cerebral ischemia (Kobayashi et al. 1995; Matsushima et al. 1996; Kawahara et al. 1997; Plumier et al. 1997; Caggiano and Kraig 1998). Several mechanisms of neuroprotection by CSD against cerebral ischemia have been proposed. For example, CSD upregulated BDNF mRNA at 4 h, followed by a delayed secondary increase at 2 to 3 d (Kawahara et al. 1997; Matsushima et al. 1998). Also, Kobayashi et al. (1995) found that 2 h of CSD 1 d prior to forebrain ischemia, protected ipsilateral cortex, but not striatum or hippocampus and that this protection was accompanied by widespread expression of c-fos mRNA. They also observed increased HSP72 expression, but this increase was restricted to the site of KCl injection. Interestingly, Plumier et al. (1997) showed that 20 min of KCl-induced CSD increased HSP72, but specifically on GFAP cells. Additional evidence linking astrocytes with preconditioning was provided recently by Caggiano and Craig (1998), who measured neuronal NOS increased immunohistochemistry in the somatosensory cortex at 6 h and 3 d following CSD, whereas iNOS was unchanged. This increase in nNOS appeared to be localized in GFAP cells, indicating that nNOS upregulation occurred in astrocytes.

The role of depolarization is further supported by findings that intra-IPC hypothermia reduced IPC neuroprotection (Taga et al. 1997). Also, Corbett and Crooks (1997) showed that IPC did not markedly affect post-ischemic brain temperature suggesting that the observed protection was not due to reduction in temperature.

2) Protein Synthesis: Cycloheximide (a protein synthesis inhibitor) eliminated IPC-induced protection if administered before IPC, but not if administered long after IPC (Barone et al. 1998).

3) Inhibition of anoxic LTP: Kawai et al. (1998) showed that preconditioning in vivo inhibits anoxic LTP. They suggested that since anoxic LTP is mediated by NMDA receptors, IPC may be protective against ischemia by inhibiting NMDA currents.

A putative common pathway

Figure 1 describes the possible biochemical common pathways by which anoxic or ischemic preconditioning promotes tolerance against such insults in both windows. At present, it is uncertain whether common pathways converge to promote neuroprotection in both IPC windows. However, studies in heart suggest that protein kinase C might be that convergence point.

During anoxic preconditioning it is expected activation of the adenosine A1 receptor, which in turn may activate the K^+_{ATP} channel. Activation of the adenosine A1 receptor will also promote PKC activation via production of diacylglycerol (DAG) and inositol trisphosphate. Also during ischemic/anoxic preconditioning a mild accumulation of cytosolic calcium and free radical production must occur. Cytosolic calcium by itself will activate PKC. Free radicals generated by mitochondrial inhibition during preconditioning insults will promote opening of the NMDA receptor and activation of phospholipase C. NMDA receptor activation will induce cytosolic calcium accumulation, which in turn will activate PKC. Phospholipase C in turn, will activate PKC by producing DAG and inositol trisphosphate.

In conclusion, even though the mechanisms of ischemic preconditioning remain undefined, a more clear picture is emerging, which includes, activation of the adenosine A1 receptor, the opening of the K^+_{ATP} channel, mild accumulation of cytosolic calcium, and perhaps the activation of PKC. Additional studies are required to thoroughly define the role of the different isoforms of PKC, and to determine

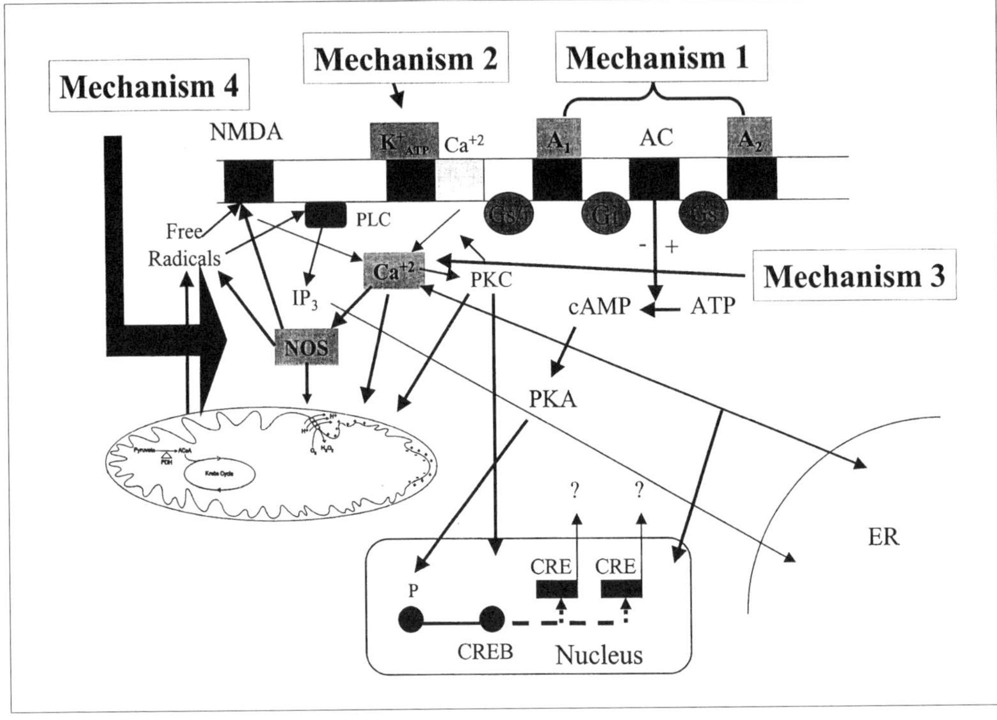

Fig. 1. Putative mechanisms of anoxic preconditioning neuroprotection. Refer to text for explanation.

whether this type of preconditioning will promote prolonged protection after brain ischemia.

Acknowledgments

These studies were supported by PHS grant NS 34773.

References

1. Alkhulaifi AM, Pugsley WB, Yellon DM (1993) The influence of the time period between preconditioning ischemia and prolonged ischemia on myocardial protection. Cardioscience 4(3):163–169
2. Aoki M, Abe K, Kawagoe J, Nakamura S, Kogure K (1993) Acceleration of HSP70 and HSC70 heat shock gene expression following transient ischemia in the preconditioned gerbil hippocampus. J Cereb Blood Flow Metab 13(5):781–788
3. Auchampach JA, Gross GJ (1993) Adenosine A1 receptors, K^+_{ATP} channels, and ischemic preconditioning in dogs. Am J Physiol 264(5 Pt 2):H1327–1336
4. Auchampach JA, Grover GJ, Gross GJ (1992) Blockade of ischemic preconditioning in dogs by the novel ATP dependent potassium channel antagonist sodium 5-hydorxydecanoate. Cardiovasc. Res 26:1054–1062
5. Auchampach JA, Maruyama M, Cavero I, Gross GJ (1991) The new K^+ channel opener Aprikalim (RP 52891) reduces experimental infarct size in dogs in the absence of hemodynamic changes. J Pharmacol Exp Ther 259(3):961–967
6. Bankwala Z, Hale SL, Kloner RA (1994) Alpha-adrenoceptor stimulation with exogenous norepinephrine or release of endogenous catecholamines mimics ischemic preconditioning. Circulation 90(2):1023–1028
7. Barone FC, White RF, Spera PA, Ellison J, Currie RW, Wang XK, Feuerstein GZ (1998) Ischemic preconditioning and brain tolerance – Temporal histological and functional outcomes, protein synthesis requirement, and interleukin-1 receptor antagonist and early gene expression. Stroke 29(9):1937–1950
8. Caggiano AO, Kraig RP (1998) Neuronal nitric oxide synthase expression is induced in neocortical astrocytes after spreading depression. J Cereb Blood Flow Metab 18(1):75–87
9. Centeno JM, Orti M, Salom JB, Sick TJ, Pérez-Pinzón MA (1999) Nitric oxide is involved in anoxic preconditioning neuroprotection in rat hippocampal slices. Brain Res 836(1–2):62–69
10. Chen J, Graham S, Chan P, Lan J, Zhou R, Simon R (1995) bcl-2 is expressed in neurons that survive focal ischemia in the rat. NeuroReport 6:394–398
11. Chen J, Simon R (1997) Ischemic tolerance in the brain. Neurology 48(2):306–311

12. Corbett D, Crooks P (1997) Ischemic preconditioning: A long term survival study using behavioural and histological endpoints. Brain Res 760(1–2):129–136
13. Das DK, Prasad MR, Lu D, Jones RM (1992) Preconditioning of heart by repeated stunning. Adaptive modification of antioxidative defense system. Cell Mol Biol 38(7):739–749
14. Downey JM, Cohen MV, Ytrehus K, Liu Y (1994) Cellular mechanisms in ischemic preconditioning: The role of adenosine and protein kinase C. Ann Ny Acad Sci 723:82–98
15. Fitzgibbons JC, Shah AR, Park TS, Gidday JM (1994) Caffeine blocks the cerebroprotective actions of preconditioning in the hypoxic-ischemic neonate. Soc Neurosci Abs 20(1):618
16. Gidday JM, Fitzgibbons JC, Maceren RG, Shah AR, Shah NR, Park TS. (1995) Inhibition of adenosine deaminase with deoxycoformycin (DCF) potentiates preconditioning cerebroprotection in a perinatal rat model of ischemic tolerance. Soc Neurosci Abs 21(1):513
17. Gross GJ, Auchampach JA (1992) Blockade of ATP-sensitive potassium channels prevents myocardial preconditioning in dogs. Circ Res 70(2):223–233
18. Gruver EJ, Toupin D, Smith TW, Marsh JD (1994) Acadesine improves tolerance to ischemic injury in rat cardiac myocytes. J Mol Cell Cardiol 26(9):1187–1195
19. Hale SL, Kloner RA (1994) Protection of myocardium by transient, preischemic administration of phenylephrine in the rabbit. Coron Artery Dis 5(7):605–610
20. Heurteaux C, Lauritzen I, Widmann C, Lazdunski M (1995) Essential role of adenosine, adenosine A1 receptors, and ATP-sensitive K^+ channels in cerebral ischemic preconditioning. Proc Natl Acad Sci USA 92(10):4666–4670
21. Hoshida S, Kuzuya T, Yamashita N, Oe H, Fuji H, Hori M, Tada M, Kamada T (1993) Brief myocardial ischemia affects free radical generating and scavenging systems in dogs. Heart Vessels 8(3):115–120
22. Inoue I, Nagase H, Kishi K, Higuti T (1991) ATP-sensitive K^+ channel mitochondrial inner membrane. Nature 352:244–247
23. Janier MF, Vanoverschelde JL, Bergmann SR (1994) Ischemic preconditioning stimulates anaerobic glycolysis in the isolated rabbit heart. Am J Physiol 267(4 Pt 2):H1353–1360
24. Kaplan LJ, Bellows CF, Blum H, Mitchell M, Whitman GJ (1994) Ischemic preconditioning preserves end-ischemic ATP, enhancing functional recovery and coronary flow during reperfusion. J Surg Res 57(1):179–184
25. Kato H, Araki T, Murase K, Kogure K (1992) Induction of tolerance to ischemia: alterations in second-messenger systems in the gerbil hippocampus. Brain Res Bull 29(5):559–565
26. Kato H, Kogure K, Araki T, Liu XH, Kato K, Itoyama Y (1995) Immunohistochemical localization of superoxide dismutase in the hippocampus following ischemia in a gerbil model of ischemic tolerance. J Cereb Blood Flow Metab 15(1):60–70
27. Kato H, Liu Y, Kogure K, Kato K (1994) Induction of 27-kDa heat shock protein following cerebral ischemia in a rat model of ischemic tolerance. Brain Res 634(2):235–244
28. Kawahara N, Croll SD, Wiegand SJ, Klatzo I (1997) Cortical spreading depression induces long-term alterations of BDNF levels in cortex and hippocampus distinct from lesion effects: implications for ischemic tolerance. Neurosci Res 29(1):37–47
29. Kawai K, Nakagomi T, Kirino T, Tamura A, Kawai N (1998) Preconditioning in vivo ischemia inhibits anoxic long-term potentiation and functionally protects CA1 neurons in the gerbil. J Cereb Blood Flow Metab 18(3):288–296
30. Kitakaze M, Hori M, Morioka T, Minamino T, Takashima S, Sato H, Shinozaki Y, Chujo M, Mori H, Inoue M et al (1994) Alpha 1-adrenoceptor activation mediates the infarct size-limiting effect of ischemic preconditioning through augmentation of 5'-nucleotidase activity. J Clin Invest 93(5):2197–2205
31. Kitakaze M, Hori M, Morioka T, Minamino T, Takashima S, Sato H, Shinozaki Y, Chujo M, Mori H, Inoue M et al (1994) Infarct size-limiting effect of ischemic preconditioning is blunted by inhibition of 5'-nucleotidase activity and attenuation of adenosine release. Circulation 89(3):1237–1246
32. Kitakaze M, Hori M, Takashima S, Sato H, Inoue M, Kamada T (1993) Ischemic preconditioning increases adenosine release and 5'-nucleotidase activity during myocardial ischemia and reperfusion in dogs. Implications for myocardial salvage [published erratum appears in Circulation 1993 May;87(5):1775 and 1993 Jun;87(6):2070] [see comments]. Circulation 87(1):208–215
33. Kobayashi S, Harris VA, Welsh FA (1995) Spreading depression induces tolerance of cortical neurons to ischemia in rat brain. J Cereb Blood Flow Metab 15(5):721–727
34. Lin B, Dietrich WD, Ginsberg MD, Globus MY, Busto R (1993) MK-801 (dizocilpine) protects the brain from repeated normothermic global ischemic insults in the rat. J Cereb Blood Flow Metab 13(6):925–932
35. Lin B, Globus MY, Dietrich WD, Busto R, Martinez E, Ginsberg MD (1992) Differing neurochemical and morphological sequelae of global ischemia: comparison of single- and multiple-insult paradigms. J Neurochem 59(6):2213–2223
36. Liu GS, Thornton J, Van Winkle DM, Stanley AW, Olsson RA, Downey JM (1991) Protection against infarction afforded by preconditioning is mediated by A1 adenosine receptors in rabbit heart. Circulation 84(1):350–356
37. Liu Y, Kato H, Nakata N, Kogure K (1992) Protection of rat hippocampus against ischemic neuronal damage by pretreatment with sublethal ischemia. Brain Res 586(1):121–124
38. Liu Y, Ytrehus K, Downey JM (1994) Evidence that translocation of protein kinase C is a key event during ischemic preconditioning of rabbit myocardium. J Mol Cell Cardiol 26(5):661–668
39. Lohse MJ, Klotz KN, Lindenborn-Fotinos J, Reddington M, Schwabe U, Olsson RA (1987) 8-Cyclopentyl-1,3-dipropylxanthine (DPCPX)-a selective high affinity antagonist radioligand for A1 adenosine receptors. Naunyn Schmiedebergs Arch Pharmacol 336(2):204–210
40. Matsushima K, Hogan MJ, Hakim AM (1996) Cortical spreading depression protects against subsequent focal cerebral ischemia in rats. J Cereb Blood Flow Metab 16(2):221–226
41. Matsushima K, Schmidt-Kastner R, Hogan MJ, Hakim AM (1998) Cortical spreading depression activates trophic factor expression in neurons and astrocytes and protects against subsequent focal brain ischemia. Brain Res 807(1–2):47–60
42. Miura T, Ogawa T, Iwamoto T, Shimamoto K, Iimura O (1992) Dipyridamole potentiates the myocardial infarct size-limiting effect of ischemic preconditioning. Circulation 86(3):979–985
43. Murry CE, Jennings RB, Reimer KA (1986) Preconditioning with ischemia: a delay of lethal cell injury in ischemic myocardium. Circulation 74(5):1124–1136
44. Nakata N, Kato H, Kogure K (1993) Inhibition of ischaemic tolerance in the gerbil hippocampus by quercetin and anti-heat shock protein-70 antibody. Neuroreport 4(6):695–698
45. Ohtsuki T, Matsumoto M, Kuwabara K, Kitagawa K, Suzuki K, Taniguchi N, Kamada T (1992) Influence of oxidative stress on induced tolerance to ischemia in gerbil hippocampal neurons. Brain Res 599(2):246–252
46. Pérez-Pinzón MA, Born JG (1999) Rapid preconditioning neuroprotection following anoxia in hippocampal slices: role of K^+_{ATP} channel and protein kinase C. Neuroscience 89(2):453–459
47. Pérez-Pinzón MA, Born JG, Centeno JM (1999b) Calcium and increase excitability promote tolerance against anoxia in hippocampal slices. Brain Res 833(1):20–26
48. Pérez-Pinzón MA, Mumford PL, Rosenthal M, Sick TJ (1996) Anoxic preconditioning in hippocampal slices: role of adenosine. Neuroscience 75(3):687–694

49. Pérez-Pinzón MA, Vitro TM, Dietrich WD, Sick TJ (1999a) The effect of rapid preconditioning on the microglial, astrocytic and neuronal consequences of global cerebral ischemia. Acta Neuropathol (Berl) 97(5):495–501
50. Pérez-Pinzón MA, Xu GP, Dietrich WD, Rosenthal M, Sick TJ (1997) Rapid preconditioning protects rats against ischemic neuronal damage after 3 but not 7 days of reperfusion following global cerebral ischemia. J Cereb Blood Flow Metab 17:175–182
51. Plumier JC, David JC, Robertson HA, Currie RW (1997) Cortical application of potassium chloride induces the low-molecular weight heat shock protein (Hsp27) in astrocytes. J Cereb Blood Flow Metab 17(7):781–790
52. Riepe MW, Esclaire F, Kasischke K, Schreiber S, Nakase H, Kempski O, Ludolph AC, Dirnagl U, Hugon J (1997) Increased hypoxic tolerance by chemical inhibition of oxidative phosphorylation: "Chemical preconditioning". J Cereb Blood Flow Metab 17(3):257–264
53. Riepe MW, Niemi WN, Megow D, Ludolph AC, Carpenter DO (1996) Mitochondrial oxidation in rat hippocampus can be preconditioned by selective chemical inhibition of succinic dehydrogenase. Exp Neurol 138(1):15–21
54. Sato T, B OR, Marban E (1998) Modulation of mitochondrial ATP-dependent K^+ channels by protein kinase C. Circ Res 83(1):110–114
55. Schultz JE, Qian YZ, Gross GJ, Kukreja RC (1997) The ischemia-selective K^+_{ATP} channel antagonist, 5-hydroxydecanoate, blocks ischemic preconditioning in the rat heart. J Mol Cell Cardiol 29:1055–1060
56. Schulz R, Rose J, Heusch G (1994) Involvement of activation of ATP-dependent potassium channels in ischemic preconditioning in swine. Am J Physiol 267(4 Pt 2):H1341–1352
57. Schurr A, Reid KH, Tseng MT, West C, Rigor BM (1986) Adaptation of adult brain tissue to anoxia and hypoxia in vitro. Brain Res 374(2):244–248
58. Schurr A, Rigor BM (1987) The mechanism of neuronal resistance and adaptation to hypoxia. Febs Lett 224(1):4–8
59. Shimazaki K, Ishida A, Kawai N (1994) Increase in bcl-2 oncoprotein and the tolerance to ischemia-induced neuronal death in the gerbil hippocampus. Neuroscience Research 20:95–99
60. Speechly-Dick ME, Mocanu MM, Yellon DM (1994) Protein kinase C. Its role in ischemic preconditioning in the rat. Circ Res 75(3):586–590
61. Stagliano NE, Pérez-Pinzón MA, Moskowits MA, Huang PL (1999) Focal ischemic preconditioning induces rapid tolerance to middle cerebral artery occlusion in mice. J Cereb Blood Flow Metab 19(7):757–761
62. Strasser RH, Braun-Dullaeus R, Walendzik H, Marquetant R (1992) Alpha 1-receptor-independent activation of protein kinase C in acute myocardial ischemia. Mechanisms for sensitization of the adenylyl cyclase system. Circ Res 70(6):1304–1312
63. Taga K, Patel PM, Drummond JC, Cole DJ, Kelly PJ (1997) Transient neuronal depolarization induces tolerance to subsequent forebrain ischemia in rats. Anesthesiology 87(4):918–925
64. Tomai F, Crea F, Gaspardone A, Versaci F, De Paulis R, Penta de Peppo A, Chiariello L, Gioffre PA (1994) Ischemic preconditioning during coronary angioplasty is prevented by glibenclamide, a selective ATP-sensitive K^+ channel blocker. Circulation 90(2):700–705
65. Tosaki A, Cordis GA, Szerdahelyi P, Engelman RM, Das DK (1994) Effects of preconditioning on reperfusion arrhythmias, myocardial functions, formation of free radicals, and ion shifts in isolated ischemic/reperfused rat hearts. J Cardiovasc Pharmacol 23(3):365–373
66. Tsuchida A, Liu GS, Mullane K, Downey JM (1993) Acadesine lowers temporal threshold for the myocardial infarct size limiting effect of preconditioning. Cardiovasc Res 27(1):116–120
67. Tsuchida A, Liu Y, Liu GS, Cohen MV, Downey JM (1994) alpha 1-adrenergic agonists precondition rabbit ischemic myocardium independent of adenosine by direct activation of protein kinase C. Circ Res 75(3):576–585
68. Tsuchida A, Thompson R, Olsson RA, Downey JM (1994) The anti-infarct effect of an adenosine A1-selective agonist is diminished after prolonged infusion as is the cardioprotective effect of ischaemic preconditioning in rabbit heart. J Mol Cell Cardiol 26(3):303–311
69. Tsuchida A, Yang XM, Burckhartt B, Mullane KM, Cohen MV, Downey JM (1994) Acadesine extends the window of protection afforded by ischaemic preconditioning. Cardiovasc Res 28(3):379–383
70. Van Winkle DM, Chien GL, Wolff RA, Soifer BE, Kuzume K, Davis RF (1994) Cardioprotection provided by adenosine receptor activation is abolished by blockade of the KATP channel. Am J Physiol 266(2 Pt 2):H829–839
71. Van Wylen DG (1994) Effect of ischemic preconditioning on interstitial purine metabolite and lactate accumulation during myocardial ischemia. Circulation 89(5):2283–2289
72. Walker DM, Walker JM, Yellon DM (1993) Global myocardial ischemia protects the myocardium from subsequent regional ischemia. Cardioscience 4(4):263–266
73. Wyatt DA, Edmunds MC, Rubio R, Berne RM, Lasley RD, Mentzer R, Jr (1989) Adenosine stimulates glycolytic flux in isolated perfused rat hearts by A1-adenosine receptors. Am J Physiol 257(6 Pt 2):H1952–1957
74. Yao Z, Gross GJ (1994) Activation of ATP-sensitive potassium channels lowers threshold for ischemic preconditioning in dogs. Am J Physiol 267(5 Pt 2):H1888–1894
75. Yao Z, Gross GJ (1994) A comparison of adenosine-induced cardioprotection and ischemic preconditioning in dogs: Efficacy, time course, and role of KATP channels. Circulation 89(3):1229–1236
76. Ytrehus K, Liu Y, Downey JM (1994) Preconditioning protects ischemic rabbit heart by protein kinase C activation. Am J Physiol 266(3 Pt 2):H1145–1152

The neuroprotective efficacy of human serum albumin therapy in focal and global cerebral ischemia and traumatic brain injury

M. D. Ginsberg, L. Belayev, W. Zhao, Y. Liu, E. Pinard*, J. Seylaz*, H. Nallet*, R. Busto

Introduction

While human serum albumin has, for some time, been considered as a possible therapeutic agent for ischemic stroke, only recently has its neuroprotective potential been rigorously evaluated. The beneficial effects of albumin have traditionally been ascribed to hemodilution and hyperosmolarity, with increased cardiac output, improved collateral circulation and decreased platelet aggregation. However, we consider it unlikely that the hemodiluting properties of albumin are solely responsible for its marked efficacy, as experimental and clinical trials of hemodilution with other agents have yielded only inconsistent results. Rather, we believe that *the multiple unique physiochemical properties of the albumin molecule itself are essential to its neuroprotective efficacy*. As a potential therapeutic agent for brain ischemia and trauma, human serum albumin possesses the considerable therapeutic advantage of already being in routine clinical use for a variety of indications.

In a series of recent preclinical studies, we have shown that moderate- to high-dose human serum albumin is markedly neuroprotective in experimental models of focal cerebral ischemia, global ischemia, and acute traumatic brain injury. Below, we summarize this evidence.

The experimental evidence

Human albumin therapy confers marked histological neuroprotection in acute focal cerebral ischemia:

First series (2 g/kg dose): In this study (Belayev et al. 1997), 18 adult male Sprague-Dawley rats were anesthetized with halothane, mechanically ventilated, and physiologically regulated. Arterial blood pressure, blood gases, plasma glucose and hematocrit were monitored, and cranial and rectal temperatures were both held at normothermic levels (37 °C). Animals received a 2-hour period of reversible middle cerebral artery occlusion (MCAo) by insertion of a poly-L-lysine-coated intraluminal suture (Belayev et al. 1996) – a technique that results in tight adherence of the suture to the vascular wall and gives rise to a highly reproducible cortical and subcortical infarction (coefficient of variation 8–9%). At 60 min of MCA occlusion, animals were awakened and tested on a standard neurobehavioral battery (Belayev

From the Cerebral Vascular Disease Research Center, Department of Neurology, University of Miami School of Medicine, PO Box 016960, Miami, FL 33101, USA and *Laboratoire de Recherches Cérébrovasculaires, CNRS, Université Paris 7, IFR6, France
e-mail: mdginsberg@stroke.med.miami.edu

et al. 1996) to confirm the presence of a high-grade neurological deficit. After the 2-h MCA occlusion period, the intraluminal suture was withdrawn. Rats were then treated with either 20% human serum albumin, administered intravenously over 3 minutes at a dose of 2 g/kg; or 0.9% saline (vehicle) solution. The neurological score was assessed daily. After 3-day survival, brains were perfusion-fixed for quantitation of histopathological infarction and brain swelling. Advanced computerized image-averaging methods developed by us (Zhao et al. 1993, 1995, 1996, 1997) were used to generate quantitative maps depicting the frequency of cerebral infarction on a pixel-by-pixel basis at nine standard stereotaxic levels.

Cortical infarct volume in saline-treated control rats was 129 ± 9 mm^3. By contrast, cortical infarct volume in albumin-treated rats was greatly reduced (by 57%), averaging 56 ± 24 mm^3 ($p < 0.01$) (Belayev et al. 1997). This effect was ecident throughout the 9 coronal levels examined. Statistical maps of the Fisher exact test generated on a pixel-by-pixel basis documented a confluent zone of neocortex showing a highly significant reduction of infarct volume in albumin-treated rats compared to saline-treated animals.

Albumin treatment was also strikingly effective in reducing the extent of brain swelling as measured by volumetric comparison of ipsilateral vs. contralateral hemispheres. The overall degree of brain edema was reduced by 81% in albumin-treated rats, and this effect was statistically significant at virtually every coronal level. The hematocrit of albumin-treated rats fell from control values of $40.1 \pm 1.1\%$ to $25.3 \pm 03.\%$ (Belayev et al. 1997).

Confirmatory series (2.5 g/kg dose). We next conducted two additional histopathological series (using the somewhat higher dose of 2.5 g/kg) in order to confirm our initial observations (Belayev et al. 1998). A remarkable degree of cortical neuroprotection was conferred by high-dose albumin therapy administered at the time of recirculation following 2 h MCA occlusion. For the overall series, the degree of cortical infarct reduction averaged 84% (Fig. 1). Total (cortical plus subcortical) infarct volume was reduce by 66% by albumin treatment. Remarkably, subcortical (caudoputamen) infarct volume was also significantly reduced (by 33%) by albumin therapy although this zone is traditionally resistant to neuroprotective interventions. Brain swelling as measured volumetrically was virtually eliminated at every coronal level by albumin therapy (Fig. 1). Total neurological score was markedly improved by albumin therapy throughout the three-day survival period. Mean hematocrit fell from 40–42% to 23–28% when measured immediately after albumin administration, but had recovered to normal levels by 1 day. As expected, plasma osmolality was not affected by albumin administration, while plasma colloid oncotic pressure was raised from 16–18 to 25 mmHg 15 min after treatment, and this elevation persisted at 1 day of recirculation (Belayev et al. 1998).

Diffusion-weighted magnetic resonance imaging studies – albumin therapy normalizes the apparent diffusion coefficient in focal ischemia:

In a small series (Belayev et al. 1998), rats with 2 h MCA occlusion treated with either albumin or saline were imaged 24 h later on a 1.5 T whole-body MRI magnet. Diffusion imaging was performed with a spin-echo technique, and the apparent diffusion coefficient (ADC) was computed from 4 diffusion-weighted images with b values of 205–825 s/mm^2. A reference (T2-weighted-type) image was also obtained. These images were exported to our laboratory's image analysis system for post-processing and averaging (Zhao et al. 1995). An extensive cortical and subcortical lesion was apparent on reference images of saline-treated rats, while albumin-treated rats had much smaller lesions confined chiefly to the basal ganglia. Saline-treated animals showed the expected extensive confluent zone of diminished ADC values at cortical and subcortical sites, corresponding to the T2-lesion seen on reference-MR images. By contrast, albumin therapy led to a remarkable *normalization of the apparent diffusion coefficient*, which was apparent not only within

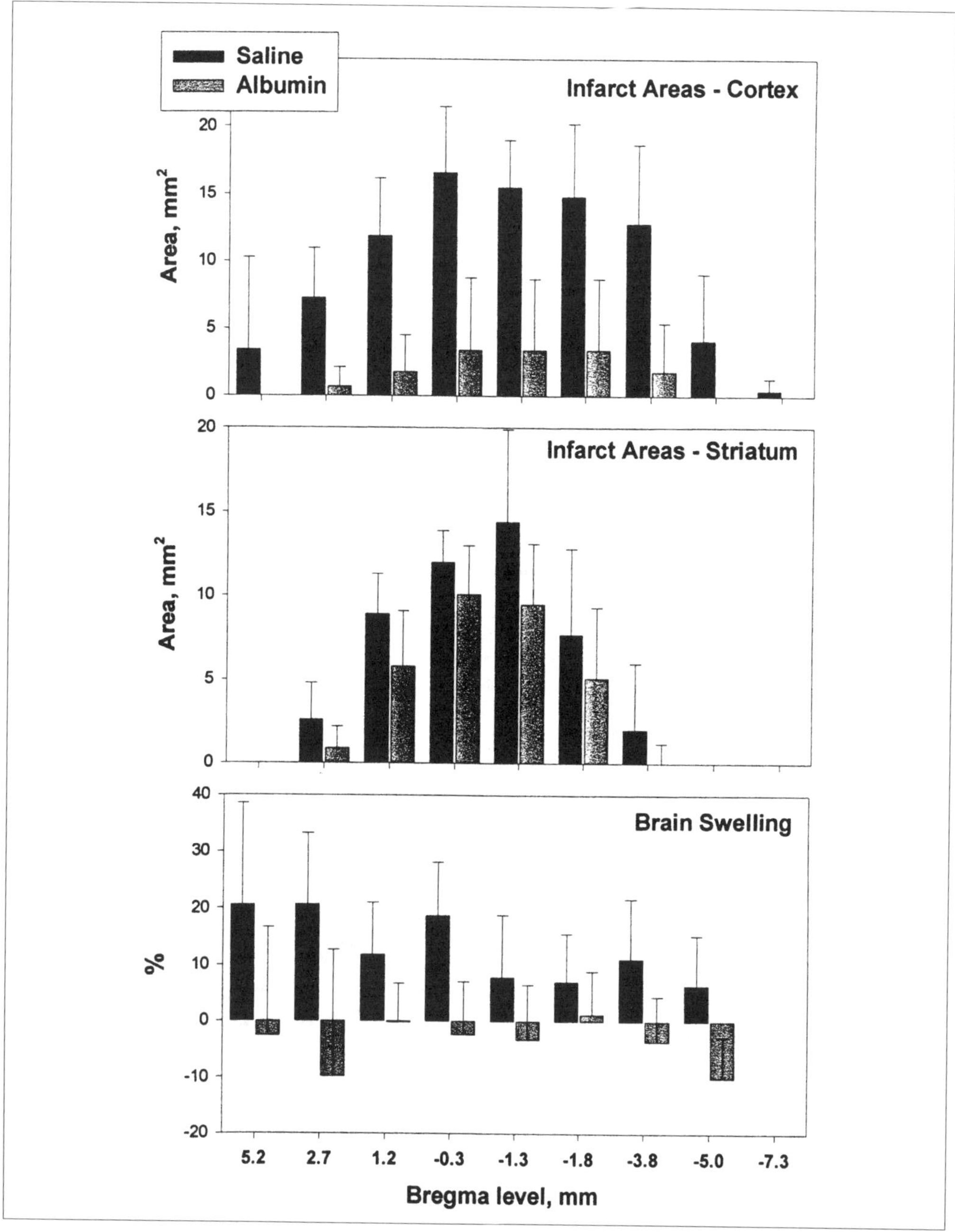

Fig. 1. Cortical and striatal infarct areas, and percent brain swelling, shown at 9 coronal levels in rats with 2-h MCA occlusion and 3-day survival, treated with either saline (n = 7) or albumin, 2.5 g/kg (n = 9) (means ± SD). The albumin-associated reductions in cortical infarct area and brain swelling are significant at virtually every level ($p < 0.05$, repeated-measures ANOVA followed by Bonferoni comparisons). Striatal infarct reduction is significant at bregma level –1.3 mm. (Data replotted from Belayev et al., Stroke, 1998; 29:2587–2599.)

brain areas histologically protected by albumin treatment, but also within the zone of residual infarction itself (Fig. 2). That is, *prior albumin therapy tended to normalize cellular water homeostasis even within zones of residual infarction.*

Albumin therapy of focal ischemia protects tisesue from pan-necrosis – microscopic observations:

The MRI observations presented above suggested the need to carry out a detailed comparison of the microscopic characteristics of the infracted zone in saline- vs. albumin-treated rats. This was performed on paraffin-embedded sections stained with hematoxylin and eosin or reacted for the histochemical visualization of activated microglia with peroxidase-labeled isolectin-B4 (Belayev et al. 1998). While the infarcted caudoputamen of saline-treated rats revealed the expected pan-necrosis affecting both neuronal, glial and vascular elements, *albumin-treated brains showed a striking preservation of microvascular endothelium.* Activated microglia were rare in the central striatal infarct of saline-treated rats while abundant activated microglia with ramified processes were present in the infarct of albumin-treated animals. These observations suggested that *albumin therapy led to partial preservation of parenchymal structure even within zones of residual infarction* (Belayev et al. 1998).

Hemodynamic and microvascular effects of albumin therapy in focal ischemia:

1. Autoradiographic LCBF studies: To ascertain the degree to which hemodynamic alterations might be responsible for the neuroprotec-

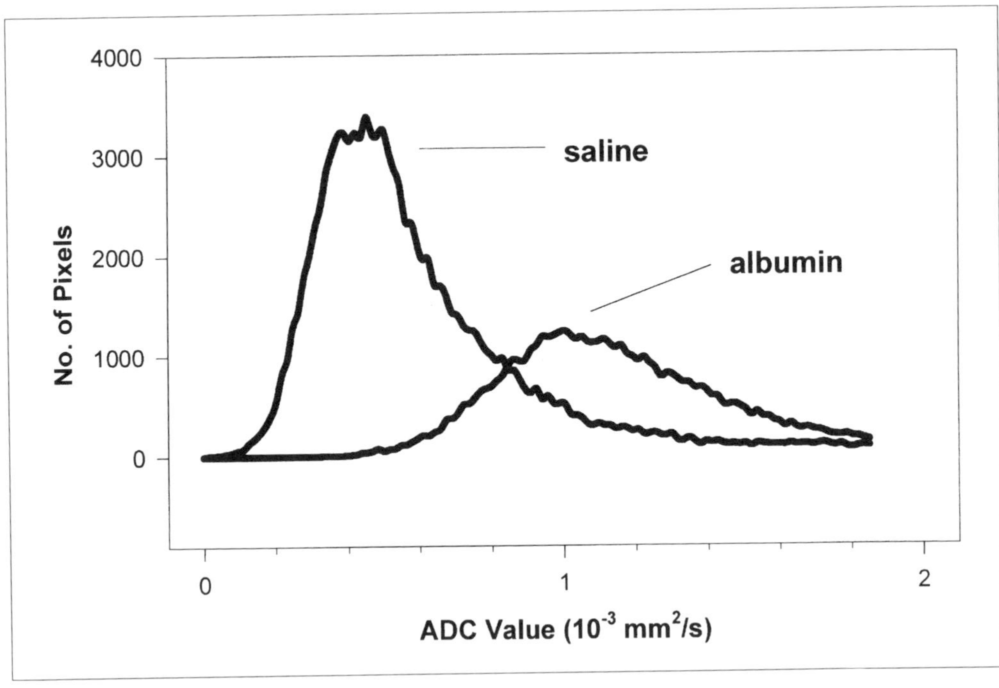

Fig. 2. Distribution of ADC values in saline- and albumin-treated rats with MCA occlusion and 24 h of recirculation. Data are taken from those pixels of the ipsilateral hemisphere that appeared infarcted on T2-weighted-type MR images. The ADC distribution of albumin-treated rats is markedly right-shifted into the normal ADC range ($p < 0.001$, Kolmogorov-Smirnov 2-sample test). (Data replotted from Belayev et al., Stroke, 1998; 29:2587–2599.)

tive effect of albumin (2.5 g/kg) in focal ischemia, we quantitated local cerebral blood flow (LCBF) auroradiographically with ^{14}C-iodoantipyrine in two series of rats subjected to 2-h MCA suture-occlusion and 1 h of recirculation (Huh et al. 1998). Image-processing methods were used to co-map average LCBF data sets against our previously accumulated infarction-frequency data sets on a pixel-by-pixel basis. Within brain regions showing albumin-associated neuroprotection, numbers of pixels having LCBF in the upper ischemic-core flow range (i.e., 0.12–0.24 ml/g/min) were reduced 8.6-fold by albumin therapy when compared to saline-treated rats; and numbers of pixels with LCBF in the lower penumbral flow range (i.e., 0.24–0.36 ml/g/min) were reduced by 3.1-fold in albumin-treated rats ($p = 0.04$ by repeated-measures ANOVA) (Huh et al. 1998). Inspection of averaged [albumin-minus-saline] three-dimensional LCBF difference images revealed a narrow circumferential zone of statistically significant albumin-associated LCBF increase within the posterior portion of the ischemic hemisphere, surrounding the core-region of prior ischemia. This study thus showed that, while albumin treatment improved local perfusion to regions of critically reduced LCBF, the spatial extent of this effect appeared too small to account fully for the marked neuroprotective efficacy of this therapy. These results thus suggested that other, non-hemodynamic mechanisms must also contribute to albumin-associated neuroprotection (Huh et al. 1998).

2. *Laser-scanning confocal microscopy of cortical microvasculature:* In collaborative studies with Drs. Elisabeth Pinard and Jacques Seylaz in the Laboratoire de Recherches Cérébrovasculaires, CNRS, Paris, we used laser-scanning confocal microscopy to image the cortical vasculature of rats through a closed cranial window placed in the dorsolateral frontoparietal cortex. Plasma was labeled with FITC-dextran, and FITC-labeled erythrocytes were also injected (Seylaz et al. 1999). Cortical DC potential was also recorded. Rats received 2-h MCA occlusion by insertion of a poly-L-lysine-coated intraluminal suture, followed by recirculation. Either saline or albumin was administered following 30 min of recirculation. Video images of cortical arterioles, capillaries, and venules were continually acquired and were digitized off-line to measure diameters and labeled erythrocyte velocities. MCA occlusion was associated with arteriolar dilatation and slowing of capillary and venular perfusion together with recurrent DC depolarizations (confirming the penumbral localization of the field). During the first 15–30 minutes of postichemic recirculation, prominent foci of vascular stasis developed within cortical venules, associated with thrombus-like stagnant foci and adherent intra-venular corpuscular structures (believed to be activated neutrophils adhering to the venular endothelium). Saline administration failed to affect these phenomena, while i.v. albumin therapy (2.5 g/kg) in most cases was followed by a prompt improvement of venular flow and partial disappearance of adherent corpuscules and thrombotic material (Fig. 3).

3. *Laser-Doppler perfusion imaging:* In related studies, we used laser-Doppler perfusion imaging (LDPI; Moor Instruments, Inc., Wilmington, Delaware) to make repeated measurements of relative cortical perfusion by scanning a low-power laser beam across a 5 x 5 mm temporal crainial window (dura intact). Rats received 2-h MCA suture-occlusion and were treated with either human albumin, 2.5 g/kg ($n = 6$), or saline ($n = 5$), at 30 min of recirculation (Belayev et al. 2000a). Albumin led to a sustained CBF increase of 17% relative to pretreatment values ($p < 0.0001$), while saline caused no change (1%, NS).

Albumin treatment of focal ischemia alters serum-protein extravasation and cellular uptake:

In this study (Remmers et al. 1999), we examined protein extravasation as a marker of blood-brain barrier disturbance in animals with 2-h MCA occlusion treated with either human serum albumin (2.5 g/kg) or saline. Immunochemistry with antibodies to rat immunoglobulins (IgG), rat albumin and (exogenous) human albumin was employed to study changes in the

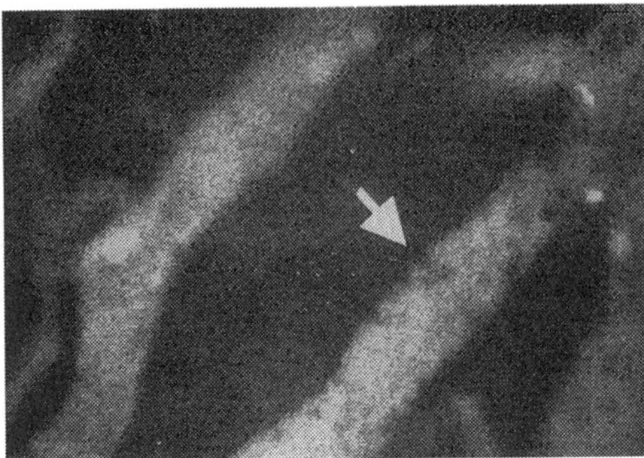
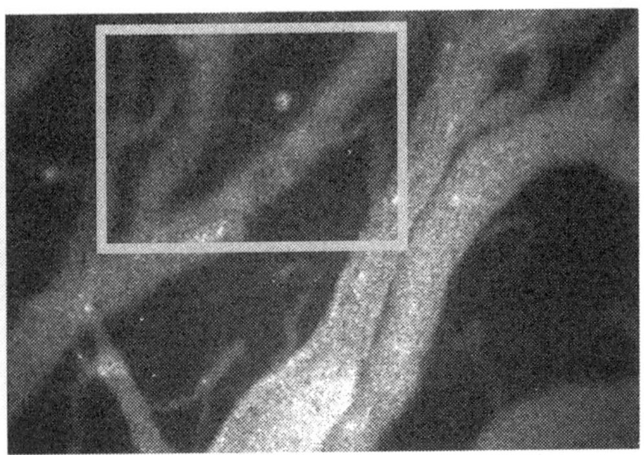

Fig. 3. Laser-scanning confocal microscopic images of dorsolateral parietal cortex of a rat with 2 h MCA occlusion that initially received 2 ml of saline i.v. following 45 min of recirculation. *Left panel:* Image at 139 min of recirculation. Cortical venule exhibits stagnant perfusion and numerous adherent cellular elements (arrow), consistent in size with polymorphonuclear leukocytes (x40). *Right panel:* Image at 240 min of recirculation, 25 min after administration of albumin, 2.5 g/kg i.v. This panel, imaged at lower magnification (x20), shows clearing of adherent cells and improved venular perfusion. (Rectangle denotes the area shown at higher power in the left panel.)

striatum and cortex after 3-day survival. By imaging methods, the area of IgG extravasation was similar in saline- and albumin-treated animals. In the striatum (a region damaged in both saline- and albumin-treated series), both groups revealed diffuse extravasation of IgG and rat albumin, and uptake into necrotic cells. In the neocortex (a region largely neuroprotected by albumin), saline-treated animals also showed diffuse IgG signals and uptake into necrotic neurons. In albumin-treated animals, however, cortical neurons with *preserved* structural features were identified, which had taken up extravasated proteins; and strong immunolabeling for human albumin was present in *normal-appearing* cortical neurons. These results thus demonstrated that, while postischemic treatment with human serum albumin does not decrease the overall degree of protein extravasation, it results in a preservation of cortical tissue and uptake of albumin into *intact-appearing (i.e., neuroprotected)* neurons. We suspect that this parenchymal uptake may contribute to the protective effect of albumin on neuronal survival (Remmers et al. 1999).

Dose-reponse study demonstrates that lower doses of human albumin are also markedly neuroprotective in focal cerebral ischemia:

In the studies described above, we employed human albumin at doses of 2.0 to 2.5 g/kg body weight. To assess whether lower doses would also be neuroprotective, we subjected Sprague-Dawley rats to 2-h of MCA suture-occlusion in a manner identical to our earlier studies (Belayev et al. 1996). Rats were then randomized to one of the following i.v. treatments:

- 25% human albumin, 1.25 g/kg (i.e., *one-half* of the previous dose, or 0.5% of body weight)
- 25% human albumin, 0.63 g/kg (i.e., *one-quarter* of the previous dose, or 0.25% of body weight)
- Control: 0.9% saline, administered in a volume equivalent to the above groups (5 ml/kg)

All treatments were given shortly after suture removal.

High-grade behavioral deficits (total neurological score 10–11 of possible 12) were present in all animals at 60 min of MCA occlusion. Saline-treated animals continued to show severe behavioral impairments throughout the 3-

day survival period. By contrast, both the 0.63 g/kg and the 1.25 g/kg albumin-treated groups showed substantial neurological recovery by the first day, which persisted throughout the survival period (repeated-measures ANOVA).

Brains were perfusion-fixed for histopathology following 3-day survival. The brains of saline-treated rats with MCA occlusion showed the expected pan-necrotic lesion involving both cortex and striatum. By contrast, *infarct size was dramatically reduced in both albumin-treated groups*. The extent of neuroprotection in the neocortex was profound (*mean tissue salvage, 96% in the 1.25 g/kg albumin group* and 66% in the 0.63 g/kg albumin group). The striatal component of the infarct was also significantly protected (by 52% and 54% in the 2 albumin dose groups, respectively) (Belayev et al. 2000b). Thus, the neuroprotective effect of lower-dose albumin (particularly, the 1.25 g/kg dose) was fully as profound as seen at the highest dose. Total infarct volume (corrected for brain swelling) was reduced by a mean of 58% and 67%, respectively, by treatment with 0.63 g/kg and 1.25 g/kg or albumin, respectively (Fig. 4). Brain swelling was diminished by three-quarters by treatment with 0.63 g/kg of albumin, and it was essentially eliminated in the 1.25 g/kg group (Fig. 4).

The histological infarct-data were also analyzed by generating infarct-frequency maps using methods previously published by our group (Zhao et al. 1996, 1997). These image-data are shown in Figure 5. Infarct frequency maps from the 3 groups were compared by Fisher exact tests on a pixel-by-pixel basis to highlight brain regions in which albumin therapy was significantly protective. Statistical maps revealed extensive areas of cortical neuroprotection at the 1.25 g/kg dose (Fig. 5).

Evidence of an extended (4-hour) therapeutic window for albumin neuroprotection in focal ischemia:

In studies currently nearing completion, the therapeutic window for human albumin-associated neuroprotection was studied in rats subjected to 2 hours of MCA occlusion by poly-L-lysine-coated intraluminal suture and treated with moderate-dose (1.25 g/kg) human albumin either at the onset of recirculation or at 1 h, 2 h, or 3 h thereafter. The following albumin-treated groups were studied (treatment times denote times after onset of MCAo): 2 h (n = 9), 3 h (n = 10), 4 h (n = 10) and 5 h (n = 8). Saline-treated rats (n = 9) were treated at 3 h.

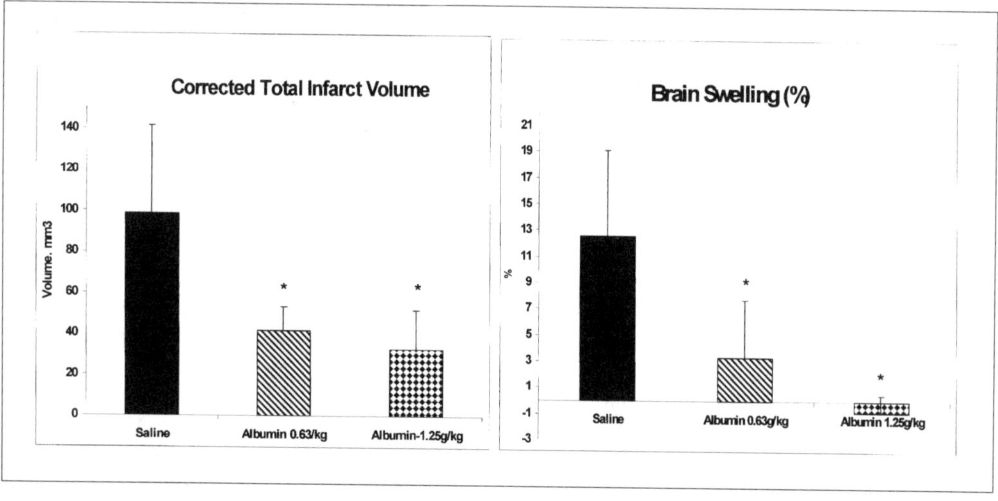

Fig. 4. Total infarct volume (corrected for swelling), and brain swelling, in rats with 2-h MCA occlusion and 3-day survival, treated with either albumin, 0.63 g/kg or 1.25 g/kg, or saline (means ± SD). *p < 0.05 vs. saline (ANOVA).

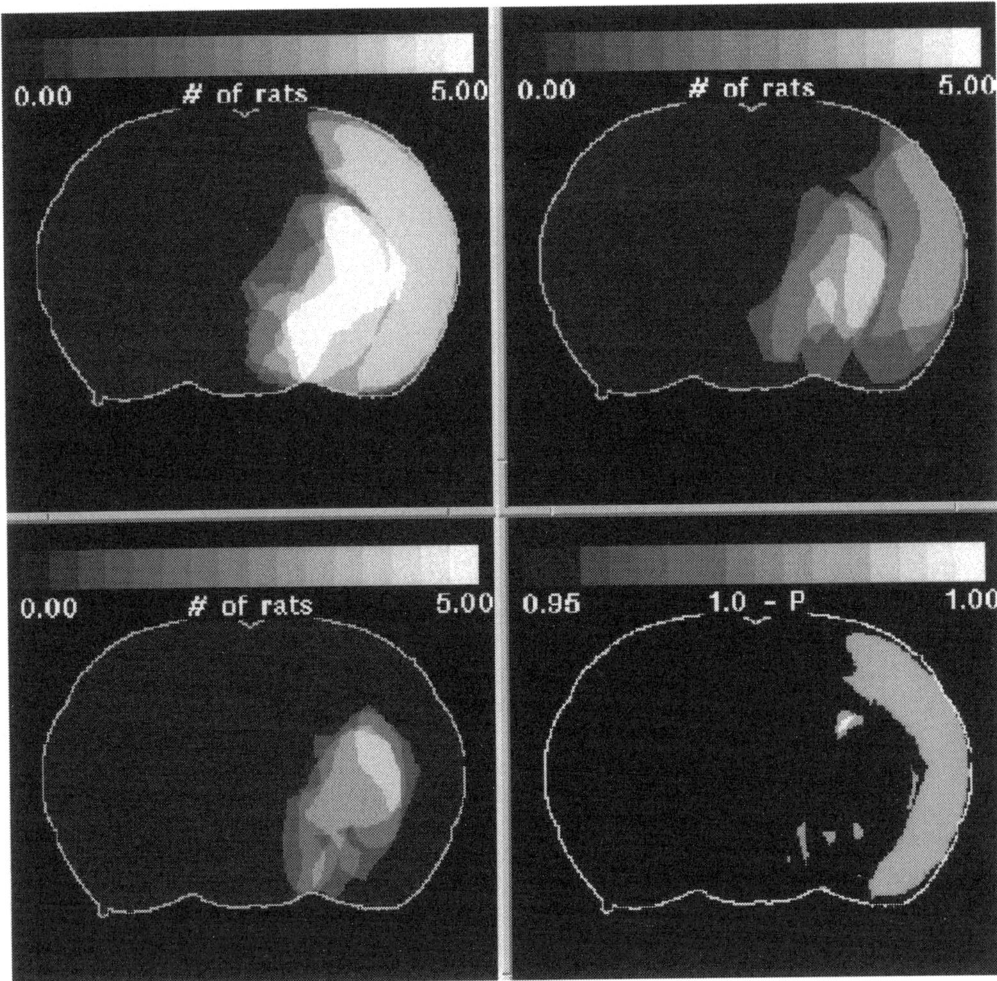

Fig. 5. Infarct-frequency maps in rats with 2-h MCA occlusion treated with saline *(upper left)*, albumin 0.63 g/kg *(upper right)*, and albumin 1.25 g/kg *(lower left)*. *Lower right* panel is a statistical map of [1-p] computed on a pixel-by-pixel basis by the Fisher exact test (thresholded to depict zones of $p < 0.05$), comparing infarct frequencies in the saline vs. 1.25 g/kg albumin group. An extensive cortical zone of albumin-induced neuroprotection is evident.

Brains were perfusion-fixed at 3 days for blinded infarct quantitation. *Albumin treatment, even when initiated as late as 4 hours after onset of MCAo, led to highly significant reductions of infarct areas in cortex (68% reduction), subcortical regions (52% reduction), and total infarct (61% reduction)* (Fig. 6).

Human albumin therapy is also neuroprotective in *permanent* focal ischemia:

In recent studies, we subjected Sprague-Dawley rats (n = 7) to *permanent* MCA suture-occlusion – an insult that results in a maximal-sized MCA-territory infarction. Four rats were treated with moderate-dose albumin (1.25 g/kg) at 2 h after onset of MCAo; another 3

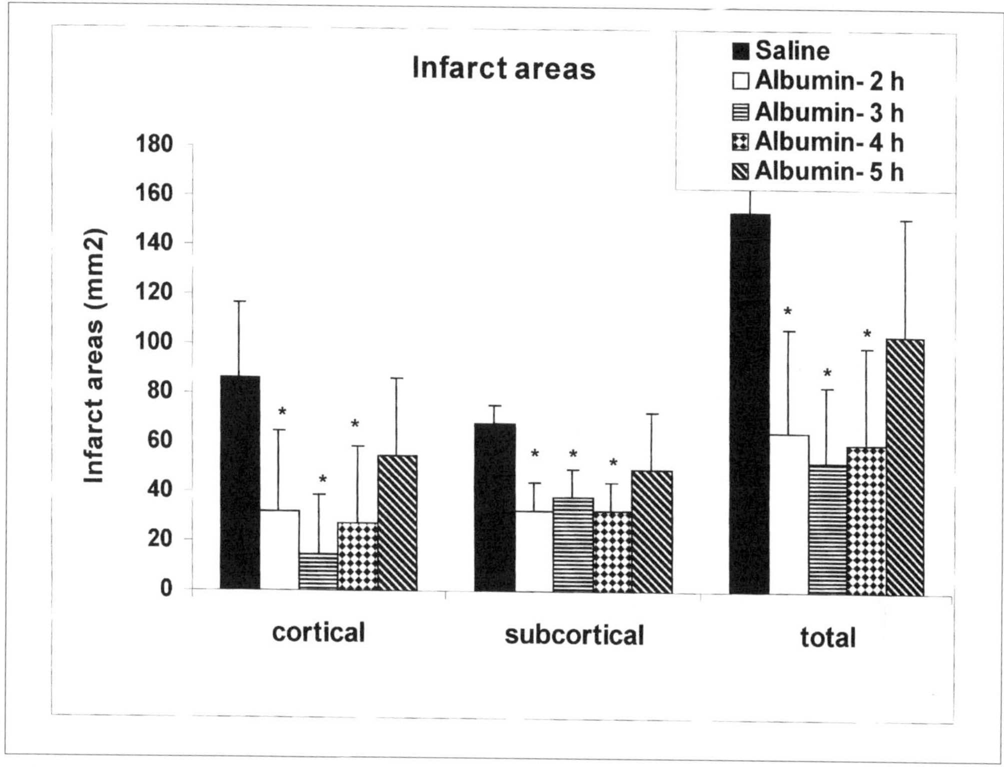

Fig. 6. Cortical, subcortical and total infarct areas in 5 groups of rats treated with either saline (at 3 h post-MCA occlusion), or with albumin, 1.25 g/kg, administered at either 2 h, 3 h, 4 h or 5 h after the onset of MCA occlusion (means ± SD). $*p < 0.05$ vs. saline.

animals received saline. Perfusion-fixation was carried out 24 h later for histological quantitation of infarct areas. In albumin-treated rats, significant reductions in infarct area were observed at 3 posterior coronal levels. The extent of infarct-area reduction at these 3 levels was 50%, 63%, and 76%, respectively. Other rats with permanent MCA occlusion were studied by laser-Doppler perfusion imaging. Animals treated with human albumin (1.25 g/kg) 2 h after onset of MCA occlusion showed improved cortical perfusion compared to saline-treated rats, amounting to a 1.8-fold increase in relative perfusion ($p < 0.05$). These exciting findings support the view that human albumin therapy at moderate doses is neuroprotective even against the extensive infarct resulting from permanent MCA suture-occlusion.

Albumin treatment is also neuroprotective in transient global forebrain ischemia:

To assess whether albumin treatment might also confer cellular protection in the context of transient *global* forebrain ischemia – an experimental setting that mimics the clinical situation of cerebral circulatory arrest with resuscitation – we used the two-vessel occlusion model of temporary bilateral common carotid occlusions plus hypotension for 10 minutes in rats, followed by recirculation (Smith et al. 1984). This insult reduces cerebral blood flow (CBF) in forebrain structures to ~2–3% of normal and gives rise to consistent ischemic neuronal alterations within selectively vulnerable brain regions (Globus et al. 1991). Five min after the onset of recirculation, animals were randomized to intravenous treatment with either 25% human serum albumin (at a dose of 2.5 g/kg i.v. over 3 minutes), or a corresponding volume of 0.9% saline. Neurological function was evaluated repeatedly by standardized testing (Belayev et al. 1995). Seven days after ischemia, brains were perfusion-fixed, and ischemic neuronal injury in the hippocampal CA1 area was assessed quantitatively. Albumin-treated rats showed a significant improvement of neurological score compared to saline-treated animals throughout the 7-day survival period (0= 0.0001). In saline-treated rats, 10 min of ischemia led to profound neuronal damage to the hippocampal CA1 sector; numbers of normal neurons were reduced to below 11% of normal. By contrast, in albumin-treated rats, normal CA1 neurons were easily detectable. Quantitative analysis confirmed that albumin treatment significantly attenuated hippocampal ischemic damage ($p = 0.02$) and led to 2.4- to 5.3-fold increases in numbers of surviving CA1 neurons compared to saline-treated animals (Belayev et al. 1999a).

Albumin treatment confers neuroprotection in traumatic brain injury and ameliorates early post-traumatic metabolism/blood flow uncoupling:

To determine whether early treatment with high-dose human serum albumin would also protect in a standard rat model of traumatic brain injury (TBI) (Belayev et al. 1999b), we subjected halothane-anesthetized normothermic Sprague-Dawley rats to right parieto-occipital parasagittal fluid-percussion injury (1.5–2.0 atm) as previously described (Dietrich et al. 1994). Human serum albumin (25% solution, 2.5 g/kg) or vehicle (0.9% saline) was administered i.v. 15 min after trauma. Neurological function was evaluated on a standardized test battery before and after TBI (at 2 h, 24 h, 48 h, 72 h and 7 days) (Belayev et al. 1996). Seven days after TBI, brains were perfusion-fixed for paraffin-embedding and light-microscopic histopathology. Coronal sections were digitized at various levels, and contusion areas in the superficial, middle and deep layers of the parieto-occipital neocortex and in the underlying fimbria were measured. Albumin therapy significantly improved the neurological score compared to saline-treated animals at 24 h after TBI (6.4 ± 0.7 vs. 8.4 ± 0.5, respectively; $p = 0.03$) and reduced contusion area by 51% (Belayev et al. 1999b).

The pathophysiology of TBI involves the actue *uncoupling* of cerebral glucose utilization (LCMRglu) and LCBF (Ginsberg et al. 1997). To establish whether human albumin therapy would influence this uncoupling, we conducted autoradiographic studies in matched groups of rats with moderate TBI followed by 60 min or 24 h recovery (Ginsberg et al. 2000). At 60 min post-TBI, vehicle-treated rats showed moderate bilateral reductions of LCBF but paradoxically normal levels of LCMRglu, resulting in marked bilateral elevations of the metabolism/flow ratio (by 3.0 fold ipsilaterally, and by 2.1 fold contralaterally). By contrast, *albumin treatment diminished by one-half the extent of metabolism/flow dissociation* (Fig. 7) (Ginsberg et al. 2000). Viewed together with the above evidence of histological neuroprotection, these findings suggest that human albumin may represent a desirable treatment modality for acute traumatic brain injury.

Discussion

The need for effective neuroprotective strategies to combat acute ischemic stroke and traumatic brain injury:

Both ischemic stroke and traumatic brain injury are common and devastating neurological illnesses. Over the past decade, impressive efforts have been expended in basic and clinical neuroscience research to elucidate the mechanisms of ischemic and traumatic brain injury and to develop neuroprotective strategies (McIntosh 1993; Ginsberg 1995; Koroshetz and Moskowitz 1996; McIntosh et al. 1998). These studies have shown that multiple pathways involving electrophysiological, biochemical, and molecular events interact in complex cascades, cul-

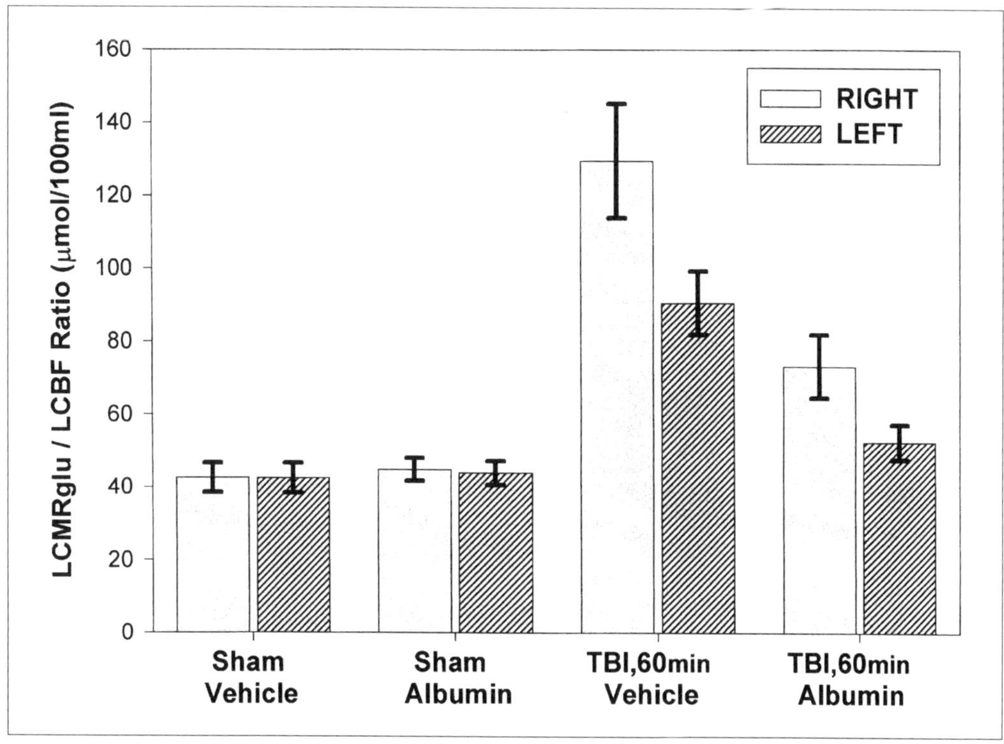

Fig. 7. Data from rats exposed to moderate fluid-percussion injury or sham-injury and studied for local cerebral glucose utilization (LCMRglu) or local cerebral blood flow (LCBF) with ^{14}C-radiotracers. Bars represent the means of 15 anatomic structures measured in each group of animals. Error bars denote 95% confidence intervals. In vehicle-treated rats with TBI, both the right hemisphere (ipsilateral to trauma) and the left (contralateral) hemisphere show marked elevations of the metabolism/flow ratio, denoting uncoupling. By contrast, the metabolism/flow ratio is more nearly normal in TBI rats treated with albumin.

minating in the death of brain cells (Siesjo 1981; Choi 1992; Hossmann 1994). Importantly, a large number of experimental studies have now conclusively established the importance of prompt intervention. To date, however, few approches have borne clinical fruit. A great variety of pharmacological strategies to protect the acutely ischemic brain have shown efficacy in preclinical studies (Ginsberg 1995), but their translation to the clinic has proven challenging (Koroshetz and Moskowitz 1996; Zivin 1997; European Ad Hoc Consensus Group 1998; Albers et al. 1998; Slyter 1998; Brott et al. 1998; Marler and Walker 1998). In the case of traumatic brain injury, the results of human clinical trials to date (e.g., pegolated superoxide dismutase (Young et al. 1996), moderate hypothermia) have been disappointing.

Clearly, a neuroprotective agent is needed that has proven efficacy, carries minimal risk of side effects or toxicity, is acceptable both to medical personnel and to patients and their families, and can be administered without the need for complicated laboratory studies or sophisticated delivery systems. On the basis of the experimental evidence presented above, we believe that human albumin offers considerable promise as a neuroprotective agent in the clinical management of acute brain ischemia and trauma.

The pluripotent characteristics of the human serum albumin molecule:

Human serum albumin is the most abundant circulating plasma protein and has a prolonged persistence in the body. With a degradative rate of 3.7% per day, the life of the average endogenous albumin molecule is 27 days; it has been estimated that the average albumin molecule undergoes ~15,000 passages through the circulation (Peters 1996)! Albumin subserves multiple crucial roles in normal homeotasis: 1) the maintenance of plasma colloid osmotic pressure; 2) the transport of fatty acids (Trigatti and Gerber 1995; Curry et al. 1998); and 3) the transfer of cholesterol between lipoproteins and cells (Zhao and Marcel 1996). In addition, albumin binds many metabolites and is responsible for the majority of drug binding in the plasma (Koch-Weser and Sellers 1976a, 1976b). Albumin possesses, as well, many other important actions:

Antioxidant effects: Albumin constitutes a major antioxidant defense against oxidizing agents generated both by endogenous processes (such as neutrophil myeloperoxidase) and by exogenous mediators (e.g., phenolic dietary compounds) (Wasil et al. 1987; Halliwell 1988; Halliwell and Gutteridge 1990; Smith et al. 1992; Hu et al. 1993). Indeed, plasma proteins, chiefly albumin, appear to account for up to three-fourths of the total radical-trapping antioxidant activity of plasma – fully 10–20 times greater than the effect attributable to vitamin E alone (Wayner et al. 1985). Albumin can also bind copper ions, thereby inhibiting copper ion-dependent lipid peroxidation and the formation of the highly reactive hydroxyl radical species (Halliwell 1988; Emerson 1989). As albumin is present in relatively high concentrations in both plasma and interstitial fluid, it is strategically situated to scavenge oxygen radicals, to bind to free fatty acids and metal ions, and to interrupt the damaging oxidative process of lipid peroxidation (Emerson 1989).

Endothelial actions: Albumin acts directly on vascular endothelium. By binding to the endothelial glycocalyx, it functions to maintain the normal permeability of microvessel walls and, by its transcytosis across endothelium, it serves as a carrier for various small molecules (Schnitzer and Oh 1992; He and Curry 1993). Microvascular endothelial cells express several specific albumin binding sites on their surface (Ghitescu et al. 1986; Schnitzer and Oh 1992; Schnitzer 1992). The binding of albumin probes to the endothelial cell surface appears to mediate their transcytosis or endocytosis (Schnitzer et al. 1992). Certain ligands such as fatty acids may increase albumin-binding to these receptors and, hence, facilitate its passage across endothelial membranes (Galis et al. 1988). Albumin exerts complex influences on erythrocyte aggregation, increasing low-shear viscosity but decreasing erythrocyte sedimentation under no-flow conditions (Reinhart and Nagy 1995). Recent work suggests that albumin may be a factor mediating the effect of blood coagulation on vascular tone and capillary permeability. Serum albumin reacts with nitric oxide to form a stable S-nitrosothiol which has endothelium-derived relaxing factor-like properties (Keaney et al. 1993). Albumin has also been shown to be a specific inhibitor of endothelial-cell apoptosis (Zoellner et al. 1996).

Metabolic effects: Albumin exerts major effects on astrocytes. When applied to cortical astrocytes in culture, albumin elicits intercellular calcium waves that can be inhibited by gap-junction blockers (Nadal et al. 1997). Albumin is also an effective mitogen for astrocytes (Nadel et al. 1995), suggesting that it may be responsible for stimulating glial scar formation in pathological states in which it is able to cross a permeable blood-brain barrier into the brain. Lactate originating in glial cells appears to be an important energy substrate for recovery of synaptic function after hypoxia/ischemia (Schurr et al. 1997a, 1997b, 1997c) as well as during neuronal activation (Schurr et al. 1999). In a recent study, albumin was shown to be a major regulator of the enzyme pyruvate dehydrogenase in astrocytes, capable of more than doubling the flux of glucose and lactate (Tabernero et al. 1999). This takes on relevance in that pyruvate dehydrogenase is inhibited by ischemia, and this inhibition promotes substrate limitation, decreasing electron flow into the mitochondiral electron-transport chain (Bogaert et al. 1994). As the entry of serum albumin into the brain is enhanced under pathological conditions (Remmers et al. 1999), it is possible that this action of albumin could be responsible for sustaining neuronal metabolism under pathological conditions by increasing the export of pyruvate to neurons for metabolism via the Krebs cycle (Tsacopoulos and Magistretti 1996).

Relevance of hemodilution: It is unlikely that albumin-neuroprotection is mediated by hemodilution alone: The traditional view of therapeutically administered albumin is that it acts solely via its oncotic, hemodiluting action. In our opinion, however, this narrow view ignores the large body of evidence, reviewed above, that albumin is in fact a unique complex molecule with multiple salutary physiochemical properties. It is difficult to draw consistent impressions from the numerous published experimental hemodilution studies owing to the great diversity of hemodiluents used (human albumin, low molecular weight dextran, hydroxyethyl starch, di-aspirin cross-linked hemoglobin, and hetastarch), obtained from various sources and administered at differing times and in diverse concentrations in differing species (dog, cat, rat) and ischemia models (permanent vs. temporary MCA occlusion, embolism), resulting in differing degrees of hematocrit reduction. The evaluation of histopathology in many of these studies lacked modern-day rigor. Another confounding factor is the use of both *isovolemic* protocols (in which the animal's blood was partially exchanged for the hemodiluent) and *hypervolemic* protocols (in which a net excess of colloid was administered, with or without partial exchange). Despite these shortcomings, several studies tend to support a beneficial effect of hemodilution, particularly in temporary rather than permanent vascular occlusion models, and with colloid agents administered in high concentrations close to the onset of the ischemic event (e.g., Tu et al. 1988; Korosue et al. 1990; Perez-Trepichio et al. 1992; Yanaka et al. 1996; Cole et al. 1996). Human serum albumin was employed as a hemodiluent in eight hemodilution studies (Sundt et al. 1967; Little et al. 1981; Korosue et al. 1990; Cole et al. 1990; Matsui et al. 1993; Cole et al. 1993, 1996; Aronowski et al. 1996). However, *high-concentration* albumin (20–25%) was assessed in only one of these studies (Little et al. 1981) – a study involving permanent MCA occlusion, inappropriately early measurement of infarct volume, and lack of rigorous histopathology.

Clinical trials of albumin therapy for ischemic stroke: The neuroprotective efficacy of albumin therapy for ischemic stroke has been studied in only one small controlled clinical trial to date (Goslinga et al. 1992). Termed "The Amsterdam Stroke Study", this was a prospective trial of 300 patients in which normovolemic hemodilution was carried out in a customized fashion by administering 20% albumin plus crystalloid solutions while monitoring pulmonary capillary wedge pressure and hematocrit; target values were 12 mm Hg and 32%, respectively. The study's small size, the individual tailoring of therapy, the insufficient reporting of detail, and various subgroup imbalances seriously compromise its interpretation. Nonetheless, there are some findings of interest. First, despite an average age of 75 among the treated patients, fewer than 1% needed to be exlcuded on the basis of cardiopulmonary insufficiency. Although the overall analysis showed no difference in clinical outcome, subgroup analysis revealed that in two-thirds of stroke patients admitted with normal hematocrit, therapy proved superior to control management. The authors' speculative conclusion is that overall reduction in mortality and increased independence with this therapy may have exceeded 50% (Goslinga et al. 1992).

Published clinical studies utilizing *high-dose* albumin administration:

Prevention of vasospasm: While there are no published clinical reports describing the rapid administration of high-dose albumin to stroke patients, the administration of large quantities of albumin over prolonged time periods, however, is a common clinical practice in patients with aneurysmal subarachnoid hemorrhage (SAH) following surgical clipping of the aneurysm, in order to prevent delayed ischemia secondary to vasospasm (Levy et al. 1993; Mori et al. 1995). In a very recent report, 82 SAH patients (mean age, 48) received crystalloids plus albumin infusions under normovolemic or hypervolemic conditions (Lennihan et al. 2000). The daily dose of albumin administered in this study was ~2 g/kg body weight. Albumin infusions were well tolerated, and congestive heart failure occurred in only one patient. (In another study, patients with cirrhosis and spontaneous bacterial peritonitis were treated with high-dose i.v. albumin (initial dose of 1.5 g/kg, followed by 1 g/kg on day 3); the treatment was tolerated, and renal impairment and mortality were reduced (Sort et al. 1999).) The albumin doses used in these published studies are in same range employed in our experimental investigations.

Treatment of brain edema: Albumin has also been used in moderate-to-high doses to combat brain edema. In patients with brain contusion, 25% albumin was administered so as to maintain elevated oncotic pressure for 2 weeks; albumin therapy safely and effectively reduced contusional edema (Tomita et al. 1994). In another study, patients with putaminal hemorrhage treated with 12.5–25 g per day of albumin for 2 weeks showed reductions of cerebral edema and improved outcome (Tone et al. 1994). Thus, in marked contrast to crystalloid-hemodilution, which *worsens* brain edema and infarction (Heros and Korosue 1989; Korosue et al. 1990), studies of high-dose albumin therapy have shown consistently beneficial effects in reducing cerebral edema.

Summary and recommendations

Human serum albumin is a unique multifunctional protein possessing neuroprotective properties. In the series of experimental studies reviewed here, we have shown that moderate-to high-dose human albumin therapy diminishes brain injury in both cerebral ischemia and traumatic brain injury. At the clinically achievable dose of 1.25 g/kg, human albumin retains its striking neuroprotective efficacy in a relevant model of focal cerebral ischemia. In our view, the striking efficacy of high-concentration (20–25%) human serum albumin therapy in experimental focal ischemia strongly supports the feasibility of initiating early-phase clinical trials of this promising agent in patients with acute ischemic stroke.

Acknowledgments

These studies were supported by Program Project grant NS 05820 of the National Institutes of Health (MDG) and by an American Heart Association Initial Investigator Award (No. 9930263V) (LB). The authors gratefully acknowledge an equipment loan from Moor Instruments, Inc., Wilmington, Delaware.

References

1. Albers GW, Zivin JA, Choi DW (1998) Ethical standards in phase 1 trials of neuroprotective agents for stroke therapy. Stroke 29:1493–1494
2. Aronowski J, Strong R, Grotta JC (1996) Combined neuroprotection and reperfusion therapy for stroke. Effect of lubeluzole and diaspirin cross-linked hemoglobin in experimental focal ischemia. Stroke 27:1571–1576
3. Belayev L, Alonso OF, Busto R, Zhao W, Ginsberg MD (1996) Middle cerebral artery occlusion in the rat by intraluminal suture. Neurological and pathological evaluation of an improved model. Stroke 27:1616–1622
4. Belayev L, Alonso OF, Huh PW, Zhao W, Busto R, Ginsberg MD (1999b) Postreatment with high-dose albumin reduces histopathological damage and improves neurological deficit following fluid percussion brain injury in rats. J Neurotrauma 16:445–453
5. Belayev L, Bar-Joseph A, Adamchik J, Biegon A (1995) HU-211, a nonsychotropic cannabinoid, improves neurological signs and reduces brain damage after severe forebrain ischemia in rats. Mol Chem Neuropathol 25:19–33
6. Belayev L, Busto R, Zhao W, Clemens JA, Ginsberg MD (1997) Effect of delayed albumin hemodilution on infarction volume and brain edema after transient middle cerebral artery occlusion in rats. J Neurosurg 87:595–601
7. Belayev L, Liu Y, Busto R, Zhao W, Ginsberg MD (2000) Sequential laser-Doppler perfusion imaging after cerebral ischemia in rats and mice; effect of albumin. Soc Neurosci Abstr 26:1032
8. Belayev L, Saul I, Huh PW, Finotti N, Zhao W, Busto R, Ginsberg MD (1999a) Neuroprotective effect of high-dose albumin therapy against global ischemic brain injury in rats. Brain Res 845:107–111
9. Belayev L, Zhao W, Busto R, Ginsberg MD (2000) Human albumin therapy, at moderate doses, is highly neuroprotective in experimental focal ischemia. Stroke 31:337

10. Belayev L, Zhao W, Pattany PM, Weaver RG, Huh PW, Lin B, Busto R, Ginsberg MD (1998) Diffusion-weighted magnetic resonance imaging confirms marked neuroprotective efficacy of albumin therapy in focal cerebral ischemia. Stroke 29:2587–2599
11. Bogaert YE, Rosenthal RE, Fiskum G (1994) Postischemic inhibition of cerebral cortex pyruvate dehydrogenase. Free Radic Biol Med 16:811–820
12. Brott T, Lu M, Kothari R, Fagan SC, Frankel M, Grotta JC, Broderick J, Kwiatkowski T, Lewandowski C, Haley EC, Marler JR, Tilley BC (1998) Hypertension and its treatment in the NINDS rt-PA Stroke Trial. Stroke 29:1504–1509
13. Choi DW (1992) Excitotoxic cell death. J Neurobiol 23:1261–1276
14. Cole DJ, Drummond JC, Osborne TN, Matsumura J (1990) Hypertension and hemodilution during cerebral ischemia reduce brain injury and edema. Am J Physiol 259:H211–H217
15. Cole DJ, Drummond JC, Patel PM, Nary JC, Applegate RL (1996) Effect of oncotic pressure of diaspirin cross-linked hemoglobin (DCLHb) on brain injury after temporary focal cerebral ischemia in rats. Anesth Analg 83:342–347
16. Cole DJ, Schell RM, Drummond JC, Reynolds L (1993) Focal cerebral ischemia in rats. Effect of hypervolemic hemodilution with diaspirin cross-linked hemoglobin versus albumin on brain injury and edema. Anesthesiology 78:335–342
17. Curry S, Mandelkow H, Brick P, Franks N (1998) Crystal structure of human serum albumin complexed with fatty acid reveals an asymmetric distribution of binding sites. Nat Struct Biol 5:827–835
18. Dietrich WD, Alonso O, Busto R, Globus MT, Ginsberg MD (1994) Post-traumatic brain hypothermia reduces histopathological damage following concussive brain injury in the rat. Acta Neuropathol 87:250–258
19. Emerson TE (1989) Unique features of albumin: a brief review. Crit Care Med 17:690–694
20. European Ad Hoc Consensus Group (1998) Neuroprotection as initial therapy in acute stroke. Third Report of an Ad Hoc Consensus Group Meeting. Cerebrovasc Dis 8:59–72
21. Galis Z, Ghitescu L, Simionescu M (1988) Fatty acids binding to albumin incerases its uptake and transcytosis by the lung capillary endothelium. Eur J Cell Biol 47:358–365
22. Ghitescu L, Fixman A, Simionescu M, Simionescu N (1986) Specific binding sites for albumin restricted to plasmalemmal vesicles of continuous capillary endothelium: receptor-mediated transcytosis. J Cell Biol 102:1304–1311
23. Ginsberg MD (1995) Neuroprotection in brain ischemia – an update – Parts I and II. Neuroscientist 1:95–103 and 164–175
24. Ginsberg MD, Zhao W, Alonso OF, Loor-Estades JY, Dietrich WD, Busto R (1997) Uncoupling of local cerebral glucose metabolism and blood flow after acute fluid-percussion injury in rats. Am J Physiol 272:H2859–H2868
25. Ginsberg MD, Zhao W, Belayev L, Alonso OF, Liu Y, Loor JY, Busto R (2000) High-dose albumin treatment diminishes metabolism/blood flow uncoupling following traumatic brain injury in rats. J Neurosurg (in press)
26. Globus MY, Busto R, Martinez E, Valdes I, Dietrich WD, Ginsberg MD (1991) Comparative effect of transient global ischemia on extracellular levels of glutamate, glycine, and gamma-aminobutyric acid in vulnerable and nonvulnerable brain regions in the rat. J Neurochem 57:470–478
27. Goslinga H, Eijzenbach V, Heuvelmans JH, van der Laan de Vries, Melis VM, Schmid-Schonbein H, Bezember PD (1992) Custom-tailored hemodilution with albumin and crystalloids in acute ischemic stroke. Stroke 23:181–188
28. Halliwell B (1988) Albumin – an important extracellular antioxidant? Biochem Pharmacol 37:569–571
29. Halliwell B, Gutteridge JM (1990) The antioxidants of human extracellular fluids. Arch Biochem Biophys 280:1–8
30. He P, Curry FE (1993) Albumin modulation of capillary permeability: role of endothelial cell [Ca^{2+}]i. Am J Physiol 265:H74–H82
31. Heros RC, Korosue K (1989) Hemodilution for cerebral ischemia. Stroke 20:423–427
32. Hossmann KA (1994) Neurological progress: Viability thresholds and the penumbra of focal ischemia. Ann Neurol 36:557–565
33. Hu ML, Louie S, Cross CE, Motchnik P, Halliwell B (1993) Antioxidant protection against hypochlorous acid in human plasma. J Lab Clin Med 121:257–262
34. Huh PW, Belayev L, Zhao W, Busto R, Saul I, Ginsberg MD (1998) The effect of high-dose albumin therapy on local cerebral perfusion after transient focal cerebral ischemia in rats. Brain Res 804:105–113
35. Keaney JFJ, Simon DI, Stamler JS, Jaraki O, Scharfstein J, Vita JA, Loscalzo J (1993) NO forms an adduct with serum albumin that had endothelium-derived relaxing factor-like properties. J Clin Invest 91:1582–1589
36. Koch-Weser J, Sellers EM (1976a) Binding of drugs to serum albumin (first of two parts). N Engl J Med 294:311–316
37. Koch-Weser J, Sellers EM (1976b) Drug therapy. Binding of drugs to serum albumin (second of two parts). N Engl J Med 294:526–531
38. Koroshetz WJ, Moskowitz MA (1996) Emerging treatments for stroke in humans. Trends Pharmacol Sci 17:227–233
39. Korosue K, Heros RC, Oglivy CS, Hyodo A, Tu YK, Graichen R (1990) Comparison of crystalloids and colloids for hemodilution in a model of focal cerebral ischemia. J Neurosurg 73:576–584
40. Lennihan L, Mayer SA, Fink ME, Beckford A, Paik MC, Zhang H, Wu Y-C, Klebanoff LM, Raps EC, Solomon RA (2000) Effect of hypervolemic therapy on cerebral blood flow after subarachnoid hemorrhage. A randomized controlled trial. Stroke 31:383–391
41. Levy ML, Rabb CH, Zelman V, Giannotta SL (1993) Cardiac performance enhancement from dobutamine in patients refractory to hypervolemic therapy for cerebral vasospasm. J Neurosurg 79:494–499
42. Little JR, Slugg RM, Latchaw JPJ, Lesser RP (1981) Treatment of acute focal cerebral ischemia with concentrated albumin. Neurosurgery 9:552–558
43. Marler JR, Walker MD (1998) Progress in acute stroke research. Stroke 29:1491–1492
44. Matsui T, Sinyama H, Asano T (1993) Beneficial effect of prolonged administration of albumin on ischemic cerebral edema and infarction after occlusion of middle cerebral artery in rats. Neurosurgery 33:293–300
45. McIntosh TK (1993) Novel pharmacologic therapies in the treatment of experimental traumatic brain injury: A review. J Neurotrauma 10:215–261
46. McIntosh TK, Juhler M, Wieloch T (1998) Novel pharmacologic strategies in the treatment of experimental traumatic brain injury: 1998. J Neurotrauma 15:731–769
47. Mori K, Arai H, Nakajima K, Tajima A, Maeda M (1995) Hemorheological and hemodynamic analysis of hypervolemic hemodilution therapy for cerebral vasospasm after aneurysmal subarachnoid hemorrhage. Stroke 26:1620–1626
48. Nadal A, Fuentes E, Pastor J, McNaughton PA (1995) Plasma albumin is a potent trigger of calcium signals and DNA synthesis in astrocytes. Proc Natl Acad Sci USA 92:1426–1430
49. Nadal A, Fuentes E, Pastor J, McNaughton PA (1997) Plasma labumin induces calcium waves in rat cortical astrocytes. Glia 19:343–351
50. Perez-Trepichio AD, Furlan AJ, Little JR, Jones SC (1992) Hydroxyethyl starch 200/0.5 reduces infarct volume after embolic stroke in rats. Stroke 23:1782–1790

51. Peters TJr (1996) *All About Albumin. Biochemistry, Genetics, and Medical Applications,* San Diego, Academic Press
52. Reinhart WH, Nagy C (1995) Albumin affects erythrocyte aggregation and sedimentation. Eur J Clin Invest 25:523–528
53. Remmers M, Schmidt-Kastner R, Belayev L, Lin B, Busto R, Ginsberg MD (1999) Protein extravasation and cellular uptake after high-dose human-albumin treatment of transient focal cerebral ischemia in rats. Brain Res 827:237–242
54. Schnitzer JE (1992) gp60 is an albumin-binding glycoprotein expressed by continuous endothelium involved in albumin transcytosis. Am J Physiol 262:H246–H254
55. Schnitzer JE, Oh P (1992) Antibodies to SPARC inhibit albumin binding to SPARC, gp60, and microsvascular endothelium. Am J Physiol 263:H1872–1879
56. Schnitzer JE, Sung A, Horvat R, Bravo J (1992) Preferential interaction of albumin-binding proteins, gp30 and gp18, with conformationally modified albumins. Presence in many cells and tissues with a possible role in catabolism. J Biol Chem 267:24544–24553
57. Schurr A, Miller JJ, Payne RS, Rigo BM (1999) An increase in lactate output by brain tissue serves to meet the energy needs of glutamate-activated neurons. J Neurosci 19:34–39
58. Schurr A, Payne RS, Miller JJ, Rigor BM (1997b) Brain lactate is an obligatory aerobic energy substrate for functional recovery after hypoxia: further in vitro validation. J Neurochem 69:423–426
59. Schurr A, Payne RS, Miller JJ, Rigor BM (1997a) Brain lactate, not glucose, fuels the recovery of synaptic function from hypoxia upon reoxygenation: an in vitro study. Brain Res 744:105–111
60. Schurr A, Payne RS, Miller JJ, Rigor BM (1997c) Glia are the main source of lactate utilized by neurons for recovery of function posthypoxia. Brain Res 774:221–224
61. Seylaz J, Charbonne R, Nanri K, Von Euw D, Borredon J, Kacem K, Meric P, Pinard E (1999) Dynamic in vivo measurement of erythrocyte velocity and flow in capillaries and of microvessel diameter in the rat brain by confocal laser microscopy. J Cereb Blood Flow Metab 19:863–870
62. Siesjö BK (1981) Review. Cell damage in the brain: A speculative synthesis. J Cereb Blood Flow Metab 1:155–185
63. Slyter H (1998) Ethical challenges in stroke research. Stroke 29:1725–1729
64. Smith C, Halliwell B, Aruoma OI (1992) Protection by albumin against the pro-oxidant actions of phenolic dietary components. Food Chem Toxicol 30:483–489
65. Smith ML, Bendek G, Dahlgren N, Rosen I, Wieloch T, Siesjö BK (1984) Models for studying long-term recovery following forebrain ischemia in the rat. 2. A 2-vessel occlusion model. Acta Neurol Scand 69:385–401
66. Sort P, Navasa M, Arroyo V, Aldeguer X, Planas R, Ruiz-del-Arbol L, Castells L, Vargas V, Soriano G, Guevara M, Gines P, Rodes J (1999) Effect of intravenous albumin on renal impairment and mortality in patients with cirrhosis and spontaneous bacterial peritonitis. N Engl J Med 341:403–409
67. Sundt TMJ, Waltz AG, Sayre GP (1967) Experimental cerebral infarction: modification by treatment with hemodiluting, hemoconcentrating, and dehydrating agents. J Neurosurg 26:46–56
68. Tabernero A, Medina A, Sanchez-Abarca LI, Lavado E, Medina JM (1999) The effect of albumin on astrocyte energy metabolism is not brought about through the control of cytosolic Ca^{2+} concentrations but by free-fatty acid sequestration. Glia 25:1–9
69. Tomita H, Ito U, Tone O, Masaoka H, Tominaga B (1994) High colloid oncotic therapy for contusional brain edema. Acta Neurochir Suppl (Wien) 60:547–549
70. Tone O, Ito U, Tomita H, Masaoka H, Tominaga B (1994) High colloid oncotic therapy for brain edema with cerebral hemorrhage. Acta Neurochir Suppl (Wien) 60:568–570
71. Trigatti BL, Gerber GE (1995) A direct role for serum albumin in the cellular uptake of long-chain fatty acids. Biochem J 108:155–159
72. Tsacopoulos M, Magistretti PJ (1996) Metabolic coupling between glia and neurons. J Neurosci 16:877–885
73. Tu YK, Heros RC, Karacostas D, Liszczak T, Hyodo A, Candia G, Zervas NT, Lagree K (1988) Isovolemic hemodilution in experimental focal cerebral ischemia. Part 2: Effects on regional cerebral blood flow and size of infarction. J Neurosurg 69:82–91
74. Wasil M, Halliwell B, Hutchison DC, Baum H (1987) The antioxidant action of human extracellular fluids. Effect of human serum and its protein components on the inactivation of alpha 1- antiproteinase by hypochlorous acid and by hydrogen perioxide. Biochem J 243:219–223
75. Wayner DD, Burton GW, Ingold KU, Locke S (1985) Quantitative measurement of the total, peroxyl radical-trapping antioxidant capability of human blood plasma by controlled peroxidation. The important contribution made by plasma proteins. FEBS Lett 187:33–37
76. Yanaka K, Camarata PJ, Spellman SR, McDonald DE, Heros RC (1996) Optimal timing of hemodilution for brain protection in a canine model of focal cerebral ischemia. Stroke 27:906–912
77. Young B, Runge JW, Waxman KS, Harrington T, Wilberger J, Muizelaar JP, Boddy A, Kupiec JW (1996) Effects of pegorgotein on neurologic outcome of patients with severe head injury. A multicenter, randomized controlled trial. JAMA 276:538–543
78. Zhao W, Belayev L, Ginsberg MD (1997) Transient middle cerebral artery occlusion by intraluminal suture: II. Neurological deficits, and pixel-based correlation of histopathology with local blood flow and glucose utilization. J Cereb Blood Flow Metab 17:1281–1290
79. Zhao W, Ginsberg MD, Prado R, Belayev L (1996) Depiction of infarct frequency distribution by computer-assisted image mapping in rat brains with middle cerebral artery occlusion. Comparison of photothrombotic and intraluminal suture models. Stroke 27:1112–1117
80. Zhao W, Ginsberg MD, Smith DW (1995) Three-dimensional quantitative autoradiography by disparity analysis: theory and application to image averaging of local cerebral glucose utilization. J Cereb Blood Flow Metab 15:552–565
81. Zhao W, Young TY, Ginsberg MD (1993) Registration and three-dimensional reconstruction of autoradiographic images by the disparity analysis method. IEEE Trans Med Imag 12:782–791
82. Zhao Y, Marcel YL (1996) Serum albumin is a significant intermediate in cholesterol transfer between cells and lipoproteins. Biochemistry 35:7174–7180
83. Zivin JA (1997) Neuroprotective therapies in stroke. Drugs 54 Suppl 3:83-88
84. Zoellner H, Hofler M, Beckmann R, Hufnagl P, Vanyek E, Bielek E, Wojta J, Fabry A, Lockie S, Binder BR (1996) Serum albumin is a specific inhibitor of apoptosis in human endothelial cells. J Cell Sci 109:2571–2580

Growth factors and cytokines

Update on growth factor treatment for stroke: 2000

S. P. Finklestein, K. Wada

In previous presentations at this Conference, we have described the rationale and preclinical studies underlying the concept of growth factor treatment for acute stroke. Within the past few years, this preclinical work led to human clinical safety trials, and, ultimately to large-scale efficacy trials. In this review, we will summarize the current status of this work.

In particular, this review will focus on the status of basic fibroblast growth factor (bFGF) treatment for stroke. In numerous preclinical studies in several species, we and others have shown that the administration of bFGF within a few hours following the onset of focal cerebral ischemia reduces infarct volume, both in models of permanent and temporary ischemia (Fischer et al. 1995; Jiang et al. 1996; Huang et al. 1996; Bethel et al. 1997). Interestingly, bFGF can be given in these animal studies either intracerebrally (esp. intraventricularly), or systemically (intravenously). bFGF is a protein of 18 kDa molecular weight and 154 amino acids. This large charged polypeptide penetrates the damaged blood brain barrier following ischemia (Fischer et al. 1995). Other recent work suggest that there may be a facilitated transport mechanism for this molecule, taking it across the intact blood brain barrier as well (Wagner et al. 1999).

bFGF is a potent survival-promoting molecule for neurons and other cell types. It protects neurons *in vitro* and *in vivo* against excitatory amino acids, free radicals, nitric oxide, hypoglycemia, anoxia, calcium ionophore, as well as other toxins and insults (Mattson and Barger 1995). Moreover, bFGF protects cultured neurons against apoptotic cell death. In recent studies, we showed that exogenously administered bFGF appears to upregulate the expression of the anti-apoptotic protein Bcl-2 in the ischemic penumbra following focal ischemia in rats (Ay et al. 2000). This may be one mechanism by which bFGF reduces infarct volume. bFGF must be given within three hours of the onset of permanent middle cerebral artery (MCA) occlusion in rats in order to reduce infarct volume (Ren and Finklestein 1997).

In other preclinical studies, we showed that bFGF also enhances neurological recovery following stroke, even when given long after stroke has occured (Kawamata et al. 1997, 1999). In this instance, it appears that the mechanism is not infarct reduction or prevention of cell death. Rather, the mechanism appears to be, at least in part, stimulation of new neuronal sprouting and synapse formation in undamaged parts of brain (Kawamata et al. 1997, 1999). In addition, bFGF is a potent mitogen for neuronal precursor cells, and may also enhance recovery by stimulation of endogenous stem cell prolifera-

CNS Growth Factor Research Laboratory, Massachusetts General Hospital and Harvard Medical School, 32 Fruit Street, WRN 408, Boston, MA 02114 USA
e-mail: finklestein@helix.mgh.harvard.edu

tion in the brain, thereby replacing some of the lost neurons due to stroke (Flax et al. 1998).

The promising preclinical data in acute stroke were followed by a Phase II safety trial of intravenous bFGF (Fiblast®) in acute human stroke (The Fiblast Safety Study Group 1998). In this randomized, double-blind, placebo-controlled study, 66 patients were enrolled within 12 hours of having suffered an acute thromboembolic stroke. Of these, 46 patients received recombinant bFGF at total doses of 3–150 mg/kg, infused over periods ranging from 3–24 hours. Twenty patients received placebo infusions. Patients were followed for three months after stroke.

In this small safety trial, no serious effects of intravenous bFGF treatment were seen, including effects on blood pressure, renal or hepatic function, neurological outcome or death. bFGF treatment was associated with a dose-dependent increase in blood leukocyte count that peaked at two days after stroke and declined thereafter. This phenomenon did not appear to be associated with infection or other adverse events. Only one patient developed anti-bFGF antibodies.

Following this encouraging small clinical safety trial, two large-scale safety/efficacy trials of intravenous bFGF for acute stroke were undertaken. The North American bFGF (Fiblast®) trial was a placebo-controlled, double-blind randomized study of an eight hour intravenous infusion of bFGF (Clark et al. 2000). Patients were enrolled with acute ischemic stroke having the onset of symptoms within six hours of enrollment, and a baseline score of four on the NIH Stroke Scale (at least two points motor). Patients were randomized either to placebo, bFGF 5 mg, or bFGF 10 mg. The primary outcome measure was the modified Rankin Scale at 90 days post-stroke.

A total of 302 patients were enrolled at 58 medical centers, when the study was stopped following an interim analysis due to safety concerns. Patients receiving 5 or 10 mg of bFGF had significantly worse neurological outcomes and mortality compared to the placebo-treated group. Specifically, mortality at 90 days was 29% in the Fiblast® 5 mg/group, 25% in the Fiblast® 10 mg/group and 13% in the placebo group ($p < 0.02$). Treatment with intravenous Fiblast® was associated with leukocytosis and decreased blood pressure. However these changes did not appear to correlate with outcome.

Concurrent with the North American trial, a trial of intravenous bFGF (Trafermin®) was also undertaken in Europe and Australia (Bogousslavsky et al. 2000). This study was similar in design to the North American trial with one notable exception. Again, this was a double-blind, placebo-controlled randomized trial of bFGF, at a dose of either 5 or 10 mg total. However, in contrast to the eight hour infusion in the North American trial, bFGF was infused in this trial over 24 hours. Again, patients were enrolled with onset of stroke within six hours or less from onset. Patients had a baseline score of seven or greater on the NIH Stroke Scale (at least two points motor). The primary outcome measure was a categorized combination of the Barthel and Rankin Scales at three months following stroke.

At interim analysis of this trial, 286 patients had been enrolled at 55 sites in 11 countries. In contrast to the North American trial, no serious adverse effects or increased mortality was found with bFGF treatment. Mortality rates at 90 days were 17% in the Trafermin® 5 mg/group, 24% in the Trafermin® 10 mg/group, and 18% in the placebo group. At this interim analysis, patients receiving Trafermin® 5 mg showed a small but nonsignificant advantage in efficacy over placebo treated patients (OR 1.2 [0.72–2.0], $p = 0.48$), but patients receiving Trafermin® 10 mg showed a nonsignificant disadvantage (OR 0.74 [0.44–1.32], $p = 0.24$). As in the North American trial, treatment with intravenous bFGF was associated with leukocytosis and decreased blood pressure. Mean decrease in diastolic blood pressure from baseline was 19 mm of mercury in the 5 mg/group, 22 mm of mercury in the 10 mg/group and 8 mm of mercury in the placebo group. The sponsor discontinued the trial at this point because no major overall trend toward efficacy was seen.

However, although no treatment effect was apparent overall, an interesting *post hoc* subgroup analysis was undertaken. As noted above, patients entering the trial suffered stroke within six hours of onset. Indeed, half of the patients were enrolled within five hours of stroke onset, and the other half were enrolled within five to six hours of stroke onset. No apparent benefit of bFGF treatment was seen in the patients receiving bFGF within five hours of the onset of stroke. However, in the patients receiving bFGF from five to six hours (half of all patients enrolled), there was an apparent advantage of bFGF treatment on the primary efficacy outcome measure. This was particularly apparent in the patients receiving the 5 mg bFGF dose (OR 2.1, $p = 0.044$, after age adjustment OR 1.9, $p = 0.08$). This significant effect was surprising, especially since it was obtained at interim analysis only one-third of the way through the projected study. (The study was initially powered for 900 patients, 300 in each treatment group. At the time of interim analysis, only 286 patients had been enrolled, i.e., 95–96 in each of the three treatment groups. There were only 47–48 patients in the subgroup in whom treatment had been initiated at 5–6 hours after stroke, and in whom significant efficacy was seen on *post hoc* analysis.)

The above clinical trials teach us some important facts concerning use of bFGF, and potentially use of any growth factor for the treatment of stroke. The first lesson, of course, is that adverse side effects can be found in large intention-to treat-studies conducted in many medical centers that are unanticipated by small preliminary safety trials conducted in just a few centers. The second lesson is that the rate of administration of bFGF may be critical to its safety. Increased mortality was seen in the North American Fiblast® Trial when total doses of 5 or 10 mg of bFGF were infused over eight hours. However, in the European/Australian Trial, no increased mortality was seen when these same total doses of bFGF were infused over 24 hours. Thus, it appears that the toxicity of bFGF may be related to the rate of infusion and consequent plasma concentrations, rather than the total dose administered.

The third possible lesson to be gleaned from the bFGF clinical trials concerns the interesting subgroup analysis done in the European/Australian trial. While such subgroup analysis is entirely *post hoc*, and cannot by any means be taken as proof of principle, it can generate interesting hypotheses. In this instance, no apparent efficacy was seen in patients receiving bFGF within the first five hours following stroke onset, but efficacy was suggested in patients receiving the drug after five hours. This was particularly apparent with the 5 mg bFGF dose. There are several possible explanations for this interesting finding. In the first place, it might be a "false positive" result due to chance. On the other hand, this finding might reflect the fact that too early an administration of bFGF might be deleterious.

Another possible interpretation for these intriguing *post hoc* findings is that bFGF may have more utility as a *stroke recovery* drug than as an *acute stroke* drug. As noted above, in preclinical studies, we showed that the *late* administration of bFGF beginning as long as 24 hours following stroke, can enhance neurological recovery *without* reduction of infarct volume. The reasons for this enhanced recovery appear to include stimulation of new neuronal sprouting and synapse formation in intact undamaged regions of brain, contributing toward the compensatory capacity of the brain to affect functional recovery following injury. Alternatively, the late administration of bFGF may stimulate andogenous neural progenitor cells in the brain to proliferate and migrate, thereby replacing some of the cells lost to stroke.

The concept of the *late* use of bFGF or indeed other growth factors as stroke recovery-promoting agents is an interesting one. Indeed, the endogenous expression of growth factors and other cytokines in the brain typically does not begin for several hours to days following stroke. This suggests that some of these factors might, indeed, be given at late times following stroke as recovery-promoting treatments. The results of the above clinical trials clearly delineate the parameters within which bFGF, in particular, can be given safely to human stroke patients. The interesting subgroup analysis of the European/Australian trial raises the hypothesis that bFGF may have particular value as a stroke recovery drug to be administered at prolonged times after stroke. This intriguing hypothesis awaits further clinical testing.

References

1. Ay I, Sugimori H, Finklestein SP (2000) Basic fibroblast growth factor (bFGF) decreases DNA fragmentation and increases bcl-2 expression following stroke in rats (abstr.). Stroke 31:282
2. Bethel A, Kirsch JR, Koehler RC, Finklestein SP, Traystman RJ (1997) Intravenous basic fibroblast growth factor decreases brain injury resulting from focal ischemia in cats. Stroke 28:609–615
3. Bogousslavsky J, Donnan GA, Fieschie C, Kate M, Ogozozo JM, Chamorro A, Victor SJ (2000) Fiblast (Trafermin) in acute stroke: Results of the European-Australian phase II/III safety and efficacy trial (abstr.). Cerebrovascular Dis 10 (Suppl 2):1–116
4. Clark WM, Schim JD, Kasner SE, Victor S (2000) Trafermin in acute ischemic stroke: Results of a phase II/III randomized efficacy study (abstr.). Neurology 54:A88
5. Fisher M, Meadows M-E, Do T, Weise J, Trubetskoy V, Charett M, Finklestein SP (1995) Delayed treatment with intravenous basic fibroblast growth factor reduces infarct size following permanent focal cerebral ischemia in rats. J Cereb Blood Flow Metab 15:953–959
6. Flax JD, Aurora S, Yang C, Simonin C, Willis AM, Billinghurst LL, Jendoubi M, Sidman RL, Wolfe JH, Kim SU, Snyder EY (1998) Engraftable human neural stem cells repsond to developmental cues, replace neurons, and express foreign genes. Nature Biotechnolgy 16:1033–1039
7. Huang Z, Chen K, Huang PL, Finklestein SP, Moskowitz MA (1996) bFGF ameliorates focal ischemic injury by blood flow-independent mechanisms in eNOS mutant mice. Amer J Physiol 272:H1401–H1405
8. Jiang N, Finklestein SP, Do T, Caday CG, Charette M, Chopp M (1996) Delayed intravenous administration of basic fibroblast growth factor (bFGF) reduces infarct volume in a model of focal cerebral ischemia/reperfusion in the rat. J Neurol Sci 139:173–179
9. Kawamata T, Dietrich WD, Schallert T, Gotts JE, Cocke RR, Benowitz LI, Finklestein SP (1997) Intracisternal basic fibroblast growth factor (bFGF) enhances functional recovery and upregulates the expression of a molecular marker of neuronal sprouting following focal cerebral infarction. Proc Natl Acid Sci 94:8179–8184
10. Kawamata, T, Ren JM, Cha CH, Finklestein SP (1999) Intracisternal antisense oligonucleotide to growth associated protein-43 (GAP-43) blocks the recovery-promoting effects of basic fibroblast growth factor (bFGF) after focal stroke. Exp Neurol 158:89–96
11. Mattson MP, Barger SW (1995) Programmed cell life: Neuroprotective signal transduction and ischemic brain injury, in Cerebrovascular Diseases: The 19th Princeton Stroke Conference, Moskowitz MA and Caplan LR, Editiors, Butterworth Heinemann: Newton, MA. p 271–290
12. Ren J, Finklestein SP (1997) Time dependence of infarct reduction by intravenous basic fibroblast growth factor (bFGF) following focal cerebral ischemia in rats. Eur J Pharmacol 327:11–16
13. The Fiblast Safety Study Group (1998) Clinical safety trial of intravenous basic fibroblast growth factor (bFGF, FIBLAST) in acute stroke (abstr.). Stroke 29:287
14. Wagner JP, Black IB, DiCicco-Bloom E (1999) Stimulation of neonatal and adult brain neurogenesis by subcutaneous injection of basic fibroblast growth factor. J Neurosci 19:6006–6016

Gene transfer of GDNF ameliorates ischemic rat brain injury after transient MCA occlusion

K. Abe[1], H. Kitagawa,[1,2] T. Hayashi[1]

Abstract

To examine a possible protective effect of exogenous glial cell line-derived neurotrophic factor (GDNF) gene expression against ischemic brain injury, a replication-defective adenoviral vector containing GDNF gene (Ad-GDNF) was directly injected into the cerebral cortex at 1 day before 90 min of transient middle cerebral artery occlusion (MCAO) in rats. 2,3,5-Triphenyltetrazolium chloride (TTC) staining showed that infarct volume of the Ad-GDNF injected group at 24 h after the transient MCAO was significantly smaller than that of vehicle or Ad-LacZ treated group. The numbers of TUNEL, immunoreactive caspase-3 and cytochrome c positive neurons induced in the ipsilateral cerebral cortex at 24 h after transient MCAO were markedly reduced by the Ad-GDNF group. These results suggest that the successful exogenous GDNF gene transfer ameliorates the ischemic brain injury after transient MCAO in association with the reduction of apoptotic signals.

Abbreviations: Ad-GDNF, replication-defective adenoviral vector containing GDNF gene; Ad-LacZ, replication-defective adenoviral vector containing E. coli lacZ gene; ANOVA, analysis of variance; CMV, cytomegalovirus; DAB, 2,3'-diaminobenzidine tetrahydrochloride; GDNF, glial cell line-derived neurotrophic factor; GFRα-1, GDNF receptor α; HSV, Herpes simplex virus; MCAO, middle cerebral artery occlusion; NAIP, neuronal apoptosis inhibitory protein; PBS, phosphate-buffered saline; Ret, c-ret proto-oncogene; TUNEL, terminal deoxynucleotidyl dUTP nick end labeling.

Introduction

Glial cell line-derived neurotrophic factor (GDNF) has a potent neuroprotective effect on a variety of neuronal damage in vitro or in vivo (Lin et al. 1993; Henderson et al. 1994; Beck et al. 1995; Li et al. 1995; Tomac et al. 1995). Our previous papers and another report have also demonstrated the amelioration of ischemic brain injury by GDNF application after middle cerebral artery occlusion (MCAO) model in rodents (Abe et al. 1997a; Wang et al. 1997; Kitagawa et al. 1998a). Therefore, GDNF could be one of the most potent candidates for acute cerebrovascular injury as well as neurodegenerative

Keywords: GDNF, gene therapy, MCAO, TUNEL, caspase-3, cytochrome c.

[1]Department of Neurology, Okayama University Medical School, 2-5-1 Shikatacho, Okayama 700-8558, Japan, [2]Second Institute of New Drug Research, Otsuka Pharmaceutical Co. Ltd., 771-0192 Tokushima, Japan,
e-mail: abek@cc.okayama-u.ac.jp

disorders such as Parkinson's disease (Lin et al. 1993; Tomac et al. 1995).

Gene delivery systems using virus vectors have been reported in many fields including not only genetic diseases but also in some acquired diseases such as cancer or cardiovascular diseases (Nabel 1995; Verma and Somia 1997). Recently, our group demonstrated successful adenovirus-mediated LacZ gene transfer into normal or ischemic rodent brain (Abe et al. 1997b, 1997c; Kitagawa et al. 1998b, 1998c). In addition, some genes have also been successfully transferred into the brain, and have shown protective effects against ischemic brain injury (Betz et al. 1995; Linnik et al. 1995; Lawrence et al. 1997; Yang et al. 1997; Yang et al. 1998; Yenari et al. 1998). Therefore, gene therapy for cerebrovascular disease would become one potential better therapy in the near future (Heistad and Faraci 1996).

The mechanism of the neuroprotective effect of GDNF is not clearly understood. Some apoptotic signals may be important in the development of ischemic neuronal cell death. Recently, it has been reported that caspases-3 and cytochrome c may play a pivotal role in apoptotic cell death after mitochondrial apoptotic signal pathways regulated by bcl-2 family genes (Kluck et al. 1997; Yang et al. 1997). Our previous reports showed an induction of caspases after ischemic injury in the rat brain and an attenuation of ischemic brain injury by GDNF associated with the suppression of caspases induction (Kitagawa et al. 1998a). Thus, we prepared an adenovirus vector containing the GDNF gene (Ad-GDNF), and a possible protective effect of the Ad-GDNF transfer into rat brain was examined after transient MCAO in association with modifications of apoptotic signals.

Materials and methods

Adenoviral vector

The recombinant adenoviral vector used in this study was based on type 5 adenovirus that was essentially the same as in previous reports (Bajocchi et al. 1993; Setoguchi et al. 1994; Abe et al. 1997b). In brief, the E3 region of the adenovirus genome was deleted, and a cassette containing cDNA for rat GDNF or E.coli lacZ gene (used as a control vector) driven by cytomegalovirus (CMV) promoter and SV40 polyadenylation signal was inserted into the E1 region of the adenovirus genome by homologous recombination. With this promotor, the rat GDNF or E. coli lacZ gene of the episomally located adenovirus vector may be transcribed as mRNA in the nucleus, and the mRNA translated into the protein in the cytoplasm. The adenoviral vector, designated as Ad-GDNF or Ad-LacZ, was propagated in 293 cells (CRL1573; American Type Collection) and purified and titered as previously described (Bajocchi et al. 1993; Setoguchi et al. 1994; Abe et al. 1997b).

In vivo adenovirus-mediated GDNF gene transfer

Male adult Wistar rats (body weight: 250–280 g) were used in this experiment. Adenovirus vector injection was performed according to our previous report with a slight modification (Abe et al. 1997b). Briefly, the animals were anesthetized with intraperitoneal injection of pentobarbital (10 mg/250 g rat), and were immobilized using a stereotactic frame (SR-5N, Narishige, Tokyo, Japan). A burr hole with a diameter of 2 mm was carefully made in the skull by an electric dental drill to avoid traumatic brain injury. The location of the burr hole was 3 mm posterior and 5 mm lateral to the right of bregma, which is located at the upper part of the MCA. Dura mater was preserved at this time. The animals were allowed to recover at ambient atmosphere.

On the next day, at about 24 h after the drilling, the rats were anesthetized by inhalation of a nitrous oxide/oxygen/halothane (68%/30%/2%) mixture, and their heads were fixed in the stereotactic frame. Ad-GDNF, Ad-LacZ (10^8 pfu in 10 µl of vector vehicle consisting of 10 mM Tris-HCl, pH 7.4, 1mM $MgCl_2$, and 10% glycerol) or vehicle solution was administered to the ipsilateral cortex via the burr hole through the dura mater at a depth of 4 mm from the surface of the skull bone at an angle of 24 ° laterally using a 10-µl sterile Hamilton syringe (the Gastight Highperformance Syringe, Hamilton, Reno, NE) and a 26-gauge needle (0.47 mm outer diameter). The injections (10 µl) were slowly completed in 10 min. During the injection, the needle was gradually withdrawn at a rate of 0.4 mm/min.

Transient MCAO

At about 24 h after the virus vector injection, the rats were again anesthetized by inhalation of a nitrous oxide/oxygen/halothane (69%/30%/1%) mixture during the surgical procedure. The right MCA was occluded by the insertion of a nylon thread through the common carotid artery as described in our previous reports (Kitagawa et al. 1998a). Body temperature was maintained at 37 ±0.3 °C during the surgical preparation for MCA occlusion using a heat pad (BWT-100, Bio Research Center Co., Ltd, Nagoya, Japan) and heating lamp. The blood flow was restored by removal of the nylon thread after 90 min of transient ischemia. Blood samples (90 µl) were collected before MCAO (–1.5 h) or at 0, 8, or 24 h after 90 min of reperfusion from ventral tail artery for measurement of PO_2, PCO_2, and pH (pH/Blood Gas Analyzer, CIBA CORNING 238, CHIRON, Tokyo Japan). Body temperature was also monitored before MCAO or at 0, 8 or 24 h after reperfusion with a rectal probe (RET-2, Physitemp Instruments Inc., Clifton, USA). The animals were allowed to recover at ambient temperature (21 to 24 °C) until the time of sampling. The experimental protocol and procedures were approved by the Animal Committee of the Okayama University Medical School.

Estimation of brain injury after transient MCAO

To examine an effect of Ad-GDNF on infarct size after transient MCAO, the rat forebrains were removed and divided into 6 coronal (2 mm each) sections at 24 h of reperfusion with vehicle (n = 9), Ad-LacZ (n = 6) or Ad-GDNF (n = 9) treatment. The coronal sections were stained with saline containing 2% 2,3,5-triphenyltetrazolium chloride (TTC) at 37 °C for 30 min, after which sections were fixed in 10% neutralized formalin, according to a technique reported previously (Bederson et al. 1986). The five infarct areas between each adjoining slice were measured by Scion Image software, version 1.62a, and then the infarct areas on each slice were summed and multiplied by slice thickness to give the infarct volume. In this experiment, regional CBF of right frontoparietal cortex region was measured before or immediately after occlusion (–1.5 h) or reperfusion (0 h) respectively, and at 8 or 24 h after the reperfusion through the burr hole using a laser blood flowmeter (Flo-C1, Omegawave).

Histological study

For the histological staining of DNA fragmentation, caspase-3 and cytochrome c, the rat forebrains were removed and quickly frozen in a powdered dry-ice at 24 h after transient MCAO (2 days after injection) of both vehicle (n = 3) and Ad-GDNF (n = 3) treated groups. Sham control samples (n = 2) were also collected in the same way without the drug injection and MCAO. Coronal sections at the caudate and dorsal hippocampal levels were cut on a cryostat at –18 °C to a 10 µm thickness and collected on glass slides.

For detection of DNA fragmentation, terminal deoxynucleotidyl dUTP nick end labeling (TUNEL) was performed with a kit (TACS TdT in situ apoptosis detection kit #80-4625-00, Genzyme, Cambridge, MA) according to our previous report (Kitagawa et al. 1998a) Staining was developed with 2,3'-diaminobenzidine tetrahydrochloride (DAB, 0.5mg/ml in 50 mmol/l Tris-HCl buffer, pH 7.4).

Immunostaining for caspase-3 and cytochrome c was performed by avidin-biotin-peroxidase method (ABC) using a kit (PK-6101 for cytochrome c, or PK-6105 for caspase-3, Vector Laboratories). In brief, the fresh-frozen sections were fixed for 10 min in ice-cold acetone and air-dried, rinsed 3 times in phosphate-buffered saline (pH 7.4) (PBS) and blocked with 10% normal serum (kit components) for 2 h. The slides were incubated for 16 h at 4 °C with a first antibody: a rabbit polyclonal antibody against cytochrome c (H-104), and a goat polyclonal antibody against caspase-3 (CPP32 p20, L-18) (Santa Cruz Biotechnology Inc. Santa Cruz CA U.S.A., cat# sc-7159, or sc-1225, respectively), diluted in PBS (1/200) containing 10% normal serum and 0.3% Triton X-100. After blocking endogenous peroxidase, the sections were incubated for 2 h with the biotinylated second antibody (1/200), in the buffer, followed by incubation with the avidin-biotin-horseradish peroxidase complex. Staining was developed with DAB, and lightly counterstained with Mayer Hematoxylin.

The sections were examined by light microscope, and the stained cells in 0.25 mm^2 of random three MCA areas were counted, summed and categorized into 4 grades as follows: no staining, small (1–10), moderate (10–100), or large (100–500) number of stained cells as (–), (±), (+), and (2+), respectively.

Statistical analyses

Statistical analysis were performed using one way analysis of variance (ANOVA) for infarct volume, two way ANOVA followed by Bonferroni post hoc test for infarct area, and ANOVA repeated measure for physiological and rCBF data, respectively.

Results

Effect of Ad-GDNF on infarction after MCAO

There were no significant differences in blood gases, pH, and rectal temperature between vehicle, Ad-LacZ, and Ad-GDNF treated groups before MCAO, or at 0, 8, or 24 h after the reperfusion (data not shown).

Regional CBF of both the vehicle, Ad-LacZ and Ad-GDNF treated groups was reduced to approximately 40% of the control immediately after MCAO, and recovered to the base line after reperfusion by withdrawing the nylon thread (Fig. 1). Although a slight increase of rCBF in case of the Ad-GDNF treated group compared to that of the vehicle or the Ad-LacZ treated group was observed, there was no significant difference among these three groups (Fig. 1). While infarction in the brain sections of the sham control group could not be observed, infarct volumes of the vehicle, Ad-LacZ and Ad-GDNF treated groups at 24 h after 90 min of transient MCAO were 209.2 ± 35.8 mm^3 (mean ± SD, n = 9), 213.3 ± 59.1 mm^3 (n = 6) and 97.6 ± 71.5 mm^3 (n = 9; $P < 0.001$ vs the vehicle and Ad-LacZ treated groups), respectively (Fig. 2A). Infarct areas of 2 or 3 coronal sections (4, 6, and 8 mm caudal from frontal pole) from the Ad-GDNF treated group were also significantly smaller than those of the vehicle or the Ad-LacZ groups (Fig. 2B), respectively.

Effect of Ad-GDNF on the changes of TUNEL, caspase-3, or cytochrome c stainings

There were no TUNEL or caspase-3 positive cells in the sham control brain (Fig. 3a, 3d), while cytochrome c stained cells were slightly detected in layers IV–V of the ipsilateral (Fig. 3g, arrowheads), or contralateral frontoparietal somatosensory cortex. TUNEL positive cells were markedly increased in ipsilateral cortex (Fig. 3b, Table 1) and caudate (Table 1) in the vehicle treated group at 24 h after transient MCAO. In the Ad-GDNF treated group, the number of TUNEL positive cells was obviously smaller, especially in the cortex (Fig. 3c, arrowhead) than that in the vehicle group (Table 1). Caspase-3 or cytochrome c positive neurons were also markedly increased in the vehicle group at 24 h after transient MCAO in both ipsilateral cortex (Fig. 3e, 3h, arrowheads) and caudate, while those positive cells were reduced in the Ad-GDNF treated group (Fig. 3f, 3i, arrowheads, Table 1). In the ipsilateral hippocampus and all parts of contralateral side,

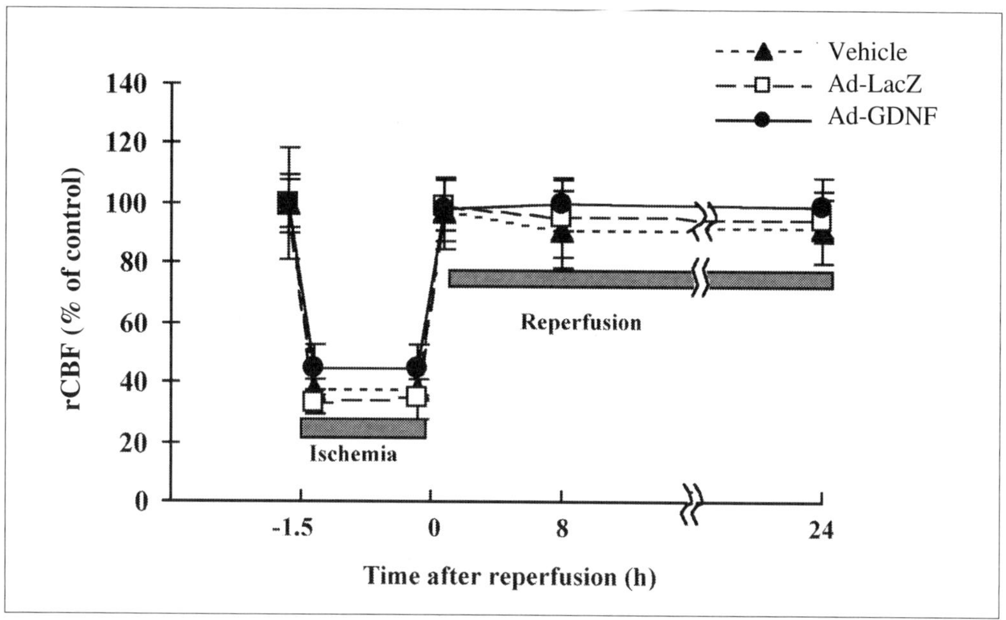

Fig. 1. Temporal profile of regional CBF after 90 min of transient MCAO. Regional CBF reduced to about 40% of basal line immediately after MCAO occlusion (–1,5 h), and restored to base line after reperfusion (0 h) in both vehicle (n = 9, —▲—), Ad-LacZ (n = 6, —□—), and Ad-GDNF (n = 9, —●—) treated groups. There was no significant difference in CBF between these three groups. Data are expressed as mean ± SD. (From Kitagawa et al. 1999 with permission).

TUNEL staining or caspase-3 immunoreactivity was not found in this experiment. Moreover, changes in cytochrome c immunoreactivity were not detected in any parts except for the ipsilateral ischemic area. No staining cells were detected in the sample treated without each primary antibody as negative control (data not shown). There was no leukocyte infiltration except for around the needle track in one vehicle treated rat, and traumatic injury was observed only around the needle track (data not shown).

Discussion

We demonstrated that Ad-GDNF used in this study had ability to infect 293 cells and produce 20 kDa GDNF in vitro (data not shown). The culture supernatant from 293 cells infected by Ad-GDNF induced the neurite growth and the survival of cultured dopaminergic neurons in primary neuronal culture (data not shown). Therefore, Ad-GDNF could produce biologically active GDNF protein. Adenovirus or adeno-associated virus-mediated GDNF gene transfer prevents dopaminergic neuron degeneration (Choi-Lundberg et al. 1997; Kojima et al. 1997; Mandel et al. 1997; Fan et al. 1998), and improves behavioral impairment in the rat model of Parkinson disease (Bilang-Bleuel et al. 1997; Lapchak et al. 1997). Neuroprotective activity of adenovirus mediated GDNF gene transfer against axotomy induced motoneuron death was also reported (Baumgartner and Shine 1997). However, it has not been reported if adenovirus-mediated GDNF gene transfer could protect more severe types of neuronal death such as with ischemia or stroke. In this experiment, we demonstrated that adenovirus-mediated exogenous GDNF gene clearly attenuated ischemic brain injury after transient MCAO model (Fig. 2).

Several reports have shown that adenovirus vector itself induces proteins such as inflamma-

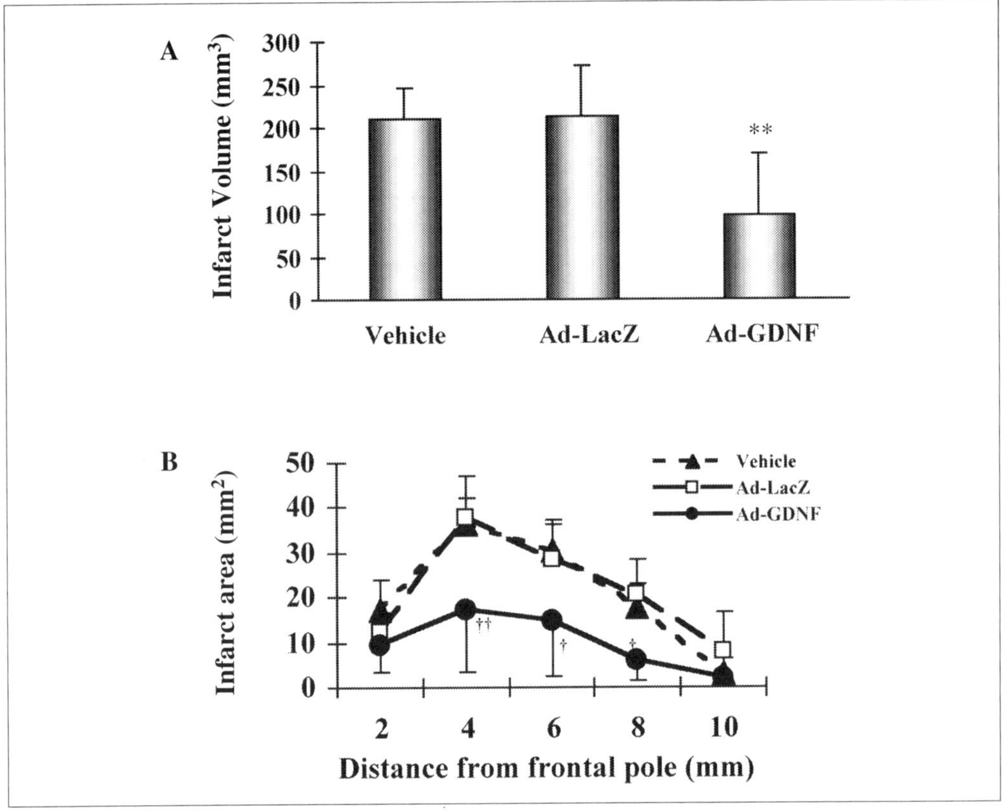

Fig. 2. Effect of Ad-GDNF on infarct volume (A) and infarct area (B) at 24 h after 90 min of transient MCAO. A; Infarct volume in the brain sections of Ad-GDNF treated group (n = 9, $^{**}p < 0.01$) was significantly smaller than that of the vehicle (n = 9) or Ad-LacZ treated group (n = 6). B; Infarct area of three coronal sections (4, 6, and 8 mm caudal from frontal pole) of Ad-GDNF (—●—) treated group ($^{**}p < 0.01$ vs vehicle group; $^{\dagger}p < 0.05$, $^{\dagger\dagger}p < 0.01$ vs Ad-LacZ group) were also significantly smaller than those of vehicle (—▲—), or Ad-LacZ (—□—) group. Data are expressed as mean ± SD. (From Kitagawa et al. 1999 with permission).

tory cytokines (Cartmell et al. 1999), adhesion molecules (Newman et al. 1995) or stress proteins (Kitagawa et al. 1998b, 1998c). There is a possibility that injection of the vector itself could influence or protect ischemic brain injury after transient MCAO. However, Ad-LacZ injection (used as a control vector) did not affect the infarction that induced after transient MCAO (Fig. 2). Therefore, the neuroprotective effect of Ad-GDNF may be due to exogenous GDNF gene product. In fact, adenovirus-mediated GDNF gene transfer into rat brain was successfully confirmed by ELISA assay or immunohistochemical study for GDNF protein (Kitagawa et al. 1999).

The protective mechanism of GDNF has not been fully understood, although previous work has demonstrated that GDNF diminished ischemia-induced nitric oxide release (Wang et al. 1997) or reduced caspase immunoreactive neurons (Kitagawa et al. 1998a). In the present study, there was no significant difference in regional cerebral blood flow (rCBF) between the vehicle, Ad-LacZ and Ad-GDNF treated group (Fig. 1), suggesting that the effect of Ad-GDNF was not associated with the improvement of

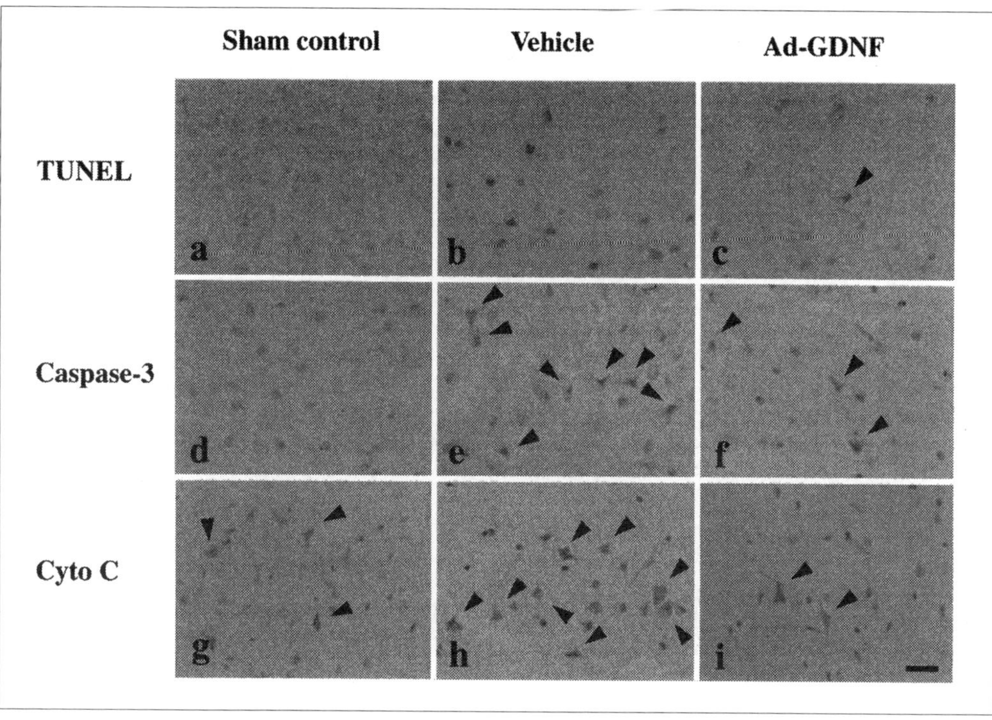

Fig. 3. Representative staining for TUNEL (a, b, c), immunoreactive caspase-3 (d, e, f), and cytochrome C (g, h, i) in the cortex at 24 h after transient MCAO. (a, d, g), Sham control; (b, e, h), the vehicle treated; (c, f, i), Ad-GDNF treated group. Note no TUNEL or caspase-3 staining cells in sham control (a, d), while large number of TUNEL (b) or caspase-3 (e, arrowheads) positive cells in the vehicle treated group. TUNEL (c, arrowhead) or caspase-3 (f, arrowheads) staining cells were markedly decreased in the Ad-GDNF treatment. Cytochrome c positive cells were detected in the lateral cortex of sham control (g, arrowheads). Large number of cytochrome c staining cells in the vehicle group (h, arrowheads), while small number in the Ad-GDNF treated group (i, arrowheads). All figures are the same magnification, x50. Bar (i): 0.04 mm. (From Kitagawa et al. 1999 with permission).

rCBF. GDNF signaling is mediated by the receptor tyrosine kinase encoded by the c-ret proto-oncogene (Ret) (Durbec et al. 1996; Trupp et al. 1996), and GFRα-1, a glycosyl-phosphatidylinositol-linked protein, assists in GDNF binding to Ret (Treanor et al. 1996; Klein et al. 1997). Distribution of Ret and GFRα-1 mRNA expressions in rat CNS was recently reported. GFRα-1 mRNA was detected in the cerebral cortex, while Ret mRNA was not seen in the normal rat brain (Trupp et al. 1997; Glazner et al. 1998). However, both GFRα-1 and Ret mRNAs were markedly induced in the pyramidal layer of the cerebral cortex 12–24 h after kainic acid treatment (Trupp et al. 1997). Therefore, GDNF/Ret/GFRα-1 interactions may also occur in the ischemic condition. Further study seems to be required to confirm that the interaction of GDNF and its receptors could be essential for its neuroprotective effect in the ischemic brain injury.

Our previous study suggested that protective effect of GDNF on ischemic brain injury was associated with the inhibition of immunoreactive caspases –1 and –3 (Kitagawa et al. 1998a). Of interest is that one of the most important pathways of neuronal death is related to mitochondrial dysfunction (Abe et al. 1995). Recently, it has been demonstrated that cytochrome c release from mitochondria to cytosol activates the caspase cascade in vitro (Kluck et al. 1997;

Table 1. Changes of TUNEL, Caspase-3 and Cytochrome c Immunoreactivities after Transient MCAO in rats

Treatment		TUNEL		Caspase-3		Cytochrome c	
		cortex	caudate	cortex	caudate	cortex	caudate
Sham control	1	–	–	–	–	+	–
	2	–	–	–	–	+	–
Vehicle	1	2+	2+	+	+	+	+
	2	+	2+	2+	2+	2+	2+
	3	2+	2+	2+	+	2+	+
Ad-GDNF	1	+	2+	+	+	+	+
	2	–	±	–	–	±	–
	3	±	+	+	+	+	+

Staining was performed at 24 h after transient MCAO, and was categorized into the following 4 grades: no staining, or a small (2-10), moderate (10–100), or large (100–500) number of stained cells into (–), (±), (+), and (2+), respectively.
Sham control, n = 2; Vehicle and Ad-GDNF treated groups, n = 3. (From Kitagawa et al. 1999 with permission).

Yang et al. 1997b). Furthermore, cytosolic redistribution of cytochrome c after transient focal cerebral ischemia in rats was demonstrated (Fujimura et al. 1998), suggesting a vital role in neuronal cell death. In the present study, both immunoreactive caspase-3 and cytochrome c were induced in the cytoplasm of neuronal cells in the penumbral cortex after transient ischemia (Fig. 3e, 3h, arrowheads), and obviously decreased in the Ad-GDNF treated group (Fig. 3f, 3i, arrowheads) with correspondence to TUNEL staining profiles (Fig. 3b, 3c). Although the TUNEL method is not specific for apoptotic neurons in the ischemic brain, the TUNEL positive neurons in the ischemic penumbral region are mainly apoptotic cells, while those in the ischemic core are necrotic (Charriaut-Marlangue et al. 1996). Therefore, some of TUNEL positive neurons observed in the present study died by apoptotic process. Thus, the apoptotic pathway via cytochrome c and caspase-3 seems to be one of the targets of protection by GDNF. In this study, we have demonstrated the change of immunoreactive caspase-3 protein after transient MCAO, but the pro- or activated form of caspase-3 has not been examined. Further study about the change of caspase-3 activity would provide us the precise information about the protective mechanism of GDNF.

Gene therapeutic study for stroke has not been tried yet in the clinical situation. Although it has been demonstrated that adenovirus-mediated neuronal apoptosis inhibitory protein (NAIP) or an interleukin-1 receptor antagonist had a protective effect against ischemic brain injury, adenoviral vectors were injected 5 days before ischemia (Betz et al. 1995; Xu et al. 1997). HSV mediated HSP72 gene transfer markedly improved striatal neuron survival in focal ischemia, but the vector was injected 8 h before occlusion (Yenari et al. 1998). In this study, adenoviral vector was also injected 24 h before MCAO, because it takes more than 8 h to express the gene product using the adenoviral vector in the normal rat brain (Abe et al. 1997b). However, gene therapy should be applied after an occurrence of stroke in the clinical situation. Therefore, therapeutic study with these vectors should be examined when delivered after ischemia. Furthermore, each vector has some disadvantages such as toxicity or efficacy of gene expression. Improvement of vectors or development of a safer vector may be necessary for more practical gene therapy. Finally, the route of administration may be of major concern for gene therapy. In the present study, we administrated the vector directly into the cerebral cortex. Of course, direct injection of the vector may not be practical in clinical application. Although intra-arterial or venous administration could be more suitable for human ischemic diseases, there may be great difficulty in how to deliver the vector specifically to the ischemic area. When these problems are successfully resolved, gene therapy could have great potential for stroke therapy in the future.

Acknowledgements

The authors would like to express their appreciation to Dr. Warita, Dr. Sakai and Dr. Sasaki for their advice and technical support. This work was partly supported by Grants-in-Aid for Scientific Research on 09470151 from the Ministry of Education, Japan.

References

1. Abe K, Aoki M, Kawagoe J, Yoshida T, Hattori A, Kogure K, Itoyama Y (1995) Ischemic delayed neuronal death: A mitochondrial hypothesis. Stroke 26:1478–1489
2. Abe K, Hayashi T, Itoyama Y (1997a) Amelioration of brain edema by topical application of glial cell line-derived neurotrophic factor in reperfused rat brain. Neurosci Lett 231:37–40
3. Abe K, Setoguchi Y, Hayashi T, Itoyama Y (1997b) In vivo adenovirus-mediated gene transfer and the expression in ischemic and reperfused rat brain. Brain Res 763:191–201
4. Abe K, Setoguchi Y, Hayashi T, Itoyama Y (1997c) Dissociative expression of adenoviral-mediated *E. coli* LacZ gene between ischemic and reperfused rat brains. Neurosci Lett 226:53–56
5. Bajocchi G, Feldman SH, Crystal RG, Mastrangeli A (1993) Direct in vivo gene transfer to ependymal cells in the central nervous system using recombinant adenovirus vectors. Nat Genet 3:229–234
6. Baumgartner BJ, Shine HD (1997) Targeted transduction of CNS neurons with adenoviral vectors carrying neurotrophic factor genes confers neuroprotection that exceeds the transduced population. J Neurosci 17:6504–6511
7. Beck KD, Valverde J, Alexi T, Poulsen K, Moffat B, Vandlen RA, Rosenthal A, Hefti F (1995) Mesencephalic dopaminergic neurons protected by GDNF from axotomy- induced degeneration in the adult brain. Nature 373:339–341
8. Bederson JB, Pitts LH, Germano SM, Nishimura MC, Davis RL, Bartkowski HM (1986) Evaluation of 2, 3, 5-triphenyltetrazolium chloride as a stain for detection and quantification of experimental cerebral infarction in rats. Stroke 17:1304–1308
9. Betz AL, Yang G-Y, Davidson BL (1995) Attenuation of stroke size in rats using an adenoviral vector to induce overexpression of interleukin-1 receptor antagonist in brain. J Cereb Blood Flow Metab 15:547–551
10. Bilang-Bleuel A, Revah F, Colin P, Locquet I, Robert J-J, Mallet J, Horellou P (1997) Intrastriatal injection of an adenoviral vector expressing glial-cell-line-derived neurotrophic factor prevents dopaminergic neuron degeneration and behavioral impairment in a rat model of Parkinson disease. Proc Natl Acad Sci USA 94:8818–8823
11. Cartmell T, Southgate T, Rees GS, Castro MG, Lowenstein PR, Luheshi GN (1999) Interleukin-1 mediates a rapid inflammatory response after injection of adenovirus vectors into the brain. J Neurosci 19:1517–1523
12. Charriaut-Marlangue C, Margaill A, Represa T, Popovici T, Plotkine M, Ben-Ari Y (1996) Apoptosis and necrosis after reversible focal ischemia: an in situ DNA fragmentation analysis. J Cereb Blood Flow Metab 16:186–194
13. Choi-Lundberg DL, Lin Q, Chang Y-N, Chiang YL, Hay CM, Mohajeri H, Davidson BL, Bohn MC (1997) Dopaminergic neurons protected from degeneration by GDNF gene therapy. Science 275:838–841
14. Durbec P, Marcos-Gutierrez CV, Kilkenny C, Grigoriou M, Wartiowaara K, Suvanto P, Smith D, Ponder B, Costantini F, Saarma M, Sariola H, Pachnis V (1996) GDNF signalling through the Ret receptor tyrosine kinase. Nature 381:789–793
15. Fan D-S, Ogawa M, Ikeguchi K, Fujimoto K, Urabe M, Kume A, Nishizawa M, Matsushita N, Kiuchi K, Ichinose H, Nagatsu T, Kurtzman GJ, Nakano I, Ozawa K (1998) Prevention of dopaminergic neuron death by adeno-associated virus vector-mediated GDNF gene transfer in rat mesencephalic cells in vitro. Neurosci Lett 248:61–64
16. Fujimura M, Morita-Fujimura Y, Murakami K, Kawase M, Chan PH (1998) Cytosolic redistribution of cytochrome c after transient focal cerebral ischemia in rats. J Cereb Blood Flow Metab 18:1239–1247
17. Glazner GW, Mu X, Springer JE (1998) Localization of glial cell line-derived neurotrophic factor receptor alpha and c-ret mRNA in rat central nervous system. J Comp Neurol 391:42–49
18. Heistad DD, Faraci FM (1996) Gene therapy for cerebral vascular disease. Stroke 27:1688–1693
19. Henderson CE, Phillips HS, Pollock RA, Davies AM, Lemeulle C, Armanini M, Simpson LC, Moffet B, Vandlen RA, Koliatsos VE, Rosenthal A (1994) GDNF: a potent survival factor for motoneurons present in peripheral nerve and muscle. Science 266:1062–1064
20. Kitagawa H, Hayashi T, Mitsumoto Y, Koga N, Itoyama Y, Abe K (1998a) Reduction of ischemic brain injury by topical application of glial cell line-derived neurotrophic factor after permanent middle cerebral artery occlusion in rats. Stroke 29:1417–1422
21. Kitagawa H, Setoguchi Y, Fukuchi Y, Mitsumoto Y, Koga N, Mori T, Abe K (1998b) Induction of DNA fragmentation and HSP72 immunoreactivity by adenovirus-mediated gene transfer in normal gerbil hippocampus and ventricle. J Neurosci Res 54:38–45
22. Kitagawa H, Setoguchi Y, Fukuchi Y, Mitsumoto Y, Koga N, Mori T, Abe K (1998c) DNA fragmentation and HSP72 gene expression by adenovirus-mediated gene transfer in postischemic gerbil hippocampus and ventricle. Metab Brain Dis 13:211–223
23. Kitagawa H, Sasaki C, Sakai K, Mori A, Mitsumoto Y, Mori T, Fukuchi Y, Setoguchi Y, Abe K (1999) Adenovirus-mediated gene transfer of glial cell line-derived neurotrophic factor prevents ischemic brain injury after transient middle cerebral artery occlusion in rats. J Cereb Blood Flow Metab 19:1336–1344
24. Klein RD, Sherman D, Ho W-H, Stone D, Bennett GL, Moffat B, Vandlen R, Simmons L, Gu Q, Hongo J-A, Devaux B, Poulsen K, Armanini M, Nozaki C, Asai N, Goddard A, Phillips H, Henderson CE, Takahashi M, Rosenthal A (1997) A GPI-linked protein that interacts with Ret to form a candidate neurturin receptor. Nature 387:717–721
25. Kluck RM, Bossy-Wetzel E, Green DR, Newmeyer DD (1997) The release of cytochrome c from mitochondria: a primary site for bcl-2 regulation of apoptosis. Science 275:1132–1136

26. Kojima H, Abiru Y, Sakajiri K, Watabe K, Ohishi N, Takamori M, Hatanaka H, Yagi K (1997) Adenovirus-mediated transduction with human glial cell-derived neurotrophic factor gene prevents 1-methyl-4-phenyl-1,2,3,6-tetrahydro pyridine-induced dopamine depletion in striatum of mouse brain. Biochem Biophys Res Commun 238:569–573
27. Lapchak PA, Araujo DM, Hilt DC, Sheng J, Jiao S (1997) Adenoviral vector-mediated GDNF gene therapy in a rodent lesion model of late stage Parkinson's disease. Brain Res 777:153–160
28. Lawrence MS, McLaughlin JR, Sun G-H, Ho DY, McIntosh L, Kunis DM, Sapolsky RM, Steinberg GK (1997) Herpes simplex viral vectors expressing bcl-2 are neuroprotective when delivered after a stroke. J Cereb Blood Flow Metab 17:740–744
29. Li L, Wu W, Lin L-FH, Lei M, Oppenheim RW, Houenou LJ (1995) Rescue of adult mouse motoneurons from injury-induced cell death by glial cell line-derived neurotrophic factor. Proc Natl Acad Sci USA 92:9771–9775
30. Lin L-FH, Doherty DH, Lile JD, Bektesh S, Collins F (1993) GDNF: a glial cell line-derived neurotrophic factor for midbrain dopaminergic neurons. Science 260:1130–1132
31. Linnik MD, Zahos P, Geschwind MD, Federoff HJ (1995) Expression of bcl-2 from a defective herpes simplex virus-1 vector limits neuronal death in focal cerebral ischemia. Stroke 26:1670–1675
32. Mandel RJ, Spratt SK, Snyder RO, Leff SE (1997) Midbrain injection of recombinant adeno-associated virus encoding rat glial cell line-derived neurotrophic factor protects nigral neurons in a progressive 6-hydroxydopamine-induced degeneration model of Parkinson's disease in rats. Proc Natl Acad Sci USA 94:14083–14088
33. Nabel EG (1995) Gene therapy for cardiovascular disease. Circulation 91:541–548
34. Newman KD, Dunn PF, Owens JW, Schulick AH, Virmani R, Sukhova G, Libby P, Dichek DA (1995) Adenovirus-mediated gene transfer into normal rabbit arteries results in prolonged vascular cell activation, inflammation, and neointimal hyperplasia. J Clin Invest 96:2955–2965
35. Setoguchi Y, Danel C, Crystal RG (1994) Stimulation of erythropoiesis by in vivo gene therapy: Physiologic consequences of transfer of the human erythropoietin gene to experimental animals using an adenovirus vector. Blood 84:2946–2953
36. Tomac A, Lindqvist E, Lin L-FH, Ögren SO, Young D, Hoffer BJ, Olson L (1995) Protection and repair of the nigrostriatal dopaminergic system by GDNF in vivo. Nature 373:335–339
37. Treanor JJS, Goodman L, Sauvage F, Stone DM, Poulsen KT, Beck CD, Gray C, Armanini MP, Pollock RA, Hefti F, Phillips HS, Goddard A, Moore MW, Buj-Bello A, Davies AM, Asai N, Takahashi M, Vandlen R, Henderson CE, Rosenthal A (1996) Characterization of a multicomponent receptor for GDNF. Nature 382:80–83
38. Trupp M, Arenas E, Fainzilber M, Nilsson A-S, Sieber B-A, Grigoriou M, Kilkenny C, Salazar-Grueso E, Pachnis V, Arumäe U, Sariola H, Saarma M, Ibáñez CF (1996) Functional receptor for GDNF encoded by the c-ret proto-oncogene. Nature 381:785–789
39. Trupp M, Belluardo N, Funakoshi H, Ibáñez CF (1997) Complementary and overlapping expression of glial cell line-derived neurotrophic factor (GDNF), c-ret proto-oncogene, and GDNF receptor-α indicates multiple mechanisms of trophic actions in the adult rat CNS. J Neurosci 17:3554–3567
40. Verma IM, Somia N (1997) Gene therapy-promises, problems and prospects. Nature 389:239–242
41. Wang Y, Lin S-Z, Chiou A-L, Williams LR, Hoffer BJ (1997) Glial cell line-derived neurotrophic factor protects against ischemia-induced injury in the cerebral cortex. J Neurosci 17:4341–4348
42. Xu DG, Crocker SJ, Doucet J-P, St-Jean M, Tamai K, Hakim AM, Ikeda J-E, Liston P, Thompson CS, Korneluk RG, MacKenzie A, Robertson GS (1997) Elevation of neuronal expression of NAIP reduces ischemic damage in the rat hippocampus. Nat Med 3:997–1004
43. Yang G-Y, Liu X-H, Kadoya C, Zhao Y-J, Mao Y, Davidson BL, Betz AL (1998) Attenuation of ischemic inflammatory response in mouse brain using an adenoviral vector to induce overexpression of interleukin-1 receptor antagonist. J Cereb Blood Flow Metab 18:840–847
44. Yang G-Y, Zhao Y-J, Davidson BL, Betz AL (1997a) Overexpression of interleukin-1 receptor antagonist in the mouse brain reduces ischemic brain injury. Brain Res 751:181–188
45. Yang J, Liu X, Bhalla K, Kim CN, Ibrado AM, Cai J, Peng T-I, Jones DP, Wang X (1997b) Prevention of apoptosis by bcl-2: release of cytochrome c from mitochondria blocked. Science 275:1129–1132
46. Yenari MA, Fink SL, Sun GH, Chang LK, Patel MK, Kunis DM, Onley D, Ho DY, Sapolsky RM, Steinberg GK (1998) Gene therapy with HSP72 is neuroprotective in rat models of stroke and epilepsy. Ann Neurol 44:584–591

The expression pattern of TGF-β1 in rat hippocampus after transient forebrain ischemia and after stimulation of β_2-adrenoceptors

Y. Zhu, J. Krieglstein

Abstract

TGF-β1 has been suggested as a neuronal survival factor in brain tissue. In this study we examined endogenous expression of TGF-β1 in the hippocampus of non-ischemic and ischemic rats. Furthermore, TGF-β1 expression was investigated in the ischemic brain after stimulation of β_2-adrenoceptors. Transient ischemia was induced for 10 min in Wistar rats by clamping both common carotid arteries and lowering blood pressure to 40 mm Hg. Bioactive TGF-β1 was exclusively determined in CA1 pyramidal neurons of non-ischemic rats. A temporary enhanced TGF-β1 immunoreactivity (ir) was detected in the hippocampal CA1 neurons in the absence of microglia and astrocyte activation after 3 h and 6 h of reperfusion. TGF-β1 ir was further elevated in the hippocampal neurons by the β_2-adrenoceptor agonist clenbuterol, as early as 3 h and 6 h, and remained at the increased level up to 48 h after ischemia. However, clenbuterol failed to increase TGF-β1 mRNA levels in the hippocampus from 3 h to 96 h after ischemia as detected by RT-PCR. Interestingly, the ir of latent TGF-β1 binding protein-1 (LTBP-1) was enhanced in the hippocampal CA1 subfield by clenbuterol. The enhancement of LTBP-1 by clenbuterol was in parallel with the changes of TGF-β1 ir. Double staining revealed that TUNEL-positive neurons did not express TGF-β1, while TUNEL-negative neurons in the CA1 subfield exhibited a distinct TGF-β1 ir. This study indicates that hippocampal CA1 neurons can express TGF-β1 under physiological conditions and upregulate its expression during the first hours after ischemia. TGF-β1 and LTBP-1 ir in the ischemic rat hippocampus are further increased by β_2-adrenoceptor stimulation.

Introduction

The transforming growth factor-beta (TGF-β) family of cytokines regulates a diverse range of cellular responses including cell proliferation, differentiation, migration and programmed cell death (Roberts and Sporn 1993). TGF-β1 is one of the most extensively studied members of this family because of its wide distribution in various tissues and its multifunction in regulation of physiological and pathological processes (Krieglstein and Krieglstein 1998; Flanders et al. 1998). In the central nervous system (CNS), TGF-β1 is mostly expressed in neurons, astrocytes, microglia and oligodendrocytes. TGF-

Keywords: TGF-β1 ir – LTBP-1 – Hippocampal CA1 pyramidal neurons – Microglia and astrocyte – β2-adrenoceptor agonist – Transient forebrain ischemia

Institut für Pharmakologie und Toxikologie, Philipps-Universität, Ketzerbach 63, D-35032 Marburg, Germany
e-mail: zhu@mailer.uni-marburg.de

β1 has been termed as injury-associated factor since its level is elevated in brain after acute injuries, e.g., stroke, seizures, and trauma, and in chronic degenerative diseases such as Alzheimer's disease and Parkinson's disease. The exact role of TGF-β1 in neurodegenerative disorders is not fully understood. However, it has been shown that exogenous TGF-β1 can prevent neuronal death induced by different pathological stimuli in vitro (Prehn et al. 1993a; Chao et al. 1994; Krieglstein and Unsicker 1994; Prehn et al. 1996; Buisson et al. 1998; Zhu et al. 2000a) and reduce the damage of brain tissue after focal and global ischemia (Gross et al. 1993; Prehn et al. 1993b; Henrich-Noack et al. 1996). These data suggest that TGF-β1 serves as a neuronal survival factor in the CNS. The beneficial effects of TGF-β1 were suggested to be associated with its capacity to maintain mitochondrial membrane potential, regulate calcium homeostasis, modulate oncoprotein expression including Bcl-2 (Prehn et al. 1994; Tomoda et al. 1996), Bcl-xl and Bcl-xs (Kim et al. 1998), and inhibit caspase-3 activation (Zhu et al. 2000a). In addition, anti-inflammation (Finch et al. 1993) and angiogenesis (Gleizes and Rifkin 1999; Kumar-Singh et al. 1999) caused by TGF-β1 may be crucial for limiting the extent of brain damage. In light of these data, we assumed that modulation of TGF-β1 expression in brain may represent a novel strategy for treatment of ischemic injury.

Clenbuterol, a lipophilic β_2-adrenoceptor agonist, has been previously shown to prevent neuronal death induced by glutamate-excitotoxicity in cultured neurons (Semkova et al. 1994, 1996) and by focal (Culmsee et al. 1999b) or global cerebral ischemia in rats (Zhu et al. 1998). Furthermore, we have demonstrated that its neuroprotective effect was mostly mediated by the induction of the growth factor NGF (Culmsee et al. 1999a; Zhu and Krieglstein 1999a).

In the present study, we attempted to examine the endogenous expression of bioactive TGF-β1 in the vulnerable hippocampus after transient forebrain ischemia in rats. Furthermore, we tested whether stimulation of β_2-adrenoceptors can influence TGF-β1 expression in ischemic hippocampus.

1. Expression of TGF-β1 mRNA and protein in the hippocampus after ischemia

The TGF-β1 ir was exclusively detected in the hippocampal CA1 subfield of non-ischemic brains and no significant TGF-β1 signal was found in other regions of hippocampus, e.g., CA3 and dentate gyrus (Fig. 1A). At high resolution, the TGF-β1 signal in the CA1 subfield could be located to the cytoplasm of pyramidal cells and was absent in the nuclei (Fig. 1B). To confirm the neuronal location of TGF-β1 under physiological conditions, the sections were double stained with TGF-β1 and the neuronal marker NeuN. The result revealed that the pyramidal cells were double labelled by TGF-β1 and NeuN.

In most of the cells, TGF-β1 is stored and secreted as a biological inactive complex (latent form) (Pircher et al. 1986; Miyazono et al. 1988,

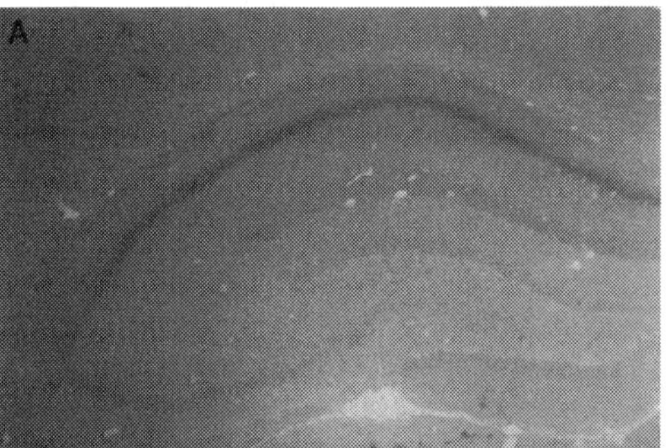

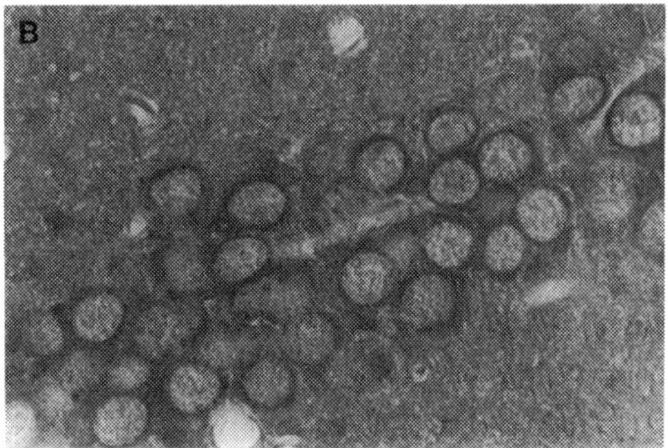

Fig. 1. The localization of TGF-β1 ir in the hippocampus. TGF-β1 ir was selectively localized in the hippocampal CA1 pyramidal neurons of non-ischemic rat (A). High power view of hippocampal CA1 subfield revealed cytoplasm location of TGF-β1 (B).

1989) which contains a latency associated peptide (LAP, ~75 kDa) and the TGF-β1 peptide (25 kDa). The latter can be generated from a latent form of TGF-β1 and possesses bioactivity (Lyons et al. 1990). To examine whether the antibody specifically recognizes the active form of TGF-β1, we compared the immunostaining pattern of TGF-β1 with that of LAP. Immunostaining showed a diffuse distribution of LAP and latent TGF-β1 in the matrix, the intracellular cytoplasm and the nuclear of the neurons in the hippocampal regions. This expression pattern is quite different from the distribution of TGF-β1 ir described before. Thus, we suggest that TGF-β1 ir detected in the hippocampal CA1 subfield is bioactive TGF-β1.

The mechanisms of TGF-β1 activation in vivo are still unclear. It has been shown in vitro that the latent TGF-β1 could be activated by acidification (Wakefield et al. 1987), proteolytic enzymes (Lyons et al. 1990), removal of carbohydrates from TGF-β1 (Miyazono and Heldin 1989) or in the presence of thrombospondin (Schultz-Cherry and Murphy-Ullrich 1993). The selective expression of TGF-β1 protein in the CA1 subfield implies special pathways for activation of TGF-β1 from the latent TGF-β1 complex.

We have previously described that neuronal apoptosis is induced in the hippocampal CA1 subfield in a rat model of transient forebrain ischemia (Zhu et al. 1998) involving upregulation of apoptosis-associated oncoproteins Bcl-2, Bcl-xl and Bax (Zhu et al. 1999b). To reveal the progressive changes of TGF-β1 expression in this vulnerable region, immunostaining and RT-PCR were used to detect TGF-β1 protein and mRNA, respectively, after ischemia.

Forebrain ischemia was induced in adult Wistar rats for 10 min by clamping both common carotid arteries and lowering the mean arterial blood pressure to 40 mm Hg by trimethaphan-camsylate (5 mg/kg, i.v.) and central venous exsanguination. The clips were removed after 10 min and the blood which had been withdrawn was rapidly re-injected. The paraffin brain sections were prepared at defined time points after onset of ischemia. TGF-β1 ir was enhanced in the CA1 region as early as 3 h and 6 h after ischemia and it returned to the basal level after 24 h of reperfusion. With the procession of neuronal damage through 2 d to 4 d after ischemia, TGF-β1 ir persisted in the morphological intact neurons, but disappeared in damaged neurons (Fig. 2, left column). As described in our previous study (Zhu et al. 1998), delayed neuronal death occurred in the hippocampal CA1 subfield 2d after ischemia. This allowed us to detect a temporary upregulation of TGF-β1 protein in CA1 region before neurons underwent damage. The transiently increased TGF-β1 ir observed at 3 h and 6 h after ischemia might be an early response of neurons to ischemic injury and may imply a role of TGF-β1 in delayed cell death after ischemic injury. The reduced TGF-β1 ir 1 d after ischemia represented the gradual exhaustion of latent TGF-β1 while new protein synthesis was limited by the impaired neuronal function. The final loss of TGF-β1 immunoreaction in damaged neurons may be caused by increased proteolysis or complete loss of the ability to synthesize new proteins in neurons.

To compare the changes of TGF-β1 ir with those of mRNA levels, TGF-β1 mRNA was detected by RT-PCR. TGF-β1 mRNA was found in the non-ischemic hippocampus (Fig. 3). It was upregulated as early as 3 h, as well as 6 h, 24 h, 48 h, and significantly increased at 96 h after ischemia. Semi-quantitative analysis showed that the intensity of TGF-β1 mRNA signals was enhanced to 155%, 148%, 148%, 123% and 166% ($p < 0.05$) of the basal level at 3 h, 6 h 24 h, 48 h and 96 h after ischemia, respectively (Fig. 3). According to this time course, we propose that the induction of TGF-β1 protein at 3 h and 6 h after ischemia could be the result of increased transcription, since it has been suggested that the injury-mediated upregulation of TGF-β1 may be a result of early activation of c-*fos* and c-*jun* transcription factors (Roberts et al. 1993). On the other hand, it is also possible that ischemia itself mediates activation of latent TGF-β1 complex in the neurons. The continuously upregulated TGF-β1 mRNA level up to 96 h after ischemia may be caused by ischemia-induced activation of glial cells.

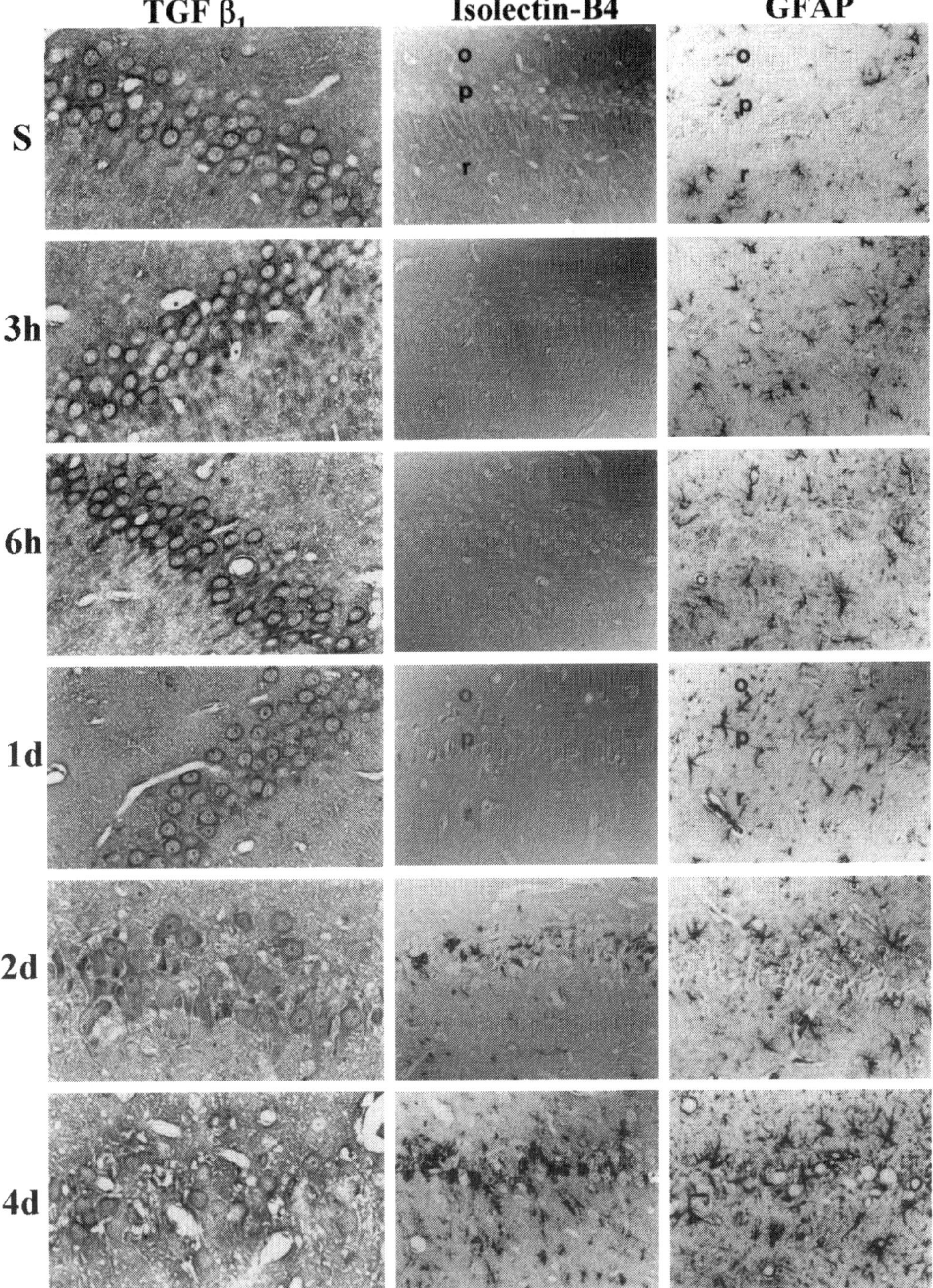

TGF β_1
Isolectin-B4
GFAP
S
3h
6h
1d
2d
4d
o
p
r
o
p
r
o
p
r
o
p
r

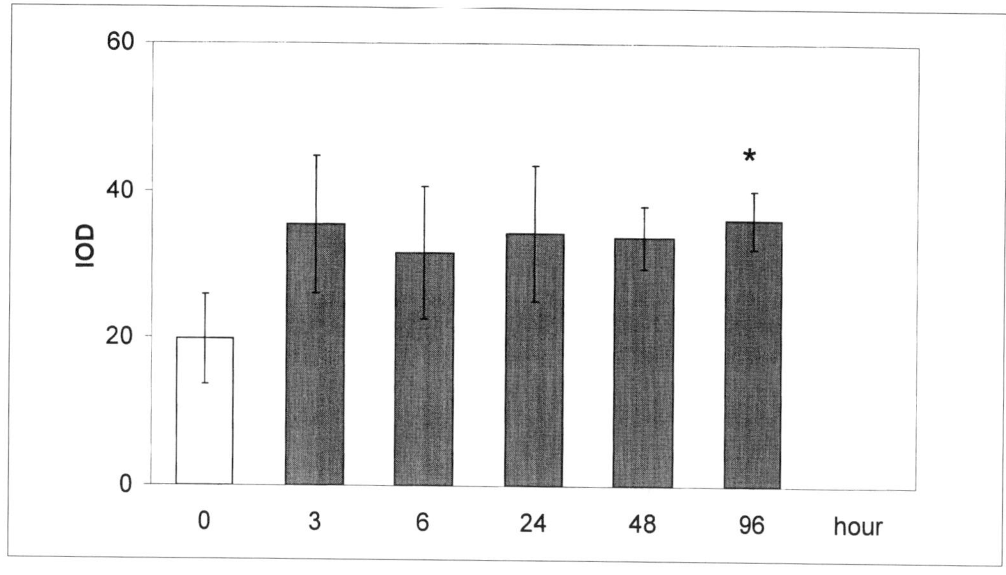

Fig. 3. The expression of TGF-β1 mRNA in the hippocampus after transient forebrain ischemia. Total RNA was extracted from the non-ischemic hippocampus (0 h), and 3 h, 6 h, 24 h, 48 h and 96 h after ischemia. TGF-β1 mRNA was measured by RT-PCR. Semi-quantification of the intensity of TGF-β1 signals revealed that an enhanced TGF-β1 signal appeared as early as 3 h and was significantly elevated at 4d after ischemia. * $p < 0.05$, compared with non-ischemic hippocampus (0 h) (Student *t* test). IOD: integrated optical density.

We have not yet directly proven what the physiological and pathological meaning of the selective expression of TGF-β1 protein in the vulnerable CA1 subfield is, and whether the loss of TGF-β1 ir in neurons results in neuronal damage. However, our previous study demonstrated neuroprotection by exogenous TGF-β1 in vitro (Prehn et al. 1993a, 1993b, 1996; Zhu et al. 2000a) as well as in vivo (Henrich-Noack et al. 1996). Similar results were reported by others (Gross et al. 1993; McNeill 1994). Therefore we suggest that such selective expression of TGF-β1 protein in the hippocampal CA1 subfield under physiological conditions and the injury-mediated early upregulation of TGF-β1 protein may play a role in the pathology of delayed neuronal death after ischemia. Although the expression of TGF-β1 protein was preserved in viable and disappeared in damaged neurons, the responsibility of TGF-β1 for neuronal survival is not proven but seems to be likely.

2. The time course of glial cell activation in the ischemic hippocampus: Comparison with TGF-β1 ir location

It has been shown that the neuronal damage induced by transient forebrain ischemia is accompanied with microglia and astrocyte activa-

Fig. 2. Comparison of the time course of TGF-β1 protein expression with that of glial cell activation in the hippocampal CA1 subfield after ischemia. Left column: time course of TGF-β1 ir in the CA1 subfield of sham-operated rat (S), and 3 h, 6 h, 1 d, 2 d and 4 d after ischemia. Middle and right columns: representation of the time courses of microglia and astrocyte activation by isolectin-B4 labelling and GFAP-immunostaining, respectively. (o): stratum oriens; (p): pyramidal cell layer; (r): stratum radiatum. (Fig. see page 388)

tion (Braun et al. 1998; Lin et al. 1998). Furthermore, the activated glial cells and brain macrophages have been suggested to be the major source of TGF-β1 (Wießner et al. 1993; Lehrmann et al. 1995; Knuckey et al. 1996). To identify whether the expression of TGF-β1 in neurons was dependent on activation of glial cells, we compared, within corresponding sections, the pattern obtained by TGF-β1 immunostaining with that of isolectin-B4 staining (microglia) and immunostaining for GFAP (astrocytes).

The microglial activation was not detectable in the hippocampus 3 h, 6 h and 1 d after ischemia, and first visible 2 d after ischemia. The staining became stronger in all pyramidal layers after 4 d of reperfusion (Fig. 2, middle column). A similar time course of astrocyte activation was revealed by GFAP staining (Fig. 2, right column). Astroglial processes were slightly visible in the pyramidal cell layer surrounding the neuronal cell bodies by 1 d after ischemia. Two days after ischemia the changes in astroglial morphology and GFAP enhancement became evident. The strongest GFAP staining was observed 4 d after ischemia and activated astrocytes entered the pyramidal cell layer.

As described above, TGF-β1 ir was exclusively detected in the CA1 neurons in the non-ischemic and sham-operated hippocampal CA1 pyramidal layers, and furthermore, it was enhanced 3 h and 6 h after ischemia. This expression is actually detected in the absence of evident microglia and astrocyte activation, suggesting that the CA1 pyramidal neurons are able to synthesize and activate TGF-β1. Neuronal synthesis and activation of TGF-β1 supports the hypothesis that TGF-β1 may act as a neuroprotectant in an autocrine manner (Chalazonitis et al. 1992; Finch et al. 1993; Krieglstein and Unsicker 1994; Krieglstein and Krieglstein 1998).

It has been noted that the star-shaped cells showing TGF-β1-positive staining were scattered in pyramidal layers, as well as in stratum oriens and stratum radiatum of the CA1 subfield 4 d after ischemia. These TGF-β1-positive, non-neuronal cells may represent activated glial cells which have been shown to be capable of expressing TGF-β1 (Wießner et al. 1993; Lehrmann et al. 1995). The persistent expression of TGF-β1 in viable neurons after long periods of reperfusion may suggest that these viable neurons still have the ability to synthesize TGF-β1, and, in addition, they may take up TGF-β1 secreted by activated glial cells.

3. The role of TGF-β1 in neuronal apoptosis

The role of TGF-β1 in apoptosis has been widely studied in non-neuronal cells and seems to be extremely dependent on the cell type, the pathological stimuli and the experimental conditions (Bechtner et al. 1999; Kuo et al. 1997). However, there were only few data showing the effect of TGF-β1 on neuronal apoptosis. We have previously demonstrated delayed neuronal death and apoptosis in the hippocampal CA1 subfield after transient forebrain ischemia (Zhu et al. 1998). Furthermore, a potential neuroprotection of exogenous TGF-β1 has been shown in the hippocampus after transient forebrain ischemia (Henrich-Noack et al. 1996). In this study we have especially chosen the brain sections from 2 d after transient forebrain ischemia to perform double-staining of TGF-β1 and DNA fragments, where the neuronal damage just started and exhibited typically apoptotic morphology (Zhu et al. 2000b). The result revealed that TGF-β1 ir was selectively localised in the hippocampal CA1 TUNEL-negative neurons, while TUNEL-positive neurons did no longer express TGF-β1, suggesting that the endogenous TGF-β1 may play a role in prevention of DNA fragmentation after ischemic insult. This hypothesis could be supported by the recent evidence that TGF-β1 inhibits caspase-3 activation and reduces the neuronal apoptosis induced by staurosporine in the primary rat hippocampal cultures (Zhu et al. 2000a). The mechanism how TGF-β1 inhibits neuronal apoptosis is not completely clear. However, it is well known that cytochrome c is an essential component of apoptosome which activates caspase-3. Bcl-2 can prevent mitochondrial release of cytochrome c and thereby inhibit activation of caspase-3. TGF-β1 was previously reported to upregulate Bcl-2 expression in cultured hippocampal cells (Prehn et al. 1994). Based on these data, we propose that the inhibition of caspase-3 activity by TGF-β1 is mediated through the upregulation of Bcl-2. Furthermore, Bcl-2 was also found to be a substrate of caspase-3. Thus, upon inhibiting caspase-3 activation, the cleavage of Bcl-2 by caspase-3 could in turn be attenuated. In view of this point, reduced activation of caspase-3 by TGF-β1 may contribute to upregulation of Bcl-2 expression. This loop would be an important mechanism for TGF-β1 to antagonize neuronal apoptosis.

4. Clenbuterol enhances TGF-β1 ir in the hippocampus without influencing TGF-β1 mRNA expression

It has been previously shown that administration of TGF-β1 protected brain tissue against ischemic damage (Gross et al. 1993; Prehn et al. 1993a; Henrich-Noack et al. 1996). Pang et al. (1999) recently reported that overexpression of TGF-β1 in mouse brain diminished the infarct volume after transient focal cerebral ischemia. Moreover, neutralisation of endogenous TGF-β1 in rat brain accelerated brain damage following excitotoxic or ischemic injury (Ruocco et al. 1999). Therefore, it is conceivable that an increase in TGF-β1 level in brain tissue may support the neuronal survival after ischemic injury.

As mentioned before, the bioactive TGF-β1 level is elevated in the hippocampal CA1 subfield during 3–6 h after transient forebrain ischemia (Zhu et al. 2000b). The temporary increase in bioactive TGF-β1 expression may function as an endogenous defensive mechanism to minimise the extent of ischemic injury. However, it did not seem to be sufficient to prevent the massive damage caused by ischemia. We assume that the TGF-β1 level in ischemic brain tissue can be enhanced by pharmacological intervention, thereby protecting neurons against ischemic damage. In this study, we attempted to test whether stimulation of β_2-adrenoceptors might influence TGF-β1 expression after transient forebrain ischemia.

Clenbuterol at the dosage of 0.5 mg/kg showed a significant neuroprotective effect in rats accompanied by an increase in the NGF protein (Zhu et al. 1998) and Bcl-2 protein levels (Zhu et al. 1999b) in the hippocampus following transient forebrain ischemia. The same treatment was applied to the rats in the present study, i.e., clenbuterol (0.5 mg/kg) or saline was intraperitoneally administered to rats 3 h before onset of transient forebrain ischemia. For immunochemistry study, the paraffin brain section were prepared 3 h, 6 h, 24 h and 48 h after ischemia.

TGF-β1 ir temporarily increased 3 h and 6 h after ischemia (Fig. 4C and E). It returned to the basal level 1d (Fig. 4G) and further decreased 2d after ischemia (Fig. 4I). Comparably, clenbuterol markedly enhanced TGF-β1 ir after 3 h and 6 h as well as 24 h of reperfusion (Fig. 4D, F and H). Furthermore, clenbuterol considerably elevated and maintained the TGF-β1 protein level up to 2d after ischemia (Fig. 4J). In the hippocampus of clenbuterol-treated rats, increased TGF-β1 ir was detected in the cell bodies, in the dendrites of the neurons, as well as in the extracellular space around the cell bodies. Notably, these pyramidal cells still kept intact morphology up to 2 d of reperfusion (Fig. 4J), whereas neurons in the hippocampal CA1 subfield of saline-treated controls became damaged at this time point (Fig. 4I). These data suggest that TGF-β1 in ischemic hippocampus elevated by clenbuterol may contribute to its neuroprotective effect.

To evaluate the influence of clenbuterol on TGF-β1 mRNA expression, RT-PCR was performed 3 h, 6 h, 24 h, 48 h and 96 h after ischemia. Surprisingly, the expression of TGF-β1 mRNA in the hippocampus was not changed by clenbuterol from 3 h to 96 h after ischemia. The semi-quantification of the TGF-β1 mRNA signals revealed no significant difference between clenbuterol-treated and saline-treated rats at all defined time points.

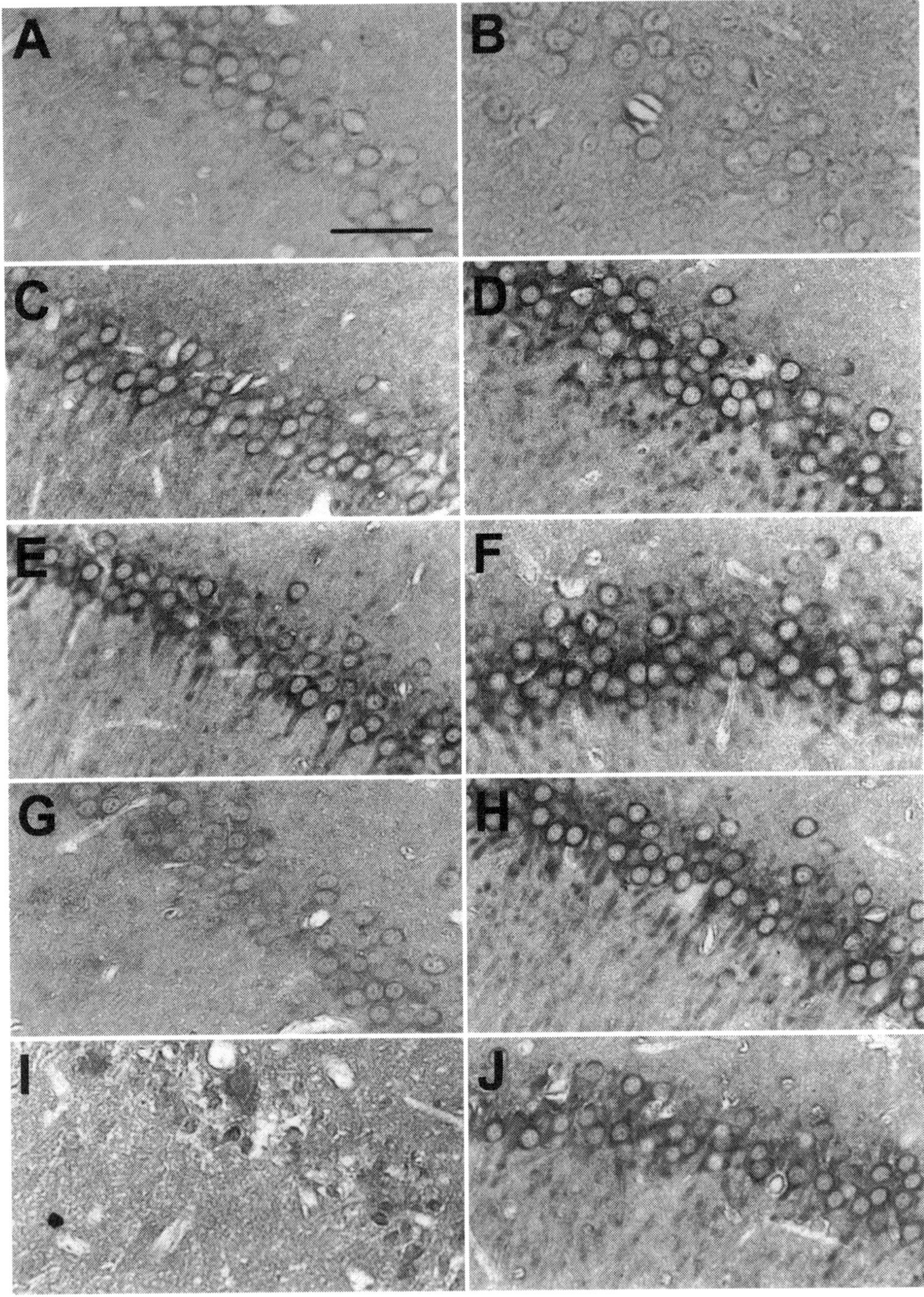
A
B
C
D
E
F
G
H
I
J

These results indicate that clenbuterol increases TGF-β1 expression at the post-transcription or post-translation level. Post-translational modulation of TGF-β1 expression, e.g., acceleration of the activation step, might be a more efficient way to increase the amount of bioactive TGF-β1, because the level of bioactive TGF-β1 mainly depends on the secretion and activation steps. TGF-β protein expression independent of its de novo synthesis has also been previously reported in hepatic parenchymal cells (Roth et al. 1998).

5. Clenbuterol increases the expression of LTBP-1 in the hippocampus after ischemia

LTBPs are multidomain glycoproteins with a molecular weight ranging from 125 to 240 kDa. Four LTBP genes (LTBP-1, -2, -3, -4) have been identified (Kanzaki et al. 1990; Morén et al. 1994; Yin et al. 1995; Saharinen et al. 1998), and all appear capable of forming a complex with TGF-β1. In addition, they may also occur in a free, uncomplexed form (Morén et al. 1994). LTBP-1 is the best characterized isoform of the LTBP family. Beside its function as a structural matrix protein (Dallas et al. 1995), it may facilitate the secretion of latent TGF-β1 from producer cells (Miyazono et al. 1991), and target the latent TGF-β1 to the extracellular matrix, thereby regulating the availability of the bioactive TGF-β1 (Managasser-Stephan and Gressner 1999). LTBP-1 has also been suggested to be involved in TGF-β1 activation processes (Flaumenhaft et al. 1993; Nunes et al.1997; Sinha et al. 1998). Abundant evidence confirms that the association of LTBP-1 with TGF-β1 is a crucial determinant of TGF-β1 activity. Based on these data, we asked whether TGF-β1 could modulate LTBP-1 expression, and thereby increase the TGF-β1 protein level in the hippocampus.

To this end, we first examined the expression of this protein in sham-operated and ischemic hippocampus of the rats either treated with clenbuterol (0.5 mg/kg, i.p.) or saline. Immunostaining of LTBP-1 was performed on the adjacent brain sections which were immunostained with TGF-β1. LTBP-1 immunosignals were located in the pyramidal cell bodies, dendrites as well as the extracellular compartments in the hippocampal CA1 region of sham-operated rats (Fig. 5A). The control did not show detectable signals (Fig. 5B). Double-staining of LTBP-1 and NeuN revealed that LTBP-1 expressing cells in the hippocampus were also stained with the neuronal marker, NeuN, indicating that LTBP-1 ir was located in the neurons.

The LTBP-1 protein level moderately increased in the hippocampus 3 h (Fig. 5C) and 6 h (Fig. 5E) after ischemia, and it returned to the basal level 24 h after ischemia (Fig. 5G). With the progressive neuronal damage 48 h after ischemia, LTBP-1 ir was further decreased, and finally disappeared in the damaged cells (Fig. 5I). In clenbuterol-treated rats, LTBP-1 ir was gradually enhanced in the hippocampus from 3 h to 24 h after ischemia (Fig. 5D, F and H). A massive increase in LTBP-1 ir was observed in the clenbuterol-treated hippocampus after 48 h of reperfusion (Fig. 5J). Evaluation of the brain sections at low magnification revealed that the enhanced LTBP-1 ir was present in the hippocampal CA1 subfield as well as in the region of the cingulum (Fig. 5L).

The effect of clenbuterol on LTBP-1 expression in the hippocampus was confirmed by Western blotting. LTBP-1 protein level was enhanced 6 h and returned to control level 24 h after transient forebrain ischemia. Clenbuterol

Fig. 4. Clenbuterol upregulates TGF-β1 ir in the hippocampal CA1 subfield after transient forebrain ischemia. Clenbuterol (0.5 mg/kg) or saline were administered (i.p.) to the rats 3 h prior to ischemia. Immunostaining of TGF-β1 was performed on the sections prepared 6 h after sham-operation (A), and 3 h (C and D), 6 h (E and F), 1 d (G and H) and 2 d (I and J) after ischemia. C, E, G and I: saline-treated control; D, F, H and J: clenbuterol-treated rats. B: control of immunostaining. Scale bar = 50 μm. (Fig. see page 392)

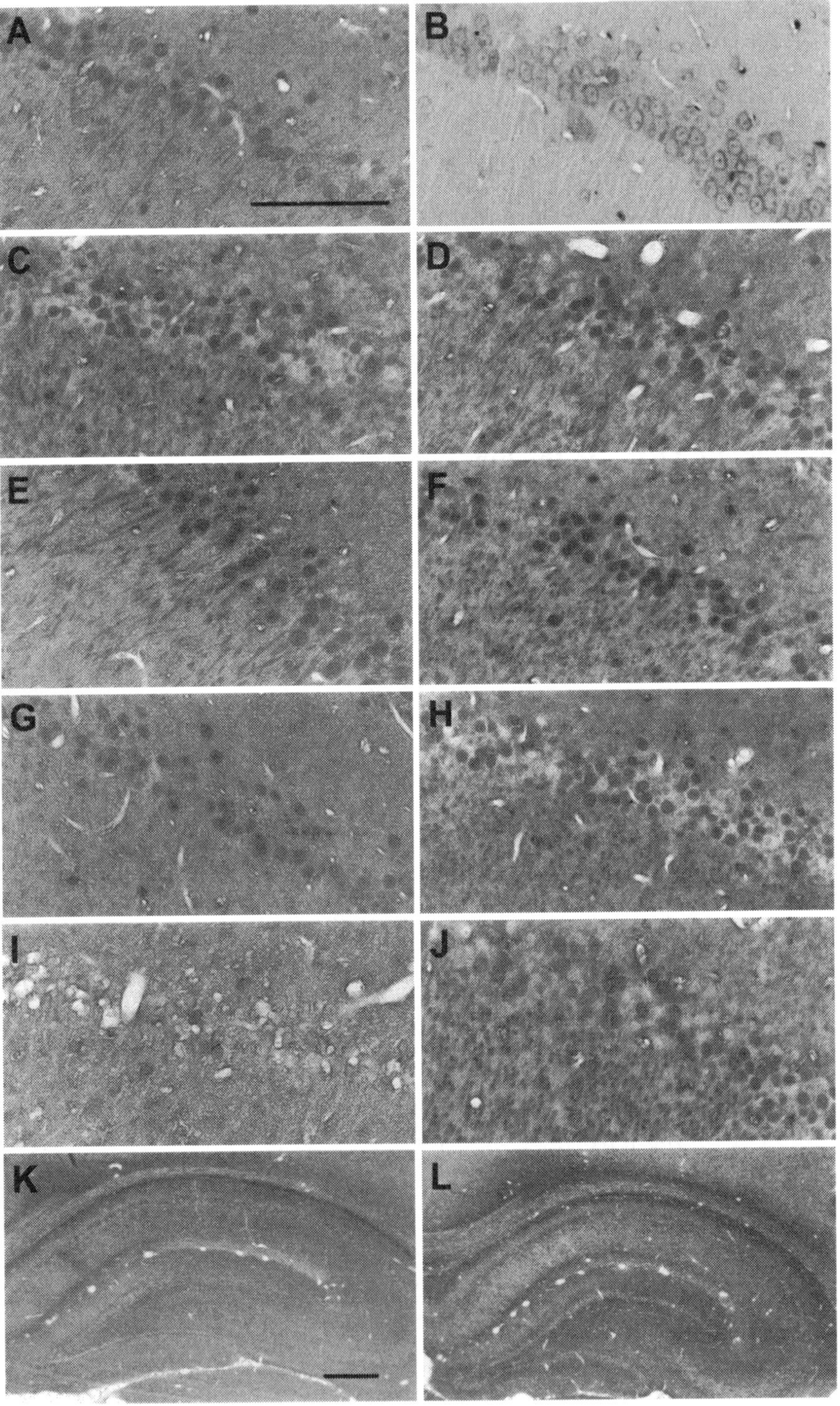
A
B
C
D
E
F
G
H
I
J
K
L

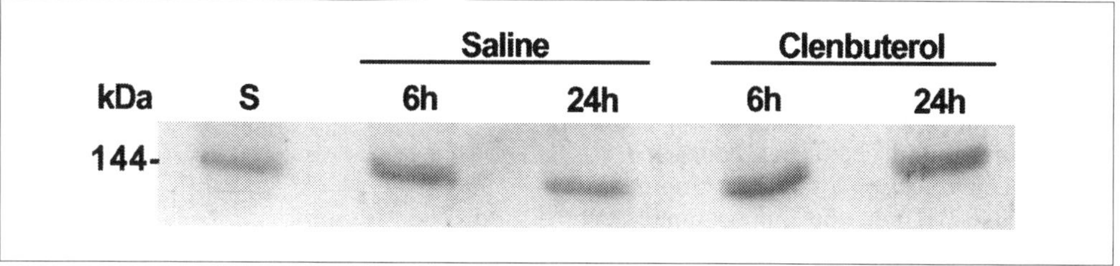

Fig. 6. Western blotting analysis of LTBP. Clenbuterol (0.5 mg/kg) or saline were administered (i.p.) to the rats 3 h prior to ischemia. The total protein was extracted from hippocampus 6 h and 24 h after ischemia and 6 h after sham-operation (S).

further increased LTBP-1 expression 6 h and maintained LTBP-1 expression at the elevated level up to 48 h of reperfusion (Fig. 6).

Comparing the effect of clenbuterol on TGF-β1 with that on LTBP-1, it has been noted that the increase in LTBP-1 expression correlates with the increase in TGF-β1 expression in the hippocampus either after ischemia or after clenbuterol treatment. More interestingly, the TGF-β1 ir in sham-operated and in saline-treated controls was mostly located in the pyramidal cytoplasm (Fig. 4A, C, E, G and I), while TGF-β1 ir in clenbuterol-treated hippocampus intensively appeared in both cytoplasm and the extracellular side of the pyramidal neurons (Fig. 4D, F, H, and J), suggesting an increased amount of available TGF-β1 protein around the cell surface after clenbuterol treatment. LTBP-1 may regulate TGF-β1 bioactivity by associating intracellularly with small latent TGF-β1 and facilitating efficient secretion, and subsequently sequestrate latent TGF-β1 to the extracellular matrix. Although the processes for activation of TGF-β1 are not well understood, LTBP-1 is suggested to play a role in the release and activation of TGF-β1 from the latent complex (Miyazono et al. 1991; Flaumenhaft et al. 1993; Nunes et al. 1997; Sinha et al. 1998; Managasser-Stephan and Gressner 1999). Therefore, we suggest that the LTBP-1 level enhanced by clenbuterol contributes to the increase in bioactive TGF-β1 expression in the hippocampal neurons.

Because of the multifunction of LTBPs and TGF-β1 the regulation of their expression is of particular interest and significance for therapeutic intervention. Krohn (1999) recently found that TGF-β1 may upregulate rat LTBP-2 homolog mRNA in C6 and cortical astrocytes, and cause self-activation and exaggeration of TGF-β signalling. Similarly, TGF-β1 was able to elevate the transcription of LTBP-1 and -2 (Dallas et al. 1994; Ahmed et al. 1998). These data imply the possible interactions between LTBP-1 and TGF-β1 after clenbuterol treatment. It is assumed that clenbuterol increases the TGF-β1 level through the upregulation of LTBP-1 expression, and that the elevated TGF-β1 in turn stimulates LTBP-1 synthesis. This loop might be an important regulatory mechanism to maintain TGF-β1 and LTBP-1 levels in a proper ratio.

Fig. 5. Expression of LTBP-1 in the hippocampus after transient forebrain ischemia. Clenbuterol (0.5 mg/kg) or saline were administered (i.p.) to the rats 3 h prior to ischemia. A-J: high power view of hippocampal CA1 subfield. Immunostaining of LTBP-1 was performed on the sections prepared 6 h after sham-operation (A), and 3 h (C and D), 6 h (E and F), 24 h (G and H) and 48 h (I and J) after ischemia. C, E, G and I: saline-treated controls; D, F, H and J: clenbuterol-treated rats; B: control for immunostaining. Scale bar = 50 μm. K and L: overview of hippocampus 24 h after ischemia in saline-treated rats (K) and in clenbuterol-treated rats (L). Scale bar = 200 μm. (Fig. see page 394)

6. Conclusions

We demonstrate a selective expression of TGF-β1 in pyramidal neurons of hippocampal CA1 subfield in the non-ischemic rat. Transient forebrain ischemia causes a temporary upregulation of TGF-β1 ir in the hippocampal CA1 subfield of the hippocampus after ischemia in the absence of evident activation of microglia and astrocytes, suggesting that the neurons in the hippocampal CA1 subfield may synthesize TGF-β1. We report for the first time that LTBP-1 expression is increased in rat brain after ischemia. Furthermore, the expression of TGF-β1 could be elevated in the vulnerable hippocampus by the lipophilic β_2-adrenoceptor agonist clenbuterol after transient forebrain ischemia without an influence in the mRNA level. Notably, this increase was associated with an enhanced LTBP-1 level in the hippocampus, suggesting a correlation of TGF-β1 and LTBP-1 after clenbuterol treatment. These results indicate that the expression of TGF-β1 and LTBP-1 in ischemic rat brain can be modulated by pharmacological intervention.

Acknowledgements

This study was supported by grants to J. K. from the Bundesministerium für Bildung, Wissenschaft, Forschung und Technologie (BMBF, Bonn, Germany) and from the DFG (Bonn, Germany).

References

1. Ahmed W, Kucich U, Abrams W, Bashir M, Segade F, Mecham R, Rosenbloom J (1998) Signalling pathway by which TGF-β1 increases expression of latent TGF-β binding protein-2 at the transcriptional level. Connect Tissue Res 37:263–276
2. Bechtner G, Fröschl H, Sachse A, Schopohl D, Gartner R (1999) Induction of apoptosis in porcine thyroid follicles by transforming growth factor beta 1 and epidermal growth factor. Biochem 81:315–320
3. Braun N, Zhu Y, Krieglstein J, Culmsee C, Zimmermann H (1998) Upregulation of the enzyme chain hydrolyzing extracellular ATP after transient forebrain ischemia in the rat. J Neurosci 18:4891–4900
4. Buisson A, Nicole O, Docagne F, Sartelet H, MacKenzie ET, Vivien D (1998) Up-regulation of a serine-protease inhibitor (PAI-1) in astrocytes mediates the neuroprotective activity of transforming growth factor-β1 (TGF-β1). FASEB J 12:1683–1691
5. Chalazonitis A, Kalberg J, Twadzik DR, Morrison RS, Kessler A (1992) Transforming growth factor β has neurotrophic actions on sensory neurons in vitro and is synergistic with nerve growth factor. Devl Biol 152:121–132
6. Chao CC, Kravitz FH, Tsang M, Anderson WR, Peterson PK (1994) Transforming growth factor-β protects human neurons against β-amyloid-induced injury. Mol Chem Neuropathol 23:159–178
7. Culmsee C, Semkova I, Krieglstein J (1999a) NGF mediates the neuroprotective effect of the β2-adrenoceptor agonist clenbuterol in vitro and in vivo: Evidence from a NGF-antisense study. Neurochem Int 35:47–57
8. Culmsee C, Stumm RK, Schäfer MKH, Weihe E, Krieglstein J (1999b) Clenbuterol induces growth factor mRNA, activates astrocytes, and protects rat brain tissue against ischemic damage. Eur J Pharmacol 379:33–45
9. Dallas SL, Miyazono K, Skerry TM, Mundy GR, Bonewald LF (1995) Dual role for the latent transforming growth factor-beta binding protein in storage of latent transforming growth factor-beta in the extracellular matrix and as a structural matrix protein. J Cell Biol 131:539–549
10. Dallas SL, Park-Snyder S, Miyazono K, Twardzik D, Mundy GR, Bonewald LF (1994) Characterization and autoregulation of latent transforming growth factor β (TGF-β) complex in osteoblast-like cell lines. J Biol Chem 269:6814–6822
11. Finch CE, Laping NJ, Morgan TE, Pasinetti N (1993) TGF-β1 is an organizer of response to neurodegeneration. J Cellular Biochem 53:314–322
12. Flanders KC, Ren RF, Lippa CF (1998) Transforming growth factor-betas in neurodegenerative disease. Prog Neurobiol 54:71–85
13. Flaumenhaft R, Abe M, Sato Y, Miyazono K, Harpel J, Heldin CH, Rifkin DB (1993) Role of the latent TGF-beta binding protein in the activation of latent TGF-beta by co-cultures of endothelial and smooth muscle cells. J Cell Biol 120:995–1002
14. Gleizes PE, Rifkin DB (1999) Activation of latent TGF-beta. A required mechanism for vascular integrity. Pathol Biol 47:322–320
15. Gross CE, Bednar MM, Howard DB, Sporn MB (1993) Transforming growth factor beta-1 reduces infarct size after experimental cerebral ischemia in a rabbit model. Stroke 24:558–562
16. Henrich-Noack P, Prehn JHM, Krieglstein J (1996) TGF-β1 protects hippocampal neurons against degeneration caused by transient global ischemia: dose-response relationship and potential neuroprotective mechanisms. Stroke 27:1609–1615
17. Kanzaki T, Olofsson A, Moren A, Wernstedt C, Hellman U, Miyazono K, Claesson-Welsh L, Heldin CH (1990) TGF-β1 binding protein: a component of the large latent complex of TGF-β1 with multiple repeat sequences. Cell 61:1051–1061
18. Kim ES, Kim RS, Ren RF, Hawver DB, Flanders KC (1998) Transforming growth factor-beta inhibits apoptosis induced by beta-amyloid peptide fragment 25–35 in cultured neuronal cells. Mol Brain Res 62:122–130
19. Knuckey NW, Finch P, Palm DE, Primiano MJ, Johanson CE, Flanders KC, Thompson NL (1996) Different neuronal and astrocytic expression of transforming growth factor-beta isoforms in rat hippocampus following transient forebrain ischemia. Mol Brain Res 40:1–14
20. Krieglstein K, Krieglstein J (1998) Transforming growth factor-β signalling and neuroprotection. In: Neuroprotective signal transduction, (Mattson MP, ed.), Totawa NJ: Humana Press Inc., pp 119–144
21. Krieglstein K, Unsicker K (1994) TGF-β1 promotes survival of midbrain dopaminergic neurons and protects them against MPP^+ toxicity. Neurosci 63:1189–1196

22. Krohn K (1999) TGF-β1-dependent differential expression of a rat homolog for latent TGF-β binding protein in astrocytes and C6 glioma cells. Glia 25:332–342
23. Kumar-Singh S, Weyler J, Martin MJH, Vermeulen PB, van Marck E (1999) Angiogenic cytokines in mesothelioma: a study of VEGF, FGF-1 and -2, and TGF-β expression. J Pathol 189:72–78
24. Kuo ML, Chen, CW, Jee SH, Chuang SE, Cheng AL (1997) Transforming growth factor-beta 1 attenuates ceramide-induced CPP32/Yama activation and apoptosis in human leukaemic HL-60 cells. Biochem J 327:663–667
25. Lehrmann E, Kiefer R, Finsen B, Diemer NH, Zimmer J, Hartung HP (1995) Cytokines in cerebral ischemia: expression of transforming growth factor-beta1(TGF-β1) mRNA in the postischemic adult rat hippocampus. Experimental Neurol 131:114–123
26. Lin B, Ginsberg MD, Busto R, Dietrich WD (1998) Sequential analysis of subacute and chronic neuronal, astrocytic and microglial alterations after transient global ischemia in rats. Acta Neuropathol 95:511–523
27. Lyons RM, Gentry LE, Purchio AF, Moses HL (1990) Mechanisms of activation of latent recombinant transforming growth factor beta 1 by plasmin. J Cell Biol 110:1361–1367
28. Mangasser-Stephan K, Gressner AM (1999) Molecular and functional aspects of latent transforming growth factor-β binding protein: just a masking protein? Cell Tissue Res 297:363–370
29. McNeill H, Williams C, Guan J, Dragunow M, Lawlor P, Sirimanne E, Nikolics K, Gluckman P (1994) Neuronal rescue with transforming growth factor beta-1 after hypoxic-ischemic brain injury. NeuroReport 5:901–904
30. Miyazono K, Heldin C (1989) Role of carbohydrate structures in TGF-β1 latency. Nature 338:158–160
31. Miyazono K, Hellman U, Wernstedt C, Heldin CH (1988) Latent high molecular weight complex of transforming growth factor β1. J Biol Chem 263:6407–6415
32. Miyazono K, Olofsson A, Colosetti P, Heldin CH (1991) A role of the latent transforming growth factor-β binding protein in the assembly and secretion of TGF-β1. EMBO J 10:1091–1101
33. Morén A, Olofsson A, Stenman G, Stahlin P, Kanzaki T, Claesseon-Welsh L, ten Dijke P, Miyazono K, Heldin CH (1994) Identification and characterization of LTBP-2, a novel latent transforming growth factor-beta binding protein. J Cell Chem 269:32469–32478
34. Nunes I, Gleizes PE, Metz CN, Rifkin DB (1997) Latent transforming growth factor-beta binding protein domains involved in activation and transglutaminase-dependent cross-linking of latent transforming growth factor-beta. J Cell Biol 136:1151–1163
35. Pang L, Yang GY, Roessler BJ, Ye W, Betz AL (1999) The protective effects of adenovirus mediated transforming growth factor beta-1 expression in ischemic mouse brain. J Cereb Blood Flow Metab 19 (Suppl. 1):137
36. Pircher R, Jullien P, Lawrence DA (1986) Transforming growth factor β-1 is stored in human blood platelets as a latent high molecular weight complex. Biochem Biophys Res Commun 136:30–37
37. Prehn JHM, Backhauβ C, Krieglstein J (1993a) Transforming growth factor beta-1 prevents glutamate neurotoxicity in rat neocortical cultures and protects mouse neocortex from ischemic injury in vivo. J Cereb Blood Flow Metab 13:521–525
38. Prehn JHM, Bindokas V, Jordan J, Galindo MF, Ghadge GD, Roos RP, Boise LH, Thompson CB, Krajewski S, Reed JC, Miller RJ (1996) Protective effect of transforming growth factor beta-1 (TGF-β1) on b-amyloid neurotoxicity in rat hippocampal neurons. Molec Pharmacol 49:319–328
39. Prehn JHM, Bindokas VP, Marcuccilli CJ, Krajewski D, Reed JC, Miller RJ (1994) Regulation of neuronal Bcl-2 protein expression and calcium homeostasis by transforming growth factor type β confers wide-ranging protection on rat hippocampal neurons. Proc Natl Acad Sci USA 91:12599–12603
40. Prehn JHM, Peruche B, Unsicker K, Krieglstein J (1993b) Isoform-specific effects of transforming growth factor beta-1 on degeneration of primary neuronal cultures induced by cytotoxic hypoxia or glutamate. J Neurochem 60:1665–1672
41. Roberts AB, Sporn MB (1993) Physiological action and clinical application of transforming growth factor-beta 1(TGF-β1). Growth Factors 8:1–9
42. Roth S, Michel K, Gressner AM (1998) (Latent) transforming growth factor β in liver parenchymal cells, its injury-dependent release, and paracrine effects on rat hepatic stellate cells. Hepatology 27:1003–1012
43. Ruocco A, Nicole O, Docagne F, Ali C, Chazalviel L, Komesli S, Yablonsky F, Roussel S, MacKenzie ET, Vivien D, Buisson A (1999) A transforming growth factor-beta antagonist unmasks the neuroprotective role of this endogenous cytokine in excitotoxic and ischemic brain injury. J Cereb Blood Flow Metab 19:1345–1353
44. Saharinen J, Taipale J, Monni O, Keski-Oja J (1998) Identification and charicterization of a new latent transforming growth factor β-binding protein, LTBP-4. J Biol Chem 273:18459–18469
45. Schultz-Cherry S, Murphy-Ullrich JE (1993) Thrombospondin causes activation of latent transforming growth factor β secreted by endothelial cells by a novel mechanism. J Cell Biol 122:923–932
46. Semkova I, Rami A, Krieglstein J (1994) Neuroprotective activity of clenbuterol against excitotoxic neuronal damage. In: Pharmacology of Cerebral Ischemia 1994 (Krieglstein J, Oberpichler-Schwenk H, eds), Stuttgart, Medpharm Scientific Publishers, pp 397–406
47. Semkova I, Schilling M, Henrich-Noack P, Rami A, Krieglstein J (1996) Clenbuterol protects mouse cerebral cortex and rat hippocampus from ischemic damage and attenuates glutamate neurotoxicity in cultured hippocampal neurons by induction of NGF. Brain Res 717:44–54
48. Sinha S, Nevett C, Shuttleworth CA, Kielty CM (1998) Cellular and extracellular biology of the latent transforming growth factor-β binding proteins. Matrix Biol 17:529–545
49. Tomoda T, Shasawa T, Yahagi YT, Ishii K, Takagi H, Furiya Y, Arai KT, Mori H, Muramatsu MA (1996) Transforming growth factor-beta is a survival factor for neonate cortical neurons: coincident expression of type I receptors in developing cortices. Devel Biol 179:79–90
50. Wakefield LM, Smith DM, Masui T, Harris CC, Sporn MB (1987) Distribution and modulation of the cellular receptor for transforming growth factor-beta. J Cell Biol 105:965–971
51. Wießner C, Gehrmann J, Lindholm D, Töppe R, Kreutzberg GW, Hossmann KA (1993) Expression of transforming growth factor-β1 and interleukin-1β mRNA in rat brain following transient forebrain ischemia. Acta Neuropathol 86:439–446
52. Yin WS, Smiley E, Germiller J, Mechan RP, Florer JB, Wenstrup RJ, Bonadio J (1995) Isolation of a novel latent transforming growth factor-beta binding protein gene (LTBP-3). J Biol Chem 270:10147–10160
53. Zhu Y, Ahlemeyer B, Bauerbach E, Krieglstein J (2000a) TGF-β1 inhibits caspase-3 activation and neuronal apoptosis in rat hippocampal cultures. Neurochem Int (in press)
54. Zhu Y, Culmsee C, Semkova I, Krieglstein J (1998) Stimulation of β_2-adrenoceptors inhibits apoptosis in rat brain after transient forebrain ischemia. J Cereb Blood Flow Metab 18:1032–1039
55. Zhu Y, Krieglstein J (1999a) β_2-Adrenoceptor agonist clenbuterol causes NGF expression and neuroprotection. CNS Drug Rev 5:347–364

56. Zhu Y, Prehn JHM, Culmsee C, Krieglstein J (1999b) The β_2-adrenoceptor agonist clenbuterol modulates Bcl-2, Bcl-xl and Bax protein expression following transient forebrain ischemia. Neurosci 90:1255–1263

57. Zhu Y, Roth-Eichhorn S, Braun N, Culmsee C, Rami A, Krieglstein J (2000b) The expression of transforming growth factor-beta1 (TGF-β1) in hippocampal neurons: A temporary upregulated protein level after transient forebrain ischemia in the rat. Brain Res. 866:286–298

Modulation of the serpin/serine proteases axis by TGF-β1 is a key element in the control of the glutamatergic neurotransmission

D. Vivien, C. Ali, O. Nicole, F. Docagne, A. Buisson

TGF-β is an endogenous neuroprotective cytokine against ischemic neuronal death

It is now well accepted that the neurotoxic overstimulation of postsynaptic glutamate receptors, which occurs following acute brain injury, is mediated by the activation of ion channel-linked glutamate receptors, especially N-methyl-D-aspartate (NMDA) receptors (Choi 1992). Considerable interest currently exists for developing effective methods to attenuate excitotoxicity in various disease states. How–ever, most of the drugs designed to directly target glutamatergic ionotropic receptors, present harmful side effects which have limited their potential use in man (Del Zoppo et al. 1997). In order to propose alternative therapeutic strategies, there is an increasing interest in determining the influence on the neurological outcome of cytokines, such as IL-1β, IL-6 or TGF-β, that can be produced in the brain parenchyma in response to acute or chronic brain injuries (review Feuerstein et al. 1998). Among these cytokines, the TGF-β family has elicited an increasing interest. *In vitro*, a number of studies has described a neuroprotective role of TGF-β1 against different metabolic and excitotoxic challenges (Unsicker et al. 1991; Prehn et al. 1993; Klempt et al. 1992). *In vivo*, several studies have described a marked increase in TGF-β1 mRNA following hypoxic-ischemic brain injury (Prehn et al. 1993; McNeill et al. 1994; Rimaniol et al. 1995; Vivien et al. 1998). While the intracerebroventricular application of TGF-β1 induces a slight reduction of the ischemic volume (Prehn and Krieglstein 1994; McNeill et al. 1994), there is no clear evidence for the influence of endogenously produced TGF-βs mainly because of the lack of a potent antagonist.

To determine the influence of endogenous TGF-βs produced following an acute brain injury on the volume of injured tissue, we injected into the brain of rats subjected to intrastriatal injection of NMDA or focal cerebral ischaemia, a molecular construct that has the ability to antagonize the binding of TGF-β1 to its native receptor: a soluble TGF-β type II receptor fused with the Fc region of a human immunoglobulin (TβRIIs-Fc) (Ruocco et al. 1999).

The intrastriatal injection of 75 nmol of NMDA in rats induced a rapid up-regulation of the expression of TGF-β1 mRNA that is observable by RT-PCR as early as 6h following the injection of the glutamatergic agonist. When we performed the same intrastriatal injection of NMDA in the presence of 1.5 μg of TβRIIs-Fc, we increased by 2.2 fold ($P < 0.05$) the size of the NMDA-induced lesion. This result reveals that excitotoxic striatal lesion is exacerbated in the presence of a TGF-β antagonist. This deleterious effect induced by blocking the influence

UMR CNRS 6551, Université de Caen, IFR 47, Centre Cyceron, Bld Henri Becquerel, 14074 Caen Cedex, France.

J. Krieglstein, S. Klumpp (Eds.) Pharmacology of Cerebral Ischemia 2000

of endogenously produced TGF-β was also present when the same strategy was applied to a model of focal cerebral ischaemia. Indeed, intracortical injection of TβRIIs-Fc in rats subjected to a 30 minute reversible cerebral focal ischaemia aggravated the infarction. In the group injected with the TGF-β1 antagonist, we measured a 3.5 fold increase in the infarction size (43.3 ± 9.5 vs 152.8 ± 46.3 mm^3; $P < 0.05$). Taken together, these experiments provide evidences that antagonizing the influence of the endogenous TGF-βs into brain tissue subjected to excitotoxic or ischaemic lesion, exacerbates the extent of the infarction. So, it can be suggested that in response to acute injury, brain tissue responds by the synthesis of a neuroprotective cytokine, TGF-β1, which in turn limits the extent of the lesion.

In a next step, we investigated by which mechanism endogenous TGF-β1 may exert its neuroprotective effect against both excitotoxic lesion and ischemic injuries.

A serine protease inhibitor mediates the neuroprotective activity of TGF-β1

By using a model of primary cortical cell culture, we have demonstrated that TGF-β1 incubation induces a selective neuroprotective effect against NMDA-induced neuronal death (Buisson et al. 1998). This effect was only observed when TGF-β1 was added to cortical cultures containing both neurons and astrocytes. In regard to these results, we hypothetized that glia mediates the TGF-β1 neuroprotective effect. Accordingly, by transfecting astrocytes with a dominant negative receptor for TGF-β1, we totally abolished the neuroprotective activity of TGF-β1 incubation against NMDA-mediated neurotoxicity. Finally, we identified a protein produced by astrocytes in response to TGF-β1 stimulation that could mediate the neuroprotective effect of TGF-β against NMDA-mediated neurotoxicity: Plasminogen Activator Inhibitor-1 (PAI-1). To validate the involvement of PAI-1 in the TGF-β1 effect in our culture model, we showed that the neuroprotection induced by TGF-β1 was prevented by the addition of an antibody raised against PAI-1 and was mimicked by the coapplication of the recombinant form of PAI-1 (Buisson et al. 1998). These data suggest that the neuroprotective activity of TGF-β1 occurs via an up-regulation of PAI-1 in astrocytes (Buisson et al. 1998).

TGF-β1 belongs to a large family of peptides including activin and bone morphogenetic proteins (BMPs) which are expressed in the CNS (Ebendal et al. 1998; Dewulf et al. 1995). Recently, two other members of the same family, termed the Glial cell line Derived Neurotrophic Factor (GDNF) (Lin et al. 1993) and neurturin (NTN) (Kotzbauer et al. 1996), have been identified in brain tissues. Although TGF-β1 and activin are able to enhance the expression of PAI-1 in astrocytes (Docagne et al. 1999), BMPs, GDNF and NTN are devoid of activity. These results provide novel insights into the regulation of the inhibitors of the serine protease and the mechanisms by which an injury-related cytokine, such as TGF-β1, may be neuroprotective in situation of induced excitotoxicity. Taken together, these results reveal a tight link between TGF-β1 and the inhibitors of serine proteases, named serpins, in the CNS.

Interaction between Serine proteases and excitotoxic lesion

The involvement of serine proteases in the physiopathology of glutamate-induced neuronal cell death was first identified in 1995 by Tsirka and collaborators. In this study the authors have described that t-PA deficient mice are resistant to an excitotoxic lesion induced by the injection of kainate into the hippocampus. They have also suggested that t-PA influences the excitotoxic neuronal death which occurs following ischemic injury (Tsirka et al. 1995). Based on the literature on this topic since 1995, it seems that the modulation of the activity of serine proteases may play a key role into the control of the extent of acute brain damage. The experimental data obtained from studies with wild type or knock out mice ($tPA^{-/-}$ or

PAI-1$^{-/-}$) have all lead to the same conclusion: t-PA participates in excitotoxic neuronal death (Tsirka et al. 1995, 1997a, 1997b; Chen and Strickland 1998) and ischaemia-induced neuronal death (Wang et al. 1998; Nagai et al. 1999).

By using either wild type or t-PA deficient cultured cortical neurons, we have demonstrated that the addition of t-PA in the extracellular medium selectively potentiates NMDA-mediated neuronal cell death by modifying the properties of a glutamatergic receptor: the NMDA receptor. We evidence that t-PA interacts with the NR1 subunit of the NMDA receptor, that leads to its cleavage and enhancement of the NMDA-mediated calcium influx.

When depolarized, cortical neurons release bio-active t-PA into the synaptic cleft that interacts and cleaves the NR1 subunit of the NMDA receptor. This modification leads to an increase in the calcium influx via the channel gated NMDA receptor. These results were confirmed *in vivo* since the intrastriatal injection of rt-PA potentiates the excitotoxic lesions induced by NMDA.

As the usual causes of stroke are related to thrombo-embolic processes in cerebral arteries, the idea that prevention of clot formation might be helpful for patients was understood as early as the 1940's. The National Institutes of Health recommanded in the 1980's the use of tissue-type plasminogen activator (t-PA) for the treatment of thrombo-embolic diseases. In 1995, the National Institute of Neurological Disorders rt-PA Stroke Study Group concluded that ischemic brain damage is reduced following t-PA administration. Clinical studies have revealed that t-PA treatment is beneficial in the treatment of acute stroke. However, since the ischemic lesion is thought to progress, largely via an excitotoxic pathway, the data that demonstrate that serine proteases may potentiate excitotoxin-induced neurodegeneration raise the question of potential risks in the use of t-PA for the treatment of acute stroke (Fig. 1). Dysruption of the blood brain barrier which occurs in

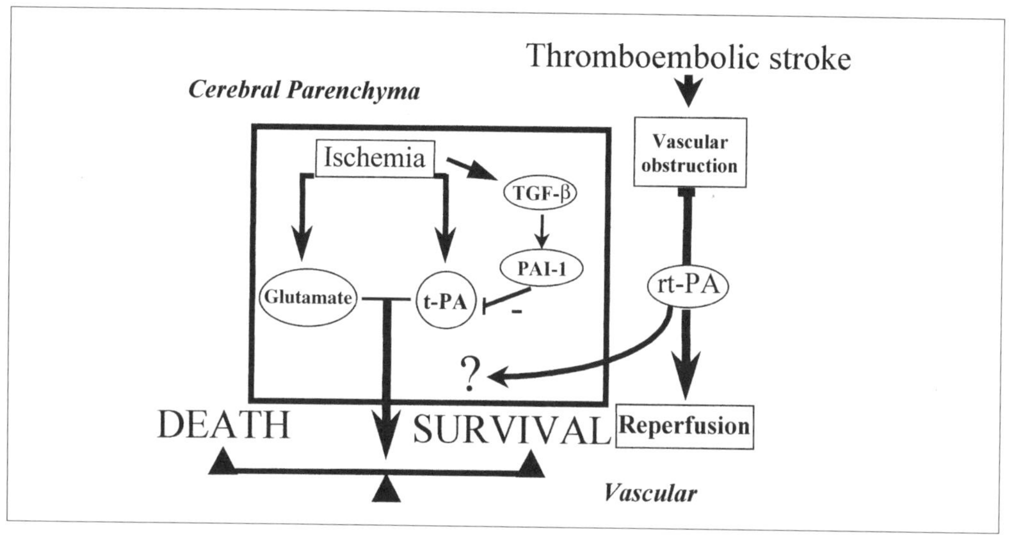

Fig. 1. Proposed mechanism for the involvement of the tissue-type plasminogen activator (t-PA)/type 1 plasminogen activator inhibitor (PAI-1) axis in the central nervous system during stroke. Intravenous injection of t-PA is used for the treatment of focal cerebral infarction in humans (thrombolysis). In the cerebral parenchyma, t-PA could be released from stressed neurons and could potentiate excitotoxin-mediated neuronal death. The expression of transforming growth factor-β1 is up-regulated after either permanent or transient cerebral ischaemia in rodents. Then, TGF-β1 induces an overexpression of PAI-1 in astrocytes, a mechanism leading to the neuroprotective activity of TGF-β against NMDA-mediated excitotoxicity. Concerning these results, we can postulate that the neuroprotective activity of TGF-β and PAI-1 could be related to their inhibitory effects on t-PA.

cerebral ischaemia, may facilitate the access of the systemically administered t-PA to neuronal tissues and may thus lead to the potentiation of neuronal death. The idea that thrombolytic agents may be used in combination with potent neuroprotective agents merits further attention. Since serine protease inhibitors specific for t-PA are neuroprotective, it is possible to suggest novel ways to counteract the neuronal death observed in acute stroke patients. The inhibition of the proteolytic activity of serine proteases into the cerebral parenchyma or the potentiation of the serpins expression in brain cells could be a potential therapeutic intervention for those disorders in which excitotoxicity is thought to play a critical role.

References

1. Buisson A, Nicole O, Docagne F, Sartelet H, MacKenzie ET, Vivien D (1998) Up-regulation of a serine-protease inhibitor (PAI-1) in astrocytes mediates the neuroprotective activity of transforming growth factor-β1 (TGF-β1). FASEB J 12:1683–1691
2. Chen ZL, Strickland S (1997) Neuronal death in the hippocampus is promoted by plasmin-catalyzed degradation of laminin. Cell 91:917–925
3. Choi DW (1992) Excitotoxic cell death. J Neurobiol 23:1261–1276
4. Del Zoppo GJ, Wagner S, Tagaya M (1997) Trends and future developments in the pharmacological treatment of acute ischaemic stroke. Drugs 54:9–38
5. Dewulf N, Verschueren K, Lonnoy O, Moren A, Grimsby S, Vande Spiegle K, Miyazono K, Huylebroeck D, Ten Dijke P (1995) Distinct spatial and temporal expression patterns of two type I receptors for bone morphogenetic proteins during mouse embryogenesis. Endocrinology 136:2652–2663
6. Docagne F, Nicole O, Marti HH, MacKenzie ET, Buisson A, Vivien D (1999) Transforming growth factor-β1 as a regulator of the serpins/t-PA axis in cerebral ischaemia. FASEB J 13:1315–1324
7. Ebendal T, Bengtsson H, Soderstrom S (1998) Bone morphogenetic proteins and their receptors: potential functions in the brain. J Neurosci 51:139–146
8. Feuerstein GZ, Wang X, Barone FC (1998) The role of cytokines in the neuropathology of stroke and neurotrauma. Neuroimmunomodulation 5:143–159
9. Klempt ND, Sirimanne E, Gunn AJ, Klempt M, Singh K, Williams C, Gluckman PD (1992) Hypoxia-ischaemia induces transforming growth factor beta 1 mRNA in the infant rat brain. Brain Res Mol Brain Res 13:93–101
10. Kotzbauer PT, Lampe PA, Heuckeroth RO, Golden JP, Creedon DJ, Johnson EM Jr, Milbrandt J (1996) Neurturin, a relative of glial-cell-line-derived neurotrophic factor. Nature 384:467–470
11. Lin LF, Doherty DH, Lile JD, Bektesh S, Collins F (1993) GDNF: a glial cell line-derived neurotrophic factor for midbrain dopaminergic neurons. Science 260:1130–1132
12. McNeill H, Williams C, Guan J, Dragunow M, Lawlor P, Sirimanne E, Nikolics K, Gluckman P (1994) Neuronal rescue with transforming growth factor beta 1 after hypoxic-ischaemic brain injury. Neuroreport 5:901–904
13. Nagai N, De Mol M, Lijnen HR, Carmeliet P, Collen D (1999) Role of plasminogen system components in focal cerebral ischemic infarction: a gene targeting and gene transfer study in mice. Circulation 99:2440–2444
14. Prehn JHM, Backhauss C, Krieglstein J (1993) Transforming growth factor-b1 prevents glutamate neurotoxicity in rat neocortical cultures and protects mouse neocortex from ischemic injury in vivo. J Cereb Blood Flow Metab 13:521–525
15. Prehn JHM, Krieglstein J (1994) Opposing effects of transforming growth factor-beta 1 on glutamate neurotoxicity. Neuroscience 60:7–10
16. Rimaniol AC, Lekieffre D, Serrano A, Masson A, Benavides J, Zavala F (1995) Biphasic transforming growth factor β production flanking the pro-inflammatory cytokine response in cerebral trauma. Neuroreport 7:133–136
17. Ruocco A, Docagne F, Nicole O, Ali C, Chazalviel L, Komesli S, Yablonsky F, Roussel S, MacKenzie ET, Vivien D, Buisson A (1999) A TGF_β antagonist unmasks the neuroprotective role of this endogenous cytokine in excitotoxic and ischemic brain injury. J Cereb Blood Flow and Metab 19:13145–13153
18. Tsirka SE, Bugge TH, Degen JL, Strickland S (1997a) Neuronal death in the central nervous system demonstrates a non-fibrin substrate for plasmin. Proc Natl Acad Sci USA 94:9779–9781
19. Tsirka SE, Gualandris A, Amaral DG, Strickland S (1995) Excitotoxin-induced neuronal degeneration and seizure are mediated by tissue plasminogen activator. Nature 377:340–344
20. Tsirka SE, Rogove AD, Bugge TH, Degen JL, Strickland S (1997b) An extracellular proteolytic cascade promotes neuronal degeneration in the mouse hippocampus. J Neurosci 17:543–552
21. Unsicker K, Flanders KC, Cissel DS, Lafyatis R, Sporn MB (1991) Transforming growth factor beta isoforms in the adult rat central and peripheral nervous system. Neuroscience 44:613–625.
22. Vivien D, Bernaudin M, Buisson A, Divoux D, MacKenzie ET, Nouvelot A (1998) Evidence of type I and type II transforming growth factor-β receptors in central neryous tissues: changes induced by focal cerebral ischemia. J Neurochem 70:2296–2304
23. Wang YF, Tsirka SE, Strickland S, Stieg PE, Soriano SG, Lipton SA (1998) Tissue plasminogen activator (tPA) increases neuronal damage after focal cerebral ischaemia in wild-type and tPA-deficient mice. Nat Med 4:228–231

Contextual actions of TGF-β and cytokine signaling pathways in mediating neurotrophic functions

N. Schuster, A. Schober, K. Krieglstein

A crucial step in the development of the nervous system is the regulation of neuronal survival during and following the period of ontogenetic neuron death, following lesion, and in neurodegenerative disease. The classic neurotrophic factor concept is based on the assumption that neurons compete for limiting amounts of neurotrophic factors synthesized and released from their target tissues, and therefore, retrogradely regulating neuronal survival (see Levi-Montalcini 1987). The amount of neurotrophic factor determines the number of surviving neurons during ontogenesis, whereas lack of neurotrophic support results in neuron degeneration (see Hamburger 1993). Research of the last decade provides lots of evidence that the neurotrophic factor concept has to be revised for a better understanding of the biological background (see Korsching 1993). Neurotrophic support is not exclusively provided retrogradely by the target cells, it also may be provided by (i) anterograde neuronal input (v Bartheld et al. 1996), (ii) axon ensheathing glial cells, (iii) in a paracrine fashion by glia located in close proximity to neuronal cell bodies in a paracrine fashion, or (iv) even by an autocrine mode by neurons themselves (Acheson et al. 1996). On the other hand, induction of apoptotic neuron death can not be viewed just as a lack of neurotrophic support, as ample evidence is available for selective apoptotic triggers using specific cascades referred to as genetically determined cell death programs. Furthermore, numbers of molecules, prejudicially grouped as neurotrophic factors, growth factors or cytokines, and thought to regulate neuron survival and differentiation are exploding (deLapeyrere and Henderson 1997). However, the cross talk, contextual actions, and mutual requirements as well as redundancies are completely not understood at present. Null mutants of a substantial number of proteins that were thought to be extremely important and essential in the context of neuronal survival often show very mild and marginal defects in the peripheral and central nervous system (see Snider 1994). In this review we would like to outline the impact of transforming growth factor beta (TGF-β) on the neurotrophic actions of the neurotrophins, glial cell line-derived neurotrophic factor (GDNF), ciliary neurotrophic factor (CNTF), and basic fibroblast growth factor (FGF-2).

1. Transforming growth factors-β

TGF-βs are multifunctional growth factors with widespread distribution (see Roberts and Sporn 1990). The TGF-β family is composed of three

Key words: TGF-β, GDNF, neurotrophin, CNTF, neuronal survival

Department of Anatomy, University of Saarland, D-66421 Homburg/Saar, Germany
e-mail: ankkri@med-rz.uni-sb.de

J. Krieglstein, S. Klumpp (Eds.) Pharmacology of Cerebral Ischemia 2000

TGF-β isoforms, TGF-β1, -β2 and -β3, each encoded by an individual gene, all acting on the same transmembrane serine-threonine kinase containing receptor complex, consisting of the TGF-β receptor type 2 (TβR-II) and TβR-I (Massage 1998; Heldin et al. 1997). TGF-β has become the prototype of a superfamily also comprising bone morphogenetic proteins (BMPs), growth/differentiation factors (GDFs), activins and members of the GDNF-family (for review see Böttner et al. 2000; Unsicker et al. 1999; Hogan 1999; Mehler and Kessler 1998; Furuta et al. 1997). Some of these factors are known to play an essential role in early morphogenesis, in dorso-ventral patterning, in the determination of neural crest derivatives, in bone formation, in the composition of the extracellular matrix, and in the induction of apoptosis. In the nervous system TGF-β is known for its role in the regulation of proliferation of neural progenitor cells, the regulation of survival and differentiation as well as its impact on axon growth (Krieglstein et al. 1995a; Krieglstein and Krieglstein 1997; Böttner et al. 2000). In the lesioned nervous system TGF-β orchestrates the immunomodulatory response (Wahl 1992) and is known for its effects on microglia and astrocytes (Flanders et al. 1998). However, one should keep in mind that all TGF-β isoforms are known for the strong contextuality of their actions (Nathan and Sporn 1991).

2. TGF-β and GDNF co-operativity

GDNF was originally discovered and purified from B49 cells by its ability to promote survival and differentiation of cultured rat mesencephalic dopaminergic neurons (Lin et al. 1993). Distribution analysis of GDNF revealed that GDNF is almost ubiquitously expressed throughout the nervous system (Pochon et al. 1997; Trupp et al. 1995), which is mirrored by the identification of increasing numbers of GDNF-responsive neuron populations (Henderson et al. 1994; Buj-Bello et al. 1995; Trupp et al. 1995). Several lines of evidence suggested that GDNF may require a co-factor for acting as a neurotrophic factor: (i) GDNF did not promote survival of most peripheral neurons in low-density cultures, run under serum-free conditions (Henderson et al. 1994; Krieglstein and Unsicker 1996a), (ii) The neurotrophic effects of GDNF on dopaminergic neurons are achieved using a highly complex culture system with high cell densities, serum exposure at the beginning of the culture period and a duration of seven days (Lin et al. 1993), raising the possibility that GDNF interacted with other growth factors in these cultures. As TGF-β is present in serum in reasonable amounts, as well as ubiquitously expressed, may therefore be a good candidate for the co-trophic and co-operative component for GDNF. Figure 1 illustrates that TGF-β is present in 10%-solutions of different batches of horse serum (HS) or fetal calf serum (FCS) typically used for tissue culture. The amount of TGF-β detectable in these culture media is in the range of 0.25 ng/ml TGF-β. Using chick ciliary ganglionic neurons as an example, Figure 2a demonstrates that GDNF supplemented with 10% HS maintains the survival of these ciliary ganglionic neurons as effectively as saturating concentrations of the established growth factor for this neuron population, CNTF (5ng/ml). However, neutralizing serum-contained TGF-β by preincubation with neutralizing antibodies to TGF-β (known to neutralize all three TGF-β-isoforms) significantly reduced the effect of GDNF, suggesting that GDNF requires TGF-β for establishing its neurotrophic effect. Consistent with this notion, if a serum-containing culture medium was replaced with a fully defined culture-medium (DMEM plus N1 supplements), both GDNF and TGF-β alone, showed no survival promoting effects (Fig. 2b). However, the combination of GDNF and TGF-β promoted ciliary ganglionic neuron survival as effectively as CNTF (Fig. 2b). This synergistic effect of GDNF and TGF-β does also apply to other populations of peripheral neurons, i.e. chick sensory dorsal root ganglionic neurons as well as paravertebral sympathetic neurons (Krieglstein et al. 1998b). As GDNF was first characterized by its pronounced trophic effects on mesencephalic dopaminergic neurons it is particularly interesting to test whether this effect was dependent or

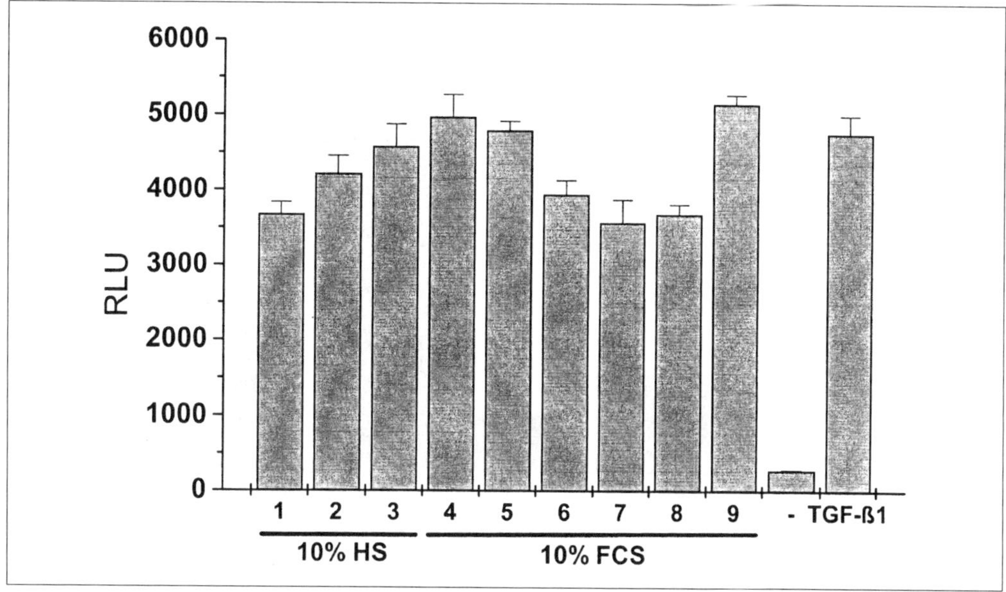

Fig. 1. TGF-β activity detected in serum containing culture medium. Cultures were treated with different batches of horse serum (HS), fetal calf serum (FCS) as 10% dilutions in DME medium, or with TGF-β1 (0.25 ng/ml in DMEM). TGF-β activity was quantified using a TGF-β-sensitive reporter gene assay (as described in Krieglstein et al. 1998a). Data are given in relative light units (RLU) as mean +/– SEM (n = 3).

independent from TGF-β. The system commonly used for culturing dopaminergic neurons is a serum-free but a quite complex culture system, as it requires a relatively high cell density (50,000–200,000 cells/cm^2) and a long culture period (usually 7 days *in vitro*). The tissue dissected for establishment of these cultures, the ventral midbrain of embryonic rats E 14, synthezises mRNA and protein for TGF-β2 and TGF-β3 and continues to do so following the dissociation procedure (Krieglstein et al. 1995b), suggesting that these cultures become conditioned by endogenous TGF-β during the experiment. As shown in Figure 3, GDNF and TGF-β each promoted the survival of dopaminergic neurons under serum-free conditions. Combination of factors further enhances survival. However, addition of neutralizing antibodies to TGF-β abolished the trophic effect of GDNF.

In summary, experiments using dissociated neuronal cell cultures, in which serum was replaced by fully defined supplements or used in the presence of neutralizing antibodies recognizing all three TGF-β antibodies provided evidence that GDNF requires TGF-β in order to promote survival of peripheral (parasympathetic ciliary ganglionic, sensory dorsal root ganglionic and paravertebral sympathetic neurons) and CNS (mesencephalic dopaminergic) neurons (Krieglstein et al. 1998b).

To elucidate the *in vivo* relevance of the GDNF/TGF-β co-operativity Schober and coworkers (1999) challanged this hypothesis using the adrenomedullectomy modell in which GDNF was shown to act as a potent neurotrophic factor in vivo (Schober et al. 1999). Chromaffin cells in the adrenal medulla receive a prominent cholinergic innervation from neurons located in the intermediolateral column of the spinal cord. Electrosurgical destruction of the adult rat adrenal medulla leads to degeneration and death of these neurons within four weeks. Implantation of a gelfoam loaded with GDNF into the adrenal cavity rescues all preganglionic neurons which otherwise die. However, the application of GDNF plus neutralising antibod-

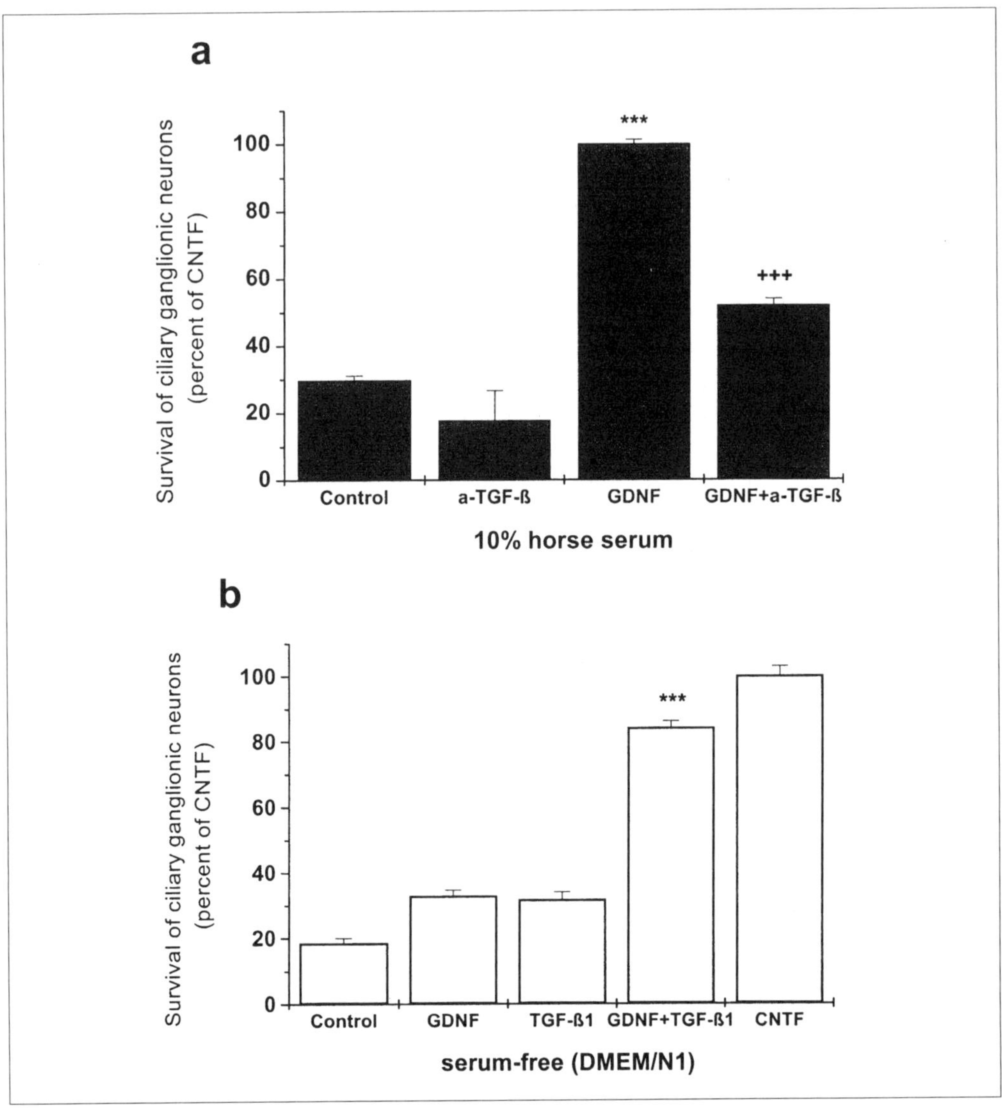

Fig. 2. Survival of ciliary ganglionic neurons by the synergistic actions of GDNF and TGF-β. Neurons from chick ciliary ganglia were isolated at E8 and maintained (a) in serum-containing medium (10% HS) or (b) in serum-free medium. Cultures were treated with GDNF, TGF-β1 (2 ng/ml), in combination of TGF-β1 and GDNF, with neutralizing antibodies to TGF-β1, -β2, -β3 (a-TGF-β, 10 µg/ml), GDNF in combination with a-TGF-β, or with CNTF (5 ng/ml). Data are given as mean +/– SEM (n = 6) relative to CNTF-dependent survival (100%). p values derived from Student's t test are $^{***}p < 0.001$ for increased survival as compared with single factors and $^{+++}p < 0.001$ for decreased survival following antibody treatment.

ies recognising all three TGF-β-isoforms completely abolished the protective effect of GDNF (Schober et al. 1999). Together, these data indicate that to exert its neurotrophic and neuroprotective functions GDNF requires TGF-β not only *in vitro*, but also *in vivo*.

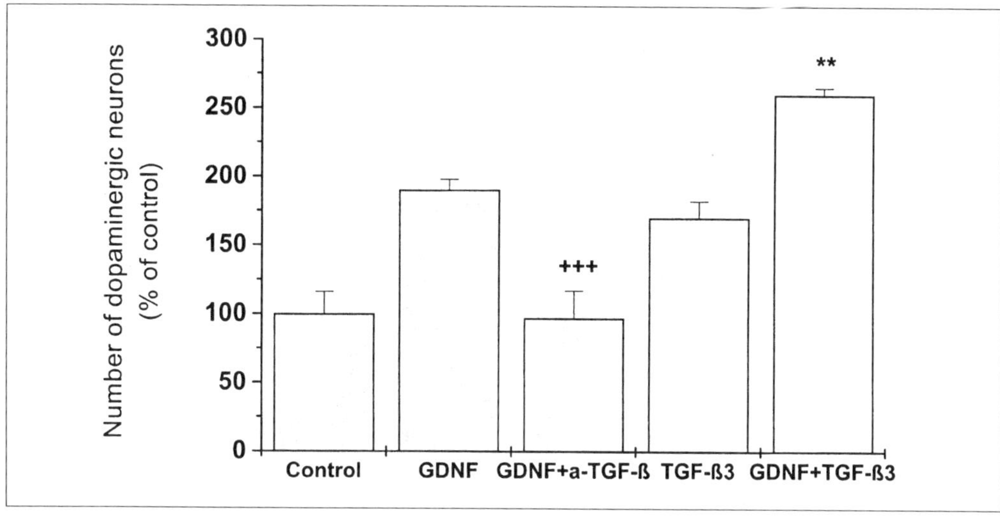

Fig. 3. Survival promoting effect of GDNF and TGF-β on rat mesencephalic dopaminergic neurons. Dissociated mesencephalic dopaminergic neurons (E14) were cultured at a density of 50,000 per cm^2 in serum-free medium (see Krieglstein et al. 1998b) and treated with GDNF (2 ng/ml), TGF-β3 (2 ng/ml), GDNF plus TGF-β3, or GDNF plus a-TGF-β antibodies (10 μg/ml). Data are gives as mean +/– SEM (n = 4) and expressed in percent of controls. p values derived from Student's t test are $^{**}p < 0.01$ for increased survival of GDNF plus TGF-β as compared to induvidial treatments and $^{+++}p < 0.001$ for decreased survival following antibody treatment.

3. TGF-β and neurotrophins

The neurotrophins nerve growth factor (NGF), brain-derived neurotrophic factor (BDNF), neurotrophin-3 (NT-3) and NT-4/5 are important for the regulation of survival and differentiation of many neuron populations, including embryonic sensory neurons located in the dorsal root ganglia (DRG). TGF-β, on the other hand, fails to maintain these sensory neuron cultures from embryonic day (E) 8 chick DRG, although DRG neurons are immmunoreactive for the ligand binding TGF-β receptor type II (Krieglstein et al. 1998b). However, in combination with various concentrations of NT-3 and NT-4, but not NGF, TGF-β3 causes a significant increase in neuronal survival (Krieglstein and Unsicker 1996b). As NGF-treatment has been shown to induce TGF-β mRNA and protein (Cosgaya and Aranda 1995) we testet whether endogenously synthesized TGF-β already contributes to the neurotrophin-dependent survival promoting effects. Treatment of DRG cultures with NGF, NT-3 and NT-4, in combination with a neutralizing antibody to TGF-β decreases neuron survival suggesting that endogenous TGF-β in these serum-free cultures affects the efficiencies of neurotrophins (Krieglstein and Unsicker 1996b). Together, these data indicate that actions and efficacies of neurotrophins are under distinct control of TGF-β.

4. TGF-β and other factors

Ciliary neurotrophic factor (CNTF) and fibroblast growth factor (FGF)-2, established neurotrophic factors for parasympathetic neurons of the ciliary ganglion (CG; Manthorpe et al. 1989; Unsicker et al. 1987) upregulate TGF-β3 mRNA and biological activity in cultures of E8 CG neurons. None of the TGF-β isoforms has a survival-promoting effect of cultured CG neurons on their own. However, all isoforms enhance CG neuron survival mediated by CNTF or FGF-2 significantly and over a wide range of concentrations (Krieglstein et al. 1998a). Immunoneutralization of endogenous TGF-β released from CG neurons significantly reduces the potency of CNTF or FGF-2 to promote CG neuron survival. Furthermore, TGF-β-treatment of CG neurons in combination with the neurotrophins NGF and NT-3, which are not neurotrophic for CG neurons, resulted in a neurotrophic activity to promote CG neuron survival (Krieglstein et al. 1998a). Together, these data suggest that para-/autocrine TGF-β signaling has an important effect on the regulation of neuron survival in a model system of peripheral neurons.

Conclusion

Data summarized in this article clearly show that TGF-β exerts a key role in the context of actions of neurotrophic factors and cytokines. This role of TGF-β may not be too surprising given the multiple lines of evidence that document the contextual and pleiotropic actions of TGF-β on non-neural cells (for review see Nathan and Sporn 1991).

Acknowledgements

Work performed in our laboratory is supported by grants from the "Deutsche Forschungsgemeinschaft".

References

1. Acheson A, Conover JC, Fandl JP, DeChiara TM, Russell M, Thadani A, Squinto SP,Yancopoulos GD, Lindsay RM (1995) A BDNF autocrine loop in adult sensory neurons prevents cell death. Nature 374:450–453
2. Böttner M, Krieglstein K, Unsicker K (2000) The TGF-βs: structure, signaling and roles in nervous system development and functions. J Neurochem (in press)
3. Buj-Bello A, Buchman VL, Horton A, Rosenthal A, Davies AM (1995) GDNF is an age-specific survival factor for sensory and autonomic neurons. Neuron 15:821–828
4. Cosgaya JM, Aranda A (1995) Nerve growth factor regulates transforming growth factor-beta 1 gene expression by both transcriptional and posttranscriptional mechanisms in PC12 cells. J Neurochem 65:2484–2490
5. deLapeyriere O, Henderson CE (1997) Motoneuron differentiation, survival and synaptogenesis. Curr Opin Genet Dev 7:642–650
6. Flanders KC, Ren RF, Lippa CF (1998) Transforming growth factor-betas in neurodegenerative disease. Prog Neurobiol 54:71–85
7. Furuta Y, Piston DW, Hogan BL (1997) Bone morphogenetic proteins (BMPs) as regulators of dorsal forebrain development Development 124:2203–2212
8. Hamburger V (1993) The history of the discovery of the nerve growth factor. J Neurobiol 24:893–897
9. Heldin CH, Miyazono K, ten Dijke P (1997) TGF-beta signaling from cell membrane to nucleus through SMAD proteins. Nature 390:465–471
10. Henderson CE, Phillips HS, Pollock RA, Davies AM, Lemeulle C, Armanini MP, Simpson LC, Moffet B, Vandlen RA, Koliatsos VE, Rosenthal A. (1994) GDNF: a potent survival factor for motoneurons present in peripheral nerve and muscle. Science 266:1062–1064
11. Hogan BL (1999) Morphogenesis. Cell 96:225–233
12. Korsching S (1993) The neurotrophic factor concept: a reexamination. J Neurosci 13:2739–2748
13. Krieglstein K, Farkas L, Unsicker K (1998a) TGF-β regulates the survival of ciliary ganglionic neurons synergistically with ciliary neurotrophic factor and neurotrophins. J Neurobiol 37:563–572
14. Krieglstein K, Henheik P, Farkas L, Jaszai J, Galter D, Krohn K, Unsicker K (1998b) GDNF requires TGF-β for establishing its neurotrophic activity. J Neurosci 18:9822–9834
15. Krieglstein K, Krieglstein J (1998) Transforming growth factor-β signaling and neuroprotection: relevance to ischemic brain injury, Alzheimer's, and Parkinson's disease. In: Neuroprotective signal transduction, ed. Mattson MP, Humana Press, Totowa, New Jersey, pp 119–144
16. Krieglstein K, Rufer M, Suter-Crazzolara C, Unsicker K (1995a) Neural functions of the transforming growth factor β. Int J Dev Neurosci 13:301–315
17. Krieglstein K, Suter-Crazzolara C, Fischer WH, Unsicker K (1995b) TGF-β superfamily members promote survival of midbrain dopaminergic neurons and protect them against MPP+ toxicity. EMBO J 14:736–742
18. Krieglstein K, Unsicker K (1996a) Proteins from chromaffinc granules promote survival of dorsal root ganglionic neurons:comparison with neurotrophins. Dev Brain Res 93:10–17
19. Krieglstein K, Unsicker K (1996b) Distinct modulatory actions of TGF-β and LIF on neurotrophin-mediated survival of developmental sensory neurons. Neurochem Res 21:849–856
20. Levi-Montalcini R (1987) The nerve growth factor 35 years later. Science 237:1154–1162
21. Lin LFH, Doherty DH, Lile JD, Bektesh S, Collins F (1993) GDNF – a glial cell line-derived neurotrophic factor for midbrain dopaminergic neurons. Science 260:1130–1132
22. Manthorpe M, Ray J, Pettmann B, Varon S (1989) ciliary neuronotrophic factors. In: Nerve growth factors. Rush RA ed Wiley, New York, pp 31–56
23. Massague J (1998) TGF-beta signal transduction. Annu Rev Biochem. 67:753–791
24. Mehler MF, Kessler JA (1998) Cytokines in brain development. Adv Protein Chemistry 52:223–251
25. Nathan C, Sporn MB (1991) Cytokines in context. J Cell Biol 113:981–986
26. Pochon NA, Menoud A, Tseng JL, Zurn AD, Aebischer P (1997) Neuronal GDNF expression in the adult rat nervous system identified by in situ hybridization. Eur J Neurosci 9:463–471
27. Roberts AB, Sporn MB (1990) The transforming growth factors-βs. In: Sporn MB, Roberts AB (eds) Handbook of Experimental Pharmacology. Springer, Heidelberg, Vol. 95, pp 419–472

28. Schober A, Hertel R, Arumäe U, Farkas L, Jaszai J, Krieglstein K, Saarma M, Unsicker K (1999) GDNF rescues target-deprived spinal cord neurons but requires TGF-β as co-factor in vivo. J Neurosci 19:2008–2015
29. Snider WD (1994) Functions of the neurotrophins during nervous system development: what the knockouts are teaching us. Cell 77:627–638
30. Trupp M, Ryden M, Jornvall H, Funakoshi H, Timmusk T, Arenas E, Ibanez CF (1995) Peripheral expression and biological activities of GDNF, a new neurotrophic factor for avian and mammalian peripheral neurons. J Cell Biol 130:137–148
31. Unsicker K, Reichert-Preibsch H, Schmidt R, Pettmann B, Labourdette G, Sensenbrenner M (1987) Astroglial and fibroblast growth factors have neurotrophic functions for cultured peripheral and central nervous system neurons. Proc Natl Acad Sci USA 84:5459–5463
32. Unsicker K, Suter-Crazzolara C, Krieglstein K Neurotrophic roles of GDNF and related factors (1999) Handbook of Exp. Pharmacology 134, "Neurotrophic Factors" (Hefti, F., Ed.) Springer, Heidelberg pp 189–224
33. v Bartheld CS, Byers MR, Williams R, Bothwell M (1996) Anterograde transport of neurotrophins and axodendritic transfer in the developing visual system. Nature 379:830–833
34. Wahl SM (1992) Transforming growth factor beta (TGF-β) in inflammation: a cause and a cure. J Clin Immunol 12:66–74

Cytokines as therapeutic targets in stroke

N. J. Rothwell

Summary

Numerous cytokines have been implicated in the aetiology and clinical outcome of stroke. Several anti-inflammatory cytokines (eg IL-1ra, IL-10, TGFβ) are neuroprotective, but other cytokines such as TNFα and IL-6, exert conflicting effects and seemingly both cause or inhibit brain damage. IL-1 is now recognised as a key mediator of experimentally induced ischaemic, excitotoxic and traumatic brain injury and offers several targets for therapeutic intervention eg actions of ATP on the P2x7 receptor which induces IL-1β release, caspase-1 which cleaves pro IL-1β, or agents which bind IL-1, block interaction with its receptor or modify signal transduction. At present the most advanced of these approaches is the naturally occurring IL-1 receptor antagonist which will soon be tested in stroke patients.

The last five years have witnessed a dramatic increase in our knowledge about, and interest in, the role of proinflammatory cytokines in ischaemic brain damage, and identification of several new therapeutic targets.

The cytokines include interleukins, tumour necrosis factors, chemokines, interferons and growth factors/neurotrophins. Members of each of these large families of polypeptides have been implicated in stroke, either as mediators of damage or as potential neuroprotective/neurotrophic factors. However, extensive review of all of these cytokines is well outside the scope of this review which will consider initially the major pro (IL-1, TNFα, IL-6) and anti-inflammatory (IL-1ra, IL-4, IL-10) cytokines, then focus primarily on the IL-1 family.

Pro- and anti-inflammatory cytokines in cerebral ischaemia

Available information on TNFα and IL-6 suggest conflicting actions of these cytokines. Both have been strongly implicated in host defense responses to injury and infection (eg fever, appetite suppression, see Rothwell and Hopkins 1995) and are recognised mediators of inflammation. TNFα and IL-6 (like most cytokines) are expressed at low levels in normal brain, but are upregulated rapidly in response to ischaemia or other insults (see Rothwell 1999).

Several studies have reported that acute administration of TNFα exacerbates ischaemic and traumatic brain damage, while inhibiting TNFα action, for example by administration of neutralising antibody or soluble receptor reduces injury (eg Nawashiro et al. 1996). However, in marked contrast to these data, mice lacking TNF receptors show increased ischaemic damage, and neuroprotective actions of TNF have

School of Biological Sciences, 1.124 Stopford Building, University of Manchester, Oxford Road, Manchester M13 9PT UK
e-mail: Nancy.Rothwell@man.ac.uk

J. Krieglstein, S. Klumpp (Eds.) Pharmacology of Cerebral Ischemia 2000

been observed (Bruce et al. 1996; Probert et al. 1997). Similar discrepancies exist for IL-6 which inhibits ischaemic and excitotoxic brain damage when injected acutely in rats (Loddick et al. 1998), yet chronic overexpression of IL-6 in the brains of transgenic mice leads to severe inflammation and neuronal loss (Campbell et al. 1993).

Injection of IL-10 reduces ischaemic brain damage (Dietrich et al. 1999; Spera et al. 1998), suggesting that this anti-inflammatory cytokine is an endogenous inhibitor of injury. Data for IL-4 are more limited and largely restricted to in vitro data (Chao et al. 1993; Omuri et al. 1996; Vannier et al. 1992).

In contrast to these conflicting data, considerable evidence now supports the role of IL-1 as a mediator of several forms of acute brain damage.

IL-1 family

The IL-1 family comprises the two ligands IL-1α and IL-1β and the naturally occurring receptor antagonist IL-1ra which blocks all known actions of IL-1 (see Dinarello 1998; Fantuzzi and Dinarello 1999; Hannum et al. 1998). All effects of IL-1 are believed to depend on binding to the IL-1RI (80kDa) receptor, which then interacts with a specific accessory protein (AcP) to recruit intracellular adaptor molecules and signal through MAP kinases and NFKβ (see Sims et al. 1993; O'Neill and Dinarello, 2000). Recently, five putative new members of the IL-1 family have been identified (Smith et al. 2000; Kumar et al. 2000), on the basis of sequence homology, though none bind to IL-1RI, and as yet their biological actions or involvement in CNS disease are unknown. IL-18 also shares homology with IL-1, acts through a related receptor (RrP) and accessory protein (AcPL), and shares common signalling mechanisms with IL-1 (Fantuzzi and Dinarello 1999). Pro-IL-18 is cleaved by the same enzyme as pro-IL-1β, caspase-1, to yield the active cytokine (see Fantuzzi and Dinarello 1999).

IL-1 in stroke

IL-1α and β, IL-1ra and caspase-1 are all upregulated rapidly after experimentally induced ischaemic brain damage in rodents (eg Davies et al. 1999; Legos et al. 2000; Touzani et al. 1999), and raised IL-1 and IL-1ra levels have been reported in human stroke patients (Touzani et al. 1999). Administration of IL-1 to the brains of normal rodents or to neurones in culture fails to cause cell death, but in vivo administration (icv) of low doses of IL-1 markedly exacerbates ischaemic and excitotoxic brain damage in the rat and mouse (see Rothwell et al. 1997; Rothwell 1999; Touzani et al. 1999).

A number of studies have now demonstrated that inhibiting the release or actions of IL-1 (eg by injection of anti-IL-1β antibody, or IL-1ra) markedly reduces damage (infarct volume and neuronal loss, oedema and neutrophil entry) in permanent or focal ischaemia in rodents (see Garcia et al. 1995; Rothwell 1999; Touzani et al. 1999). We have also found recently that in mice lacking the genes for IL-1α and IL-1β, ischaemic brain damage (reversible middle cerebral artery occlusion MCAo) is reduced by over 70% (Boutin and Rothwell, unpub data).

These data suggest that IL-1 is an important mediator of ischaemic brain damage, and a therapeutic target for clinical intervention. Since IL-1 has little role in normal brain function, it is unlikely that blocking its release or actions will have significant adverse effects.

Therapeutic targets in the IL-1 family (see Fig. 1)

Expression and release of IL-1

The major early source of IL-1 after cerebral ischaemica is microglia (Davies et al. 1999), which also express caspase-1. General inhibitors of microglial activation may prove beneficial in stroke and related conditions, through suppression of the release of IL-1 and other inflammatory and potentially neurotoxic factors.

At present the mechanisms leading to gene expression of IL-1, activation of caspase-1 and

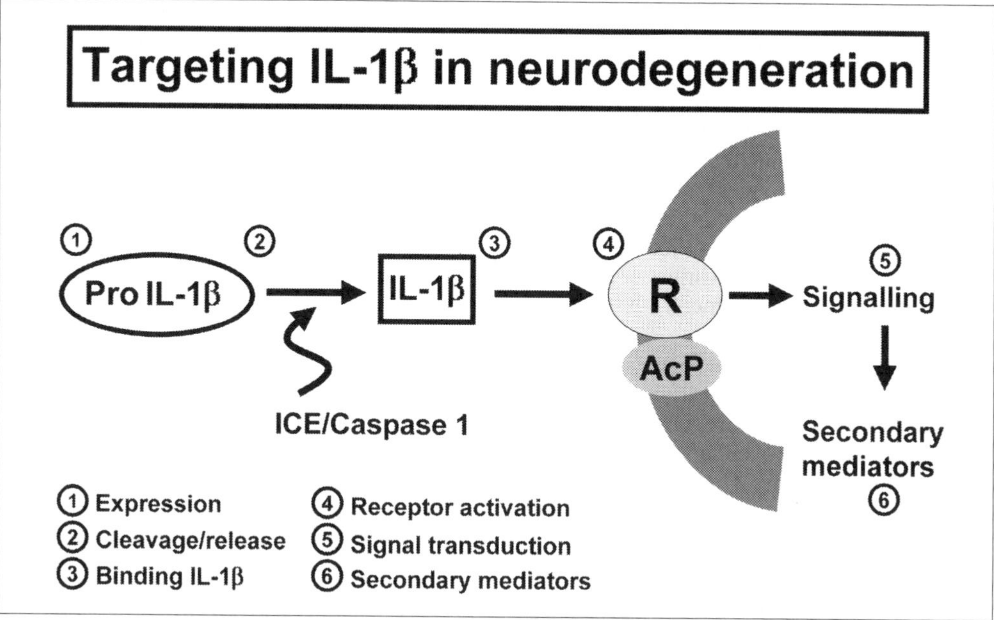

cleavage/cellular release of IL-1β are largely unknown. Neither IL-1α or β have a classical leader sequence required for cellular release, and while IL-1α remains largely intracellular, IL-1β is released from the cell (Fantuzzi and Dinarello 1999). In macrophages, activation of the purinergic P2x7 receptors by extracellular ATP leads to cleavage and release of IL-1β, and similar processes seem to operate in microglia (Ralevic and Burnstock 1998; Sanz and Virgilio, 2000). P2x7 receptor antagonists may therefore be neuroprotective.

In addition to IL-1, IL-1ra expression is also increased in response to cerebral ischaemia and acts as an endogenous inhibitor of IL-1 action and of ischaemic brain damage (Loddick et al. 1997). Thus, factors which inhibit the expression of IL-1 and/or enhance IL-1ra production are likely to be beneficial. Indeed, IL-41, IL-10 and cannabinoids may exert their reported neuroprotective effects (Louw et al. 2000; Nagayama et al. 1999, Vannier et al. 1992) through this mechanism.

Mice lacking the caspase-1 gene or expressing a dominant negative form of caspase-1 exhibit reduced ischaemic brain damage (Friedlander et al. 1997; Schielke et al. 1998). Thus, selective caspase-1 inhibition may be neuroprotective (Holtzman and Deshmukh 1997), though to date only non-selective or partially selective inhibitors have been reported (Endres et al. 1998; Hara et al. 1997; Loddick et al. 1996). However, caspase-1 also cleaves IL-18 (see above) and the actions of this cytokine in stroke are not yet reported.

IL-1 bioactivity

Both the main IL-1 signalling receptor (RI) and the second, non-signalling receptor (RII) can be shed from the membrane and bind IL-1, thus limiting its biological activity (see O'Neill and Dinarello, 2000). Such molecules, or neutralising antibodies to IL-1β, could therefore offer therapeutic benefit. However, these are very large molecules and are therefore unlikely to readily enter the brain from circulation.

IL-1 receptor blockade

The most effective means of experimentally blocking IL-1 actions and limiting stroke damage identified to date is by injection of recombinant IL-1ra (Hannum et al. 1990). This protein, which is approximately 17kDa in size, is effective when administered peripherally (Garcia et al. 1995), possibly because it can be actively transported into the brain (Gutierrez et al. 1994). IL-1ra is neuroprotective when administered up to 30–60 min after permanent focal MCAo in the rat, but for a least 6 h in other experimental forms of brain injury or ischaemia (see Relton et al. 1996; Rothwell 1999; Touzani et al. 1999).

IL-1ra has been used quite extensively in the treatment of rheumatoid arthritis with no significant adverse responses and no attenuation of biological activity (Bresnihan et al. 1998), suggesting that it is safe. However, high doses would probably be required in stroke in order to achieve brain penetration of effective doses. Thus, small molecule receptor antagonists may prove more practical in the long term.

To date the search for effective, small molecule IL-1 receptor antagonists has not been productive, probably due to the complexity of IL-1 interactions with its receptor. Molecules which block the interactions between RI and the AcP, or the recruitment of intracellular adaptor molecules such as MyD88, TRAF6 or IRAK may be effective, but would require cellular penetration.

Post-receptor targets

The signalling cascades involved in IL-1 action have been elucidated almost exclusively in non-neuronal cells, though there is some evidence for similar processes in the brain. Inhibitors of specific MAP kinases implicated in IL-1 signalling (O'Neill and Dinarello, 2000) should block IL-1 actions in the CNS. Indeed recently it has been reported that a p38 inhibitor markedly attenuates ischaemic brain damage in the rat (Barone et al. 2000).

Inhibition of downstream mediators of IL-1 action should also prove beneficial, though as yet the mechanisms of action of IL-1 have not been fully elucidated. Nitric oxide, corticotrophin releasing factor, bradykinin and free radical release have all be implicated in IL-1 actions (see Rothwell 1999; Touzani et al. 1999), and inhibition of the release or actions of each of these mediators can offer protection. However, targeting IL-1 actions downstream of its receptor inevitably means loss of specificity since the signalling pathways and putative mediators are all involved in other processes, some of which may be beneficial or necessary for normal brain function.

Clinical studies

No clinical studies on CNS disease have been conducted on agents which modify IL-1. Trials of IL-1ra in multiple sclerosis have recently begun and we will shortly commence a safety study to compare IL-1ra (administered intravenously within 6 hours of symptoms) and placebo in stroke patients. IL-1ra is undoubtedly the most advanced approach to modify IL-1 action, is safe and has been administered to patients with rheumatoid arthritis (Bresnihan et al. 1998). However, its molecular size means that second generation, small molecule inhibitors of IL-1 release or action may be more useful. As yet therapeutic targets for other cytokines remain uncertain, and some may have both protective and detrimental effects and/or may not readily gain access to the CNS.

References

1. Barone FC, Irving EA, Ray AM, Lee JC, Kassis S, Kumar S, Badger AM, Legos JJ, Erhardt JA, Ohlstein EH, Hunter AJ, Harrison DC, Philpott K, Smith BR, Adams JL, Parsons AA (2000) Inhibition of p38 mitogen-activated protein kinase provides neuroprotection in cerebral focal ischaemia. Med Res Rev, in press
2. Bresnihan B, Alvaro-Gracia JM, Cobby M, Doherty M, Domljan Z, Emery P, Nuki G, Pavelka K, Rau R, Rozman B, Watt I, Williams B, Aitchison R, McCabe D, Musikic P (1998) Treatment of rheumatoid arthritis with recombinant human interleukin-1 receptor antagonist. Arthritis and Rheumatism 41:2196–2204
3. Bruce AJ, Boling WB, Kindy MS, Paschon J, Kroener PJ, Carpenter MK, Holtsberg PW, Mattson MP (1996) Altered neuronal and microglial responses to excitotoxic and ischaemic brain injury in mice lacking TNF receptors. Nature Med 2:788–794
4. Campbell IL, Abraham CR, Masliah E, Kemper P, Inglis JD, Oldstone MB, Mucke L (1993) Neurologic disease induced in transgenic mice by cerebral overexpression of interleukin-6. Proc Natl Acad Sci USA 90:10061–10065

5. Chao CC, Molitor TW, Hu S (1993) Neuroprotective role of IL-4 against activated microglia. J Immunol 151:1473–1481
6. Davies CA, Loddick SA, Toulmond S, Stroemer RP, Hunt J, Rothwell NJ (1999) The progression and topographic distribution of interleukin-1beta expression after permanent middle cerebral artery occlusion in the rat. J Cereb Blood Flow Metab 19:87–98
7. Dietrich WD, Busto R, Bethea JR (1999) Postischaemic hypothermia and IL-10 treatment provide long lasting neuroprotection of CA1 hippocampus following transient global ischaemia in rats. Exp Neurol 158:444–450
8. Dinarello CA (1998) Interleukin-1, interleukin-1 receptors and interleukin-1 receptor antagonist. Int Rev Immunol 16:457–499
9. Endres M, Namura S, Shimizu-Sasamata M, Waeber C, Zhang L, Gomez-Isla T, Hyman B, Moskowitz MA (1998) Attenuation of delayed neuronal death after mild focal ischaemia in mice by inhibition of the caspase family. J Cereb Blood Flow Metab 18:238–247
10. Fantuzzi G, Dinarello CA (1999) Interleukin-18 and interleukin-1 beta: two cytokine substrates for ICE (caspase-1). J Clin Immunol 19:1–11
11. Friedlander RM, Gagliardini V, Hara H, Fink KB, Li W, MacDonald G, Fishman MC, Greenberry AH, Moskowitz MA, Yan Y (1997) Expression of a dominant negative mutant of interleukin-1β converting enzyme in transgenic mice prevents neuronal cell death induced by trophic factor withdrawal and ischaemic brain injury. J Exp Med 185:933–940
12. Garcia JH, Lui K-F, Relton JK (1995) Interleukin-1 receptor antagonist decreases the number of necrotic neurones in rats with middle cerebral artery occlusion. Am J Pathol 147:1477–1486
13. Gutierrez EG, Banks WA, Kastin AJ (1994) Blood-borne interleukin-1 receptor antagonist crosses the blood brain barrier. J Neuroimmunol 55:153–160
14. Hannum CH, Wilcox CJ, Arend WP, Joslin FG, Dripps DJ, Heimdal PL, Armes LG, Sommer A, Eisenberg SP,Thompson RC (1998) Interleukin-1 receptor antagonist activity of a human interleukin-1 inhibitor. Nature 434:336–340
15. Hara H, Friedlander RM, Gagliardini V, Ayata C, Fink K, Huang Z, Shimizu-Sasamata M, Yuan J, Moskowitz MA (1997) Inhibition of interleukin-1 beta converting enzyme family proteases reduces ischaemic and excitotoxic neuronal damage. Proc Natl Acad Sci USA 94:2007–2012
16. Holtzman DM, Deshmukh M (1997) Caspases: a treatment target for neurodegenerative diseases? Nature Medicine 3:954–955
17. Kumar S, McDonnell PC, Lehr R, Tierney L, Tzimas MN, Griswold DE, Capper EA, Tal-Singer R, Wells GI, Doyle ML, Young PR (2000) Identification and initial characterization of four novel members of the interleukin-1 family. J Biol Chem 275:10308–10314
18. Legos JJ, Whitmore RG, Erhardt JA, Parsons AA, Tuma RF, Barone FC (2000) Quantitative changes in interleukin-1 proteins following focal stroke in the rat. Neurosci Lett 282:189–192
19. Loddick SA, MacKenzie A, Rothwell NJ (1996) An ICE inhibitor, z-VAD-DCB attenuates ischaemic brain damage in the rat. NeuroReport 7:1465–1468
20. Loddick SA, Wong M-L, Bongiorno PB, Gold PW, Licinio J, Rothwell NJ (1997) Endogenous interleukin-1 receptor antagonist is neuroprotective. Biochem Biophys Rev Comm 234:211–215
21. Loddick SA, Turnbull AV, Rothwell NJ (1998) Cerebral interleukin-6 is neuroprotective during permanent focal cerebral ischaemia in the rat. J Cereb Blood Flow Metab 18:176–179
22. Louw DF, Yang FW, Sutherland GR (2000) The effect of delta-9-tetrahydrocannabinol on forebrain ischaemia in rat. Brain Res 857:183–187
23. Nagayama T, Sinor AD, Simon RP, Chen J, Graham SH, Jin K, Greenberg DA (1999) Cannabinoids and neuroprotection in global and focal cerebral ischaemia and in neuronal cultures. J Neurosci 19:2987–2995
24. Nawashiro H, Martin D, Hallenbeck JM (1996) Inhibition of tumour necrosis factor and amerlioration of brain infarction in mice. J Cereb Blood Flow Metab 72:1–4
25. O'Neill LA, Dinarello CA (2000) The IL-1 receptor/toll-like receptor superfamily: crucial receptors for inflammation and host defense. Imunol Today 21:206–209
26. Omuri Y, Smith MF, Hamilton TA (1996) IL-4 induced expression of the IL-1 receptor antagonist gene is mediated by STAT6. J Immunol 57:2058–2065
27. Probert L, Akassoglou K, Kassiotis G, Pasparakis M, Alexopoulou L, Kollias G (1997) TNF-α transgenic and knockout models of CNS inflammation and degeneration. J Neuroimmunol 72:137–141
28. Ralevic V, Burnstock G (1998) Receptors for purines and pyrimidines. Pharmacol Rev 50:413–493
29. Relton JK, Martin D, Thompson RC, Russell DA (1996) Peripheral administration of interleukin-1 receptor antagonist inhibits brain damage after focal cerebral ischaemia in the rat. Exp Neurol 138:206–213
30. Rothwell NJ, Hopkins SJ (1995) Cytokines and the nervous system II: Actions and mechanisms of action. TiNS 18:130–136
31. Rothwell NJ (1999) Cytokines – killers in the brain? J Physiol 514:3–17
32. Rothwell NJ, Allan S, Toulmond S (1997) Cytokines and the brain: the role of interleukin-1 in acute neurodegeneration and stroke: pathophysiological and therapeutic implications. J Clin Invest 100:2648–2652
33. Sanz JM, Virgilio FD (2000) Kinetics and mechanism of ATP-dependent IL-1beta release from microglial cells. J Immunol 164:4893–4898
34. Schielke GP, Yang GY, Shivers BD, Betz AL (1998) Reduced ischaemic brain injury in interleukin-1 beta converting enzyme-deficient mice. J Cereb Blood Flow Metab 18:180–185
35. Sims JE, Gayle MA, Slack JL, Alderson MR, Bird TA, Giri JG, Colotta F, Re F, Mantovani A, Shanebeck K (1993) Interleukin 1 signalling occurs exclusively via the type I receptor. Proc Natl Acad Sci USA 90:6155–6159
36. Smith DE, Renshaw BR, Ketchem RR, Kubin M, Garka KE, Sims JE (2000) Four new members expand the interlukin-1 superfamily. J Biol Chem 275:1169–1175
37. Spera PA, Ellison JA, Feuerstein GZ, Barone FC (1998) IL-10 reduces rat brain injury following focal stroke. Neurosci Lett 251:189–192
38. Touzani O, Boutin H, Chequet J, Rothwell NJ (1999) Potential mechanisms of interleukin-1 involvement in cerebral ischaemia. J Neuroimmunol 100:203–215
39. Vannier E, Miller LC, Dinarello CA (1992) Coordinated anti-inflammatory effects of interleukin-4: interleukin-4 suppresses interleukin-1 production but up-regulates gene expression and synthesis of interleukin-1 receptor antagonist. Proc Natl Acad Sci USA 98:4076–4080

Inflammatory and anti-inflammatory cytokines and neuronal cell death

S. A Loddick

Abstract

Cytokines are a family of polypeptide mediators associated with the immune system and inflammation in the periphery. Despite the fact that the brain was often thought of as an immune privileged site, it is now well established that cytokines are involved in various neurodegenerative conditions. Cytokines are often categorised as either pro- or anti-inflammatory, however in the brain such distinctions may prove misleading. The role of interleukin-6 and tumor necrosis factor-α in neuronal death is far from clear, with both damaging and protective actions attributed to each of these cytokines. However, it is now well established that interleukin-1 mediates neuronal death in experimentally induced brain injury in vivo, and that inhibiting the actions of interleukin-1 will reduce ischaemic brain injury.

Cytokines

Cytokines are a diverse group of polypeptides that include interleukins (IL), tumor necrosis factors (TNF), interferons, colony stimulating factors, chemokines and growth factors. Although originally thought of as intercellular messengers in the immune system, it is now recognised that cytokines have multiple cellular sources, targets and functions outside the immune system.

Cytokines are often categorised as either pro or anti-inflammatory, a classification that is based largely on their actions within the periphery. Interleukins-1 and 6 and TNF-α are generally thought of as pro-inflammatory, whereas IL-4 and IL-10 are considered anti-inflammatory (see Rothwell and Hopkins 1995).

Many members of this family have been implicated in the pathogenesis of neurodegenerative conditions, with the role of cytokines in stroke being particularly well studied. In these circumstances the classification of cytokines as either pro- or anti-inflammatory may be over-simplified since both IL-6 and TNF appear to produce conflicting actions on neurodegeneration. The present review will focus on the role of these cytokines in the ischaemic brain.

Anti-inflammatory cytokines and neuronal death

There are relatively few data describing the effects of the anti-inflammatory cytokines IL-4 and IL-10. In keeping with its anti-inflammato-

Keywords: Interleukin-1, interleukin-1 receptor antagonist, interleukin-6, tumor necrosis factor-α, cerebral ischaemia, cytokines.

School of Biological Sciences, 1.124, Stopford Building, University of Manchester, Oxford Road, Manchester M13 9PT UK
e-mail: sarah.loddick@man.ac.uk

ry actions IL-4 appears to have protective effects in the inflammatory condition experimental allergic encephalomyelitis (EAE) (Falcone et al. 1998). Mice in which the gene for IL-4 has been deleted (IL-4 knock-out mice) develop a more severe form of EAE which is associated with elevated levels of inflammatory cytokines compared to their wild-type. Interestingly the recovery rate of the IL-4 knock-out mice was no different from the wild-type (Falcone et al. 1998). Neurotrophic/neuroprotective actions of IL-4 have been described in vitro (Araujo and Cotman 1993; Chao et al. 1993), but as yet there are no published reports describing the effect of this cytokine on experimental brain damage in vivo.

The expression of interleukin-10 in the brain is increased in several experimental and clinical neurodegenerative conditions (Tarkowski et al. 1997; Bell et al. 1997; Morganti-Kossman et al. 1997; Tarkowski et al. 1999; Csuka et al. 1999). This increased expression may be of benefit to the injured brain since IL-10 prevents EAE relapses in rats (Crisi et al. 1995) and improves outcome after ischaemic and traumatic brain injury (Spera et al. 1998; Knoblach and Faden 1998; Dietrich et al. 1999).

There is considerable evidence supporting a neuroprotective role for the anti-inflammatory cytokine IL-1 receptor antagonist (see below), and in fact the protective effects of IL-4 and IL-10 may be mediated via modulation of IL-1ra expression (Vannier et al. 1992).

Most studies have focussed on the role of the pro-inflammatory cytokines in brain injury, where conflicting data still exist.

Pro-inflammatory cytokines and neuronal death

Tumor necrosis factor α

Tumor necrosis factor α is a prototypical pro-inflammatory cytokine, that mediates tissue injury and inflammation (see Rothwell and Hopkins 1995). The expression of TNF-α in the brain is increased in several experimental and clinical neurodegenerative conditions (see Barone and Feuerstein 1999). In experimentally induced cerebral ischaemia (middle cerebral artery occlusion, MCAO) in rats, elevated expression of TNF-α mRNA and protein as early as 1 h has been reported (Liu et al. 1994; Wang et al. 1994; Buttini et al. 1996; Botchkina et al. 1997). However the impact of this elevated expression of TNF-α is unclear since there are conflicting data about the role of TNF-α in the injured brain. TNF-α protects cultured rat brain neurones from various forms of excitotoxic and metabolic injury (Cheng et al. 1994; Barger et al. 1995a; Barger et al. 1995b; Bruce-Keller et al. 1999). Some in vivo studies support these findings since pre-treatment with TNF-α can induce a state of "resistance", protecting the brain from subsequent ischaemic injury (Nawashiro et al. 1997a). Further support is derived from studies using mice in which the gene for one or both of the TNF receptors has been deleted. TNF-α binds to two different receptors, the p55 and the p75 receptor, both of which are present in brain (Kinouchi et al. 1991; Cheng et al. 1994). Mice lacking the p55 receptor have increased ischaemic and excitotoxic injury compared to wild-type, or mice lacking the p75 form (Bruce et al. 1996; Gary et al. 1998). These data suggest that TNF-α may protect the brain via activation of the p55 receptor. However, these studies do not necessarily indicate the role of TNF-α per se, and there are several studies to suggest that increased expression of TNF-α may be damaging to the injured brain. Injection of TNF-α into the brain 1day before MCAO results in increased neuronal death (Barone et al. 1997) in comparison to the previous study describing protective effects with 48 h pre-treatment (Nawashiro et al. 1997a). This study and several others have also demonstrated that inhibition of the effects of endogenous TNF-α by injection of a TNF antibody, soluble receptor or binding protein result in reduced damage after ischaemic and traumatic brain injury in rodents (Shohami et al. 1996; Barone et al. 1997; Meistrell III et al. 1997; Nawashiro et al. 1997b, 1997c; Yang et al. 1998; Lavine et al. 1998; Knoblach et al. 1999; Yang et al. 1999a). Taken together these latter studies appear to indicate that TNF-α is damaging to the injured brain, apparently in direct conflict with the data from TNF receptor knockouts (Bruce et al. 1996; Gary et al. 1998). Studies utilising mice which lack the gene for TNF (TNF knock-out) suggest that *endogenous* TNF may indeed have opposing actions on neuronal injury. When subjected to cortical impact injury, the TNF knock-out mice initially perform better than their wild-type (based on tests of memory or motor function) but when assessed 2–4 weeks later the TNF knock-out mice showed less functional recovery and greater neuronal cell loss than the wild-type (Scherbel et al. 1999). These data suggest that TNF-α may initially contribute to neuronal degeneration, but in the later stages may be important in recovery. Clearly the effect of TNF on damaged neurones is very complex, and its precise role in brain injury is still unclear. Similarly controversial data exist for the role of IL-6 in neurodegeneration.

Interleukin-6

The actions of IL-6 are very similar to those of the prototypical inflammatory cytokine IL-1, and IL-6 actually mediates some of the effects of IL-1 (Rothwell and Hopkins 1995). However, in some respects IL-6 acts as an anti-inflammatory cytokine (Tilg et al 1997), and in the brain, both neurotrophic and neurodegenerative effects of this cytokine have been described. Increased expression of IL-6 occurs in a variety of CNS disorders, including clinical and experimental cerebral ischaemia (Wang et al. 1995; Tarkowski et al. 1995; Martin-Ancel et al. 1997; Loddick et al. 1998; Clark et al. 1999; Suzuki et al. 1999; Yang et al. 1999b; Ali et al. 2000). Transgenic mice over-expressing IL-6 in the brain develop profound neuropathology implicating IL-6 in the pathology of CNS disorders (Campbell et al. 1993; Steffensen et al. 1994; Chiang et al. 1994; Heyser et al. 1997). However, there are data to suggest that IL-6 may protect the brain from injury. IL-6 is a neurotrophic factor (Hama et al. 1989, 1991; Kushima et al. 1992; Kushima and Hatanaka 1992; Hirota et al. 1996; Thier et al. 1999) and it increases regeneration after peripheral nerve injury (Hirota et al. 1996). Furthermore, IL-6 reduces excitotoxin-induced neuronal death in vitro and in vivo, and prevents delayed neuronal loss after forebrain ischaemia (Toulmond et al. 1992; Yamada and Hatanaka 1994; Maeda et al. 1994; Matsuda et al. 1996; Ali et al. 2000). None of these data describe the role of *endogenous* IL-6 in brain injury, and even recent studies using IL-6 knock-out mice have yielded conflicting data. Whilst one study described a compromised inflammatory reaction and increased neuronal death after cryo injury in the IL-6 deficient mice (Penkowa et al. 1999), a separate study found the IL-6 knock-out mice were no different in their susceptibility to ischaemic brain injury after middle cerebral artery occlusion (Clark et al. 2000). Knock-out animals are not ideal for investigating the role of an endogenous cytokine, as alternative mediators may compensate for the loss. Investigations into the role of *endogenous* IL-6 have been limited by the lack of selective inhibitors of IL-6 appropriate for use in vivo. Because of this, we used an alternative approach to investigate the role of IL-6 in brain ischaemia. We measured brain IL-6 bioactivity after MCAO in order to determine an appropriate dose of recombinant IL-6 to test in ischaemic rats. Ischaemia, caused by permanent occlusion of the middle cerebral artery, resulted in a significant increase in IL-6 bioactivity as early as 2 h after the insult with further increases observed at the later time-points studied (8 and 24 h, see Fig. 1A, Loddick et al. 1998). We subsequently tested the effects of injecting IL-6 at doses similar to those detected in the ischaemic hemisphere. IL-6 caused a dramatic reduction in the lesion volume assessed 24 h after MCAO (see Fig. 1B, Loddick et al. 1998). These data taken with data from previous studies suggest that acute increases in brain IL-6 may be of benefit to the injured brain. Although our study does not indicate the role of endogenous IL-6 in brain injury, our finding that physiologically relevant doses of IL-6 reduce ischaemic brain injury (Loddick et al. 1998) suggest that IL-6 may be an endogenous neuroprotective agent.

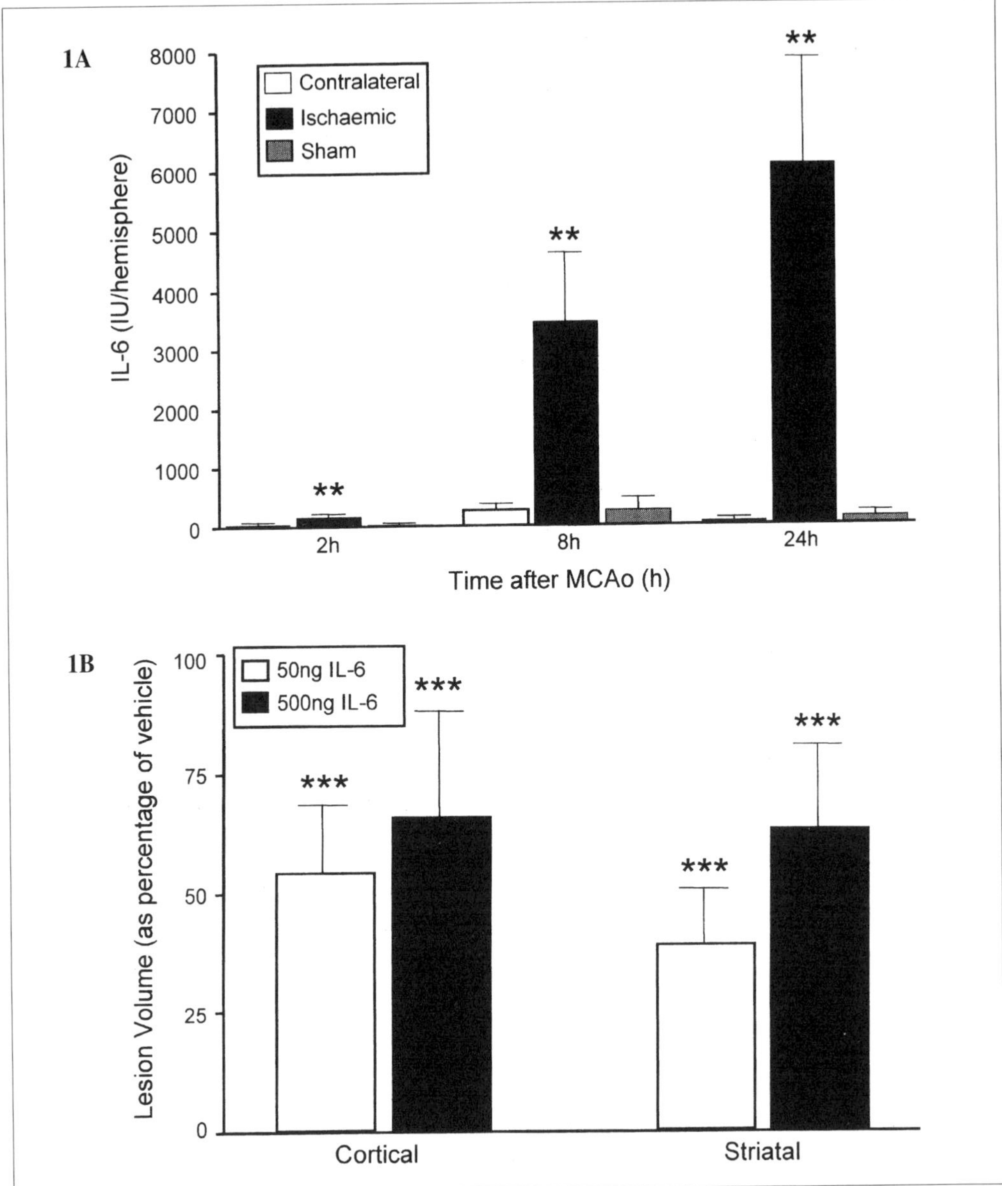

Fig. 1. The role of interleukin-6 in ischaemic brain damage.
1A: Data are presented as the amount of IL-6 biactivity (mean of 4–5 animals ± SD) detected in hemisphere homogenates at different times after MCAO or sham surgery. ** $p < 0.01$ versus the contralateral hemisphere.

1B: Data are presented as mean lesion volume (as percentage of vehicle treated animals) measured 24 h after middle cerebral artery occlusion (MCAO) in rats injected icv with either saline (4 µl, n = 9), 50 ng rhIL-6 (n = 8) or 500 ng rhIL-6 (n = 8) 30 min before and 15 min after MCAo. Values denote the mean, and error bars indicate SD.
*** $p<0.001$ versus saline-treated group.

Interleukin-1

Interleukin-1 is perhaps the most studied cytokine in terms of its role in neuronal death. The term interleukin-1 refers to a family of proteins which consists of two agonists, IL-1α and IL-1β and an IL-1 receptor antagonist (IL-1ra). The two agonists elicit very similar actions, presumably because they act on the same cell surface receptors (see Dinarello 1991). Most studies investigating the role of IL-1 in neuronal death have focused on the beta form, and expression of IL-1β is increased in response to numerous neurodegenerative conditions including cerebral ischaemia (see Rothwell and Hopkins 1995; Hopkins and Rothwell 1995; Touzani et al. 1999). IL-1 was initially thought to be of benefit to the injured brain since it elicits neuronal sprouting, neovascularisation and induction of nerve growth factor synthesis (Giulian et al. 1988; Spranger et al. 1990; Fagan and Gage 1990). Indeed, protective effects of IL-1 in neuronal cultures have been described (Strijbos and Rothwell 1995; Carlson et al. 1999). However higher doses cause time- and dose-dependent neurodegeneration, particularly when in combination with other cytokines (Chao et al. 1995; Hu et al. 1997; Jeohn et al. 1998). Consistent with these detrimental effects of IL-1 in vitro, numerous studies in vivo indicate that although injection of IL-1 appears to have minimal effects on neuronal survival in normal brain (Andersson et al. 1992; Lawrence et al. 1998), injection of IL-1β exacerbates ischaemic and excitotoxic brain damage in the rat (Yan et al. 1992; Minami et al. 1992; Yamasaki et al. 1995; Loddick and Rothwell 1996; Rothwell et al. 1997; Allan et al. 1998; Lawrence et al. 1998; Grundy et al. 1999; Allan et al. 2000). There is now considerable evidence derived from in vivo studies to indicate that *endogenous* IL-1 mediates neuronal death in a variety of CNS insults. Inhibition of IL-1 action reduces injury caused by ischaemic, hypoxic, traumatic and excitotoxic insults as well as seizure related brain damage and EAE (see Martin et al. 1998) implicating IL-1 in the progression of all these neurodegenerative conditions. Much of this evidence is derived from studies using administration of recombinant IL-1ra either by direct injection or viral delivery into the brain to inhibit IL-1 actions. Together these studies have demonstrated that IL-1ra can protect the adult mouse; gerbil and rat brain and the neonatal rat brain from global and focal (permanent and transient) brain ischaemia (see Martin et al. 1998; Touzani et al. 1999). This compelling data is further supported by our finding that endogenous brain IL-1ra is a neuroprotective agent, since IL-1ra synthesis is increased in the brain after cerebral ischaemia, and administration of an anti-IL-1ra antiserum exacerbates neuronal death (Loddick et al. 1997).

Thus, although the effects of IL-1 in the CNS are complex, and dependent on the state of activation of the CNS cells, there is clear and consistent evidence that inhibiting the effects of IL-1 can protect the brain from ischaemia. This has led to the consideration of IL-1 inhibitors as a treatment for stroke, which is discussed in more detail in a chapter by Professor Nancy Rothwell.

References

1. Ali C, Nicole O, Docagne F, Lesne S, MacKenzie ET, Nouvelot A, Buisson A, Vivien D (2000) Ischemia-induced interleukin-6 as a potential endogenous neuroprotective cytokine against NMDA receptor-mediated excitotoxicity in the brain. J Cereb Blood Flow Metab 20:956–966
2. Allan SM, Lawrence CB, Rothwell NJ (1998) Interleukin-1 beta and interleukin-1 receptor antagonist do not affect glutamate release or calcium entry in rat striatal synaptosomes. Mol Psychiatry 3:178–182
3. Allan SM, Parker LC, Collins B, Davies R, Luheshi GN, Rothwell NJ (2000) Cortical cell death induced by IL-1 is mediated via actions in the hypothalamus of the rat. Proc Natl Acad Sci USA 97:5580–5585
4. Andersson PB, Perry VH, Gordon S (1992) Intracerebral injection of proinflammatory cytokines or leukocyte chemotaxins induces minimal myelomonocytic cell recruitment to the parenchyma of the central nervous system. J Exp Med 176:255–259
5. Araujo DM, Cotman CW (1993) Trophic effects of interleukin-4, -7 and -8 on hippocampal neuronal cultures: potential involvement of glial-derived factors. Brain Res 600:49–55
6. Barger SW, Horster D, Furukawa K, Goodman Y, Krieglstein J, Mattson MP (1995b) Tumor necrosis factors alpha and beta protect neurons against amyloid beta-peptide toxicity: evidence for involvement of a kappa B-binding factor and attenuation of peroxide and Ca^{2+} accumulation. Proc Natl Acad Sci USA 92:9328–9332
7. Barger SW, Hörster D, Furukawa K, Goodman Y, Krieglstein J, Mattson MP (1995a) Tumor necrosis factor α and β protect neurons against amyloid β-peptide toxicity: evidence for involvement of a kB-binding factor and attenuation of peroxide and Ca^{2+} accumulation. Proc Natl Acad Sci USA 92:9328–9332

8. Barone FC, Arvin B, White RF, Miller A, Webb CL, Willette RN, Lysko PG, Feuerstein GZ (1997) Tumor necrosis factor-alpha. A mediator of focal ischemic brain injury. Stroke 28:1233–1244
9. Barone FC, Feuerstein GZ (1999) Inflammatory mediators and stroke: new opportunities for novel therapeutics. J Cereb Blood Flow Metab 19:819–834
10. Bell MJ, Kochanek PM, Doughty LA, Carcillo JA, Adelson PD, Clark RSB, Wisniewski SR, Whalen MJ, DeKosky ST (1997) Interleukin-6 and interleukin-10 in cerebrospinal fluid after severe traumatic brain injury in children. Journal of Neurotrauma 14:451–457
11. Botchkina GI, Meistrell ME, III, Botchkina IL, Tracey KJ (1997) Expression of TNF and TNF receptors (p55 and p75) in the rat brain after focal cerebral ischemia. Mol Med 3:765–781
12. Bruce-Keller AJ, Geddes JW, Knapp PE, McFall RW, Keller JN, Holtsberg FW, Parthasarathy S, Steiner SM, Mattson MP (1999) Anti-death properties of TNF against metabolic poisoning: mitochondrial stabilization by MnSOD. J Neuroimmunol 93:53–71
13. Bruce AJ, Boling W, Kindy MS, Peschon J, Kraemer PJ, Carpenter MK, Holtsberg FW, Mattson MP (1996) Altered neuronal and microglial responses to excitotoxic and ischemic brain injury in mice lacking TNF receptors. Nat Med 2:788–794
14. Buttini M, Appel K, Sauter A, Gebicke-Haerter PJ, Boddeke HW (1996) Expression of tumor necrosis factor alpha after focal cerebral ischaemia in the rat. Neuroscience 71:1–16
15. Campbell IL, Abraham CR, Masliah E, Kemper P, Inglis JD, Oldstone MB, Mucke L (1993) Neurologic disease induced in transgenic mice by cerebral overexpression of interleukin 6. Proc Natl Acad Sci USA 90:10061–10065
16. Carlson NG, Wieggel WA, Chen J, Bacchi A, Rogers SW, Gahring LC (1999) Inflammatory cytokines IL-1 alpha, IL-1 beta, IL-6, and TNF-alpha impart neuroprotection to an excitotoxin through distinct pathways. J Immunol 163:3963–3968
17. Chao CC, Hu S, Ehrlich L, Peterson PK (1995) Interleukin-1 and tumor necrosis factor-alpha synergistically mediate neurotoxicity: involvement of nitric oxide and of N-methyl-D-aspartate receptors. Brain Behav Immun 9:355–365
18. Chao CC, Molitor TW, Hu S (1993) Neuroprotective role of IL-4 against activated microglia. J Immunol 151:1473–1481
19. Cheng B, Christakos S, Mattson MP (1994) Tumor necrosis factors protect neurons against metabolic- excitotoxic insults and promote maintenance of calcium homeostasis. Neuron 12:139–153
20. Chiang CS, Stalder A, Samimi A, Campbell IL (1994) Reactive gliosis as a consequence of interleukin-6 expression in the brain: studies in transgenic mice. Developmental Neuroscience 16:212–221
21. Clark WM, Rinker LG, Lessov NS, Hazel K, Eckenstein F (1999) Time course of IL-6 expression in experimental CNS ischemia. Neurol Res 21:287–292
22. Clark WM, Rinker LG, Lessov NS, Hazel K, Hill JK, Stenzel-Poore M, Eckenstein F (2000) Lack of Interleukin-6 expression is not protective against focal central nervous system ischemia. Stroke 31:1715–1720
23. Crisi GM, Santambrogio L, Hochwald GM, Smith SR, Carlino JA, Thorbecke GJ (1995) Staphylococcal enterotoxin B and tumor-necrosis factor-alpha-induced relapses of experimental allergic encephalomyelitis: protection by transforming growth factor-beta and interleukin-10. Eur J Immunol 25:3035–3040
24. Csuka E, Morganti-Kossmann MC, Lenzlinger PM, Joller H, Trentz O, Kossmann T (1999) IL-10 levels in cerebrospinal fluid and serum of patients with severe traumatic brain injury: relationship to IL-6, TNF-alpha, TGF-beta1 and blood-brain barrier function. J Neuroimmunol 101:211–221
25. Dietrich WD, Busto R, Bethea JR (1999) Postischemic hypothermia and IL-10 treatment provide long-lasting neuroprotection of CA1 hippocampus following transient global ischemia in rats. Exp Neurol 158:444–450
26. Dinarello CA (1991) Interleukin-1 and interleukin-1 antagonism. Blood 77:1627–1652
27. Fagan AM, Gage FH (1990) Cholinergic sprouting in the hippocampus: a proposed role for IL-1. Exp Neurol 110:105–120
28. Falcone M, Rajan AJ, Bloom BR, Brosnan CF (1998) A critical role for IL-4 in regulating disease severity in experimental allergic encephalomyelitis as demonstrated in IL-4-deficient C57BL/6 mice and BALB/c mice. J Immunol 160:4822–4830
29. Gary DS, Bruce-Keller AJ, Kindy MS, Mattson MP (1998) Ischemic and excitotoxic brain injury is enhanced in mice lacking the p55 tumor necrosis factor receptor. J Cereb Blood Flow Metab 18:1283–1287
30. Giulian D, Woodward J, Young DG, Krebs JF, Lachman LB (1988) Interleukin-1 injected into mammalian brain stimulates astrogliosis and neovascularisation. J Neurosci 8:2485–2490
31. Grundy RI, Rothwell NJ, Allan SM (1999) Dissociation between the effects of interleukin-1 on excitotoxic brain damage and body temperature in the rat. Brain Res 830:32–37
32. Hama T, Kushima Y, Miyamoto M, Kubota M, Takei N, Hatanaka H (1991) Interleukin-6 improves the survival of mesencephalic catecholaminergic and septal cholinergic neurons from postnatal, two-week-old rats in cultures. Neuroscience 40:445–452
33. Hama T, Miyamoto M, Tsukui H, Nishio C, Hatanaka H (1989) Interleukin-6 as a neurotrophic factor for promoting the survival of cultured basal forebrain cholinergic neurons from postnatal rats. Neurosci Lett 104:340–344
34. Heyser CJ, Masliah E, Samimi A, Campbell IL, Gold LH (1997) Progressive decline in avoidance learning paralleled by inflammatory neurodegeneration in transgenic mice expressing interleukin 6 in the brain. Proc Natl Acad Sci USA 94:1500–1505
35. Hirota H, Kiyama H, Kishimoto T, Taga T (1996) Accelerated nerve regeneration in mice by upregulated expression of interleukin (IL) 6 and IL-6 receptor after trauma. J Exp Med 183:2627–2634
36. Hopkins SJ, Rothwell NJ (1995) Cytokines and the nervous system I: expression and recognition. Trends in Neurosciences 18:83–88
37. Hu S, Peterson PK, Chao CC (1997) Cytokine-mediated neuronal apoptosis. Neurochemistry International 30:427–431
38. Jeohn GH, Kong LY, Wilson B, Hudson P, Hong JS (1998) Synergistic neurotoxic effects of combined treatments with cytokines in murine primary mixed neuron/glia cultures. J Neuroimmunol 85:1–10
39. Kinouchi K, Brown G, Pasternak G, Donner DB (1991) Identification and characterization of receptors for tumor necrosis factor-α in the brain. Biochem Biophys Res Commun 181:1532–1538
40. Knoblach SM, Faden AI (1998) Interleukin-10 improves outcome and alters proinflammatory cytokine expression after experimental traumatic brain injury. Exp Neurol 153:143–151
41. Knoblach SM, Fan L, Faden AI (1999) Early neuronal expression of tumor necrosis factor-alpha after experimental brain injury contributes to neurological impairment. J Neuroimmunol 95:115–125
42. Kushima Y, Hama T, Hatanaka H (1992) Interleukin-6 as a neurotrophic factor for promoting the survival of cultured catecholaminergic neurons in a chemically defined medium. Neuroscience Research 13:267–280
43. Kushima Y, Hatanaka H (1992) Interleukin-6 and leukemia inhibitory factor promote survival of acetylcholinesterase-positive neurons in culture from embryonic rat spinal cord. Neurosci Lett 143:110–114

44. Lavine SD, Hofman FM, Zlokovic BV (1998) Circulating antibody against tumor necrosis factor-alpha protects rat brain from reperfusion injury. J Cereb Blood Flow Metab 18:52–58
45. Lawrence CB, Allan SM, Rothwell NJ (1998) Interleukin-1beta and the interleukin-1 receptor antagonist act in the striatum to modify excitotoxic brain damage in the rat. Eur J Neurosci 10:1188–1195
46. Liu T, Clark RK, McDonnell PC, Young PR, White RF, Barone FC, Feuerstein GZ (1994) Tumor necrosis factor-alpha expression in ischemic neurons. Stroke 25:1481–1488
47. Loddick SA, Rothwell NJ (1996) Neuroprotective effects of human recombinant interleukin-1 receptor antagonist in focal cerebral ischaemia in the rat. J Cereb Blood Flow Metab 16:932–940
48. Loddick SA, Turnbull AV, Rothwell NJ (1998) Cerebral interleukin-6 is neuroprotective during permanent focal cerebral ischemia in the rat. J Cereb Blood Flow Metab 18:176–179
49. Loddick SA, Wong ML, Bongiorno PB, Gold PW, Licinio J, Rothwell NJ (1997) Endogenous interleukin-1 receptor antagonist is neuroprotective. Biochemical and Biophysical Research Communications 234:211–215
50. Maeda Y, Matsumoto M, Hori O, Kuwabara K, Ogawa S, Yan SD, Ohtsuki T, Kinoshita T, Kamada T, Stern DM (1994) Hypoxia/reoxygenation-mediated induction of astrocyte interleukin 6: a paracrine mechanism potentially enhancing neuron survival. J Exp Med 180:2297–2308
51. Martin-Ancel A, Garcia-Alix A, Pascual-Salcedo D, Cabanas F, Valcarce M, Quero J (1997) Interleukin-6 in the cerebrospinal fluid after perinatal asphyxia is related to early and late neurological manifestations. Pediatrics 100:789–794
52. Martin D, Miller G, Neuberger T, Relton J, Fischer N (1998) Role of IL-1 in neurodegeneration. Pre-clinical findings with IL-1ra and ICE inhibitors. In: Neuroinflammation: mechanisms and management (Wood PL, eds), Totowa, Humana Press Inc, pp 197–219
53. Matsuda S, Wen TC, Morita F, Otsuka H, Igase K, Yoshimura H, Sakanaka M (1996) Interleukin-6 prevents ischemia-induced learning disability and neuronal and synaptic loss in gerbils. Neurosci Lett 204:109–112
54. Meistrell ME III, Botchkina GI, Wang H, Di Santo E, Cockroft KM, Bloom O, Vishnubhakat JM, Ghezzi P, Tracey KJ (1997) Tumor necrosis factor is a brain damaging cytokine in cerebral ischemia. Shock 8:341–348
55. Minami M, Yabuuchi K, Katsumata S, Tomozawa Y, Kuraishi Y, Satoh M (1992) Possible involvement of interleukin-1β in neuronal death after transient forebrain ischaemia. Soc Neurosci Abstr 18:425
56. Morganti-Kossman MC, Lenzlinger PM, Hans V, Stahel P, Csuka E, Ammann E, Stocker R, Trentz O, Kossmann T (1997) Production of cytokines following brain injury: beneficial and deleterious for the damaged tissue. Mol Psychiatry 2:133–136
57. Nawashiro H, Martin D, Hallenbeck JM (1997b) Inhibition of tumor necrosis factor and amelioration of brain infarction in mice. J Cereb Blood Flow Metab 17:229–232
58. Nawashiro H, Martin D, Hallenbeck JM (1997c) Neuroprotective effects of TNF binding protein in focal cerebral ischemia. Brain Res 778:265–271
59. Nawashiro H, Tasaki K, Ruetzler CA, Hallenbeck JM (1997a) TNF-alpha pretreatment induces protective effects against focal cerebral ischemia in mice. J Cereb Blood Flow Metab 17:483–490
60. Penkowa M, Moos T, Carrasco J, Hadberg H, Molinero A, Bluethmann H, Hidalgo J (1999) Strongly compromised inflammatory response to brain injury in interleukin-6-deficient mice. Glia 25:343–357
61. Rothwell N, Allan S, Toulmond S (1997) The role of interleukin 1 in acute neurodegeneration and stroke: pathophysiological and therapeutic implications. Journal of Clinical Investigations 100:2648–2652
62. Rothwell NJ, Hopkins SJ (1995) Interactions between cytokines and the nervous system II: Actions and mechanisms. Trends in Neurosciences 18:130–136
63. Scherbel U, Raghupathi R, Nakamura M, Saatman KE, Trojanowski JQ, Neugebauer E, Marino MW, McIntosh TK (1999) Differential acute and chronic responses of tumor necrosis factor-deficient mice to experimental brain injury. Proc Natl Acad Sci USA %20; 96:8721–8726
64. Shohami E, Bass R, Wallach D, Yamin A, Gallily R (1996) Inhibition of tumor necrosis factor alpha (TNFα) activity in rat brain is associated with cerebroprotection after closed head injury. J Cereb Blood Flow Metab 16:378–384
65. Spera PA, Ellison JA, Feuerstein GZ, Barone FC (1998) IL-10 reduces rat brain injury following focal stroke. Neurosci Lett 251:189–192
66. Spranger M, Lindholm D, Bandtlow C, Heumann R, Gnahn H, Naher-Noe M, Thoenen H (1990) Regulation of nerve growth factor (NGF) synthesis in thr rat central nervous system: Comparison between the effects of interleukin-1 and various growth factors in astrocytes cultures and in vivo. Eur J Neurosci 2:69–76
67. Steffensen SC, Campbell IL, Henriksen SJ (1994) Site-specific hippocampal pathophysiology due to cerebral overexpression of interleukin-6 in transgenic mice. Brain Res 652:149–153
68. Strijbos PJ, Rothwell NJ (1995) Interleukin-1 beta attenuates excitatory amino acid-induced neurodegeneration in vitro: involvement of nerve growth factor. J Neurosci 15:3468–3474
69. Suzuki S, Tanaka K, Nogawa S, Nagata E, Ito D, Dembo T, Fukuuchi Y (1999) Temporal profile and cellular localization of interleukin-6 protein after focal cerebral ischemia in rats. J Cereb Blood Flow Metab 19:1256–1262
70. Tarkowski E, Rosengren L, Blomstrand C, Jensen C, Ekholm S, Tarkowski A (1999) Intrathecal expression of proteins regulating apoptosis in acute stroke. Stroke 30:321–327
71. Tarkowski E, Rosengren L, Blomstrand C, Wikkelso C, Jensen C, Ekholm S, Tarkowski A (1997) Intrathecal release of pro- and anti-inflammatory cytokines during stroke. Clin Exp Immunol 110:492–499
72. Tarkowski E, Rosengren L, Blomstrand C, Wikkelsö C, Jensen C, Ekholm S, Tarkowski A (1995) Early intrathecal production of interleukin-6 predicts the size of brain lesion in stroke. Stroke 26:1393–1398
73. Thier M, Marz P, Otten U, Weis J, Rose-John S (1999) Interleukin-6 (IL-6) and its soluble receptor support survival of sensory neurons. J Neurosci Res 55:411–422
74. Tilg H, Dinarello CA, and Mier JW (1997) IL-6 and APPs: anti-inflammatory and immunosuppressive mediators. Immunol Today 18:428–432
75. Toulmond S, Vige X, Fage D, Benavides J (1992) Local infusion of interleukin-6 attenuates the neurotoxic effects of NMDA on rat striatal cholinergic neurons. Neurosci Lett 144:49–52
76. Touzani O, Boutin H, Chuquet J, Rothwell N (1999) Potential mechanisms of interleukin-1 involvement in cerebral ischaemia. J Neuroimmunol 100:203–215
77. Vannier E, Miller LC, Dinarello CA (1992) Coordinated anti-inflammatory effects of interleukin 4: Interleukin 4 supresses interleukin 1 production but up-regulates gene expression and synthesis of interleukin 1 receptor antagonist. Proc Natl Acad Sci USA 89:4076–4080
78. Wang X, Yue TL, Barone FC, White RF, Gagnon RC, Feuerstein GZ (1994) Concomitant cortical expression of TNF-alpha and IL-1 beta mRNAs follows early response gene expression in transient focal ischemia. Mol Chem Neuropathol 23:103–114
79. Wang XK, Yue TL, Young PR, Barone FC, Feuerstein GZ (1995) Expression of interleukin-6, c-fos, and zif268 mRNAs in rat ischemic cortex. J Cereb Blood Flow Metab 15:166–171

80. Yamada M, Hatanaka H (1994) Interleukin-6 protects cultured rat hippocampal neurons against glutamate-induced cell death. Brain Res 643:173–180
81. Yamasaki Y, Matsuura N, Shozuhara H, Onodera H, Itoyama Y, Kogure K (1995) Interleukin-1 as a pathogenetic mediator of ischemic brain damage in rats [see comments]. Stroke 26:676–680
82. Yan HQ, Banos MA, Herregodts P, Hooghe R, Hooghe-Peters EL (1992) Expression of interleukin (IL)-1beta, IL-6 and their respective receptors in the normal rat brain and after injury. European Journal of Immunology 22:2963–2971
83. Yang GY, Gong C, Qin Z, Liu XH, Lorris BA (1999a) Tumor necrosis factor alpha expression produces increased blood-brain barrier permeability following temporary focal cerebral ischemia in mice. Brain Res Mol Brain Res 69:135–143
84. Yang GY, Gong C, Qin Z, Ye W, Mao Y, Bertz AL (1998) Inhibition of TNFalpha attenuates infarct volume and ICAM-1 expression in ischemic mouse brain. Neuroreport 9:2131–2134
85. Yang GY, Schielke GP, Gong C, Mao Y, Ge HL, Liu XH, Betz AL (1999b) Expression of tumor necrosis factor-alpha and intercellular adhesion molecule-1 after focal cerebral ischemia in interleukin-1beta converting enzyme deficient mice. J Cereb Blood Flow Metab 19:1109–1117

Site-specific actions of interleukin-1 in neurodegeneration

S. M. Allan, L. C. Parker, R. I. Grundy*, B. Collins

Abstract

The pro-inflammatory cytokine interleukin-1β (IL-1β) mediates diverse forms of acute neurodegeneration but its precise mechanism of action is unknown. We have shown previously that exogenous and endogenous IL-1β acts specifically in the rat striatum to dramatically enhance ischaemic and excitotoxic brain damage. More specifically intrastriatal administration of IL-1β with the excitotoxin α-amino-3-hydroxy-5-methyl-4-isoxazolepropionate (S-AMPA) results in extensive cortical injury, not observed with either IL-1β or S-AMPA when injected alone.

We now show that IL-1β injected into the rat striatum with S-AMPA produced increased expression of IL-1β in the cortex, where maximum injury occurs. However, increased expression of IL-1β was also observed in the hypothalamus and injection of IL-1β into the lateral hypothalamus immediately after striatal S-AMPA resulted in widespread cell loss throughout the ipsilateral cortex. In addition, cortical cell death produced by striatal co-injection of S-AMPA and IL-1β was significantly reduced by administration of the IL-1 receptor antagonist (IL-1ra) into the hypothalamus.

These data suggest that IL-1 dependent pathways project from the striatum to the cortex via the hypothalamus that, when activated in combination with striatal AMPA receptor activation, lead to widespread cortical cell death.

1. Introduction

1.1 Interleukin-1 and neurodegeneration

The cytokine interleukin-1β (IL-1β) has a number of diverse effects in the CNS and considerable interest has focussed on its involvement in mediating various forms of acute neurodegeneration (Rothwell 1999). Injection or over-expression of the naturally occurring IL-1 receptor antagonist (IL-1ra) in experimental animals undergoing experimental ischaemia, head injury or excitotoxic insult has been shown to dramatically attenuate the resultant damage (Betz et al. 1995; Garcia et al. 1995; Toulmond and Rothwell 1995; Loddick and Rothwell 1996; Lawrence et al. 1998). In contrast intracerebral administration of IL-1β itself exacerbates these forms of injury (Yamasaki et al. 1995; Loddick and Rothwell 1996; Lawrence et al. 1998; Stroemer and Rothwell 1998). Further support of a

Keywords: interleukin-1; excitotoxicity; cytokines; cell death; S-AMPA

School of Biological Sciences, 1.124 Stopford Building, University of Manchester, Oxford Road, Manchester, UK, M13 9PT; *Schering-Plough Research Institute, San Raffaele Science Park, Via Olgettina 58, 20132 Milano, Italy
e-mail: stuart.allan@man.ac.uk

J. Krieglstein, S. Klumpp (Eds.) Pharmacology of Cerebral Ischemia 2000

role for IL-1β in acute neurodegeneration comes from numerous studies that have demonstrated increased expression of IL-1β in the brain in response to ischaemic, traumatic or excitotoxic injury (Yamaguchi et al. 1991; Yabuuchi et al. 1993, 1994; Hagan et al. 1996; Sairanen et al. 1997; Davies et al. 1999; Pearson et al. 1999). The increased expression is usually observed within the damaged region or in areas which subsequently undergo cell loss.

Precisely how IL-1β mediates its effects in neurodegeneration is still not clear, although it may be due to a number of different mechanisms and appears to involve specific sites of action within the CNS (Rothwell 1999; Allan et al. 2000).

1.2 Site-specific actions of interleukin-1

We have demonstrated that IL-1β can act at specific sites within the rat brain to affect cell death. In rats subjected to permanent middle cerebral artery occlusion (pMCAo), striatal injection of IL-1β increases damage in both the striatum and cortex, whereas cortical administration of IL-1β has no effect (Stroemer and Rothwell 1998). Similar site-specificity is observed with IL-1ra, in that striatal treatment reduces infarct volume after pMCAo while cortical injection fails to do so (Stroemer and Rothwell 1997).

Such site specific actions of IL-1β are supported by studies on excitotoxic brain damage. Intrastriatal administration of the glutamatergic agonist methanoglutamate or S-AMPA results in local injury that is significantly reduced by IL-1ra. In contrast when IL-1ra is co-infused with either of the excitotoxins in the cortex no change in the resultant lesion volume is observed (Lawrence et al. 1998).

Interestingly when IL-1β is co-injected with S-AMPA in the striatum, extensive cell death occurs throughout the ipsilateral cortex, which is not seen with either IL-1β or S-AMPA alone (Lawrence et al. 1998). The mechanisms of this potent effect of IL-1β are not clear although it appears to be an "all or nothing" response. We have observed that certain regions of the striatum appear to be more responsive to the co-injection of S-AMPA and IL-1β i.e. a greater frequency of cortical damage is observed (Grundy et al. 1998). These positive sites include the ventral striatum and lateral shell of the nucleus accumbens, both of which have connections to the limbic system and hypothalamus, the latter of which we now believe to be involved in mediating the effects of IL-1β on excitotoxic cell death (Allan et al. 2000).

2. Results

2.1 Increased IL-1 expression at sites remote from injury

Expression of IL-1β mRNA was studied within the striatum, cortex and hypothalamus in male Sprague-Dawley rats injected with vehicle, S-AMPA (7.5 nmol), human recombinant IL-1β (hrIL-1β; 10 ng) or S-AMPA (7.5 nmol) + hrIL-1β (10 ng) in the striatum (co-ordinates relative to bregma, (mm): anterior-posterior (AP) +0.7, medial-lateral (ML) –2.7, dorsal-ventral (DV) –5.5) using reverse transcription polymerase chain reaction (RT-PCR). In addition immunoreactive IL-1β levels were determined by a rat-specific ELISA (Cartmell et al. 1999).

No marked differences in striatal IL-1β mRNA expression were observed between any of the treatments 8 h after injection (Fig. 1). In contrast in the ipsilateral cortex animals treated with hrIL-1β+S-AMPA in the striatum showed almost 100-fold increases in IL-1β mRNA compared to vehicle animals and 10-fold greater amounts than those injected with S-AMPA or hrIL-1β (Fig. 1). Intrastriatal injection of hrIL-1β or hrIL-1β+S-AMPA also induced marked increases (10-fold) of IL-1β mRNA in the hypothalamus 8 h post-treatment when compared to vehicle or S-AMPA groups (Fig. 1).

There was no significant difference in striatal levels of immunoreactive rat IL-1β, measured after 8 h, between the hrIL-1β or hrIL-1β+S-AMPA treated groups and those animals injected with vehicle (Fig. 2) although levels were significantly greater than that observed in animals injected with S-AMPA alone. In the

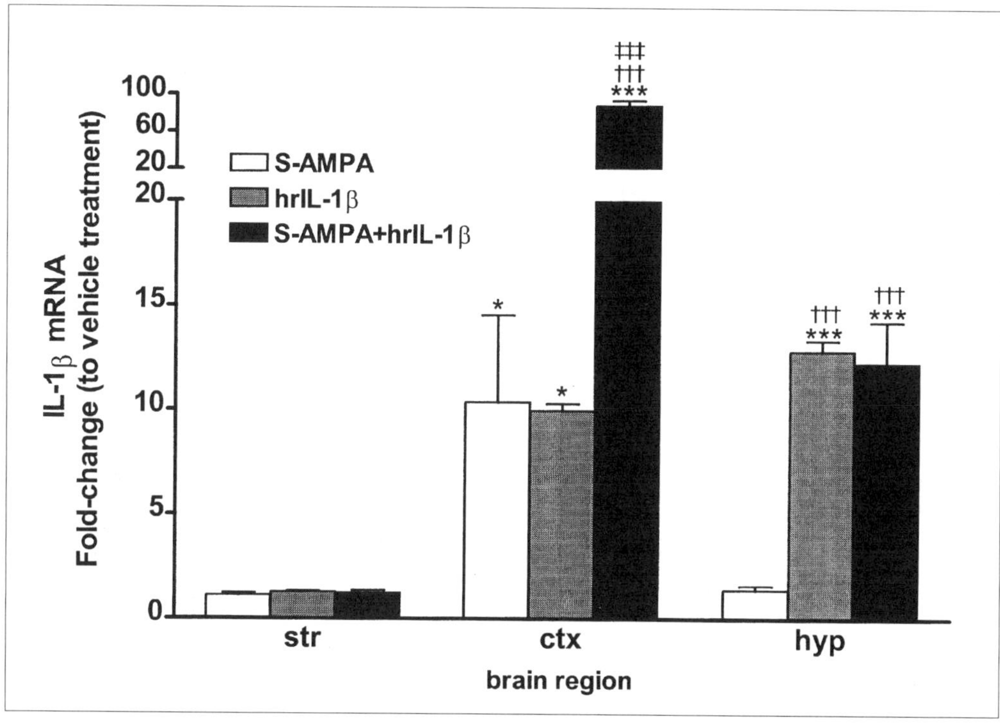

Fig. 1. Expression of IL-1β mRNA in the striatum (str), cortex (ctx) and hypothalamus (hyp) of the rat brain 8 h after intrastriatal injection of vehicle, S-AMPA (7.5 nmol), hrIL-1β (10 ng) or S-AMPA (7.5 nmol) + hrIL-1β (10 ng). Values (n = 3–4) are expressed as the mean fold-change (± SD) from the IL-1β mRNA expression levels observed after vehicle treatment. *$P < 0.05$, ***$P < 0.001$ vs. vehicle; $^{\dagger\dagger\dagger}P < 0.001$ vs. S-AMPA; $^{\ddagger\ddagger\ddagger}P < 0.001$ vs. hrIL-1β.

ipsilateral cortex 8 h after striatal injection, animals treated with hrIL-1β+S-AMPA showed markedly increased (> 6-fold) levels of immunoreactive IL-1β when compared to animals injected with vehicle, S-AMPA or hrIL-1β (Fig. 2). Eight hours after intrastriatal injection, immunoreactive rat IL-1β levels in the hypothalamus were significantly higher in animals treated with hrIL-1β alone or together with S-AMPA than those in animals injected with vehicle or S-AMPA separately (Fig. 2).

2.2 The hypothalamus mediates actions of IL-1 on excitotoxic cell death

Given that IL-1β mRNA and immunoreactivity increased in the hypothalamus following striatal co-administration of S-AMPA and hrIL-1β we studied whether direct injection of IL-1β itself in the lateral hypothalamus (LH) could affect cortical cell death in response to intrastriatal injection of S-AMPA

Therefore animals were injected with S-AMPA (7.5 nmol) in the striatum, followed by vehicle or hrIL-1β (10 ng) in the LH (injection co-ordinates: AP –3,6, ML –1.8, DV –8.4). The total lesion volume was determined from coronal cryostat sections stained with cresyl fast violet.

Hypothalamic injection of hrIL-1β alone caused no damage either at the site of injection or in distant sites (data not shown). Injection of hrIL-1β (10 ng) in the LH immediately after intrastriatal S-AMPA, resulted in extensive cortical cell death compared to the modest and localised (piriform) cortical injury caused by intrastriatal injection of S-AMPA and adminis-

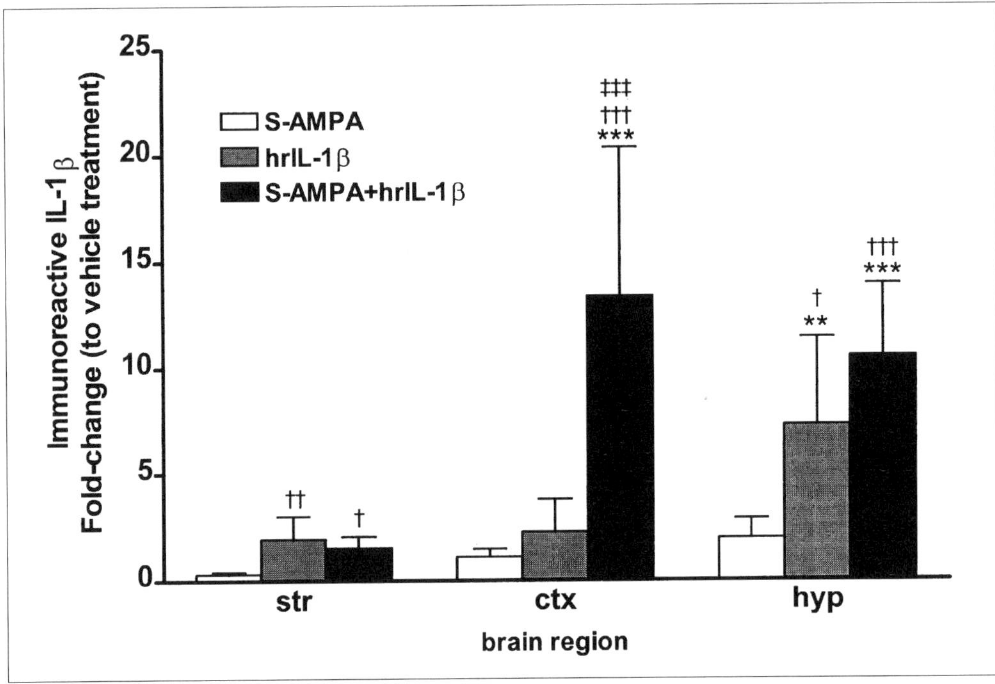

Fig. 2. Expression of immunoreactive IL-1β in the striatum (str), cortex (ctx) and hypothalamus (hyp) of the rat brain 8 h after intrastriatal injection of vehicle, S-AMPA (7.5 nmol), hrIL-1β (10 ng) or S-AMPA (7.5 nmol) + hrIL-1β (10 ng). Values (n = 5–6) are expressed as the mean fold-change (± SD) from immunoreactive IL-1β levels produced by vehicle treatment. $^{**}P < 0.01$, $^{***}P < 0.001$ vs. vehicle; $^{\dagger}P < 0.05$, $^{\dagger\dagger}P < 0.01$, $^{\dagger\dagger\dagger}P < 0.001$ vs. S-AMPA; $^{\ddagger\ddagger\ddagger}P < 0.001$ vs. hrIL-1β.

tration of vehicle in the LH (Fig. 3). Striatal damage resulting from intrastriatal injection of S-AMPA was unaffected by injection of vehicle or hrIL-1β in the LH (Fig. 3).

To determine whether increases in endogenous IL-1β in the hypothalamus mediate the cortical damage resulting from striatal injection of S-AMPA plus hrIL-1β, vehicle or IL-1ra (10 µg) was administered into the LH immediately after co-injection of hrIL-1β (10 ng) and S-AMPA (7.5 nmol) in the striatum. Intrastriatal co-injection of hrIL-1β plus S-AMPA resulted in an extensive lesion throughout the ipsilateral cortex that was reduced by injection of hrIL-1ra (10 µg) into the LH (Fig. 4). The local striatal lesion was no different between animals treated with intrahypothalamic vehicle or IL-1ra (Fig. 4).

3. Discussion

Our data demonstrates that hypothalamic IL-1β can contribute to cortical neurodegeneration. Injection of hrIL-1β+S-AMPA into the striatum increased IL-1β mRNA and protein expression at the site of distant cell death (cortex), and in the hypothalamus, where no injury was detected. In addition, application of IL-1ra directly into the hypothalamus markedly reduced the cortical damage resulting from intrastriatal co-injection of IL-1β and S-AMPA. Conversely administration of IL-1β in the LH with S-AMPA in the striatum produced extensive cortical damage. It seems therefore that the hypothalamus is a primary site of action of IL-1β which directly influences cortical cell viability after activation of striatal AMPA receptors. In further studies, we have demonstrated that cor-

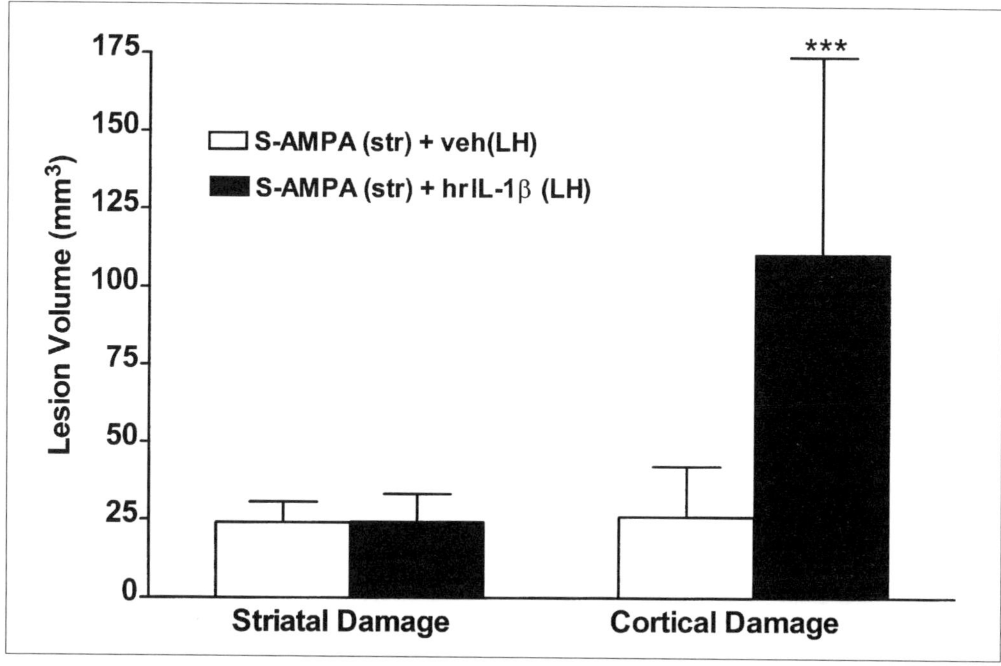

Fig. 3. Effect of hypothalamic IL-1β treatment on cell death produced by intrastriatal injection of S-AMPA in the rat brain. Groups of animals (n = 19) were injected intrastriatally (str) with S-AMPA (7.5 nmol), immediately followed by injection of hrIL-1β in the lateral hypothalamus (LH). Values are represented as the mean lesion volume (± SD) in the striatum and cortex. ***P < 0.001 vs. vehicle treatment.

tical cell death resulting from intrastriatal injection of IL-1β and S-AMPA is mediated via the activation of cortical NMDA receptors, which suggests the involvement of a glutamatergic pathway(s) from the striatum to the cortex (Allan and Rothwell 2000).

The LH was chosen as the initial site of injection within the hypothalamus because of its known connections with the cortex, ventral striatum (including the nucleus accumbens) and other major hypothalamic nuclei (Bernardis and Bellinger 1993; Risold et al. 1997). However other brain areas may contribute to the effects of IL-1β, and our preliminary data indicate that injection of hrIL-1β, after intrastriatal S-AMPA, into the basolateral amygdala also results in extensive cortical cell death (Allan et al., unpublished data).

Increased expression of IL-1β in the cortex of animals injected with IL-1β+S-AMPA in the striatum was observed 8 h after injection when injury is emerging. This supports a role for locally synthesised IL-1β in the cortical cell death resulting from the striatal co-injection. Indeed, an increase in cortical IL-1β levels appear necessary for cortical cell death to occur because direct cortical injection of IL-1ra immediately after the striatal co-injection markedly reduces the amount of cortical injury (Allan and Rothwell, unpublished data).

A marked increase in both IL-1β mRNA and immunoreactivity was observed in the hypothalamus after striatal administration of IL-1β alone. However, no obvious cortical cell death was seen in this group and we propose that raised levels of IL-1β in the hypothalamus are necessary, but not sufficient, to produce remote cell death in the cortex. It seems therefore that an additional 'priming' stimulus (i.e. striatal activation of AMPA receptors) is required to

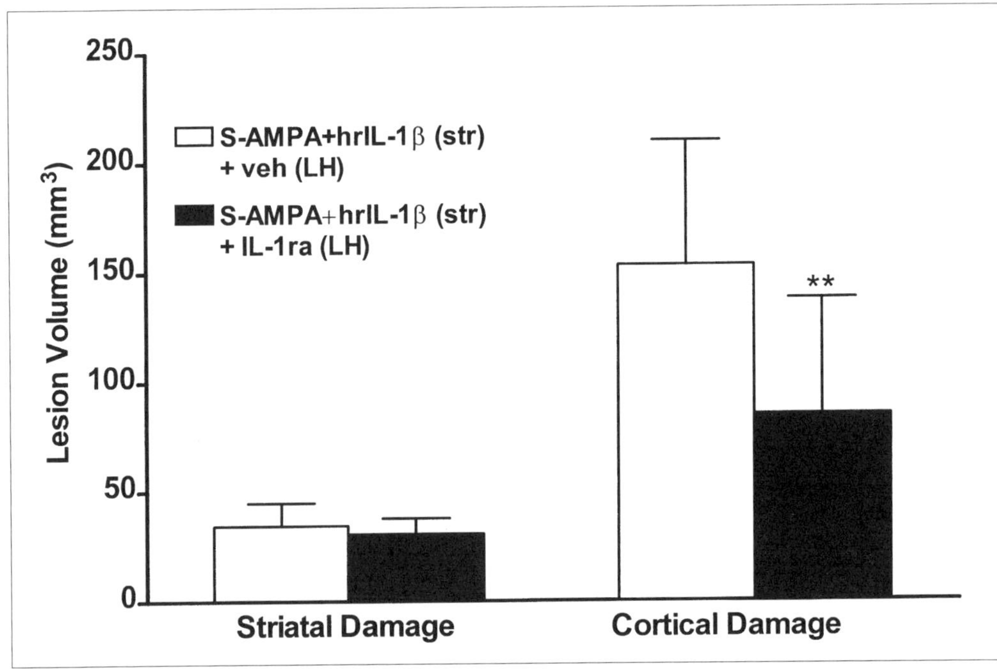

Fig. 4. Effect of hypothalamic IL-1ra treatment on cell death produced by intrastriatal injection of S-AMPA and IL-1β in the rat brain. Groups of animals (n = 14–15) were co-injected in the striatum (str) with S-AMPA (7.5 nmol) and hrIL-1β (10 ng), immediately followed by injection of hrIL-1ra (10 μg) in the lateral hypothalamus (LH). Values are represented as the mean lesion volume (± SD) in the striatum and cortex. **$P < 0.01$ vs. vehicle treatment.

produce cortical cell death. Striatal AMPA administration results in the activation of a number of neuronal pathways, particularly those associated with seizures and activation of the limbic system (Ben-Ari et al. 1980; Ben-Ari 1985) and these could play an important part in the observed effect.

Increased expression of immunoreactive IL-1β after hippocampal kainic acid injection has been reported and IL-1β was also shown to prolong seizure activity, possibly through enhanced glutamatergic neurotransmission (Vezzani et al. 1999). Indeed IL-1β has been shown to affect synaptic transmission in a number of systems (Miller et al. 1991; Yu and Shinnick-Gallagher 1994; O'Connor and Coogan 1999) although the precise effect (i.e. inhibition or potentiation) may depend on a number of factors, including the brain area and neurotransmitter involved.

In summary, IL-1β shows site-specific actions within areas of the striatum that connect directly with the hypothalamus and other brain regions that project back to the cortex (Saper 1985; Risold et al. 1997). We propose that intrastriatal IL-1β and S-AMPA can induce extensive distant injury in the cortex by activation of these complex neuronal circuits which increase local expression of IL-1β in the hypothalamus. It is possible that hypothalamic IL-1 may contribute to other forms of neurodegeneration, therefore regulation of IL-1 expression or action in the hypothalamus may yield new targets for therapeutic intervention in neurodegenerative disease.

Acknowledgements

This work was supported by the Medical Research Council.

5. References

1. Allan SM, Parker LC, Davies R, Luheshi GN, Rothwell NJ (2000) Cortical cell death induced by interleukin-1 is mediated via actions in the hypothalamus of the rat. Proc Natl Acad Sci USA 97:5580–5585
2. Allan SM, Rothwell NJ (2000) Cortical death caused by striatal administration of AMPA and interleukin-1 is mediated by activation of cortical NMDA receptors. J Cerebr Blood Flow Metab (in press)
3. Ben-Ari Y (1985) Limbic seizure and brain damage produced by kainic acid: mechanisms and relevance to human temporal lobe epilepsy. Neurosci 14:375–403
4. Ben-Ari Y, Tremblay E, Ottersen OP, Meldrum BS (1980) The role of epileptic activity in hippocampal and "remote" cerebral lesions induced by kainic acid. Brain Res 191:79–97
5. Bernardis LL, Bellinger LL (1993) The lateral hypothalamic area revisited: neuroanatomy, body weight regulation, neuroendocrinology and metabolism. Neurosci Biobehav Rev 17:141–193
6. Betz AL, Yang G-Y, Davidson BL (1995) Attenuation of stroke size in rats using an adenoviral vector to induce over expression of interleukin-1 receptor antagonist in brain. J Cerebr Blood Flow Metab 15:547–551
7. Cartmell T, Southgate T, Rees GS, Castro MG, Lowenstein PR, Luheshi GN (1999) Interleukin-1 mediates a rapid inflammatory response after injection of adenoviral vectors into the brain. J Neurosci 19:1517–1523
8. Davies CA, Loddick SA, Toulmond S, Stroemer RP, Hunt J, Rothwell NJ (1999) The progression and topographic distribution of interleukin-1β expression after permanent middle cerebral artery occlusion in the rat. J Cereb Blood Flow Metab 19:87–98
9. Garcia JH, Liu K-F, Relton JK (1995) Interleukin-1 receptor antagonist decreases the number of necrotic neurons in rats with middle cerebral artery occlusion. Am J Pathol 147:1477–1486
10. Grundy RI, Rothwell NJ, Allan SM (1998) Site of action of IL-1 on AMPA receptor mediated excitotoxicity within the rat striatum. Soc Neurosci Abstr 24:568.15
11. Hagan P, Poole S, Bristow AF, Tilders F, Silverstein FS (1996) Intracerebral NMDA injection stimulates production of interleukin-1β in perinatal rat brain. J Neurochem 67:2215–2218
12. Lawrence CB, Allan SM, Rothwell NJ (1998) Interleukin-1beta and the interleukin-1 receptor antagonist act in the striatum to modify excitotoxic brain damage in the rat. Eur J Neurosci 10:1188–1195
13. Loddick SA, Rothwell NJ (1996) Neuroprotective effects of human recombinant interleukin-1 receptor antagonist in focal cerebral ischaemia in the rat. J Cereb Blood Flow Metab 16:932–940
14. Miller LG, Galpern WR, Dunlap K, Dinarello CA, Turner TJ (1991) Interleukin-1 augments γ-aminobutyric $acid_A$ receptor function in brain. Mol Pharmacol 39:105–108
15. O'Connor JJ, Coogan AN (1999) Actions of the pro-inflammatory cytokine IL-1 beta on central synaptic transmission. Exp Physiol 84:601–614
16. Pearson VL, Rothwell NJ, Toulmond S (1999) Excitotoxic brain damage in the rat induces interleukin-1β protein in microglia and astrocytes: correlation with the progression of cell death. Glia 25:311–323
17. Risold PY, Thompson RH, Swanson LW (1997) The structural organization of connections between hypothalamus and cerebral cortex. Brain Res Rev 24:197–254
18. Rothwell NJ (1999) Cytokines-killers in the brain? J Physiol (Lond) 514:3–17
19. Sairanen TR, Lindsberg PJ, Brenner M, Siren A-L (1997) Global forebrain ischemia results in differential cellular expression of interleukin-1β (IL-1β) and its receptor at mRNA and protein level. J Cereb Blood Flow Metab 17:1107–1120
20. Saper CB (1985) Organization of cerebral cortical afferent systems in the rat. II. Hypothalamocortical projections. J Comp Neurol 237:21–46
21. Stroemer RP, Rothwell NJ (1997) Cortical protection by localized striatal injection of IL-1ra following cerebral ischemia in the rat. J Cereb Blood Flow Metab 17:597–604
22. Stroemer RP, Rothwell NJ (1998) Exacerbation of ischemic brain damage by localized striatal injection of interleukin-1beta in the rat. J Cereb Blood Flow Metab 18:833–839
23. Toulmond S, Rothwell NJ (1995) Interleukin-1 receptor antagonist inhibits neuronal damage caused by fluid percussion injury in the rat. Brain Res 671:261–266
24. Vezzani A, Conti N, De Luigi A, Ravizza T, Moneta D, Marchesi F, De Simoni MG (1999) Interleukin-1β immunoreactivity and microglia are enhanced in the rat hippocampus by focal kainate application:functional evidence for enhancement of electrographic seizures. J Neurosci 19:5054–5065
25. Yabuuchi K, Minami M, Katsumata S, Satoh M (1993) In situ hybridization study of interleukin-1β mRNA induced by kainic acid in the rat brain. Mol Brain Res 20:153–161
26. Yabuuchi K, Minami M, Katsumata S, Yamazaki A, Satoh M (1994) An in situ hybridization study on interleukin-1 beta mRNA induced by transient forebrain iscemia in the rat brain. Mol Brain Res 26:135–142
27. Yamaguchi T, Kuraishi Y, Minami M, Nakai S, Hirai Y, Satoh M (1991) Methamphetamine-induced expression of interleukin-1β mRNA in the rat hypothalamus. Neurosci Lett 128:90–92
28. Yamasaki Y, Matsuura N, Shozuhara H, Onodera H, Itoyama Y, Kogure K (1995) Interleukin-1 as a pathogenetic mediator of ischemic brain damage in rats. Stroke 26:676–681
29. Yu B, Shinnick-Gallagher P (1994) Interleukin-1β inhibits synaptic transmission and induces membrane hyperpolarization in amygdala neurons. J Pharmacol Exp Ther 271:590–600

Genes and gene therapy

Expression analysis and functional genomics for brain research: Expression profiling in a mouse model for Huntington's Disease

W. Nietfeld[1,*], J. Schuchhardt[2], A. Malik[1], N. Tandon[1], E. Rohlfs[1], E. E. Wanker[1], H. Eickhoff[1], H. Lehrach[1]

Abstract

To identify molecular mediators for Huntington's Disease (HD) we have used a transgenic mouse model for HD expressing exon 1 of the HD gene carrying a $(CAG)_{150}$ repeat expansion. Applying DNA microarray technologies and hierarchical clustering algorithms we analyzed in parallel the expression profiles of 5,376 transcripts in the cortex of 4, 8 and 12 weeks old HD transgenic and wildtype animals. Clustering of the obtained expression data resulted in the identification of about 500 differentially expressed genes. Many of these genes, which are down regulated, are encoded by mitochondrial DNA suggesting that pathways in energy metabolism are altered in the HD transgenic mouse model. In contrast, genes that are up regulated are functional in cell signaling pathways, cell cycle regulation or cytoskeleton assembly. Most of the identified differentially expressed gene have no database entry and will be further characterized to investigate their function in the formation and progression of HD.

Introduction

Automated approaches in functional genomics and proteomics are very efficient techniques to generate more knowledge about the complex network of molecular mechanisms. Several methods have been developed during the past years to gain essential information on the regulation of gene expression. These approaches rely either on counting clone numbers in libraries prepared from different tissues, cell-lines or development stages or on signal intensity measurements with probes generated from biological samples. Examples of the first approach are EST sequencing (Adams et al. 1993; Boguski and Schuler 1995) oligonucleotide fingerprinting (Meier-Ewert et al. 1998) or SAGE (Velculescu et al. 1995; Zhang et al. 1997). To the second class of methods belong complex cDNA hybridization (Lehrach et al. 1990; Lennon and Lehrach 1991; Gress et al. 1996; Duggan et al. 1999), *in situ* hybridization (Wilkinson and Nieto 1993) or differential display (Liang and Pardee 1992).

Among these techniques, the use of complex cDNA hybridization combined with high-density arrays of spotted DNA (Gress et al. 1992; Schena et al. 1995; DeRisi et al. 1996, DeRisi et al. 1997; Lashkari et al. 1997) or oligonucle-

Keywords: Huntington's disease, expression profiling, functional genomics

[1]Max-Planck-Institut für Molekulare Genetik, Ihnestr. 73, 14195 Berlin, Germany, [2]Institut für Theoretische Biologie, Humboldt Universität Berlin, Invalidenstr 42, 10115 Berlin, Germany
e-mail: Nietfeld@molgen.mpg.de

otides (Hoheisel 1997; Southern 1995; Lipshutz et al. 1999), offers a number of advantages. It combines high sensitivity with high throughput, due to the possibility of an enormous number of parallel experiments carried out on a single DNA array (Poustka et al. 1986; Lehrach et al. 1990; Schena et al. 1996; Brown and Botstein 1999). To extract the significant biological information from complex cDNA hybridization experiments, computational analysis and statistical methods are necessary, thus providing an efficient technique to group differentially expressed or functionally related genes together (Eisen et al. 1998; Iyer et al. 1999).

Changes in gene expression are very often associated with human diseases or disorders. Although many people suffer from neurodegenerative disorders like Huntington's disease, Alzheimer's disease or Parkinson's disease, their molecular mechanisms are not well characterized today. HD is an autosomal dominant progressive disorder. The disease is manifested by a complex and variable set of symptoms that have psychological, cognitive and motor components. The onset of disease occurs typically in midlife and progresses to death within fifteen to twenty years. The mutation that causes HD is a CAG/polyglutamine repeat expansion in the first exon of the HD gene encoding the huntingtin protein (Huntington's Disease Collaborative Research Group, 1993). The molecular mechanism by which the expanded polyglutamine repeats mediate the disease, is only poorly understood. Lines of mice (R/6) that are transgenic for the HD mutation have been generated (Mangiarini et al. 1996). In these mice the exon 1 of the human HD gene with a CAG repeat expansion of 115–156 units is expressed under the control of the human HD promoter. The transgenic animals exhibit a progressive neurological phenotype including trema, irregular gait, grooming movement and epileptic seizures. Neuropathological analysis showed the presence of neuronal inclusions preceding the neural dysfunction (Davis et al. 1997; Scherzinger et al. 1997) suggesting that the formation of insoluble protein aggregates is the cause of the motor symptoms. However, further studies are necessary to substantiate this hypothesis.

We have used complex cDNA hybridization to examine whether the formation of polyglutamine containing aggregates in 4, 8 and 12 weeks results in an alteration of gene expression in this transgenic mouse model. An earlier generated mouse UNIGENE subset of 5,376 cDNAs (Eickhoff et al. 2000) was arrayed on glass slides and used for expression profiling. This approach allows the simultaneous analysis of differential gene expression of 5,376 transcripts in parallel. About 500 differentially expressed genes have been identified.

Abbreviations: NMDA, N-methyl-D-aspartic acid; GABA, gamma-Aminobutyric acid; HD, Huntington's Disease; MTP, Microtiterplate; Acc. Number, Accession number;

Methods

Amplification of cDNA inserts

The inserts of 5,376 cDNA clones were amplified by PCR as described by Eickhoff and coworkers (Eickhoff et al. 2000). The primers used for the PCR reaction were 5' amino-modified derivatives of the primer described by Meier-Ewert and colleagues (Meier-Ewert et al. 1998). Prior to spotting, the PCR products were purified by ethanol precipitation in 96 well plates. To 80 µl of the PCR reactions, 4 µl of 3 M sodiumacetate pH 5,2 and 110 µl of ethanol were added. The whole reaction was centrifuged for 1 hour at 20 °C with a speed of 2800 rpm (Eppendorf Centrifuge 5810R). The pellets were washed with 70% ethanol and centrifuged again at 2800 rpm for 45 minutes at 20 °C. The supernatant was then discarded and the plates were left in a cold room over night for drying. The pellets were resuspended in 70 µl of 0.1-N-NaOH and then used for spotting. The PCR products spotted to the glass slides had a DNA concentration of 20 to 50 ng/µl. 48 PCR reactions of each 384 well plate was analyzed on a 1.2% Agarosegel. All arrays used in this publication were spotted from the same PCR reaction.

Preparation of glass slides

Normal glass was cut to a size of 9 cm x 13 cm and cleaned with 30% NH_3 at 50 °C for one hour. For coating the glass slides were boiled under reflux in Xylene containing 20% (w/v) of (3-Glycidoxypropyl)-trimethoxysilane (Sigma, Germany) and 1% (w/v) N-Ethyl-diisopropylamin for six hours. The slides were then rinsed once in methanol, ether and dried in a nitrogen stream for 3 minutes and used immediately for spotting.

Production of cDNA arrays

The PCR products were spotted onto glass slides as described earlier (Eickhoff et al. 2000). In brief, a 384-pin tool with individually spring-loaded blunt-end pins with a tip size of 250 µm was used for spotting. Two glass slides were processed in parallel. 5,376 clones were spotted in an array of 384 blocks. Each block (6 x 6 spots) contains fourteen mouse clones and two *Arabidopsis thaliana* control clones (GenBank accession numbers AF104328 and U29785, derived from the Arabidopsis Biological Resource Center and DNA stock donor at Ohio State University), all spotted in duplicate. Four spotting positions were left blank for background estimation.

Complex cDNA hybridization

Total RNA from cortex tissues of wildtype and HD transgenic mouse strain R6/2 (Mangiarini et al. 1996; Davis et al. 1997) was isolated by using the "RNAgents Total RNA Isolation System" (Promega, USA). Prior to mRNA isolation the total RNA of three animals was pooled. The mRNA was isolated using the Oligotex mRNA Kit (Qiagen, Germany). For the generation of complex probes 1.5 µg of mRNA were incubated at 70 °C for 5 minutes with 1 µl 50 A_{260} random hexamers (Pharmacia, Germany) in a total volume of 10 µl and chilled on ice for two minutes. For the reverse transcription reaction 6 µl of 5x first strand synthesis buffer (Gibco, Germany), 3 µl of 0.1 M-DTT (Gibco, Germany), 1 µl of RNase-block (Ambion, Germany), 1.5 µl of a nucleotide mix containing 20 mM dATP, 20 mM dTTP, 20 mM dGTP, 0.1 mM dCTP and 7 µl (10 µCu/µl) of alpha-^{33}P dCTP (Amersham, Germany) were added and incubated at 37 °C for two minutes, then 1.5 µl of SuperScript II (Gibco, Germany) reverse transcriptase (200u/µl) were added and incubated at 37 °C for one hour. Prior to hybridization, 10 ng of *Arabidopsis thaliana* DNA were labeled with a random priming labeling reaction (Amersham, Germany). Controls and complex probes were purified using a Sephadex G50 column. For hybridization two spotted glass slides were fixed "face-to-face" with a 0.5 mm hand-cut rubber spacer. For additional sealing all glass edges were sealed with Parafilm and put into liquid wax to form a sandwich hybridization chamber. The arrays were prehybridized for at least 30 minutes at 42 °C in 4.5 ml of hybridization solutions (DIG EasyHyb, Roche Molecular Biochemicals, Germany). The hybridization were performed in a custom-build overhead rotator overnight at 42 °C as described above, containing 0.5 µg of labeled complex probe and 2 ng of labeled *A. thaliana* probe. Washing was done at 65 °C in 0.1 x SSC, 0,4% SDS.

Image analysis and quantification of complex cDNA hybridization

After hybridization the arrays were exposed for 16 hours to Fuji BAS-SR 2025 intensifying screens (Raytest, Germany). The screens were then scanned at 25 µm resolution with a Fuji BAS 5000 phosphorimager (Raytest, Germany). The files were analyzed with a custom written image analysis system based on a Windows NT™ 4.0 platform. (Biochip Explorer, http://www.gpc-ag.com). Numerical values of spot intensities were transferred to the S-PLUS™ – spreadsheet calculation programs for normalization and analysis.

Analysis of expression profiles by hierarchical clustering algorithms

The normalization, analysis and clustering of the obtained expression profiles were performed as described earlier (Eickhoff et al. 2000). In brief, for the identification of clones with identical or similar expression patterns a hierarchical clustering algorithm was used. Hierarchic methods generate clusters as nested structures in a hierarchical fashion; the clusters of higher levels are aggregations of the clusters of lower levels. We used an agglomerative clustering method, which constructs the hierarchy from bottom to top. Agglomerative clustering can be presented in the following unified way. Let (d_{ij}) be a dissimilarity entity-to-entity matrix. Then find the minimal value d_{i*j*} in the dissimilarity matrix, and merge clusters i* and j*. Transform the distance matrix, substituting one new row (and column) $i^* \cup j^*$instead of the rows and columns i*, j* with its dissimilarities defined as

$$d_{i,i^*\cup j^*} = F\left(d_{ii^*}, d_{ij^*}, d_{i^*j^*}, h(i), h(i^*), h(j^*)\right)$$

where F is a fixed (usually linear) function and h(i) is an index function defined for every cluster recursively. As a distance function F the Euclidean distance was used. The Euclidean distance $d(x,y), x,y \in R^n$, can be defined as the norm of the difference $x - y = (x_1 - y_1, \ldots, x_n - y_n)$:

$$d(x,y) = \left(\sum_{k \in K} (x_k - y_k)^2 \right)^{1/2}.$$

Because we had no information about the nature of the expected clusters we chose the average linkage method for generating the clusters. With this hierarchical method the between-cluster distance d_{i*j*} is defined as the average of the distances d_{ij} by all $i \in i^*, j \in j^*$

$$d_{i,i^*\cup j^*} = \left(\frac{n_{i^*} d_{ii^*}}{(n_{i^*} + n_i)} + \frac{n_j * d_{ij^*}}{(n_{j^*} + n_i)} \right).$$

Results

Complex cDNA hybridization on glass arrays

We have analyzed the gene expression profiles in cortex tissue from HD transgenic (Mangiarini et al. 1996; Davis et al. 1997) and wildtype mice at 4, 8 and 12 weeks after birth. In Figure 1 is a schematic outline of a typical complex cDNA experiment shown. In the experiments described here, a normalized mouse UNIGENE set of 5,376 cDNA clones from a mouse embryonic day 9 and 12 cDNA library (Eickhoff et al. 2000) was arrayed on glass slides as schematically shown in Figure 1 (upper-right side). As indicated in Figure 1 (upper-left side) the mRNAs were isolated from cortex tissues of HD transgenic mice (Mangiarini et al. 1996; Davis et al. 1997) and wildtype mice at an age of 4, 8 and 12 weeks and used to generate probes for the complex cDNA hybridization experiments.

After hybridization with radioactive labeled probes every glass-slide was exposed for 16 hours and scanned with a phosphorimager at 25 µm resolution. Such resolution corresponds to 100 pixels per spot. Example images of obtained hybridization results are shown in Figure 2. For the quantification of signal intensities the mean pixel intensities of each spot were chosen. The background was calculated for each 6 x 6 spotting block. On each block we determined the background intensity on four empty spotting positions. The mean value of these points was used to calculate the local background and was subtracted from the spot intensities in each block (Nguyen et al. 1995; Pietu et al. 1996). For each clone an average intensity value was calculated from the duplicate pairs per slide.

Analysis of genes showing a significant alteration in expression levels

To enable comparison of the obtained expression profiles, hybridization intensities were normalized with the mean intensity of the clones on each filter after subtracting the local background (Eickhoff et al. 2000). Comparing HD

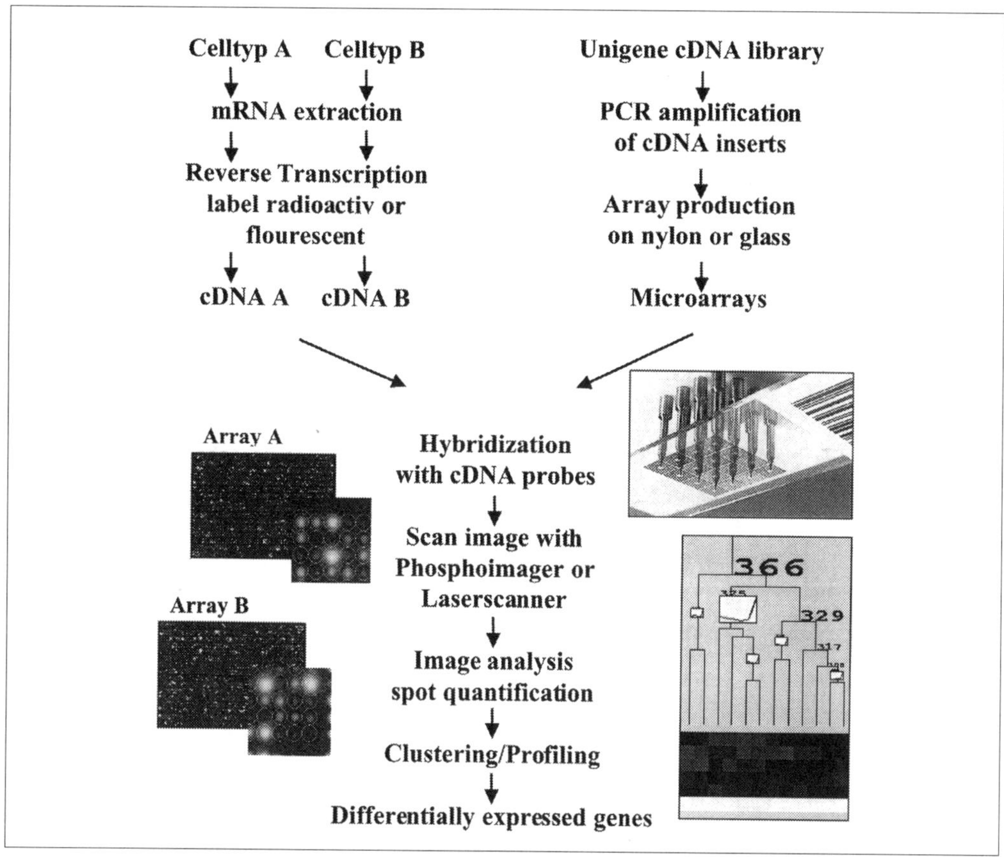

Fig. 1. Schematically illustration of complex cDNA hybridization experiments.
The mRNAs from different celltypes are used as templates for the generation of labeled celltyp specific cDNA probes, as indicated in the upper left drawing. The production of DNA arrays is indicated in the upper right part, inserts from cDNA libraries are arrayed on glass or nylon surfaces. The hybridization of DNA-arrays with complex cDNA probes, the comparison of the obtained images and clustering of the expression profiles leads to the identification of differentially expressed genes, as indicated in the lower part of the illustration. In the experiments described here, celltyp A and B would correspond to cortex tissue of wildtyp and HD transgenic mice. The UNIGENE cDNA library is a normalized mouse set of 5,376 cDNA clones (Eickhoff et al. 2000).

and wildtype gene expression profiles we identified significant expression changes. For the generation of a specific clustering-tree, only slides showing an adequate hybridization quality were selected. The main criterion for judging the slide quality was the condition of the spotting blocks, (areas that were produced by a single spotting pin). The quality of a block was calculated by comparing the constant *Arabidopsis thaliana* control clones spotted in duplicate in each block to the mean background signal of the slide. Only slides with more than 90% of the blocks above the quality threshold were used for clustering. For the identification of transcripts with identical or similar expression profiles for the three timepoints a hierarchical clustering algorithm was used.

About 500 clones with an altered expression profile during the investigated time period were identified. These clones were grouped together

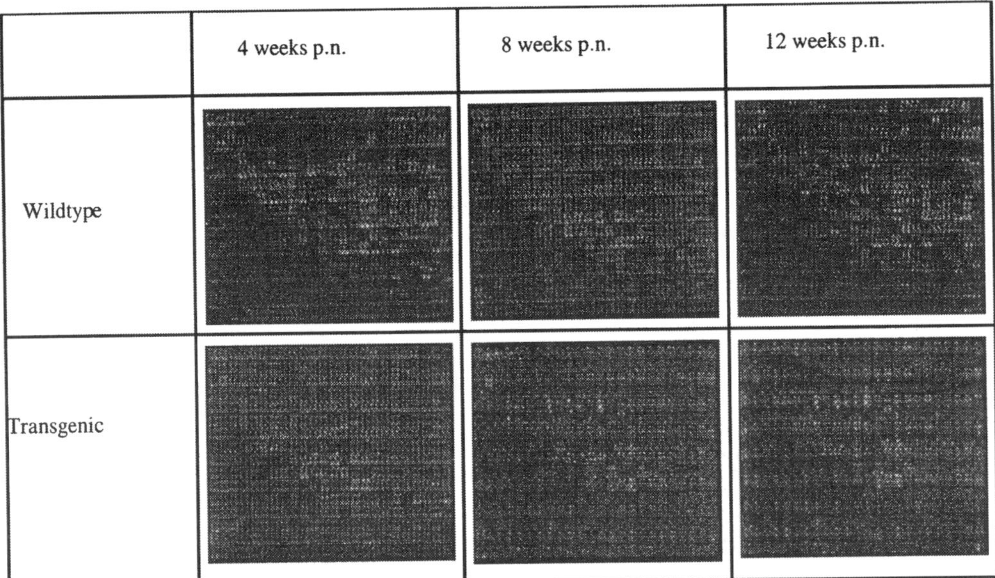

Fig. 2. Monitoring gene expression in Chorea Huntington transgenic mice.
Six arrays obtained after complex cDNA hybridization with 0.5 µg of cortex polyA+ RNA from wildtype or HD transgenic animals are shown. The RNA was isolated at 4 , 8 and 12 weeks post natal (p.n.). 5,376 cDNA inserts were arrayed on 3 x 13 cm glass slides. On this raw data image the hybridization signals detected spanned a range over at least three orders of magnitude. Prior to imaging the hybridized glass slides were exposed for 16 hours to a Fuji MP Imaging Plate.

in cluster #1042, which comprises three sub-cluster as shown in Figure 3. Cluster #1036 shows a panel of transcripts, which are up regulated in the cortex of 4, 8 and 12 weeks old mice, whereas cluster #1037 contains transcripts, that are down regulated during the same time period. Most of the identified transcripts are EST clones or clones which have no entry in GeneBank up to know. The known genes corresponding to cluster #1036 are summarized in Table 1. We could identify the up regulation of many mRNAs involved in cell signaling, cell cycle regulation and cytoskeleton assembly. Transcripts related to cell signaling are mouse cop9 and NLRR-1. Genes involved in cell cycle regulation are fizzy-related protein (Fyr), transcription factor E2F-1, TIAP or candidate tumor suppressor p33 ING1. Representatives for cytoskeleton organization are dynactin (50 kd isoform), alpha-spectrin and ralbp1 associated eps domain. The known down regulated transcripts from cluster #1037 are summarized in Table 2. The most obvious group of transcripts are genes encoded by mitochondrial DNA and involved in the energy metabolism, e.g., ARF1, cytochrome C oxidase, ATP synthase or mitochondrial transcription factor.

The cluster #985 shown in Figure 4 is a sub-cluster of cluster #1036 and shows the up-regulation of gene expression of 63 transcripts in the HD transgenic mice. The cluster #985 can be divided into two clusters #952 and #970 displaying different gene expression profiles. Cluster #952 groups transcripts together showing an almost linear increase over the analyzed period of time, whereas transcripts in cluster #970 show a weaker increase in expression level from week 8 to 12.

The down regulation of the gene expression of 32 transcripts is shown in Figure 5. This cluster #907 is a sub-cluster of cluster #1037 and can be further divided into two clusters #787 and #876. We detected an almost linear down regulation of the genes in cluster #787

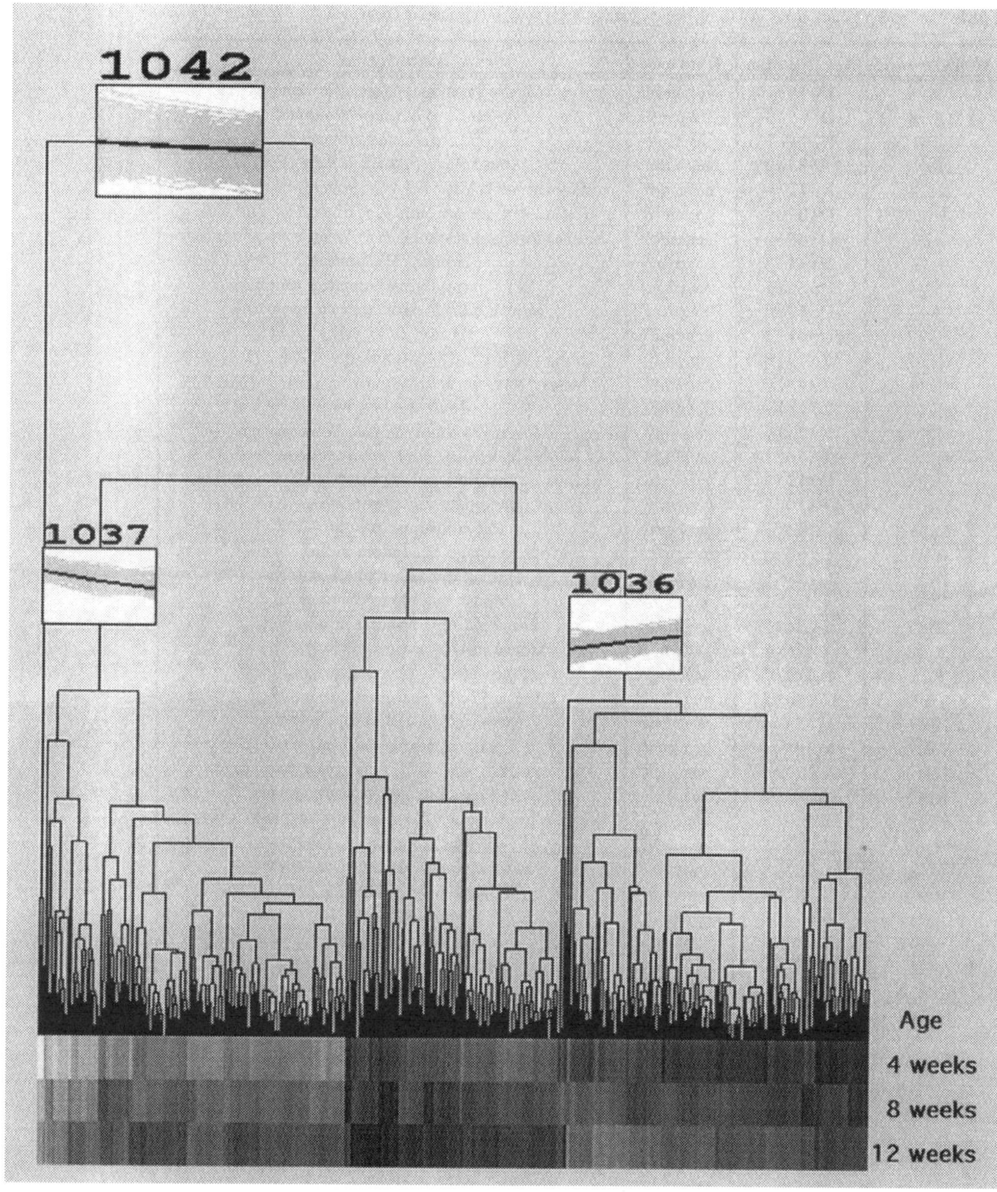

Fig. 3. Clustering of gene expression in Chorea Huntington transgenic mice.
Clustering was done by the hierarchical clustering method as described in the methods part, using a correlation-based distance measure for the clones on a slide. The numbering of the different branches is done in such a way that the numbers are unique for a sub-cluster or subtree and allow an easy identification. In the cluster #1042 about 500 transcript were identified showing an altered gene expression in 4, 8 and 12 weeks old mice. In sub-cluster #1037 down regulated genes are grouped together whereas sub-cluster #1036 shows up regulated genes. The consensus vector (bold lines) represents the mean expression values of the cluster members (faint lines). White bars indicate a high expression level, black bars a low expression level.

Table 1. Known genes up regulated in the cortex of HD mice (Cluster #1036)

MTP-Position	Acc. Number	Database	Description
1A11	U25691	genembl	Mouse lymphocyte specific helicase
1A18	O88543	swplus	Mouse cop9 complex subunit
1E01	P14413	swplus	Hamster atp synthase
2B05	AF083809	genembl	Mouse fizzy-related protein (Fyr)
2H24	X57778	genembl	Human mRNA for E-1 beta subunit of pyruvate
2J02	D10706	genembl	Rat mRNA for ornithine decarboxylase antizyme
2J20	U18869	genembl	Mouse mitogen-responsive 96 kDa phosphoprotein
2L14	Q13454	swplus	Human n33 protein
2N04	Q62625	swplus	Rat microtubule-associated protein
3A11	O54916	swplus	Mouse ralbp1 associated eps domain
3N22	U90123	genembl	Mouse HN1 (Hn1)
4B19	AF117107	genembl	Human IGF-II mRNA-binding protein 2 (IMP-2)
4B04	M34327	genembl	Mouse retinoic acid-responsive protein (MK-2)
4K20	L75940	genembl	Mouse alpha-globin
4K24	Z47088	genembl	Mouse RNA polymerase II elongation
4L24	AF086830	genembl	Mouse leukemia/lymphoma related factor LRF
4N21	U31758	genembl	Mouse transcriptional regulator RPD3 homolog
5H07	AF110645	genembl	Human candidate tumor suppressor p33 ING1
6F09	X68282	genembl	Rat ribosomal protein L13a
6J13	U30838	genembl	Mouse voltage dependent anion channel 2
7A23	Q13561	swplus	Human dynactin, 50 kd isoform
7B06	P00416	swplus	Mouse cytochrome c oxidase
7D17	Q99471	swplus	Human c-myc binding protein mm-1
7G14	X83589	genembl	Mouse mRNA expressed in E12 brain
7I11	P36578	swplus	Human 60s ribosomal protein l4
7J09	AF140348	genembl	Mouse 37kDa oncofetal antigen mRNA
7K15	M26894	genembl	Mouse beta-H1-globin mRNA
8A15	M26898	genembl	Mouse zeta-globin mRNA
8G13	AL009266	genembl	Human cDNA similar to C. elegans RNA binding
8J13	Q15324	swplus	Human alpha-spectrin (fragment)
8L13	D45913	genembl	Mouse NLRR-1 mRNA for leucine-rich-repeat protein
9G09	AB013819	genembl	Mouse mRNA for TIAP
10G22	U75358	genembl	Rat myeloma protein kinase (PAK-2)
10H06	M33024	genembl	Rat prothymosin-alpha and parathymosin
10M19	X65922	genembl	Mouse fau mRNA
10N03	X92750	genembl	Mouse red-1 gene
10N21	X05300	genembl	Rat mRNA for ribophorin I
10N22	AJ006971	genembl	Rat mRNA for DAP-like kinase
11B19	AB024303	genembl	Mouse mRNA similar to human Sua1
11J10	AF100421	genembl	Rat p80 mRNA
11J11	Y08614	genembl	Homo sapiens mRNA for CRM1 protein
11M10	Q9z1w6	swplus	Rat p80 (fragment)
12I03	U24428	genembl	Mouse mu-class glutathione s-transferase (mGSTM5)
12J08	U30828	genembl	Human splicing factor SRp55-2 (SRp55)
12K13	P03888	swplus	Mouse nadh-ubiquinone oxidoreductase
13D05	U91922	genembl	Mouse RNA helicase A (Ddx9)
13F17	U09874	genembl	Mouse SKD3
13J10	Q9z2i1	swplus	Mouse endomucin
13J04	M22432	genembl	Mouse protein synthesis elongation factor Tu
13K11	U20225	genembl	Mouse adenylosuccinate lyase (adl)
13K12	AF060090	genembl	Mouse proteasome subunit C7-I (Psmb2)
13L11	U46923	genembl	Mouse G protein-coupled receptor
14F01	Q61501	swplus	Mouse transcription factor e2f1 (e2f-1)
14G13	Q9z2x1	swplus	Rat ribonucleoprotein
14G23	X70100	genembl	Mouse mal1 mRNA for keratinocyte lipid-binding
14I13	M73436	genembl	Mouse ribosomal protein S4 (Rps4)

Table 2. Down regulated known genes in the cortex of HD mice (Cluster #1037)

MTP-Position	Acc. Number	Database	Description
2A01	D87898	genembl	Mouse mRNA for ARF1
2C22	O88297	swplus	Mouse rh blood group protein
2D04	P56480	swplus	Mouse atp synthase beta chain
2E10	X96859	genembl	Mouse mRNA for ubiquitin-conjugating enzyme
2E05	Z34918	genembl	Human mRNA for translation initiation factor
2G10	P31800	swplus	Bovine ubiquinol-cytochrome c reductase
2K03	AF093677	genembl	Mouse ATPase subunit 6 (Atpase6)
2L03	U49056	genembl	Rat CTD-binding SR-like protein rA1
2P15	X51893	genembl	Mouse fms-like gene (mflg)
2P19	P05209	swplus	Hamster tubulin alpha-1
3A16	Q61491	swplus	Mouse zinc finger protein 97
3D11	Z32519	genembl	Rat mRNA for brain myosin II
3D20	O55057	swplus	Mouse retinal rod rhodopsin-sensitive
3K09	S83456	genembl	GTP-binding protein
3M22	AF101435	genembl	Mouse Wolf-Hirschhorn syndrome candidate
3M24	X04663	genembl	Mouse mRNA for beta-tubulin (isotype Mbeta 5)
3O18	P55735	swplus	Human sec13-related protein
4A15	M33212	genembl	Mouse nucleolar protein N038
4A05	D12513	genembl	Mouse mRNA for DNA topoisomerase II
4G23	AF035683	genembl	Mouse p21 mRNA
4P13	P00848	swplus	Mouse atp synthase a chain
5G22	AF099733	genembl	Mouse proteasome subunit C3 (Psma2)
5I24	P80314	swplus	Mouse t-complex protein 1, beta subunit
5M22	AB006715	genembl	Mouse mRNA for dihydropyrimidinase related
6E24	O70579	swplus	Mouse pmp35 protein
7J06	U19893	genembl	Rat alpha actinin
7J08	AF116910	genembl	Human clone HAW100 putative ribonuclease III
7P18	Q9z2w1	swplus	Mouse ste20-like kinase
7P19	P00405	swplus	Mouse cytochrome c oxidase
8E12	X16857	genembl	Mouse mRNA for HSP86 heat-shock protein
8I11	M29793	genembl	Mouse slow/cardiac troponin C (cTnC)
8L22	X64837	genembl	Mouse Oat mRNA for ornithine aminotransferase
8P20	X79233	genembl	Mouse EWS mRNA
9E13	U77039	genembl	Mouse skeletal muscle LIM protein (FHL1)
9G15	M26897	genembl	Mouse epsilon-globin
9I05	U57692	genembl	Mouse N-terminal asparagine amidohydrolase
11D07	AF159396	genembl	Mouse cytochrome b gene
11D14	V00711	genembl	Mouse mitochondrial genome
11L09	Z47088	genembl	Mouse mRNA for RNA polymerase II elongation
11P03	X15958	genembl	Rat mRNA for mitochondrial enoyl-CoA hydratase
11P07	U81491	genembl	Mouse polyhomeotic (mPh2)
11P21	O14981	swplus	Human tbp-associated factor 170
12A09	V00711	genembl	Mouse mitochondrial genome
12E18	M62606	genembl	Mouse surfeit locus surfeit 4 protein gene
12L03	U90123	genembl	Mouse HN1 (Hn1)
12O01	AF124786	genembl	Mouse NADH-ubiquinone oxidoreductase B8 subunit
13A21	P35293	swplus	Mouse ras-related protein rab-18
13E11	M22432	genembl	Mouse protein synthesis elongation factor Tu
13E12	O54946	swplus	Mouse mrj
13F22	U76253	genembl	Mouse E25B protein mRNA
13I22	J02809	genembl	Mouse neural specific calmodulin-binding protein P-57
13J06	AF188297	genembl	Mouse TGF-beta receptor binding protein (Trip1)
13J07	S63233	genembl	Rat phosphoglycerate mutase type B subunit
13K01	Y12474	genembl	Mouse mRNA for centrin gene
13K06	M12414	genembl	Mouse apolipoprotein E mRNA
13K08	M12414	genembl	Mouse apolipoprotein E mRNA
13O17	D26610	genembl	Mouse mRNA for monoclonal nonspecific suppressor factor
14H01	AB026190	genembl	Human mRNA for Kelch motif containing protein
14I18	Y09615	genembl	Human mRNA for mitochondrial transcription factor

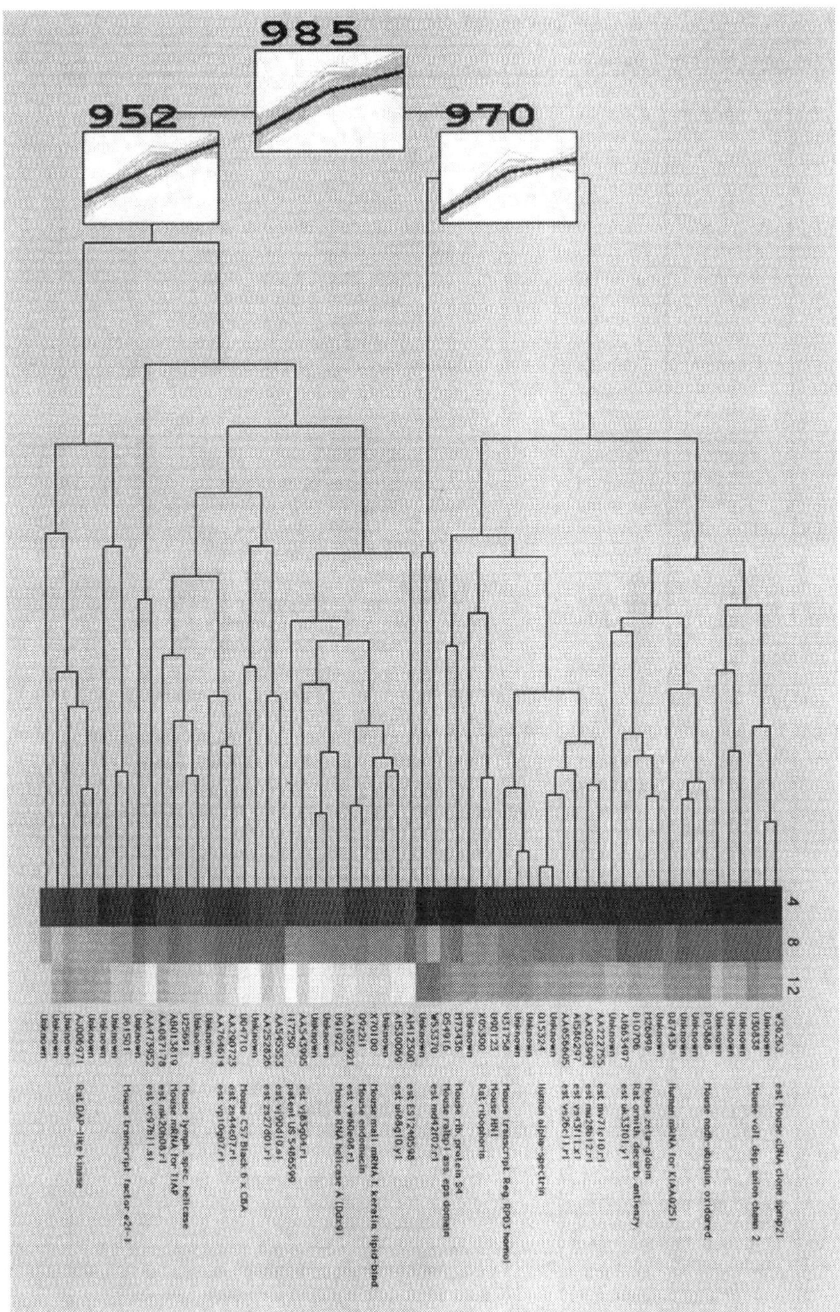

Fig. 4. Clustering of up-regulated genes in Chorea Huntington transgenic mice.
The sub-cluster #985 shows an upregulation of 63 transcripts during the time period investigated (4, 8 and 12 weeks of age). The consensus vector (bold lines) represents the mean expression values of the cluster members (faint lines). White bars indicate a high expression level, black bars a low expression level.

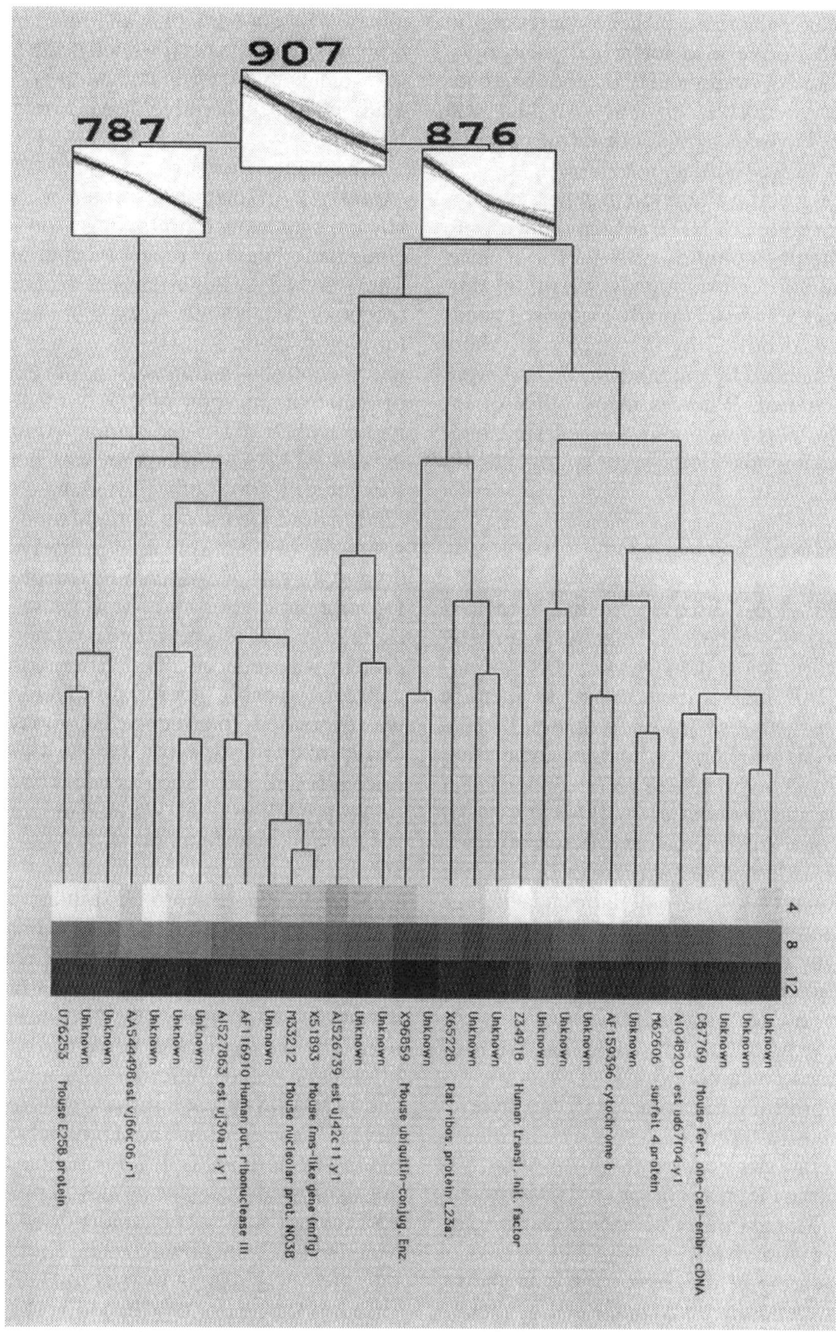

Fig. 5. Clustering of down-regulated genes in HD transgenic mice.
In sub-cluster #907 are 32 genes grouped together, which are down regulated over the period investigated. The consensus vector (bold lines) represents the mean expression values of the cluster members (faint lines). White bars indicate a high expression level, black bars a low expression level.

and a weaker decrease in gene expression in cluster #876. We also identified transcripts, which were not continuously up or down regulated. They were either up or down regulated at early age (4 to week 8) and showed the opposite from 8 to 12 weeks (data not shown).

An age-specific alteration in gene transcription in the cortex of HD transgenic mice were investigated by complex cDNA hybridization and hierarchical clustering algorithm. In summary about 500 differentially expressed genes have been identified by this approach. Many mRNAs encoded by mitochondrial DNA were down regulated. Whereas many mRNAs encoding proteins functioning in cell signaling, cell cycle or cytoskeleton were up regulated.

Discussion

The Huntington's disease gene has been well characterized, but the molecular mechanism by which neurological damage occurs is still unknown. This makes it necessary to identify molecular mediators in the formation of HD. The analysis of alteration in gene expression profiles by genome wide screenings starting at very early stages in disease will make it possible to identify such mediators. Microarray techniques provide a powerful tool to monitor gene expression profiles. Several thousands of gene representatives can be immobilized on a planar surface and their expression level can be analyzed in parallel in a single experiment (for a recent review see Young 2000).

In the experiments presented here we used glass arrays containing 5,376 cDNAs for expression profiling. By complex cDNA hybridization and clustering analysis we could identify the alteration in gene expression of about 500 transcripts in the cortex tissues of HD transgenic mice (Mangiarini et al. 1996; Davis et al. 1997) and wildtyp mice at 4, 8 and 12 weeks of age. Clustering of the expression data shows, that many genes involved in the energy metabolism and encoded by mitochondrial DNA are down regulated. Whereas many genes functioning in signaling, cell cycle control or cytoskeleton assembly were identified as up-regulated. Mitochondria play an important role in both apoptotic and necrotic cell death and there is evidence that their dysfunction is crucial in many neurodegenerative diseaes (reviewed in Beal 2000).

Cha and coworkers described an altered expression of neurotransmitter receptors in HD transgenic mice expressing exon 1 with an elongated glutamine repeat (Cha et al. 1998). They showed the down regulation of dopamine receptors, kainate receptors, glutamate receptor type 1, 2 and 3 in HD transgenic mice but not in controls. In comparison, the expression of glutamate receptor type 5, N-methyl-D-aspartic acid (NMDA) and gamma-Aminobutyric acid (GABA) – receptors was not altered (Cha et al. 1998). Luthi-Carter and colleagues (2000) described a down regulation of transcripts involved in signaling pathways, for example expression of dopamine receptor D_2 and D_4, protein kinases and phosphatases as well as retinoic acid receptors and a retinol-binding protein was reduced. Furthermore, the abundance of specific neurotransmitter receptors was decreased. In a second HD mouse model (N171-82Q) they identified in the 4-month old mice a set of genes such as adenylate cyclase or preproenkephalin, which are critical for striatal neuronal function (Luthi-Carter et al. 2000).

Many of these neurotransmitters and their receptors described by Cha and coworkers (Cha et al. 1998) and Luthi-Carter and colleagues (Luthi-Carter et al. 2000) were not present in the subset of 5,376 genes used in this investigation. The 5,376 cDNAs derived from cDNA libraries prepared from embryonic mice at day 9 and 12 and did not contain these gene representatives. These genes are most probably very low expressed during this developmental stages or are expressed later during development. The EST clones and so far unidentified cDNAs, described as "Unknown", makes it difficult to interpret these data in respect to Huntington's Disease. Currently, new experiments are performed using a mouse UNIGENE set of about 24,000 cDNA clones. Many so far not characterized transcripts have been identified and will be further characterized by functional genomics approaches like yeast two-hybrid system, *in situ* hybridization or knock out mice.

Acknowledgements

The authors would like to thank the German Ministry for Research and Education for funding this research with grant 0311018 and the HDSA.

References

1. Adams MD, Soares MB, Kerlavage AR, Fields C, Venter JC (1993) Rapid cDNA sequencing (expressed sequence tags) from a directionally cloned human infant brain cDNA library. Nature Genetics 4:373–380
2. Beal MF (2000) Energetics in the pathogenisis of neurodegenerative diseases. Trends Neurosci 23:298–304
3. Boguski M, Schuler G (1995) Establishing a human transcript map. Nature Genetics 10:369–371
4. Brown PO, Botstein D (1999) Exploring the new world of the genome with DNA microarrays. Nature Genetics 21:33–37
5. Cha J-H, Kosinski CM, Kerner JA, Alsdorf SA, Mangiarini L, Davies SW, Penney JB, Bates GP, Young AB (1998) Altered brain neurotransmitter receptors in transgenic mice expressing a portion of an abnormal human huntington disease gene. Proc Natl Acad Sci USA 95:6480–6485
6. Davies SW, Turmaine M, Cozens BA, DiFiglia M, Sharp AH, Ross CA, Scherzinger E, Wanker EE, Mangiarini L, Bates GP (1997) Formation of neuronal intranuclear inclusions underlies the neurological dysfunction in mice transgenic for the HD mutation. Cell 90:537–548
7. DeRisi J, Penland L, Brown PO, Bittner ML, Meltzer PS, Ray M, Chen Y, Su YA, Trent JM (1996) Use of a cDNA microarray to analyse gene expression patterns in human cancer [see comments]. Nature Genetics 14:457–460
8. DeRisi JL, Iyer VR, Brown PO (1997) Exploring the metabolic and genetic control of gene expression on a genomic scale. Science 278:680–686
9. Duggan DJ, Bittner M, Chen YD, Meltzer P, Trent JM (1999) Expression profiling using cDNA microarrays. Nature Genetics 21:10–14
10. Eickhoff H, Schuchhardt J, Ivanov I, Meier-Ewert S, O'Brien J, Malik A, Tandon N, Wolski EW, Rohlfs E, Nyarsik L, Reinhardt R, Nietfeld W, Lehrach H (2000) Genome Research 8:1230–1240
11. Eisen MB, Spellman PT, Brown PO, Botstein D (1998) Cluster analysis and display of genome-wide expression patterns. Proc Natl Acad Sci USA 95:14863–14868
12. Gress TM, Hoheisel JD, Lennon GG, Zehetner G, Lehrach H (1992) Hybridization fingerprinting of high-density cDNA-library arrays with cDNA pools derived from whole tissues. Mammalian Genome 3:609–619
13. Gress TM, Muller-Pillasch F, Geng M, Zimmerhackl F, Zehetner G, Friess H, Buchler M, Adler G, Lehrach H (1996) A pancreatic cancer-specific expression profile. Oncogene 13:1819–1830
14. Hoheisel JD (1997) Oligomer-Chip Technology. Trends in Biotechnology 15:465–469
15. Huntingtons Disease Collaborative Research Group (1993) A novel gene containing a trinucleotide repeat that is unstable on Huntingtons Disease chromosomes. Cell 72:971–983
16. Iyer VR, Eisen MB, Ross DT, Schuler G, Moore T, Lee JCF, Trent JM, Staudt LM, Hudson J, Boguski MS, Lashkari D, Shalon D, Botstein D, Brown PO (1999) The transcriptional program in the response of human fibroblasts to serum. Science 283:83–87
17. Lashkari DA, DeRisi JL, McCusker JH, Namath AF, Gentile C, Hwang SY, Brown PO, Davis RW (1997) Yeast microarrays for genome wide parallel genetic and gene expression analysis. Proc Natl Acad Sci USA 94:13057–13062
18. Lehrach H, Drmanac R, Hoheisel JD, Larin Z, Lennon G, Monaco AP, Nizetic D, Zehetner G, Poustka A (1990) Hybridization Fingerprinting in Genome Mapping and Sequencing. In Genome Analysis Volume 1: genetic and Physical Mapping (Cold Spring Harbor: Cold Spring Harbor Laboratory Press), pp 39–81
19. Lennon GG, Lehrach H (1991) Hybridization analyses of arrayed cDNA libraries. Trends in Genetics 7:314–317
20. Liang P, Pardee A (1992) Differential display of eukaryotic messenger RNA by means of the polymerase chain reaction. Science 257:967–971
21. Lipshutz RJ, Fodor SP, Gingeras TR, Lockhart DJ (1999) High density synthetic oligonucleotide arrays. Nature Genetics 21:20–24
22. Luthi-Carter R, Strand A, Peters NL, Solano SM, Hollingsworth ZR, Menon AS, Frey AS, Spektor BS, Penney EB, Schilling G, Ross CA, Borchelt DR, Tapscott SJ, Young AB, Cha JH, Olson JM (2000) Decreased expression of striatal signaling genes in a mouse model of Huntington's disease. Hum Mol Genet. 9:1259–1271
23. Mangiarini L, Sathasivam K, Seller M, Cozens B, Harper A, Hetherington C, Lawton M, Trottier Y, Lehrach H, Davies SW, Bates GP (1996) Exon 1 of the HD gene with an expanded CAG repeat is sufficient to cause a progressive neurological phenotype in transgenic mice. Cell 87:493–506
24. Meier-Ewert S, Lange J, Gerst H, Herwig R, Schmitt A, Freund J, Elge T, Mott R, Herrmann B, Lehrach H (1998) Comparative gene expression profiling by oligonucleotide fingerprinting. Nucleic Acids Research26:2216–2223
25. Nguyen C, Rocha D, Granjeaud S, Baldit M, Bernard K, Naquet P, Jordan BR (1995) Differential gene expression in the murine thymus assayed by quantitative hybridization of arrayed cDNA clones. Genomics 29:207–216
26. Pietu G, Alibert O, Guichard V, Lamy B, Bois F, Leroy E, Mariage-Sampson R, Houlgatte R, Soularue P, Auffray C (1996) Novel gene transcripts preferentially expressed in human muscles revealed by quantitative hybridization of a high density cDNA array. Genome Research 6:492–503
27. Poustka A, Pohl T, Barlow DP, Zehetner G, Craig A, Michiels F, Ehrich E, Frischauf AM, Lehrach H (1986) Molecular approaches to mammalian genetics. Cold Spring Harbor Symposia on Quantitative Biology 51:131–139
28. Schena M, Shalon D, Davis RW, Brown PO (1995) Quantitative monitoring of gene expression patterns with a complementary DNA microarray [see comments]. Science 270:467–470
29. Schena M, Shalon D, Heller R, Chai A, Brown PO, Davis RW (1996) Parallel human genome analysis: microarray-based expression monitoring of 1000 genes. Proceedings of the National Academy of Sciences of the United States of America 93:10614–10619
30. Scherzinger E, Lurz R, Turmaine M, Mangiarini L, Hollenbach B, Hasenbank R, Bates GP, Davies SW, Lehrach H, Wanker EE (1997) Huntingtin-encoded polyglutamine expansions form amyloid-like protein aggregates in vitro and in vivo. Cell 90(3):549–558
31. Southern EM (1995) DNA Fingerprinting By Hybridisation to Oligonucleotide Arrays. Electrophoresis 16:1539–1542

32. Velculescu V, Zhang L, Vogelstein B, Kinzler K (1995) Serial Analysis of Gene Expression. Science 270:484–487
33. Wilkinson DG, Nieto MA (1993) Detection of messenger RNA by *in situ* hybridization to tissue sections and whole mounts. Methods Enzymol 225:361–373
34. Young RA (2000) Biomedical discovery with DNA arrays. Cell 102:9–15
35. Zhang L, Zhou W, Velculescu VE, Kern S, Hruban RH, Hamilton SR, Vogelstein B, Kinzle RKW (1997) Gene expression profiles in normal and cancer cells. Science 276:1268–1272

High throughput transcript profiling: An assessment of SAGE in the context of stroke research

G. Trendelenburg, U. Dirnagl

Introduction

Brain tissue damage as a result of focal cerebral ischemia (stroke) has long been viewed as an acute passive event in which energy failure directly leads to necrotic cell death. Only recently experimental evidence is accumulating that delayed events involving gene expression, such as inflammation or apoptosis, are important contributors to ischemic cell death in the brain (Dirnagl et al. 1999) and may be used as targets for beneficial pharmacological interventions.

Candidate approaches have already identified a number of genes relevant for cerebral ischemia and their corresponding signaling pathways have been partially elucidated. It is to be expected that with the completion of the human and other mammalian genomes many related and new ischemia-relevant candidates will be discovered.

While up to now cerebral ischemia research has progressed with 'hypothesis driven' (i.e. candidate based) paradigms, the recent technological advances in generating comprehensive transcription profiles (microarrays; serial analysis of gene expression, SAGE; expressed sequence tag (EST) -sequencing etc.), together with the ever increasing availability of genomic data have made possible high throughput screening and 'question driven' (Lockhart and Winzeler, 2000) approaches, which are currently entering the cerebrovascular reseach arena.

In this paper we will first discuss some general aspects of screening approaches, which will be, or already have been applied in the neurosciences. We have recently applied transcription profiling using SAGE to focal cerebral ischemia, which we will review in some detail in the second part of the manuscript.

The rise of functional genomics

The last decade has seen an exponential rise in genomic data in public and proprietary sequence databases, a development that will probably culminate this year with the publication of the complete human genome (Macilwain 2000). In addition, the genome of a number of model organisms has been (Drosophila, C.elegans etc.) or will be (rat, mouse etc.) sequenced in the near future. From this data already functions can be assigned to uncharacterized genes based on

Keywords: Differential gene expression, DNA chip, microarray, knockout mice, screening approach, serial analysis of gene expression, stroke, SAGE, transcription profiling

Department of Neurology, Charité, Humboldt Universität Berlin, Schumannstraße 20/21, D-10098 Berlin, Germany
e-mail: ulrich.dirnagl@charite.de

J. Krieglstein, S. Klumpp (Eds.) Pharmacology of Cerebral Ischemia 2000

sequence information and comparison to homologous genes, transcripts, or protein ('data mining'). These advances have been made possible by evolutionary (e.g., sequencing) as well as revolutionary (e.g., microarrays) progress in molecular biotechnology, which stipulated the creation of the new field of 'functional genomics'.

Functional genomics analyses biological systems in a holistic and high throughput fashion, which is not necessarily hypothesis, but rather question driven. This has been critisized as 'mindless' and unscientific. However, numerous recent studies have demonstrated that comparisons of large sets of genes in different organisms and different tissues under different conditions can help to understand physiological and pathophysiological processes and unravel hitherto unknown functions of genes and proteins (Young 2000; Hughes et al. 2000; Roberts et al. 2000; Velculescu et al. 1999; Brown and Botstein 1999; Polyak et al. 1997). Whether such an approach will also be applicable to the brain, the organ with the most complex cellular composition and function, and to such processes as cerebral ischemia, in which many different pathophysiological processes interact (Dirnagl et al. 1999), has yet to be demonstrated. Another general issue of concern is the high degree of expertise (molecular biology, computing, biomathematics, etc.) and sophisticated machinery required to successfully apply functional genomics. This is a particular challenge for academic research, which suddenly has problems in competing with the multinational pharmaceutical industry and upstart biotech companies supplied with plenaty of venture capital.

Screening for differential expression: transcriptomics

The 'genetic' status of a tissue or individual is not only characterized by its structural basis, the genome, but also by the complete proteome with its modifications, as well as the corresponding RNA-pool, the transcriptome (Velculescu et al. 1997). The central dogma of 'transcriptomics' is that changes in protein expression (and abundance) is correlated with the appearance (and amount) of the corresponding transcript. At present RNA-based technologies are technically advanced compared to proteomics, therefore screening for transcriptional changes is currently more widely applied in high throughput approaches.

Methods for studying gene-expression at the transcript-level can be divided into three major groups according to the underlying principle: Hybridization-based methods (northern blotting, subtractive cloning, DNA microarrays and chips), PCR-based methods (RT-PCR, differential display) and sequencing-based methods (expressed sequence tags-approaches, SAGE).

A breakthrough in gene expression analysis was the development of the Northern-blot technique (Alwine et al. 1977), where signal intensity after hybridization between a fixed mRNA and a specific and labeled probe correlates with transcript abundance in the mRNA preparation. Even today this technique has not lost importance, as differences detected in high throughput transcript expression analysis are almost always confirmed by Northern-analysis.

Modern mircoarray or chip technologies are based on a very similar principle, but with an 'inverse' design: specific probes are spotted on a solid support, whereas the RNA pool to be examined is labelled and hybridizes with each specific transcript in the corresponding probe. This procedure has been known in principcle for several years, but the breakthrough was brought about by advances in miniaturization of spotting and readout. By slightly different ways specific DNAs can be spotted on the solid support substrate (commonly glas): either a long cDNA-fragment is fixed on the surface (Schena et al. 1995; Brown and Botstein 1999) or short oligonucleotides are synthesized directly on the substrate using photolithographic procedures, a technology derived from computer chip construction (Lockhart et al. 1996; Lipshutz et al. 1999).

PCR related techniques like differential display (DD)-RT-PCR have been applied sucessfully by several groups, but are limited by a high degree of false positive results and many primer combinations are necessary for the analysis of complete transcription profiles. Yet, since it is based on standard molecular biological technique, DD-RT-PCR can be applied even in small laboratories. RT-PCR with its need for known primer sequences has widely been applied for confirmation of differential gene expression, especially for low abundancy transcripts, but it cannot be used for gene discovery.

Further methods successfully applied in the identification of transcriptional changes like suppression subtractive hybridization (SSH) (Diatschenko et al. 1996; Zuber et al. 2000), which is based on a substraction procedure, are not further discussed here because of their focus on a selection process rather than the measurement of whole transription profiles.

All the procedures mentioned above have in common one major drawback, which has to be kept in mind: regulatory mechanisms on the posttranslational level (phosphorylation, glykosylation etc.) can not be detected by them.

Serial analysis of gene expression (SAGE)

After these more general remarks, in the second part of the manuscript we will focus on the transcription profiling technique SAGE. Since SAGE, in contrast to microarray technology is based on standard molecular biological techniques and does not necessitate specialized equipment, it has been particularly advocated for the academic setting.

Almost at the same time when the first successful microarray experiments were reported (Schena et al. 1995; Lockhart et al. 1996), serial analysis of gene expression (SAGE) was described by Velculescu et al. (1995). The principle of SAGE (Fig. 1) is based on 1) the reduction of each transcript sequence to a representative short tag (14–15 bp) and 2) the concatenating of these tags into long DNA molecules, which, when sequenced reveal the identity of multiple tags simultaneously. The number of

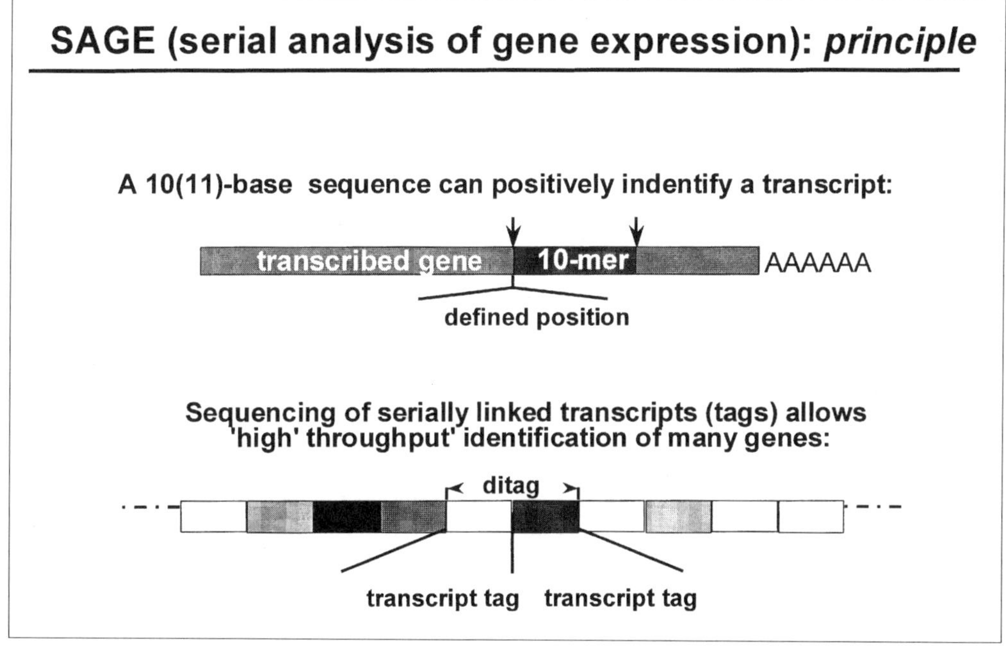

Fig. 1. Principle of SAGE

times a particular tag is detected in a SAGE library corresponds to the abundance of its transcript in the starting pool (transcriptome) and therefore provides a quantitative measure of gene expression.

In contrast to hybridization based procedures like microarray technologies, SAGE is based on a rather digital as well as procedure: like EST-sequencing projects, it relies on the counting of absolute numbers of transcripts, thereby resulting in a digital expression profile (Velculescu et al. 1995, 1997; Zhang et al. 1997). SAGE yields information of absolute expression, which can be compared with those of other SAGE-datasets to search for differentially expressed genes. In contrast to chip or other blotting technologies there is no need for sequence information before starting with SAGE. Because SAGE also includes sequence information of each analysed gene, one can benefit from EST-databases for direct gene identification, or may discover completely unknown genes by the use of classical cloning techniques.

Technical aspects

For SAGE, as well as for most other expression methods, RNA isolation as the first step is a very critical one. Especially high quality and sufficient quantity of mRNA are essential for the generation of SAGE libraries. Fresh material is superior to frozen tissue for RNA isolation and long postmortal times should be avoided in order to obtain RNA pools representative for the *in vivo* situation. Standard RNA-amounts recommended for SAGE are in the range of 1–5 μg mRNA and therefore comparable to those required for microarray experiments. Nevertheless, several methods were described which allow to reduce the RNA amount when only minor quantities of tissue are available (e.g., cell culture) (Virlon et al. 1999; Datson et al. 1999; Peters et al. 1999).

A rarely discussed problem of SAGE is related to the need for a poly-A-tail, at least when using Oligo-dT for reverse transcription. Since SAGE relies on the analysis of the 3' end of each transcript, which has to be polyadenylated according to the standard procedure (Velculescu et al. 1995), a small fraction of non-polyadenylated mRNA, which has been detected in the central nervous system (Jaber et al. 1994; Primus et al. 1992; Harris and Sherbany 1991) will be lost at the reverse transcription step. It should be noted that other expression profiling methods which use an Oligo-dT-primed reverse transcription step, are affected by this.

Modifications of the original protocol

Since the first description of SAGE 1995 (Velculescu et al. 1995), the number of variations of the original protocol is rising. One central issue already mentioned above is the aim for a reduction of the relatively high amount of starting tissue or initial mRNA recommended in the original protocol. Most improvements were based on a more efficient use of mRNA in the initial steps (reverse transcription, washing). Technical modifications rely on the use of Streptavidin-coated reaction tubes instead of paramagnetic streptavidin beads (Datson et al. 1999), or a completely modified protocol with the use of Oligo-dT primers directly fixed on the paramagnetic beads used for cDNA synthesis (Virlon et al. 1999). An alternative approach is an initial amplification step of whole cDNA before starting with SAGE (Peters et al. 1999).

To yield enough material at the concatamer stage for SAGE library construction, a PCR amplification step has been introduced. One may try to circumvent the need for a high amount of mRNA by increasing the cycle number of the SAGE-implicated PCR-amplification step. However, this will (as any additional PCR cycles) result in a poor quality of the resulting SAGE-library, as the amount of PCR-biased products will increase. Fortunately, however, PCR bias can be recognized at the analysis stage since identical 'ditags' and corresponding transcripts can be eliminated from further analysis.

Recently published modifications refer to one of the last SAGE steps, where the concatamers are ligated in the vectors of choice. One group is recommeding an additional heating step (Kenzelmann and Mühlemann 1999) while others favor the use of biotin-linked primers in the amplification step to minimize the amount of contaminating short fragments (Powell 1998). Further improvement has been described for the restriction digest by a prior purification step (Angelastro et al. 2000).

Sequence identification

Identifying corresponding transcripts for SAGE-tags sometimes is complicated, as different database entries may match to a specific tag, or no homologous entry is available at all. High quality SAGE-libraries with a high degree of tag length uniformity yield information on the 11th basepair, which simplifies proper transcript identification. Because approximately 10% of tags yield erroneous sequences (Velculescu et al. 1997; own observations), only tags occuring with a frequency of more than one should be considered for further analysis. Several strategies to identify corresponding sequences via PCR have been described (Chen et al. 1999; van den Berg et al. 1999), as well as an identification of specific transcripts by colony screening with short tags used as probes (Velculescu et al. 1995).

SAGE statistics

A major aspect of SAGE data analysis concerns the threshold in absolute tag counts which is accepted as a statistically significant expression difference. Thus, one may ask: how many tags have to be sequenced to detect differential expression of a certain gene? A detailed discussion of this problem is found in Kal et al. 1999. Their strategy has been implemented in a statistical software for SAGE called SAGESTAT (Kal et al. 1999). Other analysis tools based on Monte Carlo analysis have been incorporated in the SAGE2000 software, which is available on request from Dr. K. Kinzler (http://www.sagenet.org/home/Info.htm). Further help on SAGE statistics is given on the SAGE-pages of the NCBI (http://www.ncbi.nlm.nih.gov/SAGE/) (Lal et al. 1999). Several other statistical models have been used to analyse SAGE tag data, as presented last year by Dr. J.M. Rujiter at a SAGE symposium (Baas and Tabak 1999). In prinicple, the amount of total tags which have to be sequenced depends on 1) the significance level required, 2) the average copy per cell count and 3) the expression level of the genes of interest. For example, 315.000 tags have to be sequenced in each of two different conditions to detect a 3-fold upregulation of a specific gene normally expressed at 10 copies in a mammalian cell (assuming 300.000 transcripts per cell) when a significance level of 0.05 is required (Kal et al. 1999).

Advantages of SAGE

One of the major advantages of SAGE is based on the fact that it relies on a combination of standard procedures of molecular biology available in many laboratories, without the need for expensive, specialized equipment (such as spotter and reader in microarray technology). Since no apriori information about transcripts is needed, and because of the sequence information yielded, SAGE can be used for gene discovery and may speed up EST-sequencing projects. In contrast to hybridization based procedures it can also discriminate between different splicing variants, which may become increasingly relevant.

Disadvantages of SAGE

SAGE depends on bulk sequencing, which is necessary to yield information on medium or even low-level expression patterns. Before starting a SAGE project one should calculate the number of tags to sequence, based on the desired depth and fidelity of the transcriptional information which is desired. In contrast to SAGE, microarray technologies can be automatized, which facilitates the analysis of large sets of material from different conditions, time points, or tissues. SAGE may be of advantage where an exact, partly unknown transcriptome in an rather definite genomic context is studied, whereas microarray technology is more suited when an known subset of candidate genes is studied under various conditions (e.g., time kinetics).

Sage applications

SAGE already has been succesfully applied in various tissues, and the number of publications which apply SAGE rises exponentially. In the neurosciences, SAGE has been used to reveal differential gene expression in the context of NMDA and nitric oxide-mediated neurotoxicity (Gonzalez-Zulueta et al. 1998). Using serial analysis of gene expression (SAGE) we analysed differential gene expression after transient focal cerebral ischemia (unpublished data). After analysis of more than 60,000 transcripts, SAGE identified metallothionein II (MT-II) as the most significantly upregulated transcript 14 hours after induction of focal cerebral ischemia in the mouse.

This prompted us to further investigate the expression and functional role of MT-II and the related gene MT-I. By using a mouse knockout model we demonstrated that MT-II is a highly relevant neuroprotective gene in focal cerebral ischemia (unpublished data). Thus, a descriptive screening approach can indeed identify functionally relevant genes, which might represent future targets of pharmacological intervention in stroke.

Conclusion

We have applied SAGE successfully to differential gene expression after mouse focal cerebral ischemia. Since it is based on standard procedures of molecular biology and does not need specialized technology, SAGE appeals to gene discovery and differential gene expression projects in the academic setting. However, SAGE is a techniqually demanding method, which necessitates the sequencing of a large amount of DNA, at least when medium to low abundance transcripts are targeted. We speculate that the use of SAGE in the future will be limited to projects where gene identification is the primary goal, or where defined transcriptomes of small to medium size are compared to identify differentially regulated genes.

Acknowledgements

Supported by the Deutsche Forschungsgemeinschaft (ME 1562/1-1) and the Hermann und Lilly Schilling Stiftung. SAGE software (V 3.01) and Detailed Protocol (V. 1.0c) were kindly provided by Dr. K. Kinzler.

References

1. Alwine JC, Kemp DJ, Stark GR (1977) Method for detection of specific RNAs in agarose gels by transfer to diazobenzyloxymethyl-paper and hybridization with DNA probes. Proc Natl Acad Sci USA 74:5350–5354
2. Angelastro JM, Klimaschewski LP, Vitolo OV (2000) Improved Nla III digestion of PAGE-purified 102 bp ditags by addition of a single purification step in both the SAGE and microSAGE protocols. Nucleic Acids Res 28:e62
3. Baas F, Tabak HF (1999) A tale of tags: report on a HUGO/EU SAGE workshop, 29 January-1 February 1999, Hilversum, The netherlands. Eur J Hum Genet 7:510–512
4. Brown PO, Botstein D (1999) Exploring the new world of the genome with DNA microarrays. Nat Genet 21(1 Suppl):33–37
5. Chen J-J, Rowley JD, Wang SM (1999) Generation of longer cDNA fragments from serial analysis of gene expression tags for gene identification. Proc Natl Acad Sci USA 97:349–353
6. Datson NA, Vanderperkdejong J, Vandenberg MP, Dekloet ER, Vreugdenhil E (1999) MicroSAGE – a modified procedure for serial analysis of gene-expression in limited amounts of tissue. Nucleic Acids Res 27:1300–1307
7. Diatschenko L, Lau YFC, Campbell AP, Chenchik A, Moquadam F, Huang B, Lukyanov, S, Lukyanov K, Gurskaya N, Sverdlov ED, Siebert PK (1996) Suppression subtractive hybridization: a method for generating differentially regulated of tissue-specific cDNA probes and libraries. Proc Natl Acad Sci USA 903:6025–6030
8. Dirnagl U, Iadecola C, Moskowitz MA (1999) Pathobiology of ischaemic stroke: an integrated view. Trends Neurosci 22:391–397
9. Gonzalez-Zulueta M, Ensz LM, Mukhina G, Lebovitz RM, Zwacka RM, Engelhardt JF, Oberley, LW, Dawson VL, Dawson TM (1998) Manganese superoxide dismutase protects nNOS neurons from NMDA and nitric oxide-mediated neurotoxicity. J Neurosci 18:2040–2055
10. Harris DA, Sherbany AA (1991) Cloning of non-polyadenylated RNAs from rat brain. Brain Res Mol Brain Res 10:83–90
11. Hughes TR, Marton MJ, Jones AR, Roberts CR, Stoughton R, Armour CD, Bennett HA, Coffey E, Dai H, He YD, Kidd MJ, King AM, Meyer MR, Slade D, Lum PY, Stepaniants SB,

Shoemaker DD, Gachotte D, Chakraburtty K, Simon J, Bard M, Friend SH (2000) Functional Discovery via a Compendium of Expression Profiles Cell 102:109–126
12. Jaber M, Merlio JP, Bloch B (1994) Expression of polyadenylated and non-polyadenylated trkC transcripts in the rodent central nervous system. Neurosci 61:245–256
13. Kal AJ, van ZA, Benes V, van dB, Koerkamp MG, Albermann K, Strack N, Ruijter JM, Richter A, Dujon B, Ansorge W, Tabak HF (1999). Dynamics of gene expression revealed by comparison of serial analysis of gene expression transcript profiles from yeast grown on two different carbon sources. Mol Biol Cell 10:1859–1872
14. Kenzelmann M, Mühlemann K (1999) Substantially enhanced cloning efficiency of SAGE (serial analysis of gene expression) by adding a heating step to the original protocol. Nucleic Acids Res 27:917–918
15. Lal A, Lash AE, Altschul SF, Velculescu V, Zhang L, McLendon RE, Marra MA, Prange C, Morin PJ, Polyak K, Papadopoulos N, Vogelstein B, Kinzler KW, Strausberg RL, Riggins GJ (1999) A public database for gene expression in human cancers. Cancer Res 59:5403–5407
16. Lipshutz RJ, Fodor SP, Gingeras TR, Lockhart DJ (1999) High density synthetic oligonucleotide arrays. Nat Genet 21(1 Suppl):20–24
17. Lockhart DJ, Dong H, Byrne MC, Follettie MT, Gallo MV, Chee MS, Mittmann M, Wang C, Kobayashi M, Horton H, Brown EL (1996) Expression monitoring by hybridization to high-density oligonucleotide arrays. Nat Biotechnol 14:1675–1680
18. Lockhart DJ, Winzeler EA (2000) Genomics, gene expression and DNA arrays. Nature 405:827–836
19. Macilwain C (2000) World leaders heap praise on human genome landmark. Nature 405:983–984
20. Peters DG, Kassam AB, Yonas H, O'Hare EH, Ferrell RE, Brufsky AM (1999) Comprehensive transcript analysis in small quantities of mRNA by SAGE-Lite. Nucleic Acids Res 27:e39
21. Polyak K, Xia Y, Zweier JL, Kinzler KW, Vogelstein B (1997) A model for p53-induced apoptosis. Nature 389:300–305
22. Powell J (1998) Enhanced concatemer cloning-a modification to the SAGE (Serial Analysis of Gene Expression) technique. Nucleic Acids Res 26:3445–3446
23. Primus RJ, Jacobs AA, Gallager DW (1992) Developmental profile of polyadenylated and non-polyadenylated $GABA_A$ receptor subunit mRNAs. Mol Brain Res 14:179–185
24. Roberts CJ, Nelson B, Marton MJ, Stoughton R, Meyer MR, Bennett HA, He YD, Dai H, Walker WL, Hughes TR, Tyers M, Boone C, Friend SH (2000) Signaling and circuitry of multiple MAPK pathways revealed by a matrix of global gene expression profiles. Science 287:873–880
25. Schena M, Shalon D, Davis RW, Brown PO (1995) Qantitative monitoring of gene experssion patterns with a complementary DNA microarry. Science 270:467–470
26. Trendelenburg G, Muselmann C, Prass K, Ruscher K, Polley A, Wiegand F, Meisel A, Rosenthal A, Dirnagl U (2000) Reproducibility of serial analysis of gene expression (SAGE) and comprehensive transcript profiling in focal cerebral ischemia in the mouse. Eur J Neurosci 12 Suppl 11:307
27. Van den Berg A, van der Leij J, Poppema S (1999) Serial analysis of gene expression: rapid RT-PCR analysis of unknown SAGE tags. Nucleic Acids Res 27:e17
28. Velculescu VE, Zhang L, Vogelstein B, Kinzler KW (1995) Serial analysis of gene expression. Science 270:484–487
29. Velculescu VE, Zhang L, Zhou W, Vogelstein J, Basrai MA, Bassett Jr DE, Hieter P, Vogelstein B, Kinzler KW (1997) Characterization of the yeast transcriptome. Cell 88:243–251
30. Velculescu VE, Madden SL, Zhang L, Lash AE, Yu J, Rago C, Lal A, Wang CJ, Beaudry GA, Ciriello KM, Cook BP, Dufault MR, Ferguson AT, Gao Y, He TC, Hermeking H, Hiraldo SK, Hwang PM, Lopez MA, Luderer HF, Mathews B, Petroziello JM, Polyak K, Zawel L, Kinzler KW, et al. (1999) Analysis of human transcriptomes. Nat Genet 23:387–388
31. Virlon B, Cheval L, Buhler JM, Billon, E, Doucet A, Elalouf JM (1999) Serial microanalysis of renal transcriptomes. Proc Natl Acad Sci USA 96:15286–15291
32. Young RA (2000) Biomedical discovery with DNA arrays. Cell 102:9–15
33. Zhang L, Zhou W, Velculescu VE, Kern SE, Hruban RH, Hamilton SR, Vogelstein B, Kinzler KE (1997) Gene expression profiles in normal and cancer cells. Science 276:1268–1272
34. Zuber J, Tchernitsa OI, Hinzmann B, Schmitz AC, Grips M, Hellriegel M, Sers C, Rosenthal A, Schafer R (2000) A genome-wide survey of RAS transformation targets. Nat Genet 24: 144–152

The role of gene therapy in acute cerebral ischemia

M. A. Yenari[1,2,3], T. C. Dumas[4,5], R. M. Sapolsky[2,4,5], G. K. Steinberg[1,3,4]

Abstract

Significant advances have been made over the past few years concerning the cellular and molecular events underlying neuron death. This has allowed the design of rational therapies to protect neurons at such times. One of the most exciting arenas of such interventions is the use of viral vectors to deliver neuroprotective genes. Neuroprotection has been demonstrated against a variety of central nervous system insults with vectors overexpressing genes that target various facets of injury. These include energy restoration by the glucose transporter (GLUT-1), buffering calcium excess by calbindin, preventing protein malfolding or aggregation by stress proteins and inhibiting apoptotic death by BCL-2. This review discusses some of the progress made in this area including whether gene therapy is effective against different kinds of central nervous system insults, whether therapy can be applied after the onset of injury, and if sparing a neuron from death necessarily spares function. Finally, we consider the possibility of such gene therapy becoming relevant to clinical neurology in the near future.

Introduction

Recent scientific advances in the area of stroke and neurodegeneration has led to the discovery of specific cellular events which occur during necrosis and apoptosis. It is now possible to therapeutically target these events with the hope of rescuing brain cells from death. The past decade has seen a variety of pharmaceutical agents designed to limit excitotoxicity, inflammation and free radical generation. Another strategy utilized by a few groups is that of gene therapy, or the transfer of genetic material into host cells with the intent of expressing the protein of interest. Several studies have shown that cerebral ischemia alters gene expression and that some of the induced genes may serve a protective or damaging role. Among the many genes which have been identified to participate in ischemia, those which possess neuroprotective properties may be excellent candidates for gene therapy. Of the various candidate genes, we have shown that neurons can be rescued from various insults through the overexpression of the glucose transporter (GLUT-1), the

Keywords: gene therapy, cerebral ischemia, excitotoxin, heat shock protein, herpes virus, apoptosis

Departments of Neurosurgery,[1] Neurology,[2] and Stanford Stroke Center[3], 1201 Welch Rd., MSLS Bldg. P304, Stanford University, Stanford, CA 94305-5487
e-mail: yenari@ leland.Stanford.edu.
Stanford University Medical Center and Program in Neurosciences,[4] and Department of Biological Sciences[5]

calcium buffering protein calbindin D28K (CaBP), the antiapoptotic protein BCL-2 and the stress protein HSP70. We review our recent experience with gene transfer therapy to cerebral neurons using defective herpes simplex viral vectors.

The cellular cascade of neuron death following injury

The cascade of events mediating necrotic and apoptotic elements of neuron death (Green and Reed 1998; Sapolsky and Steinberg 1999) suggests specific points to be targeted in therapy (Fig. 1). Following the deprivation of its metabolic substrates, synaptic concentrations of excitatory amino acids (EAAs) in the brain rise into the excitotoxic range. Excessive EAAs, namely glutamate, exert their excitotoxic effects through NMDA and non-NMDA receptors, and increase influx of calcium and sodium. Further calcium accumulation results from internal release from the endoplasmic reticulum and mitochondria. This excess of free cytosolic calcium is central to the excitotoxic hypothesis, whereby calcium activates the generation of reactive oxygen species (ROS), cytoskeletal proteolysis, and the malfolding and aggregation of proteins, collectively leading to cell death. ROS are thought to be particularly damaging when reduced cerebral blood flow is followed by reperfusion.

Recently, it has become recognized that apoptotic, or programmed cell death occurs in a subset of neurons (Bredesen 1995). Whereas necrotic cell death typically involves non-specific DNA degradation, nuclear pyknosis, loss

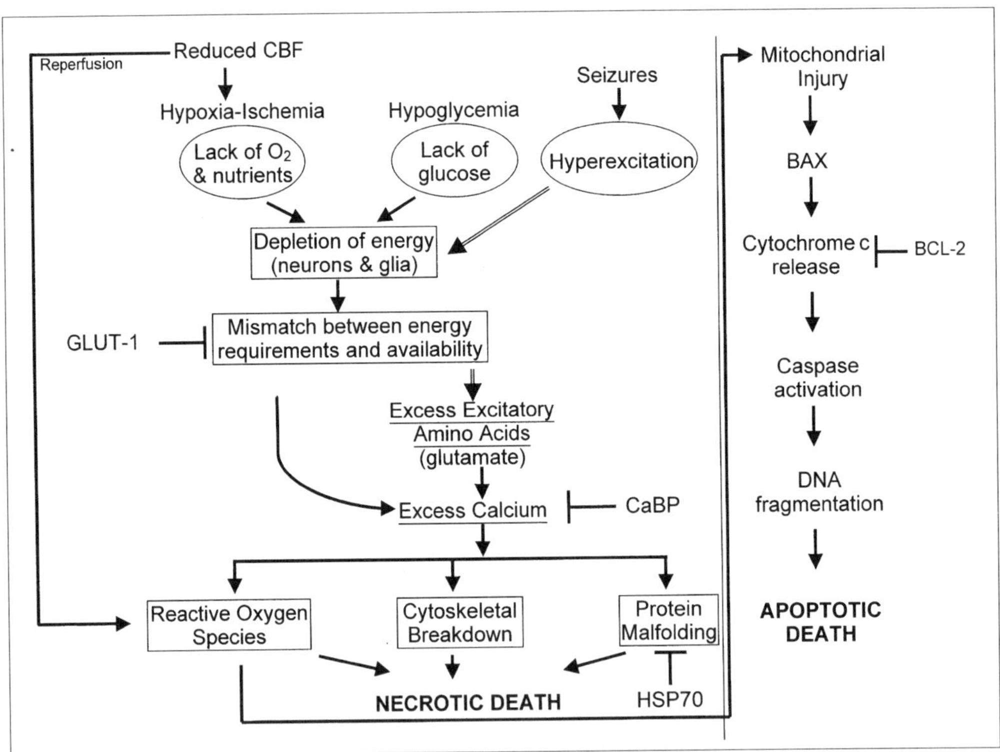

Fig. 1. Schematic representation of the pathways mediating necrotic and apoptotic death following acute neurological insults (arrows), and sites of demonstrated therapeutic efficacy of gene transfer approaches (T-squares). Abbreviations: CBF: cerebral blood flow; GLUT-1 = glucose transporter; CaBP = calbindin D28K; HSP70: heat shock protein 70.

of membrane integrity, and mitochondrial swelling, apoptosis involves chromosome condensation and DNA fragmentation at internucleosomal sites, membrane rounding and blebbing of the cell into apoptotic bodies, and changes in surface antigens. Current evidence suggests that for ischemic and excitotoxic insults, ROS-induced damage to mitochondria results in activation and dimerization of the pro-apoptotic protein BAX. This leads to cytochrome c release from mitochondria which, in turn, activates proteolytic enzymes called caspases. This eventually results in the pathway of events leading to DNA, membrane and antigenic changes noted above that characterize apoptosis. Among the various genes involved in apoptotic death, some are known to inhibit this process. One is example is the anti-apoptotic gene, BCL-2, a membrane bound protein now known to antagonize cytochrome c release (Kluck et al. 1997).

While this picture of neuron death is highly simplified, it does suggest potential targets for the genetic interventions (Sapolsky and Steinberg 1999). For example, expression of the glucose transporter (GLUT-1) could enhance transport of the neuron's metabolic substrate during a period where the availability is critically low. Intracellular calcium could be buffered by overexpressing high levels of endogenous binding proteins. Protein malfolding and aggregation could be prevented by upregulating heat shock proteins. Finally, apoptotic death could be inhibited by increasing the amount of anti-apoptotic proteins.

Viral vector construction and characterization

Viral vectors are one means by which genetic material can be transferred into host cells. Herpes simplex virus is a natural choice for gene transfer into the adult central nervous system as the virus is neurotropic (Geller et al. 1991; Glorioso et al. 1994). While herpes is known to cause devastating human illnesses, replication incompetent strains have been developed which contain mutations within genes responsible for cytotoxicity (DeLuca et al. 1985). The *d120* strain contains a 4.1 kb deletion mutation in α4, an immediate early gene essential for early and late gene induction (DeLuca et al. 1985). Without α4, the virus is incapable of performing replication, capsid synthesis and assembly (Fink et al. 1996). Our group utilizes an amplicon ("cloning amplifying") based system for vector generation. The construction of amplicon plasmids and vectors has been described in detail elsewhere (Ho 1994; Ho et al. 1995a, 1995b; Lawrence et al. 1996a; Fink et al. 1997; Yenari et al. 1998a). A plasmid containing the gene(s) of interest and a replication incompetent helper virus are cotransfected into a cell line (E5) which contains all the necessary components for virus replication and assembly. The transfected cell line produces progeny virion containing either the plasmid of interest or helper virus. After removing cellular debris, the vector, containing concatemers of the plasmid and helper virus, is said to be purified, and suitable for in vivo gene transfer study. After direct parenchymal injection, the vector is taken up almost exclusively by neurons, although ependymal cells will take up the viral vector after intraventricular injection. In fact, with direct injection into hippocampus and striatum, approximately 80% of transfected cells colocalize with neuronal markers.

The vectors used in our studies are referred to as "bipromoter." That is, 2 separate promoters drive expression of 2 different genes (Ho 1994). An advantage of this system is that both a reporter gene (e.g., the *E. coli lacZ* gene) and the gene of interest are coexpressed within targeted cells. Since many insults often induce the gene of interest within the cells themselves, transgene expression due to transfection and endogenous gene expression can be difficult to differentiate. With these vectors, the problem is circumvented because transfected cells also overexpress a reporter gene, in this case β-galactosidase (β-gal), the gene product of *lacZ*. Transgene expression begins within 4–6 h after injection and peaks at about 12–24 h (Yenari et al. 1998a). Expression is typically limited to a few days, but the duration of expression may depend on the tissue half life of the protein itself, rather than the duration of transcription and translation. For example, the tissue half life of βgal is particularly long and may persist as long as 7 days, whereas HSP70 protein persists for only one day (Yenari et al. 1998a, 1998b). For cerebral ischemia and other acute nervous system insults, the issue of long term expression from these vectors may not be so critical, since the temporal therapeutic window for stroke treatment is finite, and for most interventions, relatively brief. Therefore, stroke treatments using gene therapy may require transgene expression for only a few hours to a few days. On the other hand, recent data has also shown that ischemic injury evolves over a few days to weeks depending on the model studied (Du et al. 1996); therefore, the prolonged detection of the reporter protein, βgal may serve as an advantage in stroke models in that the "tagged" cells can be identified regardless of whether the transgene of interest is still expressing. A limitation of this vector system concerns the extent of transfection. With a transfection efficiency of approximately 10%, only a few hundred neurons can be expected to take up the plasmid, and about 80% of transfected cells are contained within a 0.5 mm radius of the injection site (Ho et al. 1993; Yenari et al. 1998a). Nevertheless, we have adapted this system for gene transfer studies using various *in vivo* models of necrotic and apoptotic injury.

Therapeutic targets for gene therapy

We now review our experience using viral vectors to alter the various steps in cell death. Because viral vector injection can only transfect a few hundred cells at best, and the genes we have studied to date act intracellularly or within the membrane, we have adapted standard injury models to accommodate this limitation. To date, we have primarily utilized the rodent suture occlusion model to study focal cerebral ischemia and kainic acid administration to study excitotoxic injury.

In the focal cerebral ischemia model (Yenari et al. 1996), a 3–0 surgical suture with the tip rounded and enlarged by flaming is inserted into the common carotid artery and advanced to occlude the ostium of the middle cerebral artery (MCA). Reperfusion can be controlled simply with withdrawing the suture. Injury to the ipsilateral striatum is consistent even after brief periods of MCA occlusion, and injection and expression of the viral vector to this brain region is consistent and reproducible (Lawrence et al. 1996b; Yenari et al. 1998b). It should first be emphasized that the injury paradigms applied here have been optimized for the purpose of hypothesis testing, and less for the purpose of clinical application. These issues will be discussed at the end of this review. The vector is stereotaxically injected into each striatum approximately 6–15 h prior to ischemia onset. Because the transgene reaches peak expression 9–12 h after injection, the rationale is to coincide gene expression and injury onset. The MCA is occluded for a relatively brief period of time (1 h) to ensure some ischemic striatal damage, but not so much as to hinder transcriptional and translational machinery of the vector and host cell. 48 h later, the brains are harvested, and coronal sections are stained with X-gal (a chromogenic substrate for β-galactosidase) and cresyl violet to identify vector targeted cells and to delineate the extent of ischemic injury, respectively. The number of X-gal positive neurons are counted in each striatum and the total number of positive cells in the ischemic striatum is normalized to the number of positive cells in the contralateral striatum (Fig. 2). Therefore, a percentage of surviving neurons receiving the vector can be determined. To ensure that any observed neuroprotection is not due to an imbalance in the overall damage between the treated and control groups, the infarct size is both measured and given a semiquantitative score (Lawrence et al. 1996a, 1996b; Yenari et al. 1998b).

For the kainic acid model, a similar logic is applied. Kainic acid administration (either by parenteral administration or direct parenchymal injection) leads to destruction of the neurons in the hippocampal formation, especially CA3/4. Vector is injected into the hippocampus followed by kainic acid administration approximately 12 h later. Because hand injection of the

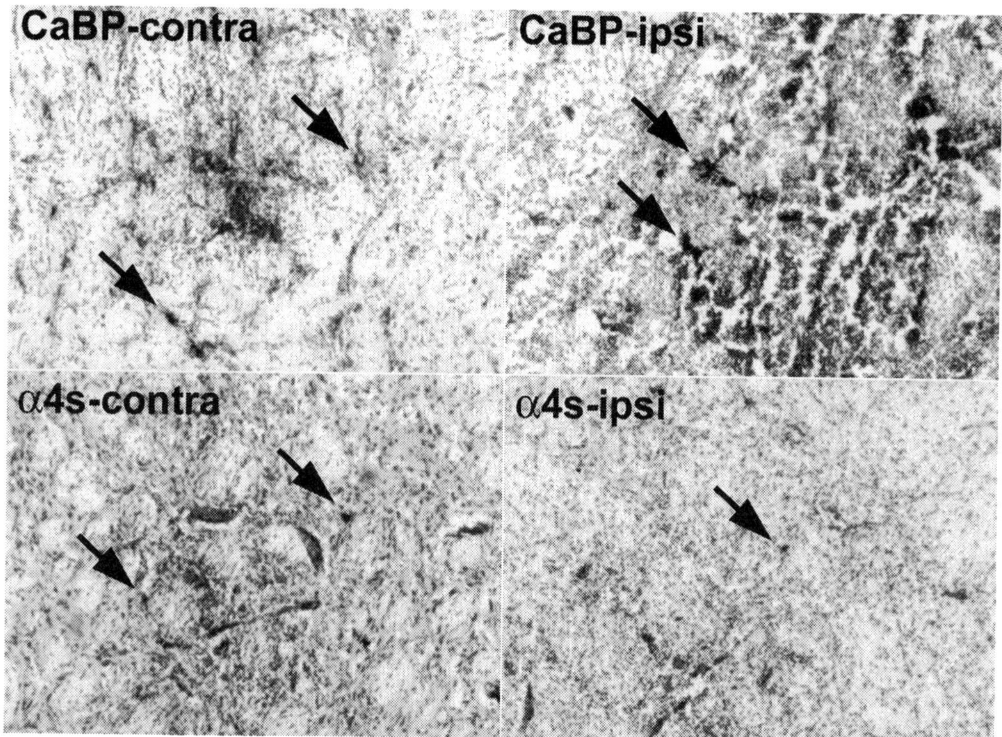

Fig. 2. Calbindin (CaBP) overexpression protects striatal neurons from a stroke. Several surviving vector targeted, X-gal stained (arrows) neurons are observed within the nonischemic (**CaBP-contra**) and ischemic (**CaBP-ipsi**) striata of an animal injected with the CaBP vector. In the striata of an animal given control vector, X-gal stained neurons are seen within targeted striatal neurons on the nonischemic side (**α4s-contra**), whereas fewer X-gal stained cells are observed on the ischemic side (**α4s-ipsi**).

vector leads to transfection of primarily dentate neurons, a higher dose of kainic acid is necessary to cause measurable damage in this subsector. To determine the percentage of surviving transfected dentate neurons, the number of remaining X-gal positive neurons is normalized to the number of transfected neurons in controls injected with vehicle. To ensure that the extent of damage is equal between control and treated groups, total cell densities are computed within the different subsectors (Lawrence et al. 1996a; Yenari et al. 1998b). Other neurotoxin models that selectively damage the hippocampus have been similarly developed.

Gene therapy to improve cellular energetics

One of the earliest attempts at neuronal gene therapy attempted to bolster neuronal energetics during insults via overexpression of the rat brain glucose transporter (GLUT-1). Using 2-deoxy glucose autoradiography, injection of this vector did lead to localized increased uptake of glucose (Ho et al. 1993). In fact, such overexpression is broadly protective, reducing neuron loss in different injury models. At the in vitro level, it protects neurons against aglycemia, excitotoxin exposure (Ho et al. 1995b) and mitochondrial toxicity by 3-nitroproprionic acid (3-NP, an irreversible inhibitor of succinate dehydrogenase) (Fink et al. 2000). At the whole animal model level, overexpression of GLUT-1 following transient focal cerebral ischemia (Lawrence et al. 1996b) resulted in 105% improvement in survival. Overexpression in the kainic acid model was also protective within dentate granule cells which received the GLUT-1 vector. Interestingly, neurons within CA3 were also protected, presumably by a transsynaptic mechanism (Lawrence et al. 1995). In a third study, GLUT-1 overexpression also protected against the electron transport uncoupler, 3-acetylpyridine (3-AP) which is preferentially toxic to the dentate gyrus in vivo (Dash et al. 1996). A few studies have examined subsequent downstream events leading to neuronal sparing. During an insult, GLUT-1 overexpression blunts the decline in ATP concentrations and metabolism, decreases glutamate release and cytosolic calcium concentrations (Lawrence et al. 1995; Robert et al. 1997).

Gene therapy to inhibit intracellular calcium excess

Several pharmacological studies have also targeted the excess of cytosolic calcium. At the gene therapy level, possible strategies would include overexpression of a calcium binding protein, or antisense targeting of a calcium channel. To date, all relevant studies have overexpressed the calcium binding protein calbindin D28K (Kindy et al. 1996; Meier et al. 1997, 1998; Phillips et al. 1999; Yenari et al. 1999c), chosen because of the correlation in a number of studies of its presence with neuronal survival (Mattson et al. 1991; Goodman et al. 1993; Mattson et al. 1995). Such overexpression protects against a variety of insults. Vector-mediated CaBP overexpression has been previously shown to alter neuronal synaptic responses, consistent with a calcium buffering function (Chard et al. 1995). In our prior in vitro studies, the CB vector has also been demonstrated to reduce intracellular calcium responses (Meier et al. 1997). Consistent with the notion that calcium overload is damaging, we then found that CaBP overexpression protected cultured hippocampal neurons from various ischemia-like insults such as hypoglycemia and excitotoxin exposure, including N-methyl-D-aspartate, kainate and glutamate; however, CaBP did not protect against cyanide toxicity, suggesting that the protective effects are not effective against mitochondrial toxins, or CaBP cannot protect against such severe insults (Meier et al. 1997, 1998). At the in vivo level, we did find hippocampal neuron protection against 3-AP (Phillips et al. 1999), a different mitochondrial toxin, suggesting that the lack of protection against cyanide in vitro was more likely due to the insult severity. More recently, we have applied this vector to the experimental stroke model and kainic acid, and found that CaBP overexpression also protected against these insults (Fig. 2, 3) (Phillips et al. 1999; Yenari et al. 1999c).

In contrast to our findings, Klapstein et al. (1998) found that CaBP deficient mice were resistant to forebrain ischemia, suggesting that CaBP might play a detrimental role in ischemic injury. These animals displayed improved electrophysiological parameters and higher CA1 cell counts. In addition, there was less TUNEL staining in the remaining hippocampal neurons, suggesting that these mice were also more resistant to apoptotic death. Interestingly, there did not appear to be any differences in the levels of other calcium binding proteins such as parvalbumin in this strain. The reasons for this discrepancy are not clear, although lifelong CaBP deficient animals may have unforeseen alterations in other systems. There are some reports where intracellular calcium buffering may be detrimental. Abdel-Hamid and Baimbridge (1997) found that artificial calcium buffers potentiated excitotoxicity in cultured hippocampal neurons by paradoxically increasing calcium influx through voltage-gated ion channels. There may also be differences in the susceptibility of neurons to ischemic injury within the hippocampus, compared to the striatum. Although we found protection in hippocampal neurons against excitotoxins and mitochondrial toxins, whether our CaBP vector might protect hippocampal neurons against similar ischemic insults is the subject of future study.

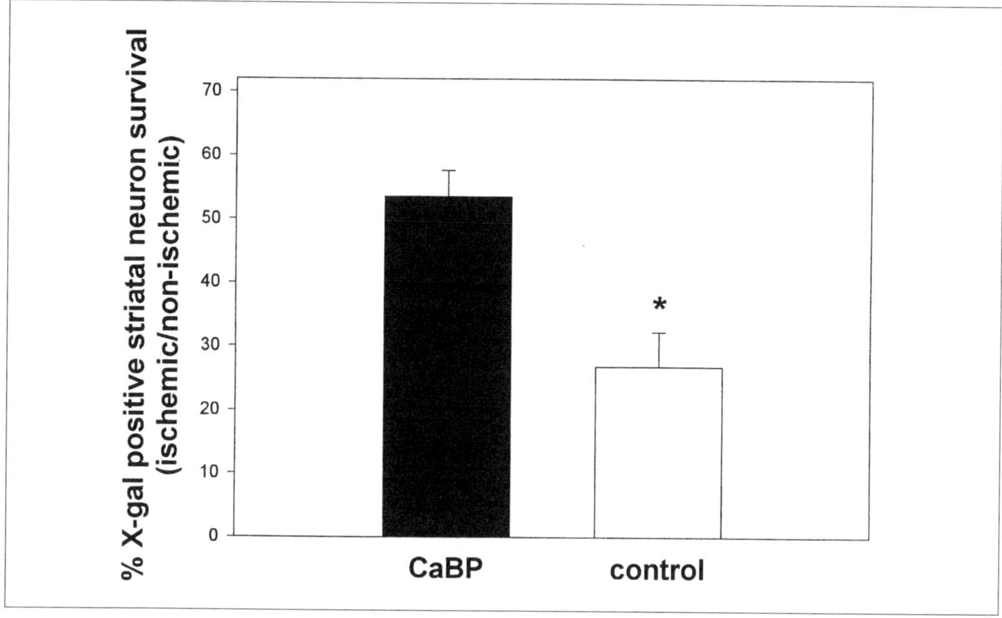

Fig. 3. Calbindin overexpression in a model of experimental stroke. 15 h prior to ischemia onset 19 rats were injected with calbindin (CaBP) or control vector. Animals were subjected to 1 h of transient focal cerebral ischemia followed by 47 h of reperfusion. Brain sections were stained with X-gal to detect vector transfected cells, then counter stained with cresyl violet to delineate regions of infarction. The bar graph shows the percentage of X-gal stained neurons remaining in the ischemic striatum relative to the contralateral nonischemic striatum. (*$p < 0.001$).

Gene transfer of stress proteins

Gene transfer therapy can also be used to address certain biological questions which cannot ordinarily be addressed by other means. Other adverse consequences of calcium excess following insults include incorrect intracellular targeting of nascent proteins, their failure to function due to malfolding, and the potential for malfolded proteins to aggregate. It is in this realm that heat shock proteins, as molecular chaperones, are most likely to have their protective actions. Thus, heat shock protein overexpression is also a potential strategy, complicated by the lack of consensus as to whether any of the expressed genes have a physiological role during these acute insults. The published reports have been concerned mainly with the inducible form of HSP70 (also referred to by HSP72), the most robustly induced of stress proteins. Some have argued that the induction of HSP70 served a protective role against ischemic insults because expression was most robust in the most resistant cell populations (Nowak and Jacewicz 1994). Induction of HSP70 was also correlated with the phenomenon of induced tolerance (Chen et al. 1996). Others found that stress proteins were expressed in cells regardless of their fate, and argued that these proteins were merely epiphenomena which served no neuroprotective role (Chopp et al. 1991). In our hands, HSP70 overexpression failed to protect against an excitotoxic insult in primary neuronal cultures, but did protect against other insults in neuronal and astrocytic cultures including heat shock (Fink et al. 1997) and ischemia-like conditions (Papadopoulos et al. 1996; Xu and Giffard 1997) as well as against ischemic and excitotoxic insults in vivo (Yenari et al. 1998b). These observations have since been replicated using transgenic animal models, but with some variability (Plumier et al. 1997; Yenari et al. 1999b; Rajdev et al.

2000). Nevertheless, the majority of data support an active protective role for the heat shock proteins, although there may be strict limits to this protection (Yenari et al. 1999a).

Gene therapy to alter apoptotic death

It is now established, that to some extent, apoptotic, or programmed, energy dependent death also occurs during cerebral ischemic injury (Bredesen 1995). Among the various genes involved include those that inhibit apoptosis. Perhaps the most studied of these anti-apoptotic genes is *bcl-2*, which encodes a 26 kD protein that is the mammalian analogue of the nematode gene, *ced-9*. A membrane bound protein, BCL-2 inhibits apoptosis by blocking cytosolic translocation of mitochondrial cytochrome c (Kluck et al. 1997; Yang et al. 1997), and subsequent activation of downstream caspases. BCL-2 may also have different sites of action given that it protects against a variety of insults (Zhong et al. 1993b), both necrotic (Behl et al. 1993; Zhong et al. 1993a; Kane et al. 1995; Jia et al. 1996) and apoptotic (Allsopp et al. 1993; Kane et al. 1993; Mah et al. 1993; Lawrence et al. 1996a). BCL-2 is induced by cerebral ischemia (Gillardon et al. 1996; Chen et al. 1997; Matsushita et al. 1998), and we and others have shown that BCL-2 overexpression protects against cerebral ischemia either by vector-mediated overexpression (Linnik et al. 1995; Lawrence et al. 1996a, 1997), or in transgenic animal models (Martinou et al. 1994). BCL-2 does not appear to protect against all insults, however. While it demonstrates marked protection by several groups against cerebral ischemia and trauma, it does not appear to be effective against the electron transport uncoupler 3-AP (Phillips et al. 2000).

Post-insult gene transfer & neuron function

In order for gene therapy to have direct clinical relevance, the various vectors should also be examined for neuroprotection when given after the insult. Furthermore, it will be increasingly important to determine whether the rescued neuron also functions normally. To these ends, our groups have begun to address these issues in our models.

Post-insult gene transfer

While we have shown that pre-insult gene therapy can ameliorate neuronal death against cerebral ischemia, most clinicians would agree that pretreatment of stroke has limited utility. Therefore, it is important to investigate whether post-insult gene therapy is also feasible. Certainly, this approach may be dependent upon the nature of the gene used. Apoptotic death may explain the observed delayed injury in ischemia; therefore, BCL-2 could be viewed as a rational choice. In fact, we first found that the BCL-2 vector applied following ischemia onset improved striatal neuron survival when vector was delayed 1.5 h, but not 5 h (Yenari et al. 1996; Lawrence et al. 1997). Given that gene expression from these vectors begins 4–6 hours following injection (Lawrence et al. 1997) with peak protein expression 12–24 hours later (Fink et al. 1997), this would imply that neuroprotection from BCL-2 is possible when overexpression is applied as late as 6.5–13.5 hours following the onset of ischemia in the rodent. A similar observation was also noted by Jia et al. (1996), who found that BCL-2 protected cultured neurons when applied 8 h after glutamate exposure.

Surprisingly, genes that interfere early in the ischemic cascade protect even when applied post-insult. In the in vivo excitotoxin model, GLUT-1 vector protected the hippocampus even when administered 30 minutes after kainic acid administration, but not 4 h (Lawrence et al. 1995). Hippocampal neuron cultures exposed to hypoglycemia were protected when GLUT-1 was applied 1 h later (Lawrence et al. 1995), but the therapeutic window for CaBP in the same model was only 30 min (Meier et al. 1997). No protection was observed for either vector when administered at 4 h, however.

The mechanisms of protection for HSP70 are only beginning to emerge (Sharp et al. 1999;

Yenari et al. 1999a). Although a widely held concept is that HSP70 protects in the early phases of injury by maintaining protein structure and preventing aggregation, other work has shown that HSP70 may also exert an anti-apoptotic effect downstream of caspase-3 (Jaattela et al. 1998). Therefore, HSP70 may also provide neuroprotection when given post-insult as well. In fact, in a preliminary study, we found that HSP70 overexpression applied 30 min after MCA occlusion in our focal cerebral ischemia paradigm did lead to improved striatal neuron counts (Fig. 4) (Ringer et al. 2000). The mechanisms and the temporal therapeutic window for HSP70 neuroprotection are currently under intensive study.

Gene transfer and neuron function

Another critical issue is whether a neuron, when saved from death because of the protective effects of some transgene, actually *functions* appropriately afterward. In the studies described to this point, however, "protection" consists of improved numbers of surviving cells, with no demonstrated preservation of neuronal function. Certainly, the hope of successful gene therapy is for naught if the rescued neuron does not work properly. Recently, our laboratories have embarked on detailed physiological (Dumas et al. 1999) testing to determine whether gene therapy results in recovery of neurological function. In an initial study, we first established that injection of the vectors themselves did not alter synaptic transmission (Dumas et al. 1999). Using the model of KA toxicity, the GLUT-1 or the BCL-2 vector was used to overexpress these respective proteins within the hippocampus. We then delivered KA with active vector to the ipsilateral hippocampus, and control vector to the contralateral hippocampus. The extent of injury was measured as the percent of the entire CA3 subregion that was lesioned. We established conditions where overexpression of either GLUT-1 or BCL-2 were equally protective, decreasing excitotoxicity to equivalent extents in hippocampal cultures and the hippoc-

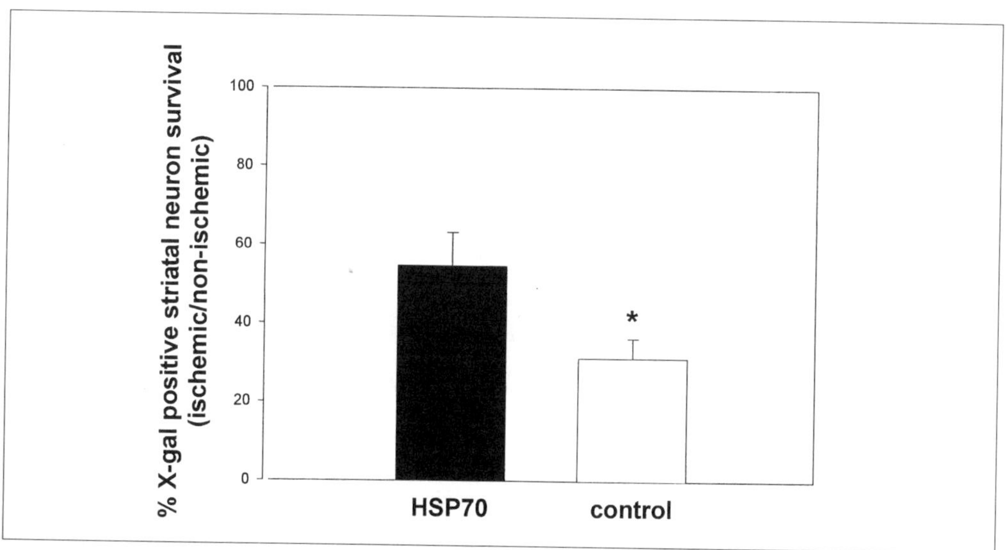

Fig. 4. HSP70 overexpression protects striatal neurons when vector is administered 20 min after ischemia onset. 21 rats were subjected to 1 h of transient focal cerebral ischemia followed by 47 h of reperfusion. HSP70 or control vector was injected into the striata 20 min after MCA occlusion. Brain sections were stained with X-gal to detect vector transfected cells, then counter stained with cresyl violet to delineate regions of infarction. The bar graph shows the percentage of X-gal stained neurons remaining in the ischemic striatum relative to the contralateral nonischemic striatum. (*$p < 0.05$).

ampus. Post tetanic potentiation (PTP) and excitatory post synaptic potentials (EPSP) were determined from the slices. PTP is one form of short-term plasticity found in the hippocampus, whereby increases in EPSP reflects an increase in transmitter release due to residual calcium in the presynaptic terminal following the high frequency stimulation. Electrophysiological function improved after GLUT-1 gene transfer, but not after BCL-2 (Fig. 5) suggesting that there are two routes of protection involving different intermediary steps (Dumas et al. 2000).

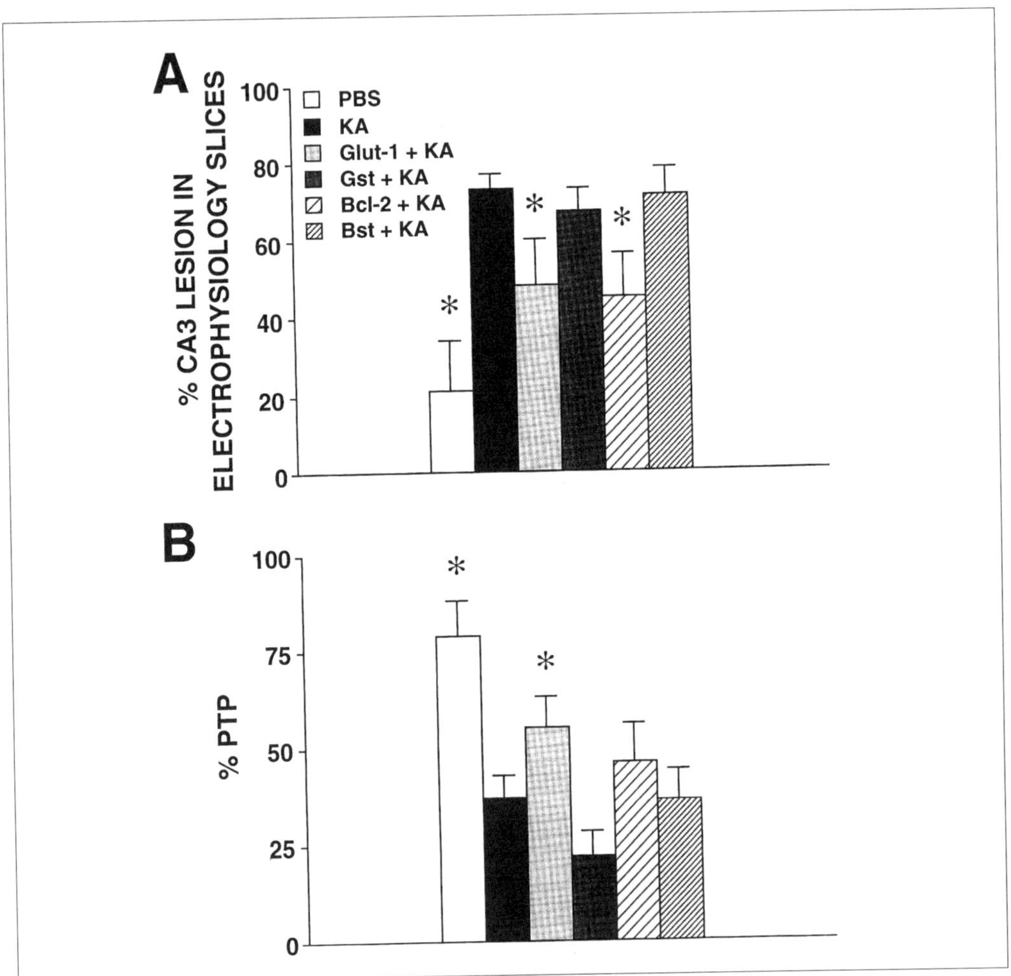

Fig. 5. Electrophysiology is preserved after gene transfer with Glut-1, but not Bcl-2. A: The upper panel shows the mean CA3 lesion size in slices used for electrophysiological recording. The extent of injury in CA3 is expressed relative to the entire length of CA3. Recordings were made 3 days after delivery of kainic acid (KA) and vector to the dentate gyrus. **B:** The lower panel shows the mean percent PTP of the mossy fiber excitatory post-synaptic potential (EPSP) slope for each group. The stimulating electrode is placed in the dentate granule cell layer and recording electrode is in the stratum lucidum of CA3. Percent PTP for each slice was measured as the average of the first two responses following tetanization (equated to the mean change in the response within the first minute after induction). (*$p < 0.05$ vs. pooled controls; PBS = phosphate buffered solution; KA = kainic acid; Glut-1 = glucose transporter vector; Gst = control vector identical to the Glut-1, but contains a stop codon early in the sequence for Glut-1; Bst = control vector identical to the Bcl-2 vector, but contains a stop codon early in the sequence for Bcl-2; PTP = post-tetanic potentiation).

GLUT-1 overexpression constituted an early intervention (in that the time-window of saving post-insult was an hour), maintained neuronal metabolism longer during the insult, and decreased ROS accumulation. In contrast, BCL-2 overexpression constituted a late intervention (with a time-window of saving post-insult of at least six hours) and had no sparing effect on metabolism or ROS accumulation (McLaughlin et al. 2000).

At the behavioral level, experiments are ongoing to determine whether gene transfer can effect improvements in behavioral scores. Like the electrophysiological data, preliminary data in the KA model suggests that, GLUT-1, but not BCL-2 gene transfer spared spatial maze learning deficits (McLaughlin et al. 2000). Thus, a gene therapy intervention which spares neurons from insult-induced death does not necessarily translate into a sparing of function.

Future directions

Saving neurons versus merely delaying death

In the studies cited, the endpoint (e.g., number of surviving neurons) was assessed at a single time point, raising the possibility that there was merely delay, rather than prevention of death. This would be analogous to other strategies that postpone neuron death, including mild brain hypothermia under certain ischemic conditions (Dietrich et al. 1993; Tasdemiroglu 1996). Despite the lack of studies quantifying neuron loss at multiple time points, in most of those discussed, the time point used was one at which maximal damage occurs and suggests that the gene therapy interventions did indeed prevent neuron death. Studying the long term effects of neuroprotection from gene therapy in the paradigms described is currently limited by the relatively brief (days) duration of reporter gene expression. More work using functional endpoints could be applied for chronic timepoints, although to date, we are limited to insults affecting primarily hippocampal function.

Gene transfer in other models of brain injury

The main in vivo models studied in our laboratories include the focal cerebral ischemia model and kainic acid model. However, we have expanded some of our work to address questions such as whether gene therapy might protect against global insults, or whether gene therapy to the ischemic penumbra is possible. These questions are valid to the extent that global ischemic injury may be different from focal. Certainly, some glutamate antagonists do not appear to be effective against global ischemia, although they are protective in focal (Yenari and Steinberg 1998c). Early clinical trials for stroke treatment have focused on targeting the ischemic penumbra, the brain region most amenable to salvage, particularly in the case of irreversible vessel occlusion (De Keyser et al. 1999).

Gene therapy in global ischemia models was limited in our laboratories due to the fact that the herpes viral vector tended to preferentially transfect dentate neurons. Although the reasons for this are not well known, it may be due to specific receptors present in the dentate, but not in other subfields. For studying gene transfer in global ischemia models, this posed a significant problem since most of the hippocampal injury occurs in CA1, and dentate is relatively resistant (Pulsinelli et al. 1982). However, by using a mechanical microinfusion pump and delivering vector at a rate of 0.5 μl/hr, we are now capable of transfecting CA1 neurons (Fig. 6 A). By applying the model of bilateral carotid artery occlusion plus hypotension (Smith et al. 1984), we can now apply a similar paradigm as the kainic acid model to study CA1 neuron survival. By injecting the vector via a microinfusion pump into CA1, animals are subjected to 8 min of forebrain ischemia followed by 72 h of reperfusion. This leads to moderate damage within CA1, and our preliminary studies suggest that the number of HSP70 transfected CA1 neurons are higher than that of control vector transfected (Fig. 6 B, C). Paralleling the kainic acid studies, future studies in this model may include the application of behavior testing to

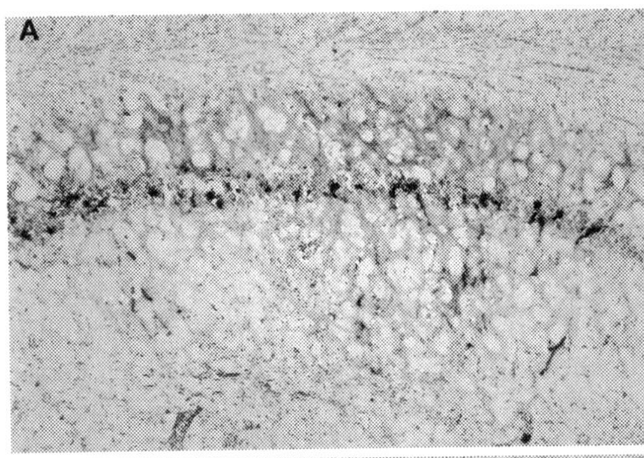

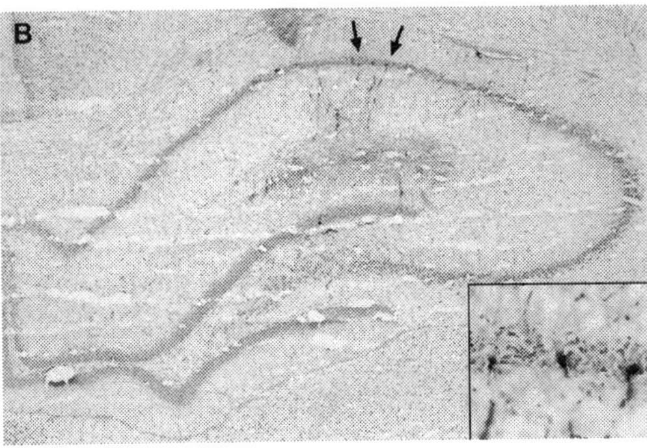

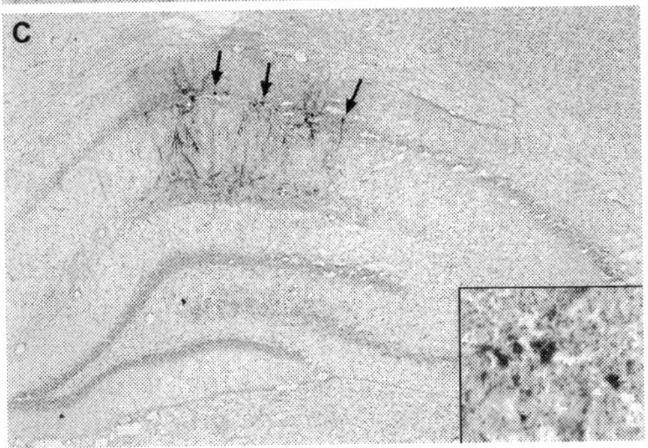

Fig. 6. Gene transfer in global cerebral ischemia: Using a micro infusion pump, vectors were injected into both hippocampal CA1 subsectors of rats. Animals were subjected to 8 min of forebrain ischemia followed by 72 h reperfusion. Sham animals received similar surgery and anesthesia, but no ischemia. A sham operated animal injected with control vector demonstrates numerous X-gal positive CA1 neurons (A). Following ischemia, a few X-gal positive neurons are visible after control vector injection (B), but more X-gal positive cells are observed in an animal injected with the HSP70 vector (C).

determine whether neuronal function is rescued with gene therapy in ischemia models.

Penumbral gene therapy makes logical sense given that a majority of pharmaceuticals are designed to target this region. In order to determine whether gene overexpression can rescue in the ischemic penumbra, we employed a model of distal MCA occlusion as described by Chen et al. (1986). In this model, a reproducible cortical infarct is produced in the territory of the MCA. Since the borderzones are quite consistent between experiments, we applied vector to this region (and a comparable contralateral area in the nonischemic cortex) and utilized permanent distal MCA occlusion plus 2 h of temporary bilateral carotid artery occlusion. From our preliminary experiments, we show that cortical penumbral vector targeting is possible (Fig. 7).

Gene transfer to human tissues

Undoubtedly, a progressive goal in these studies would be to ultimately apply this technology to humans. Although there are certain safety issues that need to be addressed before such studies in clinical stroke can commence, some preliminary ex vivo work is promising. Using fresh human brain tissue from surgical specimens, stable metabolism could be maintained for at least 24 h by incubating in artificial CSF. Using our control vectors, we were able to transfect human brain specimens within 20 minutes of removal (Bottino et al. 2000). However, long term studies and in vivo safety in humans is not yet known for these vectors. Early clinical experience with adenoviral vectors for treatment of cystic fibrosis has shown that transgene expression is transient, and patients may develop an inflammatory response (Crystal 1995). Whether defective HSV vectors can reactivate latent viral infection in humans is also not known. Retroviral vectors are being studied in patients with brain tumors, but results of these studies have yet to be published. Unfortunately, the recent decision by the FDA to terminate all clinical gene therapy trials in the United States has raised significant concerns

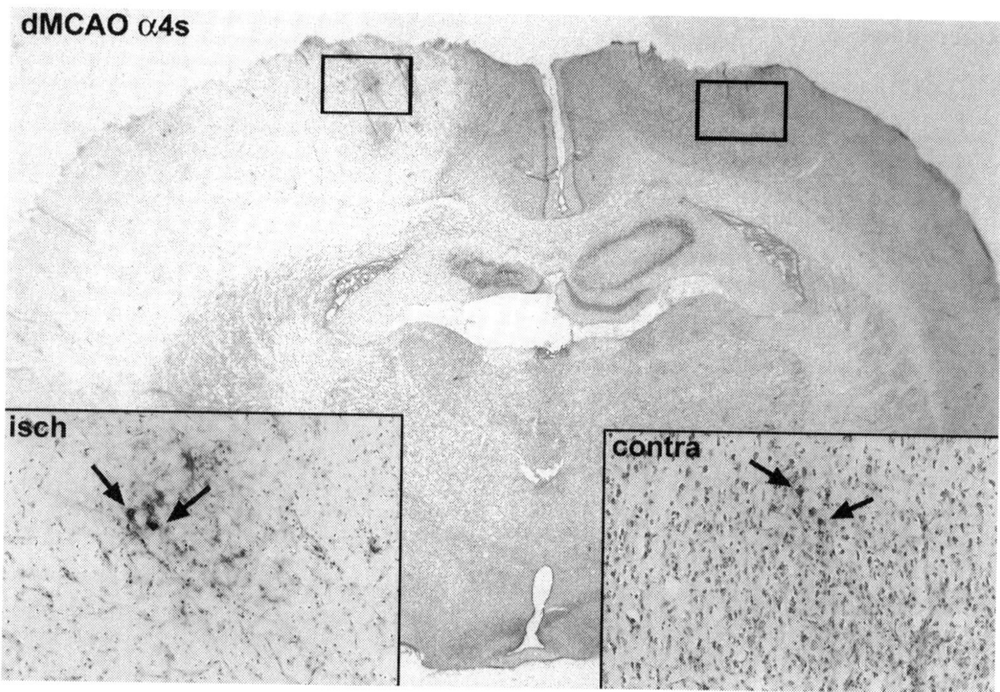

Fig. 7. Penumbral gene transfer: Control vectors (α4s) were injected into penumbral zones of the cortex supplied by the middle cerebral artery (MCA). 12–15 h later, animals were subjected to permanent distal MCA occlusion (dMCAO) plus bilateral carotid artery occlusion for 2 h. Brains were harvested 48 h later, and stained with X-gal and cresyl violet. Several transfected (arrows) neurons are visible within both the ischemic (isch) and nonischemic cortices (contra).

regarding the safety of viral vectors (Balter 2000). The future may bring effective nonviral strategies for gene transfer such as liposomes or mechanical transfer.

Conclusions

We show that gene transfer therapy in experimental stroke is feasible, although it is currently limited by the extent to which these viral vectors can infect and the route of administration. We find that these techniques provide insights into the molecular biology and pathophysiology of cerebral ischemia which are complementary to studies utilizing transgenic animals. Moreover, the finding that some of the genes induced in response to cerebral injury are neuroprotective when expressed at high levels, offer new possibilities in the development of novel pharmaceuticals. We and others are beginning to show that gene transfer therapy for treatment of cerebral ischemia and variety of other diseases has potential, although a number of questions and issues remain before it can be implemented in humans.

Acknowledgments/Support

This work was supported by NIH NINDS Grants PO1 NS 37520 (G.K.S., R.M.S., M.A.Y.) and K08 NS01860 (M.A.Y.), the Adler Foundation (R.M.S.), Bernard and Ronni Lacroute (G.K.S.), the William Randolph Heart Foundation (G.K.S.) and John and Dodie Rosekrans (G.K.S.). We would also like to extend our thanks to the many members of the Sapolsky, Steinberg and Yenari labs at Stanford University who contributed significantly to the data discussed here.

References

1. Abdel-Hamid KM, Baimbridge KG (1997) The effects of artificial calcium buffers on calcium responses and glutamate-mediated excitotoxicity in cultured hippocampal neurons. Neuroscience 81:673–687
2. Allsopp TE, Wyatt S, Paterson HF, Davies AM (1993) The proto-oncogene bcl-2 can selectively rescue neurotrophic factor-dependent neurons from apoptosis. Cell 73:295–307
3. Balter M (2000) Gene therapy on trial. Science 288:951–957
4. Behl C, Hovey Ld, Krajewski S, Schubert D, Reed JC (1993) BCL-2 prevents killing of neuronal cells by glutamate but not by amyloid beta protein. Biochem Biophys Res Commun 197:949–956
5. Bottino CJ, Howard SA, Steinberg G, Sapolsky RM (2000) Model for examining neuroprotection in human brain tissue. Soc Neurosci Abs 26:266
6. Bredesen DE (1995) Neural apoptosis. Ann Neurol 38:839–851
7. Chard PS, Jordan J, Marcuccilli CJ, Miller RJ, Leiden JM, Roos RP, Ghadge GD (1995) Regulation of excitatory transmission at hippocampal synapses by calbindin D28k. Proc Natl Acad Sci USA 92:5144–5148
8. Chen J, Graham SH, Nakayama M, Zhu RL, Jin K, Stetler RA, Simon RP (1997) Apoptosis repressor genes Bcl-2 and Bcl-x-long are expressed in the rat brain following global ischemia. J Cereb Blood Flow Metab 17:2–10
9. Chen J, Graham SH, Zhu RL, Simon RP (1996) Stress proteins and tolerance to focal cerebral ischemia. J Cereb Blood Flow Metab 16:566–577
10. Chen ST, Hsu CY, Hogan EL, Maricq H, Balentine JD (1986) A model of focal ischemic stroke in the rat: reproducible extensive cortical infarction. Stroke 17:738–743
11. Chopp M, Li Y, Dereski MO, Levine SR, Yoshida Y, Garcia JH (1991) Neuronal injury and expression of 72-kDa heat-shock protein after forebrain ischemia in the rat. Acta Neuropathol (Berl) 83:66–71
12. Crystal RG (1995) Transfer of genes to humans: early lessons and obstacles to success. Science 270:404–410
13. Dash R, Lawrence M, Ho D, Sapolsky R (1996) A herpes simplex virus vector overexpressing the glucose transporter gene protects the rat dentate gyrus from an antimetabolite toxin. Exp Neurol 137:43–48
14. De Keyser J, Sulter G, Luiten PG (1999) Clinical trials with neuroprotective drugs in acute ischaemic stroke: are we doing the right thing? Trends Neurosci 22:535–540
15. DeLuca NA, McCarthy AM, Schaffer PA (1985) Isolation and characterization of deletion mutants of herpes simplex virus type 1 in the gene encoding immediate-early regulatory protein ICP4. J Virol 56:558–570
16. Dietrich WD, Busto R, Alonso O, Globus MY, Ginsberg MD (1993) Intraischemic but not postischemic brain hypothermia protects chronically following global forebrain ischemia in rats. J Cereb Blood Flow Metab 13:541–549
17. Du C, Hu R, Csernansky CA, Hsu CY, Choi DW (1996) Very delayed infarction after mild focal cerebral ischemia: a role for apoptosis? J Cereb Blood Flow Metab 16:195–201
18. Dumas TC, McLaughlin JR, Ho DY, Lawrence MS, Sapolsky RM (2000) Gene therapies that enhance hippocampal neuron survival after an excitotoxic insult are not equivalent in their ability to maintain syaptic transmission. Exp Neurol (in press)
19. Dumas TC, McLaughlin JR, Ho DY, Meier TJ, Sapolsky RM (1999) Delivery of herpes simplex virus amplicon-based vectors to the dentate gyrus does not alter hippocampal synaptic transmission in vivo. Gene Ther 6:1679–1684
20. Fink SL, Chang LK, Ho DY, Sapolsky RM (1997) Defective herpes simplex virus vectors expressing the rat brain stress-inducible heat shock protein 72 protect cultured neurons from severe heat shock. J Neurochem 68:961–969
21. Fink DJ, DeLuca NA, Goins WF, Glorioso JC (1996) Gene transfer to neurons using herpes simplex virus based vectors. Ann Rev Neurosci 19:265–287
22. Fink SL, Ho DY, McLaughlin J, Sapolsky RM (2000) An adenoviral vector expressing the glucose transporter protects cultured striatal neurons from 3-nitropropionic acid. Brain Res 859:21–25
23. Geller AI, During MJ, Neve RL (1991) Molecular analysis of neuronal physiology by gene transfer into neurons with herpes simplex virus vectors. Trends Neurosci 14:428–432
24. Gillardon F, Lenz C, Waschke KF, Krajewski S, Reed JC, Zimmermann M, Kuschinsky W (1996) Altered expression of Bcl-2, Bcl-X, Bax, and c-Fos colocalizes with DNA fragmentation and ischemic cell damage following middle cerebral artery occlusion in rats. Brain Res Mol Brain Res 40:254–260
25. Glorioso JC, Goins WF, Meaney CA, Fink DJ, DeLuca NA (1994) Gene transfer to brain using herpes simplex virus vectors. Ann Neurol 35 Suppl:S28–34
26. Goodman JH, Wasterlain CG, Massarweh WF, Dean E, Sollas AL, Sloviter RS (1993) Calbindin-D28k immunoreactivity and selective vulnerability to ischemia in the dentate gyrus of the developing rat. Brain Res 606:309–314
27. Green DR, Reed JC (1998) Mitochondria and apoptosis. Science 281:1309–1312
28. Ho DY (1994) Amplicon-based herpes simplex virus vectors. Methods Cell Bio 43:191–219
29. Ho DY, Lawrence MS, Meier TJ, Fink SL, Dash R, Saydam TC, Sapolsky RM (1995a) Using of herpes virus vectors for protection from necrotic neuron death. In: Viral Vectors (Kaplitt MG and Loewy AD, eds), New York, Academic Press, pp 133–155
30. Ho DY, Mocarski ES, Sapolsky RM (1993) Altering central nervous system physiology with a defective herpes simplex virus vector expressing the glucose transporter gene. Proc Natl Acad Sci USA 90:3655–3659
31. Ho DY, Saydam TC, Fink SL, Lawrence MS, Sapolsky RM (1995b) Defective herpes simplex virus vectors expressing the rat brain glucose transporter protect cultured neurons from necrotic insults. J Neurochem 65:842–850
32. Jaattela M, Wissing D, Kokholm K, Kallunki T, Egeblad M (1998) Hsp70 exerts its anti-apoptotic function downstream of caspase-3-like proteases. Embo J 17:6124–6134
33. Jia WW, Wang Y, Qiang D, Tufaro F, Remington R, Cynader M (1996) A bcl-2 expressing viral vector protects cortical neurons from excitotoxicity even when administered several hours after the toxic insult. Brain Res Mol Brain Res 42:350–353
34. Kane DJ, Ord T, Anton R, Bredesen DE (1995) Expression of bcl-2 inhibits necrotic neural cell death. J Neurosci Res 40:269–275
35. Kane DJ, Sarafian TA, Anton R, Hahn H, Gralla EB, Valentine JS, Ord T, Bredesen DE (1993) Bcl-2 inhibition of neural death: decreased generation of reactive oxygen species. Science 262:1274–1277
36. Kindy M, Yu J, Miller R, al. e (1996) Adenoviral vectors in ischemic injury. In: Pharmacology of Cerebral Ischemia (Krieglstein J, ed), Stuttgart, Medpharm Scientific Publishers, pp 525–535
37. Klapstein GJ, Vietla S, Lieberman DN, Gray PA, Airaksinen MS, Thoenen H, Meyer M, Mody I (1998) Calbindin-D28k fails to protect hippocampal neurons against ischemia in spite of its cytoplasmic calcium buffering properties: evidence from calbindin-D28k knockout mice. Neuroscience 85:361–373
38. Kluck RM, Bossy-Wetzel E, Green DR, Newmeyer DD (1997) The release of cytochrome c from mitochondria: a primary site for Bcl-2 regulation of apoptosis. Science 275:1132–1136

39. Lawrence MS, Ho DY, Dash R, Sapolsky RM (1995) Herpes simplex virus vectors overexpressing the glucose transporter gene protect against seizure-induced neuron loss. Proc Natl Acad Sci USA 92:7247–7251
40. Lawrence MS, Ho DY, Sun GH, Steinberg GK, Sapolsky RM (1996a) Overexpression of Bcl-2 with herpes simplex virus vectors protects CNS neurons against neurological insults in vitro and in vivo. J Neurosci 16:486–496
41. Lawrence MS, Sun GH, Ho DY, Sapolsky RM, Steinberg GK (1997) Herpes simplex viral vectors expressing Bcl-2 are neuroprotective when delivered following a stroke. J Cereb Blood Flow Metab 17:740–744
42. Lawrence MS, Sun GH, Kunis DM, Saydam TC, Dash R, Ho DY, Sapolsky RM, Steinberg GK (1996b) Overexpression of the glucose transporter gene with a herpes simplex viral vector protects striatal neurons against stroke. J Cereb Blood Flow Metab 16:181–185
43. Linnik MD, Zahos P, Geschwind MD, Federoff HJ (1995) Expression of bcl-2 from a defective herpes simplex virus-1 vector limits neuronal death in focal cerebral ischemia. Stroke 26:1670–1674
44. Mah SP, Zhong LT, Liu Y, Roghani A, Edwards RH, Bredesen DE (1993) The protooncogene bcl-2 inhibits apoptosis in PC12 cells. J Neurochem 60:1183–1186
45. Martinou JC, Dubois-Dauphin M, Staple JK, Rodriguez I, Frankowski H, Missotten M, Albertini P, Talabot D, Catsicas S, Pietra C, Huarte J (1994) Overexpression of BCL-2 in transgenic mice protects neurons from naturally occurring cell death and experimental ischemia. Neuron 13:1017–1030
46. Matsushita K, Matsuyama T, Kitagawa K, Matsumoto M, Yanagihara T, Sugita M (1998) Alterations of Bcl-2 family proteins precede cytoskeletal proteolysis in the penumbra, but not in infarct centres following focal cerebral ischemia in mice. Neuroscience 83:439–448
47. Mattson MP, Cheng B, Baldwin SA, Smith-Swintosky VL, Keller J, Geddes JW, Scheff SW, Christakos S (1995) Brain injury and tumor necrosis factors induce calbindin D-28k in astrocytes: evidence for a cytoprotective response. J Neurosci Res 42:357–370
48. Mattson MP, Rychlik B, Chu C, Christakos S (1991) Evidence for calcium-reducing and excito-protective roles for the calcium-binding protein calbindin-D28k in cultured hippocampal neurons. Neuron 6:41–51
49. McLaughlin J, Roozendaal B, Dumas T, Gupta A, Ajilore O, Hsieh J, Ho D, Lawrence M, L. MJ, Sapolsky R (2000) Sparing of neuronal function post-seizure with gene therapy. Proc National Acad Sci (in press)
50. Meier TJ, Ho DY, Park TS, Sapolsky RM (1998) Gene transfer of calbindin D28k cDNA via herpes simplex virus amplicon vector decreases cytoplasmic calcium ion response and enhances neuronal survival following glutamatergic challenge but not following cyanide. J Neurochem 71:1013–1023
51. Meier TJ, Ho DY, Sapolsky RM (1997) Increased expression of calbindin D28k via herpes simplex virus amplicon vector decreases calcium ion mobilization and enhances neuronal survival after hypoglycemic challenge. J Neurochem 69:1039–1047
52. Nowak TS, Jr., Jacewicz M (1994) The heat shock/stress response in focal cerebral ischemia. Brain Pathol 4:67–76
53. Papadopoulos MC, Sun XY, Cao J, Mivechi NF, Giffard RG (1996) Over-expression of HSP-70 protects against combined oxygen-glucose deprivation. Neuroreport 7:429–432
54. Phillips RG, Lawrence MS, Ho DY, Sapolsky RM (2000) Limitations in the neuroprotective potential of gene therapy with Bcl-2. Brain Res 859:202–206
55. Phillips RG, Meier TJ, Giuli LC, McLaughlin JR, Ho DY, Sapolsky RM (1999) Calbindin D28K gene transfer via herpes simplex virus amplicon vector decreases hippocampal damage in vivo following neurotoxic insults. J Neurochem 73:1200–1205
56. Plumier JC, Krueger AM, Currie RW, Kontoyiannis D, Kollias G, Pagoulatos GN (1997) Transgenic mice expressing the human inducible Hsp70 have hippocampal neurons resistant to ischemic injury. Cell Stress Chaperones 2:162–167
57. Pulsinelli WA, Brierley JB, Plum F (1982) Temporal profile of neuronal damage in a model of transient forebrain ischemia. Ann Neurol 11:491–498
58. Rajdev S, Hara K, Kokubo Y, Mestril R, Dillmann W, Weinstein PR, Sharp FR (2000) Mice overexpressing rat heat shock protein 70 are protected against cerebral infarction. Ann Neurol 47:782–791
59. Ringer T, Fink SL, Ho DY, Sapolsky RM, Steinberg GK, Yenari MA (2000) HSP72 overexpression protects striatal neurons when delivered after experimental stroke. Soc Neurosci Abs 26:15
60. Robert JJ, Bouilleret V, Ridoux V, Valin A, Geoffroy MC, Mallet J, Le Gal La Salle G (1997) Adenovirus-mediated transfer of a functional GAD gene into nerve cells: potential for the treatment of neurological diseases. Gene Ther 4:1237–1245
61. Sapolsky RM, Steinberg GK (1999) Gene therapy using viral vectors for acute neurologic insults. Neurology 53:1922–1931
62. Sharp FR, Massa SM, Swanson RA (1999) Heat-shock protein protection. Trends Neurosci 22:97–99
63. Smith ML, Bendek G, Dahlgren N, Rosen I, Wieloch T, Siesjo BK (1984) Models for studying long-term recovery following forebrain ischemia in the rat. 2. A 2-vessel occlusion model. Acta Neurol Scand 69:385–401
64. Tasdemiroglu E (1996) Mild hypothermia fails to protect late hippocampal neuronal loss following forebrain cerebral ischaemia in rats. Acta Neurochir (Wien) 138:570–578
65. Xu L, Giffard RG (1997) HSP70 protects murine astrocytes from glucose deprivation injury. Neurosci Lett 224:9–12
66. Yang J, Liu X, Bhalla K, Kim CN, Ibrado AM, Cai J, Peng TI, Jones DP, Wang X (1997) Prevention of apoptosis by Bcl-2: release of cytochrome c from mitochondria blocked. Science 275:1129–1132
67. Yenari MA, Fink SL, Lawrence MS, Sun GH, McLaughlin J, Onley D, Ho DY, Sapolsky RM, Steinberg GK (1998a) Gene transfer therapy for cerebral ischemia. In: Pharmacology of Cerebral Ischemia (Krieglstein J, ed), Stuttgart, Medpharm Scientific Publishers, pp 453–465
68. Yenari MA, Fink SL, Sun GH, Chang LK, Patel MK, Kunis DM, Onley D, Ho DY, Sapolsky RM, Steinberg GK (1998b) Gene therapy with HSP72 is neuroprotective in rat models of stroke and epilepsy. Ann Neurol 44:584–591
69. Yenari MA, Giffard RG, Sapolsky RM, Steinberg GK (1999a) The neuroprotective potential of heat shock protein 70 (HSP70). Mol Med Today 5:525–531
70. Yenari MA, Lawrence MS, Sun GH, Ho DY, Kunis DM, Sapolsky RM, Steinberg GK (1996) Herpes simplex viral vectors expressing Bcl-2 are neuroprotective against focal cerebral ischemia. In: Pharmacology of Cerebral Ischemia (Krieglstein J, ed), Stuttgart, Wissenschaftliche Verlagsgesellschaft mbH, pp 537–543
71. Yenari MA, Lee JE, Emond M, Sun GH, Giffard RG, Steinberg GK (1999b) Transgenic mice which overexpress HSP70 are protected against some but not all central nervous system insults. Stroke 30:233
72. Yenari MA, Minami M, Sun GH, Meier TJ, Ho DY, Sapolsky RM, Steinberg GK (1999c) Calbindin D28K overexpression using gene transfer therapy improves striatal neuron survival following transient focal cerebral ischemia. Ann Neurol 46:479
73. Yenari M, Palmer J, Sun G, de Crespigny A, Moseley M, Steinberg G (1996) Time-course and treatment response with

SNX-111, an N-type calcium channel blocker, in a rodent model of focal cerebral ischemia using diffusion-weighted MRI. Brain Res 739:36–45

74. Yenari MA, Steinberg GK (1998c) Pharmacological Advances in Cerebrovascular Protection. In: Current Techniques in Neurosurgery (Awad IA, eds), Philadelphia, Current Science, pp 98–116

75. Zhong LT, Kane DJ, Bredesen DE (1993a) BCL-2 blocks glutamate toxicity in neural cell lines. Brain Res Mol Brain Res 19:353–355

76. Zhong LT, Sarafian T, Kane DJ, Charles AC, Mah SP, Edwards RH, Bredesen DE (1993b) bcl-2 inhibits death of central neural cells induced by multiple agents. Proc Natl Acad Sci USA 90:4533–4537

Stem cell therapy and neurogenesis

Neurogenesis and synaptogenesis in hippocampus following global ischemia

R. Bernabeu, J. Liu, F. R Sharp

Abstract

The effect of glutamate receptors on hippocampal cell proliferation and synapsin-I induction was examined following global ischemia. Cell and synaptic proliferation were assessed using BrdU and synapsin-I labeling, respectively. MK-801 and NBQX increased cell birth in the dentate subgranular zone (SGZ) of control adult gerbils (30–90%, $p < 0.05$). Two weeks following 10 minutes of global ischemia most CA1 pyramidal neurons died, whereas the numbers of BrdU-labeled cells in the SGZ increased dramatically (> 10 fold, $p < 0.0001$). Systemic and hippocampal injections of MK801 or NBQX blocked birth of cells in the SGZ and the death of CA1 pyramidal neurons at 15d following ischemia. The induction of synapsin-I in CA3 following global ischemia was also blocked by pre-treatment with systemic or intra-hippocampal MK-801 or NBQX. It is proposed that NMDA and AMPA receptors modulate neurogenesis and synaptogenesis in hippocampus following injury. The dentate neurogenesis and synaptogenesis that occur following ischemia may contribute to recovery of memory function following ischemic hippocampal injury.

Transient global cerebral ischemia causes cell injury and death in the hippocampus of all mammals – with prominent injury to hippocampal CA1 pyramidal neurons and dentate hilar neurons (Hsu and Buzsaki 1993; Gonzalez et al. 1991; Ito et al. 1975; Kirino 1982; Pulsinelli et al. 1982; Westerberg et al. 1989; Herguido et al. 1999). This hippocampal injury produces recent memory loss in animals and man (Squire and Zola-Morgan 1996; Zola-Morgan et al. 1986, 1992). The neuronal damage that follows ischemia appears to involve over stimulation of glutamate receptors (Benveniste et al. 1988; Gill et al. 1987; Westerberg et al. 1989) since AMPA receptor ($AMPA_R$) antagonists and possibly NMDA receptor ($NMDA_R$) antagonists protect hippocampal CA1 pyramidal neurons from delayed death after global ischemia (Simon et al. 1984; Sheardown et al. 1990; Buchan et al. 1991b; Gorter et al. 1997; Lazarewicz et al. 1997; Colbourne et al. 1999; Hicks et al. 1999).

Global ischemia also stimulates the birth of new neurons in the adult brain (Liu et al. 1998). Since glutamate receptors mediate ischemic injury and ischemia induces neurogenesis, we examined the role NMDA and AMPA receptors on ischemia induced neurogenesis. Since synapsin-I is induced in hippocampus follow-

Keywords: Neurogenesis; synaptogenesis; global ischemia; stroke; hippocampus; glutamate receptors; NMDA; AMPA

Department of Neurology, University of Cincinnati, 3125 Eden Avenue, Ohio 45267 and Department of Neurology, University of California at San Francisco 94143.
e-mail: frank.sharp@uc.edu

ing ischemia (Marti et al. 1999) and could be related to the birth of new cells, we also determined whether synapsin-I induction was modulated by glutamate receptors. We found that NMDA and AMPA receptor antagonists prevent the dentate neurogenesis and the dentate granule cell neuron synaptic responses that ordinarily occur following global ischemia.

Materials and methods

Adult male Mongolian gerbils (11–13 weeks of age) were used for these studies. Animal protocols were performed according to NIH guidelines under an approved local protocol from UCSF and the San Francisco VA Medical Center. Animals were anesthetized with 3% isoflurane in 30% O_2/70% N_2. After bilateral neck incisions, both common carotid arteries were exposed and occluded with aneurysm clips for 10 minutes. Rectal temperatures were maintained at 37.5 ± 0.5 °C until animals recovered from surgery. Sham-operated animals were treated similarly, except that carotids were not occluded.

MK-801 (3 mg/Kg; RBI labs; a $NMDA_R$ antagonist) and NBQX (30 mg/Kg; RBI Labs; an $AMPA_R$ antagonist) were used. MK-801 was given 30 minutes before the surgery, 6 h and 24 h after ischemia (Gill et al. 1987; Gill and Woodruff 1990). NBQX was given 10 minutes before ischemia, 6 h and 36 h after ischemia. These schedules were chosen because they protect CA1 pyramidal neurons in previous studies (Sheardown et al. 1990; Diemer et al. 1992). Control animals were treated identically except that saline (sterile 0.9% NaCl) was injected. Nine days after the ischemia, BrdU (50 mg/kg) was given i.p. daily for 4 days because this is the period of maximal cell proliferation following global ischemia in the gerbil brain (Liu et al. 1998). All animals were sacrificed 15 days after the ischemia.

A second group of gerbils was submitted to the same global ischemic injury. However, the drugs were not injected until day 7d after ischemia, when MK801, NBQX or saline were then injected on the same schedule as the first group. BrdU (50 mg/kg) was administered i.p. daily for 4 days on days 9–12 after ischemia as in all of the groups. A third group of gerbils served as drug injected controls, i.e. they were subjected to sham operations without ischemia and had glutamate antagonists or saline injected on the same schedule as the first group. Nine days after the sham surgery BrdU was administered i.p. daily for 4 days at 9–12 days after sham surgery and sacrificed 15 days after sham surgery.

To perform intracranial injections, gerbils were anesthetized with 3% isoflurane in 30% O_2/70% N_2 and placed in a rodent stereotaxic. The skin was incised and bilateral burr holes drilled manually. Bilateral microinjections of either MK801 (0.2 µl in each side, 3 µg/µl solution) or NBQX (0.2 µl in each side, 30 µg/µl solution) were performed using a Hamilton syringe (1 µl, 30 g needle, Hamilton Co.). The drugs were injected into the CA1 area of the dorsal hippocampus at coordinates A: 2.8; L: 1.9; V: 1.1

The thymidine analog BrdU (5-bromo-2'-deoxyuridine-5'-monophosphate) was given i.p. daily at 9–12 days following ischemia (50 mg/Kg, Sigma) during the peak of cell proliferation (Liu et al. 1998). All animals were sacrificed at 15 days after ischemia. Non-ischemic animals were injected with BrdU for 4 consecutive days on days 9–12 following sham surgeries, and then sacrificed 3 days later on day 15.

Gerbils were anesthetized with ketamine (80 mg/Kg) and xylazine (20 mg/Kg). They were perfused with 0.9% saline, followed by 4% paraformaldehyde (PFA) in 0.1M PBS (pH: 7.4). The brains were removed, post-fixed for 6 h, and placed in 20% sucrose overnight. Coronal frozen sections (45 µm thick) were cut on a microtome. To detect BrdU-labeled nuclei DNA was denatured by treatment with 2N HCl for 30 minutes at 37 °C. After rinsing twice, sections were then incubated overnight with primary antibody to BrdU (1/500, Boehringer Mannheim) in PBS with 1% normal serum, 0,1% BSA and 0.3% triton X-100. NeuN (1/500) immunocytochemistry was used to evaluate the loss of neuronal nuclei (Liu et al. 1998) and synapsin-I (1/800, Stressgen) immunohystochemistry was performed to evaluate synaptogenesis following ischemic injury. The same protocol used for BrdU was used for these antibodies, except that the DNA denaturation was deleted.

The numbers of BrdU immunoreactive nuclei in each dentate gyrus (DG) were counted on coronal hippocampal sections. Sections were spaced 180 μm apart. The one focal plane per section that yielded the most nuclei was used for counting. The density of BrdU stained cells in each section was calculated by dividing the number of BrdU-positive nuclei by the area of the DG (in mm^2). Differences between the mean values from each treatment group were analyzed using Krustal-Wallis ANOVA followed by Neuman-Keuls test.

Results

Bilateral carotid artery occlusions caused severe loss of NeuN stained CA1 neurons in hippocampus 15d following ischemia. Systemic injections of MK801 prevented the CA1 neuronal cell death 15d following ischemia. Injection of MK801 at 7 days after ischemia did not prevent the loss of the CA1 pyramidal neurons at 15d following ischemia. Animals microinjected with saline in the CA1 hippocampal subfield showed the typical loss of CA1 neurons 15d after ischemia. Animals microinjected one time in CA1 with MK-801 at 30 minutes before ischemia demonstrated complete neuroprotection of CA1 neurons 15 days following ischemia.

There was a basal level of BrdU incorporation into newborn cells in the subgranular zone (SGZ) of the DG as well as in the subventricular zone (SVZ, not shown) in the control animals MK-801 injected i.p. into control animals significantly increased the number of BrdU-labeled cells (Fig. 1A). At 15 days following global ischemia, BrdU incorporation into cells of DG was significantly increased (Fig. 1A). Systemic injections of MK801 blocked BrdU incorporation into DG cells, with the numbers of BrDU labeled cells being similar to those in control animals (Fig. 1A). Moreover, systemic injections of MK-801 given 7 days after ischemia had no effect on the marked increase of BrdU into cells in the DG at 9–12 days after ischemia (Fig. 1A).

Saline microinjected into hippocampus at 30 minutes before ischemia did not affect the marked increase of BrdU labeled cells in the DG (Fig. 1A-Sh) compared to ischemic, uninjected animals (Fig. 1A-I). Microinjections of MK-801 into hippocampus (Fig. 1A-Mh) at 30 minutes before ischemia produced a significant decrease of BrdU labeling at 15 days following ischemia compared to saline injected animals ($p < 0.001$).

Bilateral carotid artery occlusions (10 minutes long) resulted in severe loss of NeuN stained CA1 neurons in hippocampus 15d following ischemia. Systemic injections of NBQX prevented the CA1 neuronal cell death 15d following ischemia. Injection of NBQX at day 7 after ischemia, two days before the increased neurogenesis in the dentate gyrus , did not prevent the loss of the CA1 pyramidal neurons at 15d following ischemia. Animals microinjected with saline in the CA1 hippocampal subfield showed the typical loss of CA1 neurons 15d after ischemia. However, animals microinjected with NBQX in CA1 at 30 minutes before ischemia demonstrated complete preservation of CA1 neurons.

NBQX injected systemically (i.p.) into control animals produced a moderate increase in the number of BrdU-labeled cells (Fig. 1B). At 15 days following global ischemia, BrdU incorporation into cells in the dentate was significantly increased (Fig. 1B). Systemic injections of NBQX blocked BrdU incorporation into DG cells, with the numbers of BrDU labeled cells being similar to those in controls (Fig. 1B). Systemic injections of NBQX given 7 days after ischemia had little effect on the marked increase of BrdU into cells in the DG at 9–12 days after ischemia (Fig. 1B). The numbers of BrdU labeled cells were similar in the ischemia group (I) and in the ischemia group that received NBQX systemically (N7) at 7d following ischemia (Fig. 1B).

Saline microinjected into CA1 at 30 minutes before ischemia did not affect the marked increase of BrdU incorporation into DG com-

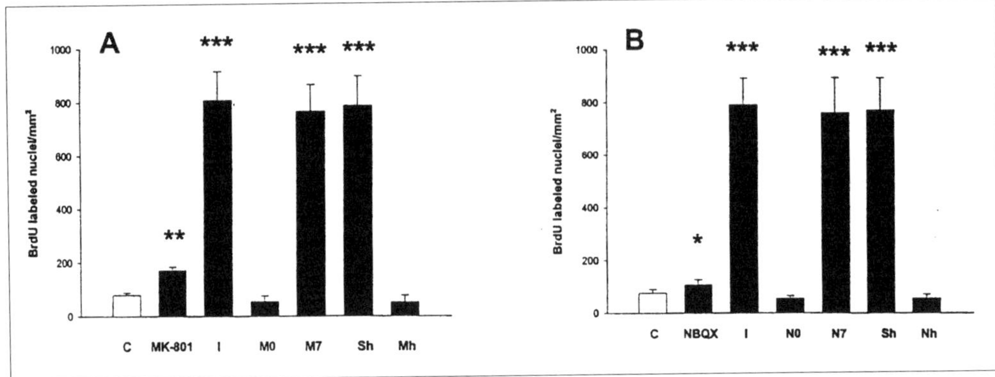

Fig. 1. MK-801 and NBQX prevent ischemia-induced neurogenesis. Gerbils were subjected to 10 minutes of global ischemia, injected daily with BrdU for four days between 9–12 days after ischemia, and sacrificed at 15 days following ischemia (3 days after the last injection of BrdU).
A. Numbers of BrdU labeled cells in the dentate subgranular zone (SGZ) in control animals or ischemic animals given MK-801. Non-ischemic animals given MK-801 had significantly more cells than animals given saline (C). Following ischemia there was a marked increase in the numbers of BrdU labeled cells (I) compared to controls (C). Treatment with MK-801 before and after ischemia (M0) decreased the numbers of BrdU labeled cells to control (C) levels. However, large numbers of BrdU labeled cells were observed in dentate when MK-801 was administered at 7d days following ischemia (M7). Injection of saline into hippocampus prior to ischemia had no effect on the increased numbers of BrdU labeled cells in dentate produced by ischemia (Sh). However, injection of MK-801 into hippocampus (Mh) prior to ischemia prevented the cell proliferation (Mh) normally produced by ischemia (I, S).
B. Numbers of BrdU labeled cells in the dentate subgranular zone (SGZ) in control animals or ischemic animals given NBQX. Non-ischemic animals given NBQX had significantly more cells than animals given saline (C). Following ischemia there was a marked increase in the numbers of BrdU labeled cells (I) compared to controls (C). Treatment with NBQX (N0) before and after ischemia decreased the numbers of BrdU labeled cells to control (C) levels. However, large numbers of BrdU labeled cells were observed in dentate when NBQX was administered at 7d days following ischemia (N7). Injection of saline into hippocampus prior to ischemia had no effect on the increased numbers of BrdU labeled cells in dentate produced by ischemia (Sh). However, injection of NBQX into hippocampus (Nh) prior to ischemia prevented the cell proliferation (Nh) normally produced by ischemia (I, S). Histogram bars indicate group mean values ± standard deviation. * $p < 0.05$; ** $p < 0.01$; *** $p < 0.001$ using Student Newman-Keuls test after ANOVA, indicate significant differences induced by ischemia.

pared to ischemic, un-injected animals (Fig. 1B). However, microinjections of NBQX into CA1 of hippocampus before ischemia produced a significant decrease of BrdU labeling at 15 days following ischemia ($p < 0.001$, Fig. 1B).

Synapsin-I immunoreactivity was observed as a fine reticular staining in the neuropil of the plexiform layers of the hippocampus. Western blots confirmed the presence of synapsin-I in CA3 of hippocampus of control animals and either MK-801 or NBQX produced a small decrease of synapsin-I protein in CA3 of non-ischemic controls. At 7 days following global ischemia and at 15 days following ischemia there was marked increase in synapsin-I immunoreactivity in stratum lucidum of CA3, as well as an increase of synapsin protein in CA3 on Western blots.

Systemic administration of MK801 and NBQX markedly decreased the induction of synapsin-I in CA3 at 15 days following ischemia as assessed using immunocytochemistry and Western blotting. Systemic administration of MK-801 and NBQX at 7d days following ischemia had little effect on the marked induction of synapsin-I in CA3 when compared to ischemia alone either by immunocytochemistry or by Western blotting.

Saline injections into hippocampus slightly decreased synapsin-I staining in CA3 of hippocampus when compared to ischemia, but the staining was still greater than in controls. Injections into hippocampus of either MK-801 or NBQX at 30 minutes prior to ischemia completely blocked the increased expression of synapsin-I protein in CA3 of hippocampus on immunocytochemically stained sections and on Western blots.

Discussion

MK801 and NBQX prevent the CA1 pyramidal neuronal cell death, the dentate cell proliferation and the induction of synapsin-I protein that occurs in hippocampus following global ischemia. We postulate that neurogenesis occurs because of decreased dentate glutamate receptor activation after acute MK-801 and NBQX administration, and because of decreased glutamate receptor activation that occurs chronically beginning days after ischemic injury. Hence, prevention of CA1 cell death following ischemia with MK-801 and NBQX could prevent glutamate receptor down regulation in CA1 and DG (Gorter et al. 1997; Aronica et al. 1998; Grabb and Choi 1999), and therefore prevent hippocampal neurogenesis. Induction of synapsin-I in granule cell mossy fiber terminals could also be a response to ischemic injury such that preventing injury with glutamate receptor antagonists prevents synapsin induction.

Systemic administration of a $NMDA_R$ antagonist to control animals stimulated cell proliferation in dentate gyrus in this study as shown previously (Gould et al. 1997; Cameron et al. 1995). The current study also shows that $AMPA_R$ antagonists also increase proliferation of dentate progenitor cells. The data imply that glutamate activation of either $NMDA_R$ or $AMPA_R$ in normal hippocampus suppresses dentate cell proliferation, which is consistent with studies that show that cell depolarization generally decreases DNA synthesis (Cui and Bulleit 1998; LoTurco et al. 1995).

The blockade of neurogenesis that occurs following ischemia by either MK-801 or NBQX was unexpected. Ischemia should acutely stimulate both $NMDA_R$ and $AMPA_R$ since there is glutamate release during ischemia (Meldrum 1995; Peruche and Krieglstein 1993) and glutamate receptor antagonists prevent injury (Buchan et al. 1991; Diemer et al. 1992; Gill et al. 1987; Lippert et al. 1994; Sheardown et al. 1990; Simon et al. 1984). The pilocarpine-induced seizures that stimulate neurogenesis (Parent et al. 1997) would also be expected to increase glutamate release and acutely activate NMDA and AMPA glutamate receptors. Though ischemia and seizure activation of glutamate receptors might increase neurogenesis, it is difficult to understand why glutamate receptor antagonists also induce neurogenesis in control animals. It seems likely, therefore, that ischemia and seizure induced neurogenesis occurs via some other mechanism other than stimulating glutamate receptors.

Ischemia, seizure and glutamate-antagonists may all increase neurogenesis because there is decreased activation or down-regulation of hippocampal glutamate receptors following chronic hippocampal injuries of any type (Gorter et al. 1997; Grabb and Choi 1999). Following global ischemia (Liu et al. 1998) there is death of CA1 pyramidal neurons, dentate hilar neurons, and some CA3 neurons and dentate granule cell neurons (Fukuda et al. 1999; Hsu and Buzsaki 1993; Li et al. 1997; Onodera et al. 1990, 1993; Sugimoto et al. 1993). Though ischemia acutely activates glutamate receptors, this cell death chronically decreases cell firing in all hippocampal circuits, decreasing the activity of dentate granule cell neurons and hippocampal CA3 and CA1 neurons (Aoyagi et al. 1998; Gao et al. 1998; Howard et al. 1998). In addition, there is down-regulation of both NMDA and AMPA receptors following ischemia in vulnerable neurons before cell death in CA1 and to some degree in DG (Pellegrini-Giampietro et al. 1992, 1997; Onodera et al. 1989; Zhang et al. 1997). Though dentate granule cell activation mediates ischemic CA1 and hilar cell loss (Johansen et al. 1986), we propose that decreased activation or down regulation of dentate glutamate receptors is the stimulus for increased neurogenesis following ischemic and other types of chronic hippocampal injury.

Neurogenesis also occurs following ischemia induced ischemic tolerance where there is no death of CA1 neurons (Liu et al. 1998). However, there is death of dentate hilar neurons, even in the ischemia induced-tolerance model (Johansen et al. 1987; Johansen 1993; Sugimoto et al. 1993; Benveniste and Diemer 1988; Benveniste et al. 1997), that provide significant input to dentate granule cells (Sugimoto et al. 1993; Johansen 1993). This could decrease dentate glutamate receptor activation, via hilar interneurons, and trigger dentate neurogenesis in ischemic tolerant animals. This would suggest the hilar cell may be directly involved in regulating neurogenesis via $AMPA_R$ or $NMDA_R$ receptors.

Seizure induced neurogenesis could also be related to cell death and glutamate receptor down-regulation since the generalized seizures produced by pilocarpine cause death of CA3 neurons (Parent et al. 1997). Seizure induced neurogenesis caused by kainate (Gray and Sundstrom 1998) is associated with CA3 and CA1 death that might be associated with decreased activation of dentate glutamate receptors following the acute seizures. Entorhinal cortical lesions (Cameron et al. 1995) and granule cell lesions that stimulate neurogenesis (Gould and Tanapat 1997) should decrease dentate glutamate receptor activation. MK-801 or NBQX given systematically would decrease stimulation of hippocampal glutamate receptors. Administration of MK-801 or NBQX prior to ischemia in this study would prevent the death of neurons that occurs following ischemia, would maintain normal hippocampal activity, and could therefore prevent ischemia induced decreases of glutamate receptor activation, and therefore prevent the increases of dentate neurogenesis.

The results confirm that synapsin-I is up-regulated in the mossy fiber layer of the CA3 region of hippocampus following global ischemia (Marti et al. 1999) and shows that the synapsin-I induction can be prevented by $NMDA_R$ and $AMPA_R$ antagonists. The stimuli for the CA3 synapsin up-regulation are uncertain, but could be similar to those that stimulate neurogenesis following ischemia.

Synapsin-I is a pre-synaptic protein involved in neurotransmitter release and regulation of axonal elongation and new synapse formation, synapsin-I phosphorylation releasing pre-synaptic vesicles from the reserve pool (Turner et al. 1999). The synapsin-I up-regulation in the CA3 region of the hippocampus following global ischemia suggests that it is induced in the pre-synaptic terminals of mossy fibers from dentate granule cell neurons that synapse on CA3 pyramidal neurons. This implies altered synaptic function and/or formation of new synapses by granule cell mossy fibers on CA3 pyramidal neurons. The stimulus for increased synapsin-I expression in dentate granule cell neuron mossy fibers could be death of some granule cell neurons with sprouting of their neighbors, and/or death of CA3 target neurons with synaptic re-organization of mossy fiber afferents onto surviving CA3 neurons (Fukuda et al. 1999; Hsu and Buzsaki 1993; Li et al. 1997; Onodera et al. 1990, 1993).

The synapsin-I induction probably occurs mainly in granule cell neurons that project to CA3. Since cell proliferation does not begin until 7 days following ischemia (Liu et al. 1998), and since newborn granule cells with neuronal phenotypes are not detected until 1–3 weeks following ischemia (Liu et al. 1998), the synapsin-I induction at 7 and 15 days is not due to synaptogenesis of neurons born following ischemia. At later times it is possible that newborn granule cell neurons contribute to mossy fiber synaptogenesis in CA3 since newborn neurons extend axons to CA3 (Stanfield and Trice 1988; Markakis and Gage 1999). The suppression of neurogenesis and synaptogenesis by glutamate receptor activation and its enhacement by $NMDA_R$ and $AMPA_R$ inactivation, may provide a means whereby natural alterations in the degree of excitatory input control the numbers of newborn neurons and the sprouting of existing neurons.

References

1. Aoyagi A, Saito H, Abe K, Nishiyama N (1998) Early impairment and late recovery of synaptic transmission in the rat dentate gyrus following transient forebrain ischemia in vivo. Brain Res 799:130–137
2. Aronica EM, Gorter JA, Groom S, Kessler JA, Bennett MV, Zukin RS, Rosenbaum DM (1998) Aurintricarboxylic acid

prevents GluR2 mRNA down-regulation and delayed neurodegeneration in hippocampal CA1 neurons of gerbils after global ischemia. Proc Natl Acad Sci USA 95 (12):7115–7120

3. Benveniste H, Diemer NH (1988) Early postischemic ^{45}Ca accumulation in rat dentate hilus. J Cereb Blood Flow Metab 8:713–719
4. Benveniste H, Jorgensen MB, Diemer NH, Hansen AJ (1988) Calcium accumulation by glutamate receptor activation is involved in hippocampal cell damage after ischemia. Acta Neurol Scand 78:529–536
5. Buchan AM, Li H, Cho S, Pulsinelli WA (1991b) Blockade of the AMPA receptor prevents CA1 hippocampal injury following severe but transient forebrain ischemia in adult rats. Neurosci Lett 132:255–258
6. Cameron HA, McEwen BS, Gould E (1995) Regulation of adult neurogenesis by excitatory input and NMDA receptor activation in the dentate gyrus. J Neurosci 15:4687–4692
7. Colbourne F, Li H, Buchan AM, Clemens JA (1999) Continuing postischemic neuronal death in CA1: influence of ischemia duration and cytoprotective doses of NBQX and SNX-111 in rats. Stroke 30:662–668
8. Cui H, Bulleit RF (1998) Potassium chloride inhibits proliferation of cerebellar granule neuron progenitors. Brain Res Dev Brain Res 106:129–135
9. Diemer NH, Jorgensen MB, Johansen FF, Sheardown M, Honore T (1992) Protection against ischemic hippocampal CA1 damage in the rat with a new non-NMDA antagonist, NBQX. Acta Neurol Scand 86:45–49
10. Fukuda T, Wang H, Nakanishi H, Yamamoto K, Kosaka T (1999) Novel non-apoptotic morphological changes in neurons of the mouse hippocampus following transient hypoxic-ischemia. Neurosci Res 33:49–55
11. Gao TM, Howard EM, Xu ZC (1998) Transient neurophysiological changes in CA3 neurons and dentate granule cells after severe forebrain ischemia in vivo. J Neurophys 80:2860–2869
12. Gill R, Foster AC, Woodruff GN (1987) Systemic administration of MK-801 protects against ischemia-induced hippocampal neurodegeneration in the gerbil. J Neurosci 7:3343–3349
13. Gill R, Woodruff GN (1990) The neuroprotective actions of kynurenic acid and MK-801 in gerbils are synergistic and not related to hypothermia. Eur J Pharmacol 176:143–149
14. Gonzalez MF, Lowenstein D, Fernyak S, Hisanaga K, Simon R, Sharp FR (1991) Induction of heat shock protein 72-like immunoreactivity in the hippocampal formation following transient global ischemia. Brain Res Bull 26:241–250
15. Gorter JA, Petrozzino JJ, Aronica EM, Rosenbaum DM, Opitz T, Bennett MV, Connor JA, Zukin RS (1997) Global ischemia induces downregulation of Glur2 mRNA and increases AMPA receptor-mediated Ca^{2+} influx in hippocampal CA1 neurons of gerbil. J Neurosci 17:6179–6188
16. Gould E, McEwen BS, Tanapat P, Galea LAM, Fuchs E (1997) Neurogenesis in the Dentate Gyrus of the Adult Tree Shrew Is Regulated by Psychosocial Stress and NMDA Receptor Activation. J Neurosci 17:2492–2498
17. Gould E, Tanapat P (1997) Lesion-induced proliferation of neuronal progenitors in the dentate gyrus of the adult rat. Neuroscience 80:427–436
18. Grabb MC, Choi DW (1999) Ischemic tolerance in murine cortical cell culture: critical role for NMDA receptors. J Neurosci 19 (5):1657–1662
19. Gray WP, Sundstrom LE (1998) Kainic acid increases the proliferation of granule cell progenitors in the dentate gyrus of the adult rat. Brain Res 790:52–59
20. Greengard P, Valtorta F, Czernik AJ, Benfenati F (1993) Synaptic vesicle phosphoproteins and regulation of synaptic function. Science 259:780–785
21. Herguido MJ, Carceller F, Roda JM, Avendano C (1999) Hippocampal cell loss in transient global cerebral ischemia in rats: a critical assessment. Neuroscience 93:71–80
22. Hicks CA, Ward MA, Swettenham JB, O'Neill MJ (1999) Synergistic neuroprotective effects by combining an NMDA or AMPA receptor antagonist with nitric oxide synthase inhibitors in global cerebral ischaemia. Eur J Pharmacol 381:113–119
23. Howard EM, Gao TM, Pulsinelli WA, Xu ZC (1998) Electrophysiological changes of CA3 neurons and dentate granule cells following transient forebrain ischemia. Brain Res 798:109–118
24. Hsu M, Buzsaki G (1993) Vulnerability of mossy fiber targets in the rat hippocampus to forebrain ischemia. J Neurosci 13:3964–3979
25. Ito U, Spatz M, Walker JT, Jr., Klatzo I (1975) Experimental cerebral ischemia in mongolian gerbils. I. Light microscopic observations. Acta Neuropathol (Berl) 32:209–223
26. Johansen FF (1993) Interneurons in rat hippocampus after cerebral ischemia. Morphometric, functional, and therapeutic investigations. Acta Neurol Scand Suppl 150:1–32
27. Johansen FF, Jorgensen MB, Diemer NH (1986) Ischemic CA-1 pyramidal cell loss is prevented by preischemic colchicine destruction of dentate gyrus granule cells. Brain Res 377:344–347
28. Johansen FF, Zimmer J, Diemer NH (1987) Early loss of somatostatin neurons in dentate hilus after cerebral ischemia in the rat precedes CA-1 pyramidal cell loss. Acta Neuropathol (Berl) 73:110–114
29. Kirino T (1982) Delayed neuronal death in the gerbil hippocampus following ischemia. Brain Res 239:57–69
30. Lazarewicz JW, Gadamski R, Parsons CG, Danysz W (1997) Protection against post-ischaemic neuronal loss in gerbil hippocampal CA1 by glycineB and AMPA antagonists. Short communication. J Neural Transm 104:1249–1254
31. Li Y, Chopp M, Powers C (1997) Granule cell apoptosis and protein expression in hippocampal dentate gyrus after forebrain ischemia in the rat. J Neurol Sci 150:93–102
32. Lippert K, Welsch M, Krieglstein J (1994) Over-additive protective effect of dizocilpine and NBQX against neuronal damage. Eur J Pharmacol 253:207–213
33. Liu J, Solway K, Messing RO, Sharp FR (1998) Increased neurogenesis in the dentate gyrus after transient global ischemia in gerbils. J Neurosci 18:7768–7778
34. LoTurco JJ, Owens DF, Heath MJ, Davis MB, Kriegstein AR (1995) GABA and glutamate depolarize cortical progenitor cells and inhibit DNA synthesis. Neuron 15:1287–1298
35. Markakis EA, Gage FH (1999) Adult-generated neurons in the dentate gyrus send axonal projections to field CA3 and are surrounded by synaptic vesicles. J Comp Neurol 406:449–460
36. Marti E, Ferrer I, Blasi J (1999) Transient increase of synapsin-I immunoreactivity in the mossy fiber layer of the hippocampus after transient forebrain ischemia in the mongolian gerbil. Brain Res 824:153–160
37. Meldrum BS (1995) Excitatory amino acid receptors and their role in epilepsy and cerebral ischemia. Ann N Y Acad Sci 757:492–505
38. Onodera H, Aoki H, Kogure K (1993) Long-term structural and biochemical events in the hippocampus following transient global ischemia. Prog Brain Res 96:271–280
39. Onodera H, Aoki H, Yae T, Kogure K (1990) Post-ischemic synaptic plasticity in the rat hippocampus after long-term survival: histochemical and autoradiographic study. Neuroscience 38:125–136
40. Onodera H, Araki T, Kogure K (1989) Excitatory amino acid binding sites in the rat hippocampus after transient forebrain ischemia. J Cereb Blood Flow Metab 9:623–628
41. Parent JM, Yu TW, Leibowitz RT, Geschwind DH, Sloviter RS, Lowenstein DH (1997) Dentate granule cell neurogenesis is increased by seizures and contributes to aberrant network

reorganization in the adult rat hippocampus. J Neurosci 17:3727–3738

42. Pellegrini-Giampietro DE, Zukin RS, Bennett MV, Cho S, Pulsinelli WA (1992) Switch in glutamate receptor subunit gene expression in CA1 subfield of hippocampus following global ischemia in rats. Proc Natl Acad Sci USA 89:10499–10503
43. Pellegrini-Giampietro DE, Gorter JA, Bennett MV, Zukin RS (1997) The gluR-2 hypothesis: Ca^{2+}-permeable AMPA receptors in neurological disorders. Trends in Neurosci 20:464–470
44. Peruche B, Krieglstein J (1993) Mechanisms of drug actions against neuronal damage caused by ischemia-an overview. Prog Neuropsychopharmacol Biol Psychiatry 17:21–70
45. Pulsinelli WA, Brierley JB, Plum F (1982) Temporal profile of neuronal damage in a model of transient forebrain ischemia. Ann Neurol 11:491–498
46. Sheardown MJ, Nielsen EO, Hansen AJ, Jacobsen P, Honore T (1990) 2,3-Dihydroxy-6-nitro-7-sulfamoyl-benzo(F)quinoxaline: a neuroprotectant for cerebral ischemia. Science 247:571–574
47. Simon RP, Swan JH, Griffiths T, Meldrum BS (1984) Blockade of N-methyl-D-aspartate receptors may protect against ischemic damage in the brain. Science 226:850–852
48. Squire LR, Zola-Morgan S (1996) Ischemic brain damage and memory impairment: a commentary. Hippocampus 6:546–552
49. Stanfield BB, Trice JE (1988) Evidence that granule cells generated in the dentate gyrus of adult rats extend axonal projections. Exp Brain Res 72:399–406
50. Sugimoto A, Shozuhara H, Kogure K, Onodera H (1993) Exposure to sub-lethal ischemia failed to prevent subsequent ischemic death of dentate hilar neurons, as estimated by laminin immunohistochemistry. Brain Res 629:159–162
51. Turner KM, Burgoyne RD, Morgan A (1999) Protein phosphorylation and the regulation of synaptic membrane traffic. Trends Neurosci 22:459–464
52. Westerberg E, Monaghan DT, Kalimo H, Cotman CW, Wieloch TW (1989) Dynamic changes of excitatory amino acid receptors in the rat hippocampus following transient cerebral ischemia. J Neurosci 9:798–805
53. Zhang L, Hsu JC, Takagi N, Gurd JW, Wallace MC, Eubanks JH (1997) Transient global ischemia alters NMDA receptor expression in rat hippocampus: correlation with decreased immunoreactive protein levels of the NR2A/2B subunits, and an altered NMDA receptor functionality. J Neurochem 69:1983–1994
54. Zola-Morgan S, Squire LR, Amaral DG (1986) Human amnesia and the medial temporal region: enduring memory impairment following a bilateral lesion limited to field CA1 of the hippocampus. J Neurosci 6:2950–2967
55. Zola-Morgan S, Squire LR, Rempel NL, Clower RP, Amaral DG (1992) Enduring memory impairment in monkeys after ischemic damage to the hippocampus. J Neurosci 12:2582–2596

Treatment of neural injury with bone marrow

M. Chopp[1,2], Y. Li[1], J. Chen[1]

Abstract

There is a great potential to treat neural injury, including stroke, as well as neurodegenerative disease using stem cell technology. In this manuscript, we describe our use of bone marrow stromal cells (MSC) in the treatment of stroke. Marrow stromal cells obtained from donor rat/ mice can be harvested, labeled and administered to rodents well after the onset of stroke. Data are presented demonstrating the efficacy of this treatment modality. Significant functional improvement, as measured by, motor, somatosensory and neurological scales is demonstrated with MSC treatment of stroke. The MSC transplanted directly to brain or injected intravascularly, migrate to sites of injury, differentiate and perhaps most important, activate the endogenous brain stem cells to proliferate, and migrate to the compromised tissue. Our data suggest that treatment of neural injury with MSC may provide important therapeutic benefit for the treatment of injury and neurodegenerative disease.

Treatment of stroke has until now focussed on the acute phase after stroke. The only available and approved treatment of stroke is that of thrombolysis, which is applicable and effective within a limited window of three hours from time of onset of ictus. In addition, substantial effort is being expended in the development of neuroprotective agents. However what has been essentially neglected and maybe forgotten has been the brain's innate ability to repair and to compensate for injury. After onset of stroke, the majority of patients show improvement in function compared to deficits experienced early at stroke onset. Although some of this benefit can be attributed to learning and functional compensation, clearly other events are present in brain which promote improved outcome. Likewise in the experimental animal, occlusion of the middle cerebral artery (MCA) brings initial neurological deficit, which over time ameliorates, even while the ischemic lesion is growing. Thus, an approach for the treatment of stroke would be to activate and enhance these endogenous compensatory and plasticity mechanisms. In this chapter, I will describe studies in which bone marrow and marrow stromal cells are employed to treat brain after stroke. The utility of this cell transplantation therapy is to primarily enhance endogenous compensatory mechanisms and to promote production of and proliferation of neural stem cells within the brain.

The underlying mechanism promoting and allowing effective transplantation of cells into brain is that injured tissue in some ways be-

[1]Henry Ford Health Sciences Center, Neurology Department, E&R 3056, 2799 West Grand Boulevard, Detroit, MI 48202
e-Mail: chopp@neuro.hfh.edu
[2]Department of Physics, Oakland University, Rochester, MI

comes developmental tissue (Cramer and Chopp 2000). It is this condition that provides the environment, the enriched environment; receptive to cellular therapy that facilitates incorporation and support of marrow stromal cells. The environment provides developmental signals to the stromal cells which allow these cells to survive, but more importantly prompts these cells to produce an array of trophic factors that promotes brain plasticity and alters the environment. There is a substantial body of literature supporting the concept of injured brain as a quasi-developing brain (for review see Cramer and Chopp 2000). After stroke or traumatic brain injury, developmental and embryonic proteins are rapidly expressed. Many of these proteins are localized to the boundaries of an ischemic or injury lesion. Among the many proteins expressed are cyclin D1 (Li et al. 1998; Timsit et al. 1999), GAP-43 (Li et al. 1998; Stroemer et al. 1995), nestin (Duggal et al. 1997; Li and Chopp 1999), neuroD (Chopp and Li 1998), and egr-1 among many others. Expression of these proteins is somewhat enigmatic. For example, cyclin proteins are in general associated with cell division. Consider that the brain has undergone an ischemic event. There is insufficient energy to provide necessities of life, ATP levels are down and protein production falls. Yet proteins associated with cell mitosis are upregulated. Teleologically, why would energy deprived tissue, expend its resources on proteins required for mitosis, particularly when neurons are post-mitotic cells? Another interesting developmental protein is nestin. Nestin is a neuroepithelial protein and a stem cell marker. It is present in large numbers in developing brain. primarily within astrocytes. Nestin is replaced by glial fibrillary protein (GFAP) after birth. In the adult brain, nestin may be found in scattered endothelial cells. After a stroke or trauma, however, there is intense nestin expression within astrocytes localized to the boundary zone of the lesion. The expression is suggestive of a reversion of these cells to a developmental state. This expression persists for at least 28 days after stroke. More remarkable is the observation, that not only astrocytes express nestin, but neurons also. This suggests that these cells are regressing to predifferentiated state. The support for the ontogeny hypothesis continues with the expression of differentiating proteins, such as neuro D. The upshot of these observations is that injured tissue is primed as developing tissue, as receptive to the influx of embryonic and stem-like cells. In our work, we capitalized on this observation and sought to implant an embryonic stem-like cell. However, we selected the marrow stromal cell and not the embryonic stem cell.

There is enormous interest and effort in the use of stem cell technology to repair the CNS. Most of this effort has been directed to the utilization of embryonic stem cells and fetal tissue. Stem cells can form new neurons and reduce behavioral deficits in damaged and compromised animal and human brain (Bjorklund and Lindvall 2000; Borlongan et al. 1998; Fisher and Gage 1993; Gage 1998, 2000; Snyder et al. 1997a). Neural transplantation using fetal human CNS tissue offers a possible therapeutic approach to the treatment of patients with Parkinson's disease (Barinaga 2000) and Huntington's disease (Peschanski et al. 1995). In hope of a clinical application, the intrastriatal fetal graft has been used to reduce behavioral deficits in animal models of focal (Borlongan et al. 1998; Goto et al. 1997) and global (Hodges et al. 1997) cerebral ischemia. However, transplantation of embryonic grafts is plagued with logistic and ethical considerations. Thus, it is reasonable to seek alternative sources of stem cells.

Stem cells have been isolated from various tissues in animals and humans, including adult bone marrow (BM) and even adult brain (Gage 1998). Two kinds of stem cells (hematopoietic and mesenchymal stem cells) localize in normal bone marrow (Prockop 1997). In the last decade, remarkable advances have been made in BM transplantation, which is now becoming a powerful strategy for supporting cells derived from hematopoietic stem cells in the treatment of life-threatening diseases such as leukemia, aplastic anemia, and congenital immunodeficiency (Ikehara 1999, 1998). In addition to hematopoietic cells, BM contains marrow stromal cells (MSCs, which includes mesenchymal stem cells) (Prockop 1997, 1998). Normally MSCs give rise to bone, cartilage, and mesenchymal cells. MSC transplantation has been employed to treat patients with severe osteogenesis imperfecta (Horwitz et al. 1999) and cancer (Lazarus et al. 1995). MSCs may be even more versatile. Cells from the BM of children and adults have properties of embryonic stem cells (Vogel 2000). These cells become liver cells, muscle cells- heart, skeletal and smooth, as well as brain cells (Ferrari et al. 1998; Vogel 2000). Within the past several years, MSCs have been investigated as vehicles for both cell therapy and gene therapy (Bruder et al. 1998; Pereira et al. 1995, 1998; Prockop 1997, 1998; Riew et al. 1998).

The fate of stem cells *in vivo* is very much influenced by contextual cues, and stem cells retain the capacity to respond to local epigenetic signals (Snyder et al. 1997b). Stem cells isolated from one region of the CNS will, when transplanted to ectopic CNS sites, differentiate with a terminal phenotype appropriate for that ectopic site (Gage et al. 1995; Snyder et al. 1992). Several lines of evidence point to BM cells as the precursor of select brain cells (de Groot et al. 1992; Hickey and Kimura 1988; Krall et al. 1994; Pereira et al. 1995, 1998; Prockop 1997; Walkley et al. 1994). Twelve percent of microglia are thought to originate from the marrow (Kennedy and Abkowitz 1997; Krall et al. 1994). A small but detectable proportion of astroglial cells also derive from marrow progenitors (Eglitis and Mezey 1997). Marrow stromal cells implanted directly into the striatum of rats result in 20% successful engraftment and migration along known pathways for neural stem cells and these cells survive and resemble astrocytes (Azizi et al. 1998). In addition, a recent study has provided evidence for preferential homing of transplanted BM cells to the site of injury after onset of permanent MCAo in irradiated rats (Eglitis et al. 1999). Some of these cells differentiate into glial fibrillary acidic protein (GFAP) positive astrocytes. These data indicate that BM, which is easily obtained from aspiration under local anesthesia, is amenable to survival and integration in the host brain. Moreover, in the soluble stroma, a number of hematopoietic cytokines are secreted by bone marrow stromal cells, which normally support hematopoietic progenitors to proliferate and differentiate (Majumdar et al. 1998). These studies support the hypothesis that transplantation of adult BM cells can be successfully used to facilitate neural repair.

The following is a brief description of ongoing studies in our laboratory using bone marrow or bone marrow derived cells as a therapy to reduce neurological deficits after neural injury. Studies were performed on rodents with allogenic transplantation of either whole bone marrow or marrow cells gleaned from donor animals.

Whole BM preparation and treatment of stroke in the adult rodent (Li et al. 2000a; Chen et al. 2000a): Adult Wistar rats received injections of bromodeoxyuridine (BrdU) i.p. daily 14-d prior harvest. Fresh BM was harvested aseptically from tibias and femurs of rats, using a syringe containing with phosphate buffered saline (PBS, 0.5 ml). There were no differences of MSC growth curves, and the numbers of colonies and cellular morphological changes in cultured medium (IMDM), between MSCs harvested from rats with or without BrdU injections. Roughly 90% of fresh BM cells show positive immunoreactivity with BrdU antibody staining prior transplantation.

Experiments were performed on rats subjected to 2 hours of MCA occlusion using the intraluminal thread model (Zea Longa et al. 1989; Chen et al. 1992). One day after stroke, whole bone marrow, approximately 1×10^6 (Bailey and Kandel 1993) BM cells in 10 μl total volume (soluble stroma and PBS) was transplanted into the boundary zone of the ischemic lesion. The cells were placed within the striatal penumbra (7 ul) and the cortex (3ul). Similar experiments were performed in an embolic model of stroke in mice (unpublished). The mice were subjected to embolic stroke, by placement of a 24-hour-old clot at the origin of the MCA. Four days after stroke, bone marrow was transplanted into the boundary zone of the mice. Placement of the cells within the penumbra was motivated by our hypothesis that ischemic tissue, particularly, tissue surrounding a lesion has developmental characteristics. Thus placement of the cells within this embryonic like tissue should facilitate survival and activate these cells to produce factors that promote tissue repair and plasticity.

In both sets of studies, the ischemic lesion was not altered by the transplantation. The endpoint in all experiments was motor function as measured by time spent on an accelerating rotarod. Bone marrow transplantation in rats resulted in (n = 8) in a significant functional recovery at 14 days after stroke on the rotarod test compared to control rats (n = 8) in which PBS was injected. Similarly in mice, significant improvement in motor function was found in bone marrow treated animals (n = 5) compared with control PBS treated animals (n = 8) at 28 days after stroke.

In an effort to refine and to hone in on the cell population responsible for the therapeutic benefit of transplantation, we performed experiments in which the bone marrow was processed and separated into hematopoetic and marrow stromal cell populations. The methods and applications of these experiments are described.

Marrow stromal cell preparation and treatment of stroke: Primary cultures of BM cells were obtained 48 h after treating rats with 5-fluorouracil (5-FU) (Gautam et al. 1995, 1998; Randall and Weissman 1997). Nucleated cells were seeded into each tissue culture flask in Iscove's Modified Dulbecco's medium (IMDM) supplemented with 10% fetal bovine serum (FBS). After 72 hours of incubation, non plastic-adherent hematopoietic cells were removed and plastic-adherent heterogeneous MSCs were collected and resuspended in fresh IMDM and were grown for several passages. As noted in previous reports (Kuznetsov et al. 1997), MSCs form single-cell-derived colonies when plated in culture. Morphologically spindle-shaped fibroblastoid MSCs were detected in cultures by hematoxylin and eosin staining. To identify cells derived from BM cells, BrdU was added into the medium at 72 h before transplantation. More than 90% of cultured MSCs show positive reactivity with BrdU antibody before intracerebral transplantation. MSCs could be induced to differentiate into neural cells under neurotrophic cell culture conditions. In preliminary experiments, HSCs derived from the bone marrow culture, i.e. non-adherent cells were transplanted within ischemic rat brain. Little or no therapeutic benefit was noted. Therefore the adherent cells were selected as the target populations for treatment of stroke.

Functional tests after MCAo and MSC transplantation: We employed the rotarod test (Hamm et al. 1994; Rogers et al. 1997), adhesive removal test (Schallert 1988; Schallert et al. 1997; Schwartz et al. 1999) and a modified neurological severity score (NSS) (Barth and Schallert 1987; Borlongan et al. 1995; Markgraf et al. 1992; Zea Longa et al. 1989) to identify the behavioral alteration of rats subjected to MCAo and MSC transplantation. MSCs were separated from hematopoietic cells and cultured in standard medium, and then transplanted into the IBZ at 1 d or 1 w after MCAo. The NSS includes motor (muscle status, abnormal movement) (Borlongan et al. 1995; Schallert et al. 1997; Zea Longa et al. 1989) sensory (visual, tactile and proprioceptive) (Barth and Schallert 1987; Markgraf et al. 1992) and reflex tests (Germano et al. 1994; Schallert et al. 1997). Our data indicate that transplantation of MSCs at 1 d after MCAo (n = 8), significantly improved functional recovery on the adhesive removal test $p < 0.05$) and NSS ($p < 0.05$) at 14 d, compared with MCAo injected with PBS (n = 8) (Li et al. 2000b; Chen et al. 2000b). Significant ($p < 0.05$) functional recovery of NSS was also observed in rats subjected to transplantation of MSCs at 1 w after 2 h of MCAo and sacrificed at 14 d, compared with MCAo injected with PBS (n = 5).

Although intracerebral transplantation of cells is viable route for treatment, a far less invasive, and a more clinically acceptable route would be transplantation of MSCs using an intravascular route. In preliminary studies, we injected 1–2 million cells intra-arterially into the carotid artery of rats 1-day after induction of 2 hours of MCA occlusion. These animals were sacrificed 2 weeks after stroke and behavioral tests and histological analysis of the tissue were performed. There was evidence of improvement of functional outcome, on neurologic (NSS) as well as somatosensory adhesive removal tests. The degree of reduction of deficit appears at least as effective as in intracranial transplantation of cells. Histological analysis of tissue revealed the presence of nearly, 20% of the BrdU labeled cells within the cerebral parenchyma two weeks after stroke. Most of the cells were localized to the ischemic boundary zone with some cells within the core and very little in contralateral tissue. The cellular localization appears similar to that of inflammatory cells "infecting" brain. Given that the cells were administered 1 day after stroke at a time with no substantial breakdown in the blood brain barrier (BBB), it is likely that the migration of cells from the vessels into the parenchyma occurs without BBB disruption. The MSC find their way to the site of the ischemic lesion. Some of the MSCs appeared to encircle blood vessels. These data indicate that intravascular administration of MSCs may be an alternate and effective route for the treatment of stroke.

What are the mechanisms responsible for the reduction of neurologic and functional deficits? There are two possibilities to consider: 1)- transplanted cells integrate into the tissue and replace damaged or dead cells. In this model, the MSCs replace or reconstruct tissue. 2) The transplanted cells produce trophic factors that promote plasticity, activate the compensatory mechanism present within brain. There are data to support both possibilities, however, as will be shown, the far more likely one is that the MSCs provide molecular resources to galvanize the endogenous repair and compensatory mechanisms within brain after stroke.

Double labeled immunohistochemical analysis of cerebral tissue subjected to stroke demonstrates that BrdU labeled cells also express proteins markers of neurons and astrocytes. 1–8% of BrdU labeled cells, the percentage dependent of the conditions of cell culture and route of administration, express these proteins. Expression of these proteins indicates a phenotypic transformation of the bone marrow cells within the developmental environment of injured brain, from a bone marrow source to a neural source. Neural proteins measured are MAP-2 and NeuN for neurons, and GFAP for astrocytes. Although there is phenotypic transformation of these cells, they are very few in number and we have no morphological or physiological evidence that these cells are integrated into the cerebral tissue, nor evidence that they form viable electrical connections. It appears highly unlikely, therefore that the MSCs replace brain cells. The more likely mechanisms are that of cellular production of a range of cytokines and trophic factors that promotes plasticity. As noted above, brain tissue after injury or stroke expresses developmental proteins, such as nestin. When bone marrow cells are transplanted into cerebral tissue there is a large and significant increase in the numbers and intensity of cells expressing the nestin protein (Li el al. 2000a). Likewise, we have morphological evidence that cells from the subventricular zone migrate to injured tissue. These migratory cells form clusters, as they do in developing brain. These clusters or rosettes move rapidly, i.e. 1–2 mm 1 day after transplantation. Thus, the brain itself responds to the implanted cells by activating stem like cells within the SVZ. These cells are remnants of neural stem cells from the developing brain. The rapid time course of functional improvement, within days after transplantation, also support a more trophic factor mediated process and not mature integration of cells within damaged tissue.

MSCs contain a variety of cells that secrete cytokines and trophic factors, e.g., interleukins (IL-1,3,6,7,8,11,12,14,15), stem cell factor (SCF), macrophage colony-stimulating factor-1 (MCSF-1) and Flt-3 ligand (Colter et al. 2000; Eaves et al. 1991; Koc et al. 2000; Majumdar et al. 1998) that might lead to behavioral recovery after MCAo. Phinney et al. (1999) demonstrate that most plastic-adherent cells express CD11 and CD45, epitopes of lymphohematopoietic cells. Bone marrow cells under different conditions both *in vitro* and *in vivo* are precursors of brain cells (de Groot et al. 1992; Hickey and Kimura 1988; Krall et al. 1994; Pereira et al. 1995, 1998; Walkley et al. 1994). Laurenzi et al.

(1998) demonstrate that human bone marrow cells consistently express mRNA for trkB (the BDNF receptor) and display variable expression of mRNA coding for trkA (the tyrosine kinase NGF receptor. Recent data (unpublished) from our laboratory also indicate that MSCs express receptors for trk, A,B,C,D. Thus, we speculate that bone marrow cells within an ischemic tissue responds to the microenvironment to produce multiple trophic factors and possible an array of cytokines that promote repair, proliferation of endogenous stem cells. This profusion of protein expression ultimately results in improved functional outcome after stroke.

Other applications: We have employed bone marrow tranplantation to investigations of traumatic brain injury (Mahmood et al. 2000; Lu et al. 2000) in the rat. Animals were subjected to controlled cortical impact injury and MSCs, and bone marrow was transplanted intracerebrally one day after injury. Functional outcome was measured daily up to 14 days after injury and statistically significant benefit in motor score as indicated in the rotorod test was evident. These studies have been followed by intra-arterial transplantation of MSCs, as in stroke. To test whether therapeutic benefit is present after MSC treatment in other forms of CNS injury, we produced a contusion injury in spinal cord by mean of the weight drop method (Chopp et al. 2000). One week after injury a laminectomy was performed and MSCs were placed at the site of injury. The Basso, Beattie, Bresnahan outcome measurement test was performed (Chopp et al. 2000). Significant improvement in function was clearly evident out to at least 5 weeks post injury. These data demonstrate that neural injury can be treated by a MSC based cellular therapy, whether the injury is stroke, traumatic brain injury and spinal cord injury. Studies are ongoing in the laboratory in models of Parkinson's disease, MS and ALS.

Potential for clinical application: We foresee the potential to harvest bone marrow from the patient and to treat the patient with this autologous marrow cells for a variety of neural injury and neurodegenerative diseases. MSC transplantation is clinically used in the cancer patient. It is considered a safe procedure with little risk or evidence of adverse effects. Additional studies in the experimental animals may provide a basis to move this therapy to the patient.

Acknowledgement

This work is supported by Program Project Grant PO1 NS 23393 and RO1 NS33504.

References

1. Azizi SA, Stokes D, Augelli BJ, DiGirolamo C, Prockop DJ (1998) Engraftment of migration of human bone marrow stromal cells implanted in the brains of albino rats-similarities to astrocyte grafts. Proc Natl Acad Sci USA 95:3908–3913
2. Bailey CH, Kandel ER (1993) Structural changes accompanying memory storage. Annu Rev Physiol 55:397–426
3. Barinaga M (2000) Fetal neuron grafts pave the way for stem cell therapies. Science 287:1421–1422
4. Barth TM, Schallert T (1987) Somatosensorimotor function of the superior colliculus, somatosensory cortex, and lateral hypothalamus in the rat. Exp Neurology 95(3):661–678
5. Bjorklund A, Lindvall O (2000) Cell replacement therapies for central nervous system disorders. Nature Neurosci 3:537–544
6. Borlongan CV, Randall TS, Cahhill DW, Sanberg PR (1995) Asymmetrical motor behavior in rats with unilateral striatal excitotoxic lesions as revealed by the elevated body swing test. Brain Res 676:231–234
7. Borlongan CV, Tajima Y, Trojanowski JQ, Lee VM, Sanberg PR (1998) Transplantation of cryopreserved human embryonal carcinoma-derived neurons (NT2N cells) promotes functional recovery in ischemic rats. Exp Neurology 149(2):310–321
8. Bruder SP, Jaiswal N, Ricalton NS, Mosca JD, Kraus KH, Kadiyala S (1998) Mesenchymal stem cells in osteobiology and applied bone regeneration. [Review] Clinical Orthopaedics & Related Research (355 Suppl):S247–256
9. Chen H, Chopp M, Zhang ZG, Garcia JH (1992) The effect of hypothermia on the transient middle cerebral artery occlusion in the rat. J Cerebral Blood Flow Metab 12:621–628
10. Chen J, Li Y, Chopp M (2000a) Intracerebral transplantation of bone marrow with BDNF after MCAo in rat NeuroPharm 39:711–716
11. Chen J, Yi L, Wang L, Zhang X, Chopp M (2000b) Therapeutic Benefit of Intracerebral Transplantation of Bone Marrow-Derived MSCs After Cerebral Ischemia in Rats. (submitted)
12. Chopp M and Li Y (1998) Protein expression: cerebral damage and opportunity for tissue repair after experimental stroke. Proceedings of the 7th International Symposium on Phamacology of Cerebral Ischemia. In Pharmacology of Cerebral Ischemia (Krieglstein J, ed.) Stuttgart, MedPharm Scientific Publishers, pp 401–405
13. Chopp M, Zhang X, Yi L, Wang L, Chen J, Lu D, Lu M, Rosenblum M (2000) Spinal Cord Injury in Rat: Treatment with Bone Marrow Stromal Cell Transplantation. NeuroReport (in press)

14. Colter DC, Class R, DiGirolamo CM, Prockop DJ (2000) Rapid expansion of recycling stem cells in cultures of plastic-adherent cells from human bone marrow. Proc Natl Acad Sci USA 97(7):3213–3218
15. Cramer S, Chopp M (2000) Recovery recapitulates ontogeny. TINS 23:265–271
16. De Groot CJ, Huppes W, Sminia T, Kraal G, Dijkstra CD (1992) Determination of the origin and nature of brain macrophages and microglial cells in mouse central nervous system, using non-radioactive in situ hybridization and immunoperoxidase techniques. GLIA 6(4):301–309
17. Duggal N, Schmidt-Kastner R, Hakim AM (1997) Nestin expression in reactive astrocytes following focal cerebral ischemiain rats. Brain Res 768:1–9
18. Eaves CJ, Cashman JD, Kay RJ, et al. (1991) Mechanisms that regulate the cell cycle status of very primitive hematopoietic cells in long-term human marrow cultures. II. Analysis of positive and negative regulators produced by stromal cells within the adherent layer. Blood 78(1):110–117
19. Eglitis MA, Dawson D, Park KW, Mouradian MM (1999) Targeting of marrow-derived astrocytes to the ischemic brain. Neuroreport 10(6):1289–1292
20. Eglitis MA, Mezey E (1997) Hematopoietic cells differentiate into both microglia and macroglia in the brains of adult mice. Proc Natl Acad Sci USA 94(8):4080–4085
21. Ferrari G, Cusella-De Angelis G, Coletta M, Paolucci E, Stornaiuolo A, Cossu G, Mavilio F (1998) Muscle regeneration by bone marrow-derived myogenic progenitors. Science 279(5356):1528–1530
22. Fisher LJ, Gage FH (1993) Grafting in the mammalian central nervous system. Physiological Reviews 73:583–615
23. Gage FH (1998) Cell therapy. [Review] Nature 392 (6679Suppl):18–24
24. Gage FH (2000) Mammalian neural stem cells. Science 287:1433–1438
25. Gage FH, Coates PW, Palmer TD, Kuhn HG, Fisher LJ, Suhonen JO, Peterson DA, Suhr ST, Ray J (1995) Survival and differentiation of adult neuronal progenitor cells transplanted to the adult brain. Proc Natl Acad Sci USA 92:11879–11883
26. Gantam SC, Noth CJ, Janakiraman N, Pindolia KR, Chapman RA (1995) Induction of chemokine mRNA in bone marrow stromal cells: modulation by TGF-beta 1 and IL-4. Exp Hematology 23(6):482–491
27. Gantam SC, Pindolia KR, Noth CJ, Janakiraman N, Xu YX, Chapman RA (1995) Chemokine gene expression in bone marrow stromal cells: downregulation with sodium salicylate. Blood 86(7):2541–2550
28. Gantam SC, Pindolia KR, Xu YX, Janakiraman N, Chapman RA, Freytag SO (1998) Antileukemic activity of TNF-alpha gene therapy with myeloid progenitor cells against minimal leukemia. J Hematotherapy 7(2):115–125
29. Germano AF, Dixon CF, d'Avella D, Hayes RL, Tomasello F (1994) Behavioral deficits following experimental subarachnoid hemorrhage in the rat. Journal of Neurotrauma 11(3):345–353
30. Goto S, Yamada K, Yoshikawa M, Okamura A, Ushio Y (1997) GABA receptor agonist promotes reformation of the striatonigral pathway by transplant derived from fetal striatal primordia in the lesioned striatum. Exp Neurology 147:503–509
31. Hamm RJ, Pike BR, O'Dell DM, Layeth BG, Jenkins LW (1994) The rotarod test: an evaluation of its effectiveness in assessing motor deficits following traumatic brain injury. Journal of Neurotrauma 11:187–196
32. Hickey WF, Kimura H (1988) Perivascular microglial cells of the CNS are bone marrow-derived and present antigen in vivo. Science 239(4837):290–292
33. Hodges H, Nelson A, Virley D, Kershaw TR, Sinden JD (1997) Cognitive deficits induced by global cerebral ischaemia: prospects for transplant therapy. [Review] Pharmacology, Biochemistry & Behavior 56 (4):763–780
34. Horwitz EM, Prockop DJ, Fitzpatrick LA, Koo WW, Gordon PL, Neel M, Sussman M, Orchard P, Marx JC, Pyeritz RE, Brenner MK (1999) Transplantability and therapeutic effects of bone marrow-derived mesenchymal cells in children with osteogenesis imperfecta. Nature Medicine 5(3):309–313
35. Ikehara S (1998) Autoimmune diseases as stem cell disorders: normal stem cell transplant for their treatment. Bioorganic & Medicinal Chemistry Letters 1(1):5–16
36. Ikehara S (1999) New strategies for allogeneic bone marrow transplantation and organ allografts. [Review] Acta Haematologica 101(2):68–77
37. Kennedy DW, Abkowitz JL (1997) Kinetics of central nervous system microglial and macrophage engraftment: analysis using a transgenic bone marrow transplantation model. Blood 90(3):986–993
38. Koc ON, Gerson SL, Cooper BW, Dyhouse SM, Haynesworth SE, Caplan AI, Lazarus HM (2000) Rapid hematopoietic recovery after coinfusion of autologous-blood stem cells and culture-expanded marrow mesenchymal stem cells in advanced breast cancer patients receiving high-dose chemotherapy. J Clin Oncol 18(2):307–316
39. Krall WJ, Challita PM, Perlmutter LS, Skelton DC, Kohn DB (1994) Cells expressing human glucocerebrosidase from a retroviral vector repopulate macrophages and central nervous system microglia after murine bone marrow transplantation. Blood 83(9):2737–2748
40. Kuznetsov SA, Krebsbach PH, Stomura K, Kerr J, Rimiucci D (1997) J Bone Miner Res 12:1335–1347
41. Laurenzi MA, Beccari T, Stenke L, Sjolinder M, Stinchi S, Lindgren JA (1998) Expression of mRNA encoding neurotrophins and neurotrophin receptors in human granulocytes and bone marrow cells – enhanced neurotrophin-4 expression induced by LTB4. J Leukocyte Biol 64(2):228–234
42. Lazarus H, Haynesworth S, Gerson S, Rosenthal N, Caplan A (1995) Ex vivo expansion and subsequent infusion of human bone marrow-derived stromal progenitor cells (mesenchymal progenitor cells): implications for therapeutic use. Bone Marrow Transplant 16:557–564
43. Li Y, Jiang N, Powers C, Chopp M (1998) Neuronal damage and plasticity identified by MAP-2, GAP-43 and cyclin D1 immunoreactivity after focal cerebral ischemia in rat. Stroke 29:1972–1981
44. Li Y, Chen J, Chopp M (2000a) Adult Bone Marrow Transplantation After Stroke in Adult Rats. Cell Trans (in press)
45. Li Y and Chopp M (1999) Temporal profile of nestin expression after focal cerebral ischemia in rats. Brain Res 768:1–9
46. Li Y, Chopp M, Chen J, Wang L, Gautam SC, Xu Y, Zhang Z (2000b) Intrastriatal transplantation of bone marrow stromal cells (MSCs) improves functional recovery after stroke in adult mice. J of Cerebral Blood Flow and Metab (in press)
47. Lu D, Li Y, Chen J, Mahmood A, Chopp M (2000) Intra-arterial transplantation of marrow stromal cells into rat brain after traumatic brain injury. Brain Research (submitted)
48. Mahmood A, Lu D, Li Y, Chen J, Chopp M (2000) Intracranial bone marrow transplantation after traumatic brain injury improves functional outcome in adult rats. J Neurosurgery (submitted)
49. Majumdar MK, Thiede MA, Mosca JD, Moorman M, Gerson SL (1998) Phenotypic and functional comparison of cultures of marrow-derived mesenchymal stem cells (MSCs) and stromal cells. Journal of Cellular Physiology 176(1):57–66
50. Markgraf CG, Green EJ, Hurwitz BE, Morikawa E, Dietrich WD, McCabe PM, Ginsberg MD, Schneiderman N (1992) Sensorimotor and cognitive consequences of middle cerebral artery occlusion in rats. Brain Research 575(2):238–246

51. Pereira RF, Halford KW, O'Hara MD, Leeper DB, Sokolov BP, Pollard MD, Bagasra O, Prockop DJ (1995) Cultured adherent cells from marrow can serve as long-lasting precursor cells for bone, cartilage, and lung in irradiated mice. Proc Natl Acad Sci USA 92(11):4857–4861
52. Pereira RF, O'Hara MD, Laptev AV, Halford KW, Pollard MD, Class R, Simon D, Livezey K, Prockop DJ (1998) Marrow stromal cells as a source of progenitor cells for nonhematopoietic tissues in transgenic mice with a phenotype of osteogenesis imperfecta. Proc Natl Acad Sci USA 95(3):1142–1147
53. Peschanski M, Cesaro P, Hantraye P (1995) Rationale for intrastriatal grafting of striatal neuroblasts in patients with Huntington's disease. Neuroscience 68:273–285
54. Phinney DG, Kopen G, Isaacson RL, Prockop DJ (1999) Plastic adherent stromal cells from the bone marrow of commonly used strains of inbred mice: variations in yield, growth, and differentiation. J Cellular Biochem 72:570–585
55. Prockop DJ (1997) Marrow stromal cells as stem cells for nonhematopoietic tissues. Science 276(5309):71–74
56. Prockop DJ (1998) Marrow stromal cells as stem cells for continual renewal of nonhematopoietic tissues and as potential vectors for gene therapy. Journal of Cellular Biochemistry – Supplement. 30–31:284–285
57. Randall TD, Weissman IL (1997) Phenotypic and functional changes induced at the clonal level in hematopoietic stem cells after 5-fluorouracil treatment. Blood 89(10):3596–3606
58. Riew KD, Wright NM, Cheng S, Avioli LV, Lou J (1998) Induction of bone formation using a recombinant adenoviral vector carrying the human BMP-2 gene in a rabbit spinal fusion model. Calcified Tissue International 63(4):357–360
59. Rogers DC, Campbell CA, Stretton JL, Mackay KB (1997) Correlation between motor impairment and infarct volume after permanent and transient middle cerebral artery occlusion in the rat. Stroke 28(10):2060–2065
60. Schallert T (1988) Aging-dependent emergence of sensorimotor dysfunction in rats recovered from dopamine depletion sustained early in life. Annals of the New York Academy of Sciences 515:108–120
61. Schallert T, Kozlowski DA, Humm JL, Cocke RR (1997) Use-dependent structural events in recovery of function. Advances in Neurology 73:229–238
62. Schwarz EJ, Alexander GM, Prockop DJ, Azizi SA (1999) Multipotential marrow stromal cells transduced to produce L-DOPA: engraftment in a rat model of Parkinson disease. Human Gene Therapy 10(15):2539–2549
63. Snyder EY, Dietcher DL, Walsh C, Arnold-Aldea S, Hartwieg EA, Cepko CL (1992) Multipotent neural cell lines can engraft and participate in development of mouse cerebellum. Cell 68:33–55
64. Snyder EY, Flax JD, Yandava BD, Park KI, Liu S, Rosario CM, Aurora S (1997a) Transplantation and differentiation of neural 'stem-like' cells: Possible insights into development and therapeutic potential. In Gage FH, Christen Y (eds): Research and Perspectives in Neurosciences: Isolation, Characterization, and Utilization of CNS Stem Cells. New York, Springer-Verlag pp 173–196
65. Snyder EY, Yoon C, Flax JD, Macklis JD (1997b) Multipotent neural precursors can differentiate toward replacement of neurons undergoing targeted apoptotic degeneration in adult mouse neocortex. Proc Natl Acad Sci USA 94:11663–11668
66. Stroemer RP, Kent TA, Hulsebosch CE (1995) Neocrotical neural spouting, synaptogenesis, and behavorial recovery after neocortical infarction in rats. Stroke 26:2135–2144
67. Timsit S, Rivera S, Ouaghi P, Guischard F, Tremblay E, Ben-Ari Y, Khrestchatisky M (1999) Increased cyclin D1 in vulnerable neurons in the hippocampus after ishemia and epilepsy; a modulator *in vivo* programmed cell death? Eur J Neurosci 11:263–278
68. Vogel G (2000) Can old cells learn new tricks? Science 287:1418–1419
69. Walkley SU, Thrall MA, Dobrenis K, Huang M, March PA, Siegel DA, Wurzelmann S (1994) Bone marrow transplantation corrects the enzyme defect in neurons of the central nervous system in a lysosomal storage disease. Proc Natl Acad Sci USA 91(8):2970–2974
70. Zea Longa E, Weinstein PR, Carlson S, Cummins R (1989) Reversible middle cerebral artery occlusion without craniectomy in rats. Stroke 20:84–91

Harnessing neural stem cell biology to compensate for cerebral ischemic injury

K. I. Park[1,2†], B. A. Tate[1†], J. M. Ren[1,3], D. Sietsma[3], A. Marciniak[1], S. P. Finklestein[3], E. Y. Snyder[1*]

Abstract

Neural stem cells (NSCs) may provide a novel approach to reconstituting brains damaged by ischemic injury. The transplantation of exogenous NSCs may, in fact, augment a natural self-repair process in which the damaged CNS "attempts" to mobilize its own pool of stem cells. Providing additional NSCs and trophic factors may optimize this response. Preliminary data in animal models of both pediatric and adult stroke lends support to these hypotheses.

Recent studies suggest that NSCs may be a substitute for fetal tissue in transplantation paradigms as well as a vehicle for gene delivery. The basic biology of NSCs appears to endow them with characteristics that make them ideal vehicles for gene therapy as well as agents of repair (Snyder and Senut 1997; Snyder and Wolfe 1996; Snyder and Fisher 1996). These biological characteristics include the ability of transplanted cells to migrate, to integrate into the neural circuitry, and to differentiate into multiple cell types. NSCs may have the ability to reestablished neural circuits that have degenerated as a result of ischemic injury. Importantly, migration of NSCs may be stimulated by neurodegenerative environments (Snyder and Macklis 1996; Snyder et al. 1997a; Rosario et al. 1997). For these reasons, there has been a growing interest in the therapeutic potential of NSCs and progenitor cells following cerebral ischemic injury.

Pediatric ischemic injury

Despite advances in perinatal monitoring, obstetrical management, neonatal care and a better understanding of some of the pathophysiology of hypoxic-ischemic (HI) injury, hypoxic-ischemic encephalopathy (HIE) (also often termed perinatal asphyxia) remains a major cause of mortality and neurodevelopmental morbidity. Current clinical management of HIE has been limited to supportive measures (Volpe 1995; Vannucci and Perlman 1997). Effective therapies have been lacking. There has been an intense search recently for new approaches that might be rooted in the growing knowledge of the molecular mechanisms that seem to mediate neural cell death and degeneration. Experimental therapies in animals have begun, for in-

[†]Equal contribution to this review: [1]Departments of Pediatrics, Neurosurgery & Neurology, Children's Hospital, Boston, Harvard Medical School, Boston, MA, USA;
[2]Department of Pediatrics and Pharmacology, Yonsei University College of Medicine, Seoul, Korea
[3]CNS Growth Factor Research Laboratory, Department of Neurology, Massachusetts General Hospital, Harvard Medical School, Boston, MA, USA
correspondence:
e-mail: Snyder@al.tch.harvard.edu

stance, to include inhibitors of oxygen free radical generation and free radical scavengers, antagonists of excitotoxic amino acids and their receptors, calcium channel blockers, nitric oxide synthase inhibitors, trophic factors with neuroprotective actions, and anti-apoptotic agents such as caspase inhibitors (du Plessis and Johnston 1997; Vannucci and Perlman 1997; see also papers in this volume). Most of these experimental therapies have not advanced to the stage of clinical trials (Tan and Parks 1999).

The growing interest in NSC biology as it might apply to HIE represents a somewhat different focus on the cellular and molecular aspects of neurodegeneration. The above-mentioned strategies seek to short-circuit cell death and/or promote neuroprotection – i.e., to combat progression of neuropathological processes. Stem cell biology focuses instead on non-pathological processes – i.e., on development and the re-invoking of developmental processes for purposes of regeneration. In other words, a putative stem cell-mediated strategy is rooted not so much in "combating" a pathological process but rather in abetting a natural self-repair process postulated – at least based on data emerging from our lab – to exist in the CNS in response to a wide range of injury and degenerative processes.

NSCs are the primordial, multipotent, self-renewing cells that are believed to have given rise to the vast array of specialized cells of the CNS. They are believed to persist all throughout life (certainly in some discrete regions but perhaps all throughout the brain) serving homeostatic and perhaps even self-repair processes. The clone of NSCs described in the following pilot experiments was initially isolated from neonatal mouse cerebellum and maintained in a proliferative state in culture with the aid of a constitutively self-regulated gene. The gene, *vmyc*, facilitates cell cycle progression, forestalls senescence, and operates within the bFGF signal transduction pathway. *Vmyc* becomes spontaneously downregulated following engraftment and in response to other environmental cues. This clone was also transduced via retroviral vector with the reporter gene, *lacZ*, transcribed from the LTR, allowing engrafted and integrated clonally-related progeny to stain blue when processed with Xgal histochemistry or to be immunoreactive to antibodies against the *lacZ* gene product, E.coli β-galactosidase (βgal) (Snyder et al. 1992, 1997a). This prototypical murine NSC clone (designated "C17.2"), because of its well-documented ability to integrate into most CNS structures, has become one of the best studied NSC clones in a number of animal models and has proved most useful for delineating the range of therapeutic possibilities for NSCs. It is well-recognized for emulating endogenous NSCs as well as NSC clones expanded and propagated by a variety of techniques by other investigators from other regions. While these NSCs, like all NSCs, are self-renewing, they become contact inhibited; never grow in soft agar; are non-tumorigenic in nude mice; fail to incorporate BrdU after 48 hrs *in vivo;* and respond to normal cues for cell cycle withdrawal, differentiation, and interaction with host cells.

The model of pediatric HIE employed entailed permanent ligation of the right common carotid artery of week-old mice followed by exposure of the animal to 8% ambient oxygen (Park et al. 1995). This combination of ischemia and hypoxia results in extensive injury to the hemisphere ipsilateral to the carotid ligation while leaving the contralateral hemisphere intact.

In an early set of experiments, C17.2 NSCs were transplanted into the cerebral ventricles of normal mice on the day of birth. The cells became stably integrated throughout the brain parenchyma, seamlessly integrated with the host endogenous neural cells. At 1 week of age, the right hemisphere was subjected to HI. When the brains are analyzed 2–5 weeks later, lazZ-expressing, donor NSC-derived cells had become densely clustered around the infarction cavity, suggesting the presence of new neural cells around the area of the injury, the result of migration or proliferation of NSCs or both. In the penumbra of the infarction, donor cells had differentiated into oligodendrocytes and neurons, the two cell types most vulnerable to asphyxia-mediated death and also classically viewed as unlikely to spontaneously regenerate. Such unexpected observations prompted subsequent careful experimental dissection of each aspect of the NSC response to asphyxial injury – proliferation, migration, and differentiation. In these experiments (Park et al. 1999), clone C17.2 NSCs serve as "reporter cells". These are well-characterized cells with known ancestry, potential, and clonal relationships that are traceable, abundant, and homogenous, and which can mirror – or "report" on – the behavior of neighboring endogenous progenitors. Such cells would also allow well-controlled experiments to proceed with minimal variability in cell population under study from experiment-to-experiment, animal-to-animal, and condition-to-condition.

To examine the proliferation of NSCs in response to HI, mice with "reporter" NSCs stably intermixed throughout their brains (following transplantation on postnatal day 0 [P0]) and subjected to HI injury at P7 as above, were pulsed with bromodeoxyuridine (BrdU), a nucleotide analogue, at various post-asphyxial time points. BrdU becomes integrated only into dividing cells. Within 24 hours of HI injury, *lacZ*+/BrdU+ cells began to appear; previously no *lacZ*+ cells incorporated BrdU suggesting that quiescent NSCs were now re-entering the cell cycle. Newly proliferative NSCs peaked at ~3–4 days after induction of HI with all NSCs returning to their quiescent state by one week after injury (i.e., no *lacZ*+ cells were also BrdU+). Endogenous cells followed a virtually superimposable pattern: new proliferation within 24 hours of HI, a peak at 3–4 days after HI, a return to quiescence at approximately a week. The first week – particularly 3–4 days – after stroke or other brain injuries would seem to be a very metabolically, biochemically, and molecularly active "window" during which a variety of mitogens, trophins, extracellular matrix molecules, and other factors are expressed. The NSC seems to reflect this pattern.

The migration of NSCs to areas of neurodegeneration was then examined in the HI mouse model. "Reporter" NSCs were transplanted into the left lateral cerebroventricular space at P0. At P7, unilateral asphyxial injury was induced in the contralateral right hemisphere in some animals, while in others the right hemisphere was left intact. In animals with an intact right hemisphere, engrafted NSCs remained stably distributed and densely integrated throughout the parenchyma of only the transplanted left hemisphere. However, in animals in which the right hemisphere had been infarcted, cells appeared to migrate across the corpus callosum and any available interhemispheric commissure into the infarcted region (Fig. 1). Not only will NSCs integrated within prior to injury migrate to areas of subsequent infarction, but NSCs transplanted *after* injury will similarly home in on infarcted regions from great distances (even from the opposite hemisphere) if implanted 3–4 days following HI. NSCs injected directly into the infarct never migrated to the contralateral intact side. Engraftment appears to be dependent on the timing of transplantation, with integration of donor NSCs most abundant within the first week following HI in the mouse (Fig. 2). If transplantation is postponed until 5 weeks after HI, virutally no engraftment is achieved.

Among the neural cell types into which these well-integrated NSCs differentiated, particularly in the penumbra, were neurons (~5%) and oligodendrocytes (~4%) – even in such "non-neurogenic" regions as the neocortex. In other words, the donor NSCs appeared to "attempt" repopulation of the damaged CNS regions by yielding those cell types most devastated by the injury. Neurons are not normally born in the intact mammalian cortex beyond fetal development (Snyder et al. 1997a; Gage et al. 1995); indeed, such neurogenesis was not observed in the intact contralateral cortex. In the context of injury, however, fetal neurogenic signals appeared to be transiently re-expressed, and the NSC – as it did during embryonic development – appeared to respond appropriately. Particularly within certain temporal windows – NSCs appeared to "shift" their normal differentiation fate to compensate for the loss of particular cell types.

That the brain does indeed attempt to "repair" itself by mobilizing pools of newly proliferative progenitors was suggested by a subsequent series of *non*-transplantation-based ex-

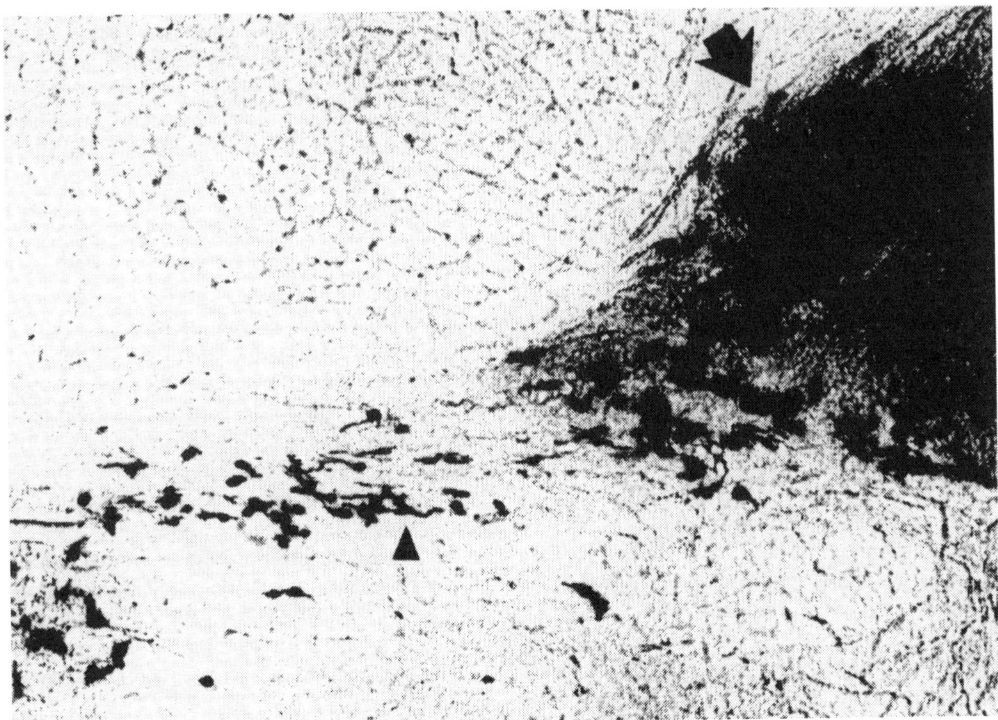

Fig. 1. Migration by transplanted "reporter" stem cells to the ischemic area of a mouse brain subjected to unilateral, focal hypoxic-ischemic brain injury. Neural stem cells (clone C17.2) were injected into the left cerebral ventricle of a mouse on the day of birth (postnatal day 0 [P0]). At 1 week of age (P7), the animal was subjected to contralateral right-sided hypoxic-ischemic injury. The animal was analyzed at maturity with Xgal histochemistry to identify *lacZ*-expressing donor-derived cells (which stain blue). Some cells appeared to migrate along the corpus callosum (**arrowhead**) throughout the cerebrum toward the highly ischemic area (**arrow**). (Reproduced from Reference 14).

periments in which *endogenous* progenitors were labeled by retroviral vectors and by BrdU administered to animals being subjected to HI. Findings similar to those described above were observed, suggesting that the "reporter" NSCs in the transplantation paradigms were, indeed, "reporting" on a genuine phenomenon. The pool of endogenous progenitors may not be sufficient for effective repair under the most devastating of asphyxial conditions; however, the process might be augmented and optimized, we believe, by providing additional exogenous NSCs in a timely fashion and in appropriate areas. This strategy is discussed in greater detail in later sections.

Adult ischemic injury

The experiments described above in models of pediatric ischemic injury have been extended to models of adult stroke with essentially similar pathology. In preliminary studies designed to examine the potential value of transplanted NSCs in enhancing recovery, focal cerebral infarcts were first produced in the right dorsolateral cerebral cortex and underlying striatum in adult rats by electrocoagulation of the proximal middle cerebral artery (MCA) (modified Tamura model). These experimental strokes, while compatible with survival, produce a reliable behavioral (sensorimotor) deficit in the contralateral limbs that recovers to some degree

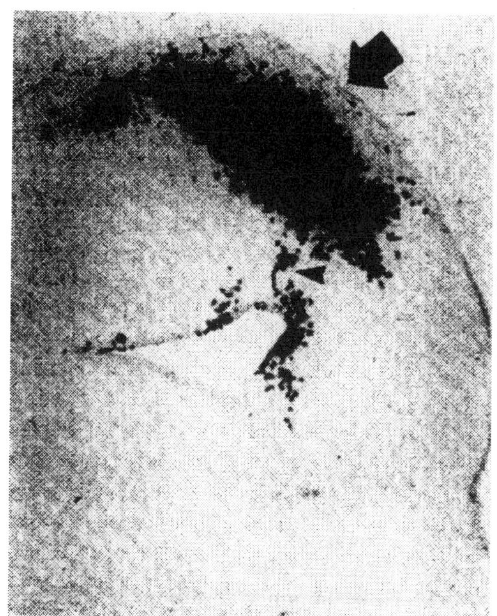

Fig. 2. Robust engraftment by transplanted neural stem cells within the ischemic region of a mouse brain subjected to unilateral focal hypoxic-ischemic injury (HI). This mouse was subjected to right hypoxic-ischemic injury on postnatal day 7 (P7). Three days later (P10), the animal receive a transplant of neural stem cells (clone C17.2) within the region of infarction. The animal was analyzed at maturity with Xgal histochemistry. A representative coronal section is shown. Robust engraftment was evident within the ischemic are (**arrow**). Similar engraftment was evident throughout the hemisphere. Even cells that implanted outside the region of infarction appeared to migrate along the corpus callosum toward ischemic area (**arrowhead**). The most exuberant engraftment was evident 3–7 days after HI. Immunocytochemical and ultrastructural analysis revealed that a subpopulation of donor-derive cells, especially those in the penumbra, differentiated into neurons and oligodendroglia, the two neural cell types most characteristically damaged by HI and the cell types least likely to regenerate spontaneously in the postnatal brain. (Reproduced from Reference 14).

spontaneously over time. In previous studies, Finklestein at al. showed that the administration of polypeptide growth factors – particularly basic fibroblast growth factor (bFGF) – can enhance neurological recovery in this model (see review by S. P. Finklestein in this volume). Growth factor treatment alone does not appear to reduce infarct volume, but does enhance behavioral recovery. Although the mechanism by which this recovery occurs remains unclear, possibilities include the stimulation of neural sprouting and new synapse formation in intact undamaged parts of the brain as well as the mobilization of endogenous progenitors and NSCs.

In more recent studies, we have begun to examine the synergistic effect of neurotrophic growth factor administration in combination with NSCs transplantation in the above-described adult MCA occlusion (MCAO) rat model. In pilot studies, anesthetized male Sprague-Dawley rats received focal infarction of the right cerebral hemisphere by proximal electrocoagulation of the MCA. One day after surgery, the rats were reanesthesized and received a percutaneous injection into the cisterna magna of a total of 50 µl containing one of the following: (a) placebo, (b) NSCs (10^6 cells), (c) bFGF (0.5 µg), or (4) NSCs + bFGF. Two days later (3 days after stroke surgery) animals received an additional intracisternal injection, identical to the injection they received previously. For the next month following stroke, animals received a series of behavioral tests, including: (a) *forelimb and hindlimb placing test* which help assay sensorimotor function of the contralateral limbs and most likely reflect cortical and subcortical function; (b) the *spontaneous limb use test,* which measures the animal's spontaneous preference for using each forelimb when rearing up to explore the inside of a narrow glass cylinder, most likely also reflects cortical and subcortical function; and (c) the *body swing test,* which measures the animal's side to side preference when held by the tail suspended above a tabletop and largely reflects basal ganglia function. All three treatment groups showed statistically significant advantage over placebo in enhancing sensorimotor recovery of the contralateral limbs on both the forelimb and hindlimb placing test, tests of cortical and subcortical function. There was a trend (though not statistically significant) in favor of a combination of NSCs and bFGF compared to either treatment alone. Similarly, a trend was seen in favor of all three treatments on the spontaneous limb use test, another test of cortical/subcortical function. These regions are the ones that, based on our pediatric stroke work, receive the greatest degree of engraftment. No significant differences were appreciated in the body swing test, which assays largely basal ganglia function. At the end of the behavioral testing, animals were euthanized and the 2% paraformaldehyde-fixed brains were sectioned and analyzed. Infarct volume was determined using image analysis of hemotoxylin-and-eosin stained 20 µm sections. There was a trend toward reduced infarct volume in NSC-treated animals, though this difference, in these pilot studies, did yet achieve statistical significance. Immunocytochemical analysis using anti-βgal antibodies to localize donor-derived βgal+ cells suggested that transplanted NSCs had, indeed, migrated from their site of administration in the cisterna magna to tissue at the margins of infarct in the forebrain, likely accounting for the somewhat smaller cortical stroke volume. Further immunohistochemical work is in progress to delineate more precisely the fate of donor mouse NSCs in the host adult rat brain, including their differentiated cell type identity and their gene expression patterns.

These preliminary experiments suggest that mouse NSCs can migrate long distances, even in the adult brain, to infarcted regions and can enhance behavioral recovery even when administered as long as a day after experimental stroke. The mechanism of this enhancement of recovery remains to be elucidated but may include the differentiation of engrafted NSCs into neurons that then form crucial new connections in the damaged brain. Alternatively, the transplanted NSCs may act as "factories" for trophic factors, neurotransmitters, and neural guidance molecules that, in turn, enhance stroke recovery. Finally, these preliminary data suggest that co-administration of exogenous to NSCs and trophic growth factors may prove be superior to either treatment alone. Considerably more work must be done on both the dose and timing parameters of these two potentially synergistic interventions.

NSC transplantation may augment normal self-repair processes; what are the signals?

Neuronal regeneration does not occur in the vast majority of the post-developmental CNS after injury or disease. However, it has been recognized for decades that specific regions of the mammalian cerebrum continue to generate neurons throughout life (Altman 1969; Altman and Das 1965; Sidman et al. 1959). These "neurogenic regions" include the olfactory bulb (OB) by way of subventricular zone (SVZ) (Goldman and Luskin 1998; Kakita and Goldman 1999; Lois and Alvarez-Buylla 1994; Lois et al. 1996; Wei et al. 1999) and the dentate gyrus (DG) of the hippocampus (Ericksson et al. 1998; Pincus et al. 1998). In experiments using a protocol similar to that previously described, HI brain injury was found to induce a significant proliferation of the SVZ neural progenitor population ipsilateral to the lesioned side. These cells were most prominent in the dorsolateral wall of the lateral ventricles adjacent to the infarction cavity. In uninjured brain most of the cells born in the SVZ migrate along the rostral migratory stream (RMS) into the OB. In contrast, in the asphyxiated brain, significantly fewer newly born cells were present in the RMS and the ipsilateral OB but appeared instead to be drawn to the area of injury. Many of the cells induced to proliferate yielded new oligodendrocytes and neurons (4.0% and 1.2%, respectively). These findings suggest that, following ischemic injury, factors are elaborated to which endogenous neural progenitors respond in a reparative fashion, promoting the establishment of new neurons even within "non-neurogenic" regions of the "post-developmental" CNS. Presumably, transplanted exogenous NSCs in the experiments described above – in which they are drawn to areas of degeneration and shift their differentiation fate – are responding to these same signals. Therefore, one strategy for assisting CNS repair following cerebral injury may be stem cell-based: using the host's own appropriately activated reserve of NSCs augmented by an exogenous supply of NSCs introduced during or shortly after injury or neurodegeneration.

The signals that are elaborated in areas of injury to which NSCs (donor and probably host) are responsive are unknown; however, preliminary data from our laboratory suggests some candidates. When NSCs, which express trkC receptors on their surface, were genetically engineered before transplantation to overexpress neurotrophin 3 (NT-3), the engineered subclone consistently differentiated into > 90% neurons for at least 3 weeks in culture. The percentage of neurons in stable cultures of the parent clone falls to < 20% over the same period. Similarly, when cells from this NT-3-overexpressing clone were implanted into the infarct of a unilaterally asphyxiated mouse brain 3 days after induction of HI at P7, the proportion of donor-derived neurons was > 15-fold greater than the parent clone; donor-derived glia became rare. One might conclude that upregulation of NT-3 expression may play a role in the neuronal differentiation observed shortly following HI. Donor and endogenous NSCs may be responding to this signal. Implanting NSCs overexpressing NT-3 may serve to augment this useful self-repair response. Other trophic factors certainly must also play a role and may be similarly augmented via exogenous administration (e.g., BDNF, GDNF, bFGF). The combination of NSC and bFGF administration in the adult rat MCAO model described above may be an another example of such a strategy.

Future prospects

Progress is proceeding in the transplantation of human neural stem cells (hNSCs) into hypoxic-ischemic brain injury. NSCs isolated from human fetal telencephelon appear to emulate many of the properties of their rodent counterparts (Flax et al. 1998; Fricker et al. 1999; Vescovi et al. 1999). They differentiate *in vitro* and *in vivo* into all three fundamental neural cell lineages; they engraftment into the developing and adult rodent brain; they express foreign genes *in vivo*; and they can replace missing neural cell types when grafted into various mutant mice. Human NSCs, in pilot studies in models of perinatal asphyxia, showed robust engraftment within the infarct and its penumbra, appeared capable of migrating to the ischemic site, and could differentiate into neurons (of multiple neurotransmitter phenotypes), oligodendrocytes, and astrocytes (Park and Snyder 1999). Such early findings suggest that human NSCs may be capable of replacing neural cell populations lost to HI injury in animal models and may ultimately play a therapeutic role in patients of all ages injured by cerebral ischemic events, particularly in the acute and subacute stages.

Acknowledgments

Supported in part by grants from the March of Dimes (EYS) and from NINDS (NS34247 and NS33852) (EYS) and NS10828 (SPF). KIP was supported in part by grant No. 981-0713-097-2 from the Basic Research Program and BDRC of the Korean Science and Engineering Foundation, and a grant HMP-98-N-1-0003 of the Ministry of Health & Welfare, R.O. Korea.

References

1. Altman J (1969) Autoradiographic and histological studies of postnatal neurogenesis: IV. Cell proliferation and migration in the anterior forebrain, with special reference to persisting neurogenesis in the olfactory bulb. J Comp Neurol 137:433–458
2. Altman J, Das GD (1965) Autoradiographic and histological evidence of postnatal hippocampal neurogenesis in rats. J Comp Neurol 124:319–335
3. du Plessis AJ, Johnston MV (1997) Hypoxic-ischemic brain injury in the newborn. Cellular mechanisms and potentialstrategies for neuroprotection. Clin Perinatol 24:627–654
4. Ericksson PS et al. (1998) Neurogenesis in the adult human hippocampus. Nat Med 4:1,313–1,317
5. Flax JD, Aurora S, Yang C et al. (1998) Engraftable human neural stem cells respond to developmental cues, replace reurons and express foreign genes. Nature Biotech 16:1,033–1,039
6. Fricker RA, Carpenter MK, Winkler C, Greco C, Gates MA, Bjorklund A (1999) Site-specific migration and neuronal differentiation of human neural progenitor cells after transplantation in the adult rat brain. J Neurosci 19:5990–6005
7. Gage FH, Coates PW, Palmer TD et al. (1995) Survival and differentiation of adult neuronal progenitor cells transplanted to the adult brain. Proc Natl Acad Sci USA 92:11,879–11,883
8. Goldman SA, Luskin MB (1998) Strategies utilized by migrating neurons of the postnatal vertebrate forebrain. Trends Neurosci 21:107–114
9. Kakita A, Goldman JE (1999) Patterns and dynamics of SVZ

cell migration in the postnatal forebrain: monitoring living progenitors in slice preparation. Neuron 23:461–472
10. Liu Y, Himes BT, Chow WY et al. (1999) Intraspinal delivery of neurotropin-3 (NT-3) using neural stem cells genetically modified by recombinant retrovirus. Exp Neurol 158:9–26
11. Lois C, Alvarez-Buylla A (1994) Long distance neuronal migration in the adult mammalian brain. Science 264:1,145–1,148
12. Lois C, Garcia-Verdugo JM, Alvarez-Buylla A (1996) Chain migration of neuronal precursors. Science 271:978–981
13. Park KI, Jensen FE, Snyder EY (1995) Neural progenitor transplantation for hypoxia-ischemic brain injury in immature mice. Soc Neurosci Abs 21:2027
14. Park KI, Liu S, Flax JD, Nissim S, Stieg PE, Snyder EY (1999) Transplantation of neural progenitor and stem cells: developmental insights may suggest new therapies for spinal cord and other CNS dysfunction. J Neurotrauma 16:675–687
15. Park KI, Snyder EY (1999) Transplantation of human neural stem cells, propagated by either genetic or epigenetic means, into hypoxic-ischemic (HI) brain injury. Soc Neurosci Abstr 25:212
16. Pincus DW, Keyoung HM, Harrison-Restelli C et al. (1998) FGF2/BDNF-associated maturation of new neurons generated from adult human subependymal cells. Ann Neurol 43:576–585
17. Rosario CM, Yandava BD, Kosaras B, Zurakowski D, Sidman RL, Snyder EY (1997) Differentiation of engrafted multipotent neural progenitors towards replacement of missing granule neurons in Meander tail cerebellum may help determine the locus of mutant gene action. Development 124:4,213–4,224
18. Sidman RL, Miale IL, Feder N (1959) Cell proliferation and migration in the primitive ependymal zone: an autoradiographic study of histogenesis in the nervous system. Exp Neurol 1:322–333
19. Snyder EY, Wolfe JH (1996) CNS cell transplantation: a novel therapy for storage diseases? Curr Opin Neurol 9:126–136
20. Snyder EY, Fisher LJ (1996) Gene therapy for neurologic diseases. Curr Opin Pediatr 8:558–568
21. Snyder EY, Macklis JD (1996) Multipotent neural progenitor or stem-like cells may be uniquely suited for therapy for some neurodegenerative conditions. Clin Neurosci 3:310–316
22. Snyder EY, Senut MC (1997) Use of non-neuronal cells for gene delivery. Neurobiol Dis 4:69–102
23. Snyder EY, Deitcher DL, Walsh C, Arnold-Aldea S, Hartwieg EA, Cepko CL (1992) Multipotent neural cell lines can engraft and participate in development of mouse cerebellum. Cell 68:33–55
24. Snyder EY, Yoon C, Flax JD et al. (1997) Multipotent neural precursors can differentiate toward replacements of neurons undergoing targeted apoptotic degeneration in adult mouse neocortex. Proc Natl Acad Sci USA 94:11,663–11,668
25. Tan S, Parks DA (1999) Preserving brain function during neonatal asphxia. Clin Perinatol 26:733–747
26. Vannucci RC, Perlman JM (1997) Interventions for perinatal hypoxic-ischemic encephalopathy. Pediatrics 100:1,004–1,014
27. Vescovi AL, Gritti A, Galli R, Parati EA (1999) Isolation and intracerebral grafting of nontransformed multipotential embryonic human CNS stem cells. J Neurotrauma 16:689–693
28. Volpe JJ (1995) Neurology of the Newborn (3rd ed), Philadelphia, PA, WB Saunders Company
29. Wei W, Wong K, Chen JH et al. (1999) Directional guidance of neuronal migration in the olfactory system by protein Slit. Nature 400:331–336

Possible transplantation strategies in stroke: Could stem cells be the answer?

C. N. Svendsen

Abstract

Transplantation therapy is emerging as a possibility for a number of different neurodegenerative diseases. Here the idea of using neural stem cells, or other types of cell line, to treat stroke victims is critically assessed. Human or rodent cells from a variety of sources can integrate into the brain, and in some cases improve function in animal models of stroke. However, the mechanisms underlying this effect are often poorly understood. The time now is for further experiments in such models to establish a correlation between cell survival and outgrowth and functional recovery. A rush to the clinic may be bad for the long term future of this potentially very exciting field.

In stroke variable types of neuronal damage occur depending on the exact duration and location of the loss of blood supply, and how efficiently, if at all, the area re-perfuses. Clearly, acute administration of pharmacological agents which prevent the immediate cell death and inflammation would be the ideal treatment. Unfortunately, although many agents have been found to be neuroprotective in animal models of stroke, few if any have translated to the clinic (DeGraba and Pettigrew 2000). Even if new acute treatments are found, this still leaves a large number of patients with permanent brain damage and little hope of restoring function above that obtained with intensive physiotherapy regimes.

Neural transplantation has been gaining momentum as a realistic approach to at least partially alleviating some of the symptoms of Parkinson's disease (Lindvall 1997). Could similar types of cell therapy work for stroke? A number of papers have highlighted the possibility of using primary foetal tissue or cell lines in rat models of stroke. These have recently been reviewed in detail (Bjorklund and Lindvall 2000). Although there are some examples of functional effects following transplantation, the mechanisms are never clear – it could be either that the cells have induced endogenous repair mechanisms or actually integrate and restore function themselves. Assuming these can be worked out over the next few years – when should we move beyond the animal models and into the clinic? As mentioned by Bjorklund and Lindvall (2000) two clinical trials are already underway by biotech companies. One with cells derived from a teratocarcinoma and another with cells derived from pig foetal tissue. The latter has been stopped due to adverse effects in

Keywords: Stroke, Stem cells, Progenitor cells, Plasticity, Transplantation

Cambridge Centre for Brain Repair, University of Cambridge, Forvie Site, Robinson Way, Cambridge CB2 2 PY, UK
e-mail: cns1000@hermes.cam.ac.uk

two patients perhaps pointing at the premature nature of the field at this stage.

The problem with transplantation for stroke patients is threefold. First, the type of brain tissue damage varies so much from patient to patient. This could be partially overcome with the latest imaging techniques, which may be able to pinpoint the most serious areas of damage. However, as mentioned above it remains to be seen in animal models whether even with focal damage, brain transplants can actually work (rather than induce host repair).

The second problem is more pragmatic. Foetal tissue is hard to collect and there are ethical complications in such studies. Although these can be worked out, only a few centres will be able to assemble the obstetrical, neurological and neuro-surgical teams required for these transplants. Furthermore, even when tissue can be collected on a regular basis, the quality will vary enormously leading to different clinical outcomes. This has been a consistent problem for the Parkinson's disease transplant programmes. The third problem is common to all stroke trials but nonetheless an issue. Unlike Parkinson's disease, which has a relatively predictable prognosis, patient outcome in stroke is far more variable. Thus large numbers of patients are required in order to get meaningful results in clinical trials. With limited amounts of foetal tissue this becomes an impossibility.

Although these are formidable challenges, there are some areas of biology which suggest at least some may be overcome in the near future. In particular the field of stem cells and brain plasticity is developing rapidly. On one hand, the adult brain appears to have pools of stem cells which may be activated and encouraged to replace damaged neurons (Gage 2000). On the other, human neural stem cells can now be effectively expanded in the culture dish while retaining the ability to generate neurons and glia (Svendsen and Smith 1999). Together these areas of research may bring brain repair via endogenous cells or transplants a step closer. By eliminating the need for foetal tissue the way is paved for large scale clinical trials. However, a number of important issues need to be addressed before this can happen. To understand these issues requires an understanding of the biology of stem cells which is outlined in the following paragraphs.

Stem cells have turned out to be remarkable in their biology. With each passing month there are new discoveries which push forward the bounderies further. Each tissue appears to harbour largely dormant pools of stem cells which generate all the cellular lineage's of that tissue. They divide rarely, unless there is injury. After damage they divide a few times to generate a separate pool of progenitors which are capable of more rapid division and the generation of large amounts of tissue. This balance between the stem and progenitor cell pool is best described in the gut where new cells are continually produced during the lifetime of the animal (Potten and Loeffler 1990). Somewhat surprisingly, the adult brain has now been shown to also harbour stem cells. These reside in two regions, the subventricular zone of the striatum (Reynolds and Weiss 1992) and the hippocampus (for review see Kuhn and Svendsen 1999). The subventricular stem cells divide again to produce progenitors which migrate along the rostral migratory stream to the olfactory bulbs where they participate in neuronal replacement throughout the life of the animal, although the function of the hippocampal stem cells is far less clear. The fact that the adult brain contains proliferating stem cells which generate neurons has changed our view of this organ. Once the dogma held that we are born with so many neurons which continually reduce with age. Now we find that certain brain regions can regenerate neurons. The discovery that astrocytes may also be able to generate neurons (Doetsch et al. 1999) and the observation that similar cells may exist outside these two "neurogenic" zones (Palmer et al. 1995), has led to the idea that many brain regions may have the capacity for self repair under appropriate circumstances. In addition to the discovery of adult stem cells, other researchers have found that stem cell lineage's may not be as fixed as once thought. Blood stem cells may be able to generate glial cells following brain penetration (Kopen et al. 1999), and neural stem cells expanded in culture have been shown to incorporate into developing check embryo's and rodent blastocyts – taking on the phenotype of the tissues they develop alongside (Clarke et al. 2000). These reports suggest that the barriers between tissue specific stem cells, the most primitive of cell types, may often be breached allowing transdifferentiation to occur.

But where does this leave the possibility of using such cells for brain repair in stroke or other diseases? To date no one has yet shown that endogenous cells within the brain can be actively recruited in large enough numbers to restore function following injury. Instead, intriguing reports have been "proof of concept" which describe a rare cell capable of repair (Magavi et al. 2000) or trans-differentiation into blood cells (Bjornson et al. 1999). Furthermore, proving these cells do the same thing in the adult human brain will be more of a challenge. Although there appear to be dividing cells in the human hippocampus and SVZ (Goldman 1998; Eriksson et al. 1998), there is no evidence yet that they are able to repair any type of brain damage. This exciting field holds great potential, but has a long way to go before therapy will be possible. An alternative approach to stimulating the brains own adult neural stem cells, is to grow them in the test tube and then transplant them into areas of damage. One possible source is the biopsy tissue from the patients own brain, from which it is possible to isolate and expand neural stem cells for short periods of time (70 days) and which appear similar to their embryonic counterparts (Palm et al. 2000; Kukekov et al. 1999). However, other groups suggest that adult neural stem cells may be different to their embryonic counterparts and in particular are difficult to grow in large numbers (Johansson et al. 1999).

Another source of neural stem cells is from post-mortem human foetal tissues. Neural stem cells isolated from the developing forebrain have a massive capacity for expansion while retaining the ability to generate large numbers of neurons. We have recently reviewed this literature in detail (Svendsen et al. 1999). Finally, it may be possible to generate neurons from embryonic stem cells derived from the inner cell mass of the blastocyts (Svendsen and Rosser 1995) even from the human (Thomson et al. 1998).

How would stem cells be an advantage to primary foetal tissues? Perhaps the most obvious advantage is that they could be fully characterised in culture and supplied at almost unlimited numbers. This is due to the exponential pattern of growth they exhibit, and the ability to freeze these cells down and store in liquid nitrogen in "stem cell banks". Other advantages are that the cells could be thoroughly tested for pathogens and possibly modified in culture to express proteins of interest. Although the immunogenic status of the human cells in culture is currently not known, it would be possible to at least haplotype the growing cultures to attempt to match them to the recipients. This is not a major issue, as patients receiving primary foetal transplants for PD currently only receive immunosupression for 6 months after which it is withdrawn. Following withdrawal the grafts continue to survive based on PET imaging (Lindvall et al. 1994). Thus the human brain appears to be imunologically protected as described previously in a number of rodent studies.

How would stem cells be used? A few studies have already been published where rat progenitor cells or human teratocarcinoma cells grown in culture have been transplanted into models of stroke. The first used a cell line derived from an immortalized mouse. These cells were then transplanted into rats or marmosets with ischemic lesions and found to reverse some of the behavioral defecits (Gray et al. 2000). However, the mechanisms of this recovery were not clear. Did the cells make new neurons or simply stimulate host repair? Work from the same group has shown that astrocytes alone transplanted to the hippocampus are sufficient to produce functional recovery following cholinergic lesions of basal forebrain (Bradbury et al. 1995) – so simply injecting astrocytes derived from theses immortal cells may be enough to alleviate various type of behavioural defects. The second study used human neuroteratocarcinoma neurons derived from at teratocarcinoma cell line and showed functional effects following transplantation into areas of ischemic damage in the rodent brain (Saporta et al. 1999). Again in this study there was no clear indication of whether the cells produced the effect, or the reaction of the host brain to xenografted tissue produced the effect. In one sense it does not matter as long as the effects are there. In another it would seem essential to correlate functional recovery with cell survival and integration – before proceeding to clinical trials.

There is far more data on the transplantation of human neural precursor cells into other disease models. Clearly, the most interest has been in models of PD where the generation of dopamine neurons would be required. But in trying to achieve this much has been learnt about how neural stem cells engraft in general, and possible problems which may be encountered. Human progenitors have been grown as monolayers for 2 weeks and then transplanted into the striatum of adult animals with 6-OHDA lesions. These studies showed that, providing large numbers of cells were grafted (greater than 1 million), mature types of transplants could be found at short survival times, and that these could carry a genetic marker (Sabate et al. 1995). The question of how passaging or growing NPCs for longer time periods may affect the differentiation of the transplants was not addressed.

In a three-part study we have systematically assessed the ability of human NPCs to mature and survive in the adult lesioned rodent brain. In the first experiments, a comparison was made between cultures grown for short periods of time in EGF or FGF-2 and not passaged (10 days) and those expanded for longer periods (21 days) with regular passaging. While the 10 days cultures generated large graft masses with a number of healthy TH positive neurons and fibres, the passaged cultures appeared thin with only a few scattered cells around the transplant. In the second experiments, we then adapted the transplant method to allow whole spheres to be grafted, whereas in our previous study the cells had been dissociated to a single cell suspension prior to grafting. This change was based on *in vitro* data showing that cell/cell contact may be important in generating high numbers of neurons (Svendsen et al. 1998). We also followed the temporal maturation of the grafts by sacrificing groups at different survival times. This study showed that although significant graft masses were present at 2 weeks after grafting (2 weeks) into the striatum of animals with 6OHDA lesions, these had thinned out to strips of surviving cells by 20 weeks (Svendsen et al. 1997). Using human-specific antibodies and bromodeoxyuridine (BrdU) labelling the majority of surviving and migrating cells were shown to be astrocytes although some neurons could be found close to the graft site. Some of these were TH positive and in two cases were able to reduce lesion induced rotational deficits. However, the generation of these cells was clearly random. We have recently shown that labelling neural stem cells with the marker BrdU can be selectively toxic to neurons (Caldwell and Svendsen, in preparation). This may have lead to the thinning of the transplants. More recently, in the third set of experiments, the grafting technique has been further refined and BrdU was omitted from the study. Furthermore FGF-2 was used as the mitogen to increase the number of neurons developing from the stem cell pool (Ostenfeld et al. 1999). NPCs expanded 100 fold in FGF-2 were taken 2 days following their final sectioning in culture to allow intact, but small and healthy spheres to be grafted. We used cell densities of 200k, 1 million or 2 million in order to establish the optimum number of cells to achieve a healthy transplant. We found that only the 200k and 1 million cell transplants produced healthy grafts at 20 weeks following transplantation, whereas the 2 million group had overt signs of rejection. The number of proliferating cells declined with time such that by 20 weeks less than 1% of the cells within the transplants were dividing. In contrast to the drop in dividing cells, the number of fibres emerging from the grafts increased dramatically with time, such that by 20 weeks the entire striatum was full of human neurofilament positive neurites. TH-positive neurons were only found transiently at 6 weeks post grafting, but had disappeared by 20 weeks. This grafting paradigm shows that expanded populations of human NPCs can survive and integrate widely into the adult lesioned CNS, and do not continue to proliferate within the host brain.

Fricker et al. (1999) used human cells isolated and expanded from the embryonic human forebrain in EGF, FGF-2 and LIF. These cells had been expanded 10^7 fold in culture (approximately 21 passages) prior to grafting into neurogenic regions of the adult rat: the subventricular zone (SVZ) and the hippocampus. The cells were also transplanted into a non-neurogenic region, the striatum. Results demonstrate that when these cells were transplanted into the SVZ they migrate along the path of endogenous progenitors toward the olfactory bulb (OB). Once these cells had reached the OB they expressed NeuN in the granule and periglomerular layers. A small population also expressed TH in the periglomerular layer, a result similar to that found with adult hippocampal progenitors (Suhonen et al. 1996). When transplanted into the hilar region of the hippocampus, these cells also migrated and expressed neuronal markers in the granule and subgranular layers and shared a similar size and shape to the intrinsic host granule neurons while, in some cases, expressing calbindin. When transplanted into the non-neurogenic region, the striatum, these cells also expressed neuronal markers, but to a much lesser degree than that seen in the neurogenic regions, and most of these neurons were also found close to the transplant core. However, some of these neurons stained positive for the striatum-specific marker DARPP-32 to an extent similar to host neurons. Cells transplanted into the striatum also expressed a high level of GFAP at a distance of up to 1.5 mm from the transplant core.

In conclusion, these human studies suggest that NPCs may be a viable source of tissue for transplantation into damaged brain regions. Much more work is now required to establish functional effects of such transplants. Clearly, for models of Parkinson's Disease, this will necessitate the generation of dopamine neurons in the culture dish prior to transplantation. However, for other disease models, such as Huntington's disease (HD), the current generation of human NPCs may be sufficient to replace primary tissues. Along these lines we have recently shown that short term expanded cortical human NPCs can survive and integrate into the excitotoxically lesioned striatum and form grafts similar to primary transplants (Armstrong et al. 2000). However, this has not yet been done for NPCs expanded for longer periods of time in culture.

Finally, how do these results relate to transplantation in stroke patients? I hope to have conveyed a note of cautious optimism. Yes the cells can be grown in large numbers, and in some cases appear to integrate into the rodent brain following transplantation. However, no study has yet correlated the numbers of neurons surviving and their connections with functional improvement in stroke models or other models for PD and HD. This should be the focus of continuing studies in this area. Rushing forward now may not be the correct approach. Well designed, careful studies are required and need to be replicated by a number of groups to establish reproducibility. Once this is achieved, the move to the clinical setting will be both exciting and, one would hope, beneficial to the patients.

Acknowledgements

I would like to thank the Wellcome Trust for providing me with a fellowship to carry out this research.

References

1. Armstrong RJ, Watts C, Svendsen CN, Dunnett SB, Rosser AE (2000) Survival, neuronal differentiation, and fiber outgrowth of propagated human neural precursor grafts in an animal model of Huntington's disease. Cell Transplant 9:55–64
2. Bjorklund A, Lindvall O (2000) Self-repair in the brain. Nature 405:892–893, 895
3. Bjornson CR, Rietze RL, Reynolds BA, Magli MC, Vescovi AL (1999) Turning brain into blood: A hematopoietic fate adopted by adult neural stem cells in vivo. Science 283:534–537
4. Bradbury EJ, Kershaw TR, Marchbanks RM, Sinden JD (1995) Astrocyte transplants alleviate lesion induced memory deficits independently of cholinergic recovery. Neuroscience 65:955–972
5. Clarke DL, Johannsson CB, Wilbertz J, Veress B, Nilsson E, Karlstrom H, Lendahl U, Frisen J (2000) Generalized potential of adult neural stem cells. Science 288:1660–1663

6. DeGraba TJ, Pettigrew LC (2000) Why do neuroprotective drugs work in animals but not humans? Neurol Clin 18:475–493
7. Doetsch F, Caille I, Lim DA, Garcia-Verdugo JM, Alvarez-Buylla A (1999) Subventricular zone astrocytes are neural stem cells in the adult mammalian brain. Cell 97:703–716
8. Eriksson PS, Perfilieva E, Bjork-Eriksson T, Alborn AM, Nordborg C, Peterson DA, Gage FH (1998) Neurogenesis in the adult human hippocampus. Nat Med 4:1313–1317
9. Fricker RA, Carpenter MK, Winkler C, Greco C, Gates MA, Bjorklund A (1999) Site-specific migration and neuronal differentiation of human neural progenitor cells after transplantation in the adult rat brain. J Neurosci 19:5990–6005
10. Gage FH (2000) Mammalian neural stem cells. Science 287:1433–1439
11. Goldman SA (1998) Adult neurogenesis: from canaries to the clinic. J Neurobiol 36:267–286
12. Gray JA, Grigoryan G, Virley D, Patel S, Sinden JD, Hodges H (2000) Conditionally immortalized, multipotential and multifunctional neural stem cell lines as an approach to clinical transplantation. Cell Transplant 9:153–168
13. Johansson CB, Svennson M, Wallstedt L, Janson AM, Frisén J (1999) Neural stem cells in the adult human brain. Exp Cell Res 253:733–736
14. Kopen GC, Prockop DJ, Phinney DG (1999) Marrow stromal cells migrate throughout forebrain and cerebellum, and they differentiate into astrocytes after injection into neonatal mouse brains. Proc Natl Acad Sci USA 96:10711–10716
15. Kuhn HG, Svendsen CN (1999) Origins, functions, and potential of adult neural stem cells. Bioessays 21:625–630
16. Kukekov VG, Laywell ED, Suslov O, Davies K, Scheffler B, Thomas LB, O'Brien TF, Kusakabe M, Steindler DA (1999) Multipotent stem/progenitor cells with similar properties arise from two neurogenic regions of adult human brain. Exp Neurol 156:333–344
17. Lindvall O (1997) Neural transplantation: a hope for patients with Parkinson's disease. NeuroReport 8:3–10
18. Lindvall O, Sawle G, Widner H, Rothwell JC, Björklund A, Brooks D, Brundin P, Frackowiak R, Marsden CD, Odin P, Rehncrona S (1994) Evidence for long-term survival and function of dopaminergic grafts in progressive Parkinson's disease. Ann Neurol 35:172–180
19. Magavi SS, Leavitt BR, Macklis JD (2000) Induction of neurogenesis in the neocortex of adult mice [see comments]. Nature 405:951–955
20. Ostenfeld T, Caldwell MA, Prowse KR, Linskens MH, Jauniaux E, Svendsen CN (2000) Human neural precursor cells express low levels of telomerase in vitro and show diminishing cell proliferation with extensive axonal outgrowth following transplantation. Exp Neuro 164:215–226
21. Palm K, Salin-Nordstrom T, Levesque MF, Neuman T (2000) Fetal and adult human CNS stem cells have similar molecular characteristics and developmental potential. Brain Res Mol Brain Res 78:192–195
22. Palmer TD, Ray J, Gage FH (1995) FGF-2-responsive neuronal progenitors reside in proliferative and quiescent regions of the adult rodent brain. Mol Cell Neurosci 6:474–486
23. Potten CS, Loeffler M (1990) Stem cells: attributes, cycles, spirals, pitfalls and uncertainties. Lessons for and from the crypt. Development 110:1001–1020
24. Reynolds BA, Weiss S (1992) Generation of neurons and astrocytes from isolated cells of the adult mammalian central nervous system. Science 255:1707–1710
25. Sabate O, Horellou P, Vigne E, Colin P, Perricaudet M, Buc-Caron M, Mallet J (1995) Transplantation to the rat brain of human neural progenitors that were genetically modified using adenoviruses. Nature Genetics 9:256–260
26. Saporta S, Borlongan CV, Sanberg PR (1999) Neural transplantation of human neuroteratocarcinoma (hNT) neurons into ischemic rats. A quantitative dose-response analysis of cell survival and behavioral recovery. Neuroscience 91:519–525
27. Suhonen JO, Peterson DA, Ray J, Gage FH (1996) Differentiation of adult hippocampus-derived progenitors into olfactory neurons in vivo. Nature 383:624–627
28. Svendsen CN, Caldwell MA, Ostenfeld T (1999) Human neural stem cells: isolation, expansion and transplantation. Brain Pathol 9:499–513
29. Svendsen CN, Caldwell MA, Shen J, ter Borg MG, Rosser AE, Tyers P, Karmiol S, Dunnett SB (1997) Long term survival of human central nervous system progenitor cells transplanted into a rat model of Parkinsons Disease. Experimental Neurology 148:135–146
30. Svendsen CN, Rosser AE (1995) Neurons from stem cells? Trends Neurosci 18:465–467
31. Svendsen CN, Smith AG (1999) New prospects for human stem-cell therapy in the nervous system. Trends Neurosci 22:357–364
32. Svendsen CN, ter Borg MG, Armstrong RJE, Rosser AE, Chandran S, Ostenfeld T, Caldwell MA (1998) A new method for the rapid and long term growth of human neural precursor cells. J Neurosci Methods 85:141–153
33. Thomson JA, Itskovitz-Eldor J, Shapiro SS, Waknitz MA, Swiergiel JJ, Marshal VS, Jones JM (1998) Embryonic stem cell lines derived from human blastocyts. Science 282:1145–1147

Predictiveness of animal models for clinical trials

Translating experimental neuroprotection to humans: Failure and successes

J. Grotta

Introduction

My assignment at this conference highlighting the cutting edge of the battle against stroke in the experimental laboratory is to describe how the results of this research might be translated into positive results in a clinical experiment. I want to emphasize that what we need to carry out in the lab *and* at the bedside are both experiments. To date, many such experiments have been positive in the laboratory, but most have been negative at the bedside. What have we learned from these experiences? It is logical to me that at the bedside we need to emulate the conditions under which the laboratory experiment turns out positive; in other words, we need to do the "rat experiment" in man. Those clinical studies that have adhered to this dictum, such as tests of rtPA (The NINDS rt-PA Stroke Study Group 1995) and Ancrod (Sherman et al. 2000) given within 3 hours of stroke onset, and of pro-urokinase given only to patients with documented MCA occlusion (Furlan et al. 1999), have been the only positive clinical trials to date.

Figure 1 depicts the general design of the rat transient middle cerebral artery occlusion model that is most often used to test neuroprotective drugs, which are the focus of this talk. It also depicts the general design of the sort of clinical trial that I postulate must be done to get positive results with such a drug in stroke patients. There are four main areas where clinical trials have departed most from this model. In rats, we take pains to produce lesions of standardized severity and location with small variability in order to better detect a treatment effect, we start our evaluations giving the drug soon after the onset of stroke and then determine how long we can wait and still see effect, we use models of temporary rather than permanent middle cerebral artery occlusion, and we increase doses of drug until we see a therapeutic effect.

These factors, all of which must be addressed in the design of future clinical trials, are listed in Figure 2 along with one other important point. We need to find drugs or drug combinations in the lab that are substantially more potent than those that have failed in clinical trials to date.

I will discuss each of these points in more detail.

Standardize stroke severity

Logically the outcome after stroke is closely related to its initial severity. In animal models, the deeper the degree of ischemia and the longer it lasts, the worse the outcome measured either histologically or functionally (Jones et al. 1981). In animal models, the depth of ischemia can be adjusted according to the number of vessels

University of Texas-Houston Medical School,
6431 Fannin St., Houston, TX 77030
e-mail: james.c.grotta@uth.tmc.edu

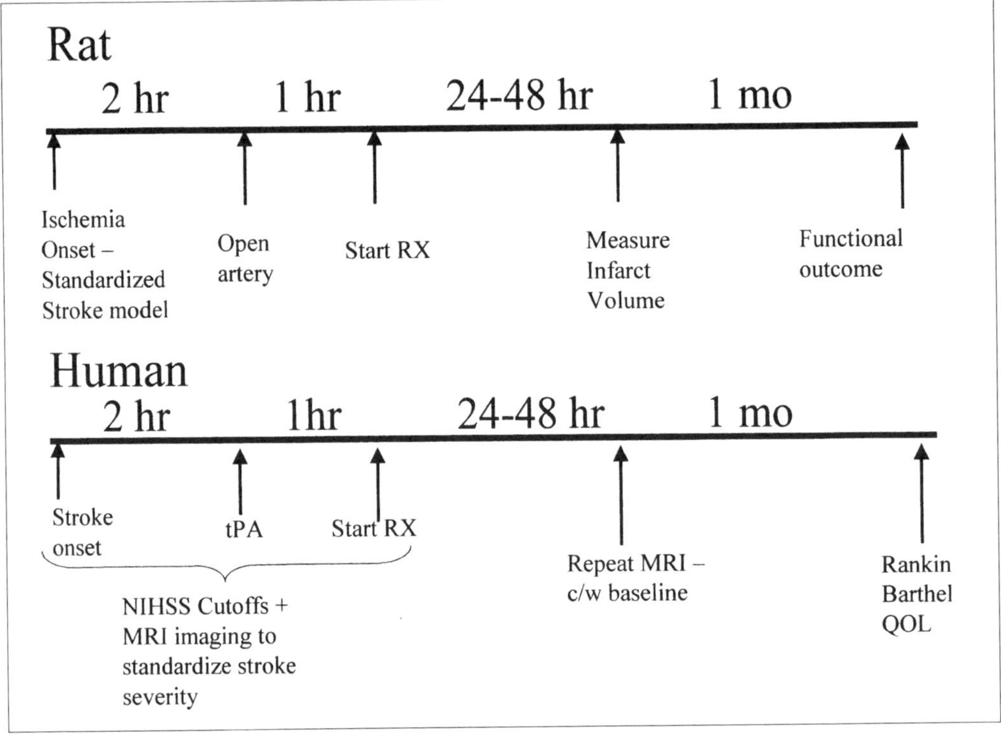

Fig. 1. Proposed algorithm for studying neuroprotective drugs in laboratory animals and human stroke patients.

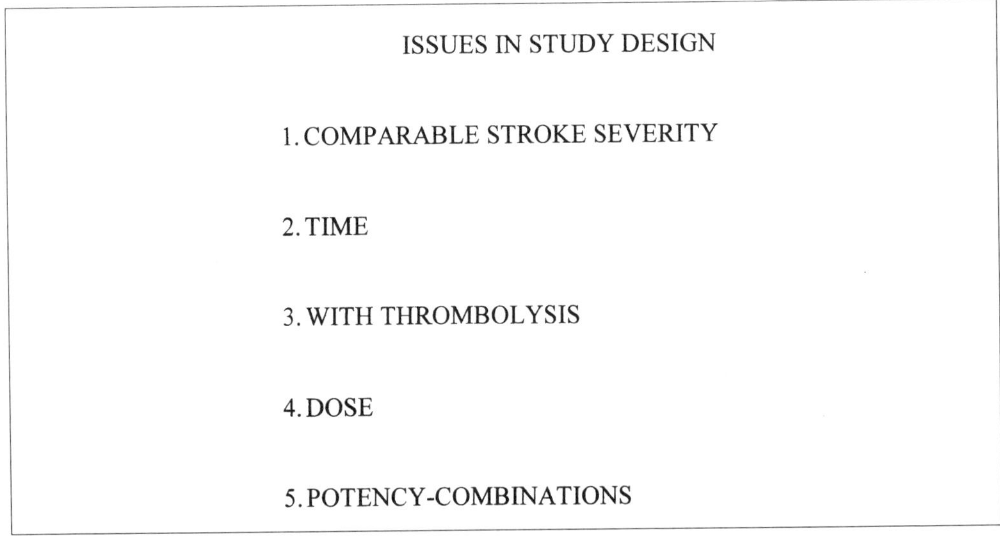

Fig. 2. Five factors important in selecting and testing a potential neuroprotective agent.

occluded and the location of the occlusion, and the duration of ischemia can be adjusted by reversing the arterial occlusion after a pre-specified interval. Stroke severity also varies according to the location of the infarct i.e. cortex or striatum, and rat strain, age and gender. Therefore, when designing an experimental evaluation of a drug in the laboratory, researchers will carefully standardize the severity of the stroke by subjecting both the treatment and vehicle groups to the same duration of ischemia and by using the same model in the same strain, age, and gender of rats.

There are two reasons why standardizing stroke severity is important in these experiments. Both relate to optimizing the ability to see a treatment effect between the drug and vehicle groups if one exists. If stroke severity is too great, then animals die whether or not they receive treatment. If severity is too mild, there is a "floor" effect where the functional deficit can't be detected, or the lesion is so small that any differences between treatment groups would be tiny. Second, if, by chance, the distribution of initial severity of the stroke varies between the treatment groups, the effect of this imbalance could be much greater than any effect of the treatment, leading to false negative or positive results.

Attempts to standardize the severity of the strokes in patients randomized into clinical trials is important for the same reasons. The severity of stroke is reflected in the neurological exam, quantified for instance in the National Institute of Health Stroke Scale (NIHSS) (Lyden et al. 1994). In most clinical studies, the baseline NIHSS is clearly the most important variable predicting outcome (The NINDS t-PA Stroke Study Group 1997). Early studies made little attempt to achieve standardization of stroke severity, using long time windows for treatment, and broad inclusion and few exclusion criteria (The American Nimodipine Study Group 1992). Many trials that included very severely affected patients were stopped, perhaps prematurely, because of high mortality in one or both groups (Hemodilution in Stroke Study Group 1989). Others arrived at equivocal or misleading results because of imbalances in the distribution of stroke severity between the groups (Albers et al. 2000). This led to attempts to find differences in subgroups based on a segment of patients with NIHSS scores matched along the severity continuum. But since these were always post-hoc analyses based on small numbers of patients, they were usually misleading. Recent studies have made more of an attempt to achieve standardization of stroke severity by using low and high NIHSS cutoffs (Davis et al. 2000), by trying to select patients with signs of cortical damage on the NIHSS (Gribkoff et al. 2000), and by ensuring that treatment groups are matched in distribution of NIHSS scores. However, the NIHSS is not a precise reflection of what is going on at the tissue level.

Might our stroke standardization be better accomplished by assessing tissue viability? This notion creates a dilemma. Just as in animal models, stroke severity should optimally be standardized by standardizing the depth of ischemia and its effect on the viability of the brain tissue at risk, *and* by including patients only within a very narrow time window (duration of arterial occlusion). The dilemma is that our ability to determine the state of tissue viability is still inexact, not available in many centers, and, most importantly, takes time. The most successful clinical strategy so far, as will be described later, is to include patients with only brief (< 3 hours) duration of ischemia. Keeping the time-to-treatment brief may itself help standardize the severity of stroke since all patients would have ischemia of relatively brief duration and consequently most would probably still have some reversibly damaged tissue. But adhering to a very narrow time window doesn't allow for ancillary tests to determine the depth of ischemia or tissue viability.

Emerging technology may provide an imaging tool to enable us to identify salvageable tissue. Such a test has, up to now, been the elusive "Holy Grail" of diagnostic studies for stroke. Initially, clinicians used measurements of cerebral blood flow (CBF) to establish the profundity of ischemia, but these methods had many disadvantages. They either lacked regional or quantitative information, or they were invasive (Lassen 1990). The only method of measuring CBF in the acute setting that is still in use is Xenon enhanced CT (Kaufmann et al. 1999). The consensus of most investigators is that the future of stroke standardization rests with magnetic resonance imaging (MRI) technology (Moseley et al. 1990). The details of how to determine tissue viability by MRI in the acute stroke setting is still uncertain, but probably rests in some correlation between diffusion and perfusion imaging (Beaulieu et al. 1999). Furthermore, just as in rats we measure the ability of a therapy to reduce infarct volume, MRI may help us compare the effect of drugs on the volume of tissue at risk that goes on to infarction. These studies are now being embodied into clinical trials. Attempts will be made to see if a certain MRI profile can help identify those patients with the severity of damage that is best targeted by neuroprotective therapy, and can help measure the effect of such therapy on eventual infarction size.

Another variable affecting severity of stroke in rats that has not been controlled in most human studies is the number of vessels occluded, which obviously affects the depth and location of ischemia. Only one study, the PROACT trial of an intra-arterially administered thrombolytic (Furlan et al. 1999), was designed to limit patients enrolled to only one type of vascular lesion. It was limited only to patients with documented middle cerebral artery occlusion of less than 6 hours duration. The results were positive, again reflecting the wisdom of designing clinical studies to closely emulate what we do in animals. Non-invasive techniques such as transcranial ultrasound, MRA or CTA may help us standardize patients enrolled into future trials by quantitating and localizing the offending arterial occlusion (Alexandrow et al. 1999).

Finally, depending on the proposed mechanism of action of the drug, we place our laboratory stroke lesions either in the cortex, striatum, or both. Although there is proportionately much less white matter in rodents than in humans, striatal lesions involve more white matter damage than do cortical strokes (Fig. 3). Many drugs work less well in the striatum (Roussel et al. 1992), not only because the depth of blood flow reduction may be greater in striatum, but also because the drug may have an effect on neurotransmitters or receptors which only are present on neuronal cell bodies. In testing such drugs in humans, we need to enrich the proportion of cortical strokes. This can be done to some extent by including only patients with cortical abnormalities on their NIHSS (Gribkoff et al. 2000), but would be far more exact if MRI imaging could be incorporated as part of the screening process.

In summary, for now we need to standardize the types of strokes we try to treat in clinical trials by controlling the time to treatment, range and distribution of the NIHSS, and exclusion of very aged patients. In the future, we need to learn how to utilize MRI to detect those patients with viable tissue at risk (and to help measure outcome). Finally, we might want to limit our trials to those with certain patterns of arterial occlusion likely to produce cortical lesions amenable to our neuroprotective therapies.

Time to treatment

In assessing the effect of a drug in the laboratory, two variables are adjusted, the time-to-treatment (TTT) and the dose of drug. As mentioned in the previous section, other variables are held constant. Seeing a gradual decrease in effect on outcome as TTT increases, and enhancing effect as the dose increases, are basic findings that confirm a pharmacologic effect on the mechanism causing the stroke. We will discuss dose later. In the lab, the investigator always starts with a brief TTT and then gradually prolongs it until an effect is no longer seen (Strong et al. 2000). This is just the opposite of what has been done in almost all clinical studies.

Researchers in the field of neuroprotection might learn important lessons by comparing results in the laboratory with clinical studies employing thrombolysis to achieve tissue reperfusion in stroke patients. In the lab, brain tissue must be reperfused within 2–4 hours, depending the model, to see a reduction of infarct size compared to animals with permanent occlusion (Kaplan et al. 1991). Clinical studies using intravenous rt-PA begun within 3 hours showed a

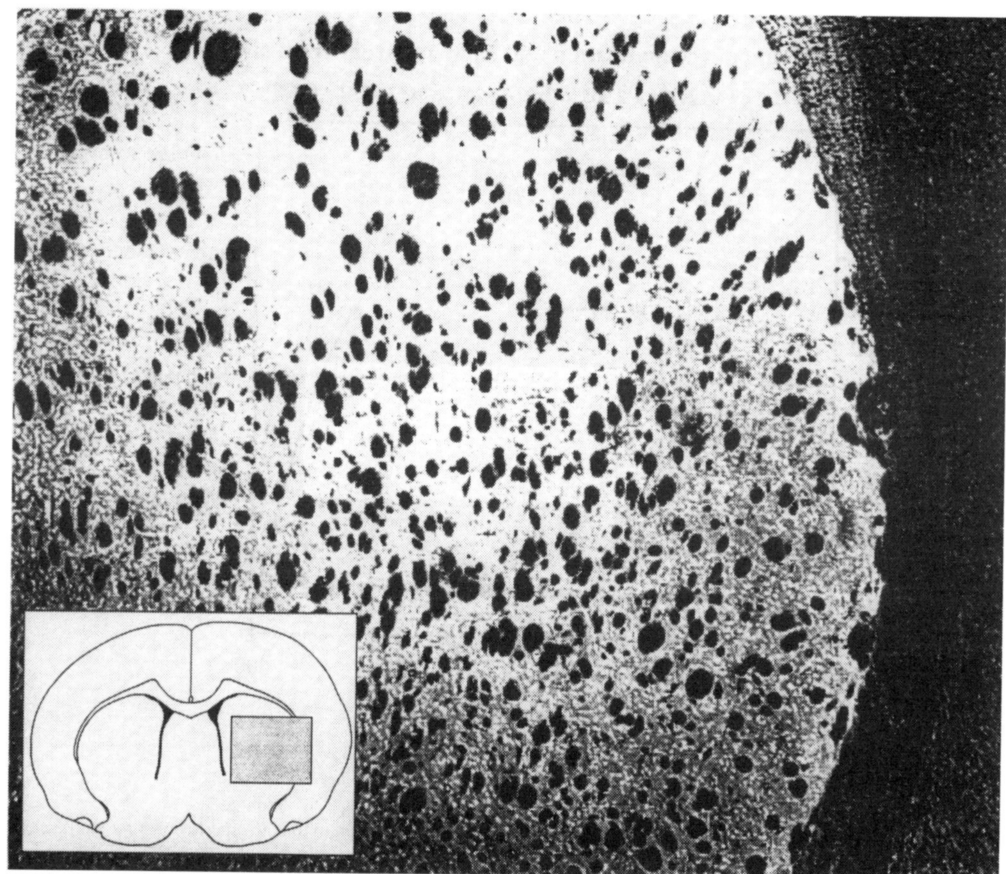

Fig. 3. Histologic section from designated area in rat caudate demonstrating white matter tracts stained with Trypan blue.

positive effect (The NINDS rt-PA Stroke Study Group 1995), with more benefit associated with earlier treatment within that window. If begun after 3 hours, rt-PA had little or no benefit (Hacke et al. 1995), though many investigators believe there may be some benefit in selected patients. Considering that it takes 30–90 minutes for a clot to dissolve after beginning IV rt-PA therapy, the TTT for reperfusion in clinical studies correlates very nicely with what has been found in laboratory models (Fig. 4). Similar laboratory results have been seen with neuroprotective drugs.

Pre-clinical studies have shown that all neuroprotective drugs are less effective the later they are given, and most are ineffective if started more than 2–4 hours after the onset of ischemia. Yet no clinical trial has included enough patients within that 4-hour time window to reach any conclusions about efficacy. The rt-PA investigators have shown that it is possible to treat patients and conduct a randomized placebo-controlled trial within this narrow TTT. Obviously, however, such a brief time window will limit the number of patients that can be treated. Seduced by imaging studies reporting "penumbral" tissue more than 6 hours after stroke onset (Baron et al. 1995), pharmaceutical companies, naturally interested in establishing the largest market for their drug, have abandoned the laboratory data, and extended the TTT in most studies to 6 hours or more.

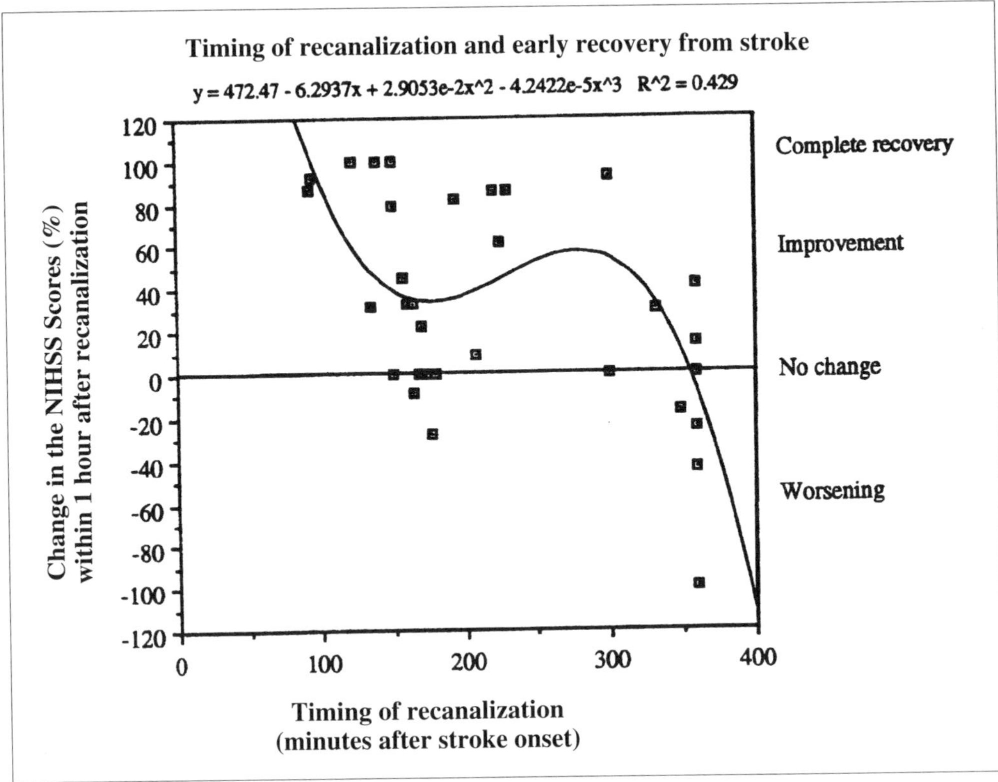

Fig. 4. Outcome (measured by change in NIH Stroke Scale Score (x axis) related to time to reperfusion after stroke onset as determined by TCD (y axis).

In summary, further clinical testing of neuroprotective agents should follow the example of pre-clinical laboratory studies and positive clinical trials of thrombolysis. Design the first efficacy experiments with very early treatment, and then work outward in prolonging the TTT. This might be a second arm of the initial study, or a separate trial, and positive results with delayed therapy might be more likely if selection of patients is based on imaging evidence of continued reversibly injured tissue. Finally, there are fewer risks associated with most neuroprotective drugs than with thrombolytics, and they might be useful in a wider spectrum of patients. Therefore, the market may be considerably larger than that of rt-PA even if the drug is only effective if given in the first few hours.

Combine neuroprotection with reperfusion

Another lesson from laboratory stroke models is that neuroprotective therapy is generally more effective if given to animals with reversible rather than permanent arterial occlusion (Zang et al. 1995). One reason for this is obvious. For a neuroprotective drug to work, it must reach the injured tissue. The fastest, safest, and most convenient way to get a drug to the brain in a stroke patient is by intravenous infusion. An occluded artery would not allow as much blood flow into the injured region than would one that is opened. Consequently, drug delivery to the target would be greater if re-perfusion of the injured tissue occurred either before or at the same time the drug is given.

An occluded artery that is opened within a certain time frame is likely to produce quantitatively less severe injury than one that is left blocked. As mentioned in the first two sections, the depth of ischemia and its duration largely determine the fate of the tissue. By lessening both of these variables, reperfusion models therefore probably produce a proportionately larger area of sub-lethal and reversible tissue damage.

In fact, it is possible that the type of tissue injury associated with reperfusion may be qualitatively different than what occurs with permanent occlusion. Reperfusion is associated with tissue reoxygenation producing free radicals that attack a variety of cellular components. It is also associated with excitotoxicity following a second wave of glutamate release. Early reperfusion may allow protein synthesis to continue or restart leading to the manufacture of proteins necessary to initiate an inflammatory response and apoptosis. These mechanisms might be quite amenable to reversal by neuroprotective drugs.

Laboratory studies support the existence of such "reperfusion injury" (Aronowski et al. 1997), a mechanism also seen with cardiac ischemia and organ transplantation. In rats, we are able to show in several models that, if the artery is opened, it actually produces *more* damage than if it were left occluded. This is seen in models of moderate severity; it is not seen after deep ischemia as occurs with arterial occlusion in Spontaneously Hypertensive Rats. We have also found that neuroprotective drugs, especially those that attack free radicals, inhibit protein synthesis, reduce inflammation, or prevent apoptosis, are particularly effective, reducing final infarct size by up to 80%.

It is possible to design a study combining reperfusion and neuroprotection? Thrombolytic therapy with IV rt-PA, according to established guidelines, is associated with at least partial recanalization in up to 70% of cases, and has been shown to increase tissue reperfusion. Even better, intra-arterial administration of a lytic drug is associated with at least partial recanalization in 80% of occluded middle cerebral arteries, and provides the advantage of possible direct administration of the neuroprotectant through the arterial catheter into the arterial blood perfusing the injured tissue. Therefore combining the neuroprotective drug with thrombolytic therapy can re-create the setting of reperfusion in which neuroprotection is most effective in the lab.

It might be difficult to randomize a patient to an investigational neuroprotective drug while at the same time determining eligibility for thrombolysis and administering both within 3 hours of symptom onset. However, this can be done. In a recent safety study of lubeluzole combined with rt-PA (Grotta 2000), all patients received IV rt-PA within 3 hours of stroke onset, and were begun on study drug within 1 hour of starting rt-PA, on average 3.3 hours after stroke onset (Fig. 5). Furthermore, patients were enrolled at a rate of more than 0.5 patients per month.

In summary, reperfusion is the best setting to see the beneficial effect of neuroprotection in the lab. Concomitant administration of a neuroprotective drug with a thrombolytic agent can reproduce this paradigm in the clinical arena.

Dose

Whether the artery is open or not, sufficient drug must reach the injured region to have the desired biological effect. Unfortunately, this has not been achieved in many clinical trials.

Side effects have been the Achilles heel limiting the doses of neuroprotective drugs given to stroke patients. Many side effects seen in humans, such as mild hypotension, sedation, and other behavioral effects can be hard to detect or don't occur in a rat. Consequently, with many drugs it is possible to dose rats until a "ceiling" is reached where no larger amount produces benefit. This is not the case with humans. Recent stroke victims seem particularly vulnerable to cardiovascular or sedative effects of a drug (The American Nimodipine Study Group 1992; Davis et al. 1997). Perhaps because of a disrupted blood-brain barrier and consequently more tissue bioavailability of the drug in the stroke patient than the same dose in normal volunteers, stroke patients often have

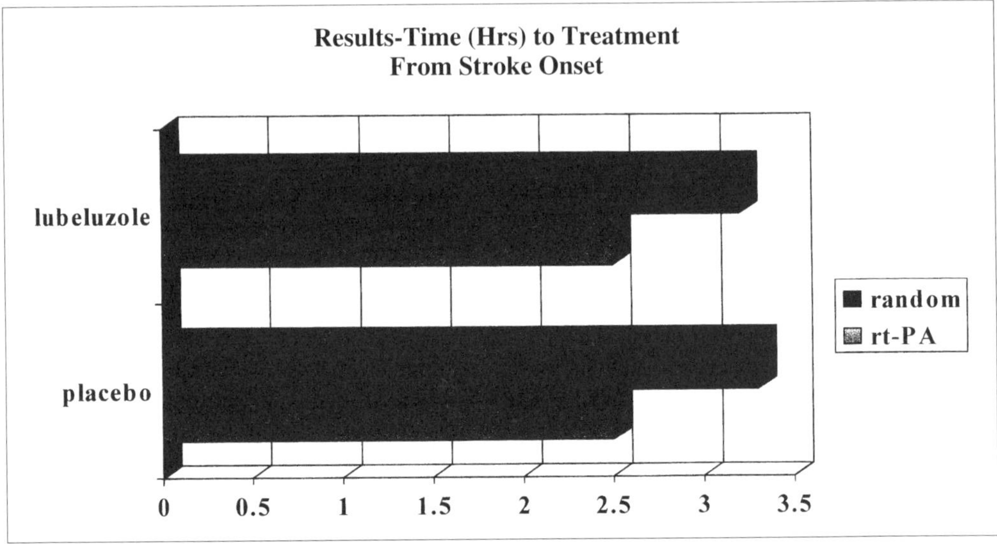

Fig. 5. Time to starting intravenous treatment with rt-PA and lubeluzole or placebo in a recently completed multicenter randomized trial of lubeluzole vs placebo in stroke patients receiving rt-PA. According to the protocol, rt-PA was given to all patients within 3 hours of stroke onset and lubeluzole or placebo had to be started before the end of the one-hour rt-PA infusion.

drug reactions not predicted by phase 1 studies in normal volunteers. Also, for any given drug there may be different rates of absorption, metabolic pathways or rates, tissue uptake mechanisms, receptor availability, and other biological differences between species. These considerations make it difficult to translate blood levels we can achieve in rats, and even in normal human volunteers, to those we can expect to reach safely in our acute stroke patients.

Even with drugs where side effects do not limit dose, many trials have used the minimal effective dose or blood level from preclinical studies when choosing the dose or target blood level for stroke patients (Grotta J for the US and Canadian Lubeluzole Ischemic Stroke Study Group 1997). Then, when the pivotal efficacy trial is carried out, it is determined that lower blood levels were achieved than expected, and most patients were therefore not exposed to a potentially therapeutic amount of drug.

In designing a clinical neuroprotective trial, it would seem logical to always begin with a dose escalation study (with blood level correlation) in stroke patients similar to those you intend to include in the pivotal trial. The highest tolerable dose should then be chosen for the pivotal trial. Ideally, the next step would be to demonstrate that the dose chosen is able to achieve a measurable beneficial effect on the target biological process. An example would be to demonstrate that the dose of thombolytic drug to be used in a study is able to lyse the clot in a sample of patients studied angiographically. Unfortunately, such tests in living stroke patients are not available for most neuroprotective drugs that have their effect on cellular mechanisms. In that case, one is forced to rely on the ability to achieve blood levels which are on the high side of the range that is effective in pre-clinical animal studies.

In summary, it is likely that effective drugs have been discarded because insufficient blood levels were achieved in their therapeutic human testing. It is also likely that futile studies have wasted time, money, energy, and the cooperation of our stroke patients by proceeding with doses that had little hope of successfully reaching therapeutic brain levels. More time should be devoted to pilot studies aimed at determining the maximal tolerated dose, and detecting if this has the desired biological effect and is able to achieve blood levels clearly in the therapeutic range determined by pre-clinical studies.

Finding a more effective drug

Most of the neuroprotective drugs subjected to clinical evaluation have been able to reduce relative infarct volume and improve behavioral outcome by about 50% compared to controls in well-standardized pre-clinical stroke models. It is possible that even if we adhere to the principles described in the preceding pages, this effect is not enough to detect in our stroke patients. Perhaps the biology of ischemic damage in the rat is so different from humans that positive results in the former cannot be extrapolated to the latter.

I think that a better explanation for our clinical failures, in addition to our failure to design trials to mimic what has been successful in the lab, is that the drugs we have chosen are too

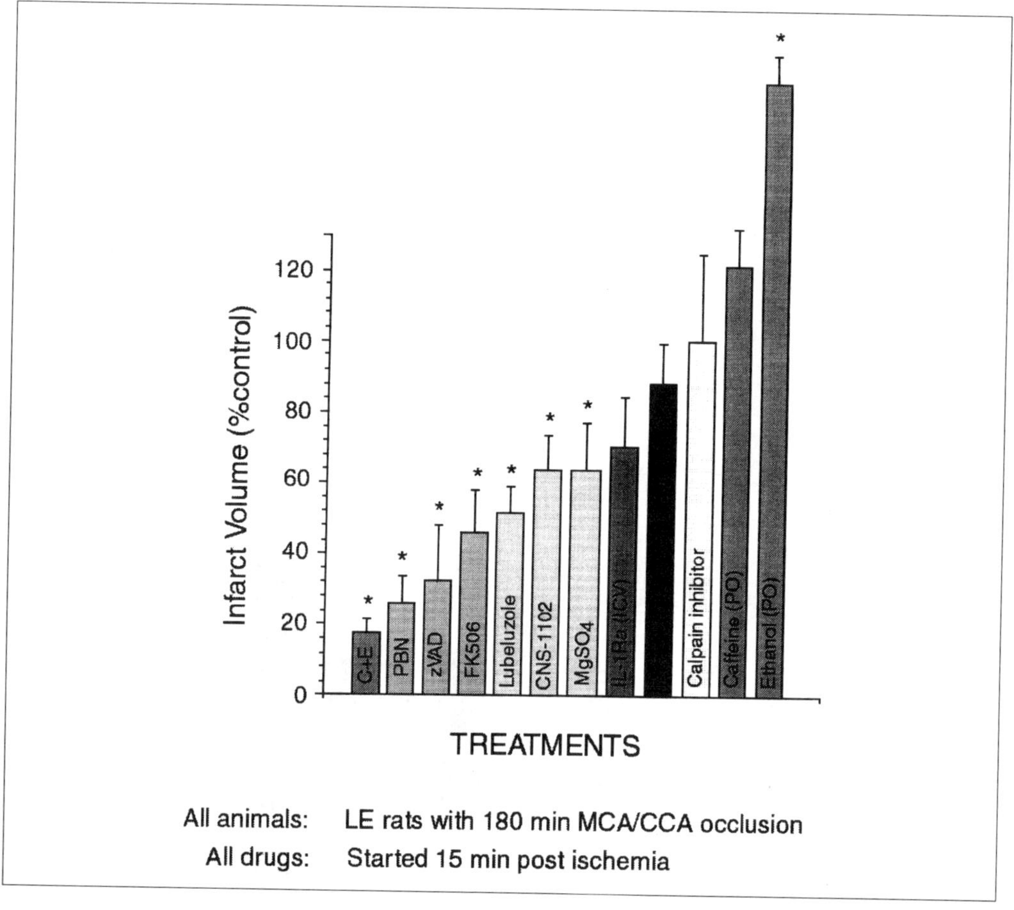

Fig. 6. Comparison of the effect of various neuroprotective drugs in a reperfusion injury model in rat. Long Evans rats were subjected to 180 minutes of reversible middle cerebral artery (MCA) occlusion followed by 24 hours reperfusion which leads to larger infarction than if the MCA is left permanently occluded (see reference #23). All treatments were given intravenously unless otherwise noted, and begun 15 minutes after the onset of MCA occlusion. Y axis is infarct volume measured as percent of control group. C+E is caffeine and ethanol, PBN is N-tert-Butyl-alpha-phenylnitrone, IL-1Ra is interleukin 1 receptor antagonist, ICV is intracerebroventricular, DCLHb is diaspirin cross-linked hemoglobin.

weak. A firm conclusion cannot be made because of weaknesses in clinical study design to date. However, based on our inability to translate pre-clinical results to the bedside, we probably should no longer move forward with clinical evaluation of a monotherapy that reduces damage by only 50% in a rat. We need to find drugs that reduce damage by 80% in these models. This is possible with some drugs we are now studying in our lab (Grotta 1999) (Fig. 6). Surprisingly, the most effective agents, particularly in our reperfusion model, are drugs that affect downstream biological consequences of ischemia such as inflammatory mechanisms and apoptosis.

Selecting a drug that affects a single pathway in the process of brain injury after stroke has scientific and regulatory purity. However, this strategy has proven ineffective clinically. It is time to look for combinations of drugs that have a stronger effect. We need to work on the regulatory and financial impediments for conducting such trials. Regulatory agencies will accept combination trials if the combination provides more effect than merely a summation of the effect of each drug alone. An example of such is our interesting finding that while caffeine has little effect on stroke outcome, and ethanol makes it worse, a combination of low doses of the combination given acutely to naïve rats is more effective than any monotherapy we have yet evaluated in our reperfusion model (Strong et al. 2000) (Figs. 6, 7). The stroke research community will need to be even more creative in designing and finding funding for such a combination trial. However, stroke is a huge public health problem. If finding a potent and safe combination therapy is the only way that neuroprotection will work, I am optimistic that eventually funding agencies and industry will support that approach.

In summary, current approaches to neuroprotection have succeeded in the lab but not at

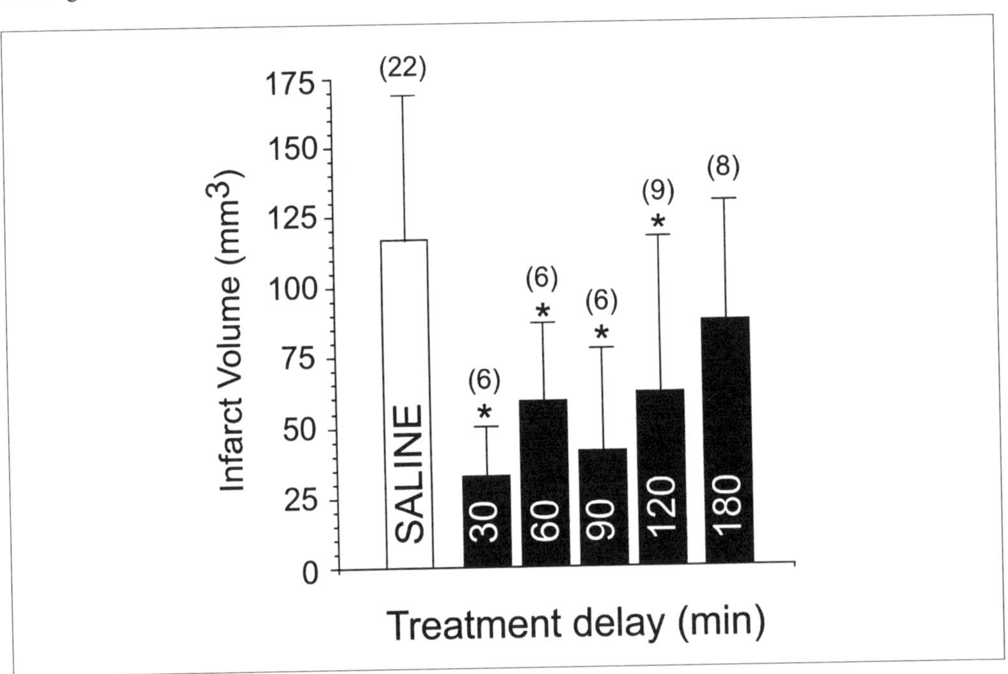

Fig. 7. Infarct volume +/– SD (mm^3) following 180 minutes of unilateral MCA/CCA occlusion in Long Evans rats after an IV bolus plus infusion that delivered a total of 0.65 g/kg ethanol (10% solution) plus 10 mg/kg caffeine initiated 30, 60, 90, 120, and 180 minutes after induction of ischemia vs saline control. Caffeine and ethanol were dissolved in 3 ml of saline. 0.5 ml was injected as a bolus and then the remaining 2.5 ml as a continuous infusion over 2.5 h. *Statistically different ($p < 0.05$) from saline treated (control) group. Numbers in parentheses represent numbers of animals per group.

the bedside. To succeed, clinicians need better trial design to reflect the conditions under which drugs work in the laboratory, and basic researchers need to discover more potent and safe therapies than those that have already been tried at the bedside.

References

1. Albers GW, Alberts MJ, Broderick JP, Lyden PD, Sacco RL (2000) Recent advances in stroke management. Stroke and Cerebrovasc Disease 9:3,95–105
2. Alexandrov A, Demchuk A, Wein T, Grotta J (1999) Yield of transcranial doppler in acute cerebral ischemia. Stroke 30:1604–1609
3. Aronowski J, Strong R, Grotta J (1997) Reperfusion injury: Demonstration of brain damage produced by reperfusion after transient focal ischemia in rats. J Cereb Blood Flow and Metab 17:1048–1056
4. Baron JC, Kummer R von, del Zoppo GJ (1995) Treatment of acute ischemic stroke: challenging the concept of a rigid and universal time window. Stroke 26:2219–2221
5. Beaulieu C, de Crespigny A, Tong DC, Moseley ME, Albers GW, Marks MP (1999) Longitudinal magnetic resonance imaging study of perfusion and diffusion in stroke: Evolution of lesion volume and correlation with clinical outcome. Ann Neurol 46:568–578
6. Davis S, Albers GW, Diener HC, Lees KR, Norris J (1997) Termination of acute stroke studies involving selfotel treatment. Lancet 349:32
7. Davis SM, Lees KR, Albers GW, Diener HC, Markabi S, Karlsson G, Norris J, for the ASSIST Investigators (2000) Selfotel in acute ischemic stroke. Possible neurotoxic effects of an NMDA antagonist. Stroke 31:347–354
8. Furlan A, Higashida R, Wechsler L, Gent M, Rowley H, Kase C, Pessin M, Ahuja A, Callahan F, Clark WM, Silver F, Rivera F, for the PROACT Investigators (1999) Intra-arterial prourokinase for acute ischemic stroke; The PROACT II Study: A randomized controlled trial. JAMA 282:2,2003–2011
9. Gribkoff VK, Starrett JE, Hewawasam P, Dworetzky SK, Ortiz AA, Kinney GG, Boissard CG, Post-Munson DJ, Trojnacki JT, Huston KM, Signor LJ, Lombardo LA, Reid SA, Hibbard JR, Myers RA, Moon SL, Yeleswaram S, Pajor LM, Johnbson G, Molinoff PB (2000) A novel maxi-K potassium channel opener, BMS-204352, reduced cortical infarct size in stringent rodent models of acute focal stroke. Neurol 54 (Suppl 3) A68
10. Grotta J (1999) Acute stroke therapy at the millennium: Consummating the marriage between the laboratory and bedside; The Feinberg Lecture. Stroke 30:1722–1728
11. Grotta J for the US and Canadian Lubeluzole Ischemic Stroke Study Group (1997) Lubeluzole treatment of acute ischemic stroke. Stroke 28:2338–2346
12. Grotta JC (2000) Combination therapy stroke trial rt-PA +/– Lubeluzole. Stroke 31:278
13. Hacke W, Kaste M, Fieschi C et al. (1995) Intravenous thrombolysis with recombinant tissue plasminogen activator for acute hemispheris stroke; the European Cooperative Acute Stroke Study (ECASS). JAMA 274:1017
14. Hemodilution in Stroke Study Group (1989) Hypervolemic hemodilution treatment of acute stroke. Results of a randomized multicenter trial using pentastarch. Stroke 20:317–323
15. Jones TH, Morawetz RB, Crowell RM et al. (1981) Thresholds of focal cerebral ischemia in awake monkeys. J Neurosurg 54:773–782
16. Kaplan B, Brint S, Tanabe J et al. (1991) Temporal thresholds for neocortical infarction in rats subjected to reversible focal cerebral ischemia. Stroke 22:1032–1039
17. Kaufmann AM, Firlik AD, Fukiu MB, Wechsler LR, Jungries CA, Yonas H (1999) Ischemic core and penumbra in human stroke. Stroke 30:93–99
18. Lassen NA (1990) Pathophysiology of brain ischemia as it relates to the therapy of acute ischemic stroke. Clin Neuropharmacol 13:S1
19. Lyden P, Brott T, Tilley B et al. (1994) Improved reliability of the NIH Stroke Scale using video training. Stroke 25:2220–2226
20. Moseley M, Kucharczyk J, Mintorovitch J et al. (1990) Diffusion-weighted MR imaging of acute stroke: correlation with T2-weighted and magnetic susceptibility enhanced MR imaging in cats. AJNR 1:423–429
21. Roussel S, Pinard E, Seylaz J (1992) Effect of MK-801 on focal brain infarction in normotensive and hypertensive rats. Hypertension Jan 19(1):40–46
22. Sherman DG, Atkinson RP, Chippendale T, Levin KA, Ng K, Futrell N, Hsu CY, Levy DE for the STAT Participants (2000) Intravenous ancrod for treatment of acute ischemic stroke: The STAT Study: A randomized controlled trial. JAMA 283:18,2395–2403
23. Strong R, Grotta JC, Aronowski A (2000) Combination of low dose ethanol and caffeine protects brain from damage produced by focal ischemia in rats. Neuro Pharma 39:515–522
24. The American Nimodipine Study Group (1992) Clinical trial of nimodipine in acute ischemic stroke. Stroke 23:3–8
25. The NINDS rt-PA Stroke Study Group (1995) Tissue plasminogen activator for acute ischemic stroke. NEJM 333:24,1581–1587
26. The NINDS t-PA Stroke Study Group (1997) Generalized efficacy of t-PA for acute stroke: Subgroup analysis of the NINDS t-PA stroke trial. Stroke 28:2119–2125
27. Zang RL, Chopp M, Jiang N, Tang WX, Prostak J, Manning AM, Anderson DC (1995) Anti-intercellular adhesion molecule-1 antibody reduces ischemic cell damage after transient but not permanent middle cerebral artery occlusion in the Wistar rat. Stroke 26(8):1438–1442

Which pathophysiologic mechanisms are relevant therapeutic targets in ischemic stroke?

W.-D. Heiss, L.W. Kracht, A. Thiel, M. Grond, G. Pawlik, R. Graf

Abstract

The efficiency of various strategies of neuroprotection is well documented in animal experiments but is thus far disappointing in ischemic stroke, for which only early reperfusion induced by thrombolysis has improved clinical outcome. This discrepancy between expectation from experimental research and clinical reality may be related to differences in the pathogenetic factors contributing to infarction. Positron emission tomography of regional cerebral blood flow and cortical flumazenil binding was used to identify various compartments of the infarct outlined on MRI 2–3 weeks after a hemispheric stroke. In 10 patients rCBF was determined within 3 hours of symptoms onset: in 9 of them hypoperfusion below the viability threshold accounted for the largest proportion (mean 70%) of the final infarct, whereas penumbral tissue (18%) and initially sufficiently perfused tissue (12%) were responsible for considerably smaller portions of the final infarct. In 10 other patients, rCBF and FMZ binding were determined 2–12 hours after the acute attack: FMZ binding at or below 3.4 times the mean in white matter was found in 74% of the final infarct. A large portion (86%) of the final infarct exhibited critically reduced flow, and only 8% of the final infarct showed FMZ binding and CBF above the critical limits.

These results indicate that early critical flow disturbance leading to rapid cell damage is the predominant cause of infarction, while secondary and delayed pathobiochemical processes in borderline or initially sufficiently perfused regions contribute only little to the final infarcts. Experimental models used in the development of therapeutic strategies for ischemic stroke should take into account the described pathophysiology.

Concepts of the pathophysiology of ischemic cell damage are mainly derived from experimental models and involve a complex cascade of molecular and biochemical mechanisms (Siesjö 1992; Pulsinelli 1992; Choi 1998) initiated by the disturbance of blood supply. Such processes might contribute also to the propagation of ischemic damage beyond the critically perfused area and might additionally be responsible for delayed growing of infarcts (Barone and Feuerstein 1999; Schulz et al. 1999; Dirnagl et al. 1999). Most of these pathophysiologic events cannot be assessed in patients and their relevance for treatment of ischemic stroke is still not proven. A necessary prerequisite for

Keywords: Ischemic stroke – Critical perfusion – Penumbra – Irreversible damage – CBF – Flumazenil – Positron emission tomography – Treatment strategies – Thrombolysis – Neuroprotection

Max-Planck-Institut für neurologische Forschung and Neurologische Universitätsklinik Köln, Gleueler Str. 50, D-50931 Köln, Germany

treatment of acute ischemic stroke, either by early reperfusion or by interference with the pathobiochemical cascade leading to ischemic neuronal damage, is the existence of functionally impaired but viable and potentially salvagable tissue. Reperfusion induced by thrombolysis is still the only clinically effective strategy but must be initiated within the first hours after onset of symptoms (systemic: 3 hours, (The NINDS rt-PA Stroke Study Group 1995), intracarotid: 6 hours, (Furlan et al. 1999)). In contrast, neuroprotective strategies thus far have been disappointing clinically and were unsuccessful with respect to improving stroke outcome (Grotta 1994; Dorman et al. 1996; Dyker and Lees 1996; del Zoppo et al. 1997; The European Ad Hoc Consensus Group 1998; Lees 1998), although significant reductions in infarct size (up to > 50%) were demonstrated in animal models with the use of strategies to antagonize the various steps in the excitotoxic cascade (Grotta 1994; Choi 1998) or free radical toxicity (Kontos 1985; Chan 1996), to inhibit harmful secondary inflammatory mechanisms (Chopp and Zhang 1996; DeGraba 1998) or to attenuate cell death by apoptosis (Endres et al. 1998; Barinaga 1998; Schulz et al. 1999). This discrepancy between experimental results and clinical efficacy may be in part due to limits of animal models concerning the complexity of clinical stroke, but may also be attributed to differences in the outcome endpoints chosen for evaluation of therapeutic effects: reductions of infarct size in a particular experimental setting may in fact be poor predictions of the functional outcome of stroke patients. Therefore, it must be questioned whether the infarct volume in animal experiments is a target relevant for the development of stroke therapy, since the relative impact of the various mechanisms contributing to the size of the final infarct has never been determined in human stroke.

Based on the assumption, that various subcompartments exist within a territory of impaired blood supply which differ with respect to their residual perfusion and consequently their ischemic compromise, final infarcts were analyzed and subcompartments were classified according to their degree of residual perfusion on early measurement. For that purpose the core of ischemia was defined as a region with flow decreased below the critical threshold usually leading to irreversible damage (Heiss and Graf 1994); in this area only immediate reperfusion before the time when cells are irreversibly damaged might prevent infarction. Bordering the core of ischemia is the penumbra zone (Astrup et al. 1981) where flow is decreased below the functional threshold but still sufficient to maintain morphological integrity for a certain time, which in turn depends on the degree of the residual perfusion. The penumbra zone as a promising target for therapy would benefit mainly from sufficient reperfusion before irreversible cell damage has occurred. However, the ischemic cell damage may be propagated to surrounding areas and thereby the final infarct may be increased into primarily sufficiently perfused regions. These regions then would mainly benefit from neuroprotective, antiinflammatory or antiapoptotic strategies. In an additional sample of stroke patients early damage was identified by a ligand of central benzodiazepine receptors which is a marker for neuronal integrity.

Subjects and methods

This report is based on 2 studies: In 10 patients with acute hemispheric stroke, regional cerebral blood flow (rCBF) was studied with the $[^{15}O]H_2O$ intravenous bolus method (Herscovitch et al. 1983) by positron emission tomography (PET) within 3 hours of symptoms (Heiss et al. 1999). Regional tracer uptake was determined voxel by voxel in gray matter structures of the affected hemisphere, and the respective ratio to the mean of the contralateral hemisphere, expressed as a percentage, was used as relative measure of perfusion. The morphological outcome was assessed on T1-weighted MRI scans acquired 2 to 3 weeks after the stroke. In the coregistered MRI-PET images gray matter infarcts, non-infarcted gray matter and the contralateral hemispheres were segmented. Within the boundaries of final infarcts outlined on the 3-dimensional coregistered MR images, 3 compartments were identified according to their perfusional state within 3 hours of symptoms onset: critically hypoperfused tissue, with a perfusion operationally set to below 50% $[^{15}O]H_2O$ uptake relative to the mean of the contralateral hemisphere; penumbral tissue with a perfusion between 50 and 70% $[^{15}O]H_2O$ uptake; and tissue with sufficient perfusion above 70% $[^{15}O]H_2O$ uptake relative to the mean of the contralateral hemisphere. These limits were chosen as representing < 12, 12–18, and > 18 ml/100 g/min in a comparative study (Löttgen et al. 1998) – values widely accepted as viability threshold and penumbra range (Baron et al. 1984; Powers et al. 1985; Hakim et al. 1989).

In another group of 10 patients with acute hemispheric stroke rCBF and binding of 11C-flumazenil (FMZ) – a central benzodiazepine receptor ligand – was studied by PET 2 to 12 hours after onset of symptoms (Heiss et al. 2000). Cortical volumes of interest were placed on coregistered CBF and FMZ images as well as on the late T1-weighted MRI scans, and categorized as infarcted or normal according to their appearance on late MRI. For all values of blood flow and FMZ binding the threshold probability integrals of final infarction or non-infarction were iteratively computed, resulting in curves predicting final outcome. From those curves the positive and negative 95% prediction limits of blood flow and FMZ binding were obtained. Subcompartments defined by morphological outcome, mean positive 95% prediction limit of FMZ binding, and mean negative 95% prediction limit of CBF were analyzed voxel by voxel to estimate the relative size of the various portions of the final infarct.

Results

Perfusion within 3 hours of ischemic stroke

As shown on Table 1, the final gray matter infarcts varied considerably in size (1.5–138.4 cm^3). All of the 3 predefined ranges of initial flow were found in each of the infarcts. However, despite large variability among individuals, in 9 patients the largest proportion by far was the subcompartment of critical hypoperfusion (51% to 92% of the final infarct), followed by penumbral tissue (8% to 34%), whereas the subcompartment initially perfused at a sufficient level was relatively small (2–25%). In only one case with a rather small final infarct of 15.6 cm^3 was the subcompartment of sufficient inital flow large (41%) and the critically hypoperfused volume relatively small (31%).

Prediction of irreversible damage and penumbra

The analysis of all the VOIs with respect to their final place within or outside the infarcts permitted to define positive and negative 95% predic-

Table 1. Volume of final infarcts and subcompartments defined by initial level of residual perfusion in 9 patients

	Compartment Volume, cm^3 Brain Tissue			Compartment Volume, % of Infarcted Volume	
	Median	Range	*P*	Median	Range
Infarcted Volume	27.7	1.5–138.4			
Critically hypoperfused tissue	21.1	0.8–126.7	< 0.05*	69.8	50.8–91.6
Penumbral tissue	5.0	0.3–19.1	< 0.05**	18.0	8.0–33.9
Sufficiently perfused tissue	1.6	0.2–19.1		12.2	2.2–24.7

*Compared with penumbral and sufficiently perfused tissue, and **compared with sufficiently perfused tissue, by Wilcoxon signed rank test.

tion limits of early cortical blood flow and early FMZ binding. The flow limits were 4.8 and 14.1 ml/100g/min, defining also the range of the penumbra between these two limits. The respective limits for FMZ binding were 3.4 and 5.5 times the mean uptake in white matter. Since the penumbral range is considerably narrower for the FMZ binding, this measure is particularly well suited for the early demonstration of cortical tissue eventually turning into necrosis.

These measurements can be combined for a more reliable definition of various tissue compartments: Using the mean positive prediction limit of FMZ binding (3.4) as the lower and the mean negative prediction limit of CBF (14.1

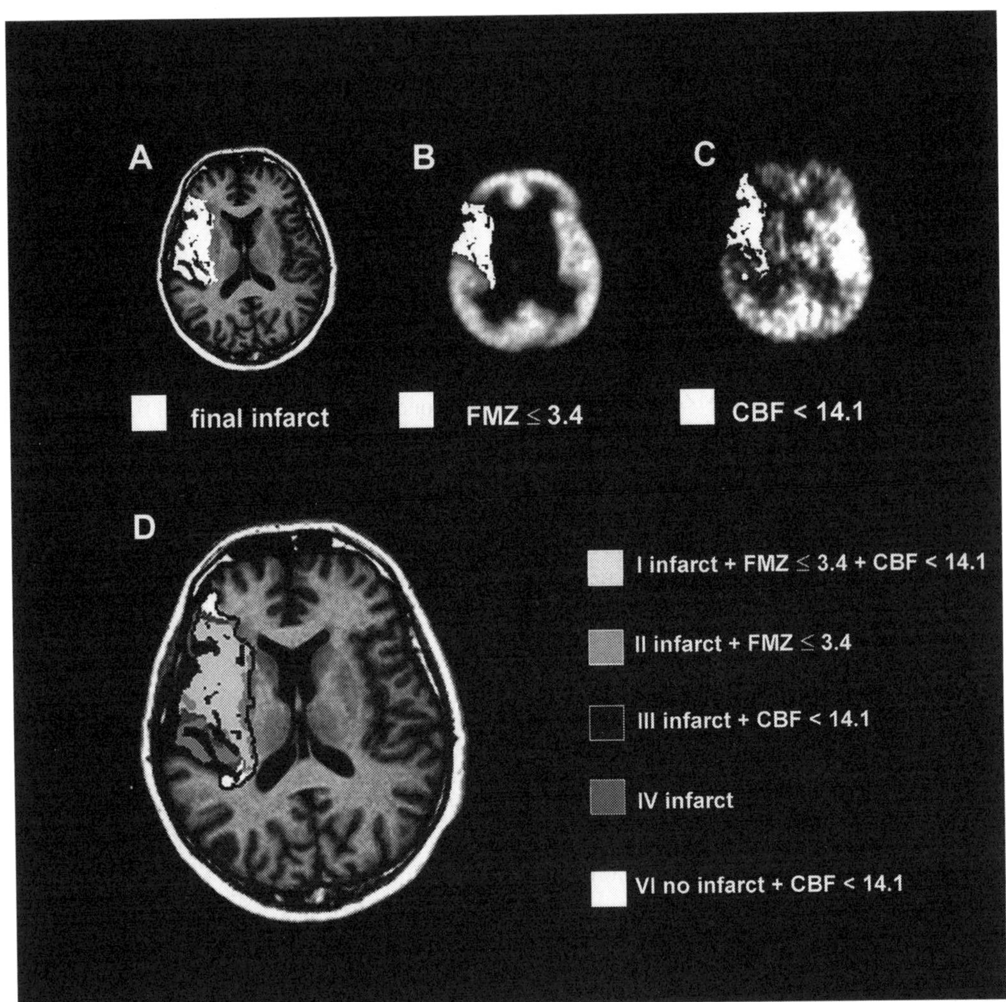

Fig. 1. Various subcompartments within and outside the final infarct:
A extension of the final infarct
B compartment with initial FMZ binding decreased to or below 3.4 times the white matter mean
C compartment with initial flow decreased below 14.1 ml/100g/min
D combination of A, B and C to show the subcompartments of decreased FMZ binding and decreased flow in relation to the final infarct

Table 2. Size (cm³, mean ± standard deviation) of cortical subcompartments I–VI

		Infarcted		**Non-Infarcted**
		CBF < 14.1 ml/100 g/min	CBF 14.1 ml/100 g/min	CBF < 14.1 ml/100 g/min
FMZ Binding	≤ 3.4	I 31.9 ± 46.97	II 2.9 ± 5.78	V not observed
	> 3.4	III 8.4 ± 8.96	IV 3.7 ± 2.49	VI 27.6 ± 30.81

Compartment I+III : 85.9% of infarcted tissue is hypoperfused
Compartment III : 17.9% of infarcted tissue is hypoperfused but still viable in early FMZ
Compartment IV : only 7.9% of final infarct is not affected in CBF and FMZ

ml/100 g/min = 54.3% of contralateral means) as the upper threshold, distinct subcompartments of cortical tissue were identified (Fig. 1, Table 2): Most (74%) of the final infarct (46.9 cm³) showed reduced FMZ binding at the early PET study (SC 1+2) whereas no region with FMZ binding initially reduced to or below 3.4 was observed outside the final infarct (SC 5). Within the eventually infarcted area, a large portion (86%) exhibited critically reduced flow (SC 1+3). The mean volume of critically perfused cortex outside the final lesion was 27.6 cm³ (SC 6). Within the volume of critical hypoperfusion finally infarcted (SC 1+3), not more than 21% had FMZ binding above the critical limit (SC 3). Only 8% of the final infarct showed FMZ binding and CBF above the defined limits (SC 4). Only in this small region the ultimate damage must be due to secondary events not related to the initial ischemia. These data support the highly predictive value for final infarction of reduced FMZ binding – this tissue compartment is irreversibly damaged already at the time of the PET study. A smaller portion (18%) of the final infarct is still viable – according to preserved function of BZR receptors – but is critically hypoperfused (penumbra).

Comment

These two sets of data indicate that except for rare cases the final infarcts are caused mainly by severe initial ischemia leading to rapid tissue damage while other mechanisms play only a minor role. Within the first 12 hours tissue damage within the critically hypoperfused area becomes more and more evident, and the finally infarcted tissue with primarily sufficient perfusion decreases its proportion. That implies that secondary and delayed effects are responsible for relatively small additional damage in most cases compared to the amount of tissue destroyed rapidly by lack of blood supply. Since the subcompartment with sufficient perfusion where the infarct is caused by delayed damage is rather small as a promising target of therapy, the benefit from treatment directed against these primary mechanisms is necessarily limited, and the disappointing results of corresponding clinical trials are not surprising. In the penumbral tissue, another rather small and over time rapidly decreasing fraction of the final infarct function is impaired as a consequence of critical hypoperfusion, but morphology is preserved; this compartment will profit from reperfusion in due time, while neuroprotective drugs alone probably do not salvage enough tissue to improve clinical outcome. When given early enough those drugs may extend the window of opportunity in the critically perfused and penumbra tissue thus enhancing the effect of reperfusion therapy; such combinations may very well form the basis of any therapeutic strategy for stroke in the future.

For the development of new treatments, it would be important to develop techniques by which the various ischemically compromised tissue subcompartments can be identified. These techniques should then be applied to the experimental model in which the treatment is developed, and then transferred to the clinical application. Only the comparative analysis of appropriate pathophysiological variables in experimental and clinical studies will improve the success in the search for a more effective therapy of ischemic stroke.

References

1. Astrup J, Siesjo BK, Symon L (1981) Thresholds in cerebral ischemia – the ischemic penumbra. Stroke 12:723–725
2. Barinaga M (1998) Stroke-damaged neurons may commit cellular suicide. Science 281:1302–1303
3. Baron JC, Rougemont D, Soussaline F, Bustany P, Crouzel C, Bousser MG, Comar D (1984) Local interrelationships of cerebral oxygen consumption and glucose utilization in normal subjects and in ischemic stroke patients: a positron tomography study. J Cereb Blood Flow Metab 4:140–149
4. Barone FC, Feuerstein GZ (1999) Inflammatory mediators and stroke: new opportunities for novel therapeutics. J Cereb Blood Flow Metab 19:819–834
5. Chan PH (1996) Role of oxidants in ischemic brain damage. Stroke 27:1124–1129
6. Choi D (1998) Antagonizing excitotoxicity: a therapeutic strategy for stroke? Mount Sinai Journal of Medicine 65:133–138
7. Chopp M, Zhang ZG (1996) Anti-adhesion molecule and nitric oxide protection strategies in ischemic stroke. Curr Opin Neurol 9:68–72
8. DeGraba TJ (1998) The role of inflammation after acute stroke: utility of pursuing anti-adhesion molecule therapy. Neurology 51:S62–S68
9. del Zoppo GJ, Wagner S, Tagaya M (1997) Trends and future developments in the pharmacological treatment of acute ischaemic stroke. Drugs 54:9–38
10. Dirnagl U, Iadecola C, Moskowitz MA (1999) Pathobiology of ischaemic stroke: an integrated view. Trends Neurosci 22:391–397
11. Dorman PJ, Counsell CE, Sandercock PAG (1996) Recently developed neuroprotective therapies for acute stroke. A qualitative systematic review of clinical trials. Cns Drugs 5:457–474
12. Dyker AG, Lees KR (1996) The rationale for new therapies in acute ischemic stroke. J Clin Pharm Ther 21:377–391
13. Endres M, Namura S, Shimizu-Sasamata M, Waeber C, Zhang L, Gomez-Isla T, Hyman BT, Moskowitz MA (1998) Attenuation of delayed neuronal death after mild focal ischemia in mice by inhibition of the caspase family. J Cereb Blood Flow Metab 18:238–247
14. Furlan A, Higashida R, Wechsler L, Gent M, Rowley H, Kase C, Pessin M, Ahuja A, Callahan F, Clark WM, Silver F, Rivera F (1999) Intra-arterial prourokinase for acute ischemic stroke. The PROACT II study: A randomized controlled trial. JAMA-Journal of the American Medical Association 282:2003–2011
15. Grotta J (1994) The current status of neuronal protective therapy: Why have all neuronal protective drugs worked in animals but none so far in stroke patients? Cerebrovasc Dis 4:115–120
16. Hakim AM, Evans AC, Berger L, Kuwabara H, Worsley K, Marchal G, Beil C, Pokrupa R, Diksic M, Meyer E (1989) The effect of nimodipine on the evolution of human cerebral infarction studied by PET. J Cereb Blood Flow Metab 9:523–534
17. Heiss W-D, Graf R (1994) The ischemic penumbra. Curr Opin Neurol 7:11–19
18. Heiss W-D, Kracht L, Thiel A, Grond M, Rudolf J (2000) Identification of targets for therapy by H_2O/FMZ-PET in early stroke. Stroke 31:276
19. Heiss W-D, Thiel A, Grond M, Graf R (1999) Which targets are relevant for therapy of acute ischemic stroke? Stroke 30:1486–1489
20. Herscovitch P, Markham J, Raichle ME (1983) Brain blood flow measured with intravenous $H_2{}^{15}O$, I. Theory and error analysis. J Nucl Med 24:782–789
21. Kontos HA (1985) Oxygen radicals in cerebral vascular injury. Circ Res 57:508–516
22. Lees KR (1998) Does neuroprotection improve stroke outcome? Lancet 351:1447–1448
23. Löttgen J, Pietrzyk U, Herholz K, Wienhard K, Heiss W-D (1998) Estimation of ischemic cerebral blood flow using [^{15}O]water and PET without arterial blood sampling. In: Quantitative Functional Brain Imaging with Positron Emission Tomography (Carson RE, Daube-Witherspoon ME, Herscovitch P, eds), pp 151–154. San Diego: Academic Press
24. Powers WJ, Grubb RLJr, Darriet D, Raichle ME (1985) Cerebral blood flow and cerebral metabolic rate of oxygen requirements for cerebral function and viability in humans. J Cereb Blood Flow Metab 5:600–608
25. Pulsinelli W (1992) Pathophysiology of acute ischaemic stroke. Lancet 339:533–536
26. Schulz JB, Weller M, Moskowitz MA (1999) Caspases as treatment targets in stroke and neurodegenerative diseases. Ann Neurol 45:421–429
27. Siesjö BK (1992) Pathophysiology and treatment of focal cerebral ischemia. Part I: Pathophysiology. J Neurosurg 77:169–184
28. The European Ad Hoc Consensus Group (1998) Neuroprotection as initial therapy in acute stroke. Cerebrovasc Dis 8:59–72
29. The NINDS rt-PA Stroke Study Group (1995) Tissue plasminogen activator for acute ischemic stroke. New Engl J Med 333:1581–1587

Pathophysiology of thrombolytic reperfusion versus reversible thread occlusion of middle cerebral artery in mice

T. Hara, R. Hata, G. Mies, K.-A. Hossmann

Introduction

Injury of brain tissue inflicted by a reduction of blood flow is mediated by complex interaction of hemodynamic and molecular mechanisms. In permanent ischemia the pathogenetic importance of hemodynamic factors is obvious whereas in transient ischemia molecular disturbances may become the dominant mechanism of injury. This is clearly exemplified by delayed tissue infarction after a brief period of vascular occlusion where irreversible injury may evolve after a delay of several weeks despite primary restoration of flow and metabolism (Du et al. 1996).

It is reasonable to assume that such delayed molecular disturbances may also contribute to tissue injury after stroke because in most patients the ischemic territory exhibits a certain degree of spontaneous reperfusion (Olsen and Lassen 1984). The importance of molecular disturbances further increases when recirculation is promoted by active therapeutic interventions such as rt-PA induced thrombolysis. A substantial amount of research, therefore, focuses on the study of reversible ischemia to understand – and possibly to treat – such disturbances.

A standard experimental model used for this purpose is transient intraluminal thread occlusion (Koizumi et al. 1986). A fine filament with a silicon-coated tip is advanced from the internal carotid artery through the carotid canal into the circle of Willis to obstruct the origin of the middle cerebral artery. After some time ranging between 30 min and 2 hours the thread is withdrawn to restore blood supply to the occluded vascular territory. The main advantage of this procedure is the rapid restoration of blood flow after the ischemic impact which prevents the masking of molecular disturbances by hemodynamic impairments. However, such sudden restitution of blood flow is rare under clinical conditions with the possible exception of neurosurgical interventions where brain arteries are temporarily clipped to avoid bleedings. Even by thrombolytic interventions blood flow is restored much more slowly because it takes some time until the clot is resolved. The difference in the reperfusion profile cannot be ignored because previous studies of global brain ischemia revealed that the recovery potential of the tissue markedly varies depending on how fast blood flow and hence energy metabolism recovers (Hossmann 1997). The evolution of ischemic injury after reversible thread occlusion may, therefore, substantially differ from the clinically more relevant type of spontaneous or drug induced reperfusion.

In the present study we address this question by comparing the evolution of tissue injury

Max-Planck-Institute for Neurological Research, Department of Experimental Neurology, Gleueler Str. 50, D-50931 Cologne, Germany
e-mail: Hossmann@mpin-koeln.mpg.de

J. Krieglstein, S. Klumpp (Eds.) Pharmacology of Cerebral Ischemia 2000

after 1 hour reversible MCA thread occlusion with thrombolysis of MCA clot embolism, induced after the same interval by intra-arterial infusion of rt-PA (for original data see Hata et al. 2000b and Hara et al. 2000). Tissue injury was assessed by a battery of pictorial methods that allow simultaneous evaluation of the parameters of interest with high regional resolution. Our observations do, in fact, reveal that the two types of reversible ischemia exhibit basically different pathophysiologies which have to be considered for the understanding of the importance of molecular mechanisms of stroke evolution.

Material and methods

Surgical interventions

Experiments were carried out in halothane anesthetized adult male C57 Black/6J mice weighing 20–30 g. Middle cerebral artery (MCA) thread occlusion was done by a modification (Hata et al. 2000a) of the technique described by Koizumi et al. (1986). The thread was withdrawn after 1 h, and brains were investigated after 1 h, 3 h, 6 h, 24 h and 3 d reperfusion. MCA clot embolism was performed by a method developed in our laboratory (Kilic et al. 1998). Cylindrical blood clots were prepared in PE10 catheters by mixing fresh arterial blood with thrombin, and four fibrin-rich segments of 4 mm length (corresponding to 0.284 µl clot material) were flushed retrogradely through the external into the internal carotid artery. Thrombolysis of clots was started 1 h after embolism by intra-carotid infusion of 10 mg/kg rt-PA (Alteplas, Boehringer-Ingelheim, Germany), and brains were investigated at 1 h, 3 h, 6 h and 24 h after start of treatment. In both thread and clot occluded animals, blood flow was monitored by laser-Doppler flowmetry and by ^{14}C-iodoantipyrine autoradiography.

Embolized animals selected for 3 d survival died intermittently between the first and the third day, and therefore could not be submitted to the full analytical protocol.

Metabolic studies

Forty-five minutes before termination of experiments, animals received an intra-peritoneal injection of L[4, 5-^{3}H] leucine (150 µCi, Amersham, Braunschweig, Germany) for autoradiographic measurement of global protein synthesis (Mies et al. 1997). The brains were frozen *in situ* with liquid nitrogen and cut into 20-µm-thick coronal cryostat sections. Pictorial ATP measurements were prepared using an ATP-specific bioluminescence assay (Kogure and Alonso 1978). For measurement of cerebral protein synthesis (CPS), brain slices were incubated in 10% trichloroacetic acid to remove labelled free leucine and metabolites other than proteins. Subsequently, slices were exposed for 14 days with ^{3}H standards to tritium-sensitive x-ray film (Hyperfilm ^{3}H; Amersham) for autoradiography of ^{3}H-labelled proteins.

Genomic expression

Pictorial assays of *c-fos, junB* and *hsp70* mRNAs were performed by *in situ* hybridization using appropriate ^{35}S-labelled oligonucleotide probes (Hata et al. 2000a). Brain sections were fixed for 15 min in 4% paraformaldehyde/phosphate-buffered saline (PBS), pH 7.4, and after overnight hybridization at 42 °C exposed to autoradiographic film (Hyperfilm β-max; Amersham).

Terminal transferase biotinylated-UTP nick end labelling (TUNEL)

TUNEL was performed by incubating paraformaldehyde/PBS-fixed cryostat sections in TDT-mix (150 U/ml terminal deoxynucleotidyl transferase, Life Technologies, Eggenstein, Germany, and 10 pmol/L biotin-16-dUTP, Boehringer-Mannheim, Germany) (Hata et al. 2000a). Incorporated biotin was visualized with the avidin-biotin peroxidase complex method (Vector Laboratories, Burlingame, CA, USA).

Image analysis

Image analysis was carried out using the National Institutes of Health image software (version 1.61). Images were digitized with a CCD camera and the volumes of ATP depletion and CPS inhibition were measured using a semiautomated method (Swanson and Sharp 1994). ATP depletion was defined as a decline to less than 30% of the value of the contralateral side. The threshold for CPS was set to the lowest CPS value of the non-ischemic hemisphere, excluding fibre tracts. The areas of ATP depletion and CPS inhibition were measured on each section by subtracting the area of the nonlesioned ipsilateral hemisphere from that of the contralateral side. The areas of preserved ATP and protein synthesis were outlined and superimposed to demarcate penumbral tissue in which protein synthesis was suppressed but ATP was preserved (Hata et al. 2000a).

To evaluate the regional reproducibility of measurements regional incidence maps were constructed (Hata et al. 2000a). The areas of biochemical disturbances were outlined on coronal brain sections at the levels of caudate-putamen and dorsal hippocampus, and superimposed to calculate the incidence of the metabolic alterations as a percentage of the number of animals per group. All values are given as means ±SD.

Results

Transient MCA thread occlusion

Blood flow

MCA thread occlusion led to the sharp decline of parietal laser-Doppler flow (LDF) to less than 15% of control (Fig. 1). When the MCA thread was withdrawn one hour later, LDF returned to normal within less than 15 min, and after 30 min overshooted by about 20%. Autoradiographic measurements of blood flow carried out at various recirculation times between 1 h and 24 h revealed longlasting hypoperfusion. In the caudate-putamen, this reduction amounted to almost 40% at 24 h after the onset of recirculation (Fig. 2).

Brain metabolism

In the sham-operated controls regional ATP content and regional cerebral protein synthesis

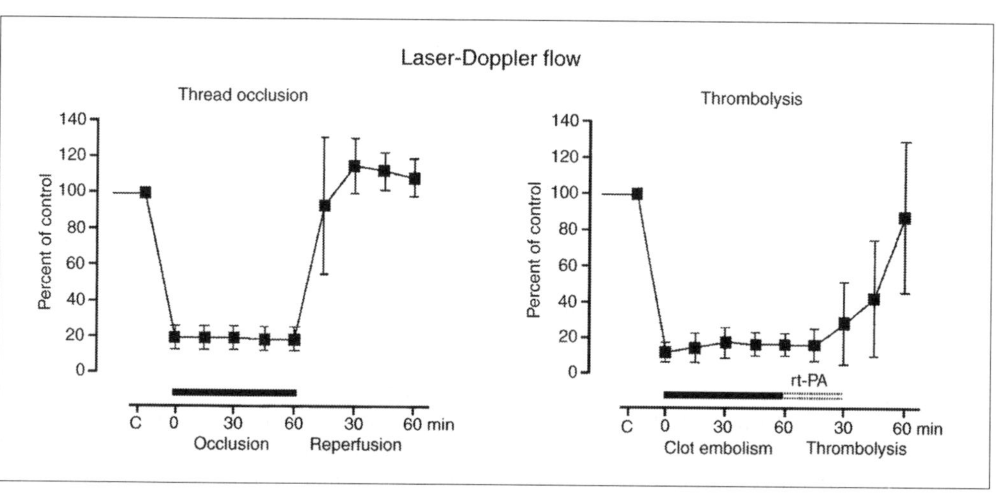

Fig. 1. Recording of Laser-Doppler flow from parietal cortex after 1 h MCA thread occlusion (left) and during rt-PA-induced thrombolysis starting 1 h after MCA clot embolism (right). Note considerably longer delay of reperfusion after initiation of thrombolysis.

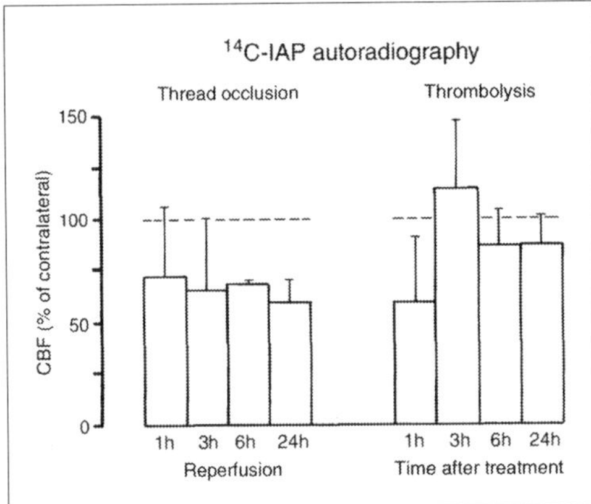

Fig. 2. Autoradiographic measurement of blood flow in caudate-putamen at various times after 1 h transient MCA thread occlusion (left) or rt-PA induced thrombolysis starting 1 h after MCA clot embolism (right). Blood flow is expressed in percent of the opposite hemisphere. Note prolonged post-ischemic hypoperfusion after transient thread occlusion.

(CPS) did not differ between hemispheres. After 1 h vascular occlusion, ATP was depleted in the fronto-parietal cortex, the lateral part of caudate-putamen and the piriform cortex (Fig. 3). Suppression of protein synthesis was present in the same areas but the changes extended distinctly more into the frontal, medial and temporo-occipital parts of the MCA territory. On coronal brain sections at the level of caudate-putamen, the ATP depleted area amounted to 40.1 ± 11% of the hemispheric cross-sectional area, and the area of CPS inhibition to 58.9 ± 5.5% (Fig. 4). When the brain was reperfused after 1 h middle cerebral artery occlusion, inhibition of CPS initially changed little. At the level of caudate-putamen the CPS-inhibited area was 54.1 ± 2.6% at 1 h, 56.9 ± 6.1% at 3 h, and 56.6 ± 4.8% at 6 h after the onset of reperfusion (Fig. 6). Later the area with suppressed CPS decreased to 48.7 ± 4.5% at 1d ($p < 0.05$) and to 37.2 ± 7.3% at 3 d ($p < 0.01$) but it never fully recovered.

In contrast to CPS, ATP transiently returned. After recirculation for 1 h, ATP was almost completely restored but with longer periods of reperfusion, ATP again deteriorated. The mean area of ATP depletion at the level of caudate-putamen thus secondarily increased from 7.2 ± 10.9% of the non-ischemic contralateral hemisphere at 3 h to 14.2 ± 10.4% at 6 h, 19.7 ± 17.9% at 1d and 34.8 ± 9.2% at 3 d after the onset of reperfusion. At this time ATP depletion had merged with the area of CPS inhibition, leading to the sharp demarcation of the brain infarct from the normal brain tissue (Fig. 3).

The reproducibility of the metabolic changes was confirmed by the injury incidence maps (Fig. 5). These maps clearly document that CPS inhibition remained virtually constant from the end of the 1 h ischemic period up to six hours after reperfusion whereas ATP transiently recovered. However, starting at 3 h after ischemia ATP secondarily deteriorated, first in the dorsal hippocampus and the central parts of caudate-putamen and later in the more peripheral parts of the MCA supplying territory. After 3 d recirculation the region of ATP depletion precisely matched the region of suppressed CPS.

Genomic expressions

Representative *in situ* hybridization autoradiograms of *hsp70*, *c-fos* and *junB* mRNAs are demonstrated in Figure 3. The outlinings of preserved ATP and normal CPS were superimposed on adjacent cryostat sections to facilitate the regional allocation of hybridization signals.

At the end of the 1 h MCA occlusion, expression of *hsp70* mRNA was slightly increased in the cortical penumbra, i.e. the region of suppressed CPS but preserved ATP located in the periphery of the MCA territory. *C-fos* and *junB* mRNAs also increased in the lateral part of the penumbra but even more so in the normal cortex outside the area of suppressed CPS, extending up to the midline but not into the opposite hemisphere.

After reperfusion *hsp70* mRNA expression sharply increased throughout the area of suppressed CPS, peaking at 3 h after the release of vascular occlusion. With longer recirculation times it gradually declined, particularly in the areas of secondary ATP failure, and completely disappeared after 3 d, i.e. at a time when the

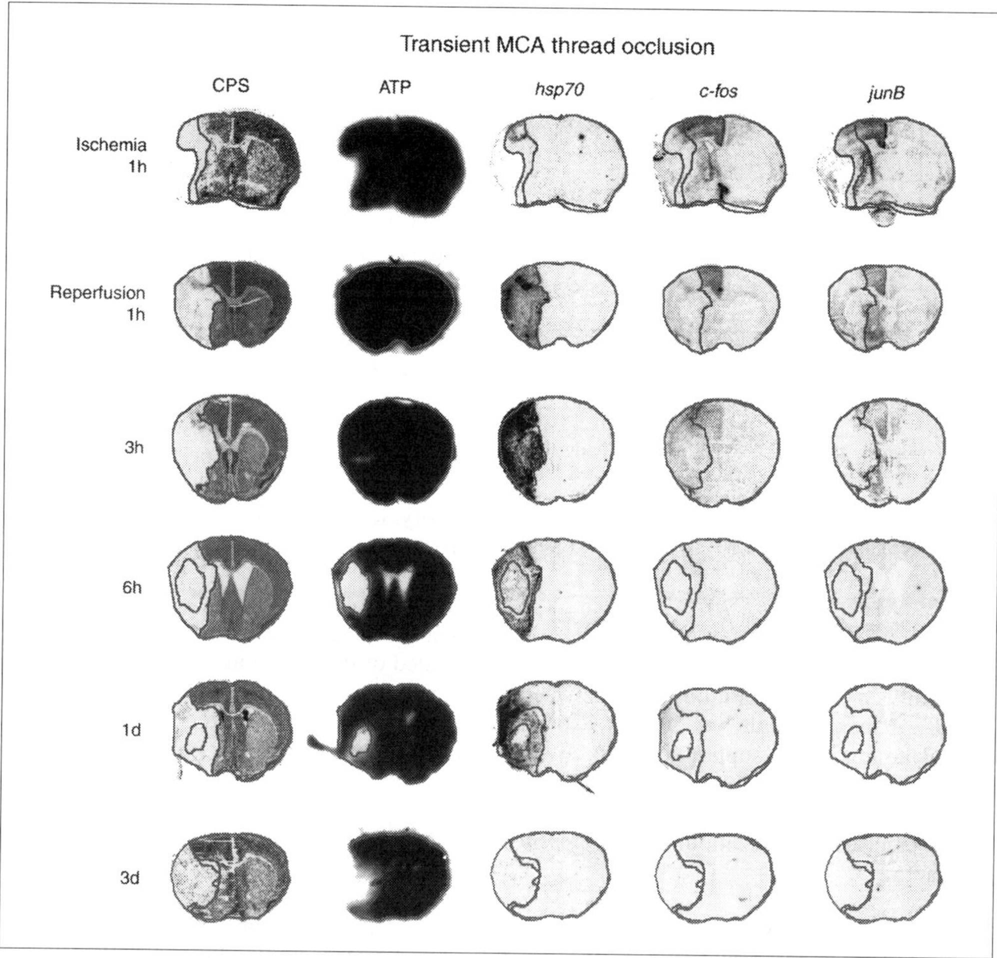

Fig. 3. Multiparametric images of cerebral protein synthesis (CPS), tissue ATP content, and of *hsp70*, c-fos and *junB* mRNAs of representative brain sections of mice at the level of the caudate-putamen at various reperfusion times following 1 h MCA thread occlusion. The outlines of preserved ATP and CPS have been superimposed on hybridization autoradiograms to demarcate the metabolically impaired areas from the normal brain tissue.

area of secondary ATP depletion had merged with that of CPS suppression. In contrast to *hsp70* mRNA, the expression pattern of the immediate early genes changed little after reperfusion, the signal intensity gradually declining to control between 6 h and 1d after the onset of reperfusion.

Terminal transferase biotinylated-UTP nick end labelling (TUNEL)

Double strand DNA breaks visualized by TUNEL could first be detected between 3 and 6 h after the beginning of reperfusion (Fig. 5). Most of the TUNEL-positive cells appeared to be neurons but the use of cryostat sections precluded precise identification. The comparison of the distribution pattern of TUNEL-pos-

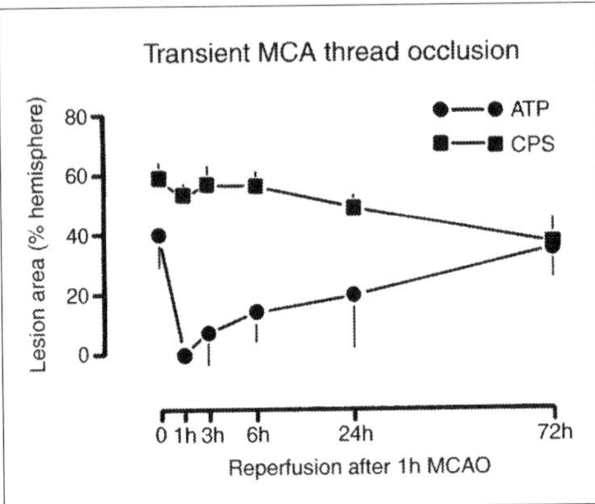

Fig. 4. Dynamics of metabolic lesions in mouse brain after 1 h MCA thread occlusion. The areas of suppressed cerebral protein synthesis (CPS) and of ATP depletion were measured at the level of caudate – putamen and expressed in percent of the opposite hemisphere. Note transient recovery of ATP followed by secondary deterioration.

itive cells with the inhibition of CPS revealed an initially central localization which between 1 and 3 d merged with but did not expand beyond the area of CPS suppression. Moreover, TUNEL-positive cells were mainly encountered in areas of secondary ATP depletion although precise co-localization was not present in all animals.

Thrombolysis of MCA clot embolism

Blood reperfusion

Restoration of LDF during thrombolysis of clot embolism was much slower than after reversible thread occlusion (Fig. 1). Thirty min after onset of therapy, parietal LDF amounted to only 30% of control, and return to baseline required 1 h. However, autoradiographic measurements of blood flow documented reactive hyperemia after 3 h and a lesser degree of subsequent hypoperfusion than after thread occlusion. In the caudate-putamen, blood flow thus stabilized above 80% of the opposite non-ischemic hemisphere and did not further decline throughout the first day of reperfusion (Fig. 2).

Brain metabolism

One hour after clot embolism, the regional pattern of metabolic impairment was similar to that observed after 1 h thread occlusion but the volume of the metabolic lesion was slightly larger (Fig. 6). At the level of caudate-putamen, the ATP depletion area amounted to 58 ±10.1%, and the CPS-impaired region to 68.0 ±6.7% of the hemispheric cross section (Fig. 7). Intra-arterial thrombolysis with 10 mg/kg rt-PA at 1 h after embolism gradually reversed these changes. ATP improved in most parts of the ischemic territory between 3 and 6 h, and fully recovered after 24 h. Interestingly, also CPS improved, initially in the peripheral and after 6 h also in the more central parts of the MCA territory, leading at 24 h to a significant reduction of the CPS suppressed area to 15.5 ±9.6% ($p < 0.05$).

Despite of this amazing recovery, animals did not survive. Between 1 and 3 days all mice – treated or not – died under the symptoms of severe brain edema, demonstrating that the here observed metabolic recovery did not prevent fatal brain damage.

Genomic expressions

The expression of *c-fos* and *junB* mRNAs resembled that after transient thread occlusion and was clearly confined to the normal cortex outside the area of suppressed CPS. Medially it extended to the midline but not to the opposite hemisphere, in accordance with the known spread of peri-ischemic depolarizations. Upregulation of immediate-early genes could be demonstrated until 3 h after the onset of thrombolysis but not after longer intervals. This is also similar to transient thread occlusion and suggests that spreading depolarizations cease after successful recirculation.

Upregulation of *hsp70* mRNA was noted from 1 h on in areas of suppressed CPS with the exception of those regions in which ATP was depleted. This pattern was particularly striking after 1 and 3 h recirculation where a sharp demarcation existed between ATP-depleted and

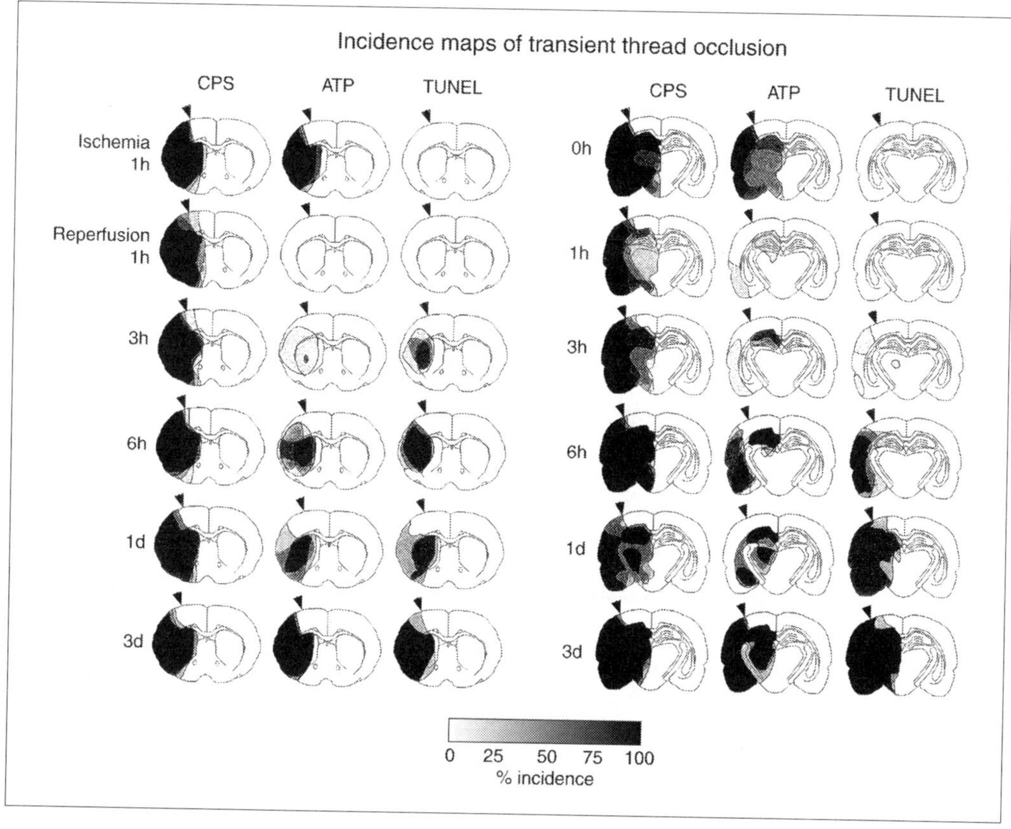

Fig. 5. Incidence maps of suppressed protein synthesis (CPS), ATP depletion and TUNEL-positive neurons on coronal sections of the mouse brain at various reperfusion times following 1 h MCA thread occlusion. Areas of disturbed metabolism were outlined in 4–5 animals per time point at the level of the caudate-putamen (left) and dorsal hippocampus (right) and superimposed to calculate the incidence of alterations in percent of the number of animals per group. The demarcation between normal and disturbed protein synthesis in parietal cortex visible at the end of 1 h middle cerebral artery occlusion was marked by the arrowheads to estimate the evolution or regression of the metabolic lesions at later time points. Note transient recovery of ATP after the beginning of reperfusion and correlation of TUNEL with secondary energy failure.

ATP-repleted parts of the MCA territory. At 24 h only small areas of increased *hsp70* mRNA persisted, corresponding to those regions in which CPS had not yet fully recovered.

Terminal transferase biotinylated-UTP nick end labelling (TUNEL)

Fragmentations of nuclear DNA were confined to neurons and occurred late during the evolution of brain injury. In untreated animals TUNEL-positive neurons were detected between 6 and 24 h after vehicle infusion. Twenty-four hours after vehicle infusion the regional distribution of TUNEL corresponded clearly to that of ATP and CPS inhibition which, in turn, colocalized with the region of critically reduced CBF (Fig. 8).

In the rt-PA treated animals the number and regional extension of TUNEL-positive neurons were distinctly reduced as compared to the untreated animals and corresponded approximately to that of persisting inhibition of CPS.

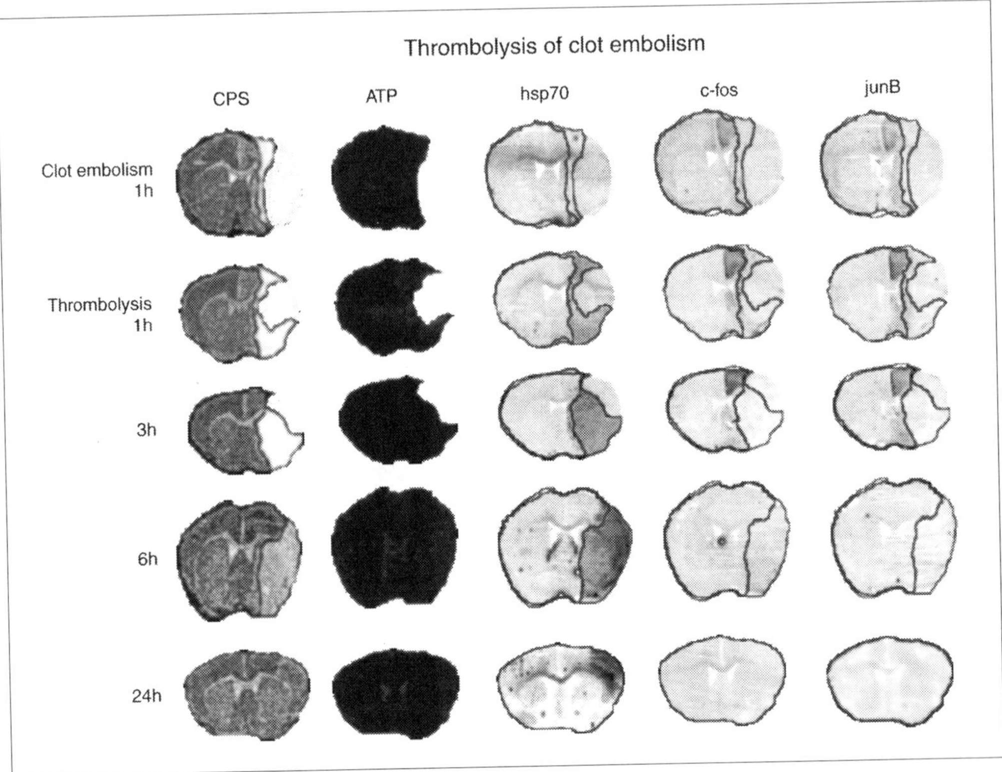

Fig. 6. Multiparametric images of cerebral protein synthesis (CPS), tissue ATP content, and of *hsp*70, c-fos and *jun*B mRNAs of representative brain sections of mice at the level of the caudate-putamen at various times after rt-PA induced thrombolysis, initiated at 1 h after MCA clot embolism. The outlines of preserved ATP and CPS have been superimposed on hybridization autoradiograms to demarcate the metabolically impaired areas from the normal brain tissue.

Interestingly, TUNEL colocalized with the areas in which ATP depletion was visible after 6 h but there was a distinct dissociation between the recovery of ATP and the progression of TUNEL at 24 h (Fig. 8).

Discussion

The comparison of the two reversible ischemia models, transient thread occlusion and thrombolysis of clot embolism, revealed differences in post-ischemic hemodynamics that were reflected by a different evolution of ischemic injury. In transient thread occlusion, instantaneous reperfusion promoted rapid recovery of energy metabolism which, however, was followed by secondary energy failure starting a few hours after the initiation of recirculation. Thrombolysis of clot embolism, in contrast, restored blood flow and energy metabolism much more slowly but during the first day of recirculation recovery was stable. Interestingly, protein synthesis never recovered after transient thread occlusion but it slowly returned after thrombolysis, demonstrating that the slow reperfusion profile in this model is not incompatible with recovery of complex metabolic functions.

This observation is surprising because previous studies of transient global ischemia suggest that non-instantaneous reperfusion impairs functional recovery, presumably because of the more severe generation of post-ischemic cytotoxic

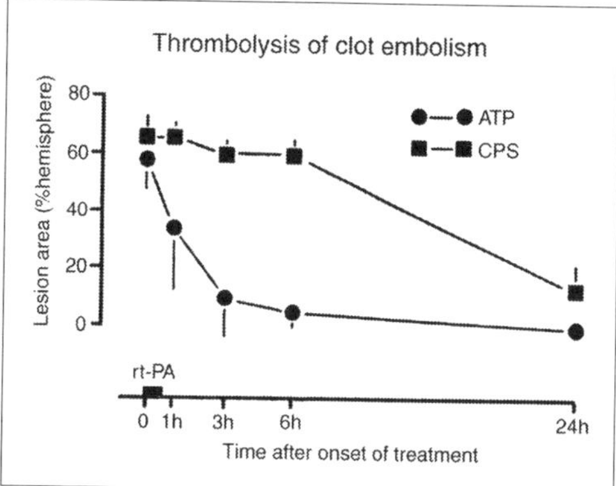

Fig. 7. Effect of rt-PA induced thrombolysis on the evolution of ischemic injury after MCA clot embolism. Hemispheric areas of suppressed ATP and CPS were measured at the level of caudate-putamen (means±SD). Thrombolysis induces gradual improvement of ATP and – after longer delays – of CPS.

brain edema (Hossmann 1997). A possible explanation for this difference is the smaller volume of injured tissue after focal ischemia. In fact, the deleterious effect of post-ischemic brain swelling has been attributed to an increase of intracranial pressure which after focal ischemia is presumably less pronounced. It is, therefore, conceivable that the higher risk of edema after thrombolysis was compensated by other, possibly beneficial side effects of delayed reperfusion. One of these might be the amelioration of free radical-induced reperfusion injury (Phillis 1994). Reactive oxygen radicals are generated by a number of pathways which include purine catabolism, activation of neutrophils and arachidonic acid metabolism. During recirculation, supply of molecular oxygen funnels free radical production but by restoring oxidative respiration the radical generating pathways are reversed. The net effect of this "oxygen paradoxon" (Hammerman and Kaplan 1998) is difficult to predict but it has been speculated that a period of reduced oxygen supply – as during early thrombolytic reperfusion – might be beneficial for the tissue.

The different evolution of ischemic injury in the two models of transient ischemia may also be explained by differences in late reperfusion. In the thread occlusion model post-ischemic hyperemia was followed by hypoperfusion which still could be detected at 24 hours after the onset of recirculation. The flow reduction was not severe enough to reach the threshold of energy failure but there is evidence from both focal and global ischemia that post-ischemic hypoperfusion is associated with a disturbance of flow regulation (Symon et al. 1975; Hossmann et al. 1973) which under conditions of increased oxygen requirements could lead to a mismatch between flow and metabolism. Such a mismatch could arise from free-radical mediated disturbances of mitochondrial membrane permeability leading to impairment of oxidative respiration (Kuroda and Siesjö 1997). Mitochondrial respiration may also suffer from excessive cytosolic calcium flooding because mitochondrial calcium accumulation diverts part of the capacity of the respiratory chain to calcium transport (Kristian et al. 1998). Both events reduce the ATP yield of mitochondrial respiration and have to be compensated by increased oxidation of glucose which, however, is limited by the disturbed flow coupling. The great number of interventions that have been shown to alleviate ischemic injury could, in fact, be explained by the improvement of such a mismatch: flow promoting interventions by increasing oxygen supply, free radical scavengers by reducing mitochondrial damage, calcium antagonists by reducing cytosolic calcium flooding and antiepileptics, hypothermia or anesthetics by reducing the energy requirements of the tissue (for a recent review of therapeutic interventions see Heiss et al. 1999).

Interestingly, slow reperfusion initiated at 1 hour after *clot embolism* by *thrombolysis* did not cause secondary deterioration of energy metabolism during the first day after onset of therapy. A more delayed manifestation of injury is unlikely because the duration of energy failure – which in this model is longer than after 1 h reversible thread occlusion – correlates inversely with the maturation interval of secondary injury (Ito et al. 1992). A straightforward explanation for the preservation of the energy state is the absence of post-ischemic hypoperfusion which apparently prevents a flow/me-

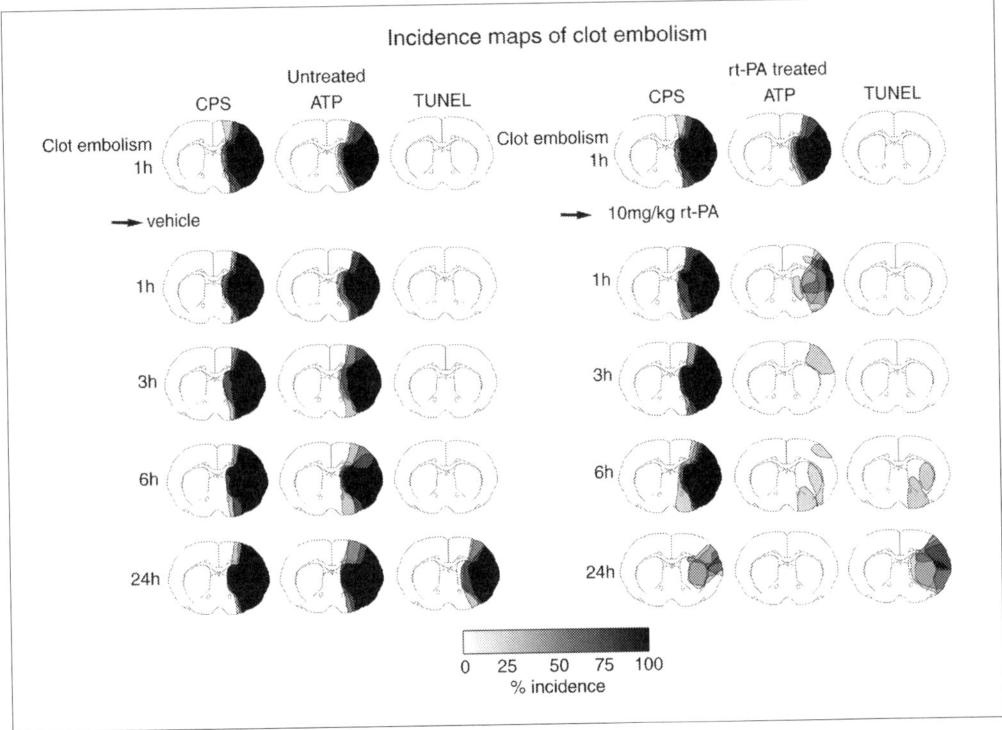

Fig. 8. Evolution of ischemic injury after clot embolism with and without rt-PA treatment. Incidence maps of suppressed cerebral protein synthesis (CPS), ATP depletion and double strand DNA fragmentations (TUNEL). Note gradual return of energy metabolism and partial restoration of protein synthesis in the rt-PA treated animals which, however, does not prevent DNA fragmentations at 24 h after initiation of thrombolysis.

tabolism mismatch, as observed in the transient thread occlusion model. The flow improvement may reflect the reversal of the post-ischemic disturbance of flow regulation, but it could also be due to a lower blood viscosity because rt-PA treatment reduces plasma fibrinogen content (Gulba et al. 1998). Prevention of a flow/metabolism mismatch also provides a plausible explanation for the recovery of protein synthesis which is particularly sensitive to transient episodes of hypoxia (Mies et al. 1991).

Compared to the obvious differences in post-ischemic hemodynamics, the role of molecular disturbances remains elusive. The expression of immediate early and stress genes was similar in the two models and mainly reflected the regional pattern of disturbed energy metabolism and protein synthesis. Immediate early genes were transiently upregulated outside the ischemic territory in accordance with the known effects of peri-focal depolarizations (Kiessling and Gass 1994). *Hsp70* mRNA was expressed within the ischemic territory but only in those parts in which protein synthesis was inhibited but ATP was preserved. Accordingly, expression was most pronounced between 1 and 6 hours after ischemia, followed by gradual decline after longer recirculation intervals. This secondary decline, however, had different reasons in the two models: after thrombolysis because of the recovery of protein synthesis, and after thread occlusion because of the secondary ATP failure.

Similarly, the evolution of DNA fragmentations may have different reasons in the two models. After transient thread occlusion neurons became TUNEL positive at the same time or shortly after secondary energy failure, supporting an unspecific effect due to cell necrosis (Charriaut-Marlangue and Benari 1995). Following thrombolysis DNA fragmentations occurred in the presence of both protein synthesis and energy metabolism. They may, therefore, reflect an active type of cell death which deserves further investigation. The elucidation of this pathophysiology may also provide an explanation why the thrombolysed animals died between the first and the third day after the onset of treatment. The severe brain edema detected in these animals could be a secondary event in response to the delayed type of injury that is heralded by the appearance of TUNEL-positive neurons. However, it may also be a complicating side effect of rt-PA treatment which is known to enhance plasmin-generated lamin degradation, matrix metalloproteinase activation and transmigration of leukocytes through the vessel walls (Hamann et al. 1999).

In conclusion, the comparison of the two models of transient focal ischemia clearly reveals that tissue injury evolves in two basically different ways. The most plausible explanation for this difference are the different rates of blood flow both during early and late reperfusion. Therapeutic interventions that improve ischemic injury in one model may, therefore, fail in the other. This raises concerns about the uncritical application of experimental treatment designs to clinical stroke and may explain why most of these interventions are unsuccessful under clinical conditions. Proper selection of animal experiments and the balanced consideration of both hemodynamic and molecular mechanisms of ischemic injury are, therefore, required to design more successful treatment strategies.

References

1. Charriaut-Marlangue C, Benari Y (1995) A cautionary note on the use of the TUNEL stain to determine apoptosis. NeuroReport 7:61–64
2. Du C, Hu R, Csernansky CA, Hsu CY, Choi DW (1996) Very delayed infarction after mild focal cerebral ischemia: A role for apoptosis? J Cereb Blood Flow Metab 16:195–201
3. Gulba DC, Bode C, Runge MS, Huber K (1998) Thrombolytic agents – an updated overview. Fibrinolysis and Proteolysis 12:Suppl. 2, 39–58
4. Hamann GF, del Zoppo GJ, von Kummer R (1999) Mechanisms for the development of intracerebral hemorrhage – what we can learn for the thrombolytic therapy in stroke. Nervenarzt 70:1116–1120
5. Hammerman C, Kaplan M (1998) Ischemia and reperfusion injury – the ultimate pathophysiologic paradox. Clin Perinatol 25:757–777
6. Hara T, Mies G, Hossmann K-A (2000) Effect of thrombolysis on the dynamics of infarct evolution after clot embolism of middle cerebral artery in mice. J Cereb Blood Flow Metab in press
7. Hata R, Maeda K, Hermann D, Mies G, Hossmann K-A (2000a) Dynamics of regional brain metabolism and gene expression after middle cerebral artery occlusion in mice. J Cereb Blood Flow Metab 20:306–315
8. Hata R, Maeda K, Hermann D, Mies G, Hossmann K-A (2000b) Evolution of brain infarction after transient focal cerebral ischemia in mice. J Cereb Blood Flow Metab 20:937–946
9. Heiss W-D, Thiel A, Grond M, Graf R (1999) Which targets are relevant for therapy of acute ischemic stroke? Stroke 30:1486–1489
10. Hossmann K-A (1997) Reperfusion of the brain after global ischemia – hemodynamic disturbances. Shock 8:95–101
11. Hossmann K-A, Lechtape-Grüter H, Hossmann V (1973) The role of cerebral blood flow for the recovery of the brain after prolonged ischemia. Zeitschrift für Neurologie 204:281–299
12. Ito U, Kirino T, Kuroiwa T, Klatzo I (Eds.) (1992) Maturation phenomenon in cerebral ischemia. Berlin, Springer-Verlag, pp 208
13. Kiessling M, Gass P (1994) Stimulus-transcription coupling in focal cerebral ischemia. Brain Pathol 4:77–83
14. Kilic E, Hermann DM, Hossmann K-A (1998) A reproducible model of thromboembolic stroke in mice. Neuroreport 9:2967–2970
15. Kogure K, Alonso OF (1978) A pictorial representation of endogenous brain ATP by a bioluminescent method. Brain Res 154:273–284
16. Koizumi J, Yoshida Y, Nakazawa T, Oneda G (1986) Experimental studies of ischemic brain edema. 1. A new experimental model of cerebral embolism in rats in which recirculation can be introduced in the ischemic area. Jpn J Stroke 8:1–8
17. Kristian T, Gido G, Kuroda S, Schutz A, Siesjö BK (1998) Calcium metabolism of focal and penumbral tissues in rats subjected to transient middle cerebral artery occlusion. Exp Brain Res 120:503–509
18. Kuroda S, Siesjö BK (1997) Reperfusion damage following focal ischemia – pathophysiology and therapeutic windows. Clin Neurosci 4:199–212
19. Mies G, Djuricic B, Paschen W, Hossmann K-A (1997) Quantitative measurement of cerebral protein synthesis in vivo - theory and methodological considerations. J Neurosci Methods 76:35–44
20. Mies G, Ishimaru S, Xie Y, Seo K, Hossmann K-A (1991) Ischemic thresholds of cerebral protein synthesis and energy state following middle cerebral artery occlusion in rat. J Cereb Blood Flow Metab 11:753–761
21. Olsen TS, Lassen NA (1984) A dynamic concept of middle cerebral artery occlusion and cerebral infarction in the acute state based on interpreting severe hyperemia as a sign of embolic migration. Stroke 15:458–468
22. Phillis JW (1994) A "radical" view of cerebral ischemic injury. Prog Neurobiol 42:441–448
23. Swanson RA, Sharp FR (1994) Infarct measurement methodology. J Cereb Blood Flow Metab 14:697–698
24. Symon L, Crockard HA, Dorsch NWC, Branston NM, Juhasz J (1975) Local cerebral blood flow and vascular reactivity in a chronic stable stroke in baboons. Stroke 6:482–492

Index

A

B

C

D

E

F

G

H

I

J

K

L

M

N

U

V

W

Z